GNRS

A Core Curriculum in Advanced Practice Geriatric Nursing

6th Edition

Geriatric Nursing Review Syllabus

CHIEF EDITOR
Barbara Resnick
PhD, CRNP, FAAN, FAANP, AGSF

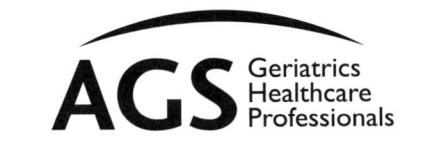

Leading Change. Improving Care for Older Adults.

As new research and clinical experience broaden our knowledge of medicine, changes in treatment and drug therapy are required. This publication is intended only to facilitate the free flow of information of interest to the medical community involved in the care of older adults.

No responsibility is assumed by the editors or the American Geriatrics Society, as the Publisher, for any injury and/or damage to persons or property, as a matter of product liability, negligence, warranty, or otherwise, arising out of the use or application of any methods, products, instructions, or ideas contained herein. No guarantee, endorsement, or warranty of any kind, express or implied (including specifically no warranty of merchantability or of fitness for a particular purpose) is given by the Society in connection with any information contained herein. Independent verification of any diagnosis, treatment, or drug use or dosage should be obtained. No test or procedure should be performed unless, in the judgment of an independent qualified physician, it is justified in light of the risk involved.

Inclusion in this publication of product information does not constitute a guarantee, warranty, or endorsement by the American Geriatrics Society (the Publisher) of the quality, value, safety, effectiveness, or usefulness of any such product or of any claim made about such product by its manufacturer or an author.

The *GNRS6* reflects care that can be provided to older adults in all settings. The words patient, resident, and older adult have been used interchangeably, as have the words provider, clinician, and primary care provider. Given the continually ongoing changes in health care today, some of the guidelines around reimbursement may have changed since publication.

The Chief Editor was Barbara Resnick, PhD, CRNP, FAANP, FAAN, FGSA, AGSF; Editors were Marie Boltz, PhD, GNP-BC, FGSA, FAAN, Elizabeth Capezuti, PhD, RN, FAAN, Deirdre M. Carolan, PhD, ANP-BC, GNP-BC, FAANP, Carolyn Clevenger, RN, DNP, AGPCNP-BC, GNP-BC, FAANP, Elizabeth Galik, PhD, CRNP, FAAN, FAANP, and Laurie Kennedy-Malone, PhD, GNP-BC, FAANP, FGSA; Medical Editor was Susan E. Aiello, DVM, ELS; Indexer was L. Pilar Wyman; and Managing Editor was Andrea N. Sherman, MS.

Many thanks to Fry Communications for all production work including typesetting, graphic design, and printing. With more than 70 years in the information industry, Fry offers printing and ancillary services to publishers and other content providers.

Citation: Resnick B, ed. *Geriatric Nursing Review Syllabus: A Core Curriculum in Advanced Practice Geriatric Nursing*. 6th edition. New York: American Geriatrics Society; 2019.

All rights reserved. Except where authorized, no part of this publication may be reproduced, stored in a retrieval system, or transmitted in any form or by any means, electronic, mechanical, photocopying, recording, or otherwise without prior written permission of the American Geriatrics Society, 40 Fulton Street, 18th Floor, New York, New York, 10038 USA.

Geriatric Nursing Review Syllabus: A Core Curriculum in Advanced Practice Geriatric Nursing. 6th edition. Cataloging in publication data is available from the Library of Congress.

Library of Congress Control Number: 2018967297

Copyright © 2019 by the American Geriatrics Society

ISBN Number: 978-1-886775-61-9

All rights reserved. Printed in the United States of America. Except as permitted under the United States Copyright Act of 1976, no part of this publication may be reproduced or distributed in any form or by any means, or stored in a database or retrieval system, without the prior written permission of the publisher, the American Geriatrics Society.

Printed in the United States of America

10 9 8 7 6 5 4 3 2 1

TABLE OF CONTENTS

GNRS6 Editorial Board ix
Original GRS10 Editorial Board xi
Authors of Original GRS10 Chapters xi
Contributing GRS10 Question Authors xv
Acknowledgments xvii
Preface xvii
Introduction xix

CURRENT ISSUES IN AGING

Chapter 1—Demography 1
Global Aging Trends and Demographics 1
United States Aging Trends and Demographics 2
Resources 4

Chapter 2—Biology 5
Theories of Aging 7
Organ System Changes with Aging 8
Normal Aging 8
Complexity, Homeostenosis, and Integrated Systems . . 8
Resources 10

Chapter 3—Ethics and Law 11
Approach to Ethical Dilemmas 11
Principles of Medical Ethics 13
Informed Consent and Decisional Capacity 13
Truth Telling 14
Surrogate Decision-Making 14
Promoting Individual Preferences for Future Care . 15
Controversial Procedures at End of Life 16
Moral Distress 17
Resources 17

Chapter 4—Financing, Coverage, and Costs of Health Care 18
Medicare Parts A and B 18
Medigap 19
Medicare Part C 20
Medicare Part D 20
Hospice 20
Medicaid 20
Dual Eligibles 21
Long-Term Care Insurance 21
Affordable Care Act (ACA) 21
Medicare Access and CHIP Reauthorization Act (MACRA) 22
Department of Veterans Affairs (VA) Benefit 22
Resources 22

APPROACH TO THE PATIENT

Chapter 5—Assessment 24
Routine Office Visit 24
Welcome to Medicare Visit 24
Annual Wellness Visit 24
Patient-Clinician Communication 24
Physical Assessment 25
Medication Assessment 25
Cognitive Assessment 25
Psychologic Assessment 26
Social Assessment 26
Functional Status 26
Acute Functional Decline 28
Quality of Life and Advance Care Planning 28
Resources 29

Chapter 6—Prognostication 30
Importance of and Barriers to Prognostication 30
Estimating Prognosis 30
Communicating Prognosis 33
Resources 33

Chapter 7—Multimorbidity 34
Approach to the Older Adult with Multimorbidity . . 34
Guiding Principles 34
Controversies and Challenges 36
Resources 36

Chapter 8—Caregiving 37
Defining Caregiving 37
Considerations in Clinical Assessment 40
Interventions and Referrals 40
Resources 41

Chapter 9—Cultural Aspects of Care 42
Use of Language and Nonverbal Communication . . . 42
History of Traumatic Experiences 44
Issues of Immigration 44
Acculturation, Tradition, and Health Beliefs 45
Approaches: The ETHNICS Mnemonic 45
Unspoken Challenges 46
Approaches to Decision Making 46
Attitudes Regarding Disclosure and Consent 46
Gender Issues 46
Spiritual and Religious Issues 47
Advance Care Planning 47
End-of-Life Issues 48
Resources 48

Chapter 10—Lesbian Gay Bisexual Transgender Health 49
Background 50

Asking About Sexual Orientation and Gender
   Identity 50
Medical Issues of LGBT Older Adults 50
Mental Health, Social, and Economic Issues
   Affecting LGBT Older Adults. 52
Resources 54

Chapter 11—Physical Activity 55
Benefits of Physical Activity 55
Recommended Amounts of Physical Activity 55
Promotion of Physical Activity 58
Resources 59

Chapter 12—Screening and Prevention 60
Cancer Screening Tests. 60
Other Screening Tests and Preventive Measures. . . . 66
Healthy Lifestyle Counseling 70
Geriatric Health Issues. 71
Immunizations. 73
Chemoprophylaxis. 73
Counseling on Cancer Screening and Preventive
   Health 74
Resources 75

Chapter 13—Pharmacotherapy 76
Age-Associated Changes in Pharmacokinetics. 76
Age-Associated Changes in Pharmacodynamics 78
Optimizing Prescribing 79
Adverse Drug Events 81
Drug-Drug Interactions 81
Drug-Disease Interactions. 82
Role of the Pharmacist 82
Principles of Prescribing 82
Discontinuing Medications 83
Nonadherence 83
Resources 84

**Chapter 14—Complementary and Integrative
   Medicine** 85
Safety Issues 85
Efficacy of CIM 85
Medical Cannabis and Cannabinoids. 88
Resources 88

Chapter 15—Mistreatment 89
Risk Factors 89
Screening 90
Observation. 90
History 90
Assessment 92
Self-Neglect 94
The Caregiver–Older Adult Dyad 94
Institutional Mistreatment 94
Intervention 95
Documentation 95
The Medical-Legal Interface 95
Resources 96

CARE SYSTEMS

Chapter 16—Perioperative Care. 97
Preoperative Assessment and Management. 97
Perioperative and Postoperative Management of
   Selected Medical Problems 102
Resources 105

Chapter 17—Palliative Care 106
Overall Care Near Death 106
Unique Populations 106
Hospice 107
Communication 108
Palliation of Symptoms. .109
Future Directions. 115
Resources 116

Chapter 18—Pain Management. 117
Assessment 118
Assessing and Treating Pain in Cognitively
   Impaired Older Adults 120
Treatment 120
Resources 125

Chapter 19—Hospital Care. 126
Hazards of Hospitalization 126
"Never Events" 128
Assessing and Managing Hospitalized Older
   Patients 130
Models of Care for Older Hospitalized Patients . . .135
Alternatives to Hospital Care 136
Hospital Compare 136
Readmission 137
Resources 138

Chapter 20—Transitions of Care. 139
The Risks of Suboptimal Care Transitions 139
Incentives, Barriers, and Responsibilities 139
Strategies and Models to Improve Transitional Care .140
Discharge Destinations and Care Venues 141
The Discharge Medication Regimen 141
Communicating with the Patient, Caregivers, and
   Receiving Team. 141
Three Steps to Improve Care Transitions. 142
Resources 142

Chapter 21—Rehabilitation 143
Conceptual Model for Geriatric Rehabilitation. . . .143
Sites of Rehabilitation Care 143
Teams and Roles 146
Impact of Comorbid Conditions 146
Elements of a Comprehensive Assessment 148
Approaches for Diagnosis-Specific Rehabilitation . . .148
Approaches for Commonly Encountered
   Rehabilitation Issues. .153
Mobility Aids, Orthotics, Adaptive Methods, and
   Environmental Modifications. 155
Resources 158

Chapter 22—Nursing-Home Care 159
The Nursing-Home Population 159
Nursing-Home Availability 159
Financing 160
Staffing Patterns 160
The Interface of Acute Care and the Nursing Home .161
Regulations 161
Medical Care 163
Special-Care Units 163
Advance Care Planning 163
Resources 164

Chapter 23—Community-Based Care 165
Home Care 165
Community-Based Services: Aging Services
 Network 167
Community-Based Services not Requiring a
 Change in Residence .168
Community-Based Services Requiring a Change of
 Residence 170
Resources 171

Chapter 24—Outpatient Care Systems 173
Geriatrics in Primary Care 173
Geriatric Specialty Care 176
Patient Selection for Outpatient Interventions 178
Resources 179

SYNDROMES

Chapter 25—Frailty 180
The Concept of Frailty 180
Evidence as to Cause 182
Assessment of Frailty 182
Prevailing Management Strategies 183
Potential Approaches for Prevention of Frailty 183
Frailty and Palliative Care 184
Resources 184

**Chapter 26—Visual Loss and Other Eye
 Conditions** 185
Common Eye Conditions Older Adults 185
Red Eye 187
Ophthalmic Corticosteroids 188
Refractive Error and Cataracts 188
Age-Related Macular Degeneration (ARMD) 189
Diabetic Retinopathy 190
Glaucoma 191
Anterior Ischemic Optic Neuropathy 191
Charles Bonnet Syndrome 192
Low-Vision Rehabilitation .192
Resources 192

Chapter 27—Hearing Loss 193
Normal Hearing and Age-Related Changes in the
 Auditory System 193
Epidemiology 193
Presbycusis 194
Clinical Presentation and Detection of Hearing
 Loss 194
Evaluation of Suspected Hearing Loss 195
Treatment 196
Resources 201

Chapter 28—Dizziness .202
Classification 202
Evaluation 204
Management 205
Resources 206

Chapter 29—Syncope 207
Natural History: Diagnosis and Prognosis 207
Pathophysiology 208
Evaluation 208
Treatment 211
Public Reporting 212
Resources 212

Chapter 30—Nutrition and Weight 213
Age-Related Changes 213
Nutrition Screening and Assessment 214
Nutrition Syndromes 217
Nutritional Interventions .218
Culturally Appropriate Nutritional Care 219
Legal and Ethical Issues 220
Resources 221

Chapter 31—Swallowing and Feeding 222
Swallowing in Health and Disease 222
Feeding 223
Resources 224

Chapter 32—Urinary Incontinence 225
Prevalence and Impact 225
Risk Factors and Associated Comorbid Conditions . .226
Pathophysiology 226
Evaluation 228
Treatment and Management 229
Evaluation and Management of UI in Nursing-
 Home Residents 231
Catheters and Catheter Care 232
Resources 233

Chapter 33—Pressure Injuries and Wound Care . .234
Chronic Wound Healing 235
Pressure Injury Definition and Classification 235
Pressure Injury Assessment and Documentation . . .236
Pressure Injury Prevention 237
Principles of Pressure Injury Treatment 238
Infectious Aspects of Pressure Injuries 241
Differential Diagnosis of Lower Extremity Wounds . .242
Palliative Care for Chronic Wounds 242
Resources 243

Chapter 34—Gait Impairment 244
Epidemiology. 244
Conditions that Contribute to Gait Impairment 244
Assessment 245
Interventions to Reduce Gait Disorders 247
Resources 249

Chapter 35—Falls. 250
Prevalence and Morbidity 250
Causes and Risk Factors. 250
Clinical Guidelines. 252
Diagnostic Approach 252
Treatment and Prevention 255
Resources 259

Chapter 36—Osteoporosis 260
Osteoporosis Definition. .260
Epidemiology and Impact 260
Bone Remodeling and Bone Loss in Aging 261
Risk Factors for Osteoporosis 261
Prediction and Diagnosis of Fractures 262
Prevention and Treatment 266
Vertebral Fracture Management 271
Resources 271

Chapter 37—Dementia .272
Epidemiology and Societal Impact. 272
Etiology. 273
Risk Factors and Prevention. 273
Assessment 273
Differentiating Between Dementia, Depression,
 and Delirium 276
Subtypes of Dementia. 276
Treatment and Management 279
Resources 283

**Chapter 38—Behavioral Disturbances in
 Dementia.** 284
Clinical Features 284
Assessment and Differential Diagnosis 285
Treatment Approach 287
Treatments for Specific Disturbances. 287
Resources 293

Chapter 39—Delirium 294
Incidence and Prognosis. 294
Diagnosis and Differential Diagnosis 294
The Spectrum and Neuropathophysiology of
 Delirium 295
Risk Factors 296
Delirium and Dementia 296
Postoperative Delirium. 297
Evaluation 297
Management 298
Quality Measures and Consensus Guidelines 303
Resources 303

Chapter 40—Sleep Issues 304
Epidemiology. 304
Changes in Sleep with Aging 304
Evaluation of Sleep 305
Common Sleep Problems 305
Changes in Sleep with Dementia 309
Sleep Disturbances in the Hospital 309
Sleep in Long-Term Care Settings 310
Management of Insomnia 310
Resources 315

PSYCHIATRY

**Chapter 41—Depression and Other Mood
 Disorders.** 316
Epidemiology. 316
Clinical Presentation and Diagnosis. 317
Treatment 319
Resources 324

Chapter 42—Anxiety Disorders 325
Classes of Anxiety Disorders. 325
Comorbidity 328
Pharmacologic Management 328
Psychologic Management 329
Resources 330

**Chapter 43—Schizophrenia Spectrum and
 Other Psychotic Disorders.** 331
Schizophrenia and Schizophrenia Spectrum
 Syndromes 331
Psychotic Symptoms Associated with Other Non-
 Schizophrenic Disorders 333
Resources 335

**Chapter 44—Personality and Somatic Symptom
 Disorders.** 336
Personality Disorders. 336
Somatic Symptom and Related Disorders. 340
Resources 343

Chapter 45—Addictions 344
Definitions of Substance Use Disorders 344
Magnitude of the Problem. 345
Risks of Substance Use. .346
Identifying Substance Use Disorders: Risk Factors
 and Screening. 348
Treatment 348
Other Addictions 351
Resources 351

**Chapter 46—Intellectual and Developmental
 Disabilities.** 352
Prevalence 352
Diagnostic and Treatment Issues 354
Psychiatric and Behavioral Disorders 354

Medical Disorders 356
Social Conditions 357
Developmental Disabilities and Comorbidity 357
Resources 359

DISEASES AND DISORDERS

Chapter 47—Dermatology 360
Aging and Photoaging 360
Inflammatory and Autoimmune Skin Conditions ... 360
Infections and Infestations 365
Benign Growths 368
Skin Cancer 369
Resources 370

Chapter 48—Dentistry and Oral Health 372
Aging of the Teeth 372
Dental Decay 372
Periodontal Disease 373
Missing Teeth and Dentures 373
Salivary Function in Aging 374
Common Oral Lesions 375
Chemosensory Perception 376
The Relationship Between Oral Health, General
  Health and the Impact of Medications on the
  Oral Cavity 377
Oral Assessment 378
Oral Hygiene in Long-Term Care Facilities 379
Resources 379

Chapter 49—Pulmonology 380
Age-Related Pulmonary Changes 380
Common Respiratory Symptoms and Complaints ... 380
Major Pulmonary Diseases 382
Resources 389

Chapter 50—Cardiovascular Disease 390
Epidemiology 390
Effects of Aging on Cardiovascular Function 390
Cardiovascular Risk Factors 390
Coronary Artery Disease 392
Acute Coronary Syndromes 393
Chronic Coronary Artery Disease 394
Valvular Heart Disease 397
Cardiac Arrhythmias 398
Peripheral Arterial Disease 404
Shared Decision Making in Cardiovascular Disease . 405
Resources 406

Chapter 51—Heart Failure 407
Epidemiology 407
Etiology and Pathophysiology 407
Clinical Features 407
Diagnosis 408
Management 408
Recurrent Hospitalization 414

Prognosis 414
End-of-Life Care 415
Resources 415

Chapter 52—Hypertension 416
Epidemiology and Physiology 416
Clinical Evaluation 417
Treatment 417
Special Considerations 421
Resources 422

Chapter 53—Gastroenterology 423
Disorders of the Esophagus 423
Disorders of the Stomach 426
Disorders of the Colon 429
Resources 434

Chapter 54—Nephrology 435
Kidney Assessment 435
Metabolic and Volume Disorders 436
Secondary Hypertension and Renal Artery Disease . 439
Hematuria 440
Acute Kidney Injury 440
Chronic Kidney Disease 443
End-Stage Renal Disease (ESRD) 445
Resources 446

Chapter 55—Gynecology 447
History and Physical Examination 447
Menopausal Symptoms 448
Genitourinary Syndrome of Menopause 449
Vulvovaginal Infection and Inflammation 449
Disorders of the Vulva 450
Pelvic Floor Disorders 451
Postmenopausal Vaginal Bleeding 453
Resources 454

Chapter 56—Prostate Disease and Cancer 455
Benign Prostatic Hyperplasia 455
Prostate Cancer 457
Prostatitis 463
Resources 464

Chapter 57—Sexuality 465
Sexuality and Aging 465
Male Sexuality 465
Female Sexuality 469
Sexuality in Long-Term Care 471
Lesbian, Gay, Bisexual, and Transgender Older
  Adults in Long-Term Care 473
Resources 474

Chapter 58—Musculoskeletal Pain 475
General Principles for Diagnosis 475
Evaluation and Management of Regional
  Musculoskeletal Complaints 476
Resources 484

vii

Chapter 59—Rheumatology 485
Osteoarthritis 485
Rheumatoid Arthritis. 487
Gout. 488
Calcium Pyrophosphate Dihydrate Deposition
    Disease. 490
Polymyalgia Rheumatica 490
Giant Cell Arteritis .491
Systemic Lupus Erythematosus. 492
Sjögren Syndrome 493
Polymyositis and Dermatomyositis 494
Fibromyalgia. 495
Resources 496

Chapter 60—Disorders of the Foot 497
The Role of the Primary Care Clinician in Foot
    Care 497
Common Deformities of the Foot. 497
Skin and Nail Disorders 503
Fall Risk and Podiatric Intervention 504
Systemic Diseases Affecting the Foot and Ankle 505
Resources 506

Chapter 61—Neurology 507
Epilepsy 507
Movement Disorders 508
Neuromuscular Disorders, Peripheral
    Neuropathy, and Myelopathy. 514
Headaches 516
Resources 517

**Chapter 62—Stroke and Cerebrovascular
    Disease** 518
Impact of Cerebrovascular Disease 518
Ischemic Stroke. 518
Hemorrhagic Stroke. 522
Resources 524

Chapter 63—Infectious Diseases. 525
Predisposition to Infection 525
Diagnosis and Management of Infections 526
Immunizations. 528
Infectious Syndromes. 531
Fever of Unknown Origin 540
Resources 541

Chapter 64—Endocrinology. 542
Thyroid Disorders 543
Disorders of Parathyroid and Calcium Metabolism. .547
Disorders of the Anterior Pituitary 551
Disorders of the Adrenal Cortex 553
Testosterone 555
Resources 557

Chapter 65—Diabetes Mellitus 558
Pathophysiology of Diabetes. 558
Diagnosis and Evaluation 558
Prevention 558

Management 559
Interventions 560
Management of Diabetes Across the Continuum of
    Care 563
Resources 566

Chapter 66—Hematology 567
Hematopoietic Stem Cells and Aging 567
Anemia 567
Platelets and Coagulation Disorders 571
Myeloid Hematologic Malignancies 572
Resources 573

**Chapter 67—Oncology and Hematologic
    Malignancies** 574
Cancer Biology and Aging 575
Principles of Cancer Management 576
Specific Cancers. 583
Hematologic Malignancies, Lymphomas, and
    Multiple Myeloma 589
Principles of Management. 590
Resources 590

Normal Laboratory Values 591
Index of Question Numbers by Primary Topic 592
Questions 593
Questions, Answers, and Critiques 627
GRS10 Editorial Board 715
Contributing *GRS10* Chapter Authors. 717
Contributing *GRS10* Question Authors 723
Disclosure of Financial Interests 728
Index 730

GNRS6 EDITORIAL BOARD

CHIEF EDITOR

Barbara Resnick, PhD, CRNP, FAAN, FAANP, AGSF, FGSA
Professor, Sonya Ziporkin Gershowitz Chair in Gerontology
University of Maryland School of Nursing
Baltimore, MD

EDITORS

Marie Boltz, PhD, GNP-BC, FGSA, FAAN
Elouise Ross Eberly and Robert Eberly Endowed Chair
Professor, Penn State College of Nursing
University Park, PA

Elizabeth Capezuti, PhD, RN, FAAN
William Randolph Hearst Foundation Chair in Gerontology
Hunter College School of Nursing
City University of New York
New York, NY

Deirdre M. Carolan, PhD, ANP-BC, GNP-BC, FAANP
Nurse Practitioner, Geriatrics
Inova Fairfax Hospital
Falls Church, VA
VANAP Project Director
Assistant Clinical Professor
The Catholic University of America
Washington, DC

Carolyn Clevenger, RN, DNP, AGPCNP-BC, GNP-BC, FAANP
Associate Dean for Clinical and Community Partnerships
Clinical Professor
Nell Hodgson Woodruff School of Nursing
Emory University
Atlanta, GA

Elizabeth Galik, PhD, CRNP, FAAN, FAANP
Professor
University of Maryland
School of Nursing
Baltimore, MD

Laurie Kennedy-Malone, PhD, GNP-BC, FAANP, FGSA
Professor of Nursing
School of Nursing
University of North Carolina at Greensboro
Greensboro, NC

GNRS6 EDITORIAL STAFF

Managing Editor
Andrea N. Sherman, MS

AGS Staff
Nancy Lundebjerg, MPA, Chief Executive Officer
Laura Banks, Customer Service Coordinator
Aimee Cegelka, Senior Manager, Education & Special Projects
Joe Douglas, Managing Editor, GeriatricsCareOnline.org and *Geriatrics At Your Fingertips*
Elvy Ickowicz, MPH, Senior Vice President, Operations
Dennise McAlpin, Senior Manager, Professional Education and Special Projects
Elisha Medina-Gallagher, Manager, Special Projects
Linda Saunders, MSW, Assistant Vice President, Education & Governance

Medical Editor
Susan E. Aiello, DVM, ELS

Indexer
L. Pilar Wyman

Fry Communications, Inc.
Melissa Durborow, Information Services Manager
Jason Hughes, Technical Services Manager
Rhonda Liddick, Composition Manager
William F. Adams, Compositor
Julie Stevens, Customer Service
Brian Judge, Graphic Designer

Cover Design
Ann Casady, Casady Design

> The *Geriatric Nursing Review Syllabus*, 6th edition, is based on the *Geriatrics Review Syllabus*, 10th edition, which was developed by the below editorial board and authors. For a complete listing of the *GRS10* contributors and their professional affiliations, please see p. 717.

ORIGINAL *GRS10* EDITORIAL BOARD AND AUTHORS

Chief Editors, Syllabus
G. Michael Harper, MD, AGSF
William L. Lyons, MD, AGSF

Syllabus Editors
Jessica L. Colburn, MD
Timothy W. Farrell, MD, AGSF
Jonathan M. Flacker, MD, AGSF
Lisa J. Granville, MD, FACP, AGSF
Melinda S. Lantz, MD
Amy M. Westcott, MD, MHPE, CMD, AGSF

Special Advisors
Kevin T. Foley, MD, FACP, AGSF
Matthew K. McNabney, MD, AGSF

Consulting Editor for Pharmacotherapy
Judith L. Beizer, PharmD, BCGP, FASCP, AGSF

Consulting Editor for Ethnogeriatrics
Sharon A. Brangman, MD, FACP, AGSF

Chief Editor, Questions
Jane F. Potter, MD, FACP, AGSF

Question Editors
Jonathan S. Appelbaum, MD, FACP, AAHIVS
Ian M. Deutchki, MD
Rachel K. Miller, MD, MsED
Gary J. Kennedy, MD
Rainier Patrick Soriano, MD

Nursing Advisor
Elizabeth Galik, PhD, CRNP, FAAN, FAANP

Student Advisor
Laura K. Byerly, MD

AUTHORS OF ORIGINAL *GRS10* CHAPTERS

CURRENT ISSUES IN AGING
Demography — Paul Scalzo, BS; Luigi Ferrucci, MD, PhD
Biology — Matthew K. McNabney, MD, AGSF; Neal S. Fedarko, PhD
Ethics and Law — Elizabeth K. Vig, MD, MPH
Financing, Coverage, and Costs of Health Care — Richard G. Stefanacci, DO, MGH, MBA, AGSF, CMD

APPROACH TO PATIENT
Assessment — Thomas M. Gill, MD
Prognostication — Daphine Lo, MD MAEd; Eric Widera, MD
Multimorbidity — Cynthia M. Boyd, MD, MPH; Matthew K. McNabney, MD, AGSF
Caregiving — Sarah H. Kagan, PhD, RN; Brianna Morgan, MSN, AGPCNP-BC
Cultural Aspects of Care — Vyjeyanthi S. Periyakoil, MD
Lesbian Gay Bisexual Transgender Health — Mark Simone, MD; Manuel A. Eskildsen, MD, MPH, CMD, AGSF
Physical Activity — Robin Marcus, PT, PhD, OCS; Paul C. LaStayo, PT, PhD, CHT
Screening and Prevention — Mara A. Schonberg, MD, MPH
Pharmacotherapy — Judith L. Beizer, PharmD, BCGP, FASCP, AGSF

xi

Complementary and Alternative Medicine   Taya Varteresian, DO, MS
    Helen Lavretsky, MD, MS
Mistreatment   Mark S. Lachs, MD, MPH
    Tony Rosen, MD, MPH

CARE SYSTEMS
Perioperative Care   Colleen Christmas, MD, FACP
    James T. Pacala, MD, MS, AGSF
Palliative Care   Grace A. Cordts, MD, MPH, MS
    Danielle J. Doberman, MD, MPH
Pain Management   Vyjeyanthi S. Periyakoil, MD
Hospital Care   Margarita Sotelo, MD
    Edgar Pierluissi, MD
Transitions of Care   Alicia I. Arbaje, MD, MPH
Rehabilitation   Kathleen T. Foley, PhD, OTR/L
    Cynthia J. Brown, MD, MSPH, AGSF
Nursing-Home Care   Suzanne M. Gillespie, MD, RD, CMD, FACP
    Timothy J. Holahan DO, CMD
Community-Based Care   Kristen Thornton, MD, FAAFP, AGSF, CWSP
    Thomas V. Caprio, MD, MPH, MS, AGSF
Outpatient Care Systems   Michael R. Wasserman, MD, CMD

SYNDROMES
Frailty   Jeremy D. Walston, MD
Visual Loss and Eye Conditions   JoAnn A. Giaconi, MD
    Pradeep S. Prasad, MD, MBA
Hearing Loss   Priscilla F. Bade, MD, FACP, CMD
    Sujana S. Chandrasekhar, MD, FACS
Dizziness   Aman Nanda, MD, CMD, AGSF
Syncope   J. William Schleifer, MD
    Win-Kuang Shen, MD
Nutrition and Weight   James S. Powers, MD, AGSF
    Maciej S. Buchowski, PhD
Swallowing and Feeding   Colleen Christmas, MD, FACP
Urinary Incontinence   Catherine E. DuBeau, MD
Pressure Injuries and Wound Care   Jeffrey M. Levine, MD, AGSF, CWSP
Gait Impairment   Neil B. Alexander, MD
Falls   Sarah D. Berry, MD, MPH
    Douglas P. Kiel, MD, MPH
Osteoporosis   Michael L. Krol, MD
    Kenneth W. Lyles, MD, AGSF
Dementia   Zaldy S. Tan, MD, MPH
    Jarrod A. Carrol, MD
Behavioral Disturbances in Dementia   Melinda S. Lantz, MD
    Priya Sharma, MD, FRCPC
Delirium   Edward R. Marcantonio, MD, SM
Sleep Issues   Cathy A. Alessi, MD, AGSF

PSYCHIATRY
Depression and Other Mood Disorders   Gary J. Kennedy, MD
    Johanna A. Cabassa, MD
Anxiety Disorders   Judith Neugroschl, MD
Schizophrenia Spectrum and Other Psychotic   Susan W. Lehmann, MD
Disorders

Personality and Somatic Symptom Disorders
Addictions

Intellectual and Developmental Disabilities

DISEASES AND DISORDERS
Dermatology
Dentistry and Oral Health
Pulmonology

Cardiovascular Disease

Heart Failure

Hypertension

Gastroenterology

Nephrology

Gynecology
Prostate Disease and Cancer
Sexuality

Musculoskeletal Pain
Rheumatology

Disorders of the Foot
Neurology
Stroke and Cerebrovascular Disease
Infectious Diseases

Endocrinology

Diabetes Mellitus

Hematology

Oncology and Hematologic Malignancies

Kecia-Ann Blissett, DO
Daniel T. McGovern, MD
Amy Swift, MD
Elizabeth Galik, PhD, CRNP, FAAN, FAANP
Andrew Warren, MB, BS, DPhil

Jane M. Grant-Kels, MD
Kevin T. Hendler, DDS, FASGD, DABSCD, FICD
Kathleen M. Akgün, MD
Margaret Pisani, MD, MPH
Jason Costa, MD
John A. Dodson, MD, MPH, FACC
Kumar Dharmarajan, MD, MBA
Michael W. Rich, MD, AGSF
Ayman Samman Tahhan, MD
Ihab Hajjar, MD, MS, FACP
Amir E. Soumekh, MD
Philip O. Katz, MD
Naomi B. Anker, MD
Josette A. Rivera, MD
Melinda Gail Abernethy, MD, MPH
Lisa J. Granville, MD, AGSF, FACP
Angela Gentili, MD
Michael Godschalk, MD
Leo M. Cooney, Jr, MD
Una E. Makris, MD, MCS
Emily A. Bowen, MD
Robert Eckles, DPM, MPH
Daniel L. Murman, MD, MS, FAAN
Daniel L. Murman, MD, MS, FAAN
Manisha Juthani-Mehta, MD
Theresa A. Rowe, DO
David A. Gruenewald, MD
Alvin M. Matsumoto, MD
Pei Chen, MD
Sei J. Lee, MD, MAS
Thomas M. Reske, MD, PhD, FACP, CMD
Scott Hebert, MD
Ronald J. Maggiore, MD
Allison Magnuson, DO

CONTRIBUTING *GRS10* QUESTION AUTHORS

Emaad M. Abdel-Rahman, MD, PhD, FASN
Kyrollis Attalla, MD
Sharon Baranoski, MSN, CWCN, APN-CCNS, FAAN
Kevin Barley, MD
Lisa C. Barry, PhD, MPH
Rachelle Bernacki, MD, MS, AGSF, FAAHPM
Michael Bogaisky, MD, MPH
Daniel C. Butler, MD
Debra L. Bynum, MD, MMEL
Johanna A. Cabassa, MD
Mirnova E. Ceïde, MD
Sujana S. Chandrasekhar, MD
Susan Charette, MD
Pei Chen, MD
Victoria Chimna, MD, MPH
Natsurang Chongkrairatanakul, MD, ABIM
Jason A. Cohen, MD
Lenise A. Cummings-Vaughn, MD, CMD
Clark DuMontier, MD
Robert Eckles, DPM, MPH
Jerome Epplin, MD, AGSF
Elisabeth Erekson, MD, MPH, FACOG, FACS
Michelle T. Fabian, MD
Mary Ann Forciea, MD, MACP
Daniel E. Forman, MD, FAHA, FACC
Shelly L. Gray, PharmD, MS, AGSF
Elizabeth N. Harlow, MD
Victoria Hornyak, PT, DPT, GCS
Peter Jin, MD
Sana F. Khan, MD
Tia Kostas, MD
Stephen Krieger, MD, FAAN
Lee A. Jennings, MD, MSHS
Karin A. Johnson, OD, DO
Theodore M. Johnson II, MD, MPH, AGSF
Deirdre Johnston, MB BCh BAO, MRCPsych
Kathleen M. Kan, MD
Fran E. Kaiser, MD, AGSF, FGSA
Anne Kenny, MD
Rashmi Khadilkar, MD
Lawrence R. Krakoff, MD

June C. Lee, DO
Pearl G. Lee, MD, MS
Milta Oyola Little, DO, CMD
Vera P. Luther, MD, FACP, FIDSA
Elizabeth Mann, MD
Sarah McGee, MD, MPH
Stephen A. McCullough, MD
Diana V. Messadi, DDS, MMSc, DMSc
Isuzu Meyer, MD
Leigh Ann Mike, PharmD, BCPS, BCGP
Ian Neel, MD
Tyson A. Oberndorfer, MD, MS
Cynthia X. Pan, MD, FACP, AGSF
Manisha Parulekar, MD, FACP, AGSF, CMD
Thomas T. Perls, MD, MPH, AGSF, FGSA
Barbara Resnick, PhD, CRNP, FAAN, AGSF
Bernardo J. Reyes, MD
Katherine Ritchey, DO, MPH
Christopher K. Rogers, MPH
Scott A. Roof, MD
Matthew Leo Russell, MD, MSc
Arunima Sarkar, MD, FACP, CMD
Jean-Pierre Schuster, MD
Himanshu S. Sharma, MD
Nina J. Solenski, MD
Margarita Sotelo, MD
Niharika Suchak, MBBS, MHS, FACP, AGSF
Winnie Suen, MD, MSc, AGSF
Dennis H. Sullivan, MD, AGSF
Kristen Thornton, MD, FAAFP, AGSF, CWSP
S.P.J. (Bas) van Alphen, PhD
Jessie VanSwearingen, PhD, PT, FAPTA
Camille P. Vaughan, MD, MS
Christina R. Whitehouse, PhD, CRNP, CDE
Supakanya Wongrakpanich, MD
Rebecca L. Wysoske, MD
Fariba S. Younai, DDS
Michi Yukawa, MD, MPH, AGSF
Raymond Yung, MD
Valerie Zamudio, MD
Phyllis C. Zee, MD, PhD

ACKNOWLEDGMENTS

It is my great pleasure to acknowledge the many people who have made the *Geriatric Nursing Review Syllabus: A Core Curriculum in Advanced Practice Geriatric Nursing, 6th Edition (GNRS6)* possible. Thanks to the *GNRS6* Co-Editors: Marie Boltz, PhD, GNP-BC; Elizabeth Capezuti, PhD, RN, FAAN; Carolyn Clevenger, RN, DNP, AGPCNP-BC, GNP-BC, FAANP; Deirdre M. Carolan, PhD, ANP, BC, GNP-BC, FAANP; Elizabeth Galik, PhD, FAAN, CRNP; and Laurie Kennedy-Malone, PhD, GNP-BC. We are all grateful to the editors and contributing *GRS10* authors of chapters and questions for lending their expertise to this publication. Thanks to Andrea Sherman, MS, GRS Managing Editor, for her guidance, organization, and coordination overseeing the administrative and editorial aspects of the program; to Susan E. Aiello, DVM, ELS, our medical editor; to L. Pilar Wyman for her comprehensive index; and to the AGS Board of Directors and AGS staff members for their support.

PREFACE

The American Geriatrics Society (AGS), with almost 6,000 members, works to improve the health, independence, and quality of life of all older adults. The AGS is committed to increasing the number of healthcare professionals using the principles of geriatrics by supporting the expansion of geriatric education in nursing and all interrelated health professions. The AGS recognizes the critically important role that nurses play as members of the team providing care to older adults, and in 2003, created the *Geriatric Nursing Review Syllabus (GNRS)* for advanced practice nurses.

The *GNRS* provides current and comprehensive clinically relevant information to nurse practitioners preparing for certification exams as adult/gerontological, adult/gerontology acute care nurse practitioners or family nurse practitioners. It is an essential resource for all providers to quickly access during their clinical day. In addition to being of value to students and nurse practitioners in practice, the *GNRS* is an invaluable resource for faculty. The comprehensive content of this new *GNRS* edition provides learners, faculty, and nurse practitioners with information on diagnosis, management, and prevention of all major health problems commonly encountered when caring for older adults as well as on the social and legal issues related to health care in the United States. Having access to the information in this book will promote our current goal of providing high-quality and affordable care to all older adults.

We are releasing the 6th edition of the *Syllabus* at a time when the population of older adults is increasing rapidly and all advanced practice nurses need to have expertise in geriatrics. The *GNRS*, given its focus on the complexities of caring for those with multiple comorbidities, can help to assure that all advanced practice nurses have the knowledge to provide optimal care to older adults across all levels of care.

Barbara Resnick, PhD, CRNP, FAAN, FAANP, FGSA, AGSF
GNRS6 Chief Editor

INTRODUCTION

The *Geriatric Nursing Review Syllabus, 6th edition (GNRS6)* is modified from the *Geriatrics Review Syllabus, 10th edition (GRS10)* and contains 67 chapters and resources that allow readers to pursue topics in greater depth, 126 case-oriented, multiple-choice questions, and the repeated questions with answers and supporting critiques to aid learner self-assessment.

The *Syllabus* is divided into six sections: Principles of Aging, Approach to the Patient, Care Systems, Syndromes, Psychiatry, and Diseases and Disorders. *GNRS6* particularly highlights developments in geriatrics since publication of the 5th edition.

Choosing Wisely® recommendations have been added to many chapters based on the American Board of Internal Medicine Foundation's Choosing Wisely® Campaign.

When discussing specific drugs, the authors and editors verified that the information provided was up-to-date at the time of publication. Any mentions of drug use not specifically approved by the U.S. Food and Drug Administration (so called "off-label" use) are tagged as ^{OL}. The majority of medications described in the text are approved in the United States, although authors occasionally note the use of medications that are approved in Europe but not in the United States.

Strength of Evidence

In support of an evidence-based approach to care, authors have included strength-of-evidence (SOE) ratings for key diagnostic, prognostic, and therapeutic information. Authors and editors also have endeavored to present measures of association (between risk factors or therapies and conditions) in terms of absolute risk or numbers needed to treat (NNT), as well as relative risk. Please see the inside cover for further explanation of the SOE rating system.

Ethnogeriatrics in *GNRS6*

The classification of individuals by race and ethnicity has a long and complex history in our country. The term African-American has been used to describe people based on ancestry that links to the continent of Africa. However, within this group are people of Caribbean descent, descendants of the U.S. slave trade, as well as those who may come from any one of the many countries of Africa. Members of groups of African-Americans may share an array of skin tones but have different ethnicities, reflected by their country of origin and cultural and religious heritage. This edition of the *GNRS* uses data that generally refer to African-Americans with ancestry related to descendants of the U.S. slave trade.

Similar designations also understate the diversity among Latino, Asian, white American, and Native American groups. Latinos may be of any race and can originate from countries across Central and South America. Asians can be from countries as different as India or Sri Lanka in South Asia, to Japan, Korea, or China in East Asia. Significant diversity also exists among those classified as white Americans who have ancestry and religious traditions from broad areas across Europe and other countries. Native Americans represent 562 recognized tribes in the United States with varied language, religious, and tribal traditions.

Our goal in this edition of the *GNRS* is to discuss topics and review research in which ethnogeriatrics is important, with the understanding that deficits and gaps exist in the available knowledge base when describing and reporting findings in diverse populations. In cases when authors have cited ethnic and racial data, the convention in *GNRS* is to maintain the designations used in the original publications, when known, in order not to inadvertently change the meaning of the data. Readers should understand this diversity and the complexity of racial and ethnic designations while avoiding stereotypes and striving to focus on the individual needs of patients.

Multiple Choice Questions

The questions are designed to complement material in the *Syllabus* chapters. The questions are case based and draw on the entire knowledge base of geriatrics, rather than just material from the *Syllabus* text. We recommend that participants prepare for answering these questions by first reading through the *Syllabus* chapters. Material addressed in the questions that is not discussed in the chapters is discussed in the critiques. The questions have been developed independently of any specialty board and will not be a part of any secure board certification examination. The *GNRS6* review questions are provided as learning aids but not as practice items for the Adult/Gerontological Advanced Practice Nurse Examination for the American Nurses Credentialing Center or the American Academy of Nurse Practitioners. We hope the *GNRS6* will meet our goal of enhancing participants' knowledge base and practice patterns when caring for older adults by providing a self-study tool that is current, concise, scholarly, and clinically relevant. We encourage your comments and suggestions, as the AGS continually strives to better serve its members and the older adults they treat.

SELF-ASSESSMENT PROGRAM

For self-assessment testing, answer sheets are available for download at www.GeriatricsCareOnline.org.

USER EVALUATION

The AGS would appreciate participants' comments about the *GNRS6* program through the User Survey located at http://www.GeriatricsCareOnline.org/. Comments and suggestions will be taken into consideration by those planning the next edition.

UPDATES AND ERRATA

Important updates, such as medication alerts, as well as errata, will be posted as necessary in the *GNRS* section of www.GeriatricsCareOnline.org. Please report any errata to info.amger@americangeriatrics.org, Attention: *GNRS* Managing Editor.

ADDITIONAL AMERICAN GERIATRICS SOCIETY RESOURCES

GNRS Teaching Slides are available as a subscription through www.GeriatricsCareOnline.org. The slide presentations in Microsoft® Power Point® are based on each of the *GNRS* chapters and suitable for faculty and students. Each presentation is designed for approximately a 1-hour seminar and may be used as a stand-alone lecture or as a complement to one's own personal teaching materials.

Geriatrics at Your Fingertips, published annually, provides quick, easy access to the specific information clinicians need to make decisions about the care of older adults. Available in print, digitally and as an App for your mobile device.

The *Geriatrics Evaluation and Management (GEM) Tools* include 20 clinical templates to support clinicians and systems that are caring for older adults with common geriatric conditions. Available digitally and as an App for your mobile device.

Doorway Thoughts: Cross-Cultural Health Care for Older Adults is a series that helps the health practitioner to understand how to best care for an increasingly multicultural patient population.

GRS10 Audio Companion includes 30-minute audio discussions on 67 topics based on the *GRS10* content with chapter authors and experts in the field. Continuing education credits can be obtained by successfully completing 35 multiple-choice questions derived from the audio content. The program offers 35 AMA PRA Category 1 Credits™.

These and other publications, including resources and clinical practice guidelines, are available at www.GeriatricsCareOnline.org.

For more information on the American Geriatrics Society, visit www.americangeriatrics.org.

CHAPTER 1—DEMOGRAPHY

KEY POINTS

- The number and proportion of older adults is increasing globally because of the increase in life expectancy and the decline in fertility and mortality.

- Less developed regions are experiencing a greater rate of population aging.

- Noncommunicable/chronic diseases are more prevalent in older adults and cause a greater financial burden than communicable diseases.

- In the United States, the aging of the baby boomer generation is causing a large increase in the number of older adults. The proportion of older adults of a minority racial and ethnic background is increasing.

- Older Americans rely greatly on public programs, such as Medicare and Social Security, and spend more on health care than younger Americans.

GLOBAL AGING TRENDS AND DEMOGRAPHICS

The recent global decline in fertility and mortality, coupled with the increase in life expectancy, has ushered the world into an era of population aging. Population aging can be defined as the change in the age composition toward older ages (≥60 years old), as the number of older adults increases relative to the number of younger people. Although population aging is a global phenomenon, substantial variability exists between geographic areas and population groups. Most of the data presented in this global section of the chapter are taken from the *World Population Prospects: The 2017 Revision* (United Nations).

In 2018, the proportion of adults ≥60 years old was estimated to be 25.0% of the population in more developed regions and 10.6% of the population in less developed regions. In 2050, 21.3% of the global population will be ≥60 years old, and about 80% of this age group will be living in less developed regions. This growth in the old age groups creates a square-shaped population pyramid (Figure 1.1). These pyramids suggest that over time, and with economic development, societies have become enriched in numbers of older individuals, but a biological age ceiling limits the maximum attainable age. In 2018, the 3 countries with the greatest number of people ≥60 years old were China (235.4 million), India (130.1 million), and the United States (71.8 million). In 2018, 25.0% of the

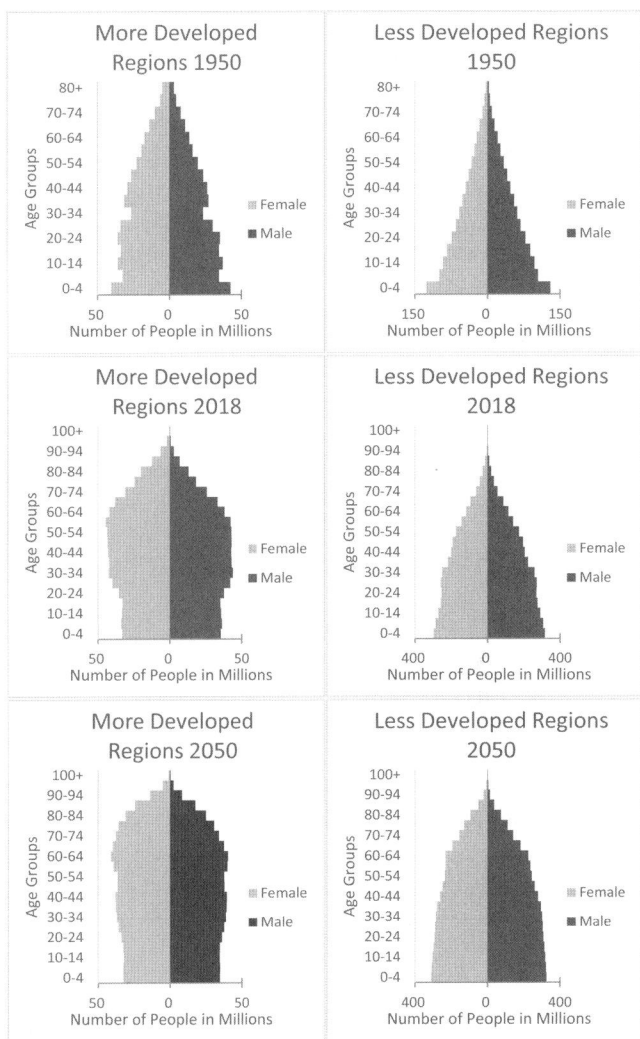

Figure 1.1—Number of People (millions) by Sex, 5-Year Age Group and Degree of Regional Development (all races)

SOURCE: Data from *World Population Prospects: The 2017 Revision*. Projections for Population by Five Year Age Group and Sex (thousands) Medium variant. 1950–2050. https://population.un.org/wpp (accessed Feb 2019). According to the United Nations' definition, more developed regions comprise Europe, Northern America, Australia/New Zealand, and Japan. Less developed regions comprise all regions of Africa, Asia (except Japan), Latin America and the Caribbean, plus Melanesia, Micronesia, and Polynesia.

population in Europe was ≥60 years old—a higher proportion than any other continent. In 2018, it was estimated that the continent of Asia had the greatest proportion of the world's elderly (57.2%), and in 2030 the proportion is expected to increase to 60.3%.

According to *World Population Aging 2017* (United Nations), the preeminent cause of the increase in the proportion of older people is a decrease in fertility and the consequent progressive reduction in the proportion of children. Increase in life expectancy also contributes

Chapter 1: Demography **1**

to global population aging. Between 2015 and 2020, the average life expectancy at birth is projected to be 79.3 years in more developed regions and 70.4 years in less developed regions. Between 2015 and 2020, it is projected that the life expectancy for those 60 years old will be 23.4 additional years in more developed regions but 19.5 in less developed regions.

Marital status does not vary considerably among developed regions. Globally, older women are more likely to be widowed than older men because of their longer life expectancy. Living arrangements depend on the social norms of the culture. Globally in 2015, 58% of adults ≥60 years old lived in urban areas; this percentage is expected to increase in the future.

Rising median age (the age that divides the population into half younger and half older) is a useful indicator of population aging. The median age of the world population has been steadily increasing and is projected to continue to increase in the future. Globally, the median age was 23.6 years of age in 1950, and 29.6 years of age in 2015; it is projected to be 30.9 years of age by 2020, 36.1 years of age by 2050, and 41.6 years of age by the end of the century.

The old-age dependency ratio is a metric used to assess the number of older persons for 100 persons of working age (15–64 years old) in the population, who are assumed to be independent and productive. The utility of this metric is controversial, because an increasing proportion of older adults work past age 65. Globally, in any case, the dependency ratio has been increasing. From 1950 to 2020, the old-age dependency ratio is projected to rise from 12 to 30 older adults (≥65 years old) per 100 productive workers in more developed regions, and it is projected to increase by an additional 16 older adults by 2050. Generally, in countries with an established pension system, the poverty rate for older people is not significantly different or may be lower than that of the population as a whole.

Because aging is a strong risk factor for most chronic diseases and because the management of chronic noncommunicable diseases is costly and long-lasting, the aging of the population is paralleled by expanding health expenditure and health care resource utilization. According to the World Health Organization's 2015 projections, noncommunicable disease accounts for 91.2% of deaths in adults ≥70 years old in developed regions, and for an average of 83.4% of deaths in the same age group in developing countries. In more developed countries, most health care costs for older adults are directly provided and financially covered by national health care systems, whereas in most of the less developed regions, older adults and their families bear most of the financial burden of care without help from the government or a structured pension system. The reform of social programs is a priority for countries with significant population aging to create a more sustainable and productive work environment for both the younger and older generations.

UNITED STATES AGING TRENDS AND DEMOGRAPHICS

Population Projections

The U.S. population is aging rapidly. The baby boomers (those born between 1946 and 1964) began turning 65 years old in 2011, and in 2029 the youngest of the individuals born during that time will turn 65 years old. The U.S. Census Bureau estimated that in July 2017, 15.6% of the U.S. population was ≥65 years old, by 2020 16.9% of the U.S. population will be ≥65 years old, and by 2030 one in five Americans, 20.6% of the U.S. population, will be ≥65 years old. In addition, the proportion of the "oldest-old" (those ≥85 years old) will grow significantly.

As the population grows older, it will also become more diverse. The U.S. Census Bureau has projected that in 2044, the aggregate minority population will surpass in number the current majority of white, non-Hispanic people. In July 2017, the racial and ethnic minority population made up about 23.1% of the population aged ≥65 years old; while about 19.9% of the population ≥85 years old was of a racial or ethnic minority. It is estimated that by 2050, "minority" individuals will account for 40.1% of the population ≥65 years old and 31.3% of the population ≥85 years old.

Because women have a longer life expectancy than men, they represent a larger proportion of the older population. In July 2017, men were 44.4% of the population ≥65 years old, and 35.2% of the population ≥85 years old.

Life Expectancy

In 2016, at the time of birth, men could expect to live an average of 76.1 years (down from 76.3 years in 2015) and women 81.1 years. In 2015, difference in life expectancy between men and women was projected to decline because of the faster rate of growth of life expectancy in men. White, native Hawaiian and other Pacific Islander men, and native Hawaiian and other Pacific Islander women will have the highest life expectancies at birth compared with other races. Black men and women will have the lowest life expectancy compared with other races. However, if ethnicity were considered, men and women of Hispanic origin have the highest life expectancy.

Health in old age is also improving, although the pace of improved health does not keep up with the increase in life expectancy. The healthy life expectancy (HALE), a statistic created by the World Health Organization, measures years of life expectancy free from morbidity and/or injury. In 2016, the HALE at birth for both sexes was 68.5 years, 70.1 years for women and 66.9 years for men. In 2016, at 60 years of age, the HALE was 17.9 years for both sexes, 19.0 years for women, and 16.7 years for men.

Marital Status and Living Arrangements

The disparity in life expectancy accounts for differences in marital status and living arrangements among older men and women in the United States. In 2017, the U.S. Census Bureau estimated that a larger proportion of men ≥65 years old (69.9%) than women (45.9%) were married and living with their spouse. Differences between sexes in marital status and living arrangements become more accentuated with aging. In 2017, at the age of ≥65 years, 20.3% of men and 34.4% of women lived alone. With increasing age, the percentage of those living alone increases.

In 2016, about 3.1% of adults ≥65 years old were living in group quarters. Group quarters are defined by the U.S. Census Bureau as places where people stay or live in a group living environment, such as noninstitutional group homes in the form of residential treatment facilities for adults, or institutional group homes such as nursing facilities. About 2.7% of the population ≥65 years old lived in institutionalized group quarters. As can be expected, the proportion of older adults who live in an institution increases dramatically with aging. About 15.4% of those ≥85 years old live in institutionalized group quarters. Women ≥65 years old make up 67.5% of the ≥65 years old nursing-home population.

The Distribution of Older Adults in the United States

The number of adults ≥65 years old varies greatly among states. In July 2017, it was estimated that about 53.6% of the total population of older adults was concentrated in only 10 states: California (5.5 million), Florida (4.2 million), Texas (3.5 million), New York (3.2 million), Pennsylvania (2.3 million), Illinois (1.9 million), Ohio (1.9 million), Michigan (1.7 million), North Carolina (1.6 million), and New Jersey (1.4 million). California had the highest number of older adults, while Alaska had the fewest. The state with the highest proportion of older adults was Florida, with 20.1% of its state population ≥65 years old.

In 2016, people ≥65 years old made up 18.4% of the population in rural areas and 14.5% of the population of urban areas. This larger proportion of elderly in rural areas is a major issue because in these geographic areas access to health care is limited and may require traveling far from the place of residence. This has a profound impact on a person's health and well-being and strongly affects prevention, life expectancy, and quality of life.

Educational Attainment

The percentages of adults ≥65 years old who have higher education has been increasing for both men and women. In 2017, 86.1% of adults ≥65 years old had completed high school or the equivalent or had a higher degree. The percentage of high school or equivalent graduates in this population varied by race. The percentage of adults ≥65 years old who had a bachelor's degree or higher was 29.7%. A higher degree usually equates to a higher income.

Income and Labor Force Participation

According to the Social Security Administration, in 2015 84% of adults ≥65 years old received some Social Security income, and such income accounted for 50% or more of the total income for 62% of the aged beneficiaries.

The median income of householders who were ≥65 years old was $39,823 (USD). However, this overall figure covers widespread situations. It was estimated that about 23.6% of householders ≥65 years old had an annual income lower than $20,000, while about 28.2% had an annual income of $70,000 and over. There is even wider disparity in the median annual income according to race.

According to the Bureau of Labor Statistics, in 2017 about 18.6% of the noninstitutionalized adult population ≥65 years old was employed. A larger percentage of men (23.1%) than women (15.1%) ≥65 years old were working.

Poverty

The poverty threshold income for a householder ≥65 years old living alone in 2016 was set at $11,511. According to the official poverty measure, in 2017 it was estimated that about 9.3% of older adults (10.6% of women and 7.6% of men) were in poverty. The proportion according to race and ethnicity were black or African-American non-Hispanic (18.8%), Asian non-Hispanic (12.0%), two or more races non-Hispanic (11.2%), American Indian and Alaska Native non-Hispanic (17.7%), white non-Hispanic (7.1%), and native Hawaiian and Other Pacific Islander non-Hispanic (6.7%). A large percentage of older adults of Hispanic origin were also in poverty (17.4%). Social Security keeps 34.8% of the older population in the United States above the poverty threshold. Medical expenses alone put 5.8% of the older population in poverty.

Health-Related Data

The CDC has found, unsurprisingly, that as people age, they are less likely to report their health as excellent or very good. About 84.6% of people <18 years old, 64.7% of people 18–64 years old, and 45.5% of those ≥65 years old reported in 2016 their health as excellent or very good.

Most chronic diseases are highly prevalent in the older population. Multimorbidity, or being affected by more than one chronic disease, could be considered the most frequent medical condition in older adults. A large proportion, 67.8% of older adults (enrolled in Medicare), had 2 or more chronic conditions.

In 2016, about 35.2% of the population ≥65 years old had some sort of disability.

In 2016, Americans ≥65 years old spent 13.1% of their total average annual expenditures on health care, in contrast to all other younger Americans, who spent an average of 6.7%. In addition, 98.8% of older adults had some type of health insurance. The majority of this proportion was accounted for by Medicare (93.0%). Private insurance covered 52.8% of the older adult population, while 1.2% had no health care coverage.

RESOURCES

- Early Release of Selected Estimates Based on Data from the 2016 National Health Interview Survey. Centers for Disease Control and Prevention, National Center for Health Statistics, National Health Interview Survey. www.cdc.gov/nchs/nhis/releases/released201705.htm (accessed Feb 2019).

- *Projections of Mortality and Causes of Death, 2015 and 2030.* World Health Organization, Health Statistics and Information Systems. Available at www.who.int/healthinfo/global_burden_disease/projections/en/ (accessed Feb 2019).

CHAPTER 2—BIOLOGY

KEY POINTS

- Aging entails a loss of homeostasis; this breakdown is the inevitable consequence of the evolved anatomy and physiology of an organism.

- There are two main types of biologic theories of aging: evolutionary (the "why" of aging) and physiologic (the "how" of aging).

- The many theories of aging are not competing or mutually exclusive; rather, the theories reflect current understanding of the multiple mechanisms that allow us to live as long as we do.

- The onset, rate, and extent of the aging process is extremely heterogeneous.

Some visible imprints of aging are loss of hair and pigmentation of hair; diminished height and muscle and bone mass; and increasingly wrinkled, thinned skin. These progressive changes have a biologic basis in altered molecular and cellular structure and function. The rate and extent of aging varies both between individuals and within an individual (eg, asymmetric changes in vision, hearing), increasing the variability with which older adults present. Thus, biologic age, based on an individual's functional capacity, and not chronologic age, is the metric for studying the biology of aging. Functional capacity is a direct measure of the ability of cells, tissues, and organ systems to function properly and optimally and is influenced by both genes and environment. Within this context, aging is defined as the progressive decline and deterioration of functional properties at the cellular, tissue, and organ level that lead to a loss of homeostasis, decreased ability to adapt to internal or external stimuli, and increased vulnerability to disease and mortality. Gradual changes in cells, tissues, and organs of the body lead to the eventual breakdown of maintenance processes—an inevitable consequence of the evolved anatomy and physiology of the organism.

THEORIES OF AGING

Evolutionary theories of aging explain historical and evolutionary aspects, addressing why aging exists in living things and how it may have evolved as a process. Physiologic theories of aging explain structural and functional age changes and elaborate a framework for translating the "what" and "where" of aging from molecules to organ systems and homeostasis.

The many theories of aging should not be viewed as competing or mutually exclusive. Rather, the theories reflect our current understanding of the individual maintenance pathways and homeostatic mechanisms that allow us to live as long as we do. The theories also provide pathways for investigating interventions that modify aging.

Evolutionary Theories of Aging

Evolution deals with the impact of natural selection (selective pressure) on the reproductive fitness of a species. There are currently two main evolutionary theories of aging: mutation accumulation theory and antagonistic pleiotropy theory.

Mutation Accumulation Theory

In this theory, aging is viewed as a nonadaptive trait. That is, traits that yield aging are neither selected for nor against. No selective pressure is brought to bear on older, postreproductive-age organisms expressing a mutation that has minimal effects on fitness. Thus, these late-acting genes accumulate over time and yield the aging phenotype.

Antagonistic Pleiotropy Theory

A single gene is described as pleiotropic if it controls or influences multiple traits. The antagonistic pleiotropic theory considers aging an adaptive trait. Genes that can influence several traits are selected for and affect individual fitness in opposite (ie, antagonistic) ways at different stages of life. Pleiotropic genes that have beneficial effects on early fitness components in the young but harmful effects on late fitness components are favored by natural selection. For example, there are inverse relationships between fecundity and life span or between longevity and brood size or metabolic rate.

Physiologic Theories of Aging

Physiologic theories address how we age. The major physiologic theories, with special emphasis on available supporting evidence, are described below.

Target Theory of Genetic Damage

Underlying the genetic theories of aging is the idea that aging is heavily influenced or caused by genes. The genome is the repository for all genetic material, and the integrity of this information is essential for reproductive fitness and survival. DNA is subject to a number of insults, including spontaneous chemical changes, environmental damage by ionizing radiation, aflatoxin, and alkylating agents, all of which modify DNA structure. Mechanisms of repair rely on the efficiency of many enzymes that in turn depend on fidelity of the information in the encoding DNA. Thus, the target theory of genetic damage states that genes are susceptible to "hits" from radiation or other damaging agents that then alter function of structural, signaling, and/or repair molecules, and that these cumulative hits give rise to an aging phenotype.

Mitochondrial DNA Damage Theory

Unlike nuclear DNA, mitochondrial DNA (mtDNA) is not protected by histone proteins and is attached to the inner mitochondrial membrane, where reactive oxygen species are produced. Thus, mtDNA damage occurs 10–20 times faster than nuclear DNA damage. In addition, mtDNA cannot repair itself, and some damaged mitochondria replicate faster than undamaged mitochondria, which gives rise to expansion of aberrant mitochondria. As a consequence, genes encoded within the mitochondria are more likely to lose their integrity over time. Damage to mtDNA has more harmful effects than damage to nuclear DNA, because each cell translates almost all its mtDNA genes but only 7% of its nuclear DNA. Nearly any adverse change in mtDNA will have deleterious effects on mitochondrial function. These effects include less energy production, more free-radical formation, reduced control of other cell processes, and accumulation of damaged harmful molecules, leading to aging and certain age-related diseases. The mitochondrial DNA theory of aging is closely allied with the free radical theory of aging.

Free Radical Theory

Reactive oxygen species are extremely unstable and are produced in mitochondria, in oxidative enzymes in the endoplasmic reticulum, in peroxisomes, and by phagocytes. Reactive oxygen species are normally policed by enzymes that inactivate them (superoxide dismutase, catalase, glutathione peroxidase), antioxidants that neutralize them (α-tocopherol, ascorbic acid, uric acid), sulfhydryl-containing compounds (cysteine, glutathione, bilirubin, ubiquinol, and carnosine), and β-carotene.

Evidence in favor of this theory include positive correlations between metabolic rate and free radical production, age and rate of free radical formation, age and amount of free radical damage, and age and the number of abnormal mitochondria. Evidence against this theory includes observations that antioxidant treatment does not reproducibly increase life span and that genetic manipulation of mice to either under- or over-express key components involved in free radical metabolism does not consistently affect life span. Reactive oxygen species can act as causative agents in other physiologic theories of aging, including DNA integrity, protein error, accumulation, and rate of living theories.

Telomere Theory

Telomeres are specialized sequences found at the ends of linear chromosomes. The DNA replication machinery cannot make a copy of the the physical end of a chromosome (because the machinery physically occupies space on the DNA). Every time DNA replicates, there is progressive shortening of the telomeres. Once telomeres are reduced beyond a threshold length, cells enter a nonreplicating state. Cellular (replicative) senescence is triggered when cells acquire critically short telomeres. Telomere length provides a mechanism for Leonard Hayflick's mid-20th century observation that mammalian cells are limited in the number of times they can divide ("Hayflick's limit"). The telomere hypothesis of aging proposes that telomere shortening causes aging through inducing replicative senescence. Evidence supporting the telomere theory includes observations that telomere length is inversely proportional to cell age, telomeres are lost faster from individuals with progerias, immortal cells such as cancerous cells have a constant telomere length, and restoring telomerase enzyme in somatic cells in vitro causes an increase in replicative life span of these cells. Evidence that is not supportive include observations that telomere length is not related to life span (mouse telomeres are much longer then those in people, for example) and that telomerase protects against replicative senescence but not cellular senescence triggered by other pathways.

Transposable Element Activation

Transposable elements, or transposons, are pieces of DNA that can move from one location in the genome to another, resulting in insertional mutagenesis. A random insertion may favor evolutionary advance, or it may lead to DNA damage and genomic instability. Cells have evolved elaborate mechanisms to repress transposons. The hypothesis that transposable elements may contribute to the aging process through somatic mutation was first proposed in 1992. Recent work has demonstrated that transposition increases in frequency with age in mammals. Activation of transposable elements is proposed to be an important contributor to the progressive dysfunction of aging cells and to induced cell senescence and cell loss. In addition, this theory provides a mechanism for age-associated deterioration in genetic stability.

Epigenetic Theory

Most cells in the human body are somatic cells. A major mechanism maintaining the appropriate, differentiated phenotype of these cells is epigenetic, dependent on DNA-protein interactions, DNA methylation, and histone acetylation. The epigenetic theory posits that phenotypic drift arising from inappropriate epigenetic modifications leads to altered gene expression and cellular function and the aging phenotype. In general, DNA methylation increases with age, but there can be variation within a tissue. The degree of hypermethylation depends on multiple factors, including age, diet, and exposure to environmental agents/insults (eg, carcinogens, epimutagens, toxins). The causal action of these changes in producing the aging phenotype has yet to be demonstrated.

Error Catastrophe Theory

The error catastrophe theory holds that damage is not to the genes themselves but to the RNA and proteins that read the genes and carry out their instructions. The damaged molecules spread, increasing the number of mistakes and causing biologic changes that are seen as "aging." For RNA, there may be issues with transcriptional accuracy, proofreading, mismatch repair, splicing, and transport. For proteins, errors in translating RNA to the correct amino acid sequence or in polypeptide folding and conformation have deleterious effects on protein function. Error catastrophe theory holds that cumulative errors in subsets of proteins involved in transfer of information from DNA to protein are normally below a threshold. Critical errors can destabilize the information transfer machinery, causing an irreversible increase in the error level and accelerating loss of function. This theory has only equivocal support.

Accumulation Theories

Accumulation theories posit that aging is associated with accumulation of cellular and extracellular components with altered structure that compromise cellular function. The components can be *molecular*, as in the clinker theory in which lipofuscin (an oxidized lipid), for example, accumulates in lysosomes compromising the organelle's capacity for catabolism. These components can be *macromolecular*, as in the protein modifications theory in which, for example, collagen cross-links in skin and bone, neurofibrillary tangles and plaque formation in the brain, and advanced glycation end products in multiple organ systems alter cellular and tissue functional capacity. Finally, components can be damaged whole organelles such as mitochondria, lysosomes, peroxisomes, and cell membranes, and the inability to remove functionally compromised organelles through autophagy leads to further loss of function.

Energetics Theories

Energy metabolism is central to normal cellular function. Two sensors of a cell's energy level are AMP kinase, a ubiquitous enzyme that gauges AMP/ATP and ADP/ATP ratios, and sirtuins, a group of enzymes that detect NAD/NADH levels. These sensors take part in highly conserved and interacting pathways that are believed to enhance longevity by stimulating autophagy, component recycling, and stress resistance. Caloric restriction, which can increase longevity in organisms from worms to mammals, activates these two pathways. The rate of living theory holds that aging is determined by the rate of metabolism, because aerobic metabolism causes damage, primarily through the production of reactive oxygen species. This theory predicts that the higher the rate of metabolism, the faster the rate of aging and the shorter the life span.

Endocrine Theory

The synthesis and secretion of many hormones change as the body ages. In addition, cell receptors on target organs can change in number and functional signal transduction. The circadian cycles of certain hormones also become irregular. The endocrine theory of aging posits that changes in hormone levels and signaling are a major cause of loss of homeostasis and that aging arises from dysregulated hormone signaling.

Immune Theory

Relatively slow-growing organisms must confront infection by rapidly reproducing pathogens or parasites, and the immune system has evolved to do this. Homeostasis of the immune system is maintained by innate or nonspecific processes such as humoral mechanisms (complement) and cellular mechanisms (macrophages, neutrophils, natural killer cells), as well as by the specific, acquired immune response involving humoral mechanisms (antibodies) and cellular mechanisms (T and B lymphocytes). The well-documented gradual decline in the maintenance of the acquired immune system ("immunosenescence") has been associated with increased morbidity and mortality in late life. The immune theory of aging posits that immunosenescence contributes to aging by limiting systemic defensive and repair responses that impact the functional capacity of other organ systems. It has been proposed that, to compensate for age-related decline in acquired immunity, the innate immune system is activated, yielding a pro-inflammatory state marked by increased levels of cytokines (eg, interleukin-6) and macrophage activation markers. Failure to resolve the repair and remodeling program of inflammation results in an altered tissue structure and cellular organization that can mar cellular and organ system function.

Stem Cell/Progenitor Cell Theory

Adult stem cells in the brain, bone marrow, and circulation maintain homeostasis by replenishing depleted reserves. Examples include satellite cells that contribute to muscle mass and repair of muscle tissue, and osteoprogenitor cells that replenish osteoblasts and form bone. Over time, precursor cells may become depleted by injury, illness, or environmental challenge, or may show phenotypic drift, failing to "keep with their program" by expressing inappropriate genes. Normally, for example, adult bone mesenchymal stem cells can produce cells in the osteoblastic, myoblastic, or adipocytic lines. Aging is associated with osteopenia and sarcopenia, yet increased fat content in bone marrow and muscle. These age-related changes may arise from a shift in the pathway commitment of bone mesenchymal stem cells away from bone and muscle cells toward the adipocytic cell line.

ORGAN SYSTEM CHANGES WITH AGING

Aging nerves, muscle, skin, hair, cartilage and bone, vasculature, and other organs exhibit changes at the molecular and cellular level. Some molecular changes with aging are shared between tissue types and organ systems, whereas others are unique. For example, in skin, bone, and cartilage, increases in cross-links (both enzymatic and nonenzymatic) alter compressibility and resiliency, and decreases in structural components (eg, proteoglycans and glycosaminoglycans) alter tissue hydration and function. In contrast, changes in the immune system (eg, diminished ability of dendritic cells to present antigen) are unique to the specific cell type, organ system, and function. A brief overview of significant age-related changes in the major organ systems follows below and is summarized in Table 2.1. These changes represent biologic processes common to everyone, although they progress at different rates.

NORMAL AGING

All of the above changes accompany advancing age but occur at different rates in individuals. Variability in onset, rates, and extent of aging suggest complex interactions between genetic predisposition, environmental exposure, and biologic and behavioral coping mechanisms in the etiology of aging. Despite these age-related changes, the different organ systems continue to maintain function, although their ability to maintain homeostatic conditions under times of stress diminishes. These changes may also be magnified by the impact of organic disease. The greater incidence of certain pathologies or diseases with increasing age (Table 2.2) reflects, in part, diminution of immune and other defense systems, increased exposure to disease-causing factors, and greater time for development of slow-progressing pathologies. Age-dependent increases in frequency of diseases such as diabetes, atherosclerosis, thrombosis, hypertension, cancer (especially of the breast, prostate, and colon), coronary heart disease, stroke, osteoporosis, and Alzheimer disease may characterize a synergy between aging and chronic disease in dysregulating homeostasis. Although age-related chronic disease can be viewed as promoting an advanced biologic age, a distinction between normal aging and pathology is that in disease, compromised function is evident in the resting (nonstressed) state. In contrast, with normal aging, physiologic effects are present only when internal or external stressors, or both, perturb homeostasis. In the language of control theory, physiologic set points do not generally change with normal aging, but the body's control systems that promote correction after perturbations are less robust, ie, older people have less ability to bounce back. The next section elaborates further on this concept.

COMPLEXITY, HOMEOSTENOSIS, AND INTEGRATED SYSTEMS

The changes that occur with aging contribute to dysregulation and loss of maintenance across physiologic systems. Additionally, the complexity in the dynamics of interacting physiologic systems decreases with age, resulting in a loss of robust and integrated homeostasis. Loss of complexity occurs both at the microscopic anatomic level (eg, in neuron structure, with more spare dendritic and axonal branching, or in progressively delicate bone trabeculae) and in the dynamics of physiologic processes (eg, heart rate or blood pressure, graphs of which show fewer harmonics with age). Reduced system complexity is associated with loss of the ability to adapt to external or internal stresses. The term *homeostenosis* is used to describe the narrowing of reserve capacity that underlies a decreased ability to maintain homeostasis under stress. As people age, there is a much greater demand on their physiologic reserve (in terms of proportion of the total capacity that is taxed) to maintain homeostasis. Sooner or later the corrective capacity is exceeded, resulting in loss of homeostasis and development of disease.

The ability to maintain the physiologic variable of body temperature can be used as an example to explore systems-wide effects of aging. With increased age, biologic changes in certain structures (loss of fat and thinning of skin, loss of sweat glands, decreased number of blood vessels and blood flow to skin surface, decreased muscle mass) contribute to decrements in the functional capacity to maintain body temperature in the face of a hot or cold environment. Adding to the problem, certain biologic changes of aging impact the body's components that effect its negative feedback pathways (eg, fewer nerve cells that monitor/sense temperature and weaker

Table 2.1—Physiologic Changes of Aging

Body System	Change	Consequences
Cardiovascular		Stressed heart is less able to respond
Heart	↑ Left ventricular wall thickness	
	↑ Lipofuscin and fat deposits	
	↑ Stiffness	
Vasculature	↓ Responsiveness to receptor-mediated agents	
Digestive	↑ Dysphagia	
	↑ Achlorhydria	↓ Iron absorption
	Altered intestinal absorption	↓ B_{12} and calcium absorption
	↑ Lipofuscin and fat deposition in pancreas	
	↑ Mucosal cell atrophy	↑ Incidence of diverticula, transit time, and constipation
Ears	↑ Thickening of tympanic membrane	↑ Conductive deafness (low-frequency range)
	↓ Elasticity and efficiency of ossicular articulation	↑ Sensorineural hearing loss (high-frequency sounds)
	↑ Organ atrophy	
	↓ Cochlear neurons	
	↓ Number of neurons in the utricle, saccule, and ampullae	↓ Detection of gravity, changes in speed, and rotation
	↓ In size and number of otoliths	
Endocrine	↑ Atrophy of certain glands (eg, pituitary, thyroid, thymus)	Changes in target organ response, organ system homeostasis, response to stress, functional capacity
	↓ Growth hormone, dehydroepiandrosterone, testosterone, estrogen	
	↑ Parathyroid hormone, atrial natriuretic peptide, norepinephrine, baseline cortisol, erythropoietin	
Eyes	↑ Lipid infiltrates/deposits	↓ Transparency of the cornea
	↑ Thickening of the lens	Difficulty in focusing on near objects
	↓ Pupil diameter	↓ Accommodation and dark adaptation
Immune	↓ Primary and secondary response	↓ Immune functioning
	↑ Autoimmune antibodies	↓ Response to new pathogens
	↓ T-cell function, fewer naive and more memory T cells	↓ T lymphocytes, natural killer cells, cytokines needed for growth and maturation of B cells
	Atrophy of thymus	
Muscle	Fibers shrink	Tissue atrophies
	↓ Type II (fast twitch) fibers	↓ Tone and contractility
	↑ Lipofuscin and fat deposits	↓ Strength
Nervous	↓ Number of neurons	↓ Muscle innervation
	↓ Action potential speed	↓ Fine motor control
	↓ Axon/dendrite branches	
Pulmonary	↓ Elastin fibers	↓ Effort-dependent and -independent ventilation (quiet and forced breathing)
	↑ Collagen cross-links	
	↓ Elastic recoil of the lung	↓ Exercise tolerance and pulmonary reserve
	↑ Residual volume	
	↓ Vital capacity, forced expiratory volume, and forced vital capacity	
Skeletal	↓ Bone density	Movement slows and may become limited
	Joints become stiffer, less flexible	
Skin	↓ Thickness	Loss of elasticity
	↑ Collagen cross-links	
Urinary	↓ Kidney size, weight, and number of functional glomeruli	↓ Ability to resorb glucose
	↓ Number and length of functional renal tubules	↓ Concentrating ability of kidney
	↓ Glomerular filtration rate	↓ Renal clearance of drugs, toxins
	↓ Renal blood flow	

Table 2.2—Organ System Age-Related Pathologies

Body System	Pathologies or Diseases that Increase in Incidence with Increasing Age
Cardiovascular	Hypertension, thrombosis, anemia
Heart	Congestive heart failure, myocardial infarction
Vasculature	Coronary artery disease, atherosclerosis, varicose veins, hemorrhoids
Digestive	Esophageal strictures, hiatal hernia Atrophic gastritis, acute gastritis, peptic ulcer, diverticulitis Fecal incontinence, cirrhosis, gall stones, pancreatitis Cancer
Ears	Presbycusis Tinnitus, dizziness, vertigo
Endocrine	Diabetes Graves disease
Eyes	Entropion, ectropion, cataracts, age-related macular degeneration, glaucoma Diabetic retinopathy
Immune	Autoimmune disorders (giant cell arteritis, myasthenia gravis) Leukemias
Muscle	Sarcopenia
Nervous	Stroke, dementias
Pulmonary	Chronic bronchitis, emphysema, pneumonia, pulmonary embolism Sleep apnea, stertorous breathing Lung cancer
Renal	Atherosclerotic renovascular disease Acute kidney injury
Skeletal	Osteoporosis Rheumatoid arthritis, osteoarthritis
Skin	Pressure injury, fungal infections (especially toenails) Neoplasms (basal and squamous cell carcinomas, melanoma)
Urinary	Urinary incontinence Benign prostatic hyperplasia

functioning of the remaining nerve cells). The net effect is that older bodies demonstrate a decreased ability to detect and respond to thermal variance, placing older individuals at greater risk of hypo- and hyperthermia.

Geriatric syndromes such as delirium, dementia, depression, dizziness, failure to thrive, malnutrition, falls, frailty, functional dependence, and gait disorders all reflect composites of dysregulation in multiple domains. For example, aging in the nervous system leads to a decreased sense of smell; altered flavor preferences lead to an altered diet which can effect glycemic balance as well as salt and water intake. Decreased sensory function and coordination, muscle weakness, and changes in cartilage and in bone mobility and stability can make it more difficult to obtain, prepare, and eat nutritionally adequate food. In the circulatory system, thicker blood vessels reduce blood flow through the digestive system, impairing digestion and absorption of various nutrients. In the respiratory system, decreased thoracic compliance and pulmonary capacity may lead to difficulty in obtaining, preparing, and eating a proper diet. All these changes lead to consumption and absorption of fewer nutrients, resulting in malnutrition. Similarly, sundry domains contributing to the geriatric syndrome of gait impairment include age-related changes in cartilage, bone, muscle, nerves, circulation, and vision.

The many biologic changes of aging affect multiple systems, tending to strain the body's homeostasis and the person's functional capacity. The prudent clinician bears in mind these aging-related physiologic changes, because they influence decision making about treatment plans (drug choice, drug dosing, whether to risk operative care, etc) constructed for the diseases of later life.

RESOURCES

- Burzynska AZ, Jiao Y, Knecht AM, et al. White matter integrity declined over 6-months, but dance intervention improved integrity of the fornix of older adults. *Front Aging Neurosci.* 2017;9:59.

- Byars SG, Huang QQ, Gray LA, et al. Genetic loci associated with coronary artery disease harbor evidence of selection and antagonistic pleiotropy. *PLoS Genet.* 2017;13(6):e1006328.

- Michalski B, Olasz E. What you didn't know about the sun: infrared radiation and its role in photoaging. *Plast Surg Nurs.* 2016;36(4):170–172.

CHAPTER 3—ETHICS AND LAW

Key Points

- Ethical dilemmas arise out of conflicts in values or from uncertainty about the right thing to do in a given situation. Clinicians should be familiar with current perspectives on ethics topics and adopt a framework for working through these situations.

- Four guiding ethical principles of American medical practice are respect for autonomy, nonmaleficence, beneficence, and justice. Ethical dilemmas often result from conflicts between these principles. No single principle is absolute, although autonomy is valued more in the United States than in some other countries.

- Decisional capacity is a patient's ability to accept or refuse a treatment. Capacity is decision-specific and may change over time. Determining if a patient has decisional capacity usually hinges on an assessment of four decision-making abilities: understanding, appreciation, reasoning, and choice.

- Patients who lack decisional capacity need others to make medical decisions on their behalf. The identified legal surrogate applies substituted judgment to make health care decisions that he or she believes the patient would have made.

- Fully informed patients with decisional capacity have the right to forgo or terminate life-sustaining treatments. Advance directives include living wills, which provide information about an individual's end-of-life care preferences, and Durable Powers of Attorney for Health Care, which designate someone to be an individual's legal decision-maker should that individual lose decisional capacity.

- Unaddressed moral distress can have devastating impacts on patient care, individual clinicians, and institutions; thus, recognition is an important first step toward mitigating its damaging effects.

Approach to Ethical Dilemmas

Health care professionals frequently encounter ethical dilemmas in working with older patients across a variety of care settings. Ethical dilemmas can be stressful and contribute to burnout for health care professionals. Clinicians should be familiar with current perspectives on ethics topics and adopt a framework for working through these situations.

See Table 3.1 for examples of some ethical dilemmas.

The first step is to identify whether the dilemma is about ethics or something else, such as the law. Ethical dilemmas stem from cases in which there is uncertainty or conflict in values between stakeholders about the right thing to do in a situation. Values are defined as an individual's strongly held beliefs or principles.

The second step is to identify what information is needed to fully understand the situation. This may include information about the patient's medical condition, the patient's values and care preferences, and the preferences of others involved such as family and clinicians. It also may involve investigation for additional relevant information such as precedent cases, published literature, clinical guidelines, legal cases, institutional policies, and professional codes of ethics.

The third step is to analyze the information gathered, evaluating the benefits and risks of each potential solution and its likely consequences.

In wrestling with difficult cases, creative solutions can often be found by considering more than 2 possible outcomes.

Another complementary approach is to evaluate the case through different ethical lenses. One commonly used approach in the United States is principlism, ie, the weighing of different ethical principles that are in conflict (see next section). The *prima facie* principles of autonomy, beneficence, nonmaleficence, and justice are often applied in this process (see Table 3.1). Other ethical lenses include casuistry (comparing the case to other similar ones), utilitarianism/consequentialism (evaluating which outcomes maximize the greatest good), and deontological/rights-based (determining which outcome honors universally held rules).

Another method is to weigh the risks and benefits of the different options from the perspectives of the different stakeholders. Although avoiding harm is preferable, there are some situations in which patients are willing to accept a risk of harm in hopes of the slim chance of a positive outcome (eg trials of new chemotherapeutic agents). If an ethical dilemma is examined through more than one lens and the same ethically justifiable option results, then this option has more ethical weight.

It can be beneficial for the clinician to share the relevant information and the analysis with others involved, providing an opportunity for further discussion.

For particularly difficult situations, a formal ethics consultation can be obtained. There is indirect evidence on the positive effects of guidance from ethics consultants. Studies have found that ethics consultation is associated with increased patient and provider satisfaction, and with decreased unwanted

Table 3.1—Sample Ethical Dilemmas in Geriatric Care, Uncertainty or Conflict in Values, and Resources

Situation	Conflicting Values (Relevant Ethical Principles)	Additional Resources
A hospitalized patient wants to go home, but the medical team feels this is unsafe and wants to discharge the patient to a skilled-nursing facility for rehabilitation.	Patient believes he or she has the right to be in his or her own home (autonomy). Medical team wants to promote patient health and safety (beneficence).	Carrese, J. Refusal of care: patients' well-being and physicians' ethical obligations "But Doctor, I Want to Go Home." *JAMA*. 2006;296(6): 691–695.
A patient does not want to start dialysis, but the medical team feels that doing so will help the patient live a better life.	Patient/family do not feel that the benefits of dialysis outweigh the burdens (autonomy). Medical team believes that dialysis will help the patient live longer and better (beneficence).	Lam DY, O'Hare AM, Vig EK. Decisions about dialysis initiation in the elderly. *J Pain Symptom Manage*. 2013;46(2):298–302.
A patient's spouse asks the patient's primary care provider (PCP) not to disclose the diagnosis of dementia to the patient.	Patient's spouse wants to protect patient from any suffering related to knowing dementia diagnosis (nonmaleficence). The PCP feels that he or she has a duty to share the diagnosis with the patient (autonomy, informed consent).	van den Dungen P, van Kuijk L, van Marwijk H, et al. Preferences regarding disclosure of a diagnosis of dementia: a systematic review. *Int Psychogeriatr*. 2014;26(10):1603–1618.
A patient who is a convicted sex offender requests a prescription for sildenafil; the PCP is concerned about the risk to others and liability if he or she writes the prescription.	Patient believes that he has a right to have his erectile dysfunction treated similarly to any other patient (justice). The PCP is concerned that giving the prescription could enable the patient to abuse new victims and create liability (nonmaleficence).	www.ethics.va.gov/docs/net/NET_Topic_20040526_Treating_ED_In_Patients_with_STDs.doc (accessed Feb 2019)
A PCP is concerned about a patient's continued ability to drive but is uncertain about reporting the patient to the Department of Motor Vehicles (DMV).	Patient believes he or she has a right to continue driving to maintain independence (autonomy). The PCP is concerned about potential risk to the patient and others, potential liability, and impairing the clinician-patient relationship if the patient is reported to the DMV (nonmaleficence, confidentiality).	*Physician's Guide to Assessing and Counseling Older Drivers*. 3rd ed. American Geriatrics Society, 2015.
Nursing home staff are frustrated that a resident who has longstanding personality issues, but has decisional capacity, at times refuses basic nursing care, such as being cleaned after having a bowel movement.	Nursing home staff want to promote the resident's health and cleanliness (beneficence, nonmaleficence). The resident wants to exert control over what happens to his or her body and does not trust some of the nursing staff (autonomy, trust).	Dudzinski DM, Shannon SE. Competent patients' refusal of nursing care. *Nurs Ethics*. 2006 Nov;13(6):608–621.
Nursing home staff want to hide a resident's medications in his or her food to ensure that the patient takes it.	Resident refuses to take medication (autonomy). Staff want to promote resident's health (beneficence).	McCullough LB, Coverdale JH, Chervenak FA, et al. Constructing a systemic review for argument-based clinical ethics literature: the example of concealed medications. *J Med Philos*. 2007;32:65–76.
An investigator wonders whether he or she can include individuals with dementia in a new research study.	Investigator wants to include individuals in a research study to see if they respond to an intervention differently than people without dementia but is uncertain about whether it is ethical to expose people who do not fully understand the risks of participating to an intervention (autonomy, informed consent, nonmaleficence, justice).	Johnson RA, Karlawish J. A review of ethical issues in dementia. *Int Psychogeriatr*. 2015;27(10):1635–1647.

treatments, leading to decreased lengths of stay. It may be difficult to obtain ethics consultation in some locations, such as nursing homes or rural areas. It may be possible for health care facilities to reach out to academic medical centers and universities to provide guidance on the ethically justifiable options in especially difficult situations.

The process of ethics consultation often takes time because the consultants need to become familiar with the case, need to talk to involved stakeholders, and may also need to review the literature. Although some ethics teams are able to respond to urgent requests, most questions coming to ethics consultants are not urgent. In the case of whether to continue life-sustaining treatments, most ethics consultants recommend continuing interventions aimed at promoting life, unless doing so is futile. As noted below, different health care institutions have different policies regarding what to do when continuing the life-sustaining treatments are thought to be futile.

PRINCIPLES OF MEDICAL ETHICS

The four guiding principles of American medical ethics most often cited are respect for autonomy, nonmaleficence, beneficence, and justice. Ethical dilemmas often arise when there is a conflict between these principles (Table 3.1). When there is an ethical dilemma, these ethical principles can be weighed against each other to help determine the ethicality of different proposed options.

The primacy of individual autonomy is a foundation of American culture. Early court cases, such as Schloendorff vs. Society of NY Hospital in 1914, Early court cases established the importance of patient autonomy by ruling that informed consent was essential prior to treatments and procedures, or they could be considered battery. Respect for individuals' autonomy includes allowing individuals to defer medical decision-making to others. In many cultures, family structure dictates who will be the decision maker for individuals within that family, and that person is deferred to even when the individual involved has the cognitive ability to make his or her own decisions. However, it is unethical to *automatically* defer decision making to another, for example, to an adult child of an older patient who is capable of making decisions and who wishes to do so.

Beneficence, doing more good than harm, is largely determined by each individual's reactions and needs as well as by culture. The weighing of benefits, risks, and burdens (ie, how much would someone be willing to endure for what chances of what outcomes) is the mainstay of decision making in older adults whose wishes are unclear or unobtainable.

Nonmaleficence is often interpreted as "do no harm" but is better represented by the phrase "do not intend to do harm." Definitions or perceptions of harm differ widely between cultures and between individuals within cultures. A frequently cited medical conflict between mainstream culture and subculture perspectives involves blood transfusions for a Jehovah's Witness. For a Jehovah's Witness, blood transfusion may be thought to cause more harm than good, even if the outcome of not having the transfusion might be death. Understanding the values of subcultures within our society may provide clues to the spectrum of values that underlie an individual's perspective on harm.

Finally, the concept of justice in the context of health care in our society remains ambiguous. The distribution of health care benefits and the use of health care technologies continue to be uneven and reflect biases regarding gender, age, race, and ethnic origin. Researchers have frequently excluded older adults in their study populations, and the lack of knowledge on the relative effectiveness of interventions when they are used for older adults can lead to the under- or overuse of interventions in this age group. Furthermore, assumptions that equate age with chronic illness and comorbidity can result in denial of beneficial treatment to healthy older adults. Patients from groups who have been marginalized or mistreated by society may be more reluctant than more historically privileged patients to step back from aggressive treatments because of a perception of continued prejudice.

INFORMED CONSENT AND DECISIONAL CAPACITY

To give informed consent, patients need to hear about the condition and the associated risks, benefits, and alternatives of each therapeutic option. Decisions are then made voluntarily without coercion. Patients who are deemed to have decisional capacity (see below) and who are fully informed of the risks, benefits, and alternatives of a given treatment have the right to refuse that treatment, even if refusal of treatment may shorten life. Informed consent arises out of the principle of respect for patient autonomy.

More recently, the concept of shared decision-making has become increasingly popular. In shared decision-making, the medical professional shares the relevant medical information with the patient, and the patient, in turn, shares information about his or her values and preferences. The clinician and patient then make the best decision together by weighing all relevant information and options.

Before undergoing procedures or treatments, patients need to give informed consent and must have decisional capacity to do so. Refusal of recommended treatments does not necessarily indicate lack of decisional capacity. Capacity can be assessed by any qualified provider. In challenging or complex situations, psychiatrists should be called on to determine decisional capacity.

Several approaches may be used to determine if a patient has decisional capacity. Table 3.2 lists 5 questions that can be used to assess decisional capacity and is consistent with a more formal approach that involves assessing 4 decision-making abilities: understanding, appreciation, reasoning, and choice.

The first step in determining if a patient can make a given medical decision is to review the decision with the patient, including the associated risks, benefits, and alternatives. The patient then explains this back to the clinician in his or her own words, which tests **understanding** of the relevant information. Patients who do not understand may not feel comfortable asking the clinician to clarify points of confusion. Efforts also should be made to engage patients with sensory deficits, such as hearing or visual loss, in this process.

The second step is to assess whether the patient has an **appreciation** of the fact that the decision being made will affect his or her body. For example, a patient in denial about a diagnosis may be able to repeat back the relevant information (and have a good understanding of matters in the abstract) but may not be able to apply this information to his or her specific situation.

The third step is to assess **reasoning**, including how well the patient is able to take in the information and weigh the options against personal values. Reasoning should generally be consistent with previous decisions that the patient made over time, and any inconsistencies should be logically explained. In clarifying the rationale for a decision, the patient describes what factors were taken into account, what priorities were incorporated, and what consequences were anticipated.

Finally, the patient makes a **choice**, consistent with his or her values and preferences and maintains this choice over time. A delirious patient may, for example, lack decisional capacity when the delirium waxes but may recover capacity when it wanes. Thus, assessing decisional capacity when cognition is at its best is important to honor patient autonomy.

Assessment of decision-making capacity can be modified based on the seriousness of the decision and its consequences. For example, before allowing a patient to stop a life-sustaining treatment such as dialysis, an in-depth assessment of capacity is needed. An assessment of capacity to refuse a routine blood draw would be appropriately much less stringent.

Patients with cognitive impairments such as dementia may still be able to make some of their own decisions and should be allowed to do so. Although lack of decisional capacity is more prevalent in those with lower scores on cognitive tests, incapacity does not automatically occur at a given test score. When patients can no longer give consent, their legal surrogates make these decisions instead. In cases in which the patient's decisional capacity is marginal or unclear, it may be beneficial to also include the legal surrogate in the discussion. Efforts can be made to encourage the patient and surrogate to make the decision together.

When a patient is deemed to lack decisional capacity, he or she cannot make the decision by himself or herself. Efforts should still be made to include that patient in the decision-making process. To honor the patient's personhood, it is preferable for that patient to *assent* to the procedure. Assent is the process of agreeing to something by someone who cannot give consent.

Patients with decisional capacity have the right to defer decision-making to others. As they have aged, some members of past generations have done this. As the baby boomers age, however, they may be less inclined to defer decision-making to others, preferring to maintain the locus of control.

Table 3.2—Sample Questions to Assess Decisional Capacity

- What's your main medical problem right now?
- What treatment has been recommended?
- If you receive this treatment, what will happen?
- If you don't receive this treatment, what will happen?
- Why have you decided to/not to receive this treatment?

SOURCE: Courtesy of Dr. Mark Siegler, used with permission.

TRUTH TELLING

Clinicians have not always routinely informed patients of serious diagnoses such as cancer. Some clinicians still do not routinely inform their patients of dementia diagnoses, believing that this information could be emotionally upsetting to patients. In the case of dementia, a clinician may be torn between fully informing a patient of the diagnosis (honoring patient autonomy) and protecting the patient from emotionally harmful information (reflecting nonmaleficence). Similarly, family members may want their loved ones protected from hearing information about disturbing diagnoses and poor prognoses.

Research has found that most patients want to be informed of diagnoses, even if effective treatments do not exist. This allows patients to attend to unfinished business and be involved in planning for future decline. Although learning that one has dementia may be distressing, people with cognitive impairments may already sense that something is wrong and be relieved that there is a reason for their difficulties.

Logistically, it is preferable to discuss patient preferences about how to share test results when testing is initiated, rather than after testing has been completed. Before sharing a new dementia diagnosis with patients, it is best to check with them about whether they want this information or whether they want it shared with someone else.

SURROGATE DECISION-MAKING

Patients who lack decision-making capacity need others to make medical decisions on their behalf. Most states and the Department of Veterans Affairs have laws or policies designating a hierarchy of legal surrogate decision-makers for incapacitated patients. A legal guardian is usually the first on the list of legal surrogates, followed by a designated decision-maker or health care agent through a Durable Power of Attorney for Health Care. If no such individual is appointed, the designated decision-maker is usually the spouse, followed by other family members. Checking with one's own state laws is recommended, because states have different hierarchies. Some states require consensus of all members of a category, such as adult children, whereas other states require only majority agreement. The oldest child is not automatically the legal decision-maker. Some states allow for non-relative surrogate decision makers who know the patient well. Table 3.3 illustrates a sample legal hierarchy of surrogates.

The identified legal surrogate is tasked with making health care decisions. Surrogates are expected to make decisions they believe the patient would have made through applying the substituted judgment standard. When a surrogate is uncertain what a patient would want, the best interest standard applies, in which the surrogate makes a decision that is felt to be in the patient's best interests.

Surrogates are often close family members who are emotionally attached to the patient. Research has shown that surrogates sometimes make decisions for others based on their own personal preferences. Although this may appear to disregard the patient's preferences, there also is research showing that patients often allow their surrogates leeway in following their preferences. Patients are concerned about burdening loved ones and recognize that their loved ones may need to make decisions that they can live with, even if these decisions go against what patients would have wanted. Thus, when surrogates appear to be making decisions that are different from what the patient would have wanted, it is best to ask surrogates for their rationale and offer support before assuming that surrogates have nefarious reasons behind their choices.

Surrogate difficulties with decision-making may stem from different reasons. Difficulties imagining life after the patient dies may paralyze the surrogate's decision-making. The surrogate may be hopeful that the patient will get better, or may be waiting for signs indicating whether the patient will improve or not. Clinicians may sometimes want decisions made faster than the surrogate can make them. In situations in which a surrogate's decision-making is in question, an ethics consultant may be able to help identify the ethically justifiable options. Options might include asking other family members to support that surrogate in decision making, and petitioning the courts to remove the impaired legal surrogate. It is not appropriate for clinicians to assess the decisional capacity of someone who is not their patient.

Although a clinician's primary duty is to his or her patients, he or she also should consider the impact of decisions and decision-making on the surrogate and other family members. Clinicians can support decision-makers by providing them with recommendations that are based on the clinician's knowledge of the patient's preferences. In doing this, the clinician shares the burden of decision-making with the surrogate.

Table 3.3—Sample Hierarchy of Surrogates (varies per state law)

- The appointed guardian of the patient, if any
- The individual, if any, to whom the patient has given a durable power of attorney that encompasses the authority to make health care decisions
- The patient's spouse or state registered domestic partner
- Children of the patient who are ≥18 years old
- Parents of the patient
- Adult siblings of the patient
- Non-relatives who show "special care and concern"

SOURCE: RCW 7.70.065. Informed consent—Persons authorized to provide for patients who are not competent. http://app.leg.wa.gov/rcw/default.

When a patient loses decisional capacity and does not have family to fill the role of decision-maker, clinicians can petition a court to appoint a legal guardian for the patient. Initially, the courts appoint a guardian ad litem, who is tasked with gathering information about the patient and his or her situation. This information is presented to the courts and, if deemed necessary, a permanent guardian is then appointed. Guardians have variable levels of experience and training requirements. State laws differ on what decisions guardians can make with and without returning to the courts for guidance and approval.

PROMOTING INDIVIDUAL PREFERENCES FOR FUTURE CARE

Advance Directives

Fully informed patients with decisional capacity have the right to forgo or terminate life-sustaining treatments.

Advance directives, also called advance care directives and advance health care directives, include living wills, which provide information about an individual's end-of-life care preferences, and Durable Powers of Attorney for Health Care, which designate someone to be an individual's legal decision-maker should that person lose decisional capacity. Durable Power of Attorney (DPOA) documents can vary by category of decision-making. Some designate a proxy for medical decisions, some identify a surrogate for financial decisions, and some establish a surrogate for both financial and medical decisions. Some DPOA documents give surrogates the power to make medical decisions even if the patient has not lost decisional capacity. Because of these differences, health care providers should review their patients' DPOA documents.

Advance Care Planning

Advance care planning is the process by which patients and their clinicians engage in discussions about future goals of care and care preferences at the end of life. As people age and develop chronic conditions, advance care planning is important to ensure they receive the type of care they desire. Advance care planning is rarely completed in one session.

The older population is heterogeneous in end-of-life care preferences, with some older adults desiring to forgo any life-sustaining treatments and others wanting any and all treatments to prolong life regardless of condition. Clinicians should not, of course, presume to know a patient's preferences without talking to the patient.

One outcome of advance care planning can be completion of a living will. Research has demonstrated the benefit of living wills in preventing patients from receiving unwanted care, especially undesired aggressive care at the end of life. Living wills have also been shown to provide surrogate decision-makers guidance in making decisions and to reduce their stress and decisional regret. Living wills, however, also have limitations and can be vague or difficult to interpret. For example, a patient with heart failure may have a living will stating that he or she does not want life-sustaining measures if "terminally ill." When that patient is admitted to the hospital with an exacerbation of congestive heart failure, it may be unclear if the patient is actually terminally ill, casting into doubt the applicability of the preferences in the living will.

In addition to engaging in advance care planning with their clinicians, patients should also be encouraged to discuss care preferences with their loved ones, especially those they have designated as their surrogate decision-makers through DPOA documents. Decision-making is easier for surrogates who are familiar with their loved ones' preferences. Individuals also can reduce stress for loved ones and surrogates by compiling important documents and information in one place.

As patients approach the end of life, many decisions need to be made, and patients should be involved in this decision-making as much as they want and can be. Engaging in discussions about the patient's preferred goals of care may be helpful in framing treatment decisions through a shared decision-making process.

Some states have passed laws authorizing forms that identify a patient's preferences about such treatments as resuscitation, feeding tubes, and antibiotics. These forms serve as physician orders that are active outside the hospital and are honored by paramedics. The POLST (Physician Orders for Life-Sustaining Treatment) form was originally developed in Oregon to help convey the preferences of nursing-home residents being transferred across health care sites. Names of these forms vary across states; variations include MOLST (Medical Orders for Life-Sustaining Treatment), MOST (Medical Orders for Scope of Treatment), and POST (Physician Orders for Scope of Treatment).

CONTROVERSIAL PROCEDURES AT THE END OF LIFE

In addition to the myriad difficult decisions that may arise as patients approach the end of life, certain procedures are considered to be controversial by some clinicians and family members. These procedures include palliative sedation, physician aid-in-dying, and euthanasia. The ethicality of these procedures has been greatly debated.

Palliative sedation is a procedure of last resort used to promote comfort at the end of life in individuals with intractable suffering. It may be an appropriate procedure for patients who are terminally ill, have comfort-focused goals, and have endured reasonable efforts by their medical teams to promote comfort using other palliative care therapies. When palliative sedation is undertaken, patients are purposely given medications, such as barbiturates or benzodiazepines, at the minimal doses to ensure their comfort, but not necessarily until they become unconscious. Although a recent systematic review indicated that palliative sedation does not hasten death, this concern remains prevalent. The use of palliative sedation for patients with intractable suffering due to existential concerns is more controversial than using it to palliate physical symptoms, such as pain or nausea. Intractable suffering may arise from such existential concerns as questions about whether one's life has any meaning/value/purpose or anger that one has outlived a prognosis. Some existential suffering may be amenable to interventions by members of the interdisciplinary team such as chaplains, social workers, and psychologists.

The doctrine of double effect often has been used to justify palliative sedation. Under this doctrine, if a procedure has both potentially good and bad effects, it can be justified if the action itself is good, if the intent is for the good effect, and if the good effect is not achieved through the bad effect.

Physician aid-in-dying (PAD), also referred to as physician-assisted suicide or physician-assisted death, is currently legal in a few states in the United States. In 1997, the Supreme Court heard 2 cases about the legality of PAD. The court ruled that suicide is not a fundamental right and that state laws prohibiting assistance with suicide are not unconstitutional. However, these rulings did not establish that the U.S. Constitution forbids all types of suicide or participation in suicide events by others. Oregon was the first state to legalize the practice in 1998. As of 2017, PAD is now also legal in Washington, California, Montana, Colorado, Vermont, and the District of Columbia.

Clinicians should recognize that some patients ask about PAD to begin a conversation about death and dying, not because they are ready to request lethal medications.

Even if a patient lives in a state where the practice is illegal, or if the physician cannot or will not participate, the physician's initial response to requests should be to inquire about the patient's intractable sources of suffering, rather than to suppress a dialogue about dying. An ensuing conversation can cover alternatives to PAD such as hospice care or referral to a chaplain, social worker, or psychologist to address existential suffering.

One legal alternative to PAD is the voluntary stopping of eating and drinking (VSED) by terminally ill patients with decisional capacity. Advocates of VSED argue that the process is superior to PAD. They argue that patients can fulfill their wishes without needing to surmount bureaucratic hurdles. Some also argue that VSED can be pursued by those who are not terminally ill or who are unable to self-administer lethal medication.

There is some evidence that challenges may arise in attempts to pursue VSED. Patients may become delirious after several days because of dehydration and begin to ask for food or water. Their loved ones are then faced with the difficult choice of whether to continue VSED despite pleas for relief or to acquiesce to their loved one's demands, thereby prolonging the process of dying.

The practice of euthanasia, in which a clinician purposely acts to cause the death of a terminally ill patient (eg, with injection of a lethal medication) is legal in Belgium and the Netherlands but not in the United States. It differs from PAD because of the role that the physician takes (administering the lethal medication versus writing the prescription). Some believe that palliative sedation is a form of euthanasia, although most literature and medical societies consider them to be different.

MORAL DISTRESS

Moral distress occurs when health care professionals are unable to do what they think is morally right because of obstacles. For example, nurses may experience moral distress when providing aggressive care that they believe to be futile to a critically ill patient. In this situation, nurses may believe that the goal of care should be to maximize patient comfort. They may believe that they are contributing to patient suffering by providing life-prolonging treatment. Different aspects of a case may cause moral distress for different clinicians. For example, one nurse might experience moral distress when trying to suction a patient who she believes is dying, whereas another might experience moral distress when observing clinicians painting an overly optimistic prognosis to the patient and family.

Although studied most in nursing, moral distress also has been noted in nearly every other health care profession, including health care managers. Unaddressed moral distress can have devastating impacts on patient care, individual clinicians, and institutions. Recognizing moral distress is an important first step toward mitigating its damaging effects.

RESOURCES

- American Geriatrics Society. Brangman S, Periyakoil VS, eds. *Doorway Thoughts: Cross-Cultural Health Care for Older Adults*; 2014. http://bit.ly/2jw1f9Y (accessed Feb 2019).

- Bernacki R, Block S. Communication about serious illness care goals: a review and synthesis of best practices. *JAMA Intern Med.* 2014;174(12):1994–2003.

- Bressler T, Hanna DR, Smith E. Making sense of moral distress within cultural complexity. *J Hosp Palliat Nurs.* 2017;19(1):7–14.

CHAPTER 4—FINANCING, COVERAGE, AND COSTS OF HEALTH CARE

KEY POINTS

- Medicare comprises 4 benefits: Medicare Parts A, B, C, and D.
  - Medicare Part A covers hospital, subacute skilled-nursing home, home health, and hospice services.
  - Medicare Part B covers physicians, nurse practitioners, social workers, psychologists, therapists, laboratory tests, and durable medical equipment.
  - Medicare Part C provides the benefits offered under Medicare Parts A and B through Medicare Advantage (MA) plans, which are managed care plans from private insurers. Most MA plans also offer Medicare Part D benefits.
  - Medicare Part D covers some of the cost of prescription medications.
- Medigap supplemental insurance plans are available from private insurers that cover Medicare Part A and Part B deductibles and co-insurance costs, as well as preventive care and other health-related goods and services.
- Medicaid is a joint federal and state program that provides health insurance to people of all ages who have low incomes and limited savings. Medicaid will pay for long-term custodial care in nursing homes among patients who reach a "spend down" threshold.
- Medicare reimbursement is shifting from a volume-based to a value-based approach.

The financial aspects of the U.S. health care system continue to undergo substantial change. Appreciation of these changes starts with an examination of the beginning of the current health care financing system for older adults. This foundation began in 1965, the year that the U.S. government passed legislation designed to improve access to acute health care for old, disabled, and poor people. During the decades that followed, the resulting Medicare and Medicaid programs expanded, evolved, and spawned thousands of supplemental commercial insurance plans. Today, a complex and often confusing array of personal payments, public programs, and private insurance plans (see Figure 4.1) pays for, and thereby determines, much of the health care that older Americans receive. This is especially confusing given the changes occurring with the expansion of Medicaid and individual insurance under the Affordable Care Act (ACA).

Medicare is undergoing significant changes as the program moves from basing reimbursement on volume of patients seen to value of services provided. Provider reimbursement is in the process of shifting from the number of patients seen in a day to how well clinical and financial outcomes are achieved for each patient and on the population being cared for. This shift is the result of the Medicare Access and CHIP Reauthorization Act of 2015 (MACRA).

Medicare is a federal insurance program run by CMS, which pays health professionals and organizations to provide health care for Americans who are ≥65 years old, disabled, or suffering from end-stage renal disease. As originally enacted, Medicare comprises two separate fee-for-service (FFS) plans, Part A and Part B, each of which pays predetermined amounts for specified health-related goods and services. More than 55.3 million Americans are covered by both plans, comprising 17% of the U.S. population. For a summary of Medicare Parts A, B, C, and D, see Table 4.1.

MEDICARE PARTS A AND B

The Medicare FFS program, the nation's largest health insurance plan, is administered by private organizations under contract to CMS. Called Medicare Administrative Contractors, these organizations enroll providers, educate them about coverage and appropriate billing, answer beneficiary and provider inquiries, and detect fraud and abuse.

Older Americans (and their spouses) who have had Medicare taxes deducted from their paychecks for at least 10 years are entitled to coverage through Part A without paying premiums. Others may be able to purchase Part A coverage (for up to $413 per month in 2017, depending on how long Medicare taxes were deducted from their paychecks).

Medicare Part B uses other regional insurance companies ("carriers") to pay physicians, nurse practitioners, social workers, psychologists, rehabilitation therapists, home-care agencies, ambulances, outpatient facilities, laboratory and imaging facilities, and suppliers of durable medical equipment for the Medicare-covered goods and services they provide.

At age 65, older adults become eligible for Part B coverage if they are entitled to Part A coverage and if they are citizens or permanent residents of the United

States. To obtain this coverage, eligible older adults must enroll in Part B and pay premiums, usually by agreeing to have these amounts deducted from their monthly Social Security checks.

Providers must choose among three options for participating in the FFS Medicare program: participation, nonparticipation, or private contracting. For each Medicare-covered service provided, a participating provider submits a claim to the Part B carrier, accepts Medicare's fee for the service (80% of its preestablished "allowed" amount with nurse practitioners receiving 85% of the physician rate), and bills the patient or the patient's secondary insurer for no more than a 20% co-insurance payment. Providers who elect nonparticipation status can bill patients directly for up to 15% more than 95% of Medicare's allowed amounts. The patients pay the providers and then submit their requests to Medicare for partial reimbursement (ie, for 80% of 95% of the allowed amounts. For services not covered by Medicare, the provider may bill the patient if the patient agrees to this arrangement in advance in writing.

A small minority (<1%) of providers choose to completely "opt out" of Medicare and enter into private contracts with their patients (also known as "concierge practice"). Such opt-out decisions apply to all their patients; they may not be made on a case-by-case or patient-by-patient basis. Under private contracts, Medicare carriers (and Medigap insurance plans) pay nothing, and patients pay physicians the full amount of the fees specified by these contracts.

Providers who opt out of Medicare can still have their patients' Medicare Part D prescriptions covered through that program. It is the office visit and related charges for services provided directly by such providers that are not covered by Medicare.

Neither Part A nor Part B of the Medicare program covers homemaking services, driving safety evaluations, routine dental or foot care, hearing aids, eyeglasses, orthopedic shoes, cosmetic surgery, or care in foreign countries. There are situations in which home health aides are covered temporarily for tasks such as homemaking services if patients qualify for other skilled home health services. Part B does cover some preventive services such as influenza and pneumococcal vaccines. Other vaccines are covered under Part D. Part D vaccines such as those for shingles cover both the cost of the vaccine and the cost associated with administration of the vaccine.

MEDIGAP

Medigap supplemental plans fill some of the holes in the insurance coverage provided by Medicare Parts A and B. Private insurance companies offer FFS Medigap plans of 12 types (A through L), classified according to the benefits they offer. For new Medicare beneficiaries at age 65, the premiums for A-level (basic) plans across the United States vary considerably. These policies cover a person's Part A and Part B co-insurance costs, eg, 20% of Medicare's allowed fees for durable medical equipment and providers' services. B-level plans cover Part A and Part B co-insurance, plus the Part A deductible. (A deductible is a charge for which the patient is 100% responsible for payment; with coinsurance, the insurance provider

Table 4.1—Key Features of Medicare Parts A, B, C, and D

	Medicare Part			
	A	B	C	D
Benefits	Inpatient care Subacute skilled nursing facility care Home health care Hospice care Blood transfusions	Clinician services Outpatient care Ambulance services Durable medical equipment Laboratory services Preventive services	Part A and B services delivered through private managed care plans Additional services (eg, vision, dental) may be included	Prescription drug benefit
Delivery	Hospitals Skilled nursing facilities Home health care services	Physicians and other providers	MA plans (eg, HMOs, PPOs, POS, PFFS, PSO, SNP, MSA)	Stand-alone prescription drug plan or MA prescription drug plans
Beneficiary cost sharing (2017)	Inpatient hospital deductible $1,316 Skilled nursing facility $164.50	Monthly premium (income adjusted) $134–$428.60 Deductible $183 20% copayment	MA monthly premiums vary depending on type of plan and state (range $0 to high $300s)	Monthly premium average $35.63

MA = Medicare Advantage, HMOs = health maintenance organizations, PPOs = preferred provider organizations, POS = point of service, PFFS = private fee-for-service, PSO = provider-sponsored organizations, SNP = special needs plan, MSA = medical savings account

Source: www.medicare.gov/pubs/pdf/10050-Medicare-and-You.pdf (accessed Feb 2019)

pays just a portion of the charge, and the patient is responsible for any remaining amount.) Each successive level of Medigap policy provides additional benefits and costs more. J-level plans cover co-insurance, deductibles, care in foreign countries, and preventive services. Less expensive Medigap coverage can be obtained by purchasing plans that require the insured to pay high deductibles (F- and J-level plans only) or plans that cover the services of only selected providers and hospitals ("Medicare SELECT" policies). Medigap policies do not cover long-term care, dental care, eyeglasses, hearing aids, or private-duty nursing. They also do not cover out-of-pocket costs for MA plans.

Within 6 months of their initial enrollment in Medicare Part B, beneficiaries are entitled to purchase any Medigap policy on the market at advertised prices. This is referred to as the Medigap open enrollment period and is the only open enrollment available for this coverage. After this period, Medigap insurers can refuse to insure individual beneficiaries or charge them higher premiums because of their past or present health problems. This limited open enrollment occurring at the beginning of beneficiaries' Medicare coverage is meant to encourage enrollment of lower-risk individuals to balance against the higher-risk individuals occupying the program later in their life. This provides for lower premiums, as these early enrolling low-risk individuals balance the costs from high-utilizers (www.medicare.gov/supplement-other-insurance/when-can-i-buy-medigap/when-can-i-buy-medigap.html).

MEDICARE PART C

As an alternative to traditional FFS Parts A, B, and D, Medicare beneficiaries can instead elect to enroll in a Medicare managed-care plan, an option known as Part C or Medicare Advantage (MA). MA plans, operated by private insurers, hold contracts with CMS specifying that for each Medicare beneficiary they enroll, they will provide at least the standard Medicare Part A, B, and D benefits in return for fixed monthly capitation payments. MA plans operate on a risk-adjusted basis for each member based on the ICD diagnoses that are provided.

To attract enrollees, most MA plans also cover additional benefits and charge low or no premiums, deductibles, and co-payments. The average premium in 2017 was just under $40 per month. The plans achieve cost savings by managing their enrollees' use of services within their networks of providers, with whom they negotiate price discounts in return for patient volume.

MEDICARE PART D

Medicare Part D was established in 2003, as part of a sweeping Medicare reform bill for beneficiaries to purchase insurance coverage for outpatient prescription medications. The Part D option is open to all Medicare beneficiaries, whether enrolled in traditional FFS or MA. Part D benefits can be purchased as stand-alone policies or as sponsored by MA plans.

As originally implemented, Part D provided no coverage when prescription drug costs exceeded a specified yearly amount, a policy known as the "coverage gap" or "donut hole." Under the ACA, Medicare gradually began closing the donut hole, including giving a $250 rebate to all Part D beneficiaries who entered the donut hole in 2010, providing discounts on brand-name drugs and generic drugs in the donut hole beginning in 2011, and phasing in additional discounts for brand-name and generic drugs to close the donut hole completely by 2020.

It is important for prescribers to appreciate that the standard Medicare Part D benefit changes each year. Some aspects (eg, the initial deductible and period of time before getting to the catastrophic point) may change, such that many patients experience an increase in their out-of-pocket expense. This could result in adherence issues as patients are forced to pay more out of pocket at different times during the year.

HOSPICE

Hospice is a benefit under Medicare Part A, providing a wide range of medical coverage for patients deemed by the patient's attending physician and the hospice physician to be within 6 months of death. Medicare hospice beneficiaries can receive medication coverage under the hospice benefit or under Part D. Hospice organizations under the Medicare Part A hospice benefit are responsible, rather than Medicare Part D, for covering all medications for palliation and management of the terminal and related conditions. Therefore, medications covered under the Medicare Part A per diem payment to a hospice program are excluded from coverage under Part D. Part D covers prescription medications for problems unrelated to the terminal condition.

Careful review of medications and communication with the hospice and Medicare Part D plan is critical to assure timely access and appropriate coverage for medications for hospice patients.

MEDICAID

Medicaid is a joint federal and state program that provides health insurance to people of all ages who have low incomes and limited savings. The exact criteria for Medicaid eligibility and the benefit packages provided by Medicaid programs vary considerably from state to state. For persons qualifying for both Medicaid and

Medicare, known as dual eligibles, most Medicaid programs pay for Medicare Part B premiums and some pay for Medicare deductibles and co-insurance costs. Most importantly, Medicaid pays for long-term custodial care in nursing homes for those who qualify. Many individuals qualify for Medicaid after a few months by spending down nearly all of their assets and resources as a long-term care resident of a nursing home, which can cost up to $100,000 per year.

The ACA established a new methodology for determining income eligibility for Medicaid, which is based on modified adjusted gross income (MAGI).

Several states offer fixed capitation payments to managed-care organizations that are willing to provide Medicaid and Medicare benefits to residents who are dually eligible (ie, for both Medicaid and Medicare).

DUAL ELIGIBLES

The two major advantages for dual eligibles are much lower out-of-pocket costs and extra benefits such as dental and long-term care.

Although eligible for benefits, many low-income individuals do not receive Medicaid. Many qualify but have difficulty navigating the application process. Poor health literacy is an especially common problem among dual eligibles, who often do not understand their plan or its benefits.

Dual eligibles tend to have more functional and cognitive limitations and correspondingly greater medical needs than beneficiaries enrolled in Medicare or Medicaid alone. As a result, they account for a disproportionate share of Medicare and Medicaid spending.

Considering the significant level of need and the limited resources of dual eligibles, it is perhaps not surprising that long-term care expenses account for a large share (70% of Medicaid dollars) of total costs. One program available for dual eligibles who qualify for nursing-home level care is the Program for All-inclusive Care of the Elderly (PACE), which provides all benefits available under Medicare and Medicaid. Research has demonstrated that nonprofit PACE provides high-quality, cost-effective community-based care to older adults who would otherwise require nursing-home level care (https://www.ncbi.nlm.nih.gov/pubmed/28085633 [accessed Feb 2019]).

LONG-TERM CARE INSURANCE

More than 3 million Americans have long-term care insurance policies, but these policies pay for <2% of all delivered nursing-home care. The high premiums for these policies, combined with consumers' uncertainty about needing long-term care in the future and their doubts about the policies' ability to cover the costs of long-term care in the future, have limited the growth of the long-term care insurance sector.

AFFORDABLE CARE ACT (ACA)

In addition to expanding insurance coverage, the ACA provides older adults new delivery models to improve quality and reduce costs. Examples of funding arrangements under the ACA include coordinated care models such as accountable care organizations (ACOs) and Comprehensive Primary Care Plus (CPC+), as well as bundled payment arrangements.

The ACA established the CMMI, charged with reducing costs in Medicare, Medicaid, and CHIP, while preserving or enhancing quality of care.

Accountable Care Organizations (ACOs)

ACOs are groups of providers, hospitals, and others who come together voluntarily to provide coordinated, high-quality patient care. The goal of coordinated care is to ensure that Medicare beneficiaries, especially the chronically ill, receive the right care at the right time, while avoiding unnecessary duplication of services and preventing medical errors. When an ACO succeeds in both delivering high-quality care and spending health care dollars more wisely, it will share in the savings it achieves for the Medicare program.

Bundled Payments for Care Improvement

Historically, Medicare made separate payments to providers for each service provided to beneficiaries during a single illness or course of treatment. This FFS approach results in fragmented care with haphazard coordination across providers and health care settings. Rather than incentivizing quality, the FFS system rewards the quantity of services offered. Bundled payments have been shown to align incentives for providers (hospitals, postacute care providers, physicians, and other practitioners). This system of reimbursement encourages providers to work closely together across all specialties and settings. As a result, in early 2013, to provide higher quality and more coordinated care at a lower cost to Medicare, CMS introduced the Bundled Payments for Care Improvement initiative.

Other ACA Changes Impacting Medicare

- Partial closure of the coverage gap in the Medicare Part D prescription drug benefit, which began in 2011, with 50% of the cost of branded pharmaceuticals covered during the coverage gap

- Extended coverage for preventive care services, as well as elimination of the co-payment requirements for some services

- Expansion of Medicaid (beginning in 2014), in which 16.7 million individuals gained coverage under Medicaid

- Changes in provider reimbursement, including decreases for MA plans and increases for primary care providers through Medicare and Medicaid

MEDICARE ACCESS AND CHIP REAUTHORIZATION ACT (MACRA)

Medicare payment prior to MACRA was based on an FFS payment system, and this FFS schedule was to be adjusted by the Sustainable Growth Rate (SGR). The SGR required Congress to pass temporary "doc fixes" each year to avert cuts so that providers receive a more predictable payment method that incentivizes value. This payment method, the Quality Payment Program (QPP), improves Medicare by helping providers focus on care quality and patient health. Providers can choose how they want to take part in the QPP based on practice size, specialty, location, or patient population. The QPP has 2 tracks to choose from: the Merit-based Incentive Payment System (MIPS) or the Alternative Payment Model (APM).

The Merit-based Incentive Payment System (MIPS)

The four components of MIPS are quality, cost/resource use, clinical practice improvement, and advanced care information. MIPS gives providers the flexibility to choose the activities and measures that are most meaningful to their practice to demonstrate performance.

The Alternative Payment Model (APM)

The APM is a payment approach that gives added incentive payments to provide high-quality and cost-efficient care. APMs can apply to a specific clinical condition, a care episode, or a population. Practices may earn a 5% incentive payment by participating in an advanced APM.

DEPARTMENT OF VETERANS AFFAIRS (VA) BENEFIT

The VA provides a medical benefits package to all enrolled veterans. This comprehensive plan provides a full range of preventive, outpatient, and inpatient services within the VA health care system. Also, once enrolled in the VA's health care system, veterans can be seen at any VA facility across the country.

Those VA facilities include a system comprising 153 medical centers, 773 ambulatory care and community-based outpatient clinics, 260 veterans centers, 136 nursing homes, 45 residential rehabilitation treatment programs, and 92 comprehensive home-based care programs—all providing medical and related services to eligible veterans. Veterans who are Medicare beneficiaries can use the Medicare system as well. In an effort to reduce delays in care that sometimes come from a closed system with limited supply and increasing demand, the VA is increasing partnerships with outside providers to extend the services available to veterans through opening access.

To support increasing access to care, Congress passed the Veterans Access, Choice and Accountability Act of 2014 ("Choice Act") that allow those veterans who are unable to schedule an appointment within 30 days of their preferred date or the clinically appropriate date, or on the basis of their place of residence, to elect to receive care from eligible non-VA health care entities or providers.

RESOURCES

Patients and Families

- CMS Medicare Prescription Drug Plan Finder: www.medicare.gov/find-a-plan/questions/home.aspx (Enrollees can enter their location and medications to compare available Part D options and identify the most appropriate Part D plan for them based on their individual needs.)

- State Medicare assistance offices: www.medicare.gov/Contacts/

- Nursing Home Compare: www.medicare.gov/nursinghomecompare/search.html?

- Medicare & You Annual Guide: www.medicare.gov/forms-help-and-resources/mail-about-medicare/about-medicare-and-you.html

- 1-800-MEDICARE (1-800-633-4227) or 1-877-486-2048 for hearing-impaired TTY users

- VA Medical Benefits: www.va.gov/healthbenefits/access/medical_benefits_package.asp

Health Care Professionals

- CMS Quality Payment Program: https://qpp.cms.gov/ (accessed Feb 2019)

- MACRA Value-Based Programs: https://www.cms.gov/Medicare/Quality-Initiatives-Patient-Assessment-Instruments/Value-Based-Programs/MACRA-MIPS-and-APMs/MACRA-MIPS-and-APMs.html (accessed Feb 2019)

- Medicare Learning Network: www.cms.gov/Outreach-and-Education/Medicare-Learning-Network-MLN/MLNGenInfo/index.html?redirect=/MLNGenInfo/ (accessed Feb 2019)

CHAPTER 5—ASSESSMENT

KEY POINTS

- Geriatric assessment is a multifaceted approach to the care of older adults, with the goal of promoting wellness and independent function.

- Assessment of function includes physical, cognitive, psychologic, and social domains.

- Time-efficient, valid tools are available for use in a variety of settings to evaluate the status of older adults in all these domains.

- Time tends to be a less important element than the skills of the clinician in successful communication with older adults.

The scope of the assessment of any individual depends on the goals of care, the site of care, the individual's level of frailty, time constraints, and the availability of an interprofessional team. The essential aspects of geriatric assessment should be performed routinely in all sites of care, including the ambulatory setting, the emergency department, the hospital, the nursing home, and the home. Whenever possible, assessments should be performance based. An informant, ideally a caregiver or family member who lives with the older adult, is often required to provide or to verify pertinent historical information about the older adult's day-to-day functioning. *Try This*, a publication of the Hartford Institute for Geriatric Nursing, covers a series of geriatric assessment tools and describes their use. Examples include the Geriatric Depression Scale, Predicting Pressure Ulcer Risk, the Geriatric Oral Health Assessment Index, and Decision Making and Dementia. Each of the more than 40 *Try This* issues can be downloaded from www.ConsultGeriRN.org.

ROUTINE OFFICE VISIT

Incorporating geriatric assessment into routine office practice requires use of efficient strategies, which can be facilitated by use of the electronic medical record through prompts, checklists, and templates. Many of the initial screens can be completed by trained office staff; some can be completed by the patients themselves while seated in the waiting area or at home before the visit. Alternatively, the use of a "rolling" assessment, which targets at least one area for screening during each office visit, should be considered. Finally, in the absence of specific target symptoms, parts of the routine examination, such as auscultation of the chest and palpation of the abdomen, can be replaced by aspects of geriatric assessment, such as observation of gait, balance, and transfers. However, office-based screening for common geriatric conditions has not been shown to improve patient outcomes (SOE=A).

WELCOME TO MEDICARE VISIT

Recognizing the need for enhanced preventive care, in 2005, Medicare began to offer a one-time initial preventive examination known as the "Welcome to Medicare" visit. The visit allows all new beneficiaries to receive a preventive examination without a copayment within 1 year of beginning coverage. The Welcome to Medicare visit provides access to a comprehensive range of preventive services, including a review of the patient's medical and family history; the measurement and recording of biometrics such as blood pressure and BMI; screening for cognitive impairment, depression, functional ability, and level of safety; establishing a written schedule for recommended screening and preventive services; planning end-of-life care; and education, counseling, and referrals for other personalized preventive services, such as colonoscopy.

ANNUAL WELLNESS VISIT

In 2011, Medicare began covering an Annual Wellness Visit (AWV), which includes a comparable array of services as the Welcome to Medicare visit, along with a health risk assessment. The AWV is provided at no cost to beneficiaries, including those with Medicare Advantage or fee-for-service coverage. Assessment and documentation of functional status, nutrition, cognitive impairment, depression, and other components of geriatric assessment are required for a visit to qualify as an AWV.

PATIENT-CLINICIAN COMMUNICATION

Because of the demands of a busy clinical practice, the time available for office visits is often constrained. However, time tends to be less important than the skills of the clinician in successful communication. To accommodate the high prevalence of sensory deficits among older adults, particular attention should be given to the environment of the examination room. The use of simple, inexpensive amplification devices with lightweight earphones can be especially effective, even for those with severe hearing impairment. During the course of the interview, the clinician should go beyond the customary clinical inquiries by asking open-ended questions such as, "What would you like me to do for you?" Finding out what the patient wants can be a prime mechanism for solving potential problems, generating trust, and improving mutual satisfaction in the patient-clinician relationship. The National Institute on Aging offers practical tips for communicating with older patients in ways that are respectful and effective: https://www.nia.nih.gov/health/understanding-older-patients (accessed Feb 2019).

Effective communication can be compromised by low health literacy—the diminished ability to obtain, process, and understand basic health information and services needed to make appropriate health decisions. Increasing evidence suggests that low health literacy, which has been documented in about one of every four community-living older adults, has deleterious effects on health and survival, at least in part because of deficiencies in self-management skills, poor adherence, and inadequate use of preventive services (SOE=A). Helpful information on low health literacy, including strategies to enhance communication, is available at http://healthlit.fcm.arizona.edu (accessed Feb 2019).

PHYSICAL ASSESSMENT

The importance of an appropriately detailed physical examination cannot be overstated. Many older adults cannot see well enough to report signs of disease, or have cognitive impairment that prevents them from being able to accurately report symptoms. The physical examination should routinely include measurement of blood pressure, weight, and BMI, followed by additional evaluations individualized based on symptoms, underlying medical conditions, effects of disease progression, and adverse effects of treatments. Gait and sensory impairment are particularly common and should be periodically assessed (described below).

Vision and Hearing

Although visual impairment from cataracts, glaucoma, macular degeneration, and abnormalities of accommodation usually worsens with age, older adults are often unaware of their visual deficits. Asking about difficulty with driving, watching television, or reading may uncover a problem with vision. A brief performance-based screen can be accomplished by asking an older adult to read (using corrective lenses, if applicable) a short passage from a newspaper or magazine (SOE=C). Significant visual impairment can be confirmed through use of a Snellen chart or Jaeger card; visual acuity worse than 20/40 is the standard criteria for visual impairment.

The high prevalence of hearing loss among older adults and its association with depression, dissatisfaction with life, and withdrawal from social activities make it an important target for assessment. Hearing loss is usually bilateral and in the high-frequency range. Older adults who acknowledge hearing loss in the absence of cerumen impaction should be referred directly for formal audiometric testing. For those who deny hearing loss, further screening with the whisper-voice test is indicated (SOE=B). Inability to perceive a letter/number combination whispered at a distance of 2 feet is considered abnormal and warrants a discussion about referral for formal audiometric testing.

Nutrition

Poor nutrition in older adults may reflect concurrent medical illness, depression, dementia, inability to shop or cook, inability to feed oneself, or financial hardship. Aside from visual inspection for signs of malnutrition, older adults should have their weight and height measured routinely. Unintentional weight loss of ≥5% in 6 months or a low BMI (ie, <20 kg/m^2) suggests poor nutrition and requires further evaluation (SOE=A).

MEDICATION ASSESSMENT

Time should be dedicated at each office visit to review both prescribed and OTC medications, and home remedies and herbal products. Polypharmacy, which is common in older adults, can be the cause of many adverse reactions and contribute to the onset of new symptoms (SOE=A). Suspected treatment failure may be related to medication nonadherence. Exploring issues around nonadherence is important to discern whether the cause is related to finances, fear of being over-medicated, or lack of understanding of the need for a medication.

COGNITIVE ASSESSMENT

The prevalence of dementia doubles every 5 years after the age of 65 and approaches 40%–50% at age 90. Many patients with dementia do not complain of memory loss or volunteer symptoms of cognitive impairment unless specifically questioned. Older adults with cognitive impairment, even in the absence of dementia, are at increased risk of accidents, delirium, medical nonadherence, and disability. Therefore, an important feature of every assessment of an older adult, especially those ≥75 years old, is a brief cognitive screen (SOE=C). Before cognitive testing, clinicians should determine the patient's native language and be aware of any vision and hearing deficits.

Because short-term memory loss is typically the first sign of dementia, the best single screening question is recall of three words after 1 minute. Anything other than perfect recall should lead to further testing. The clock-drawing test is valuable, because it assesses executive control and visual-spatial skills, two domains of cognition with profound effects on daily function. In the clock-drawing test, the patient is asked to draw the face of a clock and to place the hands correctly to indicate 2:50 (or 11:10). The clock-drawing test is combined with the three-item recall in the Mini-Cog Assessment Instrument for Dementia, a validated screening test that takes about 3 minutes to administer. The Mini-Cog has an advantage over many other instruments of being relatively uninfluenced by level of education or language differences. As another quick screen of executive function, the patient can be asked to name as many four-legged animals as possible in 1 minute. Fewer than 10 animals or repetition of the same animals is abnormal and suggests the need for further evaluation.

Because the Folstein Mini–Mental State Examination (MMSE) is now proprietary and has several limitations, other validated tools are being used more commonly to assess cognition, including the Montreal Cognitive Assessment (MoCA) and Saint Louis University Mental Status Examination (SLUMS). These two instruments assess a comparable set of cognitive domains, including memory, executive function, abstract thinking, attention, calculation, and visual-spatial skills. The MoCA, which also assesses concentration, language, and orientation, takes about 10 minutes to complete. The total possible score is 30 points; a score of ≥26 is considered normal. The SLUMS takes about 7 minutes to complete. The total possible score is 30 points; a score ≥27 or above is considered normal. Regardless of the instrument used, the results of cognitive testing should be interpreted in the context of the patient's educational attainment and literacy.

PSYCHOLOGIC ASSESSMENT

Although the prevalence of major depressive disorder among community-dwelling older adults is only about 1%–2%, the rate is much higher—up to 10%—in those seen in primary care settings. A large number of older adults, moreover, suffer from significant symptoms of depression below the severity threshold of major depression as defined by the *Diagnostic and Statistical Manual of Mental Disorders, Fifth Edition*. These subthreshold depressive symptoms, which often include somatic complaints such as poor sleep and fatigue, increase the risk of physical disability and slower recovery after an acute disabling event (SOE=A). They are also associated with a significant increase in the cost of medical services, even after accounting for the severity of chronic medical illness (SOE=A). Hence, clinicians should have a high index of suspicion for depressive symptoms and a low threshold for treatment.

The PHQ-2 is a very short, validated instrument for depression screening. An affirmative response (ie, answering "yes" to either question) warrants further evaluation of other depressive symptoms, perhaps through the use of a standardized instrument such as the 15-item Geriatric Depression Scale or the 9-item Patient Health Questionnaire (SOE=B).

Anxiety and worries are also important symptoms in older adults and are often a manifestation of an underlying depressive disorder. Finally, because older adults are particularly likely to experience the loss of a loved one, special efforts should be made to recognize and manage the consequences of bereavement.

SOCIAL ASSESSMENT

A social assessment consists of evaluation of several elements, including ethnic, spiritual, and cultural background; availability of a personal support system; need for a caregiver, his or her role, and presence of caregiver burden; safety of the home environment; economic well-being; possibility of mistreatment; and the patient's advance directives. Although a comprehensive social assessment may not be feasible in a busy office practice, clinicians caring for older adults should be mindful of these aspects of their patient's lives. Clinicians can uncover important clues to unmet needs by inquiring about the availability of help in case of an emergency. For frail older adults, particularly those who lack social support, referral to a visiting nurse or physical therapist may help assess home safety and level of personal risk.

FUNCTIONAL STATUS

Functional status refers to the person's ability to perform activities of daily living (ADLs). When assessing function, clinicians should ask whether the individual is independent or requires the help of another person to complete ADLs. Bathing is typically the self-care ADL with the highest prevalence of disability, and needing assistance with bathing is often the reason for home aide services (SOE=A). Disability in ADLs may occur when there is a gap or mismatch between personal capabilities (eg, balance, muscle strength, cognition) and environmental demands. For example, an older adult with quadriceps weakness might require assistance to stand from a deeply cushioned, low-lying chair but have no difficulty standing from a hard-back kitchen chair. To identify patients with "preclinical" disability, ie, those who do not yet require personal assistance but who are at risk of becoming disabled, clinicians should ask about perceived difficulty with the tasks and whether the individual has changed the way he or she completes the task because of a health-related problem or condition (SOE=A). Use of any assistive devices, such as a cane or walker, as well as duration and circumstances of use, should also be assessed.

Assessing life space allows clinicians to distinguish among different levels of mobility, not only in community-living older adults but also in nursing-home residents (SOE=A). Life space can be viewed rather simply as a series of concentric areas radiating from the room where a person sleeps to more distant locations, such as beyond one's town (for community-living older adults) or outside the facility (for nursing-home residents). The frequency of movement to various locations and the need for assistance are also assessed by formal life space instruments. For older adults with diminished life space, the ability to get in and out of a bed should be assessed.

Outside a rehabilitation setting, performance-based testing of most self-care and instrumental ADLs is not practical. Hence, performance-based testing of functional status focuses primarily on mobility, including transfers, gait, and balance. The person should be asked to stand from a seated position in a hard-backed chair while keeping his or her arms folded. Inability to complete this task suggests leg (quadriceps) weakness and is highly predictive of future disability (SOE=A). Once the person is standing, he or she should be observed walking back and forth over a short distance, ideally with the usual walking aid. Abnormalities of gait include path deviation; diminished step height or length, or both; trips, slips, or near falls; and difficulty with turning. The tasks of rising from the chair, walking 10 feet (3 meters), turning around and returning to the chair, turning again, and then sitting back down in the chair make up the "Timed Up and Go" test. In individuals who take >12 sec, the risk of falls is increased and further evaluation is required (SOE=B).

If time permits completion of only one performance test, gait speed should be measured. Gait speed is the single strongest predictor of future disability and death (SOE=A). A gait speed of 0.8 meters/sec allows for independent ambulation in the community; a speed of 0.6 meters/sec allows for community activity without use of a wheelchair. These norms indicate that older adults who can walk 50 feet in an office hallway in ≤20 sec should be able to walk independently in normal activities.

Balance can be tested progressively by asking the older adult to stand first with his or her feet side by side, then in semitandem position, and finally in tandem position. Difficulty with balance in these positions predicts an increased risk of falling (SOE=A). Although standardized instruments, such as the Performance-Oriented Mobility Assessment, can be used to quantify impairments in gait and balance, a qualitative assessment is usually sufficient to make recommendations about the need for an assistive device, such as a cane or walker.

Useful functional information can also be gleaned by observing older adults as they complete simple tasks such as undressing or dressing, picking up a pen and writing a sentence, touching the back of the head with both hands, and climbing up and down from an examination table.

Assessing the Older Driver

Evaluating the older driver is a difficult challenge. The automobile is the most important—and often the only—source of transportation for older adults. Yet a variety of age-related changes, chronic conditions, and medications place older adults at risk of automobile accidents. Although the absolute number of crashes involving older drivers is low, the number of crashes per mile driven and the likelihood of serious injury or death are higher than for any age group other than those 16–24 years old (SOE=A).

The vast majority of older adults make prudent adjustments in their driving behaviors by avoiding rush hour, congested thoroughfares, night driving, or driving during adverse weather conditions. Nonetheless, impaired older adults who continue to drive are a hazard not only to themselves but also to other drivers, passengers, and pedestrians. Pertinent risk factors for automobile accidents include poor visual acuity (less than 20/40) and contrast sensitivity; dementia, particularly deficits in visual-spatial skills and visual attention; impaired neck and trunk rotation; and poor motor coordination and speed of movement (SOE=A). Alcohol and medications that adversely affect alertness, such as narcotics, benzodiazepines, antihistamines, antidepressants, antipsychotics, sedatives, and muscle relaxants, can impair driving skills and increase accident risk. Hence, caution is warranted when starting or adjusting the dosage of these medications, and patients should be warned about potential adverse effects on driving safety.

Any report of an accident or moving violation should trigger an assessment of an older adult's driving ability. Safety concerns should be discussed honestly with the older driver, and ideally with a partner or other family member as well, particularly when the older driver lacks insight into his or her driving limitations. Alternative modes of transportation should be considered. Recommendations to stop driving, however, should not be proffered lightly, because driving cessation can lead to a decreased activity level and increased depressive symptoms (SOE=B). Referral for a formal driving evaluation by a skilled occupational therapist may be helpful in confirming unsafe driving behaviors, or perhaps in suggesting interventions such as adaptive equipment to correct for specific physical disabilities. However, coverage for such evaluations from Medicare, Medicaid, and private insurance companies is variable. Many state licensing agencies offer free older driver reexaminations, but poor performance may lead to restriction, suspension, or revocation of one's license. In the interest of public safety, clinicians should know their state's law on reporting impaired drivers. In most states, clinicians are encouraged, and in some states mandated, to report their concerns to the licensing agency. To assist clinicians caring for older drivers, an excellent resource has been developed by the American Medical Association in cooperation with the National Highway Traffic Safety Administration: *The Clinician's Guide to Assessing and Counseling Older Drivers, 3rd Edition* (https://geriatricscareonline.org/ProductAbstract/clinician's-guide-to-assessing-and-counseling-older-drivers/B022) (accessed Feb 2019).

ACUTE FUNCTIONAL DECLINE

An acute decline in functional status is usually precipitated by illness or injury. Most new disability episodes are attributable to illnesses or injuries leading to hospitalization (SOE=A). The most severe forms of disability commonly arise from a relatively small number of acute conditions, including hip fracture, stroke, heart failure, and pneumonia. The adverse functional consequences of hospitalization reflect not only the disabling effects of these and other serious conditions but also the hazards of immobility and hospital-acquired complications. Up to 20% of new disability episodes are attributable to less serious illnesses or injuries that lead to restriction of activity but not to hospitalization. These restrictions are usually caused by several concurrent health-related problems, although a fall or injury is most likely to result in disability. Among older adults who are physically frail, about a third of new disability episodes occur insidiously, ie, in the absence of a discernable illness or injury. These episodes may be attributable to relatively subtle perturbations in physiologic status or to the loss of compensatory strategies among highly vulnerable older adults with relatively little reserve capacity. Most older adults who become newly disabled recover independent function within 6 months (SOE=A). However, these individuals are at high risk of subsequent disability.

QUALITY OF LIFE AND ADVANCE CARE PLANNING

During the past two decades, *quality of life* has been embraced as a convenient "catch phrase" to denote important patient outcomes other than death and traditional physiologic measures of morbidity. Although

Table 5.1—Two Global Questions for Assessing Quality of Life

1. "How would you rate your overall quality of life at the present time? Would you say it is excellent, very good, good, fair, or poor?"

2. "Thinking only about your health, how would you rate the quality of your life at the present time? Would you say it is excellent, very good, good, fair, or poor?"

a gold standard does not exist, most instruments designed to measure quality of life include various aspects of physical, cognitive, psychological, and social function. Perhaps the most commonly used instrument is the Short Form-36 Health Survey (SF-36), which includes 36 items organized into 8 domains: physical function, role limitations due to physical health, role limitations due to emotional health, bodily pain, social functioning, mental health, vitality, and general health perceptions. The SF-36 has been tested extensively among community-living adults and hospitalized patients, but it may not be suitable for use among the oldest-old group, especially those who are frail, because of "floor effects" (ie, all score the same lowest number) and insensitivity to clinically important changes in health status. An alternative approach for assessing quality of life is to ask global questions. Table 5.1 provides two examples that focus on overall and health-specific quality of life.

Older adults exhibit striking heterogeneity with respect to physiologic function, health status, belief systems, cultural and ethnic backgrounds, values, and personal preferences. **Advance care planning** (ACP) may increase the chances that a person's health care incorporates the components most likely to sustain or improve quality of life. A multidisciplinary Delphi panel has defined ACP as "a process that supports adults at any age or stage of health [that is, not just at the end of life] in understanding and sharing their personal values, life goals, and preferences regarding future medical care. The goal of ACP is to help ensure that people receive medical care that is consistent with their values, goals, and preferences during serious and chronic illness."

Patients' cultural and ethnic heritages may have an important role in their understanding of their illness, its meaning in their lives, and their response to it. It may be crucial, therefore, for the clinician to have an appreciation of that heritage and the role it plays in the patient's understanding of health and illness.

Although they share certain conceptual overlap, ACP and shared medical decision making differ. ACP is most effective when it takes place before it is needed, ie, before the person, for whatever reason, has lost decision-making capacity. It brings together the person, others he or she trusts to include in decision making, and key clinicians. These discussions may be emotionally charged, and a patient is, of course, not compelled to participate. The discussions should take into account both how ready individuals are to talk about serious matters and how much information they would like to hear about their health status and prognosis.

One important component of ACP may be the designation of a trusted person, or decisional surrogate, who may help to make medical decisions if the patient loses this capacity. Although this individual is commonly a loved one (spouse, partner, family member, or friend), he or she may instead be someone with less emotional investment (such as a personal attorney). Clinicians may advise patients to consider an individual whom they trust to make difficult decisions, who can do so under possibly stressful conditions, and who can represent the patient's values and priorities well. In any event, the preparation of this surrogate to fill the role, not just being listed in a document, is crucial.

ACP may best be conceptualized as a *process* that captures evolving conversations taking place over time, not a "one and done" event. It typically reflects changes in a patient's health status, becoming more specific about medical decisions and treatment preferences as issues arise. At the start, ACP should probably focus on a person's global, even philosophical, goals related to medical care. Common—and potentially conflicting—goals and priorities a person may articulate are to remain independent and avoid institutionalization, to assure physical comfort, to maintain dignity (however defined), to avoid the burden or perception of burden on family, to adhere to religious practices, or to extend life. Over time, elicited goals and values can be incorporated by clinicians into particular deliberations with patients and surrogates about medical treatments.

RESOURCES

- Chou R, Dana T, Bougatsos C, et al. Screening for impaired visual acuity in older adults: updated evidence report and systematic review for the US Preventive Services Task Force. *JAMA*. 2016;315(9):915–933.

- Horgas AL. Pain assessment in older adults. *Nurs Clin North Am*. 2017;52(3):375–385.

- Overcash J, Momeyer MA. Comprehensive geriatric assessment and caring for the older person with cancer. *Sem Oncol Nurs*. 2017;33(4):440–448.

- Sudore RL, Lum HD, You JJ, et al. Defining advance care planning for adults: a consensus definition from a multidisciplinary Delphi panel. *J Pain Symptom Manage*. 2017;53(5):821–832.

CHAPTER 6—PROGNOSTICATION

KEY POINTS

- Prognostication includes both the prediction and communication of the probability that a particular outcome will develop in an individual over a period of time.

- Prognostication and understanding of lag time to benefit is important for framing and guiding shared clinical decision making.

- Estimating prognosis can be accomplished using one of 4 methods: clinical judgment, age-based life expectancy, referencing published studies, and prognostic indices.

- Using a structured framework to communicate prognosis can assist in the delivery of difficult news and patient-centered care.

Prognosis is the prediction of the probability that a particular outcome will develop in an individual over a period of time. Possible outcomes include time to death and time to likelihood of significant functional decline. Developing a prognosis is an important skill that can greatly inform patient-centered goal setting and shared decision making.

Prognostication is a broader term that incorporates both estimating and communicating prognosis. Estimating prognosis using patient-relevant outcomes, communicating prognosis, and incorporating lag time to benefit of potential diagnostic or therapeutic interventions can help patients and clinicians in the process of shared decision making.

IMPORTANCE OF AND BARRIERS TO PROGNOSTICATION

Prognosis can significantly impact care decisions ranging from large goals of care decisions, such as the desire for life-sustaining treatments, to whether to continue routine cancer screening. Providing patients and their families with prognoses can greatly inform their care decisions and better delineate realistic and achievable goals of care. Estimating and communicating prognosis is also crucial to determining whether a patient is eligible for additional services and benefits such as hospice care, which requires an overall life expectancy of ≤6 months. They may also desire discussion of prognoses beyond overall life expectancy in the context of goals and outcomes they feel are important, such as functional recovery, ability to maintain independent living, and ability to achieve personal milestones (eg, attending a family member's wedding or graduation).

Incorporation of the concept of lag time to benefit is important when discussing decisions around possible diagnostic or therapeutic interventions, especially when the benefits will not be immediate. Lag time to benefit is defined as the time between an intervention and when improved health outcomes may be expected. When discussing whether to pursue diagnostic or therapeutic interventions, weighing the likelihood that a patient may live long enough to benefit from the proposed intervention can greatly aid clinical decision making. If a patient's life expectancy is significantly less than the lag time to benefit of a preventive intervention, the likelihood of the patient being harmed rather than benefitting from an intervention is high, and one might consider recommending against rather than pursuing the intervention. If a patient's life expectancy significantly exceeds the lag time to benefit, the likelihood of benefitting from the intervention is now much higher, and the patient might be encouraged to pursue the intervention. In instances when life expectancy is close to lag time to benefit, further discussion of prognosis and patient goals of care may help guide clinical decision making (Table 6.1).

Despite the evidence encouraging discussions about prognosis with patients and families, practitioners continue to shy away from having these discussions because of preconceived biases and uncertainty around prognosis. Patients and families often want to discuss prognosis to help with planning and decision making; discussion of prognosis does not negatively impact hope or overall ability to cope with illness. Although estimations of prognosis may not always be completely accurate, patients and families look to practitioners for prognostic information because practitioners are best equipped and knowledgeable to make these estimations.

ESTIMATING PROGNOSIS

Practitioners can estimate prognosis by the following 4 methods: clinician judgment, age-based life expectancy, referencing published studies, and published prognostic indices. Any combination of these methods can be used to determine the most accurate prognostic prediction.

Clinical Judgment

With time and experience, individual practitioners build a set of anecdotal cases that may shape their estimation of prognosis in particular groups of patients or specific presentations. Practitioners may weigh their experience with previous patients' pathologic and clinical findings, diagnosis, comorbidities, ongoing and

Table 6.1—Lag Time to Benefit for Common Preventive Screening Tests and Clinical Interventions

Lag Time to Benefit	Common Clinical Interventions/Screening Tests
1–2 months	SSRIs for depression
6 months	Statins for secondary prevention of cardiovascular disease Finasteride for benign prostatic hyperplasia
1–2 years	Blood pressure control for primary prevention of cardiovascular disease
1–3 years	Strict blood pressure and lipid control in type 2 diabetes mellitus Statins for primary prevention of cardiovascular disease
8–10 years	Tight glycemic control for prevention of microvascular complications in type 2 diabetes mellitus
10 years	Colon and breast cancer screening for reducing cancer mortality

previous therapies, and various psychosocial factors to predict prognosis for a particular patient.

Age-Based Life Expectancy

Average life expectancy tables based on current age provide a broad estimate of median survival in the general population. While this may provide a more data-driven starting point to estimate prognosis, there is substantial heterogeneity in life expectancy among older adults within the same age category. To partially account for this, practitioners can use life tables that separate life expectancy into quartiles (Table 6.2), and then use clinical judgment to decide whether an individual is in the healthiest quartile, least healthy quartile, or one of the middle quartiles.

Published Studies

Some published studies may closely align with a particular patient's clinical characteristics such as age and comorbidities. In those cases, a practitioner may choose to apply the results of published studies to generate a prognosis. This method may provide a more accurate and individualized prognosis provided that a patient's clinical details closely match those of the study's patient population. This is especially helpful in quickly advancing fields, such as oncology, in which new therapeutics are dramatically improving life expectancy for those with cancer. Generalizability to the older adult is of concern when using this method to estimate life expectancy, because those with functional or cognitive limitations, and/or significant comorbidities are often excluded from clinical trials.

Published Prognostic Indices

Prognostic indices are validated tools that use select characteristics from a particular population such as functional status and comorbidities to calculate a prognostic estimate (Table 6.3). These are commonly used in clinical practice, whether it be to assess the risk of death and ischemic events in patients experiencing a thrombolysis in myocardial infarction (TIMI score),

Table 6.2—Average Life Expectancy Based on Estimates of Health

Age	Quartile of Life Expectancy (years)					
	Women			Men		
	75th	50th	25th	75th	50th	25th
65	26.9	21.2	14.2	24.3	18.3	11.4
70	22.2	16.9	10.7	19.8	14.4	8.5
75	17.8	12.9	7.6	15.6	10.8	6.0
80	13.6	9.3	5.1	11.8	7.7	4.0
85	9.9	6.3	3.2	8.5	5.2	2.5
90	6.9	4.1	1.9	5.9	3.4	1.6
95	4.7	2.6	1.2	4.1	2.2	1.0

SOURCE: Data from Arias E. National Vital Statistics Reports. *Natl Vital Stat Reports*. 2015;64(11):1–63.

risk of stroke from atrial fibrillation ($CHADS_2$), or risk of developing a pressure injury (Braden scale). When used for mortality predictions in older adults, tools that incorporate functional status tend to perform better than those that rely only on factors that are normally captured in an electronic medical record, such as comorbidities or demographic factors like age. A collection of these types of indices can be found at ePrognosis (https://eprognosis.ucsf.edu [accessed Feb 2019]).

Use of prognostic indices requires an understanding of the accuracy, validity, and generalizability of a specific index. For example, indices developed to estimate risk of mortality for nursing-home residents are not applicable to community-dwelling adults because they would likely underestimate prognosis. Additionally, many older adults do not have one single terminal diagnosis and often have a complex mix of medical comorbidities and functional and cognitive impairment. Using a disease-specific prognostic index in these cases disregards the interactions of the patient's multiple health factors and will provide an inaccurate prognosis. In such cases, nondisease-specific prognostic indices tailored to populations residing in different settings (community, nursing home, hospital, hospice) may be most useful. However, for those with one dominant

Table 6.3—Common Prognostic Indices

	Prognostic Index	Patient Population	Website*
Nondisease-specific examples			
	Walter 1-year index	Hospitalized adults ≥70 years old	www.ePrognosis.org
	Lee 4- and 10-year index	Community-dwelling adults ≥50 years old	
	Schonberg 5- and 9-year index	Community-dwelling adults ≥65 years old	
	Go-FAR	Hospitalized patients who experienced an in-hospital cardiac arrest	www.gofarcalc.com
Disease-specific examples			
Cancer	Palliative Performance Scale	Cancer and noncancer patients in clinics, hospitals, and hospices	www.ePrognosis.org
Heart failure	Seattle Heart Failure Model	Outpatients without significant other comorbidities. May overestimate prognosis in the old-old.	http://depts.washington.edu/shfm
	EFFECT Model	Inpatients hospitalized with acute decompensated heart failure	http://www.ccort.ca/Research/CHFRiskModel.html
COPD	BODE	Outpatients with COPD. May be more accurate in patients with severe COPD.	Reference.medscape.com/calculator/bode-index-copd
Dementia	Advanced Dementia Prognostic Tool (ADEPT)	Nursing-home residents with advanced dementia	www.ePrognosis.org

* All accessed Feb 2019.

life-limiting condition, disease-specific indices are often more valuable.

Estimating Prognosis in Common Diseases

Cancer

There is significant variability in prognosis based on types of cancer, even when restricted to advanced metastatic cancers. Furthermore, the prognosis for some cancers, such as metastatic non-small cell lung cancer, is being greatly improved by new targeted therapies. Given this, one of the most important tasks to determine prognosis is an open discussion about prognosis with specialists, such as oncologists and surgeons. Another useful method is to use published studies related to a particular cancer diagnosis to guide prognosis, with the caveat that many frail older adults with functional or cognitive limitations and multiple medical comorbidities are not included in these studies. Performance status has consistently demonstrated an association with survival, although length of survival may depend on the type of cancer. Commonly used scales to quantify performance status in cancer patients include the Eastern Cooperative Oncology Group performance status and the Karnofsky Performance Status. The Palliative Performance Scale is another tool used to calculate survival estimates based on several clinical factors such as overall function and consciousness level; it has been validated in both cancer and noncancer patients receiving palliative care in outpatient, hospital, and hospice settings.

Heart Failure

Important markers of poor prognosis for those living with heart failure include patient demographic factors, heart failure severity, need for repeat hospitalizations, comorbid diseases, physical examination findings, laboratory values (ie, hyponatremia and anemia), and functional status. Two prognostic tools that can aid in estimating prognosis in heart failure include the Seattle Heart Failure Model and the EFFECT model. The Seattle Heart Failure model is an online calculator developed and validated in over 10,000 community-dwelling outpatients without significant comorbidities. The calculator is available online and requires some time to complete. Care should be taken when using this calculator for patients with comorbid functional and cognitive decline or additional medical comorbidities.

Prognosis tends to be much worse for those who are hospitalized for heart failure. The prognosis only worsens for patients >85 years old, who have a median survival of 1 year after just a single hospitalization and of 6 months after two hospitalizations. For individuals hospitalized with heart failure, the EFFECT model combines factors such as systolic blood pressure, laboratory findings, and comorbidities to calculate 30-day and 1-year predicted mortality.

Chronic Obstructive Pulmonary Disease (COPD)

Predictions mortality in COPD can be difficult because of its natural trajectory characterized by chronic, progressive decline in pulmonary function punctuated by sudden and possibly life-threatening illness. Despite this uncertainty, several prognostic indices have been developed over the years. Airway obstruction, as measured by FEV_1, is used most commonly to assess the severity of COPD and predict survival. However, significant heterogeneity in prognosis remains among COPD patients when using only one prognostic factor such as FEV_1. The BODE index was developed from a multinational sample of outpatients with COPD and has been shown to have the most accurate short- and long-term mortality prediction when compared with FEV_1 alone. The BODE index includes weight, FEV_1, the Medical Research Council dyspnea score, and exercise capacity (6-minute walk distance).

End-Stage Renal Disease

Over the last several decades, the average age of individuals starting dialysis has progressively increased. These older individuals have a significantly worse prognosis than their younger counterparts. The prognosis is worse for individuals residing in nursing homes, which accounts for another rapidly increasing population of patients who are starting dialysis. However, age is only one factor in determining prognosis in the dialysis population. A validated prognostic index has been developed that combines several factors to calculate 6-month and 1-year mortality predictions. The model combines age, serum albumin, presence or absence of dementia, and peripheral vascular disease with the question: "would I be surprised if this patient died within the next 6 months?"

Dementia

Dementia has a progressive, prolonged period of cognitive and functional decline. Predicting prognosis in dementia can have significant implications for additional services such as hospice care. Hospice eligibility guidelines for dementia require that individuals need to meet or exceed Stage 7a on the Functional Assessment Scale and must have at least one complication of dementia that includes either aspiration, upper urinary tract infection, sepsis, multiple ulcers that are stage 3 or 4, persistent fever, or weight loss >10% within 6 months. Unfortunately, these guidelines often fail to accurately predict 6-month survival in those with advanced disease. The Advanced Dementia Prognostic Tool can be used to identify nursing-home residents with advanced dementia with an estimated life expectancy of ≤6 months with greater predictive value than general hospice eligibility criteria. The difficulty in estimating short-term survival in advanced dementia should influence how palliative care is delivered to these patients. Specifically, it should not be guided by prognosis, but rather their overall care needs and goals of care.

COMMUNICATING PROGNOSIS

Communication of prognosis can be difficult, but using communication structures that emphasize alignment with patient understanding, expectations, and emotions can greatly aid in the delivery of patient-centered care. Practitioners can make well-informed estimates of prognosis (using the tools previously discussed) and place prognosis into the context of lag time to benefit to help guide clinical decision making. Several video examples demonstrating the use of prognostication in clinical decision making can be found at https://eprognosis.ucsf.edu/communication/ (accessed Feb 2019).

The SPIKES Mnemonic

The SPIKES mnemonic was developed to provide practitioners with a structured, step-wise protocol for delivering difficult news, including poor prognoses. In 6 steps, practitioners can accomplish the 4 main goals of delivering prognosis: assess the knowledge, expectations, and readiness of patients and their surrogates; provide information in coherent, manageable quantities aligned with the needs and expectations of patients and their surrogates; support patients and their surrogates; and develop a shared plan for next steps.

RESOURCES

- Baile WF. SPIKES—A six-step protocol for delivering bad news: application to the patient with cancer. *Oncologist*. 2000;5(4):302–311.

- Bernacki RE, Block SD. Communication about serious illness care goals: a review and synthesis of best practices. *JAMA Intern Med*. 2014;174(12):1994–2003.

- Glare PA, Sinclair CT. Palliative medicine review: prognostication. *J Palliat Med*. 2009;11(1):84–103.

CHAPTER 7—MULTIMORBIDITY

KEY POINTS

- More than 50% of older adults have 3 or more chronic conditions, or *multimorbidity*.

- It is important for the clinician to consider the effect that a particular combination of conditions has on the patient in terms of symptoms, function, and likely health trajectory.

- Multimorbidity is associated with increased rates of death, disability, adverse treatment effects, institutionalization, use of health care resources, and decreased quality of life.

- Older adults with multimorbidity are heterogeneous in terms of illness severity, functional status, prognosis, personal priorities, and risk of adverse events, necessitating a flexible approach to their care.

One of the greatest challenges in geriatrics is providing optimal care (patient-centered and evidence-based) for older adults with multiple chronic conditions, or *multimorbidity*. More than 50% of older adults have ≥3 chronic diseases, with distinctive cumulative effects for each individual. A distinguishing mark of geriatric health care professionals is the ability to manage patients with complex multimorbidity.

Most clinical practice guidelines (CPGs) focus on management of a single disease, but CPG-based care for several co-occurring diseases may be cumulatively impractical, irrelevant, or even harmful for individuals with multimorbidity. Failures of CPG directives in patients with multimorbidity are not based solely on shortcomings of guideline development and implementation. Older adults with multimorbidity are regularly excluded or underrepresented in trials and observational studies. This translates to reduced representation of older adults in meta-analyses and systematic reviews and guidelines, which affects prudent interpretation of results.

Clinicians need a management approach that will consider the issues particular to each individual, including the often limited available evidence, interactions among conditions or treatments, the patient's own preferences and goals, prognosis, multifactorial geriatric issues and syndromes, and the feasibility of proposed management approaches. Tools that may be helpful include the American Geriatrics Society's Multimorbidity GEMS Mobile App (https://geriatricscareonline.org).

Older adults with multimorbidity are heterogeneous in terms of illness severity, functional status, prognosis, personal priorities, and risk of adverse events, even when diagnosed with the same list of conditions. Not only do the individuals themselves differ, but so do their treatment options, necessitating more flexible approaches to care of this population. Depending on how the definition is used, even older adults without serious illness may be considered to have multimorbidity. Older adults whose multiple chronic conditions have condition-condition, condition-treatment, or treatment-treatment interactions may benefit from the approach outlined below, even when they do not meet the criteria for serious illness. The approach described in this chapter is complementary to that used in palliative care, with some philosophical overlap.

APPROACH TO THE OLDER ADULT WITH MULTIMORBIDITY

Clinicians treating older adults with multimorbidity face many challenges, including complex clinical management decisions, inadequate evidence base, time constraints, and reimbursement structures, all of which hinder provision of efficient, high-quality care. For a useful approach for optimal management of these individuals, see Table 7.1.

Five distinct domains have been identified as relevant to the care of older adults with multimorbidity: patient preferences, interpreting the evidence, prognosis, clinical feasibility, and optimizing therapies and care plans.

GUIDING PRINCIPLES

The care of older adults with multimorbidity is challenging, and the principles described below are intended to guide clinicians toward better processes and outcomes.

Domain 1: Patient Preferences

The guiding principle of this domain is to elicit and incorporate patient preferences into medical decision-making for older adults with multimorbidity.

Care provided in accordance with CPGs may not adequately address patients' individual preferences, a key aspect of medical decision-making. Older adults with multimorbidity should be presented the opportunity to evaluate choices and to prioritize their preferences for care, within personal and cultural contexts. Clinicians can engage patients in these dialogues using an approach that emphasizes advance care planning. In this approach, clinicians ask patients to clarify values about possible outcomes of treatment, with consideration given to matters such as the ability to live independently, control of symptoms, cognitive and physical function, and life

Table 7.1—Approach to the Evaluation and Management of the Older Adult with Multimorbidity

- Inquire about the patient's primary concern (and that of family and/or friends, if applicable) and any additional objectives for visit.
- Conduct a complete review of care plan for person with multimorbidity, or focus on specific aspect of care for person with multimorbidity.
- What are the current medical conditions and interventions?
- Is there adherence/comfort with treatment plan?
- Consider patient preferences.
- Is relevant evidence available regarding important outcomes?
- Consider prognosis.
- Consider interactions within and among treatments and conditions.
- Weigh benefits and harms of components of the treatment plan.
- Communicate and decide for or against implementation or continuation of intervention/treatment.
- Reassess at selected intervals for benefit, feasibility, adherence, alignment with preferences.

SOURCE: American Geriatrics Society Expert Panel on the Care of Older Adults with Multimorbidity. Guiding principles for the care of older adults with multimorbidity: an approach for clinicians. *J Am Geriatr Soc.* 2012;60(10):E1–E25.

expectancy. Patients can be encouraged to use their own stories to clarify values and priorities, while recognizing that these may change over time.

Domain 2: Interpreting the Evidence

The guiding principle of this domain is to recognize the limitations of the evidence base and to interpret and apply the medical literature specifically to older adults with multimorbidity.

Different conditions in the same patient may interact, changing the risks associated with each condition and its treatments. Consequently, determining whether a given individual is likely to benefit from a particular treatment is complicated.

Clinicians should be aware that significant evidence gaps exist concerning condition and treatment interactions, particularly in older adults with multimorbidity.

Domain 3: Prognosis

The guiding principle of this domain is to frame clinical management decisions within the context of risks, burdens, benefits, and prognosis (eg, remaining life expectancy, functional status, quality of life) for older adults with multimorbidity.

Clinical management decisions for the multimorbid population necessitate the evaluation of prognosis to inform patient preferences and to adequately assess risks, burdens, and benefits. Important prognostic variables include remaining life expectancy, likelihood of functional disability, and future quality of life. Clinicians also need to evaluate risks for specific conditions (eg, GI hemorrhage with aspirin use for primary prevention of cardiovascular disease in men) as prognosis is considered.

The prognosis for each patient influences, but does not dictate, clinical management decisions within the context of his or her preferences. Often the time horizon to benefit for a treatment may be longer than the individual's projected life span, making the risk of drug-drug and drug-disease interactions, particularly in older adults with multimorbidity, unjustifiable. Screening tests (eg, colonoscopy) may not be beneficial or could be harmful if the time horizon to benefit exceeds remaining life expectancy, especially because associated harms and burdens increase with age and comorbidity.

A discussion about prognosis can serve as an introduction to difficult conversations, facilitating decision-making and advance care planning, and allowing exploration of patient preferences, treatment rationales, and therapy prioritization.

Domain 4: Clinical Feasibility

The guiding principle of this domain is to consider treatment complexity and feasibility when making clinical management recommendations for older adults with multimorbidity.

Some guideline organizations, such as the Grading of Recommendations Assessment, Development and Evaluation (GRADE) Working Group, now encourage routine consideration of burden of treatment when making recommendations for clinical management. However, the definition of these concepts has been inconsistent.

One practical approach is to break down treatment complexity and burden into individual components that can then be evaluated separately. This may help to identify particularly burdensome components of the process, allowing for determination of specific methods to resolve challenges.

The more complex a treatment regimen, the higher the risk of nonadherence, adverse reactions, decreased quality of life, increased economic burden, and increased strain and depression among caregivers. Medication adherence also changes according to situational factors and perceptions of need, cost, or current symptoms.

Treatment-related education and assessments must be ongoing, multifaceted, and individualized, and are best delivered via a variety of methods and settings, because patients often recall only a small fraction of what is discussed with clinicians. Cognitive impairment frequently challenges adherence as well.

Domain 5: Optimizing Therapies and Care Plans

The guiding principle of this domain is to use strategies for choosing therapies that maximize benefit, minimize harm, and enhance quality of life.

Older adults with multimorbidity are at risk of polypharmacy, suboptimal medication use, and potential harms from various interventions. Treatments and interventions must be prioritized to assure adherence to the most essential pharmacologic and nonpharmacologic therapies, to minimize risk exposure, and to maximize benefit. Polypharmacy is associated with therapeutic omissions, reduced benefit from otherwise beneficial medications, and even net harm in this population. Nonpharmacologic interventions (eg, implantable cardiac electronic devices) may prove more burdensome than beneficial if inconsistent with patient preferences.

CONTROVERSIES AND CHALLENGES

Implementing this patient-centered approach in older patients with multimorbidity is challenging, especially given the dynamic health status of such individuals and the involvement of multiple clinicians and settings. Even with appropriate decision support tools and skilled communication, the need to make multiple simultaneous decisions makes it difficult to explain information and uncertainties about benefits and harms. This may prevent individuals, families, and friends from fully participating in treatment decisions, communicating preferences, and prioritizing outcomes. Satisfactory evidence for clinical management of individuals with multimorbidity is scarce, as are reasonable prognostic measures, and different prognostic tools often yield conflicting results for the same patient. Treatments meant to improve one outcome (eg, survival) may worsen another (eg, function). Many clinical management regimens are also simply too complex to be feasible in this population, yet as clinicians attempt to reduce polypharmacy and unnecessary interventions, they may fear liability regarding underuse of therapies. Use of the strategies put forth in this chapter may help to alleviate these concerns.

Some patient-centered approaches, however, may simply be too time-consuming for an overwhelmed clinician working within the current reimbursement structure and without the support of an interprofessional team. Vigorous advocacy efforts are needed to address these resource issues.

RESOURCES

- Jones MG, DeCherrie LV, Meah YS, et al. Using nurse practitioner co-management to reduce hospitalizations and readmissions within a home-based primary care program. *J Healthc Qual.* 2017;39(5):249–258.

- Smith SM, Wallace E, O'Dowd T, et al. Interventions for improving outcomes in patients with multimorbidity in primary care and community settings. *Cochrane Database Syst Rev.* 2016 Mar 14;3:CD006560.

- Tinetti ME, Esterson J, Ferris R, et al. Patient priority-directed decision making and care for older adults with multiple chronic conditions. *Clin Geriatr Med.* 2016;32(2):261-275.

CHAPTER 8—CAREGIVING

KEY POINTS

- Caregiving is an increasingly common experience; more than 14% of all adults in the United States are caregivers.

- Varied intra- and interpersonal demographics, health conditions, functional needs, and community forces shape relationships between caregivers and care recipients.

- Giving and receiving care are not mutually exclusive. Most Americans will have one or both roles at some point during their lives.

- Different aspects of caregiving require different skills and warrant specific supportive resources. Common responsibilities of caregivers include health care decision support, care coordination or management, medical and nursing tasks (eg, medication management, wound care), physical care, emotional support, homemaking, and transportation. These responsibilities, along with other less common ones, vary widely across caregiver–care recipient dyads.

- Intervening to support caregiver–care recipient dyads and to mitigate caregiver strain and burden mandates an interdisciplinary approach to the extent possible. The interprofessional care team may include primary care physicians, nurse practitioners, physician assistants, social workers, nurses, clergy, physical and occupational therapists, and speech language pathologists.

- Resources for caregivers often exist in social care centers and not within the health care system. A variety of tools and support options for caregivers are available through web sites from reputable organizations (see Table 8.1).

Caregiving focuses on managing daily life in light of meeting needs and obtaining necessary services for care recipients. Caregiving is complex, with different roles and activities needed to match the needs of the care recipient. Common activities include health care decision support, care coordination or management, medical and nursing tasks (eg, medication management, wound care), physical care, emotional support, homemaking, and transportation. Ensuring effective caregiving assessment and intervention is key to well-coordinated health and social care for older adults.

DEFINING CAREGIVING

Caregiving is the experience of providing physical, emotional, and instrumental care to another person. In the United States, the term *caregiver* refers to a person providing any type of care to another person informally and without financial compensation. The term *carer* is a synonym more often used in the United Kingdom and elsewhere in the world. While adults of any age may require care, those receiving care are often older and may be frail with multiple morbidities.

People who provide care informally to family members, friends, and neighbors may or may not identify themselves as caregivers. Similarly, older adults receiving care may not identify themselves as care recipients—and they themselves may also be simultaneously providing care to another person.

Caregiving Statistics

The following findings from research conducted by the National Alliance for Caregiving (NAC) and The AARP Public Policy Institute on caregiving in the United States (www.aarp.org/content/dam/aarp/ppi/2015/caregiving-in-the-united-states-2015-report-revised.pdf [accessed Feb 2019]) detail the multifaceted characteristics and magnitude of caregiving today.

- About 14.3% of all American adults are caregivers for someone >50 years old, about half of whom feel as though they had no choice but to do so. Most caregivers (74%) live with or are geographically close to the care recipient.

- Hispanic adults (21%) are more commonly caregivers than those of other ethnic groups; white adults report caregiving least often (16.9%).

- Most caregivers (82%) care for only one adult, 15% care for two adults, and 3% care for three or more adults.

- Women comprise 60% of caregivers and 65% of care recipients.

- Care recipients tend to be older; 47% are ≥75 years old, 39% are 50–74 years old, and only 14% are 18–49 years old.

- The age of caregivers is more widely distributed between 18 and >75 years old. A third of caregivers (35%) are 50–74 years old, but almost half of all caregivers are 18–34 (24%) and 35–49 (23%) years old. Notably, 12% of caregivers are 50–64 years old, and 7% are ≥75 years old. These findings suggest that the oldest caregivers are more likely than their younger counterparts to be providing care by themselves, without outside resources.

- Most caregivers are supporting a family member, but 15% provide care to an unrelated individual.

- Most caregivers (73%) have been providing care for ≤5 years, but about 25% have been caring for >5 years, and 12% for >10 years.

- About 74% of caregivers provide care at least once a week or more often.

- Caregivers most often find care easy or somewhat easy to coordinate, although 18% report coordination is somewhat difficult, and 5% report coordination is very difficult.

- While most caregivers do not perceive financial strain because of their responsibilities, about 25% of caregivers reported difficulty obtaining local affordable care services.

- Employment status varies widely among caregivers, regardless of age. Employed caregivers do not always disclose their role to supervisors, although the most common benefit on which employed caregivers rely is flexible work hours.

- The costs of informal caregiving—represented by wages—have been reported to be $522 billion annually. This implies significant concerns for individual caregivers and their families, as well as societal reliance on this level of care. The cost of replacing this care with professional services is estimated to potentially total $863 billion ($221 billion for unskilled care and $642 billion for skilled services).

- Many caregivers desire policy changes. Issues such as privacy garnered considerable support. Nearly half (49%) of caregivers surveyed wanted their names to be part of the care recipient's medical record, 41% wanted health care providers mandated to notify them of major health care decisions, 43% wanted mandated instruction on hospital discharge, and one-third wanted respite care as part of health policy.

Diversity Among Caregiving Environments

Caregivers and caregiving represent a phenomenon fraught with myth and misinformation. The most common stereotype of caregivers entails women of the "sandwich generation." These women are at mid-life, caught between caring for children and caring for older family members be they parents, parents-in-law, or other older adults related by blood or marriage. Only 60% of caregivers nationally are women and, of those, not all are caring for parents or in-laws. In reality, caregivers are an extremely diverse group. Age, gender, and ethnicity are characteristics acknowledged to influence caregiving roles, responsibilities, relationships, and perceptions.

Family constellations and living arrangements increasingly affect caregiving beginning with the availability of caregivers. More adults than ever before are living alone, having never been or not presently married or in a cohabiting intimate relationship. Older people are aging and living alone without kinship networks to supply needed care. Understanding new interpretations of family, including relationships understood by the caregiver or potential caregiver and the care recipient, is crucial to successful assessment.

Current generations of older people—members of the Greatest, the Silent, and the Baby Boom Generations—are better educated than those who preceded them. Education affects function over the life course, as well as possibly altering risk of certain conditions such as dementia. Assessment targeting identification of functional illiteracy and level of health literacy among caregivers, as with their care recipients, is key to effective assessment and intervention.

Aging in place is reality for more older adults and their family and friends, whether they wish to age there or not. As a result, health care professionals are gradually becoming more familiar with various age-friendly community models. Some of these occur spontaneously as with naturally occurring retirement communities and religious communities such as Roman Catholic orders of priests and nuns. The nature of these spontaneously occurring communities presents challenges in maintaining resources for caregivers as the entire community ages and younger people join infrequently. Neighborhood organizations and religious congregations, with parish councils and other outreach groups, complement governmental and quasi-governmental resources in these aged communities. Planned models are intentionally structured and funded, providing health and social care to specific populations of older adults and their caregivers. Continuing care retirement communities and programs of all-inclusive care are among the most familiar examples.

Geographic locale (eg, urban, suburban, rural) influence caregivers' perspectives, lifeways, and culture, as well as acceptability of and access to support and resources. These community settings influence everything from the array of locally available services to expectations of caregiving relationships and needs for support held by both caregivers and care recipients.

Table 8.1—Online Resources and Tools for Caregivers

Resource	Organization/Website*	Comments
AARP Home and Family Caregiving Resource Center	www.aarp.org/home-family/caregiving/	Various planning resources for family caregivers
Alzheimer's Association online tools page	www.alz.org/care/alzheimers-dementia-online-tools.asp	A collection of online tools and resources, many of which are useful to caregivers regardless of disease or condition
American Cancer Society Caregivers and Family page	www.cancer.org/treatment/caregivers.html	Resources for caregivers and family members of people living with cancer
American Heart Association Support Network	www.heart.org/HEARTORG/Support/Support_UCM_001103_SubHomePage.jsp	Resources for caregivers supporting a person living with cardiac disease
American Psychological Association Connecting with Caregivers	www.apa.org/pi/about/publications/caregivers/consumers/index.aspx	Fact and resource compendium from the American Psychological Association
American Stroke Association/American Heart Association Support Network	www.strokeassociation.org/STROKEORG/LifeAfterStroke/ForFamilyCaregivers/For-Stroke-Family-Caregivers_UCM_308560_SubHomePage.jsp	Resources for caregivers supporting a person living after a stroke
Area Agency on Aging	http://n4a.org/about-n4a/?fa=aaa-title-VI (to find a local area agency on aging)	Family caregiver information and/or support services; family caregiver support specialists are also available.
Center for Medicare and Medicaid Services' Nursing Home Compare tool	www.medicare.gov/nursinghomecompare/search.html	Provides information about Medicare- and Medicaid-certified nursing homes with a feature that allows comparison
Chaplains on Hand	http://chaplainsonhand.org/cms/index.php	Resources from the HealthCare Chaplaincy Network for patients and caregivers
E-Care Diary	www.ecarediary.com/	Free online care diary and other resources
Eldercare Locator	www.eldercare.gov	Help in finding additional respite services for family caregivers
Family Caregiver Alliance	http://caregiver.org	Family caregiving resources and information, including online support groups
Health in Aging Caregiver Self-Assessment Questionnaire	www.healthinaging.org/resources/resource:caregiver-self-assessment/	A self-assessment tool developed by the American Medical Association, available in English, Spanish and Greek, that can be downloaded or completed online
Medline Plus	www.nlm.nih.gov/medlineplus/healthtopics.html	Health information portal
National Academy of Elder Law Attorneys Find A Lawyer	https://www.naela.org/findlawyer	Searchable data base of elder law attorneys
National Adult Day Services Association	www.nadsa.org	Help family caregivers find a local adult day service program
National Alliance for Caregiving	www.caregiving.org/resources/	Resources addressing a variety of family caregiving topics, including financial concerns
National Institutes of Health: Health Information	www.nih.gov/health-information (search using key word "caregiver" or a specific disease or condition)	Search provides currently available materials from the National Institutes of Health.
National Institute on Aging Health Information	www.nia.nih.gov/health	Health information, including caregiving topics from the National Institute on Aging
PubMed Health	www.ncbi.nlm.nih.gov/pubmedhealth/	National health information portal
Rosalynn Carter Institute for Caregiving	www.rosalynncarter.org/caregiver	Compilation of resources for professional and family caregivers, including intervention research database

Table 8.1—Online Resources and Tools for Caregivers (continued)

Resource	Organization/Website*	Comments
SAGECAP	www.sageusa.org/programs/sagecap.cfm	SAGE provides support and advocacy for lesbian, gay, bisexual, and transgender older adults. The organization launched SAGECAP to support caregivers, focusing on those in the New York City area. SAGE subsequently expanded SAGECAP to replicate the program in Baltimore, Maryland.
SAGE National Resource Center Caregiving Resource Page	www.lgbtagingcenter.org/resources/index.cfm?s=3	SAGE provides support and advocacy for lesbian, gay, bisexual, and transgender older adults, offering the National Resources Center to provide information on a variety of aging-related topics, including caregiving.

* Websites accessed Feb 2019

Caregiver Experience

Professional and ethical obligations mandate that physicians, nurses, and social work colleagues identify caregiver burden. Understanding advantages and benefits in caregiving is equally important to evaluating risks.

Many caregivers gain competence and mastery of complex skills and find emotional well-being and spiritual peace through familial respect or filial piety. They and those for whom they care often find new meaning and unexpected reciprocity in their relationships. Needs, capacity, and locations mediate both negative and positive aspects of caregiving, depending on the nature of the caregiver–care recipient relationship. Lastly, acceptability, access, and affordability of supplemental resources for the caregiver and the care recipient, from respite care to homemaker services, typically play a part in the overall experience of the caregiver.

CONSIDERATIONS IN CLINICAL ASSESSMENT

The provider who treats the care recipient is often the first health care professional to detect strain or burden because of dynamics in the caregiver–care recipient dyad. Even then, indications of need and opportunities to prevent distress mandate routine screening as a fundamental first step. Further, inquiring about self-defined caregiving and the responsibilities associated with it helps to avoid misunderstandings or misidentifying caregiver and care recipient in any encounter. Asking about daily routine—emphasizing key caregiving tasks like decision-making support, medication administration, assistance with ADLs, emotional support, and transportation—and whether the individuals consider themselves holding a role as caregiver are useful starting points.

Interdisciplinary Team Approach

Many providers are unlikely to be able to complete any assessment beyond screening during an ambulatory visit, so assessment may be completed by other members of the team. For example, social workers or nurses can continue the assessment after a positive screening result, such as "Yes, I am a caregiver for another adult" or "Yes, I am a caregiver for another adult and I feel some level of distress."

Calling on a chaplain or local clergy person is often helpful, as well as physical therapy, occupational therapy, and speech language pathology who are key partners for both assessment and intervention when functional changes present problems in caregiving or are sources of distress.

Assessment Strategies and Techniques

There are a variety of assessment tools, including the Zarit Burden Interview (www.aafp.org/afp/2000/1215/p2613.html#afp20001215p2613-f1 [accessed Feb 2019]). Many clinical settings rely on small teams and paraprofessional staff members. For example, in a practice lacking access to a social worker, immediate referral to the Area Agency on Aging with a request for specific assessment works for some caregiver–care recipient dyads who qualify. In situations when the caregiver works, he or she may have access to employee assistance program benefits for both assessment and direct support intervention.

INTERVENTIONS AND REFERRALS

Age-friendly, person- and family-centered approaches to caregivers and caregiver–care recipient dyads warrant well-sequenced introduction of interventions and referrals to resources for further support. Interventions and referrals range from online tools to make scheduling transportation or delivery of meals by family and friends more convenient to urgent interventions when clinicians suspect risk of self-harm or neglect and/or risk of harm to the care recipient.

Caregivers often benefit from conversations to screen and assess, because these interchanges promote a sense of feeling understood and prompt reflection for many. Timely connections to caregivers' primary care providers or other health and social care providers who treat them, and not the care recipients, are valuable.

RESOURCES:

- Fowler C, Kim MT. Home visits by care providers–influences on health outcomes for caregivers of homebound older adults with dementia. *Geriatr Nurs*. 2015;36(1):25–29.

- National Alliance for Caregiving and the AARP Public Policy Institute. Caregiving in the U.S. 2015. www.aarp.org/content/dam/aarp/ppi/2015/caregiving-in-the-united-states-2015-report-revised.pdf (accessed Feb 2019).

- Roth DL, Fredman L, Haley WE. Informal caregiving and its impact on health: a reappraisal from population-based studies. *Gerontologist*. 2015;55(2):309–319.

CHAPTER 9—CULTURAL ASPECTS OF CARE

KEY POINTS

- Culture and faith/spiritual beliefs have a significant impact on patients' world views, interpretation of health and illness, and their health-related behaviors.

- Clinicians should remain alert to the differences among individual patients from a given culture or faith/spiritual tradition and guard against stereotyping.

- Communication and clinical care are enhanced when health care providers make an effort to simplify medical messages and negotiate with patients a common understanding of causation, diagnosis, and treatment, while maintaining respect for the beliefs and constructs of both the provider and the patient.

As the cultural and religious/spiritual diversity of older Americans continues to grow, it is increasingly important for clinicians to develop an approach to working with older adults from a broad range of cultural and faith groups. The United States is projected to become a minority-majority nation by 2044 and by 2050, one of every three older Americans will be of "minority" status. Clinicians must be sensitive to the possibility that culture and religious/spiritual beliefs may affect relationships with individual patients and families. They also influence a patient's willingness or ability to engage in a therapeutic relationship, participate in shared decision making, and accept and adhere to the care plan.

There is no single or standard definition of cultural competence. Most definitions emphasize a careful coordination of individual behavior, organizational policy, and system design to facilitate mutually respectful and effective cross-cultural and interfaith interactions. Cultural competence combines attitudes, knowledge base, acquired skills, and behaviors that demonstrate an awareness of and respect for the patient's beliefs and behaviors. Ideally, it is a nuanced understanding of the role that culture plays in all of our lives and of the impact culture has on every health care encounter, for both the clinician and the patient.

In addition to culture, health literacy is an important consideration in providing care to older adults. It is currently estimated that more than 1 in 3 Americans has low health literacy. Data show that lower health literacy is more common in older adults than in younger adults, and in ethnic minorities than in whites. Health literacy affects the patient's ability to comprehend and act on health messages, and low health literacy is associated with poorer health outcomes.

This chapter is intended to help clinicians gain an initial understanding of the key issues in cross-cultural and interfaith patient encounters, so that they can create a self-directed training plan to develop and implement culturally competent behaviors. Clinicians should never assume that any person's cultural or religious background will dictate his or her health choices or behavior. They should remain alert to the differences among individual patients and families from a given culture or religious tradition, and guard against stereotyping older adults on the basis of their cultural or religious/spiritual affiliation. It is also neither necessary nor possible to know all the information about every cultural and faith group. Clinicians need to be able to take a learning stance to gently and respectfully elicit required information from the patient and family.

Clinicians have their own personal cultural identity and beliefs, which can implicitly or explicitly affect the manner in which they provide clinical care. Therefore, in reality, each cross-cultural and interfaith encounter is an opportunity for clinicians to engage in self-reflection on their own personal beliefs and biases and how this may potentially influence their perception of the patient. In addition to self-reflection, it is recommended that clinicians work in conjunction with the interprofessional health care team, including administrators, to promote diffusion of cultural competence in the health care organizations in which they practice.

USE OF LANGUAGE AND NONVERBAL COMMUNICATION

Preferred Terms for Cultural or Religious Identity

The terms referring to specific cultural, ethnic, or religious groups can change over time, and individuals in any one group do not always agree on appropriate terminology. It is helpful to learn the term that the individual patient prefers for his or her cultural or religious identity, and to use that terminology in conversation with the patient, as well as in his or her health records.

Formality

Attitudes regarding the appropriate degree of formality in a health care encounter differ widely among cultural groups. Learning a patient's preferences with regard to formality and allowing those preferences to shape the relationship is always advisable. Initially, a more formal approach is recommended. For example, when addressing the patient, the patient's correct title (eg, Dr.,

Reverend, Mr., Mrs., Ms., Miss) and his or her surname should be used unless and until he or she specifically requests a more casual form of address. Another important issue is to determine the correct pronunciation of the person's name, as well as the appropriate ordering of names; in a variety of countries, the family name is given first, followed by the individual's given name. Once the patient invites you to use his or her first name, it is appropriate to do so. Even in such situations, when discussing the patient with the family, it is ideal to refer to the patient in the third person with the surname, such as "Mrs. Smith told me she does not want the flu shot" instead of "Jane is refusing the flu shot."

Addressing the Health Care Provider

Learning how the patient prefers to address the clinician and to allow his or her preference to prevail is also important. In some cultures, trust in the clinician depends on the clinician assuming an authoritative role, and informality could undermine the patient's trust. This is an aspect of the clinical relationship in which the clinician's personal preferences may need to be relinquished.

Language and Literacy

The following questions should be considered before an encounter.

- What language does the patient feel most comfortable speaking?
- Will a medical interpreter be needed?
- Does the patient read and write English? Another primary language? If so, which one(s)?
- If the patient has low health literacy, does he or she have access to someone who can assist at home with written instructions?

Health messages are best delivered at a basic health literacy level, because patients may be reluctant or too embarrassed to admit to their inability to comprehend complex health messages.

These questions should be considered early in the process of establishing a therapeutic relationship to ensure that communication with the patient is effective. Even those who speak English fluently may wish to discuss complicated issues in their native language. It is the clinician's responsibility to explain medical terms and to ask the patient for explanations of any cultural or foreign terms that are unfamiliar.

Health Literacy Concerns

Health literacy is defined as "the degree to which individuals have the capacity to obtain, process, and understand basic health information and services needed to make appropriate health decisions." According to the U.S. Department of Health and Human Services, only 12% of the U.S. adult population has been determined to be at the "proficient" level of health literacy. Adults ≥65 years old were more likely to have below basic or basic health literacy skills than younger populations. More than two-thirds of older adults ≥75 years old had below basic or basic health literacy. Also, older adults who are uninsured or enrolled in both Medicare and Medicaid are at higher risk of having below basic or basic level of health literacy. It is prudent to screen all patients for level of health literacy. Ideally, clinicians should simplify their verbal communication and avoid medical jargon with *all* patients.

Key Communication Techniques

- Assess for any visual and auditory deficits. Speak clearly and slowly (many older adults may have hearing deficits but may be too embarrassed to voice their difficulties).

- Ensure that a pocket talker is readily available. A pocket talker is a portable amplifier that can be used with or without a hearing aid to reduce background noise. It is very helpful in one-on-one conversations, in a small group, or when listening to the television or radio.

- Explain things in plain English, while avoiding jargon.

- Emphasize not more than three key actionable items during each visit, and write these out in large print size in capitals and give to the patient as a handout.

- Offer to repeat the information until you are comfortable that the patient has grasped the main messages and knows exactly what he or she is supposed to do to adhere to the care plan.

- Encourage patients to ask questions; use an open-ended approach.

- Use the *"teach-back"* method to verify patient understanding. This method can be useful to confirm the patient's understanding of the medical visit by asking the patient to recall or explain in his or her own words what has been discussed. Consider use of demonstration skill, if needed. For example, the clinician may say "I always ask my patients to repeat things back to me to make sure I explained it clearly. I'd like you to tell me exactly when and how you're going to take the new medicine we discussed today."

Use of Medical Interpreters

Medical interpreters are trained professionals who can facilitate the communication between clinicians and

Chapter 9: Cultural Aspects of Care **43**

patients (and families) who speak different languages. Interpreters relay concepts and ideas between languages in a culturally sensitive way by listening attentively and then repeating the original message accurately and completely in another language. They are ethically bound to repeat everything and are obligated to maintain patient privacy and confidentiality. All clinicians caring for patients with limited English proficiency should be skilled in working with medical interpreters to communicate effectively with these patients and their families. Ideally, family members should not be asked to serve as medical interpreters, especially in situations when sensitive history is being taken or bad news is being shared.

At clinical sites of care where medical interpreters are not present in person, telephone or tablet language interpretation may be an available option. Clinicians should maintain eye contact with the patient and speak in the second person, and then pause to allow for interpretation. For specific guidelines and resources about how best to work with medical interpreters, see https://geriatrics.stanford.edu/medical-interpreters.html (accessed Feb 2019).

Respectful Nonverbal Communication

Body position and movement is interpreted differently from one cultural group to another. Specific hand gestures, facial expressions, physical contact, and eye contact can hold different meanings in different cultures. The clinician should watch for particular body language cues that appear to be significant and that might be linked to cultural norms that are important to the patient, in an effort to cultivate sensitivity to the conditions that facilitate and improve communication.

Conservative body language is advisable early in a relationship with a patient or when in doubt about a patient's background or preferences; clinicians should assume a calm demeanor and avoid expressive extremes (eg, very vigorous handshakes, a loud and hearty voice, many hand gestures, an impassive facial expression, avoidance of eye contact, standing at a distance). Clinicians should remain alert for signals of the patient's level of comfort. Directly asking the patient questions based on subtle nonverbal clues, including body language, may also help. Making negative judgments about a patient that are rooted in unconscious cultural assumptions about the meaning of his or her gestures, facial expressions, or body language should be avoided.

The physical distance from others that individuals find comfortable varies, depending in part on their cultural background. The clinician should determine what distance seems to be the most comfortable for each patient and, whenever practical, allow the patient's preference to establish the optimal distance during the encounter. Before doing a physical examination, it is prudent to request the patient's permission to do so. In doing sensitive procedures like a breast or genitalia examination, some patients may have a strong preference for a provider of the same gender. If this is not possible, it may be advisable to have a family member of the patient close at hand to support the patient while still respecting the patient's privacy.

HISTORY OF TRAUMATIC EXPERIENCES

Is the patient a refugee or survivor of violence or genocide? Are family members missing or dead? Have patients or family members been tortured? Such experiences could negatively affect the health care encounter without the clinician's knowledge unless relevant questions are included among standard questions about the patient's history. Clinicians should remember that in some historical periods and jurisdictions, health care providers have participated in torture and genocide (eg, Nazi medical personnel in World War II). The methods and tools of torture used have sometimes resembled legitimate clinical procedures and tools. Patients who have survived such experiences may not feel safe in medical or governmental settings, and contact with any clinician may invoke feelings of vulnerability, fear, panic, or anger. Great sensitivity is necessary in providing health care for these individuals.

ISSUES OF IMMIGRATION

Immigration Status

Some individuals may be living in North America without immigration documents. Clinicians may wish to assure each patient that information given within the medical encounter about immigration status will be kept confidential.

History of Immigration or Migration

The history of the movements of a large portion of a religious or cultural group can affect the attitudes and behavior of an individual in that group even when he or she has not immigrated to North America from another country. In addition, understanding an individual's specific migration history often provides insight into the key life transitions informing his or her outlook. Knowing how a person came to live in North America can be important. The time and effort the clinician invests in learning more about a cultural or religious group's history and current situation can be repaid not only in a better relationship with the individual patient but also in an enhanced appreciation of the factors affecting clinical relationships with other patients from that group.

ACCULTURATION, TRADITION, AND HEALTH BELIEFS

Acculturation is a process in which members of one cultural group adopt the beliefs and behaviors of another group. Acculturation of a group may be evidenced by changes in language preference, adoption of common attitudes and values, evolution of religious practices, or gradual loss of separate ethnic identification. Although acculturation typically occurs when a minority group adopts the habits and language patterns of a majority group, acculturation may also be reciprocal between groups.

It is essential to keep principles of acculturation in mind during any cross-cultural or interfaith health encounter. Beginning by determining how long a person has lived in North America and whether he or she was born here is helpful. However, remember that the degree to which the person is acculturated to North American customs and attitudes is the consequence of many factors and not just of the number of years since he or she immigrated. Older adults who follow the traditions of their cultural or religious group may have been born outside the United States, may be recent arrivals to the continent, or may even be lifelong North American residents.

A patient's level of cultural or spiritual shifting can impact not only his or her health behavior but also preferences in end-of-life planning and decision-making. Acculturation can also be an issue dividing family members, and a person's resistance to or ease of acculturation may be a matter of pride or of shame and guilt. Developing sensitivity about the issues of acculturation for one's older minority patients is a key element in effective cross-cultural health care. Asking patients directly about their adherence to cultural and spiritual traditions can be useful.

People from a variety of cultural groups may not conceive of illness in North American terms. Some may have highly developed concepts of the causes of health and disease that are incompatible with the concepts that form the foundations of North American medicine. Some other paradigms of wellness and illness include beliefs that illnesses have spiritual causation, are the result of imbalance among bodily humors, or are caused by a person's actions in past lives, to name but a few. Patients may make unexamined assumptions that are based on traditional beliefs, and these can cause confusion or create misunderstanding. The more the clinician knows about a patient's cultural and religious traditions, the better he or she can promote effective clinical communication. In addition, patients may use alternative treatments that are culturally important (eg, rituals, herbal preparations), which they may not mention to a physician; therefore, routinely asking patients about their use of complementary medicine as part of taking the history is important. Clinical communication and patient care is optimized when patients and health care providers work together to negotiate an understanding of causation, diagnosis, and treatment for a specific health problem, while the provider maintains respect for the patient's cultural beliefs and health constructs.

APPROACHES: THE ETHNICS MNEMONIC

To facilitate effective health interviews and care planning in cross-cultural settings, the ETHNICS mnemonic (below) provides a framework in which to ascertain a wide variety of information and to negotiate effective therapeutic next steps, all within a routine clinical session.

- **Explanation:** Ask patients to describe what they think is happening to them in their own words.

- **Treatments:** Ask patients which treatments they have used for their health problem(s). Clinicians should specifically ask about biomedical interventions, as well as any complementary and alternative treatments.

- **Healers:** Respectfully inquire about other healers involved in a patient's care; many patients seek treatment from alternative practitioners or traditional healers, as well as from conventional health care providers. Incorporating this information into the health care encounter is important to overall care planning and efficacy.

- **Negotiate:** Negotiate with each patient and/or his or her designated caregiver(s) as to which treatments the patient will accept and participate in.

- **Intervene:** Collaborate with the patient to establish the care plan. This frequently incorporates a blending of "scientific" explanations of wellness and disease, as well as each individual patient's concept of his or her health status and acceptable approaches to addressing concerns.

- **Collaborate:** Focus on building a trusting and resilient relationship with each patient. Incorporating formal and informal caregivers into a broader team alliance is also critical to the success of health care for all older adults.

- **Spirituality:** Inquire respectfully about patients' spiritual beliefs, and how these might impact their health care preferences and behavior, particularly at the end of life.

Chapter 9: Cultural Aspects of Care

UNSPOKEN CHALLENGES

Clinicians should remain alert to the possibility of issues that are critical to the success of the health care encounter that the patient may not voice, in particular for patients of color or patients from other cultural or religious groups who may have historical reasons to distrust providers and the health care system. Examples include the following:

- Lack of trust in health care providers and the health care system
- Fear of medical research and experimentation
- Fear of medications or their adverse events
- Unfamiliarity or discomfort with the Western biomedical belief system

Some patients may feel uncomfortable or uneasy in customary North American health care settings for a variety of reasons, including lack of familiarity with Western practices, dissatisfying previous encounters with the health care system, or the belief that insensitivity or discrimination is inevitable for anyone in the patient's cultural or religious group. Such feelings may result from historical treatment of the patient's cultural or religious group, or from having been stereotyped or treated insensitively or unfairly by clinicians in the past. Sensitive exploration of these issues with patients is often worthwhile and necessary. In general, sensitivity to the possibility that such issues are in play is advised in all patient encounters.

APPROACHES TO DECISION MAKING

Western bioethics emphasizes individual autonomy in all health decisions, but for many other cultures, decision-making is family or community centered. Autonomy principles allow competent individuals to involve others in their health decisions or to cede those rights to a proxy decision maker. The clinician should ask patients if they prefer to make their own health decisions or if they would prefer to involve or defer to others. Some may wish to assign the decision-making authority wholly to another individual or a group. In some cultures, the definition of family may include "fictive kin." Fictive kinship is a term used by anthropologists and ethnographers to denote deep and meaningful connections that are based on neither consanguineal (blood ties) nor affinal ("by marriage") ties, in contrast to traditional kinship ties. In families in which the degree of acculturation of the generations differs, the older adult may defer to or depend on younger relatives, even though the tradition might suggest that the reverse would occur.

Many studies have documented the impact of religious and spiritual beliefs on preferences regarding end-of-life practices and decision-making. Some religious traditions stress the religious obligation for individuals to save or extend life at almost any cost. Certain faith systems support the concept of "redemptive suffering" at the end of life; in such cases, the patient may be reluctant to take analgesics or permit withdrawal of high-intensity treatments at the end of life because health outcomes are thought to be divinely willed and acceptance in the face of adversity a mark of true faith.

Establishing an understanding of each patient's decision-making construct and preferences early in the clinical relationship will, in most instances, promote better communication and avoid the difficulties inherent in trying to address the issues at a time of crisis. When the patient's and clinician's cultural or religious backgrounds differ, careful exploration of the issues is all the more important, with specific attention to avoiding explicit and implicit biases.

ATTITUDES REGARDING DISCLOSURE AND CONSENT

Cultural attitudes toward truth telling and disclosure of terminal diagnoses vary widely. In some cultures, it is commonly believed that patients should not be informed of a terminal diagnosis, because this may hasten death or extinguish hope. Obtaining informed consent from patients with this belief may prove difficult. There is no consensus in bioethics concerning the rigorous application of full clinical disclosure in every situation. However, it is generally agreed that incorporating a patient's beliefs concerning disclosure and truth telling into clinical planning whenever possible is desirable. Some patients may prefer not to know if they are terminally ill and ask that family members or other caregivers receive all diagnostic information and make all treatment decisions. It is advisable to explore each patient's information-seeking preferences regarding disclosure of serious clinical findings early in the clinical relationship and to reconfirm these wishes periodically.

GENDER ISSUES

Culture and religion intertwine in describing traditions and structures with regard to gender roles. Societies seemingly based on the same patriarchal or matriarchal model may vary widely in their expressions of the model. A person's gender influences the sorts of experiences he or she has had, not only within the family but also in the community and health care system. Another level of complexity may be added to health care encounters when an older adult's group struggles with conflicting traditional and contemporary views on gender roles.

Cultural norms for men and women can influence their health behavior, and such norms for the genders vary widely from one culture to another. Gender-based norms may also affect how patients choose a health care provider and make health decisions, as well as how they form their preferences for disclosure and consent.

The clinician is strongly advised to explore each patient's attitudes regarding the interplay among gender, choice of health care provider, autonomy, and personal decision making early in the patient-provider relationship; to periodically confirm the patient's preferences; and to follow the individual patient's wishes whenever possible.

SPIRITUAL AND RELIGIOUS ISSUES

In some cultural groups, most individuals share one religious heritage; in others, there is a great deal of religious and spiritual diversity. As a result, the relative impact of religion and culture on health behavior and decision making for older adults may be subtle and complex, warranting respectful exploration on the part of the clinician.

Several studies have documented that most patients either prefer or would accept clinicians asking them about their spiritual beliefs and the impact such beliefs might have on their world view, health behavior, and health decision making (SOE=A). Questions regarding religion and spirituality should be incorporated sensitively and early in the patient-provider relationship and reexplored when significant health problems arise. The acronym FICA (for faith and belief, importance, community, and address in care) can help health care providers to structure questions in taking a spiritual history (https://smhs.gwu.edu/gwish/clinical/fica/spiritual-history-tool).

Religious and spiritual beliefs and practices affect how patients interpret health, illness, and suffering. Koenig and colleagues found that among 838 older hospitalized patients, religiousness and spirituality consistently predicted greater social support, fewer depressive symptoms, better cognitive and physical function, less severe illness and comorbidity, and better general health. The Joint Commission on Accreditation of Healthcare Organizations requires that both spiritual and cultural assessments be performed and integrated into care plans. Religion is "a more formal system that provides meaning to life through a common set of beliefs, rituals and practices. It provides the structure for spiritual beliefs for most people."

Spirituality has been defined "as the aspect of humanity that refers to the way individuals seek and express meaning and purpose and the way they experience their connectedness to the moment, to self, to others, to nature, and to the significant or sacred." Data show that spirituality and religion tend to play more pronounced roles in lives of older adults than in the general population. Patients use religion and spirituality to cope with illness-related suffering. More than 50% of older adults report frequent attendance at religious events (with little variation by gender or race), which has been a lifelong practice rather than a late-life development (SOE=A). A number of studies have demonstrated positive associations between religiousness, typically measured as regular attendance in organized religious activities, and a variety of health markers (eg, blood pressure) and mental health (eg, depression). There is evidence that regular attendance at religious services is associated with a lower composite measure of allostatic load among older women but not men (SOE=B). The literature suggests that religious participation may be beneficial, in part, because it promotes social interaction; however, one study suggests evidence that the effect is independent of social interaction. In addition, a number of studies have found that the beneficial effects of religious participation are not universal, and there is a suggestion that it may be most beneficial for those with the least social resources, eg, women and minorities (SOE=B).

One benefit of this growing body of literature is an increasing clarity of the distinction between the two elements. Although religion and spirituality are in no way mutually exclusive, neither do they necessarily overlap. In particular, the literature emphasizes the individualized quality of spirituality, portraying it in terms of practices through which a person seeks to establish or strengthen a link with a higher power or truth. In studies that have focused more on spirituality, findings generally indicate that such practices (eg, meditation or daily spiritual experiences) also are associated with better health and mental health (SOE=B). One study characterized the distinction between religion and spirituality as having positive associations for well-being related, in the case of religiousness, to positive social linkages and a sense of community service and, in the case of spirituality, to a sense of personal growth.

There are myriad religious and spiritual belief systems, and it is neither necessary nor feasible for clinician to be familiar with them all. However, it is very important for clinicians to recognize the important role that faith plays in the lives of many patients. It is also important that clinicians assess the patient's spiritual needs and be able to support them. Patients with complex spiritual needs should be referred to chaplains and faith leaders who may be better able to assist them.

ADVANCE CARE PLANNING

In cross-cultural situations, when discussing attitudes and beliefs regarding written directives with a patient, clinicians should be sensitive to the possibility that because of their cultappural background, some older adults will prefer to use alternatives (eg, verbal directives or directives dictated to family members or others), whereas others will avoid any such discussion so as to observe proscriptions against talking about death. In view of the fact that preferences for care intensity may also differ according to cultural and religious backgrounds, patients should also be given the opportunity to indicate the interventions they *do* want as well as those they do not want in any written or verbal directive used. For a letter directive written at a fifth-grade reading level and available in 8 languages, see http://med.stanford.edu/letter.html (accessed Feb 2019).

END-OF-LIFE ISSUES

Cultural, religious, and spiritual beliefs are an important influence in a person's formation of his or her attitudes toward supportable quality of life, approach to suffering, and beliefs about medical feeding, life-prolonging treatments, and palliative care. Some cultures and religious traditions value a direct struggle for life in the face of death, and both patients and families expect an intensive approach to treatment. Others avoid personal confrontation of death and dying and prefer to leave such decisions to the clinician. Still others take a direct approach to death and dying but reject too aggressive an approach.

Research has shown that clinicians and patients from shared cultural and religious backgrounds have similar values in these areas (SOE=B); the implications of such findings for clinicians and patients from differing backgrounds are obviously important. Both clinicians and patients bring their own attitudes and beliefs to any clinical encounter. Clinicians should be aware of their personal views, cultural values, and religious beliefs when discussing end-of-life plans with patients, and respect patients' beliefs and preferences even when different from their own.

In discussing end-of-life decisions with a patient, the clinician must listen especially carefully to the patient's goals and concerns and exert every effort to avoid making assumptions that do not apply. This may be particularly important when the clinician and the patient have different backgrounds, although clinicians should not assume that patients from the same background necessarily share the same belief system. For example, the assumption that "no one from that cultural background would want to live in that condition" or that "everyone in this faith tradition would want treatment in this situation" is likely to be faulty. To ensure that end-of-life plans and decisions reflect an individual's rights and wishes, the clinician must strive to understand an individual older adult's overall approach to life and death and, as far as possible, provide care that is consistent with that patient's personal approach.

RESOURCES

- American Geriatrics Society Ethnogeriatrics Committee. Achieving high-quality multicultural geriatric care. *J Am Geriatr Soc*. 2016;64(2):255–260.

- American Geriatrics Society. Brangman S, Periyakoil VS, eds. *Doorway Thoughts: Cross-Cultural Health Care for Older Adults;* 2014. www.GeriatricsCareOnline.org.

- Stanford Ethnogeriatrics Portal: http://geriatrics.stanford.edu (accessed Feb 2019).

- Woods DL, Mentes JC, Cadogan M, et al. Aging, genetic variations, and ethnopharmacology: building cultural competence through awareness of drug responses in ethnic minority elders. *J Transcult Nurs*. 2018;28:56–62.

CHAPTER 10—LESBIAN GAY BISEXUAL TRANSGENDER HEALTH

KEY POINTS

- Lesbian gay bisexual transgender (LGBT) older adults face many of the same health challenges as other older adults and may also have additional medical, psychological, and social needs.

- LGBT older adults are often underserved by the health care system. LGBT adults may have difficulty in disclosing sexual orientation because of prior negative experiences in the health care system and/or as a result of experiencing and fearing societal discrimination. Lack of disclosure can lead to poor access to care and sometimes inappropriate care. Health care providers may also be less likely to explore the sexual health of older adults and more likely to incorrectly assume heterosexuality.

- As transgender adults age, they may be more likely to encounter health issues that correspond to their biological sex; these patients may need help in coping with a disease or condition associated with their prior gender. Additionally, providers must be aware of hormone treatment options and adverse effects.

- LGBT older adults are more likely to live alone, be single, and not have children. They may rely more on extensive networks of friends rather than family. As they age, they may be at greater risk of isolation. As they become more reliant on others, their sense of vulnerability may enhance their fears of discrimination, especially in nursing home, assisted living and home health settings, forcing some to retreat back into the closet.

- Health care providers should provide appropriate support and resources that address and are sensitive to the needs of LGBT older adults.

LGBT older adults are at risk of experiencing disparities in physical and mental health. The cohort of LGBT older adults has specific needs and experiences different from both the general LGBT population and the general older adult population. For example, LGBT older adults report higher rates of disability, poor mental health, smoking, and excessive drinking than heterosexual older adults. Lesbian and bisexual women report higher rates of cardiovascular disease and obesity and are less likely to have screening mammography than heterosexual women. Gay and bisexual men report higher rates of poor physical health and living alone than heterosexual men. Transgender older adults are a subset of the LGBT population with distinct health concerns and disparities related to gender identity, including barriers to health services and fear of accessing health services, due to discrimination, victimization, internalized stigma, and financial barriers. They have higher rates of poverty, poor physical health, mental health needs, HIV, substance abuse, and lack of social support.

Some of these disparities are linked to the lasting effects of discrimination faced by the older LGBT generation throughout most of their lives. Although societal views about homosexuality have changed rapidly over recent years, it is important to recognize that LGBT older adults have experienced a lifetime of widespread discrimination, forcing them for much of their lives to hide their sexual orientation or transgender identity from their health care providers, their families, their employers, and sometimes even from themselves. Despite recent advances, LGBT older adults continue to be affected by past and ongoing social stigmata, governmental policies, and health care inequalities, which have important effects on their health, social supports, financial security, long-term housing options, and advance care planning. They also often lack access to clinicians trained in the health needs of and sensitivity to LGBT older adults.

BACKGROUND

Currently, an estimated 1 to 2 million LGBT older adults are living in the United States. By 2030, these numbers are expected to rise considerably along with the overall aging U.S. population. The exact number of LGBT people is unknown and probably underrepresented because of a lack of data, differing estimates by experts in related fields, and stigma that prevents LGBT people from identifying as such on surveys.

LGBT older adults came of age during a time in the United States when being a sexual or gender minority was viewed in an especially negative light. The experiences of LGBT older adults are influenced in part by whether they are part of the baby boomer generation (born 1946–1964) or were born before 1946. Those born before 1946 lived much of their lives in a society in which expression of their sexual orientation was criminalized by the government and considered pathological by the medical community. Being gay was considered not only a crime but also a mental illness until 1973, when the American Psychiatric Association stopped designating homosexuality as a disorder that could be treated and cured. As a result, LGBT persons could have been involuntarily hospitalized or treated against their will, leading to a decrease of this older generation's ability to trust the medical profession and seek psychiatric care. Given widespread discrimination, LGBT older adults are likely to have kept, and continue to keep, their sexual orientation and/or transgender identity hidden.

Society's views of homosexuality did not begin to change until the late 1960s and 1970s, and then only slowly. Baby boomers came of age during this social unrest of the 1960s and, as such, have benefited from the gay civil rights movement. To varying degrees, they have been more likely to disclose their sexual orientation than prior cohorts. Although many baby boomers have lived openly, many have still experienced acts of homophobia and transphobia. Among older adults who are open about their sexuality, some are faced with the decision to return to hiding their sexual orientation because of fear of discrimination, isolation, or mistreatment by staff or other residents when faced with the need for long-term care in an assisted-living facility or nursing home.

LGBT older adults are more likely to have experienced homophobia in health care situations and are therefore much less likely to disclose their sexual orienation with health care providers. Studies suggest that nondisclosure of sexual orientation can be associated with lower life satisfaction, lower self-esteem, depression and suicide, substance abuse, delay in seeking medical treatment, and increase in risk of illness (SOE=B). Medical mistrust is cited as a major reason why gay people, especially lesbians, do not always receive appropriate preventive care. Fear of culturally incompetent or discriminatory health care providers can also result in LGBT people avoiding care until they have reached a crisis level.

ASKING ABOUT SEXUAL ORIENTATION AND GENDER IDENTITY

To optimize care for LGBT older adults, it is important to create an environment that allows this population to feel respected and safe to disclose this information. It is important for providers to be sensitive when asking these questions. As older adults age, there is a tendency to think of them as asexual, and unless otherwise stated or obvious, assume that they are heterosexual. These assumptions can further isolate and marginalize LGBT older adults. LGBT older adults are also much less likely to self-identify as LGBT, so it is best not to use labels or force individuals to disclose such information. A helpful tip for inquiring into sexual orientation is to ask more general questions about living situation, current or past relationships, and sources of support, which can generate a conversation that often leads to this information.

MEDICAL ISSUES OF LGBT OLDER ADULTS

Although LGBT older adults can experience the same geriatric syndromes as their heterosexual counterparts, and as a result need much the same health promotion and maintenance, certain issues require particular attention.

Disease Risk in Older Gay and Bisexual Men

Cardiovascular Disease

Bisexual men are at increased risk of developing cardiovascular disease. This is likely due to higher rates of smoking, hypertension, diabetes, and hard drug use in this population in the study. Also, because gay men have an increased rate of recreational drug use and smoking, attention to traditional cardiovascular risk factors is important. The combination of smoking and HIV infection is particularly deadly; in a cohort of mostly men, all-cause mortality was 4 times higher in HIV-infected smokers than in those who had never smoked. More than 12 life-years were lost from smoking compared with 5.1 life-years lost from HIV infection alone (SOE=A).

Anal Cancer

Anal human papillomavirus infection disproportionately affects men who have sex with men (MSM) compared with the general population of men. The prevalence of anal human papillomavirus infection in HIV-positive MSM is extremely high, ranging between 72% and 90%; in HIV-negative MSM, the prevalence is 57%–61%. Risk factors for anal cancer include receptive anal intercourse and degree of immunosuppression, such as nadir CD4 count and higher HIV viral load. Although there are no recognized guidelines for routine anal cancer screening, some organizations have proposed annual anal cytology for HIV-infected MSM, and screening every 2 years for HIV-uninfected MSM (SOE=C).

Prostate Cancer

There are no data on the incidence of prostate cancer in gay and bisexual men. Prostate cancer can also affect the sexual health of gay and bisexual men in ways that are different from those in heterosexual men (SOE=C). The prostate gland is involved in the sexual response to receptive anal intercourse, and treatment options (eg, surgical vs radiation) may lead to differences in ability to maintain insertive and receptive anal intercourse. Gay and bisexual men with prostate cancer report poor communication with their health care providers about these implications, citing the incorrect assumption of heterosexuality and the lack of interest and knowledge by providers as barriers to care.

Disease Risk in Older Lesbian and Bisexual Women

Cardiovascular Disease

Higher rates of cardiovascular disease risk factors have been observed in older lesbian and bisexual women. Rates of smoking appear to be higher in the general lesbian population, and older lesbian women are twice as likely to report being heavy smokers than heterosexual women (SOE=A). Lesbian and bisexual women, on average, have a higher BMI than heterosexual women, and the risk of cardiovascular disease is more than 3 times higher in women with a BMI >29 kg/m^2 (SOE=B).

Cervical Cancer

Cervical and breast cancer screening rates have historically been lower among lesbian than heterosexual women. Fear of discrimination and not disclosing sexual orientation are associated with decreased likelihood for Pap screening. Lesbian and bisexual women remain at risk of cervical cancer, partly because many have had intercourse with a man at some point in their lives, and therefore need to be screened according to guidelines for all women.

Breast Cancer

Although some studies report that lesbian women may have greater risk factors for breast cancer, no prospective study has definitively shown an increased risk. However, older lesbian women may receive fewer mammograms than heterosexual women, and studies suggest higher rates of obesity and alcohol use among lesbian women.

Medical Needs of Older Transgender Men and Women

Cardiovascular Disease

Transgender adults have higher rates of smoking than cisgender adults, which therefore increases the risk of cardiovascular disease and other smoking-related illness. In addition, the pharmacologic use of sex hormones is thought to increase the risk of cardiovascular disease. Some studies suggest a possible increase in cardiovascular risk over time for transgender women taking feminizing hormones, although transgender men taking testosterone do not appear to have an increased risk of cardiovascular disease (SOE=C).

Cancer Screening in Transgender Older Adults

As transgender adults age, they may encounter health issues that correspond to their biological sex. For instance, a person who was born male and transitioned to a woman may develop prostate cancer if the prostate was not removed. Similarly, a person who was born female and transitioned to a man may develop uterine cancer if the female sexual organs were not removed. These patients may feel significant distress in coping with a disease or condition associated with their prior gender and the associated examinations that may be required, such as prostate examinations in transgender women (male to female) and pelvic examinations in transgender men (female to male). Hormone-related cancer in transgender persons is very rare (there are, however, case reports of breast cancer in male-to-female transgender patients).

Sexual Health of LGBT Older Adults

It is important for health care providers to address sexual function and sexual health in all LGBT older adults, most of whom can benefit from routine sexual history taking and risk-reduction counseling.

Prevention of HIV and Sexually Transmitted Infection in LGBT Older Adults

More than half of older adults 65–75 years old report being sexually active, and one quarter of those 75–85 years old are sexually active. Sexually active older adults are much less likely to use condoms than younger adults and less likely to have been tested for HIV, even in the presence of HIV risk factors. Older adults also report receiving little information about sexual health, HIV infection, and other sexually transmitted infections (STIs) from their health care providers. There are reports of increasing rates of syphilis and chlamydia in older adults and in counties with a high number of retirees.

For all these reasons, health care providers need to take routine and thorough sexual and substance use histories from their older patients, regardless of sexual orientation or gender identity. Prevention of HIV and STI transmission also requires that clinicians provide counseling on safer sex practices and offer, when appropriate, information on HIV prophylaxis (both before and after exposure).

Sexual Risk in Older Gay and Bisexual Men

Gay, bisexual, and other MSM remain the group at greatest risk of acquiring HIV infection, with MSM >50 years old accounting for over half of all new HIV infections. Older adults who are racial/ethnic minorities appear to be at greater risk of death from HIV/AIDS (SOE=A).

According to CDC guidelines, sexually active MSM who engage in high-risk sexual behavior should be routinely assessed for risk of gonorrhea, chlamydia, syphilis, herpes simplex virus, and human papillomavirus. Although the CDC's universal screening recommendations only go up to 64 years of age, providers should also screen MSM who are >65 years old based on individual risk behaviors.

Sexual Risk in Older Lesbian and Bisexual Women

Many lesbian and bisexual women have been sexually active with both women and men. Therefore, taking a complete sexual history and providing sensitive risk-reduction counseling is recommended. In addition, lesbian women have a higher incidence of bacterial vaginosis and can transmit candidiasis and *Trichomonas vaginalis* to their female partners. The use of barriers ("dental dams") is recommended for oral-vaginal and oral-anal contact.

Women who are exclusively sexually active with other women have a low risk of acquiring HIV infection. Older women who have sex with men may be at increased risk of HIV because of age-related vaginal thinning and dryness. In addition, older women starting a new sexual relationship after many years of being in a monogamous relationship may find it difficult to initiate discussions about risks and the use of barriers.

Sexual Risk in Transgender People

HIV risk is high among transgender women, and frequent screening is important. Transgender women who engage in sex work and injection drug use are at extremely high risk of STIs and HIV infection. The black American transgender community has one of the highest prevalence rates of HIV infection in the United States, highlighting the increased risk based on both racial minority status and being transgender (SOE=B).

HIV/AIDS Treatment and Care

Among older adults, HIV/AIDS tends to be diagnosed much later in the course of infection, primarily because the diagnosis is not considered and because older adults are less likely to get tested. HIV/AIDS-related symptoms and associated diseases can be easily mistaken for other problems typically seen in older adults. In addition, because aging naturally weakens the immune system and comorbid conditions are more likely to exist, AIDS may progress more rapidly in older adults.

At the same time, patients >50 years old who take antiretroviral medications seem to respond virologically as well as younger patients do, but they do not have as robust a return of their immune system. Treating older patients with HIV/AIDS is complex because many of these patients have other underlying illnesses, take several medications, and may additionally be dealing with some of the issues of aging (such as sensory loss, frailty, and dementia). The latest set of HIV treatment guidelines advises early treatment, regardless of baseline CD4 count, and that treatment protects against spread of this disease.

MENTAL HEALTH, SOCIAL, AND ECONOMIC ISSUES AFFECTING LGBT OLDER ADULTS

Mental Health

The link between mental health disorders and discrimination in LGBT populations is well documented. Discrimination is present in health care, as well as in employment, housing, civil rights, federal laws, and organizational policies, all of which must be accounted for in addressing the psychosocial needs of LGBT older adults. For an LGBT older adult, who may have lived most of his or her life in a hostile or intolerant environment, disclosing sexual orientation can induce significant stress and contribute to lower life satisfaction and self-esteem. For older adults, managing social stressors such as prejudice, stigmatization, violence, and internalized homophobia over long periods can result in higher risks of depression, suicide, risky behavior, and substance abuse. LGBT adults are one and a half to two times as likely as heterosexuals to report lifetime prevalence of mood and anxiety disorders, but little is known about the prevalence of mental health disorders in LGBT older adults (SOE=B). In studies that have been done, rates of current or lifetime mood and anxiety disorders have been increased among LGBT older adults, with rates highest among transgender people. Among MSM, depression and emotional distress were associated with being single, experiencing antigay harassment or violence, feeling alienated from the gay community, or not identifying as gay. Depression is linked to disability and poor general health, with internalized stigma and lifetime victimization predicting poor outcomes, whereas social supports and social network size have protective effects.

Suicide rates are alarmingly high in LGBT young persons, and suicidality may persist throughout adulthood into old age. Better mental health was predicted in part by a higher percentage of people who knew about the participants' sexual orientation, including their health care provider.

Transgender persons may experience mental health problems, such as adjustment disorders, anxiety disorders, post-traumatic stress disorder, depression, and substance abuse, which are similar to those experienced by other persons who endure major life changes and discrimination.

Substance Use

Although LGBT youth have higher rates of alcohol and tobacco use than their heterosexual peers, some of those behaviors differ on the basis of sexual orientation and may not persist in older age. For instance, older lesbian women and bisexual men are more likely to be current smokers than heterosexuals of the same gender after age 50, whereas there is no difference in smoking for older gay men and bisexual women than for heterosexuals. Alcohol use in LGB older adults is similar to that in heterosexuals, with the caveat that binge drinking behavior is more common in older lesbian women and less likely in gay men than in heterosexuals. In contrast, a different survey found that all LGB older adults, regardless of gender, were more likely to smoke and drink excessively than older heterosexuals. Transgender adults also have higher rates of alcohol, smoking, and substance abuse.

Concerns About Aging

LGBT adults may approach the aging process differently from their peers, and this approach may also differ by gender. Younger and older gay men feel that gay society views aging as a negative process. Lesbian women, however, feel that lesbian society views aging in a positive manner. These differences may be because of the influence of youth and physical attraction in gay male subculture, thus subjecting older gay men to ageism from within their own community.

Lesbian and gay older adults generally have the same concerns about aging (eg, loneliness, health, and income) as their heterosexual counterparts, with the additional fears of rejection by their children and grandchildren, uncertain support, and concerns of discrimination in health care, employment, housing, and long-term care. LGBT communities and extended family networks are often a source of support and resilience, and there is fear that access to this support will be less available with aging.

Palliative Care Needs

Minority stress, internalized homophobia, stigma, and misconceptions can all affect the mental health needs of LGBT older adults at the end of life. These issues may be magnified if the LGBT older adult is struggling with issues of disclosure of sexual orientation, fear of discrimination, and estrangement from family when approaching death. Disenfranchised grief, another important concern, refers to the ignored and unrecognized needs of a surviving same-sex spouse if that relationship is not recognized and validated by family, health care providers, or the legal system.

Social Supports and Family Structure

LGBT older adults often find themselves without traditional spousal, familial, and social supports to help with age-related needs. Compared with heterosexual older adults, gay or bisexual men are twice as likely to be living alone, and lesbian or bisexual women are one-third more likely to be living alone. Moreover, LGBT older adults are half as likely to have a significant other, half as likely to have close relatives to call for help, and 3 to 4 times more likely to not have children (SOE=B). LGBT older adults may also have strained relationships with their extended family or children as a result of either the lack of acceptance of their sexuality or the attempt to continue to conceal their sexual orientation.

These diminished social connections lead to higher rates of isolation and loneliness among LGBT older adults than among their non-LGBT peers, and LGBT older adults are likely to have unmet needs for basic support.

LGBT adults are sometimes able to rely on "nontraditional" family structures. For example, some form "families of choice," a term used to describe diverse family structures that include close friends, partners, or significant others who are a source of social and caregiving support although not biologically or legally related. However, families of choice pose some difficulties, because they are not recognized by law.

Housing, Home Care, and Long-Term Care

Surveys show that LGBT older adults fear rejection and discrimination by both staff and other older adults in long-term care facilities. LGBT older adults report an increased frequency of mistreatment incidents, including verbal or physical harassment from other residents and/or staff, refused admission or attempted discharge from facilities, denial of medical treatment, restriction of visitors, staff refusal to accept medical power of attorney, and/or staff refusal to refer to transgender residents by preferred name or pronoun.

Some surveys of LGBT older adults indicate that they prefer to age alongside other LGBT older adults if unable to age in place at home, citing safety as the main reason. However, not all LGBT older adults wish to live in an LGBT-targeted facility, and some residential settings for older adults have sought training in providing LGBT culturally competent care so that LGBT older adults' real and perceived fears of mistreatment may be alleviated.

Challenges with Financial Security

LGBT older adults are more likely to live in poverty than their heterosexual counterparts. The rate of poverty is 4.6% among older heterosexual couples, compared with 4.9% for older gay male couples and 9.1% for older lesbian couples (SOE=C). Surveys of men and women who identify as bisexual have found significantly greater rates of people living at or below 200% of the federal poverty level. Similarly, a study of transgender older adults found that nearly half (47.5%) of those identified as transgender had household incomes at or below 200% of the federal poverty level compared with 29.4% of non-transgender (LGB) individuals in the study.

LGBT older adults were more likely to have lived their productive years during a time when discrimination was more common, potentially equating to lower earnings and reduced savings compared with their heterosexual peers. Older lesbian couples are likely poorer than older gay couples, in part because of gender wage disparities in the general population.

Historical unequal access to benefits programs can also affect the financial security of LGBT older adults. Some of this has changed recently with landmark Supreme Court rulings, most notably the 2015 decision in Obergefell v. Hodges granting equal marriage rights to all LGBT adults throughout the nation. In 2013, the Supreme Court repealed a key portion of the Defense of Marriage Act (DOMA), allowing for federal recognition of same-sex marriage where recognized at the state level, thus allowing same-sex married couples to receive protections such as Social Security survivor and spousal benefits, Department of Veterans Affairs spousal benefits, and preferred tax treatment of health insurance and retirement savings. Because the states and the federal government jointly administer Medicaid, states without marriage equality could impose unequal treatment to LGBT couples, affecting the ability of LGBT partners to pass along property, negatively affecting their ability to become eligible for Medicaid. It is also important to note that many LGBT older couples may have never had the opportunity to legally marry, perhaps because of advanced illness or the death of a spouse before marriage became legal, therefore denying the surviving spouse access to protections and benefits such as social security, pensions, and other spousal benefits.

RESOURCES

- Emlet CA. Social, economic, and health disparities among LGBT older adults. *Generations*. 2016;40(2):16–22.

- Fredriksen-Goldsen KI, Cook-Daniels L, Kim HJ, et al. Physical and mental health of transgender older adults: an at-risk and underserved population. *Gerontologist*. 2014;54(3):488–500.

- Kwong J, Bockting W, Gabler S, et al. Development of an interprofessional collaborative practice model for older LGBT adults. *LGBT Health*. 2017;4(6):442–444.

CHAPTER 11—PHYSICAL ACTIVITY

KEY POINTS

- Regular physical activity provides numerous and substantial health benefits for older adults.

- The health benefits of physical activity accrue independently of other risk factors. Greater amounts of physical activity, within limits, have greater health benefits.

- To obtain substantial health benefits of physical activity, older adults should do at least 30 minutes of moderate-intensity aerobic activity on ≥5 days each week. If they cannot do this intensity or amount of activity, they should do the amount that is possible according to their abilities, in order to avoid inactivity.

- Older adults should also engage in progressive muscle-strengthening activity on at least 2 nonconsecutive days each week and include balance training regularly.

- When possible, obese people and those with osteoarthritis or balance problems should perform aerobic and resistance exercise using water.

- Promoting physical activity is one of the most important and effective preventive and therapeutic interventions in older adults. The clinician's recommendation for exercise (and other lifestyle habits) for their patients carries more weight than any other source of advice. Counseling by a health care provider is an important way of promoting physical activity in clinical settings. Referral of patients to community resources, particularly evidence-based programs, is also important.

Physical activity in the context of public health refers to all muscular activity either at work or during leisure time, ranging from light to high vigorous. Its benefits arise from the adaptation of multiple body systems to the muscular demand for oxygen; generally, these benefits may be considered proportional to the absolute intensity of the exercise or the mass of muscle activated by the exercise coupled with the duration of the exercise. The term *relative exercise intensity* refers to the percentage of the individual's maximal capacity that is utilized. Thus, a weaker person will activate fewer muscle fibers than a stronger person at the same relative intensity.

Another important concept is the exercise volume, which in population studies is defined as the product of exercise intensity in METS and duration in hours. Thus, a person who walks briskly (4–5 METS) for 30 minutes 4 times a week achieves an exercise volume of 8–10 MET-hours, which is considered medium volume. See Table 11.1. Gait speed is also an important temporal variable of walking activity that has been found to be associated with life expectancy.

BENEFITS OF PHYSICAL ACTIVITY

Preventive Health Benefits

Regular physical activity in adults of all ages improves cardiorespiratory and muscular fitness (SOE=A). It reduces the risk of many diseases, including coronary heart disease, stroke, hypertension, some lipid disorders, type 2 diabetes, colon cancer, breast cancer, osteoporosis, and depression (SOE=A). It also reduces the risk of unhealthy weight gain and assists in weight loss (SOE=A). In older adults, physical activity reduces the risk of falls (SOE=A) and sarcopenia, and regularly active older adults have a lower risk of hip fracture (SOE=B). The evidence that physical activity reduces the risk of cognitive impairment is substantial and growing (SOE=B). There is some evidence that physical activity can reduce the risk of lung cancer, endometrial cancer, osteoarthritis, sleep problems, and anxiety disorders (SOE=B).

Consistent with its broad physiologic effects, regular physical activity is associated with decreases in both cardiovascular and noncardiovascular mortality in older adults. This benefit is large.

The health benefits of physical activity accrue regardless of the presence of risk factors. For example, sedentary smokers experience health benefits of increasing physical activity even if they continue to smoke. The health benefits of physical activity are also generally independent of body weight: overweight and obese adults obtain benefits from physical activity even if it does not promote weight loss.

Robust, consistent observational evidence indicates that regularly active older adults are at reduced risk of moderate or severe functional limitations and limitations in work or family responsibilities (SOE=B).

Economic Benefits

Regularly active adults are consistently reported to have lower medical expenditures than sedentary adults (SOE=B).

RECOMMENDED AMOUNTS OF PHYSICAL ACTIVITY

Aerobic Activity

An older adult can achieve recommended levels of aerobic activity by doing either moderate-intensity aerobic physical activity for at least 150 minutes each week, or vigorous-intensity activity for at least 75 minutes each week. This corresponds to a walking pace of 20–24 minutes per mile. However, overweight and older adults should judge their effort at 5 or 6 out of 10 (on a 10-point scale) while being able to talk but not sing or feel breathless. Doing a combination of moderate- and vigorous-intensity activity is also acceptable. Aerobic activity should be spread throughout the week, preferably on ≥3 days per week. Doing at least 30 minutes of aerobic activity on ≥5 days each week remains an appropriate way for older adults to obtain the health benefits of activity. Studies using objective measures of physical activity have shown that most adults do not adhere to these recommendations, suggesting that an approach based on reducing inactivity may be more beneficial than one that requires moderate or higher level physical activity on most days of the week.

Several comments help clarify these recommendations. First, episodes of moderate-intensity activity of ≥10 minutes count toward meeting the recommendation. Second, the recommendation does not refer to just leisure activity or exercise. Occupational activity (eg, carpentry), domestic activity (eg, mowing the grass), and transportation activity (eg, walking to the store) all count toward meeting recommendations. Third, participation in physical activity above the minimum recommended levels results in greater health benefits. Some physical activity is clearly preferable to none for those who are unable to meet these targets. Older adults should be strongly encouraged to avoid an inactive lifestyle, even if they do not (or cannot) attain recommended amounts of activity. Finally, the recommended activity is in addition to routine (baseline) activity of light-intensity or of short duration (<10 minutes).

Muscle-Strengthening Activity

ACSM/AHA recommendations and the *2008 Physical Activity Guidelines for Americans* state that older adults should perform muscle-strengthening activities of the major muscle groups (arms, shoulder, legs, hip, back, chest, and abdomen) on ≥2 days each week that provide sufficient mechanical overload to promote muscle growth and adaptation. Importantly, muscle strengthening programs should consider frequency, duration, sets, exercise type, intensity, repetitions, and progression.

Specific exercises may vary depending on available equipment; however, exercises should span most major muscle groups (chest, back, arms, shoulders, and upper and lower legs). Intensity refers to the relative amount of weight being lifted and is an important factor in providing adequate stimulus for muscle growth and adaptation. Many studies have reported that high

Table 11.1—Exercise Intensity and Exercise Volume

Exercise intensity, in METS	
Light	= 2.5; walking (approx ~2.2 mph)
Moderate	= 4–5; brisk walking (3.4–3.9 mph)
Moderate–vigorous	= 6.5; jogging (4 mph)
High vigorous	= 8.5; running (5.4 mph)
Duration of physical activity (also known as exercise volume, ie, intensity × duration), in MET-hours per week	
Inactive	<3.75
Low volume	3.75–7.5
Medium volume	7.6–16.5
High volume	16.6–25.5
Very high volume	>25.5

1 MET = 3.5 mL O_2/kg/min = 210 mL O_2/kg/hr = 1 kcal/kg/hr (1 L O_2 = 5 kcal)

intensity strength training (eg, 80%+ of the repetition maximum) is tolerated in older adults (SOE=B); hence, it is recommended that to achieve maximum benefit, intensity should be progressed to high intensity as ability permits. Repetitions are the number of times an exercise is completed and are inversely related to the exercise intensity. When prescribing an appropriate training load, it is generally accepted that performing an exercise to task failure in 10 to 15 repetitions is consistent with an intensity of 70%–85% of maximum strength.

These activities can be done at home or in the community, but it is suggested that older adults who are starting a new strengthening program receive proper instruction and supervision by an appropriately trained exercise professional, such as a physical therapist or exercise physiologist, with knowledge of the older adult's medical limitations. To support exercise progression, increases should be gradual and can include changes in frequency, duration, volume, and intensity.

Flexibility Activity

Flexibility activity is recommended for older adults as a means of maintaining the range of motion needed for regular physical activity and daily life. Stiffness of ligaments, tendons, and other connective tissue occurs after soft-tissue injury and through the gradual glycosylation of collagen fibers with age. This process can be ameliorated with thrice weekly static stretching to the point of tightness and holding the position for a few seconds. Evidence for the long-term effects of stretching in older adults is lacking. Because some studies suggest that static stretching before activity may be detrimental to strength and athletic performance, older athletes should consider dynamic stretching before activity, a type of active movement that causes muscle to stretch but that is not held in the end position.

Yoga is a salutary activity for older adults because it combines strengthening and stretching. Classes for all abilities are widely available. To avoid injury, older adults are advised not to attempt attaining positions that are too difficult.

Balance Training

Balance can be thought of as any other motor skill, which requires practice, muscle coordination, and adequate strength. Balance training is recommended for all older adults and especially for those at risk of falls, including older adults with mobility problems.

Several falls-prevention interventions that included balance training on ≥3 days per week have been studied and found to be effective. It is preferable that older adults use standardized balance exercises from a program demonstrated to reduce falls.

There is moderate evidence that Tai Chi exercise is effective in fall prevention, although the optimal amount and forms of Tai Chi needed to reduce fall risk are unclear (SOE=B).

Management of Body Weight

Most weight-loss studies conclude that exercise enhances the effectiveness of dietary restriction in achieving a healthy body weight beyond what might be expected from calculations of caloric balance. Five miles of daily walking, which for most older adults would take 2 hours, is required to lose 1 lb of fat per week. This fact emphasizes the need for other forms of energy expenditure throughout the day, and especially to minimize the time spent sitting.

Overweight and obese older adults should first achieve minimal recommended levels of physical activity (150 minutes of moderate-intensity aerobic activity per week). If a healthy weight is not achieved with this level of activity, then caloric intake should be reduced, physical activity increased gradually, and body weight monitored. When older adults lose weight, they lose not only fat mass but also muscle mass and bone mass. Because physical activity, particularly muscle-strengthening activity, acts to preserve bone and muscle mass, older adults should not attempt to lose weight by diet alone.

Screening Before Participation

The current ACSM exercise pre-participation health screening process seeks to remove unnecessary barriers to beginning and maintaining a structured exercise program, a lifestyle of habitual physical activity, or both. Evidence suggests the risk of acute exercise-related cardiovascular events is highest among sedentary individuals with known or occult cardiovascular disease who participate in unaccustomed vigorous intensity physical activity. Because of this, the pre-participation health screening is based on 1) the individual's current level of physical activity; 2) presence of signs or symptoms and/or known cardiovascular, metabolic, or renal disease; and 3) desired exercise intensity. The goal of this screening process is to identify individuals 1) who should have an examination to assess risks of physical activity before initiating or increasing the frequency, intensity, and/or the volume of their current program; 2) who may have clinically significant disease but who might benefit from participating in a medically supervised exercise program; and 3) who have medical conditions that may require exclusion from exercise programs until those conditions are eliminated or better controlled. Further reduction of exercise-related cardiovascular events may be more likely to occur with a safe and effective exercise prescription that assures a gradual progression of exercise duration and intensity over 2–3 months, includes appropriate warm-up and cool down procedures, promotes education of warning signs and symptoms (eg, chest pain or pressure, lightheadedness, unusual shortness of breath, heart palpitations), encourages sedentary individuals to engage in regular brisk walking, and counsels physically inactive individuals to avoid unaccustomed vigorous physical activity. Exercise specialists and physical therapists are trained to provide this type of exercise prescription for older adults. It is also appropriate for providers of exercise programs to ask new participants (who are not referred after an examination by a health care provider) to complete a symptom checklist. People with undiagnosed symptoms should seek medical care before starting an exercise program.

The clinician should assess whether and how the patient should limit his or her activity because of chronic conditions. Most, if not all, studies of exercise in people with disabilities have assessed potential participants to ensure the exercise intervention is appropriate. These study populations have included adults with osteoarthritis, lower limb loss, cerebral palsy, multiple sclerosis, muscular dystrophy, Parkinson disease, spinal cord injury, stroke, traumatic brain injury, dementia, intellectual disability, and mental illness.

The U.S. Preventive Services Task Force (USPSTF) does not recommend any type of routine pre-exercise screening of healthy asymptomatic adults. Specifically, for adults at increased risk of coronary heart disease, the USPSTF finds insufficient evidence for and routine screening with resting ECG, exercise treadmill test, or electron-beam CT scanning for coronary calcium for adults at low risk of heart disease.

Promotion of Physical Activity

The public health approach to promotion of physical activity is based on a socioecologic model that recognizes the interrelationship that exists between the individual and his or her environment. To illustrate the logic of the model, consider that counseling an older adult to walk regularly (individual level intervention) is more effective if the person lives in a neighborhood with good access to parks and other safe places to walk (a community level intervention). A referral to an exercise program (an individual level intervention) is more likely to succeed if the costs of the exercise program are subsidized by a health plan (organizational level intervention).

Clinical Settings

A system is needed in each clinical setting for routinely assessing levels of physical activity in patients, for providing patients with a recommendation about physical activity, for helping patients achieve recommended levels, and for evaluating the effectiveness of the system in promoting physical activity.

Integrating Exercise into Daily Life

Engagement in structured physical activity programs is not always feasible or desirable for all older adults. A preference for lifestyle activities such as gardening or house cleaning has been reported in this population, and integrating exercises into daily living may be a promising alternative to structured exercise programs to promote engagement in daily exercise. This approach can include replacing driving time with walking or incorporating balance and strengthening into daily functional activities. Examples include standing from a chair to promote lower extremity strength and stepping over and around objects in the daily environment to promote balance.

Assessing Physical Activity and Sedentarism

Routine assessment of physical activity should include assessing the amounts of both aerobic activity and muscle-strengthening activity.

Emerging evidence indicates that how we spend our time during daily living may be important. In a meta-analysis of 47 studies of outcomes for cardiovascular disease and diabetes, cancer, and all-cause mortality, prolonged sedentary time was associated with deleterious health outcomes independent of physical activity. Older adults should strive to reduce total sedentary time, break up prolonged periods of sedentary time, and move more. Though the specific manner in which sedentary time should be interrupted is not yet known, trading off 2 minutes every hour of sedentary time for 2 minutes of light activity has been suggested as a starting point. Caregivers should be aware that doing too much for those in their care may promote sedentarism and therefore might not be in the best interests of the older adult.

Providing an Activity Prescription

For older adults, especially those with chronic conditions, the ACSM/AHA recommends development of individualized activity plans in consultation with primary care providers. Activity plans should integrate public health preventive recommendations (summarized above) with any therapeutic use of physical activity recommended, eg, by clinical practice guidelines. Older adults should understand whether, and how, chronic conditions limit the amounts and types of activity they can do.

The activity prescription is considered part of a broader approach of developing the physical activity plan. The plan considers individual preferences, individual abilities and fitness, chronic conditions and activity limitations, risk of falls, strategies for decreasing risk of injury, and behavioral strategies to increase adherence to the plan. Essentially, the plan provides specific guidance on how to meet physical activity guidelines. A resource for developing the plan is ACSM's *Exercise Management for Chronic Diseases and Disabilities*. This book covers issues in exercise management for some 40 different conditions. Some guidelines for developing a plan include the following:

- The plan will commonly emphasize walking, which is a popular and safe activity in older adults. However, for many people with knee osteoarthritis, swimming, pool exercise, and non-weight-bearing activities such as cycling and rowing, which can be done on machines, may be preferred. Individuals with osteopenia and osteoporosis should engage in weight-bearing exercises if possible.

- The plan should emphasize the importance of gradually increasing physical activity over time. It can be appropriate for older adults to spend weeks or months at activity levels below recommended levels before advancing.

- The less active an adult is currently and the less experience he or she has with physical activity, the more appropriate it is to recommend starting in a supervised, evidence-based program.

- Providing social support for physical activity is important. Social support can be provided by classes, formal mall walking groups, telephone counseling, and informal arrangements in which people simply meet to go for a walk.

Providing Assistance in Increasing Physical Activity

Behavioral approaches often include motivational interviewing, self-efficacy promotion, and education, combined with group or individual physical activity.

Particularly for adults with some functional limitations, an appropriate way to provide assistance is to make a referral to an evidence-based program. Resources, such as the National Council on Aging (www.ncoa.org),

Management of Risks of Physical Activity

Appropriate pre-participation screening and gradual progression of strength training exercises are the most important recommendations for avoiding activity-related injuries (SOE=B). Observational evidence is strong that the risk of injury is directly related to the size of the gap between a person's usual level of activity and his or her new level of activity. A series of small increments in activity, each followed by a period of adaptation, is associated with lower rates of musculoskeletal injury. The safest method for increasing activity has not been established by intervention studies.

When recommending home exercise using equipment such as treadmills, consideration should be given to whether the patient is at increased risk of falls because there has been steady increase since 2002 in injuries treated in emergency departments related to exercise equipment.

Older Adults with Low Fitness or Low Functional Ability

Older adults with functional impairments can achieve benefits from exercise (SOE=A). Similarly, a study of resistance exercise in frail nursing-home residents demonstrated improvements in strength and function (SOE=A).

Matching the abilities of older adults who have a low level of fitness or physical function with types and amounts of activity can be challenging. Sometimes referrals can be made to specific rehabilitation programs, such as pulmonary rehabilitation, for assessment, exercise prescription, and medically supervised exercise. Assessment by a physical therapist is generally appropriate, because the therapist can design and tailor an exercise program to the specific limitations of the patient. This assessment can also confirm that a patient is capable of participating in a specific community exercise program (eg, a water exercise program designed for adults with arthritis). Given that the care of such patients often involves a geriatric team and consultants, steps should be taken to ensure the activity recommendation is communicated to all the health care providers.

RESOURCES

- King A, Powell KE. *2018 Physical Activity Guidelines Advisory Committee Scientific Report*. www.health.gov/paguidelines/second-edition/report/pdf/pag_advisory_committee_report.pdf

- Miller JM, Sabol VK, Pastva AM. Promoting older adult physical activity throughout care transitions using an interprofessional approach. *J Nurs Pract*. 2017;13(1):64–71.

- Riebe D, Franklin BA, Thompson PD et al. Updating ACSM's recommendations for preparticipation health screening. *MSSE*. 2015;47(11):2473–2479.

- Weber M, Belala N, Clemson L, et al. Feasibility and effectiveness of intervention programmes integrating functional exercise into daily life of older adults: a systematic review. *Gerontology*. 2018;64(2):172–187.

CHAPTER 12—SCREENING AND PREVENTION

KEY POINTS

- Considering a patient's remaining life expectancy, comorbidities, and cognitive and functional status is important when deciding which preventive health measures to offer. If the lag time to benefit from a preventive health intervention (ie, the amount of time between undergoing an intervention until benefits [eg, mortality reduction] are seen in randomized controlled trials) is greater than the individual's expected life span, then the preventive health measure is not indicated.

- Many preventive health measures are underused among older adults, including immunizations (eg, flu shots, pneumococcal vaccinations), exercise counseling, depression screening, and counseling on geriatric health issues (eg, safety, falls prevention, incontinence), whereas cancer screening tests are overused among older adults with short remaining life expectancy.

- Tools are available to help clinicians estimate life expectancy to appropriately target cancer screening to those with adequate remaining life expectancy.

- Medicare is increasingly covering preventive services and wellness visits.

Many preventive health measures are available to older adults, including screening tests (eg, colonoscopy), counseling about a healthy lifestyle (eg, exercise) and/or geriatric health issues (eg, incontinence), immunizations (eg, flu shot), and prevention medications (eg, aspirin). Ideally, older adults should receive preventive health measures from which they are most likely to benefit based on their health and remaining life expectancy. A person-centered practice approach should also incorporate patient preferences.

Remaining life expectancy decreases uniformly with age, but it can vary from one individual to the next according to illness burden and functional status. Predicted remaining life expectancy, cognition, and function are important determinants to consider when offering preventive services to older adults, as is the lag time to benefit from the medical intervention. Lag time to benefit is defined as the time between the preventive intervention (when complications and harms are most likely) to the time when improved health outcomes are seen. If a patient is unlikely to live longer than the lag time to benefit from a medical intervention, then performing that intervention may only cause that patient harm. In vulnerable older adults, screening and prevention should focus on evidence-based interventions that minimize functional limitations and increase the number of healthy years lived.

This chapter reviews the preventive health measures available to older adults and discusses which measures are appropriate based on remaining life expectancy. Table 12.1 provides an overview of measures available and their recommended use in different populations of older adults, including those with ≥10 years of remaining life expectancy, those with 5–10 years of remaining life expectancy, those with moderate dementia, and those near the end of life. The recommendations given in Table 12.1 are based on reports from geriatric expert panels, as well as on guidelines from the American Geriatrics Society (AGS) and the United States Preventive Services Task Force (USPSTF), and include information on whether each service is cost-effective.

Several criteria should generally be met before recommending disease screening: 1) The condition being screened for must be serious and prevalent in the population being tested. 2) The disease should have a significant asymptomatic phase that can be detected by the screening test. 3) The screening test must be safe, sensitive, and specific to limit false-positive and false-negative tests. 4) Effective treatment must be available for use early in the natural course of the disease that results in lower morbidity and mortality than treatment given after symptoms develop. 5) The costs of screening should be acceptable. 6) Ideally, the screening test should have been found effective in a randomized controlled trial (RCT). Few older adults have been included in RCTs that evaluate screening measures, especially frail older adults; therefore, recommendations are often based on indirect evidence.

CANCER SCREENING TESTS

The ultimate goal of screening is to identify cancers that will lead to morbidity and mortality within an adult's lifetime if not found early and treated. Harms of screening include anxiety, complications from unneeded diagnostic evaluation, false reassurance from false-negative test results, and overdiagnosis (detection of tumors that will not affect life span because of competing mortality or nonprogressive disease) leading to overtreatment. Overtreatment is concerning because burdens of cancer treatment increase with age.

Cancer screening research is subject to 3 main types of bias: lead time, length, and selection biases. These biases can make a test appear to be effective when it actually is not. Lead-time bias occurs when screening results in earlier identification without altering the time to death. Thus, the person spends more time as a patient, but the course of the disease is basically unaltered.

Length bias occurs when screening increases the number of identified clinically slowly progressive or nonprogressive diseases that would never have affected an individual's longevity. The extreme case of length bias is overdiagnosis or the detection of "disease" that is of no consequence.

Selection bias is based on the observation that people willing to be screened for cancer may not reflect the population as a whole. Volunteers may be more health conscious or have other personal habits that favorably influence prognosis. Thus, their outcome from screening may be better than what would be seen in a random population.

Breast Cancer

Breast cancer is the most common life-threatening cancer in women and is the second leading cause of cancer death in U.S. women. The incidence of breast cancer increases with age, peaking between ages 75–79 years, with 451 cases per 100,000 women. While 31% of breast cancer diagnoses are in women ≥70 years old, 47% of deaths from breast cancer occur in women ≥70 years old. Mammography screening reduces breast cancer mortality by 19% in women 40–74 years old; however, whether it helps women >74 years old live longer is not known, because none of the randomized trials of mammography screening included women >74 years old. Therefore, the USPSTF states that there is insufficient evidence on whether to screen women ≥75 years old. The American Cancer Society (ACS) and the AGS Choosing Wisely® list states not to recommend breast cancer screening to older women without considering their life expectancy, because women with <10 years of remaining life expectancy are exposed to immediate harms of screening with little chance of benefit. These recommendations are based on a 10-year remaining life expectancy, because a meta-analysis of the RCTs on mammography screening found that on average it takes approximately 10 years before one death from breast cancer is prevented for 1,000 patients screened (SOE=A). Simulation models have found that the chance of older women benefitting from screening depends on their health. Screening has been found to be associated with breast cancers being diagnosed at an earlier stage when they may be easier to treat, and the sensitivity of mammography screening increases with age, leading to fewer false-positive tests.

Unlike the benefits of mammography screening, many of the harms are frequent and immediate and include anxiety resulting from false-positive tests, false reassurance from a false-negative test, overdiagnosis, and complications from evaluation and/or treatment of breast cancer. Among women ≥75 years old who undergo biennial screening, the cumulative probability of a false-positive mammogram over 10 years ranges from 12% to 27%. Although follow-up tests such as diagnostic mammograms and breast ultrasounds are generally low-risk procedures, approximately 10%–20% of older women who have a false-positive test undergo an unnecessary breast biopsy, which can be stressful and uncomfortable. Overdiagnosis is a particularly concerning harm, because the risks of breast cancer treatment increase as women age. However, quantifying overdiagnosis remains challenging, and estimates vary from 0 to 50% of screen-detected breast cancers; most estimates tend to average around 30%. In addition, overdiagnosis likely increases with age, because older women tend to have more indolent tumors and more competing mortality risks.

Ideally, older women will consider their risk of breast cancer, life expectancy, and their preferences around the benefits and harms of screening in deciding whether to continue mammography screening. A promising peer-reviewed decision aid to help women ≥75 years old decide whether or not to continue being screened is being tested in a larger trial. As for breast self-examination (BSE) and clinical breast examinations (CBEs), two large RCTs of women of all ages found no benefit of BSE compared with no breast cancer screening, and no trials have compared CBE alone to no screening. The USPSTF found insufficient evidence to recommend for or against CBEs and recommends against teaching BSE, because BSE may lead to unnecessary biopsies and is not associated with a survival benefit (SOE=B). The ACS recommends against CBEs for women at average risk of breast cancer who have regular mammograms.

Colorectal Cancer

Colorectal cancer (CRC) is the third most common cancer in adults >70 years old and the second leading cause of cancer death in older adults. The prevalence of adenomatous polyps increases with age from 20% to 25% at age 50 to nearly 50% by ages 75–80, with 1%–10% of these polyps progressing to cancer in 5–10 years. Fortunately, several tests are considered effective for CRC screening among adults 50–75 years old, including colonoscopy every 10 years, annual home-based high-sensitivity fecal occult blood tests (FOBT) and/or immunochemical-based fecal occult blood testing (FIT), flexible sigmoidoscopy every 5 years with high-sensitivity FOBTs every 3 years, fecal DNA testing every 3 years, and/or CT colonography every 5 years. A blood-based screening for colon cancer (mSEPT9) has been FDA approved; however, its ability to predict colon cancer is worse than that of FIT.

Table 12.1—Preventive Health Measures Available for Older Adults and Recommended Use

Procedure	≥10 years remaining life expectancy	5 to <10 years remaining life expectancy	Moderate dementia	Near end of life	SOE	Cost-effectiveness[a]
Cancer screening						
Mammography	Every 2 years if <75 years old; consider stopping if ≥75 years old	Not recommended	Not recommended	Not recommended	A/C[b]	Somewhat cost-effective for women <80 years old, may be cost-effective for women ≥80 years old in top quartile of life expectancy.
Pap smear	Stop after age 65	Not recommended	Not recommended	Not recommended	B	Cost-effective to stop
Prostate-specific antigen	Consider discussing pros/cons if remaining life expectancy >10 years; stop at age 70	Not recommended	Not recommended	Not recommended	B	Uncertain
Colon cancer screening Fecal occult blood test or Fecal immunochemical test	Yearly up to age 75, stop at age 86, shared decision making ages 76–85	Not recommended	Not recommended	Not recommended	A/C[c]	Cost-effective
Colonoscopy	Every 10 years up to age 75, stop at age 86, shared decision making ages 76–85	Not recommended	Not recommended	Not recommended		
Low-dose CT for lung cancer screening	Consider annually in those at risk[d], stop at age 75–80	Consider in those at risk[d], stop at age 75–80	Not recommended	Not recommended	A	Uncertain
Other screening tests						
Blood pressure	Consider each visit	Consider each visit	Consider each visit	Consider each visit	A	Uncertain
Height	Once a year	Once a year	Consider	Consider	C	Uncertain
Weight	Each visit	Each visit	Each visit	Each visit	C	Uncertain
DEXA screening for osteoporosis	At least once after age 65 in women, or age 60 if high risk	Consider if not done previously	Not recommended	Not recommended	A	Cost-effective
Cholesterol screening	Screen to allow for risk assessment; shared decision making after age 75	Consider	Not recommended	Not recommended	C	Uncertain
Diabetes screening	Screen if patient likely to benefit; consider stopping at age 70	Not recommended	Not recommended	Not recommended	C	Uncertain
Thyrotropin	Consider	Consider	Consider	Consider	C	Uncertain
Ultrasonography for abdominal aortic aneurysm	Once for men 65–75 years old who ever smoked; consider in men who never smoked	Consider	Not recommended	Not recommended	A	Cost-effective
HIV	Consider for those at high risk	Consider for those at high risk	Consider for those at high risk	Not recommended	A	Cost-effective
Hepatitis C	One time for those born between 1945–1965	One time for those born between 1945–1965	One time for those born between 1945–1965	Not recommended	B	Cost-effective
Hepatitis B	Consider for those at high risk	Consider for those at high risk	Consider for those at high risk	Not recommended	C	Uncertain
Immunizations						
Influenza	Annually	Annually	Annually	Annually	A	Cost-effective
Pneumococcal series	Once after age 65[e]	Once after age 65[e]	Once after age 65[e]	Once after age 65[e]	A	Cost-effective
Tetanus	Booster every 10 years	Booster every 10 years	Booster every 10 years	Not recommended	C	Cost-effective (a single booster at age 65)
Herpes zoster	Once after age 60	Once after age 60	Once after age 60	Once after age 60	A	Cost-effective

Table 12.1—Preventive Health Measures Available for Older Adults and Recommended Use (continued)

	Every visit	Every visit	Discuss with caregiver	Not recommended		
Healthy lifestyle counseling						
Smoking cessation	Every visit	Every visit	Discuss with caregiver	Not recommended	A	Telephone quit lines and counseling are cost-effective.
Exercise	Annually	Annually	Consider annually	Consider	C	Uncertain
Alcohol use disorder	Annually	Annually	Annually	Recommended initially, then if symptomatic	A	Screening and brief behavioral counseling interventions for alcohol abuse are cost-effective.
Driving assessment	Annually	Annually	Annually	Annually	A	Uncertain
Sexual function	Annually	Annually	Consider annually	Not recommended	D	Uncertain
Geriatric health issues						
Urinary incontinence screening	Annually	Annually	Annually	Annually	C	Uncertain
Visual acuity testing[f]	Consider annually	Consider annually	Consider annually	Not recommended	C	Population screening is not cost-effective; however, targeted screening of high-risk groups may be.
Hearing impairment screening[f,g]	Consider annually	Consider annually	Consider annually	Not recommended	C	A simple systematic screen, using an audiometric screening instrument, may be cost-effective for those 55–74 years old.
Cognitive impairment screening[g,h]	If symptomatic	If symptomatic	If symptomatic	If symptomatic	C	Uncertain
Gait and balance screening	Annually	Annually	Annually	Annually	C	Uncertain
Depression screening[f,g]	Annually	Annually	Annually	Annually	C	Uncertain
Falls risk assessment[g]	Annually	Annually	Annually	Annually	C	Uncertain
Advance directives completion[i]	Complete and update as needed	Complete and update as needed	Complete and update as needed	Complete and update as needed	C	Uncertain
Chemoprevention						
Vitamin D and calcium	Consider vitamin D at 1,000 IU with calcium at 500–1,200 mg/d in adults ≥65 years old	Consider vitamin D at 1,000 IU with calcium at 500–1,200 mg/d in adults ≥65 years old	Consider vitamin D at 1,000 IU with calcium at 500–1,200 mg/d in adults ≥65 years old	Consider vitamin D at 1,000 IU with calcium at 500–1,200 mg/d in adults ≥65 years old	A	Uncertain
Multivitamin	Not recommended	Not recommended	Not recommended	Not recommended	D	
Hormone therapy (women)	Not recommended	Not recommended	Not recommended	Not recommended	A	

SOURCE: Adapted with permission from Flaherty JH, Morley JE, Murphy DJ, et al. The development of outpatient clinical glidepaths. *J Am Geriatr Soc.* 2002;50(11):1886–1901.

[a] Cost-effectiveness is the ratio of costs of a test/procedure compared with the benefits of the test/procedure. It is expressed as the cost per year of life saved or the cost per quality-adjusted-life-year saved. Less than $50,000 per life-year gained is considered cost-effective.
[b] A for women up to age 74 years, C otherwise
[c] A remaining life expectancy >10 years, C otherwise
[d] Adults aged 55–80 years old who have a 30 pack-year smoking history and currently smoke or have quit within the past 15 years. www.uspreventiveservicestaskforce.org/Page/Document/UpdateSummaryFinal/lung-cancer-screening (accessed Feb 2019)
[e] If vaccinated with the 23-valent pneumococcal polysaccharide vaccine (PPSV23) before age 65, PPSV23 should be administered again 5 years later and at least 1 year after the 13-valent pneumococcal conjugate vaccine (PCV13).
[f] Required element of Medicare Initial Preventive Physical Examination
[g] Required element of Medicare first Annual Wellness Visit
[h] Required element of Medicare subsequent Annual Wellness Visits
[i] With patient's consent, end-of-life planning is a required element of the Medicare Initial Preventive Physical Examination.

In 4 trials of FOBT screening, mortality was reduced (ranging from 11% to 53%) in adults 70–80 years old, but false-positives were common; 86%–98% of trial participants had a negative colonoscopy after a positive FOBT (SOE=A). Before screening older adults with FOBT, clinicians should ask if the patient is willing to consider colonoscopy, because one study found that 58% of veterans ≥70 years old did not receive a complete colon evaluation within 1 year after a positive FOBT. In 43% of these patients, there was a lack of acknowledgement of the positive FOBT, 26% refused colonoscopy, 10% were in poor health, and the others had scheduling difficulties or difficulties with the bowel preparation. In one large RCT of sigmoidoscopy (the Prostate, Lung, Colorectal, and Ovarian [PLCO] Cancer Screening Trial) that included adults >65 years old, CRC mortality was reduced by 35% in adults 65–74 years old who were screened every 3–5 years (SOE=A). Sigmoidoscopy requires less bowel preparation than colonoscopy and it can be done without sedation, but technical challenges with achieving adequate depth are more common at older ages and there is a risk of perforation (0.1 per 1000 sigmoidoscopies).

Colonoscopy is the definitive test for detection of adenomas and CRC, and it is the most sensitive (95%) and cost-effective screening test for CRC. However, rates of procedure-related risks can increase with age. Among Medicare enrollees >65 years old, 0.6 per 1,000 experienced perforation after colonoscopy, 2.1 per 1,000 experienced GI bleeding (even when no polypectomy was performed), and 10 per 1,000 experienced cardiovascular events. Challenges with bowel preparation in older adults are common and include dizziness, abdominal pain, incontinence, and nausea; individuals can also have challenges with sedation after the procedure.

USPSTF recommends screening adults 50–75 years old, not screening those >85 years old, and making individualized screening decisions for those 76–85 years old considering patient health, life expectancy, and past screening. The Choosing Wisely® campaign recommends not screening adults with <10 years of life expectancy, because this population is thought to have little chance to benefit. These recommendations do not apply to adults who have had previous adenomas on colonoscopy and are undergoing surveillance.

Cervical Cancer

Although screening for cervical cancer with cytology is recommended every 3 years or every 5 years if combined with human papilloma virus (HPV) testing (a test for the presence of >2 high-risk or carcinogenic types), or every 5 years with HPV testing alone, guidelines recommend stopping screening after age 65 for women who have had adequate prior screening *regardless of sexual history or new sexual partners* and who are not otherwise at high risk of cervical cancer (no history of a high-grade precancerous cervical lesion in the past 20 years, no exposure in utero to diethylstilbestrol, not immunocompromised). Three consecutive negative cytology results or 2 consecutive negative HPV results within 10 years before cessation of screening, with the most recent test within 5 years, is considered adequate prior screening. These recommendations are based on evidence that shows that the incidence of high-grade cervical lesions significantly declines after middle age (SOE=A) and that the risk of false-positive tests resulting in invasive procedures is increased. Of note, positive screening results are more common with screening strategies that include HPV testing; 2.6% of women 60–65 years old will be HPV positive despite normal cytology, and follow-up testing is recommended. Older women who have undergone total hysterectomy with removal of the cervix and who do not have a history of cervical intraepithelial neoplasia grade 2 or 3 or cervical cancer should not be screened (SOE=A).

Prostate Cancer

Prostate cancer is the most common non-skin cancer affecting men >70 years old; it affects approximately 1 in 10 men and is the second leading cause of cancer-related deaths in this age group. The rate of intermediate- and high-risk prostate cancer increases substantially with age, with one study estimating 33% of men >80 years old with prostate cancer having high-risk disease compared with 6% of men <55 years old. Prostate cancer screening, by the prostate-specific antigen (PSA) test, is usually done annually. Most organizations do not recommend routine use of a digital rectal examination for screening.

Two large RCTs have evaluated the effectiveness of measuring PSA levels for prostate cancer screening. The PLCO Cancer Screening Trial was a multisite U.S. trial that included men 55–74 years old without a history of prostate, colon, or lung cancer. Men randomized to the intervention were screened annually with PSA for 6 years and a digital rectal examination for 4 years. Because men in the control group received standard care, there was high contamination of the controls (80% underwent PSA screening compared with 85% of those in the intervention group), which may explain why no reduction in mortality was found for PSA screening after 7–10 years follow-up. In the European Randomized Study of Screening for Prostate Cancer (ERSCP) trial, men 50–74 years old were randomized to PSA screening every 2–4 years. In this study, the control group did not receive PSA screening. Results showed a 20% reduction in prostate cancer mortality at 9 years for men 55–69 years old in the intervention group but no reduction in mortality for men ≥70 years old and no overall reduction in mortality for men of any age. The ERSCP researchers concluded that 1,410 men 55–69 years old would need to be screened and 48 treated to prevent one death from prostate cancer. However, men who were screened in this trial were more likely to be treated with radical prostatectomy than those who were not screened, which may explain the reduction in mortality found. Both trials documented detection of numerous clinically insignificant tumors (17%–50% of all cancers detected). The ACS recommends that clinicians discuss the potential benefits of PSA screening (modest reduction of morbidity and mortality from prostate cancer) and the possible harms (false-positive results [80% of positive PSAs are false-positives when thresholds of 2.5–4 mcg/L are used], unnecessary biopsies [15%–20% of those screened longer than 10 years], overdiagnosis/overtreatment, and possible complications of treatment [eg, erectile dysfunction, urinary incontinence, and even death from surgery]) among men ≥50 years old with at least 10 years remaining life expectancy. The USPSTF (2017) recommends that clinicians discuss the benefits and harms of PSA screening with men 55–69 years old and recommends against screening men ≥70 years old. (SOE=A).

Lung Cancer

Lung cancer is the second most common cancer and the leading cause of cancer death in the United States, accounting for 1 in 4 cancer deaths; 66% of lung cancers are diagnosed in adults >65 years old. Smoking results in 85% of U.S. lung cancer cases, and 37% of U.S. adults are current or former smokers. Annual screening for lung cancer with low-dose computed tomography (LDCT) is now recommended in adults 55–74 years old (ACS) or 55–80 years old (USPSTF) who have a 30 pack-year smoking history and currently smoke or have quit within the past 15 years (SOE=A). Screening should stop when a patient has not smoked for 15 years or life expectancy has declined such that curative lung surgery would not be performed. In addition, the USPSTF recommends smoking cessation counseling delivered with lung cancer screening, because smoking cessation is the most effective intervention to reduce the risk of lung cancer. Following the recommendations of the USPSTF, in 2015, Medicare began covering lung cancer screening with LDCT for adults 55–74 years old who meet USPSTF criteria and have engaged in shared decision-making with their clinicians. Shared decision making around lung cancer screening is reimbursed annually but not required after initial LDCT screening.

The USPSTF recommendations are based on data from the National Lung Screening Trial (NLST), which indicated that 3 annual LDCTs resulted in a 20% reduction in lung cancer mortality (which translates to 3 or 4 fewer lung cancer deaths per 1,000 participants who had LDCT screening over 6 years) and a 6.7% reduction in all-cause mortality after 6.5 years follow-up. The NNS to prevent one death from lung cancer was 320 (245 in adults 65–74 years old, and 364 in adults 55–64 years old). LDCT was found to have a sensitivity of 93.8% and a specificity of 73.4%. The overall average effective radiation dose used in the NLST was 1.5 millisievert (mSV) compared with 7 mSV for a standard-dose diagnostic chest CT examination. In 3 small European trials, no benefit of LDCT was found, but they were not powered to detect a survival difference; additional trials are underway.

Harms of LDCT include false-positive tests (39% of participants who had 3 annual LDCTs had at least one positive test, and 96% of these results were false-positive, but further imaging can usually resolve most false-positive results; 2.5% require invasive diagnostic procedures), overdiagnosis (9%–25% of tumors detected by screening), and radiation exposure. Both the benefits (more lung cancer deaths avoided) and harms of lung cancer screening (eg, false-positive tests) were greater in the NLST among adults 65–74 years old than among adults 55–64 years old. LDCT may be of most benefit to adults at the highest risk of lung cancer who are not at high risk of competing causes of death. A decision tool for lung cancer screening based on patient risk is available at http://nomograms.mskcc.org/Lung/Screening.aspx (accessed Feb 2019). Strategies for implementing lung cancer screening are being tested; however, a recent VA trial found that implementation of lung cancer screening was challenging and resource intensive and that only 58% of eligible patients chose to participate.

Other Cancers

The USPSTF states there is insufficient evidence to recommend whole-body skin examination by a primary care provider for early detection of skin cancer or to counsel older adults about sun protection. There is also insufficient evidence to assess the benefits and harms of screening for cancer of the mouth, bladder, or thyroid. In addition, screening for ovarian cancer with CA-125, transvaginal ultrasound, or pelvic examination did not reduce ovarian cancer mortality in a large RCT of women 55–74 years old at average risk; therefore, it is not recommended. Screening pelvic examinations in asymptomatic women are also not recommended, because the examination is not associated with improved health outcomes.

OTHER SCREENING TESTS AND PREVENTIVE MEASURES

Thyroid Disease

Early detection and treatment of asymptomatic adults with abnormal serum thyroid-stimulating hormone (TSH) levels with or without abnormal thyroxine (T_4) levels may be beneficial because it may prevent longer-term morbidity and mortality from fractures, cancer, or cardiovascular disease (CVD). However, widespread screening and treatment of subclinical thyroid dysfunction can also result in harms due to labeling, false-positive results, and overdiagnosis and overtreatment. *Subclinical hypothyroidism* is defined as an asymptomatic condition in which a patient has a serum TSH level exceeding the upper threshold of a specified laboratory reference interval (usually 4.5 mIU/L) but a normal T_4. However, TSH levels rise with age, fluctuate, and are sensitive to acute illness and certain medications. On the basis of expert opinion, a TSH level >10 mIU/L (on two separate occasions 6–12 months apart) is generally considered the threshold for initiation of treatment. However, in a recent RCT of 737 adults ≥65 years old with subclinical hypothyroidism, there was no benefit of treatment with levothyroxine on hypothyroid symptoms or fatigue. The USPSTF states there is insufficient evidence to recommend for or against screening for thyroid disease in older adults.

Hypertension

Hypertension is a prevalent condition, affecting 67% of adults >60 years old and is a major contributing risk factor to heart failure, heart attack, stroke, and chronic kidney disease. Moderate- to high-quality RCTs demonstrate the efficacy of treatment of the general population of people ≥60 years old to a target blood pressure of 150/90 mmHg in reducing the incidence of stroke, heart failure, and coronary heart disease events (SOE=A); some experts believe the target should be <140 mmHg for all adults regardless of age. The USPSTF recommends screening adults for high blood pressure. However, because 15%–30% of the population thought to be hypertensive may have lower blood pressure outside the office setting, the USPSTF recommends confirming the diagnosis with blood pressure measurements outside the clinical setting (with the most convincing evidence for ambulatory blood pressure monitoring) before starting treatment.

Type 2 Diabetes Mellitus

The incidence of type 2 diabetes increases with age until about 65 years and then levels off. Although a history of retinopathy is more common in older adults with middle-age onset diabetes than those with older-age onset, there is no difference in prevalence of CVD or peripheral neuropathy by age of onset. Older adults are at high risk of development of type 2 diabetes due to increasing insulin resistance and impaired pancreatic islet cell function with aging. However, no RCT of screening for diabetes has been performed, and the magnitude of benefit of initiating tight glycemic control during the preclinical phase of diabetes is unknown. In one RCT, intensive lifestyle modification in people with prediabetes delayed progression to clinical diabetes, particularly for adults ≥60 years old. Another RCT of adults with prediabetes found that 6 years of intensive lifestyle modification was associated with reduced mortality but only after 23 years follow-up. Based on indirect evidence on the benefits of treatment of type 2 diabetes, the American Diabetes Association recommends that all adults ≥45 years old be screened in the clinical setting every 1–3 years with a fasting plasma glucose, hemoglobin A_{1c} (HbA_{1c}), or oral glucose tolerance test (SOE=C). A consensus panel recommends screening older adults for diabetes if the individual is likely to benefit, noting that adults with <10 years of remaining life expectancy are unlikely to benefit from intensive glucose control and are subject to harms associated with hypoglycemia. The USPSTF recommends screening adults 40–70 years old who are overweight or obese.

The diagnosis of diabetes is confirmed if two consecutive HbA_{1c} levels are ≥6.5%, two consecutive fasting plasma glucose levels are ≥126 mg/dL (7 mmol/L), or if both the HbA_{1c} and fasting plasma glucose are above their diagnostic thresholds.

Abdominal Aortic Aneurysm

Abdominal aortic aneurysms (AAAs) are found in approximately 7% of older men and in 2% of older women who have smoked and in 2% of men and <1% of women who have never smoked. In addition to male sex and smoking history, strong risk factors for AAA include age and family history. The risk of rupture varies greatly by aneurysm size; however, rupture is associated with death in 75%–90% of cases. Four large, population-based RCTs showed that invitation to one-time screening for AAA is associated with reduced AAA-specific mortality in men (50% reduction over 13–15 years) and lower risk of AAA rupture and emergency surgery. Only one RCT on screening for AAA included women. It detected no difference in the rate of AAA rupture, AAA-specific mortality, or all-cause mortality between women invited for screening and the control group; however, the trial was ultimately underpowered to detect differences in health outcomes by sex.

Because of the higher prevalence of AAAs in men who have smoked, the USPSTF recommends 1-time screening of men 65–75 years old who have ever

Table 12.2—Components of Medicare Wellness Visits

	Initial Preventive Physical Examination (IPPE)[a]	First Annual Wellness Visit[b]	Subsequent Annual Wellness Visits[c]
History			
Past medical/surgical history	✓	✓	✓
Current medications and supplements (including calcium and vitamins)	✓	✓	✓
Family history	✓	✓	✓
Alcohol, tobacco, and illicit drug use	✓	HRA	HRA
Diet	✓	HRA	HRA
Physical activities	✓	HRA	HRA
Review risk factors for depression (eg, past history) and depression screen	✓	✓	✓
Review functional ability (ADLs)	✓	✓	✓
Fall risk	✓	✓	
Home safety	✓	✓	
Hearing impairment	✓	✓	
Examination			
Vital signs, including weight, height, blood pressure, BMI	✓	✓	✓
Visual acuity screen	✓		
Other based on history	✓	✓	✓
Counseling and referral			
Based on history and examination	✓		
End-of-life planning, provide verbal or written information[d]	On agreement of beneficiary	At discretion of beneficiary	At discretion of beneficiary
Preventive services plan			
Includes a brief written plan of appropriate screenings and other preventive services (eg, checklist) to be given to the beneficiary	✓	Establish a written schedule based on USPSTF and ACIP[e]	Update written schedule
Laboratory tests			
	None included	None included	None included
Health risk assessment (HRA)[f]			
Demographic data (age, gender, race, ethnicity)		✓	Update
Self-assessment of health status		✓	Update
Psychosocial risks (depression, life satisfaction, stress, anger, loneliness/social isolation, pain, and fatigue)		✓	Update
Behavioral risks (tobacco use, physical activity, nutrition and oral health, alcohol consumption, sexual health, motor vehicle safety [seat belt use]), and home safety		✓	Update
ADLs and IADLs		✓	Update
List of providers/suppliers			
		Establish list	Update
Cognitive function			
Direct observation combined with patient report and concerns of family and others		✓	✓

Table 12.2—Components of Medicare Wellness Visits (continued)

	Initial Preventive Physical Examination (IPPE)[a]	First Annual Wellness Visit[b]	Subsequent Annual Wellness Visits[c]
Establish list of risk factors and conditions for which primary, secondary, or tertiary interventions are recommended or underway			
	For example: mental health conditions	For example: mental health conditions, or conditions identified through IPPE	Update
Provide personalized advice and referral to health education or preventive counseling services			
Examples: weight loss, physical activity, tobacco cessation, fall prevention, nutrition	✓ (include screening ECG if appropriate)	✓	✓

NOTE: HRA = health risk assessment; ADLs = activities of daily living; IADLs = instrumental activities of daily living
[a] Initial Preventive Physical Examination (IPPE) is available to all newly enrolled Medicare beneficiaries within the first 12 months after the effective date of their first Medicare Part B coverage period (a one-time benefit); it is also known as the "Welcome to Medicare" preventive visit.
[b] Medicare covers an Annual Wellness Visit (AWV) for beneficiaries who are no longer in the first 12 months of their Part B coverage period. Medicare pays for only one *first* AWV per lifetime.
[c] Medicare pays for one subsequent AWV per year.
[d] End-of-life planning includes the beneficiary's ability to prepare an advance directive and whether the provider is willing to follow the beneficiary's wishes as expressed in the advance directive.
[e] May be a checklist for the next 5–10 years as appropriate, based on recommendations of the USPSTF and the Advisory Committee on Immunization Practices (ACIP) and the individual's health status, screening history, and age-appropriate preventive services covered by Medicare.
[f] For an example HRA, see www.howsyourhealth.org/MEDICAREAAFPPACKAGE.pdf (accessed Feb 2019).

smoked (defined as ≥100 cigarettes in lifetime) with a conventional abdominal duplex ultrasonography (sensitivity 94%–100% and specificity 98%–100%). The USPSTF recommends that clinicians selectively offer screening for AAA in men 65–75 years old who have never smoked. The USPSTF concludes that the current evidence is insufficient to assess the balance of benefits and harms of screening for AAA in women 65–75 years old who have ever smoked and recommends against screening women who have never smoked. Medicare offers coverage of this screening test only as part of a "Welcome to Medicare" preventive visit for all men and for women with a family history of AAA.

Osteoporosis

Four of every ten white U.S. women ≥50 years old will eventually experience a hip, spine, or wrist fracture. Over half of women ≥80 years old have osteoporosis (T score less than or equal to –2.5). No clinical trials have evaluated the effectiveness of screening older women for osteoporosis. However, age-based screening is supported by prevalence data. The NNS to prevent one hip fracture ranges from 731 for women 65–69 years old to 143 for women 75–79 years old. Routine screening (ie, measurement of BMD through dual x-ray absorptiometry) is recommended by the USPSTF for all women ≥65 years old and for women ≥60 years old at high risk (as determined by the FRAX tool, www.sheffield.ac.uk/FRAX/ [accessed Feb 2019]). An appropriate interval for screening has not been determined; however, a study found that osteoporosis would develop in 10% of women >65 years old with normal BMD or mild osteopenia (T score –1.01 to –1.49) within 15 years follow-up, within 5 years for women with moderate osteopenia (T score –1.50 to –1.99), and within 1 year for women with advanced osteopenia (T score –2.00 to –2.49). In another study, among women (mean age 75) untreated for osteoporosis, a second bone density test did not meaningfully improve the prediction of hip or major osteoporotic fracture after 4 years. Medicare currently reimburses BMD screening every 2 years regardless of previous test results. When to stop screening is also a matter of controversy. In the Fracture Intervention Trial, the benefit of treatment emerged 18–24 months after initiation of treatment.

The USPSTF concludes that the evidence is insufficient to assess the balance of benefits and harms of screening for osteoporosis in men. However, screening men ≥65 years old with a prior clinical fracture and all men ≥80 years old has been shown to be cost-effective. Several organizations recommend that clinicians assess older men, such as those undergoing androgen therapy, for osteoporosis risk and screen those at increased risk who are candidates for drug therapy. The National Osteoporosis Foundation recommends screening all men ≥70 years old.

Hyperlipidemia

Cardiovascular disease (CVD) is the leading cause of morbidity and mortality in the United States, accounting for 1 of every 3 deaths among adults. Low- or moderate-dose statin use has been associated with a reduced risk of all-cause mortality (pooled risk ratio [RR] 0.86; 95% CI, 0.80–0.93), cardiovascular mortality (RR 0.69; 95% CI, 0.54–0.88), and ischemic stroke (RR 0.71; 95% CI, 0.62–0.82), heart attack (RR, 0.64; 95% CI, 0.57–0.71), in a pooled analysis of 19 RCTs of adults 40–75 years old without CVD. However, few of these trials included adults >75 years old. When data were combined from the 3 trials (PROSPER, JUPITER, and HOPE-3) that included adults ≥75 years old, statins were associated with a modest reduction of CVD but no benefit on overall mortality in adults >75 years old. The estimated lag time to benefit from statins for primary prevention is 1–2 years. The majority of current guidelines on use of statins for primary prevention of CVD are based on patient risk rather than on treating to LDL targets. However, high-intensity statin therapy is generally recommended for adults with LDL-C ≥190 mg/dL. The 10-year CVD risk-threshold at which patients 40–75 years old are considered to be high risk and for whom guidelines recommend statin therapy for primary prevention vary by organization from >7.5% (ACC/AHA) to >10% (USPSTF) to >12% (Department of Veterans Affairs [VA]). These guidelines also note that clinicians may consider statins for primary prevention in adults at moderate risk (5–7.5% ACC/AHA; 7.5–10% USPSTF; 6–12% VA). For adults >75 years old, guidelines state that there is insufficient evidence to recommend for or against statin use for primary prevention. Of note, risk calculators often overestimate risk in real-world populations, and the 10-year risk for individuals >75 years old, including those with an optimal risk factor profile, always exceeds 7.5% using the 2013 ACC/AHA calculator (http://tools.acc.org/ASCVD-Risk-Estimator [accessed Feb 2019]). Because there are risks of statin therapy, including statin myopathy, drug-drug interactions, and possibly increased risk of diabetes, shared decision making about when to start statin therapy for primary prevention is generally recommended. Decision aids, such as Statin Choice from the Mayo Clinic may help (https://statindecisionaid.mayoclinic.org [accessed Feb 2019]).

To screen for hyperlipidemia, RCT evidence supports use of an initial fasting lipid panel (total cholesterol, triglycerides, HDL-C and calculated LDL-C). Direct LDL-C testing, which does not require a fasting sample measurement, is available; however, calculated LDL (which requires fasting) is the validated measurement used in trials for risk assessment and treatment decisions.

Hepatitis C

Hepatitis C virus (HCV) is the most common chronic blood-borne pathogen in the United States and a leading cause of complications from chronic liver disease, and HCV-related end-stage liver disease is the most common indication for liver transplant in U.S. adults. The prevalence of the anti-HCV antibody in the United States is ≥50% in high-risk persons (eg, those with past or current injection drug use) and is 3%–4% in U.S. adults born between 1945 and 1965 (which may be from blood transfusions before screening was implemented in 1992). Most with chronic HCV are unaware. In patients at high-risk, anti-HCV antibody testing is associated with high sensitivity (>90%) and NNS of <20 persons to identify one case of HCV infection. Identifying infected patients at earlier stages of disease may reduce complications from liver damage, because antiviral regimens are effective. Therefore, the USPSTF recommends offering one-time screening for HCV infection to adults born between 1945 and 1965 and those at high risk.

Hepatitis B

Approximately 700,000 to 2.2 million persons in the United States have chronic hepatitis B virus (HBV) infection. Persons considered at high risk of HBV infection include those from countries with a high prevalence of HBV infection, HIV-positive persons, injection drug users, household contacts of persons infected with HBV, and men who have sex with men. The natural history of chronic HBV infection varies but can include the potential long-term sequelae of cirrhosis, hepatic decompensation, and hepatocellular carcinoma. An estimated 15%–25% of persons with chronic HBV infection die of cirrhosis or hepatocellular carcinoma. Those with chronic infection also serve as a reservoir for person-to-person transmission of HBV infection. Therefore, the USPSTF recommends screening adults at high risk of infection with hepatitis B surface antigen testing.

Other Diseases

The USPSTF does not recommend routine screening for chronic kidney disease, asymptomatic carotid artery stenosis, celiac disease, COPD, obstructive sleep apnea, or peripheral artery disease (Table 12.2). The USPSTF also recommends against a resting or exercise ECG in asymptomatic patients at low risk of CVD and states the evidence is insufficient for adults at intermediate or high risk. However, Medicare covers a once-in-a-lifetime screening ECG, as appropriate, as part of an Initial Preventive Physical Examination, also known as the "Welcome to Medicare" preventive visit (www.cms.gov/Outreach-and-Education/Medicare-Learning-

Network-MLN/MLNProducts/Downloads/MPS_QRI_IPPE001a.pdf).

HEALTHY LIFESTYLE COUNSELING

Physical Activity

Physical inactivity is recognized as a risk factor for many diseases (eg, coronary artery disease, diabetes, and obesity). Increasing physical activity in sedentary older adults reduces morbidity and mortality and improves psychological health, promotes functional independence, and prevents falls. Almost all older adults can engage safely in a program of moderate physical activity (such as walking) or lifestyle modification, without special screening. Stress testing is recommended for any older adult who intends to begin a vigorous exercise program (eg, strenuous cycling, jogging). The U.S. Department of Health and Human Services recommends that older adults get at least 150 minutes per week of moderate-intensity or 75 minutes per week of vigorous-intensity aerobic physical activity, as well as muscle-strengthening activities (eg, weight training) twice per week and balance training (eg, Tai chi, dance) ≥3 times per week for those at high risk of falls. Clinicians are encouraged to counsel patients about the importance of exercise and to consider patient-specific goals and barriers for exercise, as well as encourage patients to expand current exercise habits as needed. An exercise prescription should address the type, frequency, duration, and intensity of physical activity for each fitness component.

Nutrition

The weight of older adults should be obtained at each visit, and height measured annually and BMI (in kg/m^2) calculated. The USPSTF recommends that obese (BMI ≥30) adults be offered intensive counseling and behavioral interventions to promote sustained weight loss. However, ideal BMI may be higher for older adults than middle-aged adults. In fact, BMIs between 25–29 are associated with the lowest mortality risk for adults ≥70 years old, which may be because of benefits from greater nutritional reserve. In general, higher BMI values are associated with lower relative mortality risk in older adults than in younger adults. However, weight loss, especially when combined with exercise, may improve physical function and ameliorate frailty among obese older adults (SOE=A). On the other end of the spectrum, malnutrition and undernutrition are common yet frequently unidentified problems in the geriatric population; 15% of older outpatients are malnourished. Nutritional health screens generally include questions on meal frequency, unintentional weight loss, dental health, alcohol intake, availability of money for food, and on the ability to shop, cook, and feed oneself. However, limited data are available on the effectiveness of nutritional screening in primary care. The 2015–2020 Dietary Guidelines for Americans recommends that Americans follow a healthy eating pattern across the life span and notes that all food and beverage choices matter. The guidelines recommend that adults choose a variety of nutrient-dense foods across and within all food groups in recommended amounts. They also recommend limiting calories from added sugars and saturated fats and reducing sodium intake.

Alcohol Use Disorder

Approximately half of the population ≥65 years old drinks alcohol, and many may experience health risks from consuming alcohol or from the combination of alcohol use with medications; approximately 2%–4% have alcohol use disorder. Conversely, light to moderate alcohol consumption in middle-aged or older adults has been associated with some health benefits, such as reduced risk of coronary heart disease. Moderate drinking is defined as 1 drink or less per day for adults >65 years old.

The AGS recommends that all adults ≥65 years old be asked annually about their alcohol use. Those who report using alcohol should be screened for alcohol use disorder using a validated screening instrument. The Alcohol Use Disorders Identification Test (AUDIT) and the Short Brief Michigan Alcoholism Screening Test-Geriatric Version (SMAST) can be self-administered and are effective in identifying problem drinking in older adults. The well-known CAGE questionnaire has lower sensitivity than these instruments in detecting risky or hazardous drinking in older adults. Adults who report use disorder may benefit from behavioral counseling interventions (eg, behavioral strategies such as action plans, drinking diaries, stress management, or problem solving).

Smoking Cessation

Smoking cessation at any age decreases rates of COPD, many cancers, and coronary artery disease. Clinicians should ask all adults about tobacco use. If an adult uses tobacco, he or she should be counseled to quit. Once he or she is ready to quit, there should be documentation of a quit date, discussion of therapies to aid cessation, and follow-up in person or by phone within 3–7 days of the quit date and monthly for the first 3 months (SOE=A).

Sexually Transmitted Infections

Increasingly, Americans ≥50 years old are afflicted with sexually transmitted infections (STIs) and HIV. Nationally, approximately 20% of patients with HIV are >50 years old. The USPTSF recommends routine screening of adults up to age 65, and screening adults >65 years old who are at increased risk. A cost-effectiveness analysis found that one-time HIV screening is cost-effective for patients age 65–75 years old (<$60,000 per quality-adjusted life-year gained) if the tested population has an HIV prevalence ≥0.1%, the screened patient has a partner at risk, and counseling is streamlined (abbreviated pretest counseling).

Although the prevalence of sexual activity declines with age (73% among adults 57–64 years old versus 26% among adults 75–85 years old) and is significantly less common among women than men, many older adults are sexually active. The USPSTF recommends high-intensity behavioral counseling to prevent STIs for all sexually active adults at increased risk. Screening for syphilis infection is recommended in adults at increased risk.

Latent Tuberculosis Infection

The prevalence of latent tuberculosis infection (LTBI) in the United States is 5%, and 5%–10% of those individuals will later reactivate and progress to active disease. Treatment of LTBI reduces progression to active tuberculosis. Therefore, to reduce the transmission, morbidity, and mortality of active tubercular disease, the USPSTF recommends screening for LTBI in persons at increased risk (eg, those born in, or who are former residents of, countries with increased tuberculosis prevalence and persons who live in, or have lived in, high-risk congregate settings [eg, homeless shelters and correctional facilities]).

GERIATRIC HEALTH ISSUES

Although there are few data examining the effectiveness of screening or counseling about geriatric health issues, expert panels generally recommend that clinicians screen for these conditions annually. The elements of a comprehensive geriatric assessment (CGA) include assessment of medications, cognitive status, functional status, nutritional status, hearing, vision, affect, social support, gait, and balance. CGA has been most successful when the geriatrics team directly oversees the care. In these circumstances, CGA has been associated with improvements in general well-being, life satisfaction, IADLs, and fewer clinic visits (SOE=A). Although the benefits of cancer screening tests may not be achieved for 10 years, the benefits of diagnosing and treating older adults with geriatric health issues can be immediate. Therefore, screening for these conditions should be of high priority in frail older adults with limited remaining life expectancy. Assessing for geriatric health issues is also an essential component of Medicare's Annual Wellness Visit (AWV), which Medicare began covering in 2011 for adults who have had Part B coverage for >12 months (www.cms.gov/Outreach-and-Education/Medicare-Learning-Network-MLN/MLNProducts/downloads/AWV_chart_ICN905706.pdf). Medicare also covers an Initial Preventive Physical Examination, or "Welcome to Medicare" preventive visit, that must be completed within the first 12 months of enrollment. To date, participation in these visits has been low, with only 16% of eligible beneficiaries receiving an AWV in 2014.

Falls

Falls are the leading cause of injury in adults ≥65 years old, and the AGS recommends that clinicians ask patients annually about falls, balance, or gait problems. Approximately 30%–40% of noninstitutionalized older adults fall each year, and the annual incidence of falls approaches 50% in those >80 years old. Increasing age, a history of falls, mobility problems, and poor performance on the "Timed Up and Go" test are important risk factors for falls. Extrinsic factors that contribute to falls include poor lighting, obtrusive furniture, inadequate footwear, slippery floors, loose floor coverings, and bathrooms without handrails or grab bars. A multifactorial risk assessment for falls, which incorporates a focused medical history, physical examination, functional assessments, and review of extrinsic factors, is recommended by AGS for older adults with two falls in the past year or one fall if combined with gait or balance problems assessed by a standardized gait and balance test. The AGS recommends several primary care–based interventions to prevent falls (eg, exercise and physical therapy, vitamin D supplementation, adaptation or modification of home environment, withdrawal or minimization of psychoactive or other medications, management of postural hypotension, and management of foot problems/footwear).

Incontinence

Incontinence is estimated to affect 15%–30% of older community-dwelling women. Continence problems, which have major social and emotional consequences, are frequently treatable, but only 30%–45% of women with incontinence seek care. Because of the high prevalence of undiagnosed incontinence, older women should be specifically asked about urinary incontinence as part of a review of systems, particularly those who have had children, who have comorbid conditions associated with increased risk of urinary incontinence (ie, diabetes, neurologic disease, obesity), and who are >65 years old. The following screening questions have been suggested: Do you ever leak urine when you don't want to? Do you ever leak urine when you cough, laugh, or exercise? Do you ever leak urine on the way to the bathroom? Do you ever use pads, tissue, or cloth in your underwear to catch urine?

Cognitive Status

The USPSTF states that evidence is insufficient to recommend screening older adults for dementia. However, early detection and diagnosis of dementia through assessment of patient-, family-, or clinician-recognized signs and/or symptoms was not considered screening by the USPSTF and was not the focus of that group's recommendations. Meanwhile, a Medicare AWV must include detection of cognitive impairment by direct observation with due consideration of concerns raised by the patient, family, or others. Medicare does not require use of a standardized tool for assessment of cognitive function. However, brief assessment tools, such as the Mini-Cog (clock drawing test combined with a three-item recall test), the Memory Impairment Screen, and the General Practitioner Assessment of Cognition may be helpful. All require <5 minutes to administer; are easily administered by non-physician staff; and are relatively free of educational, language, and/or cultural bias (all are available at www.nia.nih.gov). Subjective cognitive complaints have also been shown to be a reliable indicator of objective cognitive impairment. Early detection of dementia may lead to improved symptom control, help patients maintain independence, and help reduce caregiver stress and depression. In addition, the Institute of Medicine (IOM) recommends 3 actions that everyone can take to maintain their cognitive health: 1) Be physically active. 2) Reduce and manage CVD risk factors. 3) Regularly discuss and review health conditions and medications that might influence cognitive health with a health care professional. The IOM also notes that being socially and intellectually engaged and getting adequate sleep and/or treatment for sleep disorders may have positive effects on cognitive health.

Depression

Studies report a 1%–2% prevalence of a major depressive disorder, 2% prevalence of dysthymia, and 13%–27% prevalence of subsyndromal depression among community-dwelling older adults. However, depression is often missed by primary care providers. The USPSTF recommends that clinicians screen adults for depression as long as the practice setting is equipped to treat and follow patients with this disease; annual screening is covered by Medicare. The Geriatric Depression Scale, the one-question screen "Do you often feel sad or depressed?", or the Patient Health Questionnaire-2 ("Over the past 2 weeks, have you felt down, depressed, or hopeless?" and "Over the past 2 weeks, have you felt little interest or pleasure in doing things?") are effective screening tools. A positive response should be followed by a fuller assessment of severity and duration of symptoms. Because of high suicide rates, particularly in older white men, older adults who screen positive should be specifically asked about these symptoms.

Vision

Approximately 9% of adults ≥60 years old have impaired visual acuity (best-corrected vision of 20/40 or worse). The most common causes are presbyopia, cataracts, glaucoma, diabetic retinopathy, and age-related macular degeneration. Data from 3 RCTs show that screening for vision impairment in older adults in primary care settings is not associated with improved visual or other clinical outcomes. Based on these data, the USPSTF found insufficient evidence to recommend for or against visual acuity screening by primary care clinicians. However, a visual examination is a necessary component of a Medicare Initial Preventive Physical Examination. The USPSTF also found insufficient evidence to recommend screening adults for primary open-angle glaucoma; however, Medicare does cover annual glaucoma screening for those at high risk.

Hearing

The prevalence of hearing impairment is 20%-40% in adults ≥50 years old and more than 80% in those ≥80 years old. Causes of hearing impairment in older adults include presbycusis, genetic factors, exposure to loud noises or ototoxic agents, history of ear infections, and presence of systemic diseases (eg, diabetes). In one large (N=2,305) randomized trial, screening for hearing impairment was associated with increased hearing aid use at 1 year, but it was not associated with improvement in hearing-related function. The USPSTF states there is insufficient evidence to assess the balance of benefits and harms of screening for hearing impairment. However, screening for hearing impairment is a necessary component of Medicare's initial AWV. Although pure-tone audiometry is the gold standard for screening hearing, a whispered voice test at 2 feet has a positive predictive value of approximately 75%.

Mistreatment of Older Adults

Estimates of mistreatment of older adults range from 3% to 14%. Older adults who present with contusions, burns, bite marks, genital or rectal trauma, pressure injury, or BMI ≤17.5 kg/m^2 with no clinical explanation should be asked about possible mistreatment or referred to social work for assessment. Although multiple instruments have been developed to test for different types of mistreatment in older adults (eg, psychological, physical, and/or financial abuse), few have been tested in primary care. The paucity of data led the USPSTF to conclude there is insufficient evidence to recommend routine screening for mistreatment of older adults.

Safety and Preventing Injury

Older adults should be advised to keep a list of emergency numbers by each phone, to check their smoke detectors and carbon monoxide detectors, and to not set their hot water heaters >120°F. Because older adults do not adjust as well to sudden changes in temperature (sometimes because of illness or medicines that impair the body's ability to regulate its temperature), it is important to remind older adults to take precautions against heat stroke. Recommendations include drinking cool/nonalcoholic beverages, resting, taking a cool bath or shower, seeking an air-conditioned environment, and wearing lightweight clothing when the weather is hot. Older adults are also encouraged to develop an advance directive and identify a health care proxy.

In addition, older adults should be encouraged to wear seat belts and to undergo regular driving tests. One study found that 75% of adults 75–84 years old and 70% of adults ≥85 years old were current drivers. Drivers >75 years old have more traffic violations and nonfatal collisions than younger drivers, and some states are considering legislation that would tighten license renewal requirements for older drivers. However, older adults who are forced to stop driving rely more on their families, reduce their social activities, and often become depressed. There is not currently one effective, easily administered test (or series of tests) to evaluate driving competence. However, the Clinical Assessment of Driving-Related Skills (CADReS) is a toolbox of evidence-based, practical, office-based functional assessment tools in the key areas of vision, cognition, and motor/sensory function related to driving (http://bit.ly/2pbFxLW). Driving refresher courses and on-the-road evaluations of older adults are available in many communities. Specific questions about driving should be included in the social history and in the AWV health risk assessment (eg, How did the older patient get to the primary care visit? How often and under what circumstances does he or she drive? Any traffic violations, accidents, or close calls within the past 6 months, 1 year, 2 years? Any episodes of getting lost while driving? Does the patient feel comfortable and want to continue driving?) AGS *Clinician's Guide to Assessing and Counseling Older Drivers* provides helpful suggestions for assessing and improving the safety of older adults when driving (http://bit.ly/2FxUZw8 [accessed Feb 2019]).

IMMUNIZATIONS

Several immunizations are currently recommended for older adults. An annual influenza vaccination is recommended for adults ≥50 years old without contraindications (eg, egg allergy). Despite these recommendations, many older adults, especially those of racial and ethnic minorities, do not receive the influenza vaccine. Adults ≥65 years old may receive the standard or high-dose influenza vaccine; however, the intranasally administered live-attenuated influenza vaccine has not been approved for adults ≥50 years old. Although the CDC has not made a recommendation favoring the high-dose influenza vaccine over the standard-dose influenza vaccine, the high-dose vaccine has been demonstrated in an RCT to reduce the rate of laboratory-confirmed influenza by 24.2% compared with the standard-dose influenza vaccine. The rates of serious adverse events were similar in both groups.

Adults ≥65 years old should also receive immunization against pneumococcus (*Streptococcus pneumoniae*). The CDC recommends administering the 13-valent pneumococcal conjugate vaccine (PCV13) and 23-valent pneumococcal polysaccharide vaccine (PPSV23) in series. Immunocompetent adults ≥65 years old who have never received PPSV23 should first receive PCV13, followed at least 1 year later by PPSV23. Those who have previously been vaccinated with PPSV23 should receive PCV13 at least 1 year after their most recent dose of PPSV23. For those who received their first dose of PPSV23 before the age of 65 and who will require a second dose, PPSV23 should be administered at least 1 year after PCV13 is given and at least 5 years after the most recent PPSV23.

The Td (tetanus, diphtheria) booster is recommended every 10 years. Adults ≥65 years old may get the Tdap (tetanus, diphtheria, and acellular pertussis) instead. The Tdap is specifically recommended for adults ≥65 years old who have close contact with an infant <12 months old. A live attenuated herpes zoster vaccine (Zostavax) is recommended for adults ≥60 years old. In an RCT, the vaccine reduced the incidence of post-herpetic neuralgia by 67% after 3 years in patients ≥60 years old; however, vaccine efficacy was only about 38% in adults ≥70 years old. A recombinant, adjuvanted, subunit, candidate vaccine (Shingrix) that combines glycoprotein E, a protein found on the varicella zoster virus that causes shingles, with an adjuvant system ($AS01_B$), to enhance the immune response to the antigen has been approved by the FDA. Two doses of Shingrix administered 2 months apart was 97% effective against herpes zoster (shingles) in adults ≥50 years old and 89.8% effective in adults ≥70 years old.

CHEMOPROPHYLAXIS

Aspirin

Cardiovascular disease (CVD) and colorectal cancer (CRC) are major causes of death in U.S. adults. Aspirin lowers the risk of CVD and CRC, and 40% of adults

>50 years old use aspirin for primary or secondary prevention of CVD. Major risk factors for CVD are older age, male sex, race/ethnicity, abnormal lipid levels, high blood pressure, diabetes, and smoking. Risk factors for GI bleeding with aspirin use include higher dose and longer duration of use, history of GI ulcers or upper GI pain, bleeding disorders, renal failure, severe liver disease, and thrombocytopenia. Other factors that increase risk of GI or intracranial bleeding with low-dose aspirin use include concurrent anticoagulation or NSAID use, uncontrolled hypertension, male sex, and older age. There is no evidence that enteric-coated or buffered formulations reduce the risk of serious GI bleeding.

The USPSTF recommends initiating low-dose aspirin for primary prevention of CVD and CRC in adults 50–59 years old who have a 10% or greater 10-year CVD risk, are not at increased risk of bleeding, have a remaining life expectancy of at least 10 years, and are willing to take low-dose aspirin for at least 10 years. Because on average the overall benefit of aspirin compared with the risk of GI bleeding is lower for adults 60–69 years old, the USPSTF recommends that the use of aspirin in adults 60–69 years old with 10% or greater 10-year CVD risk be individualized. Although adults ≥70 years old are at increased risk of CVD, they are also at increased risk of GI bleed, and the benefits of aspirin in reducing CRC are lower in adults ≥70 years old because this benefit can take 10–20 years to manifest. Therefore, the USPSTF states that there is insufficient evidence to assess the balance of benefits or harms of initiating aspirin use for the primary prevention of CVD and CRC adults ≥70 years old. In general, treatment decisions should involve an assessment of the individual's risk of CVD, bleeding risk, life expectancy, and preferences. The optimal dose of aspirin to prevent CVD events is not known; however, a dose of 81 mg seems as effective as higher doses and may be associated with lower risk of GI bleed.

Calcium, Vitamin D, and Multivitamins

An AGS consensus statement advises clinicians to recommend vitamin D supplementation of at least 1,000 IU/d as well as calcium supplementation of 500–1,200 mg/d to community-dwelling older adults ≥65 years old to reduce risk of fractures and falls. This consensus statement included the following 4 recommendations: 1) The recommended average vitamin D intake is 4,000 IU/d from all sources (diet, supplements, sunlight). 2) Routine laboratory testing for serum 25(OH)D concentrations before supplementation is not necessary in the absence of underlying conditions that increase the risk of hypercalcemia (eg, advanced renal disease, certain malignancies, sarcoidosis). 3) Similarly, routine monitoring of serum 25(OH)D concentrations is not necessary. However, serum 25(OH)D concentrations of 30 ng/mL (74 nmol/L) should be a minimum goal to achieve in adults ≥65 years old, particularly in frail adults who are at higher risk of falls, injuries, and fractures. 4) If clinicians choose to monitor 25(OH)D, levels should be measured after 4 months of vitamin D_3 supplementation to confirm that appropriate levels have been achieved.

The USPSTF concludes that there is insufficient evidence to recommend a multivitamin for prevention of CVD or cancer.

Postmenopausal Hormone Therapy

Postmenopausal hormone therapy for primary prevention is not recommended, because the Women's Health Initiative Trial showed that it (ie, estrogen plus progesterone increased the risk of ischemic stroke, coronary artery disease, venous thrombosis, pulmonary embolism, decline in cognitive function, urinary incontinence, and invasive breast cancer among older women. Fortunately, recent analyses have found that use of postmenopausal hormone therapy for 5–7 years is not associated with an increased risk of all cause, cardiovascular, or cancer mortality within 18 years follow-up. For breast cancer prevention, the USPSTF recommends that clinicians engage in shared, informed decision making with women ≥35 years old with a 5-year projected risk of breast cancer of ≥3% (calculated using the Breast Cancer Risk Assessment Tool [www.cancer.gov/bcrisktool, accessed Feb 2019] or other models) for whom the potential benefits of risk-reducing medications (eg, tamoxifen, raloxifene) outweigh the potential risks (considering a woman's age [data on risk–benefit ratio available for women up to age 79], comorbid conditions, presence of a uterus, and risks of thromboembolic or medication-related adverse events).

COUNSELING ON CANCER SCREENING AND PREVENTIVE HEALTH

Delivery of preventive health services to older adults can be challenging for many reasons. First, many preventive health services are available, and primary care clinicians are often relied on to deliver or at least discuss most of these services. Second, time during clinic visits often needs to be spent caring for older adults' acute or chronic medical conditions rather than counseling about screening tests or geriatric health issues, for which there is little reimbursement. Third, experts increasingly recommend that clinicians consider a patient's remaining life expectancy and the lag time to benefit from a preventive health intervention when deciding which measures to recommend; however, estimating remaining life expectancy may be difficult, and discussing remaining life expectancy with patients may be uncomfortable. While few studies have addressed ways to discuss life expectancy with older adults in the context of clinical decision-making around preventive services, recent data suggest that discussions about discontinuing certain preventive health interventions should focus on how the harms of the test/intervention outweigh the benefits. Older adults are more receptive to hearing that a test would not help them live longer rather than that they may not live long enough to benefit, which is a more negative message. In addition, many older adults suffer from comcomitant disorders that encompass multiple risk factors; this presents a challenge to clinicians to synthesize the evidence and in turn make individual patient recommendations for primary, secondary, and tertiary screening measures.

Several tools are available to help clinicians estimate patients' remaining life expectancy to guide screening decisions, including the Lee-Schonberg index (available at www.ePrognosis.org [accessed Feb 2019]), which can provide a probability of a patient living 5, 10, or 14 more years. Patients who have >50% risk of mortality during a specific time frame are generally thought to have a remaining life expectancy less than that time frame. Other experts have proposed using U.S. life table data adjusted for an individual's comorbidity to estimate older adults' life expectancy.

When discussing cancer or other screening tests with older adults, clinicians should indicate whether any data suggest that the screening test improves quality or quantity of life and the lag time to benefit. Clinicians should also discuss that the harms of screening are often immediate and include discomfort from undergoing the test itself, anxiety, potential complications from diagnostic procedures resulting from a false-positive test, false reassurance from a false-negative test, and overdiagnosis (diagnosis of tumors that are of no threat) that may result in overtreatment. Furthermore, clinicians may want to explain that overdiagnosis is thought to increase with age because of decreasing remaining life expectancy, competing mortality risks, and slower-growing tumors among older adults. Older adults should be asked how they view the potential benefits and harms of different screening tests, so that their values and preferences are considered. Health maintenance discussions among older adults with limited remaining life expectancies should focus on measures that have benefits likely to be achieved in a short time frame (eg, counseling on home safety, falls prevention, immunizations).

Choosing Wisely® Recommendations

Prevention

- Do not use PET/CT for cancer screening in healthy individuals.

- Do not recommend screening for breast, colorectal, or prostate cancer (with the PSA test) without considering life expectancy and the risks of testing, overdiagnosis, and overtreatment.

- Measurement of PSA is controversial but should not be measured if remaining life expectancy is <10 years.

- Do not repeat colorectal cancer screening (by any method) for 10 years after a high-quality colonoscopy is negative in average-risk individuals.

- Do not perform routine cancer screening for dialysis patients with limited life expectancies without signs or symptoms.

RESOURCES

- The ABCs of the Annual Wellness Visit. Available at www.cms.gov/Outreach-and-Education/Medicare-Learning-Network-MLN/MLNProducts/downloads/AWV_chart_ICN905706.pdf. (accessed Feb 2019)

- Gray-Miceli D. Impaired mobility and functional decline in older adults: Evidence to facilitate a practice change. *Nurs Clin North Am.* 2017;52(3):469–487.

- Schoenborn NL, Lee K, Pollack CE, et al. Older adults' views and communication preferences about cancer screening cessation. *JAMA Intern Med.* 2017;177(8):1121–1128.

- Scott J, Mayo AM. Instruments for detection and screening of cognitive impairment for older adults in primary care settings: A review. *Geriatr Nurs.* 2018;39(3):323–329.

CHAPTER 13—PHARMACOTHERAPY

KEY POINTS

- Risk factors associated with inappropriate prescribing and overprescribing include having more than one prescriber, poor record keeping, and using more than one pharmacy.

- Underprescribing of indicated medications for older adults is a bigger problem than the prescribing of inappropriate medications.

- Cardiovascular drugs, diuretics, NSAIDs, antidiabetics, second-generation antipsychotics, anticoagulants, and antiplatelet agents are the drug classes most often associated with preventable adverse drug events.

- Collaboration with pharmacists and access to up-to-date drug information can help to minimize the total number of medications and dosages prescribed for individual patients and to avoid important drug-drug and drug-disease interactions.

Adults ≥65 years old are prescribed the highest proportion of medications relative to their percentage of the U.S. population. Currently, approximately 14% of the U.S. population is ≥65 years old; this age group purchases 33% of all prescription drugs. These figures are expected to increase to 25% and 50%, respectively, by the year 2040.

Drugs are the most common treatment for acute and chronic diseases. They are also used to prevent many diseases and disorders experienced by older adults. Successful pharmacotherapy requires the correct medication at the correct dosage, for the correct disease or condition, for the correct patient. Unfortunately, achieving these goals is not simple or easy. Many other factors come into play, including the patient's other disease states, other medications, adherence, beliefs, functional status, physiologic changes due to aging and disease, and ability to afford the medication. The basic principle of prescribing for older patients—briefly, "start low, go slow"—is repeated often. However, even when this principle is adhered to, some patients will have negative outcomes from one or more of their medications.

Over the years, the principles of pharmacotherapy have not changed significantly; however, drug treatment has become much more complex. More medications are available every year, some with a new pharmacologic profile or mechanism of action. In addition, many available agents have expanded indications, some of which are approved by the FDA and some of which are off-label. Additional complicating factors include frequent changes in insurance formularies, scientific advances in the understanding of drug-drug interactions, the change of many medications from prescription to nonprescription, and the boom in an unregulated third class of medications called nutriceuticals, including nutritional supplements, complementary medicines, and herbal preparations. Finally, very little information is available about use of these unregulated medications in older adults, particularly in older patients with multiple comorbidities and on other medications.

AGE-ASSOCIATED CHANGES IN PHARMACOKINETICS

Pharmacokinetic studies define the time course of a drug and its metabolites throughout the body with respect to absorption, distribution, metabolism, and elimination. The usual effects of aging on each of these parameters should be incorporated into the principles of prescribing for older adults. (Table 13.1)

Absorption

Aging does not affect the extent of drug absorption via the GI tract to any clinically significant degree, although the rate of absorption may be slowed. Consequently, the peak serum concentration of a drug in older patients may be lower and the time to reach it delayed, but the overall amount absorbed *(bioavailability)* does not differ in younger and older patients.

Factors that have a greater impact on drug absorption include the way a medication is taken, what it is taken with, and a patient's comorbid illnesses. For example, the absorption of many fluoroquinolones (eg, ciprofloxacin) is reduced when they are taken with divalent cations such as calcium, magnesium, and iron, which are found in antacids, sucralfate, dairy products, or vitamins. Enteral feedings interfere with the absorption of some drugs (eg, levothyroxine, phenytoin). An increase in gastric pH from proton-pump inhibitors, H2 antagonists, or antacids can increase the absorption of some drugs, such as nifedipine and amoxicillin, and decrease the absorption of other drugs, such as the imidazole antifungals, ampicillin, cyanocobalamin, and calcium carbonate. Agents that promote or delay GI motility, such as stimulant laxatives and metoclopramide, can, in theory, affect a drug's absorption by increasing or decreasing the time spent in the segment of the GI tract necessary for dissolution or absorption. Another mechanism that can increase or decrease drug absorption is the inhibition or induction of enzymes in the GI tract (see drug interactions, below).

Table 13.1—Age-Associated Changes in Pharmacokinetics and Pharmacodynamics

Parameter	Age Effect	Disease Factor Effect	Prescribing Implications
Absorption	Rate and extent are usually unaffected	Achlorhydria, concurrent medications, tube feedings	Drug-drug and drug-food interactions are more likely to alter absorption
Distribution	Increase in fat:water ratio; decreased plasma protein, particularly albumin	Heart failure, ascites, and other conditions increase body water	Fat-soluble drugs have a larger volume of distribution; highly protein-bound drugs have a greater (active) free concentration
Metabolism	Decrease in liver mass and liver blood flow decrease drug clearance; may be age-related changes in CYP2C19, while CYP3A4 and 2D6 are not affected	Smoking, genotype, other medications, alcohol, and caffeine have more effect than aging on metabolism	Lower dosages may be therapeutic
Elimination	Primarily renal; age-related decrease in glomerular filtration rate	Acute and/or chronic kidney impairment, decreased muscle mass can result in misleadingly low serum creatinine (Cr) levels	Serum Cr not a reliable measure of kidney function; best to estimate Cr clearance using formula
Pharmacodynamics	Less predictable and often altered drug response at usual or lower concentrations	Drug-drug and drug-disease interactions may alter responses	Prolonged pain relief with opioids at lower dosages; more sedation and postural instability from benzodiazepines; altered sensitivity to β-blockers

More medications are being formulated into topical products such as gels or transdermal patches. Aging skin atrophies and becomes thinner, and blood flow to the dermal layer may be reduced. These factors may alter the systemic absorption from topical products.

Distribution

Distribution refers to the locations in the body a drug penetrates and the time required for the drug to reach those locations. Distribution is expressed as the volume of distribution (Vd), with units of volume (eg, liters) or volume per weight (eg, L/kg).

Age-associated changes in body composition can alter drug distribution. In older adults, drugs that are water soluble *(hydrophilic)* have a lower volume of distribution, because older adults have less body water and lean body mass. Digoxin, which distributes and binds to skeletal muscle, has been reported to have a reduced volume of distribution in older adults because of their reduced muscle mass. Drugs that are fat soluble *(lipophilic)* have an increased volume of distribution in older adults, because fat stores are greater in older than in younger people. Thus, in older adults, lipophilic drugs take longer to reach a steady-state concentration and longer to be eliminated from the body. Examples of fat-soluble drugs include diazepam, flurazepam, and trazodone.

The extent to which a drug is bound to plasma proteins also influences its volume of distribution. Albumin, the primary plasma protein to which drugs bind, is often decreased in older adults; thus, a higher proportion of drug is unbound (free) and pharmacologically active. Drugs that bind to albumin and that have an increased unbound fraction in older adults include ceftriaxone, diazepam, lorazepam, phenytoin, valproic acid, and warfarin. Normally, additional unbound drug is eliminated; however, age-related decreases in the organ systems of elimination can result in accumulation of unbound drug in the body. Phenytoin provides an example of the way an increase in unbound drug can lead to an unnecessary and potentially harmful dosage increase. A patient with a low serum albumin (≤3 g/dL) whose phenytoin dosage is increased because his or her total phenytoin concentration is subtherapeutic can develop symptoms and signs of phenytoin toxicity after a dosage increase, because the concentration of free phenytoin is increased.

Metabolism

The liver is the most common site of drug metabolism, but metabolic conversion also can occur in the intestinal wall, lungs, skin, kidneys, and other organs. Aging affects the liver by decreasing hepatic blood flow as well as by decreasing hepatic size and mass. Consequently, the metabolic clearance of drugs by the liver may be reduced in older adults. Drug clearance is also reduced with aging for drugs that are subject to the phase I pathways or reactions, which include hydroxylation, oxidation, dealkylation, and reduction. Most drugs metabolized through phase I pathways can be converted to metabolites of lesser, equal, or greater pharmacologic effect than the parent compound (eg, diazepam). Drugs metabolized through the phase II pathways are converted to inactive compounds through glucuronidation, conjugation, or acetylation (eg, lorazepam), which are not affected by aging. Medications subject to phase II metabolism are generally preferred for older adults, because their metabolites are not active and do not accumulate. Drugs that undergo an extensive first-pass effect (eg, nitrates) tend to have higher serum concentrations or increased bioavailability, because less drug is extracted by the liver as a consequence of decreased hepatic size and blood flow.

Age and gender differences also have been reported. Zolpidem's peak serum concentrations and exposure (area under the curve) have been reported to be 44.6% and 40.4% greater in older women, respectively, with only modest differences found between older and younger men.

In drug metabolism, factors other than aging can exaggerate or override the effects of aging. For example, hepatic congestion due to heart failure decreases the metabolism of warfarin, resulting in an increased pharmacologic response. Smoking stimulates monooxygenase enzymes and increases the clearance of theophylline, even in older adults.

Elimination

Elimination refers to a drug's final route(s) of exit from the body. For most drugs, this involves elimination by the kidneys as either the parent compound or as a metabolite(s). Terms used to express elimination are a drug's *half-life* and its *clearance*.

A drug's half-life is the time it takes for its plasma or serum concentration to decline by 50% (eg, from 20 mcg/mL to 10 mcg/mL). Half-life is usually expressed in hours. Steady state is reached when the amount of drug entering the systemic circulation is equal to the amount being eliminated. For a drug administered on a regular basis, 95% of steady state in the body is achieved after 5 half-lives of the drug.

Clearance is usually expressed as volume per unit of time (eg, L/h or mL/min) and represents the volume of plasma or serum from which the drug is removed (ie, cleared) per unit of time. Clearance can also be expressed as volume per weight per unit of time (L/kg/h). Half-life and clearance can also refer to metabolic elimination.

The effects of aging have been studied to a greater extent on kidney function than on liver function. Glomerular filtration declines as a consequence of a decrease in renal size and blood flow and a decrease in functioning nephrons. On average, kidney function begins to decline when people reach their mid-30s, with an average decline of 6–12 mL/min/1.73 m^2 per decade. Renal tubular secretion also declines with age. Frailty may be responsible for a fraction of reduced renal clearance of medication.

Serum creatinine is not an accurate reflection of creatinine clearance in older adults. Because of the age-related decline in lean muscle mass, production of creatinine is reduced in older adults. The decrease in glomerular filtration rate (GFR) counters the decreased production of creatinine, and serum creatinine stays within the normal range, not revealing the change in creatinine clearance.

The conservative approach in treating older adults is to calculate the appropriate dosage for renally eliminated medications as if the patient's kidney function actually has declined with aging. Measuring a patient's 24-hour creatinine clearance is the most accurate way to determine the appropriate dosage, but doing so is unrealistic because it requires an accurate 24-hour urine collection. An 8-hour urine collection time has been shown to be accurate but has not been widely accepted.

The Cockcroft-Gault equation (C-G) can be used to initially estimate a patient's creatinine clearance (CrCl) (SOE=B in older adults for dosage adjustment):

$$CrCl = \frac{(140 - age)(weight\ in\ kg)(0.85\ if\ female)}{72(stable\ serum\ creatinine\ in\ mg/dL)}$$

It is also important to consider that FDA-labeled dosing is based on the C-G estimated CrCl and the drug's pharmacokinetic characteristics. Therefore, substituting eGFR for estimated CrCl can potentially result in suboptimal dosing, especially in patients with stage 2 chronic kidney disease as their GFR approaches 60 mL/min/1.73 m^2.

In cases in which the patient's kidney function may be impaired but estimates of function are uncertain, the clinician should consider the following:

- Avoid drugs that depend entirely on renal elimination and for which accumulation would result in toxicity (eg, imipenem).

- If the use of such an agent cannot be avoided, directly measure kidney function (eg, an 8- or 24-hour urine collection for creatinine clearance).

- Monitor serum or plasma concentrations of the drug (eg, aminoglycosides, vancomycin).

AGE-ASSOCIATED CHANGES IN PHARMACODYNAMICS

The pharmacodynamic action of a drug, ie, its time course and intensity of pharmacologic effect, can change with increasing age. Older adults may have altered pharmacodynamics due to changes in receptor affinity or numbers, postreceptor alterations, and/or impairment of homeostatic mechanisms. An excellent example of such pharmacodynamic changes in older adults has been demonstrated with the benzodiazepines. For nitrazepam, an intermediate-acting benzodiazepine similar to lorazepam, the pharmacokinetics were found to be no different in young and older individuals after a single 10-mg dose; yet, 12 hours and 36 hours after a 10-mg dose, older adults made significantly more mistakes on a psychomotor test than when they had taken placebo. Even with short-term use, young older adults can experience impaired balance and posture after a single dose of a benzodiazepine (SOE=A).

It is uncertain whether the age-associated pharmacokinetic changes of morphine account for the increased level and prolonged duration of pain relief experienced by older adults. Morphine has a smaller volume of distribution, higher plasma concentrations, and longer clearance in older adults than in younger adults. Older adults experience pain relief at least equivalent to that experienced by younger patients at half the intramuscular dose, and the pain relief lasts longer. Thus, the dose or frequency, or both, of morphine given intramuscularly or by intravenous infusion should be lower, at least initially, in older adults.

Pharmacodynamic and pharmacokinetic changes, alone or together, generally result in an increased sensitivity to medications in older adults. In some patients, particularly those who are frail, the use of lower doses, longer intervals between doses, and longer periods between changes in dose are ways to successfully manage drug therapy and to decrease the chances of medication intolerance or toxicity. Disease- and drug-specific monitoring are also necessary to ensure a successful outcome.

OPTIMIZING PRESCRIBING

Optimizing drug therapy for older adults means achieving the balance between prescribing what is indicated to treat the patient's diseases and symptoms, while being consistent with the patient's goals and avoiding adverse effects. The term "potentially inappropriate medication" (PIM) is often used when discussing prescribing in older adults. Although there is no official definition, PIMs can be considered to be medications in which there is an unfavorable balance of risks and benefits either when used by themselves or when considering alternative available treatments. Polypharmacy is another term often used and can be defined as the use of more medications than is clinically indicated. The cut point is usually 5 or more medications at any one time. Overprescribing of drug therapies refers to the use of multiple medications coupled with a lack of appropriateness in medication selection, dosage, or use. In one survey, 40% of nursing-home residents had an order for at least one PIM. Analyses of national medication use surveys in the ambulatory setting have consistently shown that >30% of older adults received at least one PIM, with at least one PIM prescribed at approximately 8% of office visits. Furthermore, nearly 4% of office visits and 10% of medical hospital admissions resulted in a prescription for one or more medications classified as "never" or "rarely appropriate" for older adults. Identification of a PIM in a patient's regimen is a signal for additional prescribing problems with other medications not considered potentially inappropriate. The potential consequences of overprescribing include adverse drug events, drug-drug interactions, duplication of drug therapy, decreased quality of life, nonadherence, and unnecessary costs. Medications frequently deemed unnecessary based on lack of indication, lack of efficacy, or therapeutic duplication are often from the same

Table 13.2–Common Inappropriate/ Overprescribed and Underprescribed Medications or Classes

Inappropriate/Overprescribed
Androgens/testosterone
Anti-infective agents
Anticholinergic agents
Urinary and GI antispasmodics
Antipsychotics
Benzodiazepines and nonbenzodiazepine hypnotics (eg, zolpidem, zaleplon, eszopiclone)
Digoxin (not a first-line drug for atrial fibrillation or heart failure)
Dipyridamole
H_2-receptor antagonists
Fecal softeners
Insulin, sliding scale
NSAIDs
Proton-pump inhibitors
Sedating antihistamines (H_1-receptor antagonists, eg, diphenhydramine)
Skeletal muscle relaxants
Tricyclic antidepressants
Vitamins and minerals
Underprescribed
ACE inhibitors for patients with diabetes and proteinuria
Angiotensin-receptor blockers
Anticoagulants
Antihypertensives and diuretics as evidenced by uncontrolled hypertension
β-blockers for patients after myocardial infarction or with heart failure
Bronchodilators
Proton-pump inhibitors for GI protection from NSAIDs
Vitamin D and calcium for patients with or at risk of osteoporosis

Table 13.3—American Geriatrics Society Beers Criteria® for Non-Anti-Infective Medications That Should Be Avoided or Have Their Dosage Reduced in Older Adults with Chronic Kidney Disease

Medication Class and Medication	Creatinine Clearance (mL/min) at Which Action Is Required	Rationale	Recommendation
Cardiovascular or hemostasis			
Amiloride	<30	Increased potassium and decreased sodium	Avoid
Apixaban	<25	Increased risk of bleeding	Avoid
Dabigatran	<30	Increased risk of bleeding	Avoid
Edoxaban	30–50 <30 or >95	Increased risk of bleeding	Reduce dose Avoid
Enoxaparin	<30	Increased risk of bleeding	Reduce dose
Fondaparinux	<30	Increased risk of bleeding	Avoid
Rivaroxaban	30–50 <30	Increased risk of bleeding	Reduce dose Avoid
Spironolactone	<30	Increased potassium	Avoid
Triamterene	<30	Increased potassium and decreased sodium	Avoid
Central nervous system and analgesics			
Duloxetine	<30	Increased GI adverse effects (nausea, diarrhea)	Avoid
Gabapentin	<60	CNS adverse effects	Reduce dose
Levetiracetam	≤80	CNS adverse effects	Reduce dose
Pregabalin	<60	CNS adverse effects	Reduce dose
Tramadol	<30	CNS adverse effects	Immediate release: reduce dose Extended release: avoid
Gastrointestinal			
Cimetidine	<50	Mental status changes	Reduce dose
Famotidine	<50	Mental status changes	Reduce dose
Nizatidine	<50	Mental status changes	Reduce dose
Ranitidine	<50	Mental status changes	Reduce dose
Hyperuricemia			
Colchicine	<30	GI, neuromuscular, bone marrow toxicity	Reduce dose; monitor for adverse effects
Probenecid	<30	Loss of effectiveness	Avoid

medication classes as those considered inappropriate or overprescribed (Table 13.2).

Simply limiting the number of medications for a given patient is not always possible or desirable. For example, a patient with heart failure may be appropriately treated with 3 or 4 drugs: a diuretic, an ACE inhibitor, a β-blocker, and perhaps digoxin. If this patient has hyperlipidemia and diabetes mellitus, another 2 or 3 medications could be required. Hence, such a patient would be taking 5 to 7 indicated medications for major medical conditions alone.

One source to identify PIMs has been the American Geriatrics Society (AGS) Beers Criteria®. The intent of the AGS Beers Criteria® is to improve drug selection and reduce exposure to PIMs in older adults. Recommendations are evidence based and appear in 5 categories: drugs to avoid, drugs to avoid in patients with specific diseases or syndromes because the drug can worsen the disease or syndrome, drugs to use with caution, selected drugs whose dose should be adjusted based on kidney function (Table 13.3), and selected drug-drug interactions (DDIs) that have been associated with harmful outcomes in older adults. A detailed description of the AGS Beers Criteria® for potentially inappropriate medication use in older adults, including evidence tables, useful clinical tools, and patient education materials, is available at the GeriatricsCareOnline website (www.GeriatricsCareOnline.org).

The underprescribing of medications to older adults is also of concern. Underprescribing can result from an

Table 13.4—Risk Factors for Adverse Drug Events in Older Adults

- Age >85 years
- Low body weight or BMI
- Six or more concurrent chronic diagnoses
- An estimated CrCl <50 mL/min
- Nine or more medications
- Twelve or more doses of medications per day
- A prior adverse drug event

effort to avoid overprescribing, a complex medication regimen, or adverse events. It can also result from the thinking that older adults will not benefit from medications intended as primary or secondary prevention, or from aggressive management of chronic conditions, such as hypertension and diabetes mellitus. Medications to treat cardiovascular conditions (including hypertension, anticoagulants, and lipid-lowering agents), GI conditions, diabetes, osteoporosis, and COPD are commonly omitted. For other medications often cited as underprescribed in older adults, see Table 13.2.

ADVERSE DRUG EVENTS

An adverse drug event (ADE) is defined as an injury resulting from the use of a drug. Preventable ADEs are among the most serious consequences of inappropriate drug prescribing among older adults. An adverse drug reaction (ADR) is a type of ADE; it refers to harm that is directly caused by a drug at usual dosages. For a listing of risk factors for ADEs in older patients, see Table 13.4.

ADEs are estimated to be responsible for 5%–28% of acute geriatric medical admissions; the estimated annual incidence rate is 26 per 1,000 beds for hospitalized patients. One study estimated there were nearly 100,000 emergency hospitalizations of older adults for ADEs annually in the United States. Adults ≥80 years old accounted for 48% of hospitalizations. Two-thirds of hospitalizations were attributed to warfarin, oral antiplatelet agents, insulin, and oral hypoglycemic drugs. The most common type of ADE was an unintentional overdose (67%). Another study found that adults ≥65 years old made up 34.5% of emergency department visits for ADEs. Anticoagulants, antidiabetic agents, and opioid analgesics were implicated in 59.9% of these visits. It has been estimated that in the nursing home, for every dollar spent on medications, $1.33 in health care resources is consumed in the treatment of drug-related morbidity and mortality. A cohort study of all long-term care residents in 18 nursing homes in Massachusetts demonstrated that ADEs are common and often preventable in nursing homes. During 28,839 resident-months of observations, 546 ADEs were identified. Overall, 51% of these ADEs were judged to have been preventable. Most of the errors occurred at the ordering and monitoring stages. In a cohort study of residents of 2 long-term care facilities, the overall rate of ADEs was 9.8 per 100 resident-months. Second-generation antipsychotics, anticoagulants, and diuretics were the drug classes most frequently associated with ADEs.

In the ambulatory setting, the ADE rate has been reported to be 50.1 per 1,000 person-years, and the preventable ADE rate to be 13.8 per 1,000 person-years. Cardiovascular drugs, diuretics, NSAIDs, hypoglycemics, and anticoagulants are the drug classes found to be most often associated with preventable ADEs. Again, errors occurred most often at the time of prescribing or were related to inadequate monitoring. Most ADEs (≥95%) experienced by older adults are considered to be predictable.

A common pathway for ADEs and polypharmacy has been described as the "prescribing cascade." One form of this cascade occurs when a medication results in an ADE that is mistaken as a separate diagnosis and treated with more medications, which puts the patient at risk of additional ADEs and more medications. Examples that have been studied include metoclopramide-induced parkinsonism and the subsequent prescribing of antiparkinson medications, and calcium channel blockers that result in peripheral edema and subsequent use of diuretics.

DRUG-DRUG INTERACTIONS

A drug-drug interaction (DDI) is defined as the pharmacologic or clinical response to the administration of a drug combination that differs from that anticipated from the known effects of each of the two agents when given alone. DDIs can take many forms. For example, absorption can be altered, drugs with similar or opposite pharmacologic effects can result in exaggerated or decreased effects, and drug metabolism can be inhibited or induced. DDIs are important because they may lead to ADEs. The likelihood of DDIs increases as the number of medications a patient is taking increases. Among prescription drugs, cardiovascular and psychotropic drugs are most commonly involved in DDIs. A positive correlation exists between the number of potential DDIs and the number of adverse events experienced by hospitalized older patients. The most common adverse events are neuropsychologic (primarily delirium), arterial hypotension, and acute kidney injury. Risk factors associated with DDIs include the use of multiple medications, receiving care from several prescribing clinicians, and using more than one pharmacy.

Table 13.5—Principles of Prescribing for Older Adults

The basics:
- Start with a low dosage.
- Titrate the dosage upward slowly, as tolerated by the patient.
- Try not to start two medications at the same time.
- When necessary, consult a board-certified geriatric pharmacist

Determine the following before prescribing a new medication:
- Is the medication necessary? Are there nonpharmacologic ways to treat the condition?
- What are the therapeutic end points, and how will they be assessed?
- Do the benefits outweigh the risks of the medication?
- Is one medication being used to treat the adverse effects of another?
- Is there one medication that could be prescribed to treat two conditions?
- Are there potential drug-drug or drug-disease interactions?
- Will the new medication's administration times be the same as those of existing medications?
- Do the patient and caregiver understand what the medication is for, how to take it, how long to take it, when it should start to work, possible adverse effects that it might cause, and what to do if such effects occur?
- Can the patient afford the new medication?

At least annually:
- Ask the patient to bring all medications (prescription, OTC, supplements, and herbal preparations) to the office; for new patients, conduct a detailed medication history.
- For prescription medications, determine whether the label directions and dosage match those in the patient's chart; ask the patient how he or she is taking each medication.
- To assess refill adherence, call the patient's pharmacy.
- Ask about medication adverse effects.
- Note if other medications are being prescribed (by other health care providers) for the patient, and what the medications are and their indications.
- Look for medications with duplicate therapeutic, pharmacologic, or adverse effect profiles.
- Screen for drug-drug and drug-disease interactions.
- Eliminate unnecessary medications; confer with other prescribers if necessary.
- Simplify the medication regimen; use the fewest possible number of medications and doses per day.
- Always review any changes with the patient and caregiver; provide the changes in writing.

DRUG-DISEASE INTERACTIONS

Drug-disease combinations common in older adults can affect drug response and lead to ADEs, including exacerbation of existing conditions. Obesity and ascites alter the volumes of distribution of lipophilic and hydrophilic drugs, respectively. Patients with dementia can have increased sensitivity or paradoxical reactions to drugs with CNS or anticholinergic activity. Patients with renal insufficiency or impaired hepatic function due to cirrhosis or hepatic congestion have impaired detoxification and excretion of drugs.

ROLE OF THE PHARMACIST

In geriatric care, it is essential to include a pharmacist as part of the team. Since 1997, pharmacists have had the opportunity to become board certified in geriatric pharmacy and carry the designation BCGP. These pharmacists practice in a variety of settings, including nursing homes, hospitals, community pharmacies, and private practice. BCGP pharmacists can assist in designing appropriate medication regimens, including choice of medication, dose, dosage form, and in monitoring parameters. They can provide information on adverse events and drug interactions, assess adherence, and advise about cost issues. For a listing of BCGP pharmacists, see www.bpsweb.org or www.ascp.com/mpage/care_pharmacist.

PRINCIPLES OF PRESCRIBING

For principles of prescribing for older adults, see Table 13.5. This basic approach applies primarily to medications that are used to treat chronic conditions for which an immediate, complete therapeutic response is not necessary. Dosage adjustments may still be needed for medications used to treat conditions requiring an immediate response (eg, when prescribing antibiotics for a patient with impaired kidney function). Medications that have been newly approved by the FDA should be used cautiously in treating older adults. Such medications are likely to be more expensive, and information about their use in older adults is often limited.

Overprescribing can be prevented by reviewing a patient's medications on a regular basis and each time a new medication is started or a dosage is changed. A medication review or medication reconciliation should be done at each transition of care to ensure that appropriate medications and doses are continued, and unnecessary ones discontinued. The importance of maintaining accurate records of all medications taken by the patient cannot be overemphasized. Many patients do not consider topical agents (even prescription ones), vitamins, herbal preparations, or OTC medications (even aspirin) to be medications, so clinicians should be specific when inquiring about a patient's use of other medications. Patients should be encouraged to carry a complete, up-to-date list of their medications at all times.

It is best if the patient brings all medications to the review, including OTC medications, vitamins, and any herbal preparations or other types of supplements (a "brown-bag" evaluation). Examining the containers and labels and asking what each medication is for and how and when it is taken can provide insight into the patient's understanding and adherence to his or her medication regimens. Any medication for which there is no longer an indication for its continued use should be stopped. A new complaint or worsening of an existing condition should prompt consideration of whether or not it could be drug-induced.

Before prescribing a new medication or renewing a prescription, the clinician should consider the patient's life expectancy, time required to achieve therapeutic benefit, goal of treatment, and treatment targets.

DISCONTINUING MEDICATIONS

Discontinuing medications or de-prescribing is as complicated as starting a new medication, sharing many of the same tasks: recognizing an opportunity such as a care transition or annual review; planning; communicating and coordinating the change with the patient, caregiver, and other healthcare providers; and adequate monitoring and follow-up for withdrawal reactions, disease worsening, and adverse effects.

NONADHERENCE

Adherence is the extent that medication administration coincides with instructions. Nonadherence and poor adherence to medication regimens is a huge and often unrecognized problem. It is estimated that nonadherence among older adults may be as high as 50%. Patients may be reluctant to admit they are not taking medications or not following directions. Because there are many possible reasons for nonadherence, there is no simple screen. Predictors of nonadherence include asymptomatic disease, inadequate follow-up, patient's lack of insight or perception of the value of treatment, missed appointments and transportation difficulties, low literacy, complicated dosing regimens, and a poor provider–patient relationship. If nonadherence is suspected, clinicians should inquire about difficulties taking medication and adverse events; they should also ask (in a nonjudgmental manner) patients to review which medications they are taking and how they are taking them. Measuring a drug's serum concentration is one way to assess adherence, but assays are available for only a small percentage of medications. Measuring a physiologic or therapeutic response such as blood pressure, heart rate, intraocular pressure, hemoglobin A_{1c}, or a change in hormone concentration is possible for many medications to treat chronic conditions. Other measures include pill counts, calling the patient's pharmacy for a refill history, and confirmation by a caregiver. All these measures have limitations, and none is foolproof. The clinician needs to consider the patient's financial, cognitive, and functional status, as well as his or her beliefs about and understanding of medications and diseases. Clinicians should avoid prescribing expensive new medications that have not been shown to be superior to less expensive generic alternatives.

Medication reviews and counseling can be used to identify individual barriers, simplify regimens, and provide education. Telephone call reminders have demonstrated improved adherence in patients with heart failure or cognitive impairment. Reminder charts and calendars have been shown to be less effective. Interactive technology, such as automated pill dispensers, is available in some areas to supervise, remind, and monitor drug adherence.

Combination products, ie, those containing more than one medication, offer the advantages of decreased pill burden and increased adherence. Potential disadvantages include exposure to higher dosages than necessary, patients not recognizing that there is more than one medication in the product, and increased cost. Before starting a combination product, it needs to be determined that both medications are necessary and that the fixed doses in the product are appropriate for the patient.

Cognitive impairment can also cause nonadherence, because patients may forget to take medications or confuse them. Simplifying the regimen and involving a caregiver to oversee medication management can be helpful approaches. Weekly pill boxes or blister packs also can help with organization, and they are very useful for patients who have difficulty remembering when they last took a medication.

The older adults' ability to read labels, open containers, or pour medications or even a glass of water may be impaired, so functional assessment can be useful This is particularly true when prescribing inhalers or insulin. Older patients should be observed for proper technique in administering these medications. Some patients may need additional education or reinforcement about the purpose of a medication, especially those used to treat conditions that are usually asymptomatic, such as hypertension and diabetes mellitus. Older adults also may need reassurance regarding the safety and possible adverse events of certain medications, particularly newly prescribed medications or those associated with serious adverse events, such as anticoagulants.

CHOOSING WISELY® RECOMMENDATIONS

Pharmacotherapy

- Do not prescribe a medication without conducting a drug regimen review.

RESOURCES

- The 2019 American Geriatrics Society Beers Criteria® Update Expert Panel. The 2019 American Geriatrics Society Beers Criteria® for potentially inappropriate medication use in older adults. *J Am Geriatr Soc.* 2019. [Published online ahead of print Jan 2019]

- O'Mahoney D, O'Sullivan D, Byrne S, et al. STOPP/START criteria for potentially inappropriate prescribing in older people: version 2. *Age Ageing.* 2014;44(2):213–218.

- Thompson W, Lundby C, Graabaek T, et al. Tools for deprescribing in frail older persons and those with limited life expectancy: a systematic review. *J Am Geriatr Soc.* 2019;67(1):172–180.

CHAPTER 14—COMPLEMENTARY AND INTEGRATIVE MEDICINE

KEY POINTS

- The growing older population is increasing not only in numbers but also in diversity, and the next cohort of older adults is showing increasing acceptance and use of complementary and integrative medicine (CIM) treatments.

- There is a growing body of evidence to support the use of CIM, especially in terms of mind-body approaches, as well as natural supplements and products; however, high-quality research that includes older adults is needed to quantify the benefits and the risks.

The use of CIM among older adults is growing, as is evidence of its efficacy and effectiveness in chronic disorders. Both clinicians and the public need accurate information about evidence-based support for the use of diverse CIM practices. Many CIM therapies are not accessible to all older adults because of limitations of insurance reimbursement. In general, most natural products and supplements are not covered by insurance, although acupuncture can sometimes be covered with visit limitations. As the evidence for safety and efficacy accumulates, CIM may become a helpful option in management of multiple disorders associated with aging because of improved tolerability and adverse effect profile; nevertheless, a risk-benefit analysis must be done for each individual patient in choosing whether to add a CIM intervention.

The National Center for Complementary and Integrative Health (NCCIH) defines terms for CIM. Alternative medicine refers to a non-mainstream practice of medicine that is used in place of conventional medicine, whereas complementary medicine refers to non-mainstream practice that is used together with conventional medicine. Integrative medicine refers to use of conventional and complementary approaches in a coordinated way. Although evidence is growing for CIM practices, more evidence is still needed.

NCCIH has 3 categories for CIM:

- Natural products, including herbal medicines, botanicals, vitamins, minerals, probiotics, and other dietary supplements

- Mind and body practices, such as massage therapy, meditation, yoga, acupuncture, chiropractic/osteopathic manipulation, hypnotherapy, Tai Chi, qi gong, healing touch, and relaxation exercises

- Other complementary health approaches, including indigenous healing practices, Chinese medicine, Ayurvedic medicine, homeopathy, and naturopathy

Roughly 40% of U.S. adults had used at least one CIM therapy within the past year, thus spending billions of dollars out of pocket. A higher proportion of baby boomers used CIM (27.7%) than pre-boomers (16.4%). Those with stroke, cancer, obesity, breathing problems, and arthritis, are more likely to use herbal supplements.

SAFETY ISSUES

Patients rarely use alternative treatments exclusively. They often combine traditional medication with complementary approaches and, therefore, it is essential that health care providers ask about CIM to monitor for interactions between prescription medications and natural products and supplements as well as to evaluate the efficacy of treatments (Table 14.1). A growing body of evidence is showing that various mind-body interventions such as yoga and meditation demonstrate an improvement in neuroplasticity and resiliency, leading to the possibility of prevention of certain age-related diseases. Unfortunately, some older adults are still reluctant to disclose information regarding their CIM use to traditional providers, sometimes due to fear of being criticized and other times due to the belief that CIM treatments do not matter to traditional providers.

EFFICACY OF CIM

Osteoarthritis

Because of adverse effects, chronic opioid use and NSAIDs have limitations and constraints, which can necessitate alternative or adjunctive treatments for many older adults suffering from osteoarthritis (OA).

These treatments include chondroitin, a component of cartilage; curcumin, a compound found in the spice tumeric with anti-inflammatory and antioxidant properties (SOE=C); and S-adenosylmethionine (SAM-e), an amino acid metabolite that is a necessary precursor for multiple neuronal functions (SOE=B).

Low Back Pain

Acupuncture, spinal manipulation therapy (including muscle energy techniques) or massage, and herbal medicine are all used in treatment of lower back pain. Although the examined studies were of limited quality, acupuncture appeared to provide clinically meaningful

Table 14.1—Safety Issues Related to Natural Products and Supplements Used by Older Adults

Supplement	Adverse Effects	Interacts With
Cannabis	Drowsiness, dizziness, ataxia, dry mouth, headache, increased appetite, derealization, hallucinations, anxiogenesis	Potential induction or inhibition at high dosages of CYP450 2C19, 3A4, 2C9 isoenzymes
Coenzyme Q_{10}	Infrequent nausea, emesis, epigastric pain, headaches >300 mg/d linked to increased liver transaminases	Warfarin
Curcumin	Nausea, diarrhea, allergic skin reactions, increase calcium oxalate kidney stones	Anticoagulants, immunosuppressants, induction CYP3A4
Dehydroepiandrosterone (DHEA)	Women: weight gain, voice changes, facial hair, headaches Men: prostatic hyperplasia, possible increase in hormone-sensitive tumors	Calcium channel blockers, sildenafil
Echinacea	Allergic reactions, hepatitis, asthma, vertigo, anaphylaxis (rare)	Immunosuppressants
Ginkgo biloba	All rare: serious bleeding, seizures, headaches, dizziness, vertigo	Anticoagulants
Glucosamine	Nausea, diarrhea, heartburn	Hypoglycemic drugs (reduce effectiveness)
Melatonin	Daytime sleepiness, headache, dizziness	Anticoagulants, immunosuppressants, diabetes medications, birth control pills
Omega-3 fatty acids	Belching, halitosis, increased blood glucose	Antiplatelets, anticoagulants, antihypertensives
SAM-e (S-adenosyl-methionine)	Nausea, vomiting, diarrhea, anxiety, restlessness	Tricyclics, SSRIs
Saw palmetto	All rare: constipation, diarrhea, decreased libido, headaches, hypertension, urine retention	Anticoagulants
St. John's wort	Nausea, allergic reactions, dizziness, headache, photosensitivity (rare)	Anticoagulants, antivirals, SSRIs

and significant reduction in self-reported chronic pain when compared with sham acupuncture and improved function when compared with no treatment (SOE=B). Reduction of acute lower back pain with acupuncture is more inconsistent (SOE=B). RCTs using spinal manipulation therapy and massage have been of low quality and have produced little evidence to support these modalities.

A Cochrane collaborative review found that topical *Capsicum frutescens* (cayenne) probably reduces chronic lower back pain better than placebo (SOE=B). This review also reported that, although study quality was limited, short-term pain improvements were found for orally administered *Harpagophytum procumbens* (devil's claw), *Salix alba* (white willow bark), and topical *Symphytom officinale L.* (comfrey root extract) (SOE=C). These herbal remedies were well tolerated with reported adverse effects being mild GI upset or skin irritations.

Cardiovascular Disorders

Because of the high prevalence of cardiovascular disease in the U.S. population, CIM interventions for hypertension are important to evaluate. The most abundant and effective interventions have been diet and exercise, including the Mediterranean diet, which includes unsaturated fats (such as olive oil), whole grains, and fruits and vegetables, as well as the DASH diet (Dietary Approaches to Stop Hypertension).

Physical activity such as exercise and mind-body interventions have also shown promise for cardiovascular disease. A large study of >5,000 individuals of mixed ages with coronary heart disease showed that physical activity improved survival. Furthermore, for patients suffering from congestive heart failure (CHF) (New York Heart Association class III or IV), aerobic exercise improved survival and minimized subsequent hospitalizations secondary to CHF. However, excessive exercise (running >7.1 miles/day or walking briskly for >10.7 km/day) has been shown to increase mortality.

In a Cochrane database review that included 6 RCTs and >500 participants, horse chestnut seed improved symptoms of leg pain, edema, and pruritus associated with chronic venous insufficiency. Because horse chestnut has anticoagulant effects, monitoring for excessive bleeding is essential. Alternatively, a Cochrane database review that examined 14 RCTs showed that hawthorn extract could be used as an adjunctive treatment for CHF, because it improved exercise tolerance. In an RCT, coenzyme Q10 (CoQ10), also called ubiquinone, demonstrated some improvement in hypertension, at a dosage of 60 mg twice daily; the average reduction in systolic blood pressure was 17.8 ± 7.3 mmHg.

Consumption of fatty fish in the diet, is thought to reduce cardiovascular disease. Furthermore, the consumption of omega-3 fatty acids has demonstrated improvements in outcomes.

Benign Prostatic Hyperplasia

In recent decades, men in the United States have been using saw palmetto to self-treat benign prostatic hyperplasia, resulting in it becoming the fifth leading medicinal herb consumed in the United States. A review of randomized controlled trials comparing saw palmetto to placebo or other conventional medications found no evidence of efficacy. Other supplements (eg, *Hypoxis rooperi*, stinging nettle, pumpkin seed extracts, rye pollen, African plum) have been studied but need more rigorous scientific investigation. The American and European Associations of Urology do not currently recommend plant extracts in treatment of benign prostatic hyperplasia.

Psychiatric Disorders

In addition, or sometimes as an alternative, to prescription antidepressant medications, many older adults look to natural products and supplements to alleviate their mental suffering. Studies have revealed some benefit for mild to moderate depression; however, for more severe forms of depression, a more traditional approach to pharmacotherapy or electroconvulsive therapy is generally recommended.

Hypericum perforatum, also referred to as St. John's wort, has been demonstrated in general adult populations to be more effective than placebo and as effective as antidepressants in the treatment of mild to moderate depression (SOE=A). However, few studies have evaluated the effect and safety of St. John's wort in older adults (SOE=C) such as the potential drug-drug interactions with St. John's wort and warfarin, methadone, cyclosporine, and tacrolimus, thereby possibly reducing the efficacy of these important therapeutic drugs.

Multiple studies using various formulations of SAM-e have demonstrated efficacy in treating depression and showed comparable effects to traditional antidepressants. Many of the studies include mixed-age populations but not exclusively older adults. SAM-e is also used to treat depression in Parkinson disease patients treated with levodopa; however, it can still contribute to GI adverse effects and serotonin syndrome.

Omega-3 fatty acids have been implicated in depression; however, they show benefits as augmentation strategies with traditional antidepressants in dosages ranging from 1,000–2,000 mg (SOE=C).

Mind-body interventions are a growing alternative to treating depression and anxiety disorders. One meta-analysis demonstrated positive outcomes of Tai-Chi on overall psychological well-being, but there were insufficient studies to assess the effect of Tai-Chi on clinical depression.

Neurocognitive Disorders

Mild Cognitive Impairment

Yoga has been shown to benefit patients with neurocognitive disorders, especially when used with traditional approaches such as memory enhancement training in terms of verbal memory and showed evidence of neuronal changes on MRI.

Both *Ginkgo biloba* and huperzine may have beneficial effects on cognition in older adults.

Alzheimer Disease

Taking an integrative approach for both the patient and the caregiver, such as recommending a mind-body intervention, can improve outcomes for both parties. Various studies have been conducted regarding mind-body interventions, such as yoga, Tai Chi, and various types of meditation, that have revealed improvements regarding cognitive decline. Furthermore, yogic meditation was associated with increase in telomerase activity, representing a reduction in cellular aging. Furthermore, yoga has been successfully adapted for use by older populations. Nevertheless, studies have a low-strength of evidence (SOE=C) for mind-body interventions in preventing cognitive decline in Alzheimer disease. Generally, physical activity, diet, and cognitive training are more effective.

The consumption of green tea has been linked with cognitive-enhancing effects; thus, consumption of green tea has been recommended to prevent development of dementia (SOE=C).

Ginkgo biloba has demonstrated some improvement in subjective memory complaints.

There is no definitive evidence for coconut oil or a derivate of coconut oil, a medium-chain triglyceride, as a medical food for treating AD.

Sleep Disorders

When insomnia is a primary disorder, or the concurrent disorder has been treated and the insomnia persists, alternative treatments such as melatonin or valerian root may be helpful. Tai chi has demonstrated improvements in sleep quality, fatigue, and depressive symptoms compared with the control group, which received education only; however cognitive-behavioral therapy outperformed both the control and Tai Chi groups in all areas, including a reduction in chronic inflammation often associated with insomnia.

Cancer

In particular, the most commonly offered therapies included acupuncture, massage, meditation, yoga, nutrition, dietary supplements, and herbs.

Cancer CIM therapies purportedly can be used to strengthen the body's innate immune systems as well as to manage the adverse effects of conventional treatments, such as chemotherapy and radiation. One of the most important benefits for many cancer patients who use CIM modalities is the experience of being more empowered while dealing with the challenges of cancer.

Biologic agents, herbal preparations, and vitamins have all been tried by patients; however, most of these modalities have not undergone much scientific study. In contrast, lifestyle changes, including exercise and stress management techniques, have helped manage mood and energy changes associated with breast cancer.

Prostate cancer usually develops slowly in older men, and CIM use in combination with conventional treatment has been reported to reduce associated discomforts and improve the quality of life.

Dietary changes as well as mind-body interventions may assist patients with lung cancer to manage emotional distress and the adverse effects of treatment. Cancer patients using relaxation and stress-management techniques have been able to manage cravings when pursuing tobacco cessation. These mind-body techniques are also effective in managing the emotional and physical distress associated with both diagnosis and the adverse effects of treatment.

Currently, no herbal preparations or botanical supplements appear to be useful in prevention or management of colon cancer.

MEDICAL CANNABIS AND CANNABINOIDS

The medicinal use of marijuana (*Cannabis sativa*) is allowed by law in 29 states as well as the District of Columbia, Puerto Rico and Guam; 8 states have legalized recreational marijuana use.

Marijuana exerts its psychoactive and therapeutic effects through cannabinoids, which act predominantly on receptors in the CNS. Two synthetic cannabinoids (dronabinol and nabilone) are FDA approved for treatment of chemotherapy-induced nausea and vomiting that has not responded to other antiemetics. Dronabinol has an additional indication for AIDS-related anorexia and weight loss. Studies of herbal cannabis and cannabinoids have demonstrated effectiveness in treatment of chronic pain, neuropathic pain, and spasticity caused by multiple sclerosis (SOE=A).

Marijuana use is prevalent in patients with psychiatric disorders. Although marijuana use is prevalent among individuals suffering from mental illness and some studies show some potential benefit, marijuana is not without potential adverse effects, and patients should be educated by health care professionals.

However, most studies to date have included very few older adults, limiting the ability to generalize findings to the geriatric population. Especially pertinent to older adults is the analgesic effect of marijuana (SOE=A) without the risk of respiratory depression; however, there is significant risk of increased falls and altered cognition and motor performance, including during driving tasks. Furthermore, the dosing of medical marijuana for analgesia is still unclear. Therefore, similar to other natural products and supplements, medical cannabis must be used with caution.

RESOURCES

- Groden S, Woodward AT, Chatters LM, et al. Use of complementary and alternative medicine among older adults: differences between baby boomers and pre-boomers. *Am J Geriatr Psychiatry*. 2017;25(12):1393–1401.

- McFeeters S, Pront L, Cuthbertson L, et al. Massage, a complementary therapy effectively promoting the health and well-being of older people in residential care settings: a review of the literature. *Int J Older People Nurs*. 2016;11(4):266–283.

- National Academy of Sciences. The health effects of cannabis and cannabinoids: the current state of the evidence and recommendations for research. Washington DC: National Academy of Sciences; 2017.

CHAPTER 15—MISTREATMENT

KEY POINTS

- Elder mistreatment is a common phenomenon that has serious medical and social consequences, but it is dramatically underrecognized by clinicians and often not reported to authorities.

- Mistreatment affects as many as 10% of community-dwelling older adults and includes physical abuse, sexual abuse, neglect, psychological/emotional abuse, and financial exploitation.

- Although some presentations of elder mistreatment are dramatic on cursory evaluation, mantypes of mistreatmenuire a high index of suspicion and careful assessment. Implementing formal screening protocols may be valuable.

- Clinical assessment should include observation of patient-caregiver interactions, obtaining history from the patient alone, and head-to-toe physical examination. When available, laboratory and imaging tests may be helpful.

- When concerned about elder mistreatment, clinicians should ensure a patient's immediate safety, document findings in detail, and report to the appropriate authorities. Clinicians should know how to access and be familiar with the role and duties of Adult Protective Services and long-term care ombudsman in their local area.

Elder mistreatment is a common phenomenon that has serious medical and social consequences, and clinicians may play a critical role in identifying it and initiating intervention. Although no universally accepted definition of mistreatment exists, the definition proposed by the 2014 Elder Justice Roadmap, a report prepared by a large, multidisciplinary team of stakeholders inside and outside the U.S. government, captures current understanding of the phenomenon as "physical, sexual, or psychological abuse, as well as neglect, abandonment, and financial exploitation of an older person by another person or entity that occurs in any setting (eg, home, community, or facility) either in a relationship where there is an expectation of trust and/or when an older person is targeted based on age or disability." Table 15.1 defines and provides examples of types of mistreatment. Unfortunately, many victims suffer from multiple types of mistreatment.

As many as 10% of community-dwelling older adults suffer from abuse, neglect, or exploitation each year. Rates among nursing-home residents are even higher, with research suggesting >20%. Neglect, psychological abuse, and financial exploitation occur more frequently, while physical and sexual abuse are less common. This mistreatment can have serious medical consequences, leading to increases in exacerbations of chronic illness, depression, and significantly higher mortality. In a pooled logistic regression analysis that adjusted for demographics, chronic disease, functional status, social networks, cognitive status, and depressive symptoms, the risk of death remained higher for cohort members experiencing mistreatment or self-neglect (SOE=A). Victims of mistreatment are more likely than other older adults to present to the emergency department, be hospitalized, and need nursing-home placement. The direct medical cost of elder mistreatment is many billions of dollars, which will likely increase substantially as the geriatric population grows.

Unfortunately, elder mistreatment is infrequently detected, with as few as 1 in 24 cases reported to the authorities. A medical office visit might be the only time that a mistreated older adult ever leaves his or her home. For clinicians who perform house calls, the in-home evaluation allows for an even more comprehensive assessment for mistreatment. Despite this, clinicians very seldom identify or report elder mistreatment. This is likely because of many factors, including: inadequate training, lack of time to conduct a complete evaluation, and desire to avoid involvement in the legal system. Also, although some presentations of elder mistreatment are dramatic on cursory evaluation, many are subtle and require a high index of suspicion and careful assessment. Patients may have a variety of chief complaints and findings may be nonspecific. The victim may be unable or unwilling to report the mistreatment, and the perpetrator may be with the patient, actively trying to avoid detection.

RISK FACTORS

Familiarity with the risk factors (Table 15.2) for victims and perpetrators of elder mistreatment may be helpful in clinical assessment (SOE=B). Particularly strong risk factors are cognitive impairment and functional dependence or disability. Frail, debilitated older adults may need a level of care that at times exceeds caregiver ability. In particular, the person with dementia who exhibits disturbing behaviors (eg, hitting, spitting, screaming) poses immense challenges to caregivers. While caregiver stress does not excuse abusive behavior, it may contribute to emotional volatility or impaired judgment. A careful assessment of caregiver stress may identify opportunities for prevention of mistreatment.

Table 15.1—Types of Elder Abuse and Neglect

Type	Definition	Examples
Physical abuse	Intentional use of physical force that may result in bodily injury, physical pain, or impairment	■ Slapping, hitting, kicking, pushing, pulling hair ■ Use of physical restraints, force-feeding ■ Burning, use of household objects as weapons, use of firearms and knives
Sexual abuse	Any type of sexual contact with an older adult that is not consensual, or sexual contact with any person incapable of giving consent	■ Sexual assault or battery, such as rape, sodomy, coerced nudity, and sexually explicit photographing ■ Unwanted touching, verbal sexual advances ■ Indecent exposure
Neglect	Refusal or failure to fulfill any part of a person's obligations or duties to an older adult that may result in harm (may be intentional or unintentional)	■ Withholding of food, water, clothing, shelter, medications ■ Failure to ensure older adult's personal hygiene or to provide physical aids, including walker, cane, glasses, hearing aids, dentures ■ Failure to ensure older adult's personal safety and/or appropriate medical follow-up
Emotional/psychological abuse	Intentional infliction of anguish, pain, or distress through verbal or nonverbal acts	■ Verbal berating, harassment, or intimidation ■ Threats of punishment or deprivation ■ Treating the older adult like an infant ■ Isolating the older adult from others
Financial/material exploitation	Illegal or improper use of an older adult's money, property, or assets	■ Stealing money or belongings ■ Cashing an older adult's checks without permission and/or forging his or her signature ■ Coercing an older adult into signing contracts, changing a will, or assigning durable power of attorney against his or her wishes or when the older adult does not possess the mental capacity to do so

Adapted from National Center on Elder Abuse. Types of abuse. Available at: https://ncea.acl.gov/faq/abusetypes.html (accessed Feb 2019).

Additionally, some risk factors may actually be proxies for other variables. For example, lower socioeconomic status is often associated with fewer resources to meet caregiving demands; mistreatment may be as high as 47.3% in this group. Recently, it has been suggested that subpopulations of older adults, including military veterans and lesbian/gay/bisexual/transgender older adults may be at higher risk (SOE=C), but additional research is needed to confirm this.

SCREENING

Given the frequency and serious consequences of elder mistreatment, routine screening within primary care may be appropriate for older adults.

Several elder abuse screening instruments exist, but many are not applicable to all clinical environments, and few have been validated. The Elder Abuse Suspicion Index (EASI) (www.mcgill.ca/familymed/research/projects/elder [accessed Feb 2019]) is a short instrument that has been validated for cognitively intact patients in primary care settings with a sensitivity of 0.47 and a specificity of 0.75. The EASI tool identifies older adults at risk of mistreatment and includes 5 questions for the patient and 1 for the clinician, with 1 or more "yes" responses suggesting the need for further assessment.

OBSERVATION

Observations of interactions between an older adult and others, particularly caregivers, may offer important clues about the presence of or potential for mistreatment (Table 15.3). If the patient is accompanied by others, clinicians should carefully observe these interactions, looking for any suggestions of a strained relationship.

HISTORY

Obtaining a comprehensive medical and social history is critical to assess for elder mistreatment. For elements from the history that may suggest the possibility of mistreatment, see Table 15.4.

Many victims are reluctant to report abuse or neglect because of guilt, shame, or fear (eg, of loss of independence or reprisal). Whenever possible, the older adult should be interviewed alone so that he or she can speak freely and frankly. If responses indicate that mistreatment may be occurring, progressively focused follow-up questions are indicated. For example, the clinician might first ask, "Is there any difficult behavior in your family you would like to tell me about?" If the answer is positive, possible questions to follow include the following: "Has anyone tried to hurt or hit you?" "Has anyone made you do things that you did not want

Table 15.2—Potential Risk Factors for Elder Abuse

For becoming a victim
- Functional dependence or disability
- Poor physical health
- Cognitive impairment/dementia
- Poor mental health
- Low income/socioeconomic status
- Social isolation/low social support
- Previous history of family violence
- Previous traumatic event exposure
- Substance abuse

For becoming a perpetrator
- Mental illness
- Substance abuse
- Caregiver stress
- Previous history of family violence
- Financial dependence on older adult

SOURCES:

Acierno R, Hernandez MA, Amstadter AB, et al. Prevalence and correlates of emotional, physical, sexual, and financial abuse and potential neglect in the United States: the National Elder Mistreatment Study. *Am J Public Health*. 2010;100:292–297.

Amstadter AB, Zajac K, Strachan M, et al. Prevalence and correlates of elder mistreatment in South Carolina: the South Carolina elder mistreatment study. *J Interpers Violence*. 2011;26:2947–2972.

Laumann EO, Leitsch SA, Waite LJ. Elder mistreatment in the United States: prevalence estimates from a nationally representative study. *J Gerontol B Psychol Sci Soc Sci*. 2008;63:S248–S54.

Pillemer K, Burnes D, Riffin C, et al. Elder Abuse: Background Paper for the World Report on Ageing and Health, 2015.

Table 15.3—Observations from Older Adult/Caregiver Interactions that Should Raise Concern for Elder Mistreatment

- Older adult and caregiver provide conflicting accounts of events
- Caregiver interrupts/answers for the older adult
- Older adult seems fearful of or hostile toward caregiver
- Caregiver appears unengaged/inattentive in caring for older adult
- Caregiver appear frustrated, tired, angry, or burdened by older adult
- Caregiver appears overwhelmed by older adult
- Caregiver appears to lack knowledge of older adult's care needs
- Evidence that caregiver and/or older adult may be abusing alcohol or illicit drugs

Table 15.4—Indicators from the Medical History of Possible Elder Abuse or Neglect

- Unexplained injuries
- Past history of frequent injuries
- Older patient referred to as "accident prone"
- Delay between onset of medical illness or injury and seeking medical attention
- Recurrent visits to the emergency department for similar injuries
- Using multiple clinicians and emergency departments for care rather than one primary care provider ("doctor hopping or shopping")
- Noncompliance with medications, appointments, or clinician directions

---

to do?" "Has anyone taken your things?" Obtaining such information requires sensitive clinical interviewing skills similar to those needed when asking about sexual orientation, alcoholism, or substance abuse.

Obtaining a reliable mistreatment history from older adults with cognitive impairment may be difficult. Clinicians should still try to interview these patients as they would others, because research has shown that older adults with dementia who are victims of crime have the ability, in certain circumstances, to provide testimony about criminal events, such as the etiology of bruises or other injuries (SOE=B). Although comprehensive investigation of cases is typically the responsibility of law enforcement and protective services, health care providers should consider seeking collateral from other sources besides caregivers (eg, other family members, neighbors, visiting nurses) when it will impact clinical decision-making or immediate safety.

Studies suggest that abuse and neglect may be defined very differently within different cultures of racial and ethnic groups; thus, cultural sensitivity is important. The older adult or caregiver from a culture different than the clinician's may be offended by some mistreatment screening questions; wording questions carefully can avoid alienating the older adult or caregiver, which could abolish any further opportunity to help the patient and family.

Private interviews with caregivers can detect not only abusive or neglectful behavior but also signs of stress, isolation, or depression in the caregiver. Caregivers may be reluctant to discuss their own problems in the presence of the older adult who depends on their care. Given the relevance for the health and care of the older adult, providers may consider conducting these interviews regardless of whether the caregiver is also the provider's patient. Providers may counsel and offer resources to overwhelmed or stressed caregivers.

Because caregivers can range from registered professionals to well-intended neighbors, it is important to know and document the caregiver's skill level, as well as his or her understanding of the situation. The latter is an essential factor in evaluating the underlying intention of any mistreatment of a dependent older adult. For example, a registered nurse in a nursing home is held to a different level of accountability than a frail spouse providing care in the home setting. Also, neglect may be active, in which a caregiver intentionally withholds basic necessities,

Table 15.5—Physical Signs Suspicious for Potential Elder Mistreatment

Physical Abuse

- Bruising in atypical locations (not over bony prominences/on lateral arms, back, face, ears, or neck)
- Patterned injuries (bite marks or injury consistent with the shape of a belt buckle, fingertip, or other object)
- Wrist or ankle lesions or scars (suggesting inappropriate restraint)
- Burns (particularly stocking/glove pattern suggesting forced immersion or cigarette pattern)
- Multiple fractures or bruises of different ages
- Traumatic alopecia or scalp hematomas
- Subconjunctival, vitreous, or retinal ophthalmic hemorrhages
- Intraoral soft-tissue injuries

Sexual Abuse

- Genital, rectal, or oral trauma (including erythema, bruising, lacerations)
- Evidence of sexually transmitted disease
- Neglect
- Cachexia/malnutrition
- Dehydration
- Pressure injuries/ulcerss
- Poor body hygiene, unchanged diaper
- Dirty, severely worn clothing
- Elongated toenails
- Poor oral hygiene

SOURCES:

Chang AL, Wong JW, Endo JO, et al. Geriatric dermatology: Part II. Risk factors and cutaneous signs of elder mistreatment for the dermatologist. *J Am Acad Dermatol*. 2013;68:533 e1–10.

Collins KA. Elder maltreatment: a review. *Arch Pathol Lab Med*. 2006;130:1290–1296.

Gibbs LM. Understanding the medical markers of elder abuse and neglect: physical examination findings. *Clin Geriatr Med*. 2014;30:687–712.

Palmer M, Brodell RT, Mostow EN. Elder abuse: dermatologic clues and critical solutions. *J Am Acad Dermatol*. 2013;68:e37–42.

or passive, in which a caregiver with good intentions neglects an older adult because of inadequate caregiving skills, experience, or resources.

Identification of shortcomings in the older adult's care can be the most elusive aspect of a comprehensive assessment. The symptoms and signs of incomplete, inadequate, or neglectful caregiving can be subtle (eg, when an older adult does not do as well as expected on a given regimen) or attributable to the older adult's physical or emotional disorders (eg, weight loss in an older adult with a history of depression). Effective assessment detects mistreatment without placing undue suspicion on well-meaning caregivers or undermining a family's ability to care for an older adult with appropriate support and counseling. (Some caregivers, it should be recognized, can be both well meaning and abusive or neglectful.)

ASSESSMENT

Physical Examination

Performing a complete head-to-toe physical examination is critical in evaluation for mistreatment. Physical findings suspicious for physical abuse, sexual abuse, and neglect are shown in Table 15.5, and the presence of more than one suggestive finding should raise a provider's index of suspicion. Clinicians should focus on a full skin examination, including fingernails and toenails as well as intra-oral examination.

When assessing older adults who have sustained injuries, clinicians should always consider whether the physical findings are consistent with the reported injury mechanism. A patient sustaining more than three upper rib fractures after rolling off a bed 2 feet above the ground should raise suspicion. However, differentiating between intentional and unintentional injuries, such as fall-related contusions or fractures, may be challenging. Researchers have begun to identify differences that may assist clinicians (SOE=B). In one study, bruises from physical abuse were often large (>5 cm) and found on the face, lateral right arm, or posterior torso. In other studies, physical abuse and assault-related injuries were most commonly found on the head, neck, and upper extremities. Recent research suggests that injuries to the left cheek/zygoma, neck, and ulnar forearm may be much more common in abuse than accident.

When sexual abuse is reported or suspected, particularly if evidence of trauma or vaginal bleeding is found on genitourinary examination, clinicians should consider sending the patient to the emergency department for a comprehensive sexual assault evaluation, which may include evidence collection by a trained sexual assault forensic examiner.

The emergency department is an important setting for assessment of mistreatment. Emergency department personnel may see older adults in crisis, and every effort should be made not to simply treat and release patients whose domestic situation merits further assessment. Astute emergency personnel can identify cases in which there may be serious safety problems in the caregiving situation.

Laboratory Testing

Laboratory tests cannot definitively diagnose or exclude elder mistreatment, but specific findings may increase concern. Anemia, dehydration, malnutrition, hypo- or hyperthermia, and rhabdomyolysis all have possible alternative explanations but may suggest neglect. Multiple abnormal findings should arouse more suspicion than a single one. Prescription medication and illicit drug levels may also be useful. Low levels of medications prescribed to the patient may indicate intentional or unintentional withholding by a caregiver, with diversion of narcotic pain medications a particular concern. Increased levels of prescribed drugs may indicate intentional or unintentional overdose, and the presence of toxins or drugs not prescribed raises the potential for poisoning.

Imaging Studies

Co-occurring old and new fractures, fractures with a radiologic appearance inconsistent with the explanation offered for the injury, distal ulnar diaphyseal fractures, and small-bowel hematomas should increase suspicion of elder mistreatment (SOE=C). If concern for elder mistreatment exists, the clinician should communicate this to the radiologist and ask him or her to focus on whether imaging findings are consistent with the purported mechanism. Clinicians may also consider additional screening imaging tests, including maxillofacial CT scan and chest radiograph, to evaluate for acute and chronic fractures, analogous to the skeletal survey routinely performed for potential child abuse victims.

Psychological Assessment

Mistreatment can be more than corporal. Psychological abuse or neglect is generally more difficult than physical abuse to detect and confirm, but it can be equally dangerous to the mistreated older adult. The behavior of both the older adult and the caregiver can provide important clues about the quality of their relationship and of the care the older adult is receiving. Factors that suggest a poor or deteriorating social and emotional situation are an important focus of assessment for mistreatment.

Psychological abuse includes threats, taunting, name-calling, promoting regressive behaviors by infantilization, making painful jokes at the expense of the older adult, or other demeaning activities, such as making fun of an older adult for needing to "wear diapers" or teasing an older adult for enjoying daytime television. The caregiver's style of communication can provide important clues. Impatience, irritability, and demeaning statements may indicate a pattern of verbal abuse. However, psychological neglect or mistreatment by the caregiver can also take more subtle forms. For example, not providing social or emotional stimulation, or restricting or preventing normal activities can result in total social isolation of the older adult.

The older adult's demeanor and emotional status can suggest the presence of psychological neglect or abuse. For example, ambivalence or high levels of anxiety, fearfulness, or anger toward the caregiver indicate the need for further assessment. Unexpected depression (ie, no obvious pathophysiologic or psychological reason for new onset, such as death in family) or uncharacteristic withdrawal also merits follow-up. Other behaviors that may indicate neglect include lack of adherence with treatment recommendations, frequent requests for sedating medication, or frequently canceled appointments.

Changes in cognitive function or mood may be psychological manifestations of abuse. Cognitive impairment, dementia, and depression are prevalent in older adults referred for evaluation for possible mistreatment. It is therefore appropriate to check any older adult presenting with cognitive impairment, dementia, or depression for symptoms and signs of neglect or mistreatment. Aggressive behaviors associated with dementia can trigger abusive responses in caregivers.

Assessment of Financial Situation

Financial exploitation includes unauthorized use of the older adult's funds, possessions, or property. This exploitation is estimated to have a prevalence of 5.2%. Often, financial exploitation is associated with neglect, when a family member or other caregiver fails to use an older adult's funds and resources to provide for his or her needs. Signs that an older adult is being mistreated financially include the following (SOE=C):

- A recent marked disparity between the older adult's living conditions or appearance and his or her assets
- A sudden inability to pay for health care or basic needs
- An unusual interest on the part of caregivers in the older adult's assets
- The sudden acquisition of expensive possessions by a caregiver who has apparently limited financial assets
- Unwillingness of a caregiver to allow access to the home of an older adult

Encouragingly, banks and other financial institutions have increased efforts to prevent fraud and other financial exploitation of older adults and to identify it and intervene when it occurs. These include developing programs to search for suspicious activity in older adults' accounts, training bank employees, and educating older consumers. Providers concerned about financial exploitation should report to protective services and potentially also to law enforcement. Additional resources include the Consumer Financial Protection Bureau (http://consumerfinance.gov), the Federal Trade Commission's Bureau of Consumer Protection (www.ftc.gov/bcp/index.shtml), and the Elder Financial Protection Network (www.elderfinancialprotection.org/).

Self-Neglect

For some older adults, especially those who live in isolation or who choose (assuming they have the capacity to choose) to endure mistreatment, self-neglect may become an issue. Self-neglect occurs when an older adult's health or safety is threatened because he or she does not perform or refuses assistance with essential self-care. Self-neglecting behaviors include not eating, not taking necessary medications, not attending to personal hygiene, not maintaining a safe home environment, and hoarding. Patients with self-neglect frequently have cognitive impairment and may also suffer from other mental disorder(s), including depression, psychosis, and substance abuse disorders. As a result, they may not appreciate that their health and safety are at risk.

Reports of self-neglect to social services are increasingly common and exceed reports of mistreatment by others. Lower levels of social network and social engagement are risk factors for self-neglect. Further, self-neglect is associated with an increased rate of 30-day hospital readmissions and increased mortality.

Clinicians may play an important role in identifying self-neglect. Self-neglect is similar to other types of elder mistreatment in that the older adult often has limited contact outside the home other than with a medical provider. Whenever possible, evaluating the patients' home environment may offer clues to this diagnosis and increase concern. Clinicians making a house call may note an empty refrigerator, expired pill bottles, extreme clutter, broken windows, extreme heat or cold, or vermin infestation.

Successful management in such cases requires an assessment of the older adult's capacity to understand the risks and benefits of the situation, as well as the consequences of allowing the circumstances to continue. Clinicians should keep in mind that capacity is decision-specific, and it may become necessary to assess multiple domains: capacity to make decisions about health care, capacity to make financial decisions, and capacity to determine with whom one associates. These are complex situations, but when appropriate, the older adult's right to autonomy and self-determination must be honored. Paternalistic viewpoints regarding what the older person "should do" need to be avoided. In self-neglect cases, the clinician may need support when coming to terms with the requirement to respect the decisionally capable older adult's wishes when this involves his or her choosing to remain in a precarious situation.

The Caregiver–Older Adult Dyad

The relationship between an older adult with caregivers can be very complex, and a dysfunctional relationship between a dependent older adult and a caregiver may not be one in which blame or fault can be fairly assigned. To approach such situations with the idea that the older adult is inevitably the victim infantilizes the patient and is unfair to caregivers. Situations in which older adults are mistreated fall along a spectrum from victimization to mutual abusiveness to relationships in which the older adult is intentionally provocative. Of course, in many cases, the older adult and his or her caregivers are making the best of a difficult situation.

To determine the best possible approach for ameliorating, if not solving, a dysfunctional relationship, professionals (not necessarily clinicians) need to make every effort to determine the facts in the situation and the perspectives of each involved party. Consultation with social workers, psychologists, or psychiatrists can be useful. Detailed investigation is the role of Adult Protective Services, an ombudsman, or the police.

Legal reporting requirements are not limited in any way by considerations of relationship difficulties or contextual subtleties. If, for example, an older man hits his son and the son strikes back, clinicians in most states are mandated to report the son's action.

Institutional Mistreatment

Mistreatment in the setting of home care by family or friends has been the focus of much of the discussion so far, but detecting and intervening to prevent mistreatment in the institutional setting is also important. Nursing-home residents are at higher risk of mistreatment than community-dwelling older adults. Several factors in this setting may increase the likelihood of mistreatment, including poor working conditions, low salaries, and inadequate staff training and supervision, resulting in poor motivation and prejudiced attitudes. Disruptive or insulting behavior by the older adult can also be a factor. Signs and symptoms suggesting mistreatment in this population are similar. Although uncommon, staff members who are sociopaths or serial sexual abusers may victimize multiple residents, and clinicians should consider this when encountering several patients from the same institution with similar presentations.

The Omnibus Budget Reconciliation Act of 1987 set a new standard for care in nursing homes. Recently, CMS issued new rules to protect the rights of long-term care facility residents, including prohibiting facilities from forcing residents into arbitration. Removing the arbitration requirement is intended to protect older adults from mistreatment and negligent care. This change would allow residents or their families to sue nursing homes. Although often more expensive than arbitration, lawsuits offer the opportunity for residents and families to have disputes with facilities settled in court, with results more available to prospective residents. Clinicians who are alert to the possibility of abuse and neglect in any institutional setting play an important role in protecting vulnerable older adults. Equally important is clinicians' readiness to use the resources available through the institution itself or through state regulatory agencies to investigate and intervene when appropriate. In cases of suspected institutional mistreatment, the challenge is to balance the rights of staff members with the rights of residents.

Each state maintains a long-term care ombudsman program. Long-term care ombudsmen are advocates for residents of nursing homes and work to resolve problems related to the residents' health, safety, welfare. They identify, investigate, and resolve complaints made by or on behalf of residents.

Evidence is growing (SOE=B) regarding the phenomenon of resident-to-resident mistreatment in long-term care facilities, which warrants careful attention. In such cases, residents may assault, rob, or psychologically abuse other residents.

INTERVENTION

Clinicians who suspect mistreatment can use the following questions to guide intervention:

- How safe is the older adult if he or she returns to the current setting?
- Does the older adult need to be removed to a safe environment?
- Does the older adult have the capacity to choose to stay?
- What services or resources are available locally to support the care of the older adult and caregivers?
- Are there any caregivers who have health problems of their own that need attention?
- Does this situation need the expertise of others (eg, medicine, nursing, social work), and if so, who would best serve the older adult's needs?
- Should the situation be reported?

Successful intervention in cases of mistreatment can become complex. Factors governing clinicians' course of action include the exact nature and degree of the mistreatment, and whether the patient and/or caregiver(s) can or will cooperate with evaluation and intervention. Social workers and case managers may be very helpful in clinical settings where they work, because they may provide counseling, safety planning, and appropriate resources to the patient and caregiver, including home health services, Meals-on-Wheels, medical transportation services, adult day care, senior centers, substance abuse treatment options, and respite care.

Local resources in support of interventions for mistreatment vary, but information is readily available. Consultation with the health department can be a useful early step. Each state's Adult Protective Services (APS) can provide relevant information as well as direct assistance. However, this essential service has limitations, given that older adults cannot be compelled to engage with APS and the constraints on available resources. Websites of the National Adult Protective Services Association (www.napsa-now.org [accessed Feb 2019]) and the National Center on Elder Abuse (https://ncea.acl.gov [accessed Feb 2019]) both provide a convenient starting point in the search for information and resources. The website of the Elder Justice Roadmap (www.justice.gov/elderjustice/research/roadmap.html [accessed Feb 2019]) is also exceptionally helpful for identifying resources, support, evidence for interventions, and ongoing efforts to eradicate mistreatment. State departments of public health are usually responsible for investigating cases of abuse and neglect in nursing homes.

DOCUMENTATION

Documenting completely and accurately is a critical component of caring for potential victims of elder mistreatment. Clinicians should be mindful that the medical record may be used for investigation and prosecution, and the documentation may affect whether justice is served. The patient's responses to questions should be comprehensively documented, and the patient's own words should be used whenever possible. Clinicians should comprehensively report the physical examination and include the general appearance of the patient. Potential signs of neglect, including dirty clothing, poor dental hygiene, and untrimmed nails should be noted. All injuries should be described in detail, including size, location, stage of healing, and whether it is consistent with the reported mechanism. Using a body diagram, available as part of many electronic medical records, may increase accuracy. Clinicians should consider photographing physical findings and add these photographs to the medical record when possible. These images may be helpful forensically in the future.

THE MEDICAL-LEGAL INTERFACE

It is important for clinicians to know their own state laws applicable to cases of mistreatment of older adults; 49 states require clinicians to report elder mistreatment, either through Adult Protective Services or state agencies associated with aging. Clinicians need to be familiar with the reporting mandates in their area. In some states, neglect by others must be reported, whereas reports of self-neglect are not required. Adult children can be charged with neglect of the older parent if it can be proved that a caregiving relationship exists and that care has been precipitously withdrawn without substitute services. In states where self-neglect is reportable, this category represents the largest number of cases. Finally, states can mandate reports for self-neglect but may not provide any services unless the older adult agrees to accept them. State-by-state responsibilities may be found at www.napsa-now.org/wp-content/uploads/2014/11/Mandatory-Reporting-Chart-Updated-FINAL.pdf (accessed Feb 2019).

Although APS is typically the agency that initially investigates these cases, it is important to understand the scope of their duties. In most states, APS may only respond to cases in which an older adult has functional or cognitive impairment (ie, the agency will not act on reports if in the agency's judgment, the older adults does not meet these criteria. Also, APS is not a police force but rather tasked with identifying older adults needing services and implementing appropriate services. Further, APS typically has ≥72 hours before being obligated to initiate an investigation. At that time, if APS has concern that a crime has been committed, the APS will contact the police. As a result, clinicians should also consider contacting the local police department when concerned about a patient's immediate safety.

If mistreatment in nursing homes is identified or suspected, clinicians should report to the state department of public health, APS, or to the long-term care ombudsman in their state (www.ltcombudsman.org/).

Although clinicians may be wary of reporting concern for mistreatment based on suspicion alone, these reports are often the only way that this life-threatening syndrome is identified. Penalties can be assessed against a non-reporter in some regions. Reports of mistreatment of older adults are confidential, and as is the case with reports of child abuse, the clinical reporter is protected from litigation unless it can be proved that the report was made maliciously.

Cases of mistreatment are often extremely complicated, and experts in several fields will need to work with clinicians to optimize identification, intervention, reporting, and response to provide the best outcomes for mistreatment victims.

RESOURCES

- Daly JM, Butchner HK. Evidence-based practice guideline: Elder abuse prevention. *J Gerontol Nurs* 2018;44(7):21–30.

- Dong XQ. Elder abuse: systematic review and implications for practice. *J Am Geriatr Soc*. 2015;63(6):1214–1238.

- *The Elder Justice Roadmap: A Stakeholder Initiative to Respond to an Emerging Health, Justice, Financial and Social Crisis.* (www.justice.gov/file/852856/download [accessed Feb 2019]).

- Wangmo T, Nordstrom K, Kressig RW. Preventing elder abuse and neglect in geriatric institutions: Solutions from nursing care providers. *Geriatr Nurs*. 2017;38(5):358–392.

CHAPTER 16—PERIOPERATIVE CARE

KEY POINTS

- Operative therapy is an important option for many health problems affecting older adults.

- The preoperative evaluation should include an appraisal of the patient's medical conditions, functional status, and risk of cardiac and other perioperative complications, as well as recommendations for preoperative testing and therapy to minimize surgical risk.

- Risk indices and practice guidelines for common cardiac, pulmonary, and neuropsychiatric problems assist in decision making and management of older surgical patients.

- Although age is a risk factor for perioperative and postoperative complications, these problems can be minimized with appropriate proactive assessment and management.

Surgery is a common form of treatment for older adults; currently >55% of all operative procedures are done in patients ≥65 years old, and this proportion is expected to grow. Many of the chronic conditions that increase in prevalence with advancing age—cataracts, arthritis, vascular occlusions, and cancers—are amenable to surgery. Over half of all malignancies are seen in patients ≥65 years old, and the primary treatment for many tumors is surgical. Advances in surgical, anesthetic, and medical care have lowered surgical risks and shifted the risk-benefit ratio to favor surgery in increasingly older patients with more complex conditions. Nevertheless, although older patients account for just over half of all surgical procedures, they suffer three-quarters of the postoperative mortality, as well as a disproportionate majority of the postoperative morbidity.

Many of the physiologic changes accompanying normal aging impact the perioperative management of older surgical patients. For example, altered body composition, and decreased kidney function, hepatic blood flow, and hepatic enzyme activity all contribute to changes in the pharmacokinetics of drugs. Cardiac and vascular stiffening complicate fluid management and optimization of intravascular volume. Both volume overload and volume depletion occur commonly in the perioperative setting and are poorly tolerated by many older adults. Stiffening of the thoracic cage and diminished ciliary function contribute to decreases in pulmonary reserve and heightened risk of postoperative pneumonia. Because of decreased thermoregulation, the older surgical patient is at particular risk of perioperative hypothermia. Finally, by mechanisms that are not yet fully elucidated, changes in the brain that accompany aging make older adults exquisitely susceptible to postoperative cognitive changes.

It is well recognized that the aging process is extremely variable from person to person and that even within one individual not all organ systems age at the same rate, producing dramatic heterogeneity even among healthy older adults. Older individuals may have several chronic conditions that can impact on perioperative care, either directly or through the medications being used to treat those conditions. The heterogeneity in physiologic aging combined with the potential for multiple comorbidities means that older patients require a more comprehensive and individualized preoperative evaluation. They often benefit from a multidisciplinary approach to perioperative care and recovery.

PREOPERATIVE ASSESSMENT AND MANAGEMENT

Clinicians are commonly asked to perform preoperative evaluations with the goals of reducing complications and death and optimizing patient outcomes. The goal of such a consultation should not be to "clear" the patient for surgery but rather to maximize the possibility of a good outcome from surgery. This consultation should appraise the patient's medical, cognitive, and functional status, assess risk of perioperative and postoperative complications, and provide recommendations for preoperative interventions to minimize potential complications. Preoperative assessment should include evaluation of the patient's cardiovascular, respiratory, renal, metabolic, and neuropsychiatric status, as well as the patient's risk of iatrogenic problems, all within the context of the patient's overall functional status. Usually, the preoperative assessment can be accomplished with only a history and physical examination for low-risk procedures, eg. breast, cataract, dermatologic, endoscopic, or superficial surgery (SOE=B). For patients undergoing procedures that are not low risk, or in whom the history and physical examination have uncovered other potential risks, further assessment and testing are indicated.

Cardiovascular System

It is estimated that 25%–30% of postoperative deaths are from cardiac causes, and the likelihood of postoperative cardiac events is directly related to age. Cardiac risk assessment is the most fully developed and widely investigated portion of the preoperative medical assessment. The American Society of Anesthesiologists (ASA) classification of patient physical status relies heavily on clinical judgment and is not specific for cardiovascular morbidity and mortality (see Table 16.1). This system has been used by anesthesiologists for years and has consistently been shown to be useful in predicting postoperative outcomes. Several indices and algorithms for specifically assessing cardiac risk in noncardiac surgery have been published since the 1970s. Risk assessment is based on patient factors and type of surgery. Non-low-risk surgeries include open aortic or other vascular, intrathoracic, intra-abdominal, major orthopedic, and major genitourinary procedures. In 2014, the American College of Cardiology and the American Heart Association (ACC/AHA) published an algorithm for preoperative cardiac assessment (Figure 16.1). The guideline calls for consideration, in order, of the following clinical factors:

1. Urgency of surgery; if emergent, proceed to surgery if consistent with patient's overall goals (SOE=C). Depending on those goals, broaching the subject of a palliative approach may be appropriate.

2. Presence of active major cardiac risk factors, eg, unstable angina or recent MI, decompensated heart failure, dyspnea, or moderate or severe valvular disease; if present, assess and correct these conditions before reconsidering surgery (SOE=B).

3. Type of surgery; if low-risk procedure, proceed to surgery (SOE=B).

4. Patient's exercise capacity; if ≥4 METs (eg. can perform heavy housework or climb a flight of stairs), proceed to surgery (SOE=B).

5. Poor or unknown functional capacity; if present, assess utility of further quantification of cardiac risk and patient willingness to undergo testing for cardiac ischemia before surgery (SOE=B).

6. Calculation of cardiac risk and preoperative testing for cardiac ischemia; perform if they will change management (SOE=B). Several scales for further quantification of cardiac risk are available including the Revised Cardiac Risk Index (www.mdcalc.com/revised-cardiac-risk-index-for-pre-operative-risk/) and 2 risk calculators from the American College of Surgeons (www.riskcalculator.facs.org and www.surgicalriskcalculator.com/miorcardiacarrest [accessed Feb 2019]).

Aside from a careful history and physical examination to determine the presence of active major cardiac risk factors and to assess functional capacity, supplemental cardiac testing or therapy should be considered in only a few specific circumstances. ECG testing is not necessary in asymptomatic patients undergoing low-risk procedures (SOE=B).

Table 16.1—American Society of Anesthesiologists Classification of Physical Status

Class	Description of Patient
I	Healthy
II	Mild systemic disease
III	Severe systemic disease
IV	Severe systemic disease that is a constant threat to life
V	Moribund; not expected to survive without surgery
VI	Declared brain-dead; organs being removed for donor purposes

NOTE: There is no additional information to help further define these categories.
SOURCE: Data from American Society of Anesthesiologists. ASA Physical Status Classification System. Available at: https://www.asahq.org/standards-and-guidelines/asa-physical-status-classification-system (accessed Feb 2019).

A preoperative ECG can provide useful information, mostly as a baseline for comparing postoperative cardiac complications, in patients with known coronary artery disease, significant arrhythmia, peripheral arterial disease, prior stroke or transient ischemic attack (TIA), or significant structural heart disease who are undergoing non-low-risk surgery (SOE=B). ECG findings suggestive of ischemia, left ventricular hypertrophy, QT prolongation, or bundle-branch blocks portend a higher risk of cardiac complications and death. Measurement of left ventricular function using echocardiography, radionuclide studies, or contrast ventriculography should be considered in patients with dyspnea of uncertain cause (SOE=C). When newly diagnosed heart failure is determined to be the cause of unexplained dyspnea, it should be maximally treated before surgery. The utility of detecting and treating asymptomatic heart failure preoperatively is unknown. A preoperative echocardiogram should be obtained in patients with moderate or worse valvular stenosis or regurgitation who have not had an echocardiogram in the previous year (SOE=C).

If noninvasive cardiac stress testing will change management, eg, postponement or cancellation of surgery, it should be considered in patients with clinical risk factors who are undergoing intermediate- or high-risk procedures and have unknown or poor functional capacity (SOE=B). It is under comparatively rare circumstances that coronary revascularization (with coronary artery bypass graft surgery or percutaneous coronary intervention) should be performed before noncardiac surgery to decrease risk of cardiac complications (SOE=A), and as medical therapies continue to advance, the benefit of surgery relative to medical therapy even for these indications has narrowed. For indications for perioperative revascularization, see Table 16.2 (SOE=A).

Certain medications given before or after surgery reduce cardiac and vascular complications of surgery.

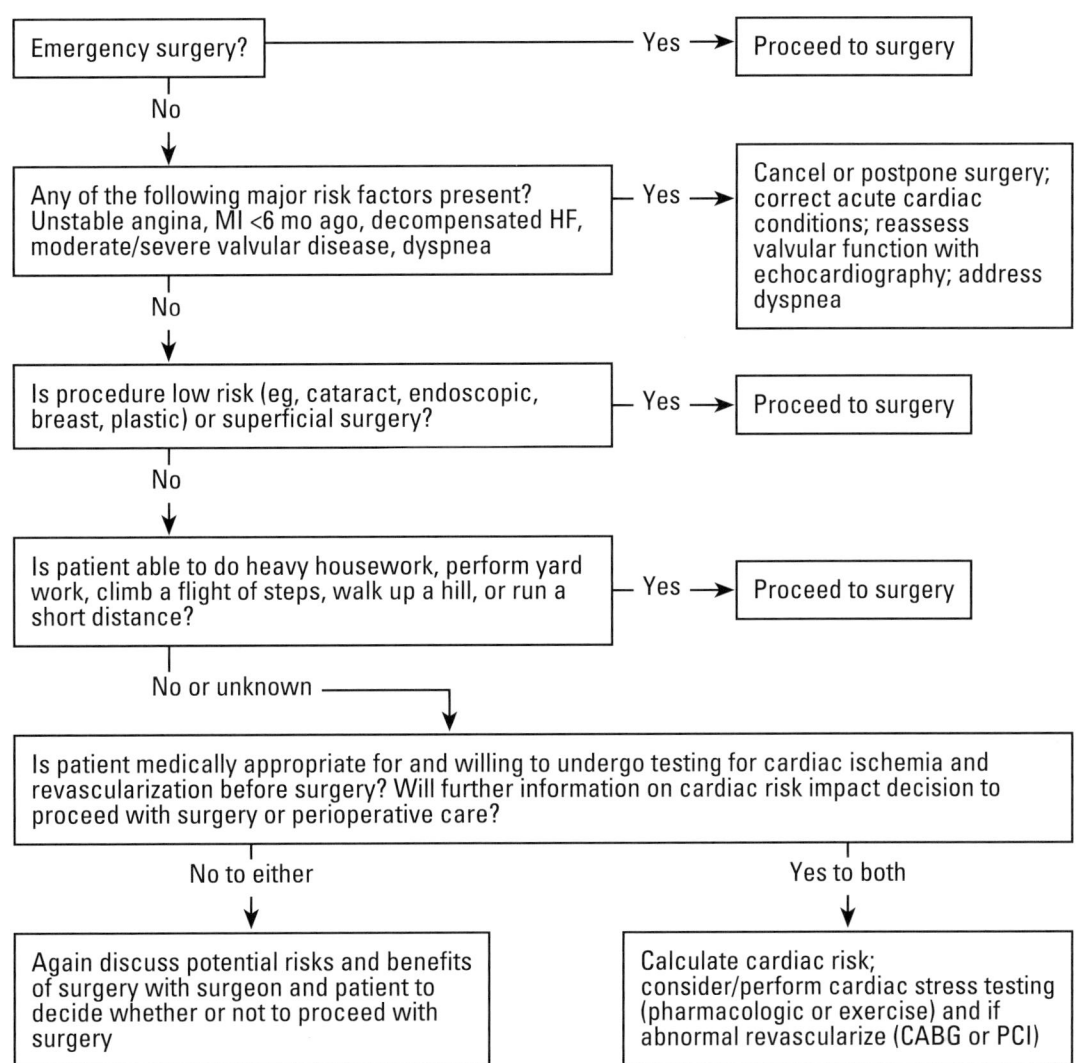

Figure 16.1—Assessing Cardiac Risk in Noncardiac Surgery

SOURCE: Fleisher LA, Fleischmann KE, Auerbach AD, et al. 2014 ACC/AHA Guideline on Perioperative Cardiovascular Evaluation and Management of Patients Undergoing Noncardiac Surgery: Executive Summary: A Report of the American College of Cardiology/American Heart Association Task Force on Practice Guidelines. *J Am Coll Cardiol*. 2014;64(22):2373–2405.

Table 16.2—Major Indications for Revascularization in the Perioperative Period (2011 ACC/AHA Guidelines)

- Significant unprotected left main vessel disease
- 3-Vessel disease
- 2-Vessel disease with proximal left anterior descending artery disease
- Survivors of sudden cardiac death with presumed ischemic ventricular tachycardia

In general, prior aspirin and other antiplatelet therapies can be safely continued in patients undergoing cutaneous surgery, dental procedures, diagnostic endoscopy, ophthalmologic procedures, and peripheral vascular surgery, and aspirin may safely be continued for neuraxial anesthesia (SOE=C). Antiplatelet therapy should be stopped before procedures that place the patient at high risk of bleeding, which include coronary artery bypass graft; abdominal, thoracic, or orthopedic surgery; spinal puncture; liver or kidney biopsy; transurethral resection of the prostate; or placement of a spinal/epidural catheter. Aspirin, clopidogrel, and prasugrel should be stopped 5 days before these procedures, and ticagrelor 1 day before.

For patients already on an anticoagulant, its protective benefits need to be weighed against the risk of perioperative hemorrhage. Anticoagulation therapy does not need to be withheld (as long as the INR is therapeutic) for cutaneous surgery (SOE=C), dental extractions and minor oral procedures (SOE=B), or cataract surgery (SOE=C). For other surgical procedures, cessation of warfarin or direct-acting oral anticoagulants, with or without bridging therapy with low-molecular-weight heparin (LMWH), can be based on the patient's risk factors for thromboembolism (Table 16.3). Warfarin is generally withheld 5 days

Table 16.3—Cessation of Anticoagulation Before Elective Surgery in Older Adults[a]

Thromboembolic Risk	Patient Conditions Determining Risk	Recommendations for Cessation of Anticoagulation
Low	No VTE in past 12 months; AF with $CHADS_2$ score of 0–2; bileaflet mechanical aortic valve without AF, prior TIA/stroke, or stroke risk factors	If INR therapeutic, stop warfarin 5 days before surgery or DOAC 1–3 days before, earlier if INR is supratherapeutic or >3.
Moderate	VTE in past 3–12 months; recurrent VTE; active malignancy (treated within 6 months or palliative); AF with $CHADS_2$ score of 3 or 4; bileaflet mechanical aortic valve with AF, prior TIA/stroke, or any stroke risk factors; nonsevere thrombophilia	Stop warfarin 5 days before surgery or DOAC 1–3 days before and begin LMWH 3 days before surgery at therapeutic (preferred) or prophylactic (optional) dosage; give last preoperative dose of LMWH 24 hours before surgery.
High	VTE within past 3 months; TIA/stroke within 6 months with mechanical heart valve or within 3 months with AF; rheumatic heart disease with AF; AF with $CHADS_2$ score of 5 or 6; mechanical mitral valve or ball/cage or tilting disc mechanical aortic valve; severe thrombophilia	Stop warfarin 5 days before surgery or DOAC 1–3 days before and begin LMWH 3 days before surgery at therapeutic dosage; give last preoperative dose of LMWH 24 hours before surgery.

VTE = venous thromboembolism; AF = atrial fibrillation; TIA = transient ischemic attack; INR = international normalized ratio; DOAC = direct-acting oral anticoagulant (apixaban, edoxaban, rivaroxaban, dabigatran); LMWH = low-molecular-weight heparin; $CHADS_2$ score = 1 point each for heart failure, hypertension, age >74 years, diabetes; 2 points for history of stroke

[a] SOE=C

SOURCE: Data from Douketis JD, Berger PB, Dunn AS, et al. The perioperative management of antithrombotic therapy. American College of Chest Physicians Evidence-Based Clinical Practice Guidelines. *Chest.* 2012;141(2Suppl);e326S.

before surgery. Apixaban and rivaroxaban can be stopped 1–2 days before surgery, and dabigatran 1–3 days before. For patients receiving bridging therapy, LMWH can generally be restarted 24 hours after surgery, longer in cases of major surgery with increased risk of major bleeding. The indications for infective endocarditis prophylaxis were dramatically reduced with the publication of guidelines by the American Heart Association in 2007, rendering the indications for endocarditis prophylaxis quite rare.

β-Blockers should be continued in patients who are already on a β-blocker for medical indications and should be considered in patients with ≥3 cardiovascular risk factors or evidence of myocardial ischemia who are not already on a β-blocker. Evidence does not support the initiation of β-blockers in the perioperative period for other indications. If β-blocker therapy is initiated, it should be started 2–30 days before surgery, titrated to a heart rate of 60 to 70 beats per minute, and the patient should be carefully monitored for hypotension and bradycardia, both of which could increase perioperative cardiac risk.

Finally, management of patients with coronary stents requires particular attention. Cohort studies identify substantially increased risk of major adverse cardiac events when surgery is performed soon after a coronary stent is placed, particularly for drug-eluting stents. The optimal timing for elective surgery is not before 30 days after a bare metal stent is placed and not before 365 days after a drug-eluting stent is placed (SOE=B). Urgent or emergent surgeries that must be performed before those time frames require careful consideration of the added adverse cardiac risks they entail. Similarly, continuation of antiplatelet medications given to reduce stent thrombosis must be carefully weighed against the risk of significant postoperative bleeding, and consideration of individual risk factors and preferences related to those competing risks must be considered.

Respiratory System

Postoperative pulmonary complications, most commonly atelectasis, pneumonia, and prolonged mechanical ventilation, occur more often in older adults than in younger age groups. The impact of these complications is more costly than the cardiovascular complications of surgery in older adults (SOE=A). Pulmonary complications are predictive of increased short- and long-term mortality in older adults and have been reported to prolong the hospital stay by an average of 1–2 weeks in this age group. A comprehensive review published by the American College of Physicians (ACP) in 2006 found that age is a powerful independent risk factor for postoperative pulmonary complications (SOE=A). Other patient-associated major risk factors include COPD, ASA Class II or greater (see Table 16.1), heart failure, deficit in ADLs, and a serum albumin <3.5 g/dL (SOE=A). Minor patient-associated risk factors include acute confusion or delirium, alcohol use, smoking, weight loss, pulmonary findings on physical examination, and an increased BUN concentration (SOE=B). The following procedures are associated with increased pulmonary complications: emergency surgery; prolonged (>3 hour) surgery; repair of abdominal aortic aneurysm (AAA); neurosurgery; and thoracic, abdominal, head and neck, or vascular surgery (SOE=A). General anesthesia is also a risk factor (SOE=A).

In 2007, the ACP published a guideline for risk assessment and perioperative management of pulmonary complications associated with noncardiothoracic surgery. It calls for preoperative assessment of pulmonary risk by appraising the above predictive factors through history, physical examination, and modest laboratory testing. Routine chest radiography is not recommended, but imaging can be helpful for detection and management of pulmonary conditions in patients with known cardiac or pulmonary disease who are undergoing thoracic, upper abdominal, or surgery for AAA. Spirometry should be reserved for evaluating lung function in patients suspected of having undiagnosed COPD after history and physical examination, based on findings such as dyspnea or wheezing. The question of whether treatment of newly discovered COPD changes outcomes after surgery has not been well studied. Preoperative pulmonary function testing is also routine before lung reduction surgeries. In recent years, several tools to predict the risk of postoperative respiratory failure and postoperative pneumonia have been published. The type of surgery, whether the surgery is emergent, the albumin level, BUN level, functional status, presence of COPD, and age are all components of the Veterans Administration Surgical Quality Improvement Program respiratory failure risk index (SOE=B). The same group validated a risk index to predict postoperative pneumonia using largely clinical information (SOE=B).

The ACP guideline primarily recommends postoperative lung expansion therapy, which has been associated most consistently with reduced pulmonary complications of atelectasis, pneumonia, bronchitis, and severe hypoxemia (SOE=A). Lung expansion therapy can be accomplished through deep breathing exercises, incentive spirometry, and/or continuous positive-airway pressure. Use of a nasogastric tube for management of postoperative nausea and vomiting, inability to tolerate oral feeding, or abdominal distention can also be helpful for minimizing pulmonary complications (SOE=B). The evidence is also good for using short-acting neuromuscular blocking agents (as opposed to long-acting agents) to reduce complications (SOE=B). Less clear are the benefits of preoperative smoking cessation, use of laparoscopic versus open procedures, epidural versus general anesthesia, and epidural analgesia.

Kidneys and Metabolism

Glomerular blood flow decreases with age as does muscle mass, such that an apparently normal serum creatinine can be misinterpreted as indicating normal kidney function. The glomerular filtration rate (GFR) can be estimated by calculating the creatinine clearance using the Cockcroft-Gault equation or by relying on the Modification of Diet in Renal Disease study (MDRD method) or the newer Chronic Kidney Disease Epidemiologic Collaboration (CKD-EPI) method that some laboratories use to automatically calculate the estimated GFR. Which method most accurately estimates GFR in older adults remains a significant area of debate. Because many drugs administered during the perioperative period may require dosage adjustments in patients with diminished renal function, accurate estimation of GFR is important.

Also, because of decrements in the ability of the kidney to appropriately conserve salt or to maximally concentrate or dilute urine in response to intravascular volume or osmolality, the use of intravenous fluids needs to be monitored carefully. The combination of receiving nothing by mouth while receiving intravenous 5% dextrose in 0.45% normal saline may result in hyponatremia.

Neuropsychiatric Concerns

Delirium is a common event in the postoperative period. The type of surgery appears to be an important determinant of delirium, with incidence rates ranging from about 4%–5% in cataract or urologic procedures to 50%–60% in some series of patients with infrarenal AAA repair or hip fracture surgery. Both preoperative and intraoperative factors have been evaluated as risk factors for delirium. Preoperative assessment is focused on identifying factors in patients undergoing surgery that predispose to postoperative delirium, including age ≥70 years; cognitive impairment; limited physical function; a history of alcohol abuse; abnormal serum sodium, potassium, or glucose; intrathoracic surgery; and AAA surgery. Preoperative assessment should include clear assessment and documentation of mental status, so that postoperative assessments have a baseline for comparison. The most important intraoperative factor found to be associated with delirium is volume of intraoperative blood loss. Patients with a postoperative hematocrit <30% have an increased risk of delirium irrespective of the presence or absence of preoperative risk factors (SOE=B). Undertreatment of pain postoperatively is a significant risk factor for the development of delirium, at least in patients who were cognitively intact at baseline (SOE=B). When preoperative risk factors are present, the clinician can identify patients at greatest risk of developing delirium and can be vigilant about correcting fluid, electrolyte, and metabolic derangements; optimizing replacement of blood loss; maintaining circadian rhythms (by getting patients out of bed during the day and minimizing sleep interruptions at night); and prescribing medications cautiously while assuring adequate pain control. In particular, medications with CNS effects and especially those with anticholinergic adverse effects should be used with caution in the perioperative period, because they may precipitate delirium.

Functional Status and Frailty

Patients who require help with IADLs or ADLs are at increased risk of poorer surgical outcomes. Functional decline after surgery can be substantial, and cognitive impairment confers a high risk of functional decline. Frailty also has been associated with poorer outcomes, with several studies showing a 3- to 13-fold increase in being discharged to a facility rather than to home, and higher rates of delirium, cognitive impairment, functional decline, and death. The Sinai Abbreviated Geriatric Evaluation (SAGE) is one tool that can be used easily in a clinic setting for assessment of cognition, frailty, and functional status to predict surgical outcomes beyond organ-based systems risk assessment. It involves a modified Mini-Cog (3-word recall and the clock-draw test), gait speed test (timed walking of 15 feet with 7-second cutoff considered as positive), and functional status ADL assessment (4 questions covering most ADLs). Each unit decrease in score was associated with an increase in odds of a complication, postoperative delirium, increased length of stay, readmission, or discharge to a higher level of care. Multiple other assessments of frailty exist, but none has been demonstrated to be superior to any other in predicting and managing surgical patients. It is important for patients and family members to understand the risks associated with frailty or poorer functional status when considering surgery and to consider whether alternatives may be appropriate, depending on a patient's goals of care. Whether targeted interventions, such as preoperative exercise or nutritional supplementation, can improve surgical outcomes in frail individuals is unknown.

Iatrogenic Complications

Untoward effects of well-intentioned interventions are common among older hospitalized adults. Some of the more common pitfalls to be avoided include mobility restriction, excessive use of catheters, inattention to nutrition and hydration status, and inappropriate use of medications. Few disease states benefit from bed rest. It is important to maintain mobility and function as much as possible by encouraging time out of bed and avoiding restraints. The risks of skin breakdown, muscle atrophy, joint stiffness, and bone loss can be reduced by preserving mobility (SOE=C). Although bladder catheters can sometimes be critical in accurately measuring urine output, prolonged use of an indwelling catheter carries substantial risk of infection. Indwelling catheters can also contribute to restricted mobility and should be removed as soon as possible. Restricted diets and lack of access to water can contribute to compromise in nutrition and hydration. Studies demonstrate that the traditional practice of nothing-by-mouth beginning the night before surgery to reduce the risk of aspiration is not more beneficial than nothing by mouth for 6 hours except water, with the latter approach more comfortable for the patient and less likely to cause volume depletion (SOE=B). Conversely, continued administration of intravenous fluids after the patient is able to maintain hydration orally can result in volume overload and impaired oxygenation. A regular review of medication administration can avoid unnecessary drug use and inappropriate dosing.

PERIOPERATIVE AND POSTOPERATIVE MANAGEMENT OF SELECTED MEDICAL PROBLEMS

Surgery in older adults often results in destabilization of chronic, coexistent medical conditions. Additionally, because of the diminished physiologic reserve common in older adults, new medical problems can arise in the postoperative period. Some of the most common medical issues to contend with postoperatively are discussed here.

Cardiovascular Problems

The most common cardiovascular problems that arise in older adults after surgery are hypertension, rhythm disturbances, and heart failure. Postoperative hypertension should initially prompt a search for a noncardiovascular cause, such as pain or urinary retention. Next, it is important to assess volume status, review fluid administration records, and note whether antihypertensive medications were mistakenly omitted before the procedure. To treat uncontrolled essential hypertension, parenteral formulations are available in several classes of medications: β-blockers, calcium channel blockers, ACE inhibitors, and drugs that block both α- and β-adrenergic receptors. Topical agents, such as topical nitroglycerin, could also be considered useful when the patient is unable to take medications by mouth.

Cardiac rhythm disturbances are a concern, because they can lead to myocardial ischemia and heart failure. Supraventricular tachycardia, commonly seen in older adults, is associated with a history of prior supraventricular dysrhythmias, asthma, heart failure, and premature atrial complexes on a preoperative ECG. This rhythm disturbance is also more common in patients who have had vascular, abdominal, or thoracic procedures. Early restoration of sinus rhythm, or at least controlling the ventricular rate, can be attempted with an infusion of adenosine, a β-blocker, or a calcium channel blocker. If the rhythm is atrial fibrillation, conversion to sinus rhythm can be attempted with electrical cardioversion or by an infusion of amiodarone if the atrial fibrillation is poorly tolerated and the risk of thromboembolism is low. Because spontaneous reversion to sinus rhythm often occurs by 6 weeks after surgery, long-term use of an antidysrhythmic such as amiodarone may not be necessary. Persistent atrial fibrillation beyond 24–48 hours is associated with an increased risk of thromboembolism, and consideration should be given to anticoagulation therapy to reduce the risk of stroke (SOE=A).

Cardiac reserve is often compromised among older adults, especially those with chronic hypertension or coronary artery disease. Heart failure can develop as a result of excessive fluid administration, new cardiac ischemia, or a rhythm disturbance. It can be extremely challenging to ensure optimal ventricular filling pressures based on the clinical assessment of volume status in older adults by physical examination and standard laboratory parameters alone. Although some have recommended the use of pulmonary artery catheters in high-risk patients, studies have not shown a decreased mortality rate for this intervention, and most authorities advise against this approach (SOE=C).

Most older adults who are undergoing surgery should receive prophylaxis for deep venous thrombosis and pulmonary embolism.

Kidney and Electrolyte Disorders

Impaired preoperative kidney function increases the risk of postoperative kidney failure. The impaired reserve makes the aging kidney more susceptible to the effects of even transient reductions of cardiac output or brief exposure to nephrotoxic medications. When kidney damage has been sustained, early clinical manifestations include oliguria, isosthenuria, and an increase in serum creatinine. When impaired renal blood flow is the cause, the urine sodium will typically be <40 mEq/L and the urine-to-plasma creatinine ratio will be greater than 10:1. In contrast, if acute tubular necrosis is the mechanism of injury, the urine sediment may have granular or epithelial cell casts, and the urine sodium will be >40 mEq/L with a urine-to-plasma creatinine ratio of less than 10:1. When acute tubular necrosis is suspected, vigorous efforts should be made to preserve kidney function by withholding all potentially nephrotoxic medications and meticulously maintaining a euvolemic state.

Another important mechanism of postoperative kidney failure is obstructive nephropathy, especially in older men with prostatic hyperplasia. The partial outflow obstruction combined with immobility, frequent constipation, and exposure to medications with anticholinergic effects compromising detrusor function can easily precipitate acute urinary retention. In addition to oliguria and an increase in serum creatinine, the bladder is typically palpable because of distention. Treatment consists of insertion of a bladder catheter to reduce the risk of hydronephrosis and lasting kidney dysfunction. Commonly, men with prostatic hyperplasia who develop postoperative obstruction are unable to void immediately after catheter removal and may need α-blocking medications and continued use of the catheter for 2–4 weeks, when another voiding trial can be attempted (SOE=C).

Gastrointestinal Concerns

Constipation is quite common postoperatively, as a consequence of the combined effects of altered diet, immobility, and frequent use of opioids and other constipating medications. At times, ileus and obstipation can be severe and produce significant anorexia, nausea, delirium, and even vomiting. Postoperative iron therapy, commonly prescribed for anemia, is an unproven but likely contributor to postoperative constipation. Given the common co-occurrence of these risk factors for constipation in the postoperative period, a reasonable approach is to simultaneously order a laxative and a fecal softener every time an opioid is prescribed, particularly if the patient has a history of constipation or if it is reasonably anticipated that mobility will be reduced for longer than a day. Prunes or prune juice, applesauce, and bran can all also have promotility effects.

Postoperative diarrhea should increase concern for fecal impaction and antibiotic-associated or *Clostridium difficile* diarrhea in the setting of recent antibiotic use. Checking manually for fecal impaction and testing fecal specimens for leukocytes and *C difficile* toxin may be appropriate. Management must focus carefully on volume resuscitation and treating the underlying cause. Use of antimotility agents, while effective in reducing fecal incontinence from diarrhea, is very risky in older adults in the postoperative period, because they significantly increase the risk of delirium, constipation, and toxic megacolon.

Finally, nausea is not uncommon in the postoperative period, often as a result of opioid, anesthetic, and other medications; new infection; or slowed gut motility. In managing nausea, first steps are to ensure that the patient is having sufficient bowel movements and to review medications to reduce or eliminate any that may be impairing GI motility or contributing to GI irritation, such as opioids and NSAIDs. Antiemetics should be considered only after these approaches have failed to identify a reversible problem. Particularly if the patient has recently received antibiotics, remaining vigilant for *C difficile* infection causing nausea is essential.

Managing Common Endocrine Abnormalities

Type 2 diabetes mellitus is a common comorbid condition of many older adults. Usually, given the long half-life of oral hypoglycemic agents and the nothing-by-mouth status for surgery, oral diabetes medications are withheld the day of surgery. It may be especially important to withhold metformin, given the potential (although quite low) additional risk of metabolic acidosis arising from use of this medication during a time of stress. To optimize glucose control, an intravenous solution containing glucose can be administered at a constant rate while blood glucose by fingerstick assay is closely monitored; subcutaneous insulin should be administered as necessary to control glucose concentrations until the patient is able to resume eating. For a patient with type 2 diabetes who uses insulin, insulin should be withheld on the day of surgery and sliding-scale insulin given (SOE=C). Once the patient is able to start eating, usually half the outpatient dosage of diabetes medications is administered the first day of oral intake, with additional sliding-scale insulin coverage as needed; full doses are resumed as the patient consumes a usual diet.

Perioperative hyperglycemia among diabetic and nondiabetic patients is associated with morbidity and mortality in medical and surgical ICU patients (SOE=B), and in patients undergoing coronary artery bypass grafting (SOE=C) or carotid endarterectomy (SOE=B). Maintaining glucose concentrations of <150 mg/dL with intravenous insulin in the perioperative period for patients undergoing vascular or major noncardiac surgery with planned ICU admission has reduced morbidity and mortality (SOE=B). However, maintaining tight glycemic control (≤110 mg/dL) among ICU patients has been associated with increased occurrence of hypoglycemia and no reduction in mortality (SOE=B); therefore, moderate glucose control in these patients is advised. The value of strict glycemic control in other surgical or medical inpatient populations has not been demonstrated.

Patients taking supplemental corticosteroids require special consideration during the perioperative period. Those taking prednisone at dosages >20–30 mg/d for longer than a week or with known adrenal insufficiency should be given "stress doses" of steroids after surgery (SOE=C). A single preoperative measurement of cortisol, if increased, is useful to assess the hypothalamic-pituitary axis (HPA) in patients who chronically use steroids when the function of the HPA is in question. If the cortisol level is not high, a 30-minute adrenocorticotropic hormone (ACTH) stimulation test may be useful. The dosage of steroids to use is debated, but some experts advise 25 mg of hydrocortisone equivalents only on the day of surgery for minor procedures, 50–75 mg of hydrocortisone equivalents daily (eg, hydrocortisone 20 mg q8h IV) for 1–2 days for moderate surgical stress, and 100–150 mg of hydrocortisone equivalents daily (eg, hydrocortisone 50 mg q8h IV beginning within 2 hours of surgery) continuing for 2–3 days after surgery for high surgical stress. Other experts simply recommend continuing usual dosages of steroids for elective, uncomplicated surgeries, or doubling or tripling the outpatient dosage by giving hydrocortisone at dosages up to 100–150 mg/d IV for higher-risk or anticipated complicated operations.

Delirium and Postoperative Cognitive Decline

Delirium is one of the most common postoperative complications. In a randomized study, a multicomponent intervention that focused on reducing sleep interruptions, minimizing medications and immobility, enhancing sensory input, and reducing dehydration reduced the rate of developing delirium by one-third over standard care for hospitalized medical patients (SOE=A). This approach, although not specifically studied in the postoperative setting, is likely to be beneficial for these patients as well (SOE=C). For the postoperative geriatric surgical patient, undertreated pain, constipation, electrolyte abnormalities, and perioperative myocardial infarction must be particularly considered as possible precipitants of delirium.

Postoperative cognitive dysfunction, characterized by abnormalities in learning and memory, can be subtle or dramatic and is considered to be a syndrome distinct from delirium. It has been reported most commonly after cardiac surgery but is experienced by patients undergoing procedures that do not involve extracorporeal circulation. Although the symptoms are often short-lived, they persist for many months in 10%–30% of patients. Efforts to define the cause of the syndrome have not yet been successful; studies have not been able to demonstrate links with hypotension, hypoxemia, or type of anesthesia. Because a better understanding of the pathophysiology is lacking, treatment efforts are supportive.

Pain Management

Management of postoperative pain remains a challenge, particularly in patients with dementia, delirium, or both. The oldest-old and cognitively impaired patients appear to be at highest risk of undertreatment of pain, so they deserve particular attention. Undertreatment of pain, at least in nondemented individuals, appears to be a more powerful predictor for development of postoperative delirium than opioid use (SOE=A).

Most postsurgical pain requires opioid analgesia, but as with any older patient, opioids should be used at the lowest effective dose for the shortest time necessary to reduce the risks associated with long-term use. Cognitively intact patients may have improved pain relief and overall lower use of opioids if administered by patient-controlled analgesia pump (SOE=A). Individuals with less severe pain may be able to tolerate scheduled acetaminophen (not to exceed 4 g/d) with only as-needed use of opioid analgesics, if they are able to ask for them. Patients with pain who are unable to communicate effectively should be given standing orders for opioid analgesics, with guidelines as to when to withhold the medications, and should be frequently assessed for medication effect. NSAIDs are best avoided because of the potential for GI bleeding, delirium, fluid retention, nephrotoxicity, and cardiovascular risks. Because opioid analgesics can precipitate constipation, concomitant use of laxatives and fecal softeners is generally advised, and patients discharged to home on opioid analgesia should be given a prescription for naloxone with instructions for its use. For comprehensive, up-to-date information on pain medications and dosing, see *Geriatrics At Your Fingertips* at www.GeriatricsCareOnline.org.

Nonpharmacologic therapies, such as ice packs, heating pads, massage, and relaxation techniques, can be useful adjuncts to therapy and are often underused.

CHOOSING WISELY® RECOMMENDATIONS

Perioperative Care

- Do not perform stress cardiac imaging or advanced noninvasive imaging as a preoperative assessment in patients scheduled to undergo low-risk noncardiac surgery.
- Patients who have no cardiac history and good functional status do not require preoperative stress testing before noncardiac thoracic surgery.
- Do not perform preoperative medical tests for eye surgery unless there are specific medical indications.
- Avoid echocardiograms for preoperative/perioperative assessment of patients with no history or symptoms of heart disease.
- Do not order coronary artery calcium scoring for preoperative evaluation for any surgery, irrespective of patient risk.
- Do not initiate routine evaluation of carotid artery disease before cardiac surgery in the absence of symptoms or other high-risk criteria.
- Before cardiac surgery, there is no need for pulmonary function testing in the absence of respiratory symptoms.
- Do not obtain preoperative chest radiography in the absence of clinical suspicion for intrathoracic pathology.

RESOURCES

- Colburn JL, Mohanty S, Burton JR. Surgical guidelines for perioperative management of older adults: what geriatricians need to know. *J Am Geriatr Soc.* 2017;65(6):1339–1346.

- Deal K, Schofield DL. Preoperative evaluation of aortic stenosis patient. *J Nurs Pract.* 2019;15(1):41–46.

- Oster KA, Oster CA. Special needs population: Care of the geriatric patient population in the perioperative setting. *AORN J.* 2015;101(4):443–456.

CHAPTER 17—PALLIATIVE CARE

KEY POINTS

- Palliative care, an interdisciplinary activity, aims to relieve physical and emotional suffering, optimize function, and assist with decision making for patients with serious illness and their families. Palliative services may be provided regardless of whether the patient is receiving curative or disease-modifying treatment. It is distinct from hospice. Hospice is a comprehensive care system for patients expected to live ≤6 months; its sole focus of care is on comfort and relief of suffering for individuals at life's end.

- For many older adults, dying is characterized by inadequately treated physical distress; fragmented care systems; poor or absent communication among clinicians, patients, and families; and enormous strain on family caregivers and support systems.

- The experiences of dying individuals are affected by geographic variations in practice patterns and services available, religious beliefs, economic status, medical diagnoses, gender, and cognitive function.

- Loss of appetite is an almost universal symptom at the end of life; often it is more distressing to loved ones than to the patient.

In the United States, the overwhelming majority of deaths occur among the older adult population. Older adults typically die slowly of chronic diseases, with multiple coexisting problems, progressive dependency on others, and heavy personal care needs, which are met mostly by family members. Many of these deaths become protracted processes for patients, family members, and clinicians, who must make difficult decisions about the use or discontinuation of life-prolonging treatments. Abundant evidence indicates the quality of life during the dying process is often poor. For many older adults, dying is characterized by inadequately treated physical distress; fragmented care systems; poor or absent communication among clinicians, patients, and families; and enormous strains on family caregivers and support systems.

Although Americans usually spend most of their final months at home, their deaths typically occur in the hospital or nursing home. The experience of dying varies greatly from one part of the country to another. For example, in Portland, Oregon, 35% of adult deaths occur in hospitals, but in New York City >80% occur there, a difference associated in part with variations in regional hospital bed supply and availability of community support for the dying. Social and medical variations also account for these differing patterns. The need for paid caregivers or institutionalization in the last months of life is much higher among poor individuals and women. Similarly, older adults suffering from cognitive impairment are much more likely than cognitively intact individuals to spend their last days in a nursing home.

OVERALL CARE NEAR DEATH

The Hospitalized Elderly Longitudinal Project (HELP) and the Choices, Attitudes, and Strategies for Care of Advanced Dementia at the End-of-Life (CASCADE) are two studies that examined the end of life for older adults. The HELP study characterized the last 6 months of life and dying in 1,266 adults ≥80 years old. Patients who died within 1 year of enrollment had significant functional impairment in activities of daily living (ADLs) and expressed strong preferences for no resuscitation attempts and for comfort care (SOE=A). The number of patients reporting severe pain increased toward the end of life, with one in three reporting severe pain within 3 months of death (SOE=A). The CASCADE study described the course of 323 nursing-home residents with advanced dementia. Researchers showed that pneumonia, eating problems, and fevers were the events most associated with 6-month mortality (SOE=A). Patients with advanced dementia were underrecognized to be at high risk of death and received suboptimal palliative care. The results of these two studies highlight the need for clinicians to talk with patients early about their preferences and to provide better symptom control and palliative measures at the end of life.

One of the challenges in providing excellent end-of-life care stems from the difficulty to accurately prognosticate, particularly for patients with chronic diseases such as heart failure and COPD, in which exacerbations and remissions are common and unpredictable. Various online tools and smart phone applications are available to help providers to prognosticate. The online site http://eprognosis.ucsf.edu is a repository of validated geriatric prognostic indices helpful in clinical practice. *"Hospice in a Minute"* is a free application for smart phones that includes a section on hospice eligibility criteria for several diseases.

UNIQUE POPULATIONS

No group of people is exempt from having serious illness. Ethnographic studies show that a patient's and family's ethnic, cultural, and religious heritage can influence their responses to disease, desire for aggressive care, death, grief, and mourning (SOE=B). Other special populations may have needs that present challenges to providing excellent end-of-life care.

Discussions of death may be thought to bring it about or speed its advance, so clinicians may wish to be careful when entering into discussions about end-of-life issues. Families may request the diagnosis not be shared directly with patients. Health care decisions may be viewed as family decisions, so it is especially important for clinicians to determine who should be present for delivery of bad news or discussion of care goals.

It is important to remember that not all patients and families from a particular background will respond and make choices in a similar manner. Assuming patients and families will do so can lead to misunderstanding. One useful way to introduce the subject is for the clinician to begin by asking, "Is there anything about your culture or your beliefs that would be helpful for me to know as we plan together for the future?"

Special Populations

Veterans who served in WWII, the Korean War, and the Vietnam War are aging and in need of end-of-life care. Veterans have unique physical and emotional health care needs. Old traumas related to war can resurface or surface for the first time. The Department of Veterans Affairs (VA) provides palliative care consultation at all of its medical centers and inpatient hospice care at many of its nursing homes. The VA contracts with local community-based hospices to provide care when needed. The VA and the National Hospice and Palliative Care Organization have partnered and developed the "We Honor Veterans" program. This national program helps community hospice providers to better understand and address veterans' needs at the end of life.

It is estimated that there are at least 1.5 million LGBT people who are ≥65 years old in the United States. LGBT people often face specific psychological, emotional and legal issues at the end of life. The LGBT community experience disparities in both health care and health status (SOE=A). Providers of end-of-life care to the LGBT community need training to address these issues.

A recent scoping review of the literature on culturally and spiritually sensitive end-of-life care found that most of the literature in this area focuses on decision making and not on the experience of end-of-life care for traditionally marginalized groups of people and their families. This lack of knowledge makes it difficult to ensure that clinicians are providing end-of-life care that fully meets the needs of all patients. Unfortunately, a lack of focus on developing effective programs to help clinicians become culturally and spiritually competent currently exists (SOE=A). Despite the lack of research in this area, guidelines are needed to promote culturally and spiritually competent care that incorporates the experience of all people.

HOSPICE

Palliative care is interdisciplinary care that aims to relieve physical and emotional suffering, improve quality of life, optimize function, and assist with decision making for patients with serious illness and their families. It is offered simultaneously with all other disease-modifying medical treatments, either by the primary medical team or in conjunction with a palliative care consultant. In contrast, hospice is specialized palliative care limited to patients who meet two criteria: their life expectancy is <6 months if their disease takes its natural course, and they (or their proxies) have elected to focus on comfort measures and forgo curative treatment.

Hospice, established as a Medicare benefit in 1982, can be provided at home or in institutional settings such as assisted-living environments or nursing homes. Initially, hospice coverage was made available through an expanded Medicare benefit; now it is supported through Medicare and Medicaid, the Veterans Affairs Medical System, and most commercial insurance policies. Hospice is primarily a home-health care program, with access to skilled inpatient beds for the infrequent management of acute problems, such as severe pain, dyspnea, or agitation. Hospice programs receive one of four daily rates for reimbursement, based on four levels of care: routine home care (RHC), general inpatient care, continuous care (short term, nursing-intensive crisis management of symptoms), and respite care. For a summary of the services hospice provides compared with palliative care, see Table 17.1.

To enroll in hospice services, two physicians—the hospice medical director and the patient's referring physician—must certify that they believe the patient has a remaining life expectancy of ≤6 months if the disease runs its expected course. Both physicians must sign a "Certificate of Terminal Illness" attesting to this assessment. Medicare guidelines require that the patient be recertified hospice-eligible every few months. This is similar to the recertification required for Medicare skilled rehabilitation and skilled home-care services. However, prognostication is challenging, and accuracy increases with experience. If the patient is no longer judged to have a remaining life expectancy of <6 months, then he or she must be discharged from hospice. The patient can also revoke the hospice benefit at any time, for example, if a decision is made to resume curative treatments. Patients may remain under hospice care for >6 months, as long as with each reevaluation they continue to meet the Medicare standard of being terminally ill with a *likely life expectancy* of ≤6 months.

On January 1, 2011, CMS enacted a new regulation on hospices requiring a "face-to-face" visit for all patients entering their third certification period (at

Table 17.1—Comparison of Hospice and Palliative Care

Characteristic	Hospice	Palliative Care
Patient population	People with a prognosis of ≤6 months to live and have decided to forgo curative treatments	Any person with serious illness regardless of prognosis and care being provided
Composition of interdisciplinary team	Must include a physician, registered nurse, social worker, chaplain, bereavement specialist, volunteers, and others	May include a physician, advanced practice nurse, social worker, chaplain and other staff
Care setting	Primarily a person's residence with access to inpatient hospice unit if needed	Primarily hospitals with a growing number of outpatient services available
Payment for services	Medicare, Medicaid, VA, and most common commercial insurance carriers; Medicare services are defined by law.	Insurance pays only professional fees (eg, Medicare Part A reimburses providers); there is no mechanism to reimburse other interdisciplinary team members.
Coverage	All medications and durable medical equipment related to hospice diagnosis	No coverage for these services

6 months of hospice services) and every 60-day certification period thereafter. These face-to-face visits may only be completed by a physician affiliated with the hospice or by a nurse practitioner who is a W2 employee of the hospice. The purpose of this bedside evaluation is for a trained clinician to assess the patient's ongoing eligibility for hospice services and to deliberately reevaluate a patient's prognosis. Anecdotal evidence suggests the face-to-face visit has not resulted in a dramatic increase in live discharges from hospice.

Concurrent Care

The phrase "concurrent care" is commonly applied to a patient's care plan that combines therapies aimed at illness modification with hospice services. The ability for a hospice to accommodate this dual approach is directly related to its funding sources. For example, the VA system wholeheartedly embraces a concurrent care model, as do most major commercial insurance companies. In other situations, the hospice agency itself might elect to underwrite a medical therapy not historically covered by the Medicare Hospice Benefit, such as radiation therapy for a painful bony metastasis, because it is the optimal treatment for a given patient, despite its cost.

Grief and Bereavement

Provision of bereavement care is required as part of the Medicare Hospice Benefit. For a minimum of 1 year after the death of a hospice patient, typically past the first anniversary of the patient's death plus 1 month, grieving families and friends of hospice patients are offered bereavement support. These supports vary widely from hospice agency to agency and may include follow-up emails, phone calls, office or home visits, and support groups. In some communities, hospices open their bereavement services as a community benefit to anyone grieving, regardless of prior hospice participation. In other models, hospice might offer outreach to families of those who died under an associated palliative care program at home, or under care of an affiliated hospital-based palliative team, both before hospice enrollment.

COMMUNICATION

Skillful communication by clinicians is essential to the delivery of high-quality palliative care. Most patients under care are dying from a progressive chronic illness (or more than one) like heart disease, cancer, cerebrovascular disease, chronic lung disease, dementia, or chronic liver disease. Many face recurrent exacerbations of illness and have to make difficult decisions about treatment options. To accompany patients and families through the process of diagnosis, evaluation of treatment options, and eventual death, clinicians need skills in discussing serious news, prognosis, and transitions of care; clarifying treatment goals; dealing with emotions of patients and families; and facilitating family meetings. Effective communication in end-of-life care improves patients' and families' satisfaction and experience of care (SOE=B).

A systematic approach to communication can foster collaboration among the patient, the family, and the clinician (SOE=C). Effective discussions can enhance the patient's and the family's ability to plan for the future, set realistic goals, and support one another emotionally. Several programs, such as VitalTalk and the Serious Illness Care Program by Ariadne Labs, are examples of programs developed to educate providers in communication skills for conversations about serious illness (SOE=B).

A key skill to enhance communication is recognizing and responding to emotions. Patients' emotional responses may interfere with their ability to digest information and thus impede decisions about next steps. Patients often report not hearing anything more after receiving notice of a life-threatening condition. Responding to emotions may help patients to process them, a step that often must precede the assimilation of information about prognosis or treatment options. Clinicians' response to emotions also demonstrates empathy and openness to further discussion, and signifies to patients they are understood. One recommended approach to responding to emotions is, first, to recognize that the patient has had an emotional response; next, to name the emotion; and finally to explicitly respond to the patient in a way that acknowledges the emotion. The recognition can be verbal or nonverbal. Data show that how patients are told about serious information (such as a new cancer diagnosis) impacts patient outcomes (SOE=B).

Communication about serious illness is enhanced when clinicians spend sufficient time getting to know their patients and adopting a goal of exploring their patients' life values and aims. Clinicians need to understand what is important to the patient, including determining if and how they want information given to them, and how they want to participate in decision making about their care. Although most Americans say they want to be fully informed about their illnesses, a minority may not want to know the full details or may prefer to have another family member informed. Although data suggest that these preferences may vary among certain ethnic groups, there is no way to know how much a given patient wants to know or be involved in decision making without asking directly. Patients with serious illness and their families also may have different communication needs from each other, and it is important to determine this early. Asking, "Are you the type of person who is comforted by details and test data?" or "Would it be helpful to discuss prognosis now?" both allows the patient to remain in control as well as determines the amount of information to which they are exposed.

Discussing serious news with patients may provoke anxiety in the clinician. The literature offers several frameworks, all with similar steps, and each based on a shared decision-making paradigm. Use of a framework can minimize stress by serving as a procedural checklist. The SPIKES framework is helpful for "breaking bad news," which encompasses many of these serious conversations (Table 17.2). One key to these dialogues is determining if patients, their families, or both, understand the current medical situation. It is then important to assess patients' and families' willingness to talk about what to do next. A clinician might first inquire if the patient has thought about what he or she would do at this point in the disease, or what he or she is hoping for or worried about. Based on these discussions, a provider may offer to make a recommendation for care that is seen as consistent with the goals and values a patient has expressed. This often will include the suggestion to enroll in hospice or make a referral to palliative care. After making the recommendation, the clinician may explore what the patient and family think about the proposal. The provider might emphasize the expertise of a palliative care team to improve symptom management and to help address the physical and practical changes brought on by the disease. When discussing hospice, it is important to specifically describe what hospice can do to meet the patient's articulated goals and needs. Providers should also emphasize their continued involvement with the patient regardless of hospice and/or palliative care involvement, because patients with advanced illness often fear abandonment by their providers at end of life. Patients and families also often have misconceptions about hospice and palliative care, which should be elicited and addressed to ensure that the goals and procedures of hospice and palliative care are understood.

After patients' preferences for end-of-life care are elicited (perhaps through surrogates), they must be faithfully communicated. Often, these preferences are documented in advance directives or written orders about cardiopulmonary resuscitation. Studies show that these documents are often ineffective in determining end-of-life treatment (SOE=B). The Physician Orders for Life Sustaining Treatment (POLST) program was developed initially in Oregon to address the inadequacies of communicating end-of-life preferences, and over the past decade use of these forms has spread to many other states. The forms may go by slightly different names, depending on the jurisdiction. These forms constitute medical orders reflecting preferences for cardiopulmonary resuscitation, medical interventions, antibiotics, and artificial hydration. Importantly, these orders transfer across care settings. For example, a patient with widely metastatic colon cancer who elects a "do-not-attempt-resuscitation" status at his or her cancer center can have a POLST form completed for his ambulance ride to a local hospice facility. The POLST orders would be immediately active on arrival, before evaluation by the receiving hospice clinician. If a cardiac arrest were to transpire en route or on arrival, the POLST would exempt emergency personnel from attempting "heroic measures." Research on the POLST program has shown a decreased rate of unwanted hospitalization and better documentation of preferences (SOE=B).

PALLIATION OF SYMPTOMS

As with all clinical evaluations in geriatric medicine, the first step in a palliative-focused, symptom assessment is determination of the patient's goals of care. Next, the clinical evaluation incorporates an assessment of the patient's functional status, physical ability to tolerate different treatment modalities and routes of medication administration, and overall prognosis. Clinical data are then merged with patient and family goals, values, and

Table 17.2—SPIKES Mnemonic

Step	Specific Tasks
Set up Interview	■ Have a unified message: obtain key prognostic data and communicate with team members before the meeting. ■ Prepare for emotional responses to difficult information and questions. ■ Control the setting: set up a private room, have enough chairs, ensure strategic seating, avoid interruptions.
Assess **P**erception	■ Begin with an open-ended question: "What have your doctors told you about your medical situation so far?" ■ Refine with specific questions: "What specific concerns do you have about...?" ■ Tailor prognostic information according to the patient's level of understanding.
Obtain **I**nvitation	■ Gain permission to share prognosis: "Many people have questions about prognosis and wonder about how long do I have? I'm wondering if you have those questions." ■ Explore how much information should be given: "Some patients like all of the information. Would you like me to discuss it all, or try to summarize for you?"
Impart **K**nowledge	■ If needed, begin with a warning statement: "I'm afraid that what I have to tell you is bad news." ■ Use small pieces of information (1 or 2 sentences), avoid jargon, pause frequently, and assess understanding. ■ Address uncertainty: use ranges, best or worst scenarios, and most likely case scenarios.
Address **E**motions	■ Observe and internally identify emotions. If unclear, clarify: "Can you tell me what you are worried about?" ■ Validate your understanding of the emotion by making an empathetic statement and/or gesture.
Summarize and **S**trategize	■ Assess understanding and address gaps in knowledge: "Before we move on, I want to make sure I communicated well. What have you heard from me today? What questions do you have?" ■ Set a specific timeline for what specific treatment or diagnostic decisions need to be made, when they need to be made, and who will communicate decisions to whom.

DATA FROM: Baile WF, Buckman R, Lenzi R, et al. SPIKES—A six-step protocol for delivering bad news: application to the patient with cancer. *Oncologist.* 2000;5(4):302–311.

cultural norms through a process of shared decision making to develop a care plan that is individualized to each patient. For example, medications that may ordinarily be eschewed elsewhere in geriatric care, such as benzodiazepines, may have their use in the care of a dyspneic patient whose life expectancy is <72 hours and whose family is gathered at bedside, sitting vigil, and hoping for a peaceful death.

Pain

Pain management in older adults with serious and life-limiting illness is no different than it is for other patients. It begins with a thorough assessment of the pain, formulation of the causes of the pain, and deliberation of management strategies to treat the pain. The key to good pain management is reassessment of interventions for their effectiveness in providing relief. It is often helpful to conceptualize pain as acute versus chronic, and with qualities that define it as somatic, visceral, or neuropathic. This is helpful in guiding what treatments might be effective. Patients who have cognitive impairment have not been shown to feel pain any less acutely than others, but they may exhibit their discomfort by withdrawing from surroundings (eg, lack of appetite or participation) or by increasing agitation and resistance to daily care. In patients at the very end of life, oral administration of medication may not be possible, and alternative routes of delivery (eg, via suppositories, transmucosal formulations, or subcutaneous injection) may need to be explored.

Constipation

Constipation is one of the most common and distressing symptoms seen in terminally ill patients. Many medications, including opioid pain medications, significantly contribute to constipation, which is further exacerbated by the reduced mobility and poor fluid intake that accompanies most life-limiting illnesses. Although other unwanted effects of opioids generally diminish over time, constipation usually persists, requiring ongoing bowel management as long as opioid therapy is used (SOE=D). Patients on opioids should receive prophylactic laxatives consisting of a bowel stimulant (eg, senna, bisacodyl), unless diarrhea has already been a problem. If these measures are not effective, then an osmotic laxative (eg, sorbitol, lactulose, or polyethylene glycol) should be added. If a patient has had no bowel movement for ≥4 days, an enema should be considered. Patients presenting with constipation should be evaluated for bowel obstruction or fecal impaction. In cases of impaction, manual removal of the impaction or enemas should be used before starting laxative therapy.

An increasing number of medications have been approved by the FDA specifically for opioid-induced constipation. It is appropriate to consider using these medications when prophylactic and first-line interventions fail (SOE=C).

Two peripherally acting mu-opioid antagonists (PAMORAs) are available, methylnaltrexone bromide and naloxegol. PAMORAs antagonize opioid binding to the peripheral mu-opioid receptors in the GI tract. The medications do not cross the blood-brain barrier and have no effect on the central analgesic effects of opioids, meaning patients do not experience a reduction in their levels of pain control. PAMORAs are contraindicated in known or suspected mechanical intestinal obstruction. Lubiprostone is a chloride channel activator also approved for use in opioid constipation, as well as idiopathic constipation. Like PAMORAs, it is contraindicated in bowel obstruction.

Nausea and Vomiting

The incidence of nausea and vomiting is estimated to be 40%–70% in patients with advanced cancer (SOE=B). Nausea has a significant impact on quality of life and can lead to complications, including dehydration, electrolyte imbalance, weight loss, and emotional distress. Nausea is a subjective sensation mediated through the stimulation of the GI lining, the chemoreceptor trigger zone, the vestibular apparatus, and the cerebral cortex. Vomiting is a neuromuscular reflex. Symptoms can be caused both by disease and its treatment. Because nausea involves multiple neurotransmitters, numerous agents are used for treatment, and often more than one medication is needed for control. The key to successful management involves identifying the likely cause of the nausea, reversing what can be reversed, identifying what area is being stimulated (GI tract, chemoreceptor trigger zone, vestibular apparatus, and /or the cerebral cortex), selecting a medication that works on the cause, and giving around-the-clock medication if the nausea is constant (SOE=D). For medications useful in treatment of nausea, see Table 17.3. Although many providers have used topical lorazepam, diphenhydramine, and haloperidol gel (aka "ABH") for treatment of nausea, evidence has shown it is not effective and should not be used to treat nausea (SOE=A). This is a recommendation of The Choosing Wisely® Campaign.

Diarrhea

Diarrhea affects 7%–10% of patients with cancer who are admitted to hospice (SOE=C). Diarrhea is defined as the passage of more than three unformed bowel movements within a 24-hour period. A common cause of diarrhea in palliative medicine is excessive laxative administration, especially after upward dose adjustments intended to clear an impaction. These diarrheal episodes respond to temporary cessation of laxatives, and delayed reintroduction at a lower dosage.

The clinician should be alert to the possibility of fecal impaction that presents as watery diarrhea, particularly in immobile older adults on opioids. The treatment of impaction should begin with manual disimpaction and tap water enemas, followed, if unsuccessful, by high colonic enemas. Laxatives should not be administered until the impaction is cleared because of the risk of bowel perforation. Untreated fecal impaction can be life threatening.

Radiotherapy involving the abdomen and pelvis commonly causes diarrhea, peaking during the second or third week of therapy. This typically responds to cholestyramine^{OL} at 4–12 g q8h (SOE=C). Cholestyramine is also helpful in treating diarrhea occurring as a complication of ileal resection. Diarrhea caused by fat malabsorption (eg, from pancreatic insufficiency or small-bowel disease) responds to pancreatic enzymes such as pancreatin (SOE=B). Secretory diarrhea generally responds to octreotide. Profuse, watery diarrhea can also be seen in both infectious colitis, and as an adverse effect of immunotherapy agents. Careful diagnostic assessment is needed for the success of targeted treatment.

Gastrointestinal Obstruction

In older adults, causes of bowel obstruction include direct intraluminal obstruction by tumor, malignant infiltration of the bowel wall, external compression of the bowel wall (eg, from bulky lymphadenopathy), dysmotility, fecal impaction, adverse effects of radiation treatment, volvulus, and adhesions from previous surgeries. The upper portions of the GI tract, such as the esophagus, stomach, and duodenum, and portions of the pancreaticobiliary systems can also become obstructed directly by tumors or infiltrating masses or externally compressed by malignancy or abscess. Patients diagnosed with malignant bowel obstruction have a poor prognosis, with a median survival of 3 months. The incidence of bowel obstruction can be up to 50% in ovarian and gastrointestinal cancers.

The symptom burden from bowel obstruction is significant and can include hyper-salivation, nausea, vomiting, colicky abdominal pain, and anorexia and weight loss. The evaluation and management of bowel obstruction depends on the functional status of the patient, goals of care, and expected survival. General treatment options include radiation therapy, surgical correction (palliative versus definitive), stenting, venting gastrostomy or jejunostomy tubes, and pharmacologic management. There is a scarcity of randomized control trials to guide optimal treatment.

Surgical management to resect the site of blockage has limited evidence for benefit in terms of quality of life and survival for most patients with bowel obstruction and limited life expectancy (ie, ≤3 months). Surgery may be beneficial for patients with a good performance status, an operable lesion, and an expected survival of 2–6 months. Advances in endoscopic techniques and self-expanding metallic stents have allowed for a nonsurgical approach to bowel obstruction. Stents have been used for

Table 17.3—Medications for Nausea

Class	Predominant Site of Action	Examples	Comments
Dopamine antagonists	Chemoreceptor trigger zone	Haloperidol[OL] 0.5–2 mg po, IV, or SC q6h, then titrate Prochlorperazine 10–20 mg po q6h, or 25 mg pr q12h, or 5–10 mg IV q6h Promethazine 12.5–25 mg IV, or 25 mg po or pr q4–6h Perphenazine 2–8 mg po q6h	Haloperidol is an effective antinausea medication. Promethazine and perphenazine can cause sedation, urinary retention, and delirium in frail older adults.
Serotonin antagonists	Chemoreceptor trigger zone, GI tract	Ondansetron 8 mg po q8h Granisetron 1 mg po q24h or q12h	Effective for chemotherapy-induced nausea; expensive
Neurokinin-1 receptor antagonist	Chemoreceptor trigger zone	Aprepitant 125 mg po then 80 mg/d po	Recommended for resistant cases of chemotherapy-induced nausea
Prokinetic agents	GI tract	Metoclopramide 5–20 mg po q6h	Useful if nausea is secondary to dysmotility
Antacids	GI tract	H_2-receptor antagonists: cimetidine, famotidine, ranitidine Proton-pump inhibitors: pantoprazole, omeprazole, lansoprazole	Useful if nausea is caused by gastritis
Corticosteroids	GI tract, cerebral cortex	Dexamethasone 6–10 mg po loading dose followed by 2–4 mg po q6–12h Prednisone 4–10 mg/d po	Useful for nausea from hepatic capsular distention and increased intracranial pressure; monitor for adverse effects, including altered mood, psychosis
Synthetic somatostatin analogue	GI tract	Octreotide 100–200 mcg SC bid to qid or a continuous infusion	Useful in nausea from bowel obstruction
Antihistamines	Vestibular	Diphenhydramine 25–50 mg po q6h Meclizine 25–50 mg po q6h Hydroxyzine 25–50 mg po q6h	Can cause sedation, urinary retention, and delirium in frail older adults
Anticholinergics	Vestibular	Scopolamine 0.1–0.4 mg SC or IV q4h, or 1 to 3 transdermal patches q72h, or 10–80 mcg/h by continuous IV or SC infusion	Useful when cause of nausea is from vestibular apparatus
Benzodiazepines	Cerebral cortex	Lorazepam up to 2mg po night before chemotherapy and up to 2 mg po after chemotherapy	Helpful for anticipatory nausea and vomiting from chemotherapy; can cause agitation in older adults
Cannabinoids	Cerebral cortex	Dronabinol 2.5 mg po to a maximum total dose of 50 mg po qd in divided doses	Can cause dysphoria, hallucinations; evidence is poor for effectiveness

esophageal, gastric outlet, small-bowel, and colonic obstructions, as well as in the pancreaticobiliary system. Radiation treatments may be considered in conjunction with stent placement, especially in esophageal cancers, or as a sole therapeutic option.

The mainstay of treatment for bowel obstruction is medical management. In most patients, symptoms can be alleviated by combination therapy with opioids, antispasmodic medications, antiemetics, antisecretory agents, and corticosteroids. Opioids can be given subcutaneously, intravenously, sublingually, and transdermally, and should be titrated for relief of abdominal pain. For antispasmodic and antisecretory medications helpful in bowel obstructions, see Table 17.4. Corticosteroids have been used for bowel obstruction as antiemetics and as analgesics, and to reduce peritumor edema. Generally, they are given for a trial period of 4–5 days and discontinued if there is no response. If medical management is not effective, a venting gastrostomy may be considered.

Nasogastric tubes are often placed when a patient is admitted to the hospital with a bowel obstruction. These tubes should be temporary measures only while a decision about surgery is considered or medications to control symptoms are started. Caution is advised because nasogastric tubes are associated with pain, sinusitis, aspiration, and erosions in the nose and esophagus.

Anorexia and Cachexia

Loss of appetite or anorexia is an almost universal symptom of patients with serious and life-limiting illness. Anorexia in those who are actively dying and

Table 17.4—Medications Used for Bowel Obstruction

Drug	Dosage	Comments
Glycopyrrolate	0.2–0.4 mg SC q2–4h	Antisecretory; less centrally mediated adverse events because does not penetrate blood-brain barrier
Scopolamine	0.1–0.2 mg SC or IV q6–8h Transdermal patch every 3 days	Antispasmodic and antisecretory; transdermal patch does not have immediate effect
Hyoscyamine	0.125 mg SL q4–8h	Antispasmodic; may cause urinary retention and confusion
Octreotide	12.5 mcg/h SC or IV continuous infusion, or 200–600 mcg SC or IV intermittently; maximum of 900 mcg in 24 hours	Antisecretory; well tolerated and effective in decreasing GI secretions

who do not express a desire to eat need not be treated. Families and significant others, however, can be very distressed when their loved one does not eat; providing food is often equated with showing love. The clinician needs to evaluate for and treat reversible causes of anorexia and cachexia (eg, thrush, nausea) if the patient's goals and prognosis warrant. Symptoms of dry mouth can be alleviated with ice chips, popsicles, moist compresses, or artificial saliva. Lemon glycerin swabs should not be used, because they irritate dry and cracked mucosa. Megestrol acetate and corticosteroids[OL] have been found to enhance appetite, cause weight gain (primarily fat), and improve quality of life in some patients with anorexia (SOE=B). However, these agents do not prolong survival or improve function or treatment tolerance of cancer therapies, and are associated with adverse events (SOE=B). The Choosing Wisely® Campaign does not recommend using prescription appetite stimulants or high-calorie supplements to treat anorexia or cachexia in older adults based on these findings. In general, patients should be encouraged to eat whatever is most appealing without regard to dietary restrictions. Often, it is preferable to provide patient and family education regarding the normalcy of anorexia as a part of the end-of-life process.

Enteral feedings are often used in chronically ill and dying patients because of families' and clinicians' perceived need to provide nutrition to a loved one. There is no evidence to support the use of such feedings in this situation. Enteral feedings are not associated with improved quality of life or survival in this context and are associated with increased frequency of aspiration and other complications. An inability to maintain oral nutrition in patients with chronic life-limiting disease is best regarded as a marker of dying, not a problem solvable by artificial nutrition. The Choosing Wisely® Campaign does not recommend the placement of enteral feeding tubes in patients with advanced dementia but instead recommends offering oral-assisted feeding.

Nevertheless, enteral feeding may enhance quality and quantity of life in a few situations; examples include patients with good functional status and proximal gastrointestinal obstruction; patients receiving chemotherapy or radiation involving the proximal gastrointestinal tract; and patients with amyotrophic lateral sclerosis (SOE=B).

Delirium

Delirium is common in seriously ill older patients and is distressing to both patients and family members. Early recognition of delirium is important. It is thought that up to 50% of delirium in palliative care is reversible. Efforts to identify potentially reversible causes (eg, infection, impaction, uncontrolled pain, urinary retention, medications, dehydration, and hypoxia) should be based on the patient's current goals of care and disease trajectory. Traditionally, both nonpharmacologic and pharmacologic approaches have been recommended to treat delirium. Nonpharmacologic approaches include minimizing noise, using an orientation board, mounting a visible clock in the room, using simple communication, having family present, educating family caregivers, and minimizing disruptions. Antipsychotics such as haloperidol[OL] or risperidone[OL] in low dosages have been the recommended medications for treatment of both hypoactive and hyperactive delirium. However, in a recent randomized control trial, the use of antipsychotic medications in palliative care worsened symptoms of delirium and were associated with lower survival rates in mild to moderately severe delirium (SOE=A). Benzodiazepines have also been used to treat delirium, but they are often associated with paradoxical agitation and worsening of the delirium in older adults; careful consideration should precede their use.

Dyspnea

Dyspnea, the subjective experience of breathlessness, is one of the most distressing symptoms experienced by dying individuals and families. Self-reporting by the patient is the only reliable measure of dyspnea. Respiratory rates, pulmonary congestion, hypoxia, or hypercarbia do not correlate with breathlessness. Clinicians may mistakenly fear that treating dyspnea in patients close to the end of life is associated with unacceptably high risks, leading some to withhold treatment and others to prescribe inadequate dosages of medications.

Because breathlessness has many causes (eg, anxiety, airway obstruction, bronchospasm, hypoxemia, pneumonia, cachexia from advanced disease), symptomatic management should begin immediately while the underlying cause is being investigated. Like pain, dyspnea is mediated through the interaction of complex pathophysiologic processes with poorly defined psychologic factors. The goal of treatment is the subjective improvement of breathlessness, rather than lowering the respiratory rate to normal. Often, patients report improvement in breathlessness yet still breathe rapidly.

The most effective agents for treatment of dyspnea are opioids[OL]. Opioids are believed to act centrally by decreasing the perception of dyspnea, and peripherally on opioid receptors in the lung without affecting respiratory drive. Nebulized opioids for intractable dyspnea have been used, but evidence of benefit is scarce. Nebulized morphine has not been shown to be helpful, but small studies of fentanyl have shown effectiveness (SOE=C). The theoretical advantages of nebulized opioids include the avoidance of systemic absorption (with resulting constipation, hypotension, sedation, respiratory depression, and hypercapnia), rapid and efficient absorption because of the large surface area of the lung parenchyma, and ease of administration. This route of administration should be reserved for patients who experience intolerable adverse effects from opioids administered by other routes.

Oxygen is considered by many to be an important component of any regimen for dyspnea. Unlike other Medicare benefits, hospice agencies will use and pay for oxygen regardless of a patient's oxygen saturation. Cool air moving across the face (eg, from fans or an open window) can treat dyspnea by stimulating the second branch of the fifth cranial nerve, which has a central inhibitory effect on the sensation of breathlessness (SOE=C).

Benzodiazepines are beneficial in controlling anxiety associated with dyspnea, but they did not improve breathlessness in randomized controlled trials in which nonanxious persons with COPD were enrolled (SOE=A). These medications should be used only in breathless patients with accompanying anxiety. Bronchodilators and corticosteroids are useful in patients with bronchospasm. Diuretics can help in care of patients with pulmonary congestion.

Cough

The prevalence of cough has been reported in the palliative care literature as ranging from 29% to 83%. Normally, cough maintains the patency and cleanliness of the airways and thus should be treated only when it causes distress. Cough can be caused by the production of excessive amounts of fluids (eg, blood, mucus), inhalation of foreign material, or stimulation of irritant receptors in the airway. Additionally, patients with neuromuscular disorders may be unable to swallow saliva because of the involvement of bulbar cranial nerves. Pooling saliva then triggers cough as it trickles into the larynx or trachea.

When feasible, underlying causes of cough should be investigated and treated (eg, with diuretics for heart failure, antibiotics for infection, anticholinergics for aspiration of saliva resulting from motor neuron disease). However, resolving the underlying cause may be impossible. Opioids can be useful in these situations.

Dextromethorphan is structurally related to opioids and has central cough-suppressant action with few sedative effects (SOE=D). Codeine and hydrocodone, usually in the form of elixirs, are also good first-line choices (SOE=D). Methadone syrup can also be helpful when taken as a single daily dose because of its longer duration of action (SOE=D).

Cough due to a pharynx irritated by local infection or malignancy may be helped by nebulized anesthetics (SOE=D). Nebulized lidocaine up to four times daily has been reported, anecdotally, to offer relief. For some patients, cough has neuropathic origins and responds to gabapentin and other similar agents (SOE=D).

Loud Respiration

Inability to clear secretions from the oropharynx often results in noisy or "rattling" respirations at the end of life. This occurs as secretions oscillate up and down during inspiration and expiration. Although there is no indication that this causes discomfort for patients, it often produces anxiety in family and caregivers. Best management includes preparing the family and caregivers for its occurrence and meaning. Anticholinergic medications reduce secretions and may be used if this symptom is distressing to the family. Because anticholinergic agents do not dry up secretions already present, it is important to ask the family to notify clinicians at the first sign of rattling. Scopolamine[OL] patches can be effective and also have a sedative effect. Hyoscyamine, glycopyrrolate, or sublingually administered atropine eye drops[OL] also effectively dry up secretions; unfortunately, these drugs contribute to dry mouth, constipation, delirium, and mucous plugging, so careful monitoring is necessary.

Depression

Depression is underrecognized and undertreated, both in older adults and seriously ill patients. It may be underdiagnosed because of clinicians' mistaken belief that it is either a normal consequence of aging or appropriate in the context of an advanced illness. Depression must also be distinguished from anticipatory grief and routine emotional response to bad news. Depression and psychological distress diminish quality of life, amplify pain and other symptoms, and impair a patient's ability to deal with the emotions involved in saying good bye. Depression is a major risk factor for suicide and for requests to clinicians to hasten death.

The diagnosis of depression in palliative care settings presents challenges. Standard neurovegetative symptoms described in the *Diagnostic and Statistical Manual of Mental Disorders* (eg, insomnia, anorexia, weight change, fatigue) are often not reliable indicators for depression near life's end, because their cause is often the terminal disease itself. Instead, clinicians should watch for change in mood, hopelessness, helplessness, worthlessness, loss of interest, and suicidal ideation. Suicidal ideation should be openly discussed, including any symptoms that are contributing to the patient's suffering, which may be influencing his or her consideration of suicide. Suicidal thoughts should be assessed immediately, and appropriate referrals considered. Aggressive treatment of symptoms, antidepressant therapy, cognitive-behavioral therapy, and psychiatric consultation are all appropriate initial responses. Involvement of clergy or pastoral care representatives may be helpful. Continued discussion with the patient about a wish to hasten death often reveals a change of mind over time.

Standard antidepressant therapy is effective, but most agents have a delayed onset of action of 2–6 weeks. Psychostimulants (eg, methylphenidate[OL], dextroamphetamine[OL]) are well-tolerated, safe, and effective short-term treatments for medically ill, depressed patients (SOE=B). Additionally, they can have a rapid onset and beneficial effect on energy, mood, appetite, and mental alertness. Methylphenidate is started at 2.5 mg in the morning and given concurrently with standard antidepressants; it should not be taken in the evening hours because of its detrimental effect on sleep. Electroconvulsive therapy is an effective, safe method of rapidly treating depression and may be considered for those who are severely depressed. The American Psychiatric Task Force Report advocates consideration of electroconvulsive therapy as a first-line treatment when rapid response is needed (SOE=D). The presence of space-occupying CNS lesions is a contraindication.

Cognitive-behavioral therapy and active listening are helpful for patients and families at end of life, whether the cause of distress is anticipatory grief, depression, or the mental fatigue of early dying. One form of brief, focused psychotherapy is dignity therapy. This therapy invites patients to reflect and discuss what is important to them, and how they wish to be remembered. The sessions are transcribed and edited. The final version is presented back to the patient who may wish to distribute it to family and/or friends.

The chaplain and social work members of hospice and palliative care teams typically serve to assist patients and families in working toward closure and resolution. Palliative care physician Ira Byock has written that dying patients need to say and hear four things to feel complete before death: "please forgive me, I forgive you, thank you, and I love you."

FUTURE DIRECTIONS

New Models of Hospice and Palliative Care

As medicine becomes more complex and funding is increasingly bundled, so too have the organizations and funding for palliative services become more sophisticated. In the past few years, palliative care services have moved from an almost exclusively inpatient, hospital-based offering underwritten by the health system itself, to the outpatient environment. Novel palliative care models now exist, including free-standing and embedded palliative clinics, home-based palliative care teams, triggered consults in skilled-nursing and long-term care facilities, and palliative care units within hospitals. Palliative services—even those in the hospital—are now offered by both for-profit and not-for-profit palliative agencies, hospices, and the health systems themselves. Perhaps some of the more exciting models to evolve are those being initiated by select health plans and accountable care organizations. Programs such as the Compassionate Care Program, a Medicare Advantage Plan, carefully select patients to offer additional services such as psychosocial supports, disease management, and care coordination as overlays to usual care. Research has shown improved symptom control, reduced emergency room and acute care use, and greater patient and family satisfaction with these "concurrent care" models. Ultimately, these programs have also shown an increase in hospice enrollment. Other innovative partnerships between palliative care clinicians and other specialists (eg, neurology, trauma surgery, etc) and evolving financing mechanisms (eg, Oncology Care Models) as well as a health care system increasingly focused on rewarding quality and value at the population level will likely result in ongoing opportunities for hospice and palliative medicine providers.

Issues on the Horizon

In the upcoming years, the current challenge of identifying quality metrics at the provider level and the agency level will become more pronounced, especially as reimbursement is increasingly linked to outcome measures. The Joint Commission began offering an advanced certification to hospitals in palliative care in 2011, and it is a rigorous standard few institutions have achieved. At the political level, laws surrounding medical marijuana and physician-assisted dying have sparked controversy and significant coverage in the press; they are no less relevant for an aging population as they are for any other group needing palliative care. The opioid epidemic is impacting pain management and will impact hospice and palliative care providers. It will take a partnership between patients, their families and caregivers, and a long-term commitment by clinicians to rationally prescribe opioids with attempts at tapering.

Choosing Wisely® Recommendations

Palliative Care and Hospice

- Do not use topical lorazepam, diphenhydramine, or haloperidol gel for nausea.

- Do not recommend percutaneous feeding tubes in patients with advanced dementia; instead offer oral assisted feeding.

- Avoid using prescription appetite stimulants or high-calorie supplements for treatment of anorexia or cachexia in older adults; instead, optimize social supports, provide feeding assistance and clarify patient goals and expectations.

RESOURCES

- Cain CL, Surbone A, Elk R, et al. Culture and palliative care: preferences, communication, meaning, and mutual decision making. *J Pain Symptom Manage*. 2018;55(5):1408–1419.

- Center to Advance Palliative Care (CAPC). https://www.capc.org

- Hospice Policy Compendium: The Medicare Hospice Benefit, Regulations, Quality Reporting and Public Policy. National Hospice and Palliative Care Organization. January 4, 2016. www.nhpco.org/sites/default/files/public/public_policy/Hospice_Policy_Compendium.pdf (accessed Feb 2019).

CHAPTER 18—PAIN MANAGEMENT

KEY POINTS

- Effective management of pain begins with a thorough assessment to determine its source, severity, and impact on functioning and well-being.

- Persistent pain constitutes a distinct pathology and causes changes throughout the nervous system that may worsen over time. It has significant psychological and cognitive correlates as well.

- Multiple pain scales are available to help quantify the severity of pain. The selection of a pain scale should be based on the cognitive and communication abilities of the patient.

- A stepped approach to the treatment of pain is advised, especially incorporating local therapies and nonpharmacologic approaches.

- Physical tolerance generally develops to the respiratory depression, fatigue, and sedating effects of opioid analgesics but not to their constipating effect.

- Given the diverse effects of persistent pain, interprofessional assessment and multimodal treatment may produce the best results for older adults who continue to have moderate or severe persistent pain despite optimal medical management.

- Clinicians should carefully monitor and document opioid usage in older adults for drug-drug interactions, impact on cognition, and aberrant usage patterns.

Relief of pain and suffering, and promotion of functional status and quality of life are primary tenets of geriatric medicine. Pain is a distressing symptom that is not just physical but also and influences the mood and even the personality of a person, thereby affecting behavior, social life, and interactions. Dame Cicely Saunders, the founder of the modern hospice movement, coined the term "total pain" to describe the multifaceted effect of pain on the "whole person including the bio-psycho-socio-spiritual-cultural impact." The contribution of each of these facets is both dynamic (varies over time) and specific to each patient.

Pain is particularly common in older adults and estimated to affect 79% of patients ≥ 85 years old. Common causes of pain in older adults include osteoarthritic pain, degenerative bone diseases, postsurgical pain, nocturnal leg pain, and pain associated with various chronic illnesses. Shingles and resultant post-herpetic neuralgia are more common in older adults, with half the cases of shingles occurring in adults ≥60 years old. Pain in older adults can lead to decreased functional status, increased falls, interrupted sleep, anxiety, agitation, delirium, and poor quality of life.

Pain among the older population is probably undertreated because of a variety of factors. Some older adults tend to underreport or do not report their pain because of cognitive impairment, limited health literacy, or an erroneous perception that pain is a part of the normal aging process. Pain is commonly underdiagnosed and undertreated in older adults who are cognitively impaired, a group shown to receive less analgesic therapies than younger, cognitively intact cohorts. Clinicians may be overwhelmed in caring for older adults who frequently have several comorbid illnesses, and thus do not regularly and systematically assess for and manage pain during busy clinic visits. Even when pain is identified, clinicians may be reluctant to manage it effectively because of the lack of adequate knowledge of pain management strategies, as well as misperceptions about opioid medications. Patients, too, may fear addiction to opioid analgesics, and commonly choose to live with pain to avoid taking these agents.

Beyond individual factors, the current national concerns about opioid-related deaths have greatly influenced the terrain of pain management. Opioids (including prescription opioids, heroin, and fentanyl) resulted in >42,000 fatalities in 2016, more than any year on record. Of all opioid overdose deaths, 40% involve a prescription opioid.

Pain is an unpleasant sensory and emotional experience associated with actual or potential tissue damage, or described in terms of such damage. Pain is subjective and idiosyncratic, beyond objective measure; its intensity and character are what the patient says they are. Pain is certainly a sensation in a part or parts of the body, but it is also by definition unpleasant and therefore also an emotional experience. *Acute pain* is of sudden onset and expected to last a short time and is clearly linked to a specific bodily insult or injury. *Chronic* or *persistent pain*, by contrast, is defined as pain without apparent biologic purpose that has persisted beyond the normal tissue healing time, variously defined as 3–6 months. Persistent pain endures as the pain signals keep firing in the nervous system for weeks, months, or even years after the initial insult or injury. Some people suffer persistent pain even in the absence of any past injury or evident body damage. Persistent pain can become so debilitating that it affects basic and instrumental ADLs, causes psychological distress (depression or anxiety), disturbs sleep, and negatively impacts social and personal relationships.

Risk factors for transition from acute to persistent pain in older adults include lower socioeconomic status, vivid memory of childhood trauma, obesity, low level of physical fitness, overuse of joints and muscles, chronic illnesses, lack of social support, and abuse.

ASSESSMENT

A thorough assessment is necessary to formulate a plan to successfully treat persistent pain. The International Association for the Study of Pain has developed a helpful taxonomy for the classification of pain that identifies 5 axes:

- Axis I: anatomic regions
- Axis II: organ systems
- Axis III: temporal characteristics, pattern of occurrence
- Axis IV: intensity, time since onset of pain
- Axis V: etiology

Beyond the limited scope of the above 5 axes, assessment should also include an exploration of the effects of pain on functional status and sleep, as well as on emotional and social well-being. Because of its subjective nature, clinicians must rely on the patient's or caregiver's description of the pain, in addition to the findings of a thorough physical examination. Assessment is complicated by several factors, including underreporting of symptoms by many older adults, the existence of multiple medical comorbidities exacerbating the pain and impairing function, and the increased prevalence of cognitive impairment with age.

When conducting a pain assessment, clinicians should concurrently assess ADLs and IADLs, assess depression, and also ask questions about underlying psychosocial and spiritual distress, both of which may serve as exacerbating factors.

Pain intensity can be quantified using pain intensity scales. Three commonly used, validated scales are the Numeric Rating Scale, the Faces Pain Scale (www.iasp-pain.org/Education/Content.aspx?ItemNumber=1519 [accessed Feb 2019]), and the Verbal Descriptor Scale. These scales are referred to as one-dimensional, because they ask the patient to rate the intensity of a single characteristic of the symptom—in this case the intensity of the pain. The patient is asked to rate his or her pain by assigning a numerical value (with 0 indicating no pain, and 10 representing the worst pain imaginable), a verbal description ("no pain" to "pain as bad as it could be"), or a facial expression corresponding to the pain. The choice of scale depends on the preference of a particular language or presence of sensory impairment. Scales such as the McGill Pain Questionnaire and the Pain Disability Scale measure pain in a variety of domains, including intensity, location, and affect. Although time intensive, such scales measuring multiple domains can provide a wealth of information about the patient's unique experience of pain. However, patients in pain may be unable or unwilling to use scales that take much time.

Other questions to consider asking in pain evaluation include the following: Is the pain interfering with your ability to complete activities like bathing, toileting, or eating? Is the pain interfering with your ability to drive, shop, cook, etc? Is the pain stopping you from doing pleasurable activities? Is the pain interfering with your sleep? Is the pain limiting your social activities?

When assessing pain in patients with cognitive impairment, it is important to remember that such patients may be unable to report their pain, much less its history. They may instead present with depression or agitation, and these secondary behaviors often serve as important clues to the presence of underlying untreated pain. Patients with cognitive impairment may not be able to use complex subjective pain assessment tools. The Pain Assessment in Advanced Dementia PAINAD can be used for measurement of pain in in those with limited ability to communicate. In patients with breathing problems, the PAINAD may overestimate the level of pain, because it uses hyperventilation and noisy breathing as proxy indicators of pain.

Before the physical examination, the patient can be asked to describe the location of the pain using a drawing of a human figure, called a pain map. The patient indicates the locations on the figure that correspond to his or her pain. Pain maps may enhance reliability in repeated assessment of pain in cognitively intact patients. In some cultures, it may be easier for patients to use a pain map to indicate pain in sensitive areas like the genitalia.

If the patient's pain pattern is erratic and diffuse, or does not conform to an anatomic distribution, a referral to a mental health specialist may help in uncovering an underlying disorder that is complicating or contributing to the complex pain presentation.

The physical examination should include careful scrutiny of the reported site of the pain and any part of the body that may be a source of referred pain. (For example, occipital pain should prompt examination of the neck, and knee pain, examination of the hip and lumbar region.) The initial evaluation should include a complete musculoskeletal examination, recognizing the common findings of musculoskeletal disorders such as fibromyalgia, osteoarthritis, and myofascial pain, as either the primary source of pain or exacerbating processes. Accurate diagnosis of these disorders is a critical part of formulating the correct therapeutic

Table 18.1—Types of Pain, Examples, and Treatment

Type of Pain and Examples	Source of Pain	Typical Description	Effective Drug Classes and Nonpharmacologic Treatments (SOE)
Nociceptive: somatic			
Arthritis, acute postoperative, fracture, bone metastases	Tissue injury, eg, bones, soft tissue, joints, muscles	Well localized, constant; aching, stabbing, gnawing, throbbing	Acetaminophen (A), opioids (B), NSAIDs (A) Physical and cognitive-behavioral therapies (B)
Nociceptive: visceral			
Renal colic, constipation	Viscera	Diffuse, poorly localized, referred to other sites, intermittent, paroxysmal; dull, colicky, squeezing, deep, cramping; often accompanied by nausea, vomiting, diaphoresis	Treatment of underlying cause, acetaminophen (C), opioids (B) Physical and cognitive-behavioral therapies (C)
Neuropathic			
Cervical or lumbar radiculopathy, post-herpetic neuralgia, trigeminal neuralgia, diabetic neuropathy, post-stroke syndrome, herniated intervertebral disc, drug toxicities	Peripheral or central nervous system	Prolonged, usually constant, but can have paroxysms; sharp, burning, pricking, tingling, electric shock–like; associated with other sensory disturbances, eg, paresthesias and dysesthesias; allodynia, hyperalgesia, impaired motor function, atrophy, or abnormal deep tendon reflexes	Tricyclic antidepressants (A), serotonin-norepinephrine reuptake inhibitor antidepressants (A), anticonvulsants (A), opioids (B), topical anesthetics (C) Physical and cognitive-behavioral therapies (C)
Undetermined			
Myofascial pain syndrome, somatic symptom pain disorders, fibromyalgia	Poorly understood	No identifiable pathologic processes or symptoms out of proportion to identifiable organic pathology; widespread musculoskeletal pain, stiffness, and weakness	Antidepressants (B), antianxiety agents (C) Physical (B), cognitive-behavioral (B), and psychological therapies (B)

SOURCE: Adapted with permission. Reuben DB, Herr KA, Pacala JT, et al. *Geriatrics At Your Fingertips*, 20th ed. New York: American Geriatrics Society; 2018:247.

plan. Fibromyalgia, which may be underrecognized in older adults, is characterized by multiple tender points, sleep disturbance, fatigue, generalized pain (often with a strong axial component), and morning stiffness. Myofascial pain is present in many patients with persistent pain and is diagnosed by the presence of taut bands of muscles and *trigger points* (ie, pain that may radiate distally when firm pressure is applied to a muscle, as opposed to *tender* points, in which radiation of pain is absent).

Pain syndromes can be divided into at least 3 types: nociceptive, neuropathic, and undetermined (Table 18.1). Nociceptive pain describes pain due to the activation of nociceptive sensory receptors by noxious stimuli resulting from inflammation, swelling, and injury to tissues. It can be defined further as either somatic or visceral pain.

Neuropathic pain derives from the irritation of components of the central or peripheral nervous systems. Confusion between neuropathic pain and myofascial pain is possible, because patients may describe both as "burning." Careful physical examination may help to differentiate these disorders (ie, taut bands and trigger points with myofascial pain, and allodynia or hyperalgesia with either disorder); both may be present in the same patient.

Mixed or unspecified pain has characteristics of both nociceptive pain and neuropathic pain, such as chronic headache of unknown cause. Older adults often have mixed pain syndromes, the complexity of which frequently poses management challenges. Lower back pain, for example, often results from a combination of spinal malalignment, myofascial pathology, and neurologic impingement. Complex regional pain syndrome is characterized by pain or sensory changes (allodynia or hyperalgesia), with some combination of edema, regional sweating abnormality, changes in blood flow to the skin, and trophic features (shiny, thin skin; altered hair or nail growth on an extremity). Treating patients with mixed or unspecified pain syndromes with trials of different medications or with combinations of medicines may be necessary, and interprofessional collaboration (physical therapy, occupational therapy, psychology) is often beneficial.

ASSESSING AND TREATING PAIN IN COGNITIVELY IMPAIRED OLDER ADULTS

Although able to speak, patients with dementia may be unable to report and localize their pain. Patients with severe cognitive impairment who are unable to verbally express pain pose a challenge to the clinicians who care for them. Not only are such patients unable to describe their pain or request analgesia, but clinicians may be hesitant to administer pain medications, fearing that pharmacologic treatment will worsen the patients' mental status. Clinicians must rely on observing these patients for pain-related behaviors, as well as on eliciting observations from caregivers. For common pain behaviors in cognitively impaired older adults, see Table 18.2. Experts suggest empirically providing analgesic therapy during procedures and conditions known to be painful. Trials of analgesia should also be considered for patients exhibiting potentially pain-related behaviors, which might include otherwise unexplained "agitation."

TREATMENT

Nonpharmacologic Therapy

Nonpharmacologic therapies must be considered in all patients with pain. A comprehensive review of nonpharmacologic therapies for persistent pain is beyond the scope of this chapter, but specific therapies are worth mentioning. Many of the strategies mentioned below are appropriate considerations for treatment plans for all patients, and they highlight the importance of an interprofessional approach to pain treatment.

Patient education and involvement in treatment decisions are essential components of all treatment plans for persistent pain. Patients should be taught how to take medications properly and how to use assessment instruments. Studies also suggest that providing partner-guided pain management training to caregivers can decrease discomfort and improve psychological and social function experienced by older adults (SOE=B).

Psychological interventions such as cognitive-behavioral therapy (CBT) can be important tools for treatment of persistent pain (SOE=B). Recognition of depression, anxiety, or other mood disturbances should prompt early consultation with a mental health professional. In CBT, patients are asked to track their pain and record the thoughts associated with the pain experience to identify maladaptive coping strategies. By consciously replacing maladaptive coping strategies with constructive ones, patients can increase control over pain and self-efficacy, leading to decreased perception of pain. CBT can be particularly useful in helping patients learn to cope with the stresses of persistent pain. When possible, family members and other caregivers should be included in the therapy.

Regular physical activity has been shown to decrease pain scores, improve mood, boost functional status, and stabilize gait (SOE=A). Referral to the Arthritis Foundation or to community resources such as senior centers for exercise, Tai Chi, and water aerobics (for continent patients) classes can be beneficial for many patients. Yoga, Tai Chi, and hydroaerobics and other exercises adapted to the functional ability of the individual are important tools that can help alleviate pain. These strategies are particularly helpful in older adults with chronic low back pain and other nonmalignant causes of pain. In a randomized clinical trial, a mind-body program for chronic low back pain improved short-term function and long-term current and most severe pain.

Table 18.2—Common Pain Behaviors in Cognitively Impaired Older Adults

Behavior	Examples
Facial expressions	Slight frown; sad, frightened face Grimacing, wrinkled forehead, closed or tightened eyes Any distorted expression Rapid blinking
Verbalizations, vocalizations	Sighing, moaning, groaning, grunting, chanting, calling out Noisy breathing Asking for help Verbal abusiveness
Body movements	Rigid or tense body posture, guarding Fidgeting Increased pacing, rocking Restricted movement Gait or mobility changes
Changes in interpersonal interactions	Aggressive, combative, resists care Decreased social interactions Socially inappropriate, disruptive Withdrawn
Changes in activity patterns or routines	Refusing food, appetite change Increase in rest periods Change in sleep or rest pattern Sudden cessation of common routines Increased wandering
Mental status changes	Crying or tears Increased confusion Irritability or distress

NOTE: Some patients demonstrate little or no specific behavior associated with severe pain.

SOURCE: American Geriatrics Society Panel on Persistent Pain in Older Persons. The management of persistent pain in older persons. *J Am Geriatr Soc.* 2002;50(6 Suppl):S211. Reprinted with permission.

Table 18.3—Topical Agents for Pain

Medication	Formulations and Dosage	Comments
Menthol and methylsalicylate (eg, Bengay)	Methyl salicylate 30%, menthol 10%, camphor 4%, q6h; patch applied daily directly over site of pain	Some people cannot tolerate the odor.
Lidocaine	3% cream apply q8–12h; 5% patch on 12 h and off 12 h, apply directly over site of pain; 4% patch OTC	No more than 3 patches at a time; caution advised with hepatic impairment.
Diclofenac	1%, 3% gel, 1.5% solution, apply q6h directly over site of pain	Caution advised with hepatic impairment.
Capsaicin	0.025%, 0.075% cream, apply q6–8h	Avoid applying to broken skin.

Frail older adults may require closely monitored rehabilitation services. For patients with advanced illness who are bedbound, regular repositioning, passive range-of-motion exercises, and gentle massage are key interventions. Treatment goals (beyond reduced pain) should include improved flexibility, strength, endurance, function, and overall quality of life.

Data support the use of many physical modalities such as massage therapy, acupuncture, heat/cold therapy, and transcutaneous electrical nerve stimulation (TENS) units (SOE=B). Interprofessional team members may also incorporate cognitive techniques into the treatment plan, such as hypnosis, aromatherapy, biofeedback, music and pet therapy, and systematic desensitization. A subset of patients may require referral for major interventions, such as radiation therapy for bone metastases or palliative surgical procedures for bowel obstruction. Suboptimal treatment response should not be viewed as a permanent condition but as an opportunity for input from specialists who have additional expertise in treating these difficult problems.

Pharmacologic Therapy

Pharmacologic therapy for patients with persistent pain should be viewed not only as a means to reduce suffering but also as a method to promote improved function and enhanced adherence with rehabilitation efforts. When starting pharmacologic therapy in older adults, the risks and benefits of the treatment should be considered and balanced carefully. If appropriate, nonsystemic therapies should be tried first. For example, patients with isolated knee pain may respond to intra-articular corticosteroid injections, avoiding the need for systemic analgesics. (However, convincing data supporting the use of intra-articular injections for knee pain are lacking.) Patients with myofascial pain often respond to local treatments such as massage, gentle stretching exercises, ultrasound, and trigger-point injections (SOE=B). Topical preparations such as capsaicin or diclofenac gel[OL] or lidocaine patches can be effective as primary or adjunctive therapy for treating neuropathic or myofascial pain syndromes (SOE=C) (Table 18.3).

If these local therapies are ineffective and a decision is made to begin systemic therapy, older adults need to be monitored closely to ensure that the treatment is effective and to minimize adverse effects.

For cancer patients, the pain ladder from the World Health Organization illustrates an excellent approach toward stepwise analgesic management. (www.who.int/cancer/palliative/painladder/en/ [accessed Feb 2019]). According to the WHO ladder, the first step in treating pain is to start the cancer patient on nonopioid medications with or without adjuvants. If the pain persists or increases, the next step is to start a weak opioid (eg, hydrocodone with acetaminophen) and adjuvants. If the pain still persists or increases despite these efforts, then the patient will likely need strong opioids (eg, morphine, hydromorphone, or others) with or without nonopioid analgesics and adjuvants. Choice of initial dose and rate of titration depends on the individual patient's physiology, which varies considerably among older adults. When using acetaminophen for alleviating chronic pain, it is most effective if scheduled regularly rather than as needed. Acetaminophen provides adequate analgesia for many mild to moderate pain syndromes, particularly musculoskeletal pain from osteoarthritis, and is recommended as first-line therapy for persistent pain.

Acetaminophen is typically a very safe analgesic. However, acetaminophen-induced hepatotoxicity can be fatal in older adults. Unintentional overdose can occur in older patients who may already be using OTC products containing acetaminophen (eg, cold medicines) who are started on scheduled acetaminophen for pain relief. Knowledge of all medications that a patient is taking is critical to avoiding acetaminophen toxicity. Patients at risk of liver dysfunction, particularly those who have a history of heavy alcohol intake, should be treated cautiously; in these patients, the dosage should be decreased by 50%, or acetaminophen should be avoided entirely. In older adults, the recommended maximal dose is 2–3 grams/24 hr. While acetaminophen is cleared by the liver, caution should be exercised in patients with kidney disease. Acetaminophen should be administered every 6 hours for patients with a creatinine clearance of 10–50 mL/min, and every 8 hours for patients with a creatinine clearance of <10 mL/min.

NSAIDs tend to be more effective than acetaminophen in chronic inflammatory pain but pose significant hazards to older adults. They must be used judiciously if at all, should be used only after acetaminophen has been tried, and then only in highly select individuals. Significant adverse events, including renal dysfunction, GI bleeding, platelet dysfunction, fluid retention, exacerbation of hypertension or heart failure, and precipitation of delirium, limit the use of NSAIDs in treatment of persistent pain in older adults. The FDA has issued a particular caution against using ibuprofen with aspirin, owing to an interaction that blocks the antiplatelet effect of the aspirin. COX-2 inhibitors were developed to decrease the risk of GI bleeding by acting on a more selective receptor, but the risk of renal complications and hypertension remains the same as with other NSAIDs, and the degree to which longer-term GI toxicity is reduced is not clear. Several studies have confirmed increased cardiovascular risks associated with COX-2 inhibitors, which is now believed to be a class effect. Thus, use of COX-2 inhibitors should be considered with great caution, if at all, in older adults. Misoprostol, a prostaglandin analogue, or a proton-pump inhibitor can be co-prescribed to reduce the risk of NSAID-induced GI bleeding, but these drugs do not reduce the risks of renal disease, hypertension, fluid retention, or delirium. Alternatively, nonacetylated salicylates such as salsalate and trisalicylate may have less renal toxicity and antiplatelet activity than other NSAIDs and therefore may be preferable in older adults, but evidence supporting this theory is sparse. Topical NSAIDs appear to be safe and effective in the short term, but longer-term studies are lacking.

Moderate to severe pain, or pain that requires chronic treatment, often requires opioid medications for sufficient relief, although evidence evaluating their role in managing persistent noncancer pain is scant. In general, it is prudent to start opioid therapy at the lowest dosage possible and to titrate up slowly. That said, opioid dosing should be titrated progressively to achieve the level of analgesia needed, and aggressively rapid titration with frequent monitoring is required for patients in a pain crisis.

Continuous pain, especially cancer pain, should generally be treated with medications in long-acting or sustained-release formulations after total opioid requirements have been estimated by an initial trial of a short-acting agent. Fast-onset medications with short half-lives may be added to the long-acting regimen to cover episodes of breakthrough pain. Typically, a patient is offered approximately 5%–15% of the total daily dose every 2–4 hours orally for breakthrough pain.

In general, different opioids provide similar analgesic efficacy. Cost and route of delivery can help guide the choice of medication.

Most opioids are metabolized by the liver and excreted by the kidneys. In renal dysfunction, the active metabolites of morphine, including morphine-6-glucuronide and morphine-3-glucuronide, can accumulate, increasing the risk of prolonged sedation and possible neurotoxicity. When using morphine to treat patients with kidney disease, the dosing intervals should be increased and the dosage decreased to reduce this risk. Hydromorphone has fewer adverse effects in patients with renal failure and, therefore, is many experts' first choice for this population (SOE=C). Some experts and limited data suggest that oxycodone is also safer than morphine in patients with kidney failure because its metabolism results in fewer active metabolites, but this remains controversial (SOE=C).

Special Considerations for Using Opioids in Older Adults

Older adults may have concerns about long-term opioid use that keep them from accepting adequate treatment for their pain. They may fear that taking opioid therapy for their current level of pain will result in the medication losing its effectiveness in the future when pain becomes more severe. Fear of addiction is another major obstacle to prescribing medications for older adults. A frank discussion and careful monitoring of these concerns may help alleviate these fears.

Providers should be aware that patients who use pharmacies in urban neighborhoods may have difficulty accessing opioids, because many urban pharmacies do not routinely keep these medications in stock. Several studies indicate that there are opioid treatment disparities in black Americans. Cultural barriers also exist when evaluating pain, especially in patients who do not speak English. Providers should become familiar with the patient's cultural and religious context for pain, how pain is expressed, and expectations for treatment.

Physical dependence is an expected change in a patient's physiology that develops while a patient is taking opioid medications for an extended period. If opioids are discontinued suddenly, patients who are physically dependent experience a withdrawal syndrome that may include restlessness, tachycardia, hypertension, fever, tremors, and lacrimation. Symptoms of withdrawal can be avoided by tapering opioids carefully over days to weeks. *Tolerance* refers to a change in physiology resulting in the need to increase opioid dosages over time to achieve adequate analgesic effect. Experts note that tolerance to analgesia, as opposed to tolerance to sedation and respiratory depression, develops slowly in stable disease. If medicines must be titrated rapidly to reduce pain, a search for the cause of the exacerbation should be undertaken, and nonphysical contributors should be considered as well.

Psychological dependence, or true addiction, refers to a state defined by compulsive drug seeking and drug using with disregard for adverse social, physical, and economic consequences. Patients who have persistent pain due to chronic or serious illness must be be appropriately assessed and skillfully managed to avoid opioid-related problems. The potential for abuse should be carefully discussed with patients who have a prior history of addiction and who now need maintenance opioids for persistent pain. Patients with cognitive impairment who are on opioids for persistent pain should be monitored carefully. The action of oral opioids peaks about 1 hour after ingestion. Cognitively impaired patients in pain may take several opioid pills in a short time interval when they do not experience immediate pain relief or because they have forgotten taking the pill. Family caregivers should be trained to identify signs of opioid overdose and call 911 for emergent help if they suspect opioid overdose in these patients.

Clinicians prescribing opioids in older adults should also be watchful for patterns such as repeated requests for dosage increases (especially in noncancer diagnoses), early refill requests, opioid prescriptions from multiple providers, and preference for short-acting opioids that may indicate opioid diversion, ie, family members misusing opioids prescribed for the patient. Opioid overdoses are another concern in older adults and are life-threatening. The prescription medication naltrexone, an opioid antagonist, is often used in overdose situations, and more prescriptions are being given concurrently with opioids for safety reasons.

Adverse Effects of Opioids

The most common adverse effect of opioid treatment is constipation, and tolerance to this toxicity does not occur. Opioid-induced constipation is due to multiple mechanisms, including dehydration, decreased GI tract secretions, and decreased intestinal motility. Because constipation usually complicates opioid use for the duration of treatment, education regarding the probable need for long-term laxative treatment is recommended for all patients when opioid therapy is started. Many experts recommend starting therapy with a stimulant laxative (such as bisacodyl or senna); however, these should be avoided in any patient with signs or symptoms of bowel obstruction. Bulking agents such as fiber and psyllium should be avoided in inactive, seriously ill patients and frail older adults with poor oral fluid intake because of the risk of fecal impaction and obstruction. All patients should be encouraged to exercise, as they are able, and to stay well hydrated. For patients who develop opioid-induced constipation despite laxative therapy, treatment with methylnaltrexone (a mu-opioid-receptor antagonist) or lubiprostone (a chloride channel activator) may relieve constipation without precipitating withdrawal symptoms or pain crisis (SOE=B).

Nausea and vomiting are common adverse effects of opioids. These agents have a direct effect on the chemoreceptor trigger zone, the part of the brain associated with the sensation of nausea. Other common causes of nausea and vomiting in patients taking opioids include gastroparesis, constipation, and metabolic disorders such as renal and hepatic failure. Although opioid-induced nausea and vomiting usually resolve spontaneously after the first few doses, some patients experience chronic nausea. After evaluation for reversible causes of nausea such as constipation, some patients benefit from changing to an alternative opioid (SOE=D). Others may need to be treated with scheduled antiemetics, although the high prevalence of adverse events, including drowsiness, delirium, and other anticholinergic effects, needs to be recognized in older adults treated with these medications.

Respiratory depression is the most serious potential adverse effect associated with opioid use, but tolerance to this effect develops quickly. Older adults and individuals with a history of respiratory dysfunction are at particular risk when opioid dosages are increased rapidly or when another sedative is taken concomitantly. Naloxone, an opioid-receptor antagonist, can reverse opioid-induced respiratory depression; however, when given to a patient who has been treated chronically with opioids, it can precipitate a pain crisis and acute withdrawal symptoms. Experts suggest withholding naloxone and placing the patient under careful observation unless respiratory rate decreases to <8 breaths per minute or the oxygen saturation drops to <90%. When needed, naloxone should be titrated carefully, using the lowest dosage possible.

Older adults can experience sedation, fatigue, and mild cognitive impairment with opioid treatment. These symptoms are common during dosage adjustment. Patients typically overcome the fatigue and sedation within days to weeks as they become tolerant to the medication. They need to be warned of the risks of increased falls and counseled not to drive or operate heavy equipment when the medication is started. A small subset of patients treated with opioids experience incessant fatigue or excessive sedation that significantly limits their function. A limited course of a stimulant such as low-dose methylphenidate may justifiably be tried in this situation (SOE=D). Rotation to a different opioid is an alternative strategy used to alleviate opioid-induced fatigue.

Nonopioid Adjuvant Analgesics

A nonopioid or adjuvant medication can be used as the sole agent or in combination with opioids. These medications can be particularly useful in treating patients with neuropathic pain or mixed pain syndromes.

Although tricyclic antidepressants (TCAs) are the most extensively studied medications for neuropathic pain, none has been FDA approved for this purpose, and their inclusion on the AGS Beers Criteria® list signals their potential for excessive risk when prescribed to older adults. Their efficacy in treatment of post-herpetic neuralgia and diabetic neuropathy has been shown in numerous placebo-controlled studies (SOE=A). Unfortunately, they are associated with significant anticholinergic adverse events in older adults, including constipation, urinary retention, dry mouth, cognitive impairment, tachycardia, and blurred vision. Of note, desipramine[OL] and nortriptyline[OL] may have fewer adverse events than amitriptyline[OL]; thus, amitriptyline should be avoided in older adults.

Clinical depression in patients with persistent pain requires treatment to achieve optimal analgesia and quality of life. Other classes of antidepressants (eg, SSRIs) have generally been less studied than TCAs as analgesics, but older adults typically tolerate these agents better than TCAs when used in antidepressant doses. Duloxetine, a serotonin-norepinephrine reuptake inhibitor (SNRI), is approved both as an antidepressant and for treatment of pain from diabetic neuropathy, and it may offer a more favorable adverse-event profile than the TCAs. Venlafaxine[OL], another SNRI, has been used in similar applications.

Anticonvulsant medications such as carbamazepine, gabapentin, pregabalin, and clonazepam[OL] are commonly used as treatments for neuropathic pain. Gabapentin and pregabalin have demonstrated clinical efficacy in treatment of post-herpetic neuralgia and have fewer adverse events than TCAs. The main adverse events of gabapentin and pregabalin are sedation and dizziness, which frequently limit dosage increases, and peripheral edema commonly occurs as well. Gabapentin doses must be limited in patients with renal dysfunction. Chronic low back pain, osteoarthritis of the knee, fibromyalgia, and diabetic neuropathy can be treated with duloxetine (30 mg/d for 1 week, then increased to 60 mg/d as tolerated); this SNRI also alleviates depression and generalized anxiety disorder. Duloxetine should be avoided in patients with chronic kidney disease and in those with a creatinine clearance <30 mL/min or with end-stage renal disease. When duloxetine is discontinued, the dosage must be tapered slowly over several days.

Corticosteroids are useful adjuvants to treat pain associated with swelling, inflammation, and tissue infiltration, as well as neuropathic pain (SOE=C). In addition to their analgesic properties, they also can increase appetite and improve energy, although weight gained is predominantly fluid and fat rather than muscle. Adverse effects seen with short-term use of steroids include psychosis, fluid retention, hair loss, loss of skin integrity, hyperglycemia, insomnia, and immunosuppression. Corticosteroid use should be limited to treatment of inflammatory conditions and metastatic bone pain; even then, these agents should be used with caution.

Intravenous bisphosphonates can substantially reduce pain from malignant bone metastases (SOE=B). Bisphosphonates have been associated with the rare occurrence of osteonecrosis of the jaw, particularly when administered to patients undergoing dental surgery.

Tramadol both binds to opioid receptors and inhibits the reuptake of norepinephrine and serotonin. It can lower the seizure threshold and is therefore not recommended for patients who have a history of seizures or who take other medications known to lower the seizure threshold. Caution should also be exercised in patients taking other medications that have serotonergic properties, to avoid precipitating serotonin syndrome (characterized by myoclonus, agitation, abdominal cramping, hyperpyrexia, hypertension, and potentially death). Tapentadol is a synthetic, oral mu-opioid-receptor agonist approved for management of moderate to severe acute pain and chronic pain in adults. Tapentadol also has SNRI properties and is structurally and pharmacologically similar to tramadol. It is cleared by the liver and excreted by the kidney and consequently should be avoided in patients with severe renal and hepatic impairment. Significant adverse effects include nausea, vomiting, constipation, dizziness, and somnolence. Because patients may experience withdrawal, the extended-release formulation should be titrated downward gradually.

Medications to Avoid

In prescribing analgesics for older adults, it is important to "start low and go slow." Most often, the dosage of analgesics is limited by adverse effects and drug-drug interactions. In older adults who live alone, it is important to regularly assess cognitive status, because this may influence their ability to take analgesics as prescribed. Mixed agonist-antagonists such as nalbuphine and butorphanol have the potential to cause restlessness and tremulousness and, therefore, should be avoided in older adults.

CHOOSING WISELY® RECOMMENDATIONS

Pain Management

- Do not prescribe opioid analgesics as first-line therapy to treat chronic noncancer pain.
- Do not prescribe opioid analgesics as long-term therapy to treat chronic noncancer pain until the risks have been considered and discussed with the patient.
- Avoid imaging studies (MRI, CT, or radiographs) for acute low back pain without specific indications.
- Do not use intravenous sedation for diagnostic and therapeutic nerve blocks, or joint injections as a default practice.
- Avoid irreversible interventions for noncancer pain that carry significant costs and/or risks.

RESOURCES

- Dowell D, Haegerich TM, Chou R, et al. CDC Guideline for Prescribing Opioids for Chronic Pain — United States, 2016. *MMWR Recomm Rep*. 2016;65(1):1–49.

- McDonald DD. Predictors of gastrointestinal bleeding in older persons taking nonsteroidal anti-inflammatory drugs: Results from the FDA adverse events reporting system. *J Am Assoc Nurse Pract*. 2018 Dec 26. [Epub ahead of print].

- Palliative Care Curriculum 2015 (a joint project of the U.S. Veterans Administration and Stanford University Medical School). Available at: https://palliative.stanford.edu/opioid-conversion/ (accessed Feb 2019).

CHAPTER 19—HOSPITAL CARE

KEY POINTS

- Adults ≥65 years old make up 14% of the population and account for 35% of acute care hospital admissions and 50% of hospital expenditures for all adults.

- Older adults experience high rates of adverse events during hospitalization, including loss of activities of daily living (ADLs) and development of delirium; they are also at high risk of adverse drug events.

- Older hospitalized adults should be routinely assessed for a limited number of common geriatric problems regardless of their admission diagnosis.

- Specific system changes in providing care to hospitalized older adults have resulted in improved patient outcomes.

Older adults are at disproportionate risk of becoming seriously ill and requiring hospital care, whether in an emergency department, on a medical or surgical ward, or in a critical care unit. Adults ≥65 years old make up 14% of the U.S. population but account for 35% of all hospital stays and nearly 50% of hospital expenditures for adults. The most common principal diagnoses in hospitalized older adults are heart failure, pneumonia, cardiac dysrhythmia, and sepsis.

Disparities in hospital care exist. Minority patients are significantly less likely than white patients to be treated at high-volume hospitals for services for which high volume is associated with better outcomes. The differences were largest for cancer surgeries and cardiovascular procedures. Hospitals in the bottom quintile on most quality measures served a significantly higher percentage of minority patients than hospitals in the top quintile.

During hospitalization, older adults tend to receive less costly care than younger patients. For example, in the Study to Understand Prognoses and Preferences for Outcomes and Risks of Treatments (SUPPORT), seriously ill patients in their 80s received fewer invasive procedures and less resource-intensive, less costly hospital care than similarly ill younger patients (SOE=A). This preferential allocation of hospital services to younger patients was not based on differences in severity of illness or general preferences for life-extending care. A more recent prospective study of 490 patients (18–96 years old) mechanically ventilated for acute lung injury examined the association between age and new limitations in life support. Primary outcome was defined as clinical documentation or an order for no cardiopulmonary resuscitation (CPR), do not reintubate, no vasopressors, no hemodialysis, or do not escalate care. After accounting for covariates that can influence decisions regarding life support, the study reported a 24% greater risk of new limitation for each decade increment in age. The addition of daily organ dysfunction status to the model only partially explained the association between age and new life support limitation. Moreover, patients' families and clinicians commonly underestimate older patients' desire for aggressive care (SOE=A). The best guides to assessment and management of any older hospitalized patient are the clinical circumstances and the patient's preferences, irrespective of age.

In a study of vulnerable older adults hospitalized on the medical service of an academic medical center, the quality of care provided was examined by measuring adherence to the third phase of Assessing Care of Vulnerable Elders (ACOVE-3) quality indicators. Adherence to indicators was significantly greater for general medical care (such as for heart failure or diabetes) than for geriatric conditions (such as delirium or pressure injury) (SOE=A). Yet, adherence to 16 ACOVE geriatric-specific quality indicators in the acute care setting may be associated with lower 1-year mortality in vulnerable older hospitalized patients. This chapter is intended to assist providers in the acute setting to adhere to effective geriatric care processes, regardless of the general medical problems of their patients.

HAZARDS OF HOSPITALIZATION

Hospital-Associated Disability

Once hospitalized, older patients are at high risk of loss of independence and institutionalization. Among hospitalized medical patients ≥70 years old, approximately one-third are discharged with a disability that was not present 2 weeks before admission, a condition referred to as hospitalization-associated disability (SOE=A). In addition, hospitalization accounts for 50% of new-onset disability in frail older adults. A validated clinical index identified risk factors (age, number of dependencies in ADLs and instrumental activities of daily living [IADLs], mobility 2 weeks before admission, metastatic cancer or stroke, severe cognitive impairment, and hypoalbuminemia) for new-onset disability in hospitalized patients ≥70 years old. Higher risk scores predicted more severe disability, greater likelihood of nursing-home placement, and worse survival. In a cohort of 449 adults ≥70 years old discharged after hospitalization for medical illness with new ADL dependence, 36% fully recovered at 1 year, 27% remained dependent, and 37% died.

Determining an older adult's ability to perform ADLs and IADLs at the time of admission can serve as a useful baseline. If functional dependence is found, the causes should be explored (eg, dependence in IADLs is often associated with dementia), and strategies to maintain and improve functional ability can be started (eg, physical and occupational therapy). The clinician plays a critical role in educating patients and families regarding the harmful effects of limited activity and the need to engage in function-promoting activity to avoid functional decline.

Delirium

Delirium occurs in 29%–64% of patients admitted to general medical and geriatric wards but is underrecognized, with recognition rates of 12%–35% (SOE=A). Certain subgroups of hospitalized older patients have higher incidence of delirium. The incidence of delirium is higher in patients in intensive care, postoperative, and palliative care settings. Significant risk factors in acute medical units are dementia, severe illness, visual impairment, urinary catheterization, hypoalbuminemia, and lengthy hospitalization.

The diagnosis of delirium should be considered when any of the following is observed: acute onset of change and/or fluctuation in mental status or behavior, inattention, disorganized thinking, and altered consciousness. The Confusion Assessment Method (CAM), and the briefer 3D-CAM, are screening tools that incorporate these features. Three psychomotor behavioral subtypes are currently recognized: hypoactive, hyperactive, and mixed. Hyperactive delirious patients are restless, agitated, and hyperalert (and this diagnosis is rarely missed), whereas hypoactive delirious patients often have decreased movement, paucity of speech, and reduced responsiveness. Hypoactive patients are often not identified in the hospital or are misdiagnosed as having depression or dementia. Delirium arising during the course of hospitalization is associated with prolonged hospital stay, functional decline, nursing-home placement, increased mortality, and worsening cognitive function. Symptoms of delirium can persist for months after hospital discharge.

Prevention is the best strategy; roughly one-third of cases of delirium can be prevented by appropriately managing 6 risk factors for delirium: cognitive impairment, sleep deprivation, immobility, visual impairment, hearing impairment, and dehydration (SOE=A). Although there is strong evidence that multifactorial interventions targeting modifiable risk factors reduce incident delirium in non-ICU hospital patients, medication prophylaxes have not shown clear benefit (SOE=B. Interventions for treating established delirium have not demonstrated improved outcomes (SOE=C). Once the diagnosis is made, measures should be taken to identify the medical condition causing the delirium by reviewing recently added medications and by investigating for likely causes such as infection, electrolyte abnormalities, and ischemia. Measures to prevent or ameliorate delirium include avoiding medications associated with delirium (such as benzodiazepines, anticholinergics, and opiates) whenever possible; treating pain and infection; detecting and correcting urinary retention, fecal impaction, and metabolic abnormalities; frequently orienting patients with cognitive or sensory impairment; limiting room changes; and avoiding excessive bed rest, restraints, and unnecessary tethers (eg, in-dwelling bladder, oxygen lines, and telemetry leads).

Suboptimal Pharmacotherapy

Pharmacotherapy involves prescribing, communicating orders, dispensing, administering, and monitoring. There is potential for error at each step. Other factors that contribute to the complexities of pharmacotherapy for older patients in the acute care setting include polypharmacy, multiple prescribing providers, restrictive hospital formularies that require careful medication reconciliation during care transitions, barriers to medication reconciliation, and significant turnover of the medication regimen with many old medications discontinued and new ones introduced.

Adverse drug events (ADEs) are a significant source of hospital hazard for older patients. A substantial number of ADEs are potentially preventable, up to 54% in one prospective study. In a review of 4 ADE risk prediction models, the proportion of older adults who suffered an in-hospital ADE ranged from 6.7% to 39%. None of the models was found to have sufficient predictive ability for clinical use.

Inappropriate medication use likely contributes to the risk of ADEs. The AGS Beers Criteria® and the STOPP/START criteria are two common-sense, evidence-based approaches to reducing inappropriate prescribing.

A hospital admission is an ideal time to completely review a patient's medication regimen and to discontinue or change medications that are unnecessary, have low therapeutic value (eg, sedative-hypnotics), are prescribed at the wrong dose or frequency, are duplicative, interact with another medication, or are prescribed despite a known allergy. In addition, a medication review at admission can evaluate whether medical conditions are being maximally treated. Review of medications should include both prescription and nonprescription medications. Changes should be undertaken in consultation with the outpatient provider. In-hospital medication review may reduce future emergency department contact during short-term follow-up. Involvement of clinical pharmacists in interprofessional teams improves pharmacotherapy outcomes.

Successful hospital medication reconciliation interventions target high risk subgroups, including older patients with polypharmacy and ≥3 comorbid conditions.

Sleep Disturbance

Over one-third of older patients have difficulty sleeping in the hospital. Sleep deprivation is important to prevent, recognize, and address, because it is associated with increased risk of delirium. Sources of sleep disruption in hospitalized older adults include intrinsic (eg, underlying medical illness, medications, drug withdrawal) and extrinsic factors (eg, noise, measuring vital signs, phlebotomy, medication administration). Sedative-hypnotic medications are prescribed to one-third of older hospitalized patients despite the associated risks of delirium, falls, hip fractures, and rebound insomnia, as well as their poor benefit-to-harm ratio (SOE=A). Therefore, sleep deprivation in the hospital is best managed nonpharmacologically. One protocol using nighttime noise reduction strategies, including warm drinks, soothing music, massage treatments, and rescheduled medication administration and measurement of vital signs to avoid sleep interruption, significantly reduced the use of sedative-hypnotics in the hospital. A review of studies of nonpharmacologic interventions that included relaxation techniques, promotion of good sleep habits, minimizing sleep interruption, and daytime bright light exposure concluded that evidence was insufficient to demonstrate improvements in sleep quality and quantity.

Nutritional Problems

The prevalence of malnutrition in older hospitalized patients worldwide is 39%. Moreover, 25% of older patients suffer further nutritional depletion during hospitalization. Even after controlling for underlying acute illness, its severity, and comorbid illnesses, malnutrition is associated with increased risk of complications, longer hospital stays, readmission, dependence, institutionalization, and death. In addition, deficiencies of vitamins (especially vitamin D) and electrolytes are common among older hospitalized patients.

Although screening for malnutrition in all hospitalized adults is mandated by the Joint Commission, a validated screening tool is used only 38% of the time. Patients who receive nutritional assessment in the hospital are less likely to experience short-term functional decline or die 1 year after hospital discharge. Beyond considering supplements, clinicians should assess malnourished older hospitalized patients for remediable factors such as difficulty chewing, need for dentures, dysphagia, medications that impair appetite, overly restrictive prescribed diet, unwarranted nothing-by-mouth orders, depression, or insufficient time or physical ability to eat.

Another potential contributor to poor oral intake in the hospital is constipation. Elimination records should be reviewed regularly, and patients who have not moved their bowels in more than a couple of days may benefit from an oral or rectal stimulant (eg, senna, bisacodyl) or an osmotic (eg, polyethylene glycol) laxative, in addition to provision of adequate fluid and fiber intake and mobility.

The maintenance of water and electrolyte balance requires special attention in older adults during and after fluid administration because of their decreased ability to achieve and maintain homeostasis. Initial efforts can be directed toward achieving euvolemia and correcting electrolyte abnormalities. Subsequent efforts to maintain fluid and electrolyte balance are based on estimates of daily metabolic requirements.

Older adults are at risk for inability to recover from malnutrition after discharge. Ensuring access to adequate food is an essential component of discharge planning.

"NEVER EVENTS"

Medicare payment for inpatient care is based on diagnoses and procedures that are assigned diagnosis-related group (DRG) codes. Prior to October 2008, hospitals received greater reimbursement for the care of a patient who developed complications that led to a costlier DRG. Concerned that this was a disincentive to improving patient safety, in October 2008, the CMS mandated non-payment for so-called "never events," conditions that met 3 criteria: 1) are high cost and/or high volume, 2) result in reassignment to a higher reimbursed DRG when designated as secondary diagnosis, and 3) are reasonably preventable through application of evidence-based interventions. This rule originally applied to eight conditions but was revised in 2011 to include 29 events in 6 categories: surgical, product or device, patient protection, care management, environmental, radiologic, and criminal.

Some stakeholders argue that the rule may penalize hospitals that treat high-risk patients, such as frail older adults. Three conditions designated "never events" for which older hospitalized adults are known to be at greater risk of developing are Stage 3 or 4 hospital-acquired pressure ulcers (HAPUs), injurious falls, and catheter-associated urinary tract infections (CAUTI).

Injurious Falls

The falls rate in the hospital range from 3 to 13 per 1,000 patient-days. Among older adults, the rates are higher at 6 to 15.9 per 1,000 patient-days. A fall leads to an incremental cost of approximately $4,000 per hospitalization. Although hospital falls meet the first 2 criteria for conditions that ought never to develop after admission, evidence-supported strategies that prevent falls in the acute care setting are limited, and falls with or without injury occur despite delivery of appropriate care.

No screening tool has sufficient accuracy for predicting falls in older adults in the hospital. The initial interview is a good time to assess a patient's risk of falling by inquiring about a history of falls (SOE=A). It is helpful to assess the patient's gait, balance, lower extremity strength, ability to get up from bed, cognition, and mood during the initial physical examination. Individuals able to walk independently should be encouraged to do so frequently during hospitalization. Immobility during hospitalization leads rapidly to diminished strength and subsequent difficulty walking (SOE=A). Those able to walk but unable to do so safely and independently should receive assistance from hospital staff while walking several times daily.

Strategies to promote mobility and reduce falls include avoiding restraints and tethers, decluttering the environment, minimizing use of medications associated with falls, providing walking assistance for those who walk with difficulty, attending to patient's toileting needs, addressing sensory impairments, and providing physical therapy for those with weakness or gait abnormalities. Bed or chair alarms as a single intervention strategy have not been shown to be effective in reducing falls and can curtail mobility.

Delirium has been implicated as a risk factor for falls. In 4 studies, reduced rates of falls were associated with multifactorial, nonpharmacologic preventive interventions for delirium. Of note, most of these included strategies for enhancing mobility.

During the 27-month period before implementation of the "Never Events" rule, analyzing data from 1,263 National Database of Nursing Quality Indicators (NDNQI) hospitals nationwide, rates of total and injurious falls were trending downward at −0.4% per quarter and −1% per quarter, respectively. A follow-up analysis of data from 1,381 NDNQI hospitals showed no change in the rate of decline in injurious falls from July 2006 to November 2010 after policy implementation.

Stage 3 or 4 Hospital-Acquired Pressure Ulcers

Although there has been an overall decrease in HAPUs since 2004, studies of frail older adults or high-risk individuals report the median incidence of pressure ulcers (PU) in the acute care setting to be 15.7%. Within the first 2 days of hospitalization on a medicine service, as many as 6.2% of patients ≥65 years old will develop one or more PUs. Most PUs are on the sacrum and heels; they are painful, associated with longer hospitalizations and delayed return of function, and costly ($37,800–$70,000 per case, or an estimated $11 billion nationally in 2009). Older age, low body weight, physical and sensory impairment, incontinence, malnutrition, and conditions that impair circulation are risk factors for developing PUs. Several assessment scales are available (Braden, Norton, Ramstadius, Waterlow) and can help identify patients at increased risk, although with low sensitivities and specificities. Patients at risk should have their skin inspected at least daily, focusing on areas of bony prominences.

Most trials on preventive interventions focused on evaluating support surfaces. For patients at higher risk, more advanced static mattresses and overlays were better than standard mattresses for preventing PUs. Repositioning is often used with other preventive strategies, but further research is required to determine the most effective position and frequency.

In an analysis of data from 1,381 NDNQI hospitals, from July 2006 to December 2010, there was no change in the rate of decline in stage 3 or 4 HAPUs associated with the introduction of the "Never Events" rule.

Urinary Catheter Use and Catheter-Associated Urinary Tract Infection

Urinary catheters (UC) are often inappropriately inserted and are associated with adverse outcomes. UCs are 1 of 5 precipitating factors for delirium identified in a prospective study of medical inpatients ≥70 years old. A similar cohort of patients admitted to a general medicine service with no medical indication for a UC were followed prospectively for insertion of a catheter within 48 hours of hospital admission. A catheter was inserted in 14% of the cohort who had no indication for the catheter. Although these patients were older and more likely to have been admitted because of a "geriatric condition" ("altered mental status," fall without hip fracture, urinary tract infection, "failure to thrive"), their admission characteristics were, otherwise, not different from those of matched controls. After adjusting for potential confounders, those who had a UC were more likely to die during hospitalization and within 90 days of discharge. UC use was also associated with longer hospitalization but not with new decline in function or admission to a nursing home.

Older age is a risk factor for urinary catheter–associated bacteriuria. The most important modifiable risk factor is duration of indwelling catheterization; the reported incidence of bacteriuria is 3%–8% per catheter-day. Accordingly, the most effective way to reduce CAUTI is to limit urinary catheterization to those who have a clear indication and to remove the catheter as soon as it is no longer necessary. Appropriate indications for a bladder catheter include acute urinary retention or bladder outlet obstruction, perioperatively for selected procedures, open sacral or perineal wounds in incontinent patients, prolonged immobility due to unstable thoracic, lumbar, pelvic fractures, and for comfort at end-of- life as needed. Inserting a catheter to measure urinary output is inappropriate in most cases. Reminder systems are useful; more than 25% of the time, clinicians are unaware that their patients have an indwelling catheter, and those catheters that have no indication are more likely to be overlooked. Evidence-based practices for CAUTI prevention include education and training of health care personnel, appropriate insertion and care, consideration of alternatives to catheter use, and early removal through reminder systems. It has been estimated that 25%–75% of CAUTI cases are preventable with use of multimodal strategies.

The "Never Events" rule was associated with a 10% reduction from January 2008 to October 2010 in the rate of change in CAUTIs in the ICU, based on an analysis of data from 1,381 NDNQI hospitals.

ASSESSING AND MANAGING HOSPITALIZED OLDER PATIENTS

Assessment on Admission

Many of the serious illnesses disproportionately experienced by older adults require hospital care for optimal management. The benefits of hospitalization can be remarkable: correcting serious physiologic derangements, repairing vascular obstructions and broken bones, and using highly technical biomedical advances to treat life-threatening illnesses. However, while in the hospital, older adults also commonly experience deteriorating functional status, adverse events from medication, or delirium. A systematic approach to assessing and managing hospitalized older adults offers the best chance of reducing the risk and consequences of these common problems.

The initial assessment should include an evaluation of function at the level of the organ system, the whole person, and the person's environment. This assessment can identify needs for which targeted interventions can improve function or reduce risk of adverse outcomes. This approach complements the traditional medical assessment by highlighting problems that are common in hospitalized older patients, and it is similar in concept to geriatric assessment conducted in other settings.

For suggestions on when assessment of these common geriatric problems can be incorporated into the routine of a hospital admission history and physical examination, see Table 19.1.

For commonly overlooked hazards and opportunities in older hospitalized patients, see Table 19.2. These problems have been selected based on their importance relative to other clinical issues, the quality of relevant evidence, and their specificity to older adults.

Daily Evaluation

Hospitalized older adults should be evaluated daily using a systematic approach to ensure that essential geriatric issues are not overshadowed by disease-specific or technologic concerns. For patients who are expected to recover mobility, progress toward that goal should be assessed. Time out of bed (eg, in a chair for meals) and ambulation (with assistance, if needed) should be encouraged. Progress on ADL recovery should be tracked, and patients encouraged and coached toward functional independence.

Daily physical examination should include identifying the devices attached to, or inserted in, each patient. Many of these devices can cause injury if used inappropriately, and a daily assessment of risks and benefits is wise. Central venous catheters, for example, allow for convenient blood draws and delivery of medications and parenteral nutrition, but they are also associated with infection, restricted mobility, deep venous thrombosis (DVT), and air embolism.

Cognitive Impairment

Adults >65 years old with dementia are hospitalized at more than 3 times the rate of those without dementia. In a systematic review, the prevalence of dementia among older patients in the acute hospital ranged from 13% to 63%. Patients with dementia were older and more undernourished before hospitalization. In hospital, they required more hours of nursing care, had longer hospitalizations, and were more likely to suffer delirium and functional decline and to be discharged to a nursing home than patients without dementia. Preexisting cognitive impairment is also a risk factor for falls, use of restraints, nonadherence to therapy, feeding tube placements, and decision-making incapacity.

Despite its importance, documentation of a dementia diagnosis is often absent in hospital records. In a cohort of 997 older patients hospitalized in a university-affiliated public hospital, 43% were cognitively impaired on admission; 61% had no documentation of impairment.

Recognizing an underlying cognitive impairment early enables the health care team to implement preemptive measures to prevent these hazards. Cognitive function can be assessed by use of an established test of cognitive function, such as the Montreal Cognitive Assessment or the Mini-Cog test. Exposure to the hospital environment may be disorienting for patients with cognitive impairment because of frequent room changes, noise, and poor way-finding cues. Creating a

Table 19.1—Systematic Assessment of Older Adults on Hospital Admission

Step	Assessments
Past medical history	Ask about vaccination history.
Medications review	Assess indications for each medication, appropriateness of dosing, potential interactions. Assess for medication effects contributing to acute illness. Determine patient's or caregiver's method for assuring adherence (eg, pill boxes).
Social history	Ask about help needed (and who provides) for ADLs and IADLs. Ask about social support. Ask if patient feels safe. Ask about treatment goals and preference in event of cardiorespiratory arrest.
Review of systems	Ask about weight loss in preceding 6 months. Ask about dietary change. Ask about anorexia, nausea, vomiting, diarrhea. Ask about incontinence. Ask about problems with memory or confusion. Ask about falls or difficulty walking. Ask about difficulties with vision or hearing.
Physical examination	Take pulse (confirm arrhythmias with ECG). Check orthostatic blood pressures in patients with falls, presyncope, syncope. Assess for weight change, loss of subcutaneous fat, muscle wasting, edema, ascites, prevalent pressure ulcer. Screen for cognitive function. Assess vision and hearing. Assess gait. Use a depression screen.

Table 19.2—Common Hazards and Opportunities to Address During an Older Adult's Hospital Stay

Problem	Possible Interventions
Functional impairments	Assess ADLs on admission consider referral to physical therapy, occupational therapy, engage social resources.
Immobility and falls	Avoid restraints, remove in-dwelling bladder catheters, encourage ambulation in hospital and physical therapy, avoid sedating medications.
Sensory impairment	Use eyeglasses, hearing aids; remove cerumen impaction.
Depression	Treat with pharmacotherapy, cognitive therapy, or both.
Cognitive impairment	Evaluate for dementia or delirium, assess social environment, implement nonpharmacologic prevention strategies.
Suboptimal pharmacotherapy	Review all medications at admission and discharge, involve clinical pharmacists as medical team members, consider use of explicit appropriateness criteria.
Nutrition	Supplement water, calories, protein; assess social environment and medical factors that contribute to poor oral intake.
Immunization status	Vaccinate against influenza, pneumococcus.
Pressure ulcers	Reposition frequently and use specialized support surfaces, manage moisture and incontinence, encourage ambulation.
Sleep disturbance	Address intrinsic and extrinsic causes, use nonpharmacologic protocols.
Venous thromboembolism	Use prophylactic anticoagulation for at-risk patients, mechanical thromboprophylaxis for high bleeding risk, encourage ambulation.

unit with a home-like ambiance that allows unrestricted mobility, provides meaningful daytime activities, encourages the presence of family, provides orientation cues, addresses sensory impairment, promotes sleep through nonpharmacologic protocols, and meets nutritional needs are prudent ways of making the hospital environment safer for patients with dementia.

Cognitive impairment may complicate the assessment and treatment of pain in the hospital. Consequently, pain is often undertreated. Most patients with mild to moderate dementia can comprehend at least one pain assessment scale, but fewer than half of those with severe dementia can do so. Cognitively impaired patients may be unable to recognize their pain trajectory or to differentiate improving pain from new or worsening symptoms. Orders for patient-controlled analgesia pumps and as-needed pain medication should be avoided in patients with impaired recall. Scheduled analgesia should be considered, especially if pain occurs frequently. Nonpharmacologic approaches to pain should be part of the treatment plan. Patients may be unable to report adverse effects from the analgesics, and detection of complications (eg, fecal impaction or delirium) may be delayed. Anticipating and preventing common adverse effects (eg, initiating a bowel regimen whenever opiates are prescribed) is one way of avoiding complications. When patients with dementia develop delirium, looking for untreated pain as a possible cause is appropriate.

The question of capacity is often raised when a patient with dementia wishes to be discharged home to live independently. A common scenario is a patient with self-neglecting behavior resulting in repeated hospitalizations and who declines in-home assistance because of impaired insight and judgment. The clinician is required to assess both the person's capacity to make decisions about daily tasks and the ability to execute them. This entails solving problems encountered while performing tasks. Because living independently requires intact abilities in multiple domains (cognitive, affective, physical), a comprehensive, multidisciplinary assessment enables identification of impairments and prediction of impact on the person's ability to cope in the home environment. Knowledgeable informants are useful, albeit imperfect, sources of information on the person's functional status. Psychometric cognitive testing is often used to estimate capacity to live independently. Performance-based functional instruments, wherein the patient is asked to demonstrate performing IADLs to a trained observer, are often used.

Trial discharge to home with supportive services, if possible, is the least restrictive option. Social, medical, and environmental adaptations can mitigate the impact of cognitive impairment. An in-home multidisciplinary team visit is useful to assess a person's ability to execute the care plan.

Sensory Deficits

Most hospitalized older adults have impairments in vision or hearing, which are risk factors for falls, incontinence, delirium, and functional dependence. The combination of both sensory impairments is associated with IADL loss. Although eyeglasses or hearing aids readily correct most visual and hearing impairments, they are often forgotten or inaccessible in the hospital.

Hospitalized older adults can be screened for sensory impairment by routinely asking if they have difficulty with seeing or hearing and whether they use eyeglasses or hearing aids. Physical examination, including a test of visual acuity (eg, with a pocket card of the Jaeger eye test) and the finger rub, watch tick, or whisper test of hearing are the next appropriate steps in evaluation. For people with visual or hearing impairments, it is important to provide the appropriate assistive devices (eyeglasses or hearing aids brought from home or voice amplifiers provided by the hospital), and staff may need to be instructed in the use of appliances to communicate more effectively.

Depression

Depressive symptoms in hospitalized older adults are common (prevalence 8%–45%), prognostically important, and potentially ameliorable, but often unrecognized. The presence of depressive symptoms is associated with increased risk of dependence in ADLs, nursing-home placement, and shortened long-term survival, even after controlling for baseline function and the severity of acute and chronic illness. The natural course of depression is one of rare remission.

All hospitalized older patients should be assessed for depression. Loss of motivation and energy, somatization, anxiety, and desire for death may be more pronounced than sadness. Simply asking patients whether they feel down, depressed, or hopeless, or whether they have lost interest or pleasure in doing things, is a good place to start. In a review of 14 studies of older medical inpatients that evaluated a depression rating scale compared with a gold standard diagnostic criteria, the Geriatric Depression Scale was found to be the only instrument that has been adequately studied. Scores of ≥5 on the GDS-15 and ≥10 on the GDS-30 were associated with the best screening performance.

Beginning pharmacotherapy during hospitalization for a medical or surgical condition may not be necessary, but follow-up shortly after discharge is critical. Those with persistently high numbers of depressive symptoms are especially at risk of functional decline and death in the year after discharge. If pharmacotherapy is started, SSRIs are generally considered first-line agents. Cognitive-behavioral therapy immediately after discharge has been shown to be effective in reducing depressive symptoms.

Deep Venous Thrombosis (DVT) Prophylaxis

Pulmonary embolism is a common preventable cause of death in hospitalized patients. Because of diminished physiologic reserve, older adults are less able to compensate for the hemodynamic and respiratory demands of a pulmonary embolism. Furthermore, numerous risk factors, comorbidities, and atypical presentations in older adults can lead to more challenging diagnosis of and worse outcomes from venous thromboembolic disease. Older adults are less likely to present with typical symptoms (eg, chest pain, extremity discomfort, or difficulty ambulating) and are more likely to complain of dyspnea. Patients hospitalized for illness other than DVT who subsequently developed DVT were more likely to be elderly than nonelderly. Despite this, older patients receive DVT prophylaxis <50% of the time. The 2012 Guidelines from the American College of Chest Physicians recommend thromboprophylaxis with low-molecular-weight heparin, low-dose unfractionated heparin, or fondaparinux for acutely ill medical patients at high risk of venous thromboembolism. Risk can be assessed using tools such as the Padua, IMPROVE, and GENEVA; all take into account increased age. Mechanical thromboprophylaxis should be used primarily for patients with high bleeding risk (active peptic ulcer disease, recent bleeding, and platelet count $<50 \times 10^9$). Ensuring proper use and maximal adherence are key to effectiveness of mechanical prophylaxis.

Code Status Discussions

Half of all patients with cardiac arrests receiving resuscitation efforts in the United States occur in people >65 years old. Because resuscitation is an emergency procedure needed by those who at the moment of arrest are incapable of expressing treatment preference, consent is presumed and treatment administered immediately. Two scenarios are generally accepted as exceptions to this presumption: the patient's previous expression of preference that CPR be withheld and the treating physician's clinical judgment that an attempt to resuscitate would be futile.

From 2000 to 2009, rates of survival to hospital discharge of patients who had in-hospital cardiopulmonary arrests and underwent attempts at resuscitation increased from 13.7% to 22.3%. Lower rates of survival to discharge and poorer outcomes were associated with increasing age. Of those >65 years old who survive to discharge, about half have clinically significant neurologic disability. Of patients with no, mild, moderate, or severe disability, or who are in a vegetative state, 27%, 39%, 58%, and 90%, respectively, died in the year after discharge.

Clinicians should solicit the wishes for resuscitation of patients who are at risk of suffering cardiac or respiratory failure. Ideally, these discussions will take place nonemergently in the clinic setting in the context of asking about the patient's general treatment preferences. The strongest predictor of whether a code discussion was documented was the presence of preexisting documentation of care wishes. However, only 25% of patients have such documentation. Many states now have programs (eg, Physician Orders for Life-Sustaining Treatment [POLST]) that allow for patients to have their wishes for care translated by a health care provider into actionable medical orders (eg, "Do not attempt resuscitation"). In the absence of previous outpatient discussion or completed POLST forms, the patient's wishes should be determined early in the hospitalization. Subsequent discussions are necessary as the patient's condition and treatment options change. In addition, any decisions made should be periodically reevaluated. When older patients with "Do not attempt resuscitation/Do not intubate" (DNR/DNI) orders are asked about specific hypothetical situations, many would choose to have a trial of cardiac resuscitation or intubation. Fewer than half would reject these interventions under any circumstance.

Essential elements of the discussions include ensuring that the 1) patient understands his or her prognosis and the likelihood of requiring CPR; 2) patient's values and treatment goals are understood; 3) patient understands the nature of CPR and the risks, benefits, and likely outcomes; and 4) physician offers a recommendation about CPR based on the patient's prognosis and treatment goals.

Information about an individual's likelihood for surviving an in-hospital cardiac arrest (IHCA) neurologically intact or with minimal deficits is useful when making informed decisions about DNR/DNI orders. The Good Outcome Following Attempted Resuscitation (GO-FAR) calculator (www.gofarcalc.com) uses data from a population of 51,240 adults who suffered index IHCA to predict survival to discharge with good neurologic performance (alert, although possibly with mild neurocognitive deficits but able to work).

Special Hospital Populations

Intensive Care

Adults >65 years old account for 42%–52% of the ICU admissions and for almost 60% of total ICU days in the United States. Many of those who survive do so with greater disability than they had on admission. In a prospective study of older adults who survived a critical illness with greater disability, half fully returned to prior function at a median of 3 months. Survivors with greater functional self-efficacy and BMI were more likely to recover, while sensory impairments were associated with poor recovery.

Respiratory failure is the most common reason for medical ICU admission and, because advanced age is associated with higher prevalence of chronic and acute pulmonary conditions, the number of older patients admitted to the ICU requiring mechanical ventilator support is rising. Patients with acute respiratory distress syndrome appear to have higher mortality with advancing age. Interestingly, in 3 separate studies of >1,500 patients, older patients recovered from their pulmonary physiologic abnormalities at a rate equal to that of their younger counterparts after acute lung injury; however, they required nearly twice as long to be successfully liberated from the ventilator and discharged from the ICU (SOE=A). Prolonged mechanical ventilation is likely an indicator not only of the severity of the initial illness that led to the respiratory failure but also of impairments in multiple organ systems.

Mortality in very old (>85 years) patients is 30%–70% for those with single organ failure and 80%–100% for those with multiple organ failure. Patients requiring renal replacement therapy have an extremely poor prognosis. Approximately 40% of older adults are alive 3 months after an ICU stay. Sepsis (defined as life-threatening organ dysfunction caused by a dysregulated host response to infection) increases the odds of developing cognitive deterioration and new ADL dependence in older survivors, and the deterioration in cognition and function after sepsis persists up to 8 years later.

ICUs provide care at end-of-life for a significant number of decedents; 1 in 5 Americans who die receive ICU services before death. Establishing goals of care in older critically ill patients is of paramount importance. In caring for critically ill patients, it may become apparent to the patient, family, and clinician that further intervention would not likely be of substantial benefit, depending on the individual patient's goals, values, and hopes. Many older patients with life-limiting illness are most concerned about maintaining function (as opposed to prolonging physiologic life) when weighing the burdens and potential outcomes of treatment options.

Defining *futility* is often difficult. The American Medical Association recommends a standardized "fair process" rather than a strict definition of futility. This approach consists of deliberation and negotiation between all parties, steps to secure alternatives in the setting of irreconcilable differences, and a final step of closure when all alternatives have been exhausted. As much as possible, clinicians should base futility decisions on factors such as clinical efficacy of treatment, likelihood of mortality, and subsequent quality-of-life considerations rather than on chronologic age alone.

Emergency Department

The emergency department (ED) is an important treatment site for acute illness and injury in older adults and is frequently a path of entry to hospital care. Older adult patients made up 15.9% of all ED visits in the United States in 2012–2013. Older adults are more likely to be transported to the ED by ambulance and are 2.5–4.6 times more likely to be hospitalized. They use more staff time and resources because of longer ED stays and are more likely, when admitted, to require a critical care bed. ED diagnoses tend to be less accurate despite greater use of diagnostic tests and procedures.

After discharge from the ED, older adults are at greater risk of future hospitalization, repeat ED visits, functional decline, and mortality. In an analysis of 172,927 older adults discharged from Quebec EDs to the community, over the next 30 days, 1% died, 5% returned to the ED and were admitted, 16% returned to the ED but were not admitted, and 29% were prescribed a potentially inappropriate medication.

Although changes in functional capacity have been inconsistently defined, approximately 10%–45% of older adults decline in functional ability during the 3 months after an ED visit.

Commonly identified risk factors for adverse outcomes are baseline functional dependence, advanced age, recent hospitalization or ED visit, lack of social support, and living alone.

Impaired cognition is common in older adult ED patients and is a risk factor for poor outcomes. Of 297 ED patients >70 years old seen in an urban teaching hospital, 26% had evidence of mental status impairment, 16% had cognitive impairment without delirium, and 10% had delirium. A small minority of cases had any documentation by the physician of mental status impairment. This is concerning, because undetected delirium is associated with higher 6-month mortality compared with when there was no delirium or when delirium was detected.

Given the prevalence of geriatric syndromes in the ED and their association with poor outcomes, older adults, particularly the highest-risk patients, would benefit from comprehensive geriatric assessment (CGA) and targeted interventions in the ED. However, the rapid pace of the ED poses a barrier to systematic performance of CGA; therefore, simplified geriatric-specific screening tools have been developed to more efficiently identify at-risk individuals discharged from the ED. Five nurse-administered screening tools have been validated in the ED: Score Hospitalier d'Evaluation du Risque de Perte d'Autonomie (SHERPA), Runciman, Rowland, Triage Risk Stratification Tool (TRST), and Identification of Seniors at Risk (ISAR). For a summary of characteristics of screening tools, see Table 19.3.

Since 2008, geriatric EDs are increasingly being developed in hospitals across the United States. Although the criteria for defining a geriatric ED are not completely established, a consensus-based guideline is available through a collaboration of the American College of Emergency Physicians, the American Geriatrics Society, the Emergency Nurses Association, and the Society for Academic Emergency Medicine. The guideline provides recommendations in the domains of staffing, staff education, policies and procedures, follow-up, performance measures, and environmental modifications. It aims to improve resource allocation and to reduce adverse outcomes and unnecessary admissions and readmissions. A survey of representatives of 24 existing and 6 planned geriatric EDs completed before the publication of this guideline revealed significant variation in the services offered, environmental modifications, and outcomes measured;

Table 19.3—Emergency Department Validated Risk-Screening Tools

Tool	Cut-off	Performance (Sensitivity, Specificity)	Outcomes Measured
Score Hospitalier d'Evaluation du Risque de Perte d'Autonomie (SHERPA)	≥3.5/11.5	85%, 45%	Functional decline, hospitalization, death at 3 months
Runciman test	≥2/8	86%, 38%	Emergency department readmission at 28 days
Rowland test	≥4/7	85%, 28%	Emergency department readmission at 14 days
Triage Risk Stratification Tool (TRST)	≥2/6	64%, 63%	Emergency department readmission and institutionalization at 30 days
Identification of Seniors at Risk (ISAR)	≥2/6	72%, 58%	Death, institutionalization, functional decline at 6 months

Data from: Graf CE, Zekry D, Giannelli S, et al. Efficiency and applicability of CGA in the ED: a systematic review. *Aging Clin Exp Res*. 2011;23:244–254.

80% served 5,000–20,000 older patients annually. The most frequently reported physical changes made were in beds, lighting, flooring, visual/hearing aids, corridor safety, and sound level. Selection of patients for treatment in the geriatric ED was based mostly on an age cutoff of 65 years and acuity of illness; only 17% used a risk screening tool for this purpose. Specialized training of geriatric ED staff was reported by 80% of respondents. Common protocols implemented addressed falls prevention, medication evaluation, delirium management, and urinary catheter use. Frequently reported targeted interventions were coordination of community resource services (eg, home aids, durable medical equipment), pharmacology review, discharge planning, communication with the primary care physician, and referral to clinical services (eg, skilled-nursing facility, physical therapy, primary care providers, geriatric clinics). The most frequently measured outcomes were hospital admissions, patient satisfaction, hospital readmissions, and ED visits.

MODELS OF CARE FOR OLDER HOSPITALIZED PATIENTS

Systematic approaches have been demonstrated in controlled trials to improve hospital care of older adults. These models involve comprehensive multicomponent assessment and interventions. Two of the models are implemented on designated medical units. CGA in the hospital was found in a review of 29 randomized trials to increase the likelihood that older patients will be alive and in their own homes at 3–12 months. The analysis was insufficiently powered to detect a difference between CGA delivered in wards and by mobile teams.

Geriatric Evaluation and Management Units

Geriatric evaluation and management (GEM) units for older adults who have stabilized during an acute hospitalization were developed and pioneered in Veterans Affairs medical centers. These units incorporate CGA (including screening for geriatric syndromes, and assessment for and treatment of functional, cognitive, affective, and nutritional problems) with interprofessional team–based care. In a meta-analysis of 13 studies, admission to a GEM unit resulted in less functional decline at discharge and a lower risk of institutionalization 1 year after discharge. No benefit was found in outcomes of mortality, readmission, or length of stay (SOE=A).

Acute Care for Elders

Acute Care for Elders (ACE), adopted in many acute care hospitals, involves a system of care designed to help acutely ill older patients to maintain or achieve independence in ADLs and IADLs. ACE programs adopt a proactive, "prehabilitative" approach, comprising 4 components:

- A prepared environment to promote mobility and orientation (eg, carpeting, raised toilet seats, low beds, clocks, calendars, and pictures)

- Interprofessional, team-based, patient-centered care with nursing-initiated protocols for independent self-care, nutrition, sleep hygiene, skin care, mood, and cognition

- Early planning to go home, with social work intervention to mobilize family and other resources at home

- Medication review to promote optimal prescribing

This approach resulted in greater independence in ADLs at discharge, less frequent discharge to a nursing home, and somewhat shorter and less expensive hospitalization (SOE=A). In addition, ACE was associated with substantial differences in the satisfaction of patients, family members, physicians, and nurses but with only modest differences in ADL function (SOE=A). These findings demonstrate that ACE is a proven approach to improve outcomes and reduce hospital costs for acutely ill older general medical patients, but the effects of ACE on patient outcomes are likely sensitive to factors that depend on the function of the interprofessional team.

Hospital Elder Life Program

The Hospital Elder Life Program (HELP) involves a multicomponent intervention to prevent delirium in hospitalized older patients. The intervention consists of protocols to manage 6 risk factors for delirium: cognitive impairment, sleep deprivation, immobility, visual impairment, hearing impairment, and dehydration. Older patients receiving this intervention are not segregated on a special hospital ward or unit. The program makes extensive use of hospital volunteers. In one prospective controlled study, incidence of delirium was reduced by one-third, from 15.0% to 9.9% (SOE=A). Severity and duration of delirium episodes appeared not to be affected by HELP. The intervention was also associated with significantly improved cognitive function among patients with cognitive impairment at admission and with reduced use of sleep medications among all patients. A meta- analysis of 14 multicomponent, nonpharmacologic preventive interventions, 9 of which were HELP adaptations, showed the odds of delirium in the intervention group to be 53% lower than in controls.

Surgical Co-Management

Increasingly, hospitalized surgical patients are being co-managed by surgeons and hospitalists or geriatric providers. One of the more well-studied models in geriatrics is the co-management of hip fracture patients by orthopedic surgeons and geriatricians. Successful models have demonstrated reduced length of stay, complication rates, readmissions, mortality rates, and cost. Key components of this model include standardized protocols and order sets, frequent communication between the surgeon and geriatrician, early discharge planning, and clear delineation of responsibilities.

Nurses Improving Care of Health System Elders (NICHE)

NICHE is a national program of the Hartford Institute for Geriatric Nursing at New York University College of Nursing, the goal of which is to improve the care of hospitalized older patients through change programs and nursing protocols.

The Geriatric Resource Nurse (GRN) Model is the foundation of the NICHE program. After receiving specialized education in nursing care of older adults, the GRN receives ongoing mentorship and clinical support from an advanced practice nurse through clinical rounds and structured learning activities. GRNs serve as the unit's resource on geriatric best practices, engage in quality and research initiatives, and educate other staff regarding geriatric care.

NICHE has grown into a national hospital network for sharing lessons and collaborating in development of inpatient geriatric nursing-care resources. After implementing the NICHE GRN model, hospitals have reported improved clinical outcomes, enhanced nurse knowledge and perceptions of quality, and increased compliance with protocol application.

ALTERNATIVES TO HOSPITAL CARE

It is often assumed that older adults would prefer to be treated for acute illness at home rather than in the hospital whenever possible. However, older adults' preferences for care at home rather than in the hospital vary widely. In a study of community-dwelling older adults, virtually all preferred care in the site that would provide the higher probability of survival. When home care and hospital care provide equivalent probabilities of survival, roughly half preferred care in each site, with those preferring home care more likely to be white, better educated, living with a spouse, deeply religious, and dependent in ≥2 ADLs. The major difference perceived by older adults between home care and hospital care was feeling safer in the hospital than at home.

Studies suggest that hospital-at-home care can provide safe, economical, and efficacious care for some older adults with selected medical conditions, eg, heart failure, community-acquired pneumonia, cellulitis, COPD (SOE=A). Common features of the home-hospital models are the provision of care by an interprofessional team, availability of 24-hour coverage (including physician coverage), and a safe home environment. In one trial, patients with dementia in the intervention group had fewer problems with sleep, feeding, and aggression. Fewer patients were prescribed antipsychotics. A review of 16 trials concluded that hospital-at-home care makes no significant difference in 6-month mortality or in the likelihood of hospital transfer or readmission but may reduce the likelihood of living in a residential care facility at 6 months. Patients receiving care in a home hospital were more satisfied with their care, but few studies reported on caregiver satisfaction.

HOSPITAL COMPARE

Hospital Compare is a CMS quality initiative that mandates reporting of hospital compliance with selected process measures and outcomes of patients treated for acute myocardial infarction (AMI), heart failure, or pneumonia. In April 2005, CMS began reporting hospital's performance on the Hospital Compare website. Publicly reported outcomes include risk-standardized 30-day mortality and, in 2013, risk-standardized unplanned readmission. Hospital Compare was designed to accomplish 2 goals: to guide patients who seek nonemergent care with relative performance among different hospitals and to spur hospital quality improvement. CMS aims to raise the performance level of as many hospitals as possible to the level set by the highest-performing hospitals.

Between 2004 and 2006, all process measures improved, particularly in baseline low-performing hospitals, whereas most high-performing hospitals maintained performance level. Concurrently, there were improvements in risk-adjusted outcomes only for AMI. Across all hospitals, a 10-point increase in performance was associated with declines in AMI-associated mortality rate of 0.6%, in length of stay of −0.19 days, and in readmission rate of 0.5%. Changes in outcomes for heart failure and pneumonia were smaller and less consistent. To date, the effect of reporting 30-day risk-adjusted mortality rates for pneumonia, heart failure, and AMI seems to have been negligible.

Hospital Compare started reporting hospital mortality performance in 2007, rating hospitals as better, worse, or no different than national average. Very few hospitals were rated as differing from average, which may have partly explained why this study found no evidence that patients shifted to higher-performing hospitals. Patient's access to higher-quality hospitals may also be constrained by other factors such as the distance to the nearest high-performing hospital, selective contracts between hospitals and insurers, and hospital crowding.

In sum, public reporting of process and outcome measures seems to be associated with significant improvement in process measures and minimal changes in mortality.

READMISSION

Readmission is costly and often considered to be a quality-of-care indicator. Although one-fifth of Medicare beneficiaries discharged from the hospital from 2003 to 2004 were readmitted within 30 days, rehospitalizations are only modestly related to age. There is significant geographic variability in readmission rates; the difference between the 5 states with the highest and lowest rates is 45%. The cost of unplanned readmissions is estimated at over $26 billion per year.

The U.S. Patient Protection and Affordable Care Act (ACA) has targeted several initiatives at reducing readmission rates. The common theme running through these strategies is incentivized coordination of care across transitions. Reducing readmissions is also a goal of public reporting through Hospital Compare. Since 2013, hospitals with high Risk-Standardized-Readmission Rates (RSRR) are penalized through reductions in Medicare reimbursement.

In 2009, CMS began reporting hospital-specific 30-day RSRR for 3 conditions: AMI, heart failure, and pneumonia. An analysis of Medicare claims data from 2006 to 2012 for discharges after hospitalization for any of these diagnoses found no improvement in the trends in 30-day readmission rates or 30-day mortality after discharge following public reporting. However, there was a reduction in the trend in heart failure care after discharge, specifically in heart failure–associated ED visits and observation stays.

The diagnosis at readmission frequently differs from the index admission diagnosis. From 2007 to 2009, 30-day readmissions for the same condition of Medicare fee-for-service patients occurred in only 35% of heart failure, 10% of AMI, and 22% of pneumonia admissions. Two-thirds of readmissions occurred within 15 days of discharge. No association was identified between readmission diagnoses or timing of readmission and age, sex, or race.

A review of interventions to prevent early readmissions reports greater efficacy in multi-component care bundles, involving more individuals in care delivery, and supporting patient's self-care capacity There is also evidence from randomized trials that integrating informal caregivers into discharge planning results in fewer readmissions at 90 days and 180 days, shorter rehospitalization, and lower care costs after discharge.

CHOOSING WISELY® RECOMMENDATIONS

Eating and Feeding

- Do not recommend percutaneous feeding tubes in patients with advanced dementia; instead offer oral assisted feeding.

- Avoid using prescription appetite stimulants or high-calorie supplements to treat anorexia or cachexia in older adults; instead, optimize social supports, provide feeding assistance and clarify patient goals and expectations.

Delirium

- Avoid physical restraints to manage behavioral symptoms of hospitalized older adults with delirium.

- Do not use benzodiazepines or other sedative-hypnotics in older adults as first choice for insomnia, agitation, or delirium.

RESOURCES

- Alberti TL, Nannini A. Patient comprehension of discharge instructions from the emergency department: A literature review. *J Am Assoc Nurs Pract*. 2013;25:186–194.

- American College of Emergency Physicians; American Geriatrics Society; Emergency Nurses Association; Society for Academic Emergency Medicine; Geriatric Emergency Department Guidelines Task Force. Geriatric Emergency Department Guidelines. *Ann Emerg Med*. 2014;63(5):e7–e25.

- Boltz M, Resnick B, Chippendale T, et al. Testing a family-centered intervention to promote functional and cognitive

- Hshieh T, Yue J, Oh E, et al. Effectiveness of multicomponent nonpharmacological delirium interventions: a meta-analysis. *JAMA Intern Med*. 2015;175(4):512–520.

- Ramirez E, Schumann L, Agan D, et al. Beyond competencies: Practice standards for emergency nurse practitioners—A model for specialty care clinicians, educators, and employers. *J Am Assoc Nurs Pract*. 2018;30(10):570–578.

CHAPTER 20—TRANSITIONS OF CARE

KEY POINTS

- Older adults undergoing care transitions have increased risk of experiencing suboptimal care and adverse events.

- Clinicians play an important role in implementing effective solutions to improve care during transitions, which requires a team-based approach to coordinate care.

- Successful care transitions can result in more effective implementation of care plans, reduced adverse events, faster restoration of older adults' functioning, and improved satisfaction among patients, caregivers, and health care providers.

THE RISKS OF SUBOPTIMAL CARE TRANSITIONS

A care transition is defined as the movement of a patient from one set of providers, level of care, or health care setting to another. Related terms include "handoffs," "handovers," or "transfers"; these other terms are limited in scope and suggest provider-to-provider communication alone, whereas the term "care transition" generally reflects a broader interaction among patients, caregivers, providers, and health care systems. Although care transitions are generally well intended, they are a time when older adults are vulnerable to receiving suboptimal or potentially unsafe care.

Fragmentation in the U.S. health care system has contributed to the rise in awareness of the importance of optimal transitional care.

Care transitions are common, complicated, and costly. Almost 40% of older adults experience two or more care transitions within 30 days of hospital discharge. About half of these transitions involved a single hospitalization followed by return to the original residence, but the other half involved a complex sequence of other transitions. This has profound implications for organizations and individuals involved in caring for older adults. This heterogeneity of transition patterns of older adults challenges approaches to improving care transitions, because it is onerous and inefficient to plan for all possible care patterns when many apply to a small number of individuals.

There is increasing recognition of "post-hospital syndrome"—an acquired, transient condition of vulnerability—in which older adults who have been recently hospitalized are at risk of a range of adverse health events in addition to recovering from their acute illness. Although intrinsic patient factors, admitting diagnoses, and hospital care processes likely affect risk of post-hospital syndrome, strategies to improve hospital discharge transitions should reduce the vulnerability.

Suboptimal care transitions that result in rehospitalizations can be costly. One in five older adults discharged from the hospital are rehospitalized within 30 days, and one in three are rehospitalized within 90 days. Beyond their economic implications, suboptimal care transitions increase the risk of adverse events resulting from poor care coordination among providers and health care entities.

Suboptimal care transitions across care settings can pose a significant threat to patient safety. Common hazards related to transitions include medication errors and inaccurate or incomplete information transfer, including delayed diagnosis, duplicative medical services, and reduced provider and patient satisfaction. Lack of availability of discharge summaries during follow-up clinician visits is common and can lead to duplicate testing and preventable rehospitalizations.

Although suboptimal care transitions adversely affect patients of all ages, older adults have higher rates of iatrogenic complications, greater frequency of admission through the emergency department (ED), and longer lengths of stay than their younger counterparts. Further, older adults are more vulnerable to the hazards of hospitalization: functional decline, delirium, adverse drug events, pressure injury, bowel and bladder dysfunction, malnutrition, and dehydration. Because of these hazards, older adults are more likely to experience complications and therefore to require complex care after discharge. Older adults also have a greater prevalence of functional deficits and cognitive impairments at baseline, and therefore may experience more difficulty with self-care after hospital discharge. Older adults are also more likely not to return to their previous baseline functional status after a complex hospitalization. Adults >65 years old have a higher prevalence of "below basic" health literacy. These risk factors can further challenge older adults' ability to participate in the care-transition process and to understand discharge and self-care instructions.

INCENTIVES, BARRIERS, AND RESPONSIBILITIES

Improving care transitions for older adults, especially between hospital and home, is an attractive target for improving health care quality and reducing medical and liability expenditures. Interventions to improve care transitions are a high priority under the Affordable Care Act of 2010, which attempts to realign financial incentives to improve care transitions and reduce rehospitalization rates. Care-transition programs are now expected to be implemented in many health care systems. Care-transition programs are intended to facilitate the communication that may be lacking among older adults, caregivers, hospital providers, and primary care providers during transitions. Currently, there are medicolegal liability concerns related to suboptimal care transitions. Hospital medicine providers and PCPs share liability during care transitions.

Several barriers exist to executing safe care transitions. Common ones include the following:

- Diverse older adult and caregiver transitional care needs depending on illness, social situation, and type of transition

- Lack of provider education and feedback on execution of care transitions, including preparation of timely and effective discharge summaries and understanding the capabilities of different types of postacute care settings

- Difficulty communicating with colleagues at the previous or next site of care

- Lack of time or financial resources to address transitional care issues

STRATEGIES AND MODELS TO IMPROVE TRANSITIONAL CARE

Transitional care entails a broad range of time-limited services designed to ensure the coordination and continuity of health care as patients transfer between different locations or different levels of care. Transitional care contains elements of care coordination, discharge planning, and disease or case management. Many successful interventions designed to improve transitional care share core components, such as assigning a care-transition coach, guide, or navigator to monitor the older adult during a care transition. Cost-effective transitional care is focused on the highly vulnerable and chronically ill population and includes numerous components (Table 20.1).

Specific Care Models to Improve Transitional Care

Transitions from Hospital to Home

Transitions-of-care programs for home care after hospitalization using directed discharge planning and follow-up protocols have shown promise in reducing early repeat hospitalizations.

Table 20.1—Components of Effective Transitional Care

Accurate and timely transfer of information to the next set of providers
Empowerment of the older adult to assert his or her own preferences
Comprehensive assessments of older adult and caregiver needs
Comprehensive medication review and management
Logistical arrangements related to executing the care transition
Education to prepare both older adults and caregivers for what to expect at the next site of care
Support for self-management of medical conditions
Coordination among medical and community resources
Follow up and support after discharge

One systematic review evaluating the effectiveness of hospital-initiated care-transition strategies found that a "bridging" strategy, incorporating pre- and post-discharge interventions with a dedicated transitions provider, reduced rehospitalization or ED visit rates. There was insufficient evidence to reach conclusions on the effectiveness of specific strategies that were components of these interventions; however, others have found that effective transitional care interventions use more than one modality, eg, phone calls and home visits, and that single-component transitional care interventions were not effective.

Other Transitions

Some models exist for transitions other than hospital to home. Guided Care is an outpatient-based interprofessional team model of care led by a specially trained registered nurse in partnership with PCPs and caregivers to support a practice's most complex patients. A major goal of the program is to refine transitions between sites of care. Patients participating in Guided Care tended to use less home health services, but there was no difference in hospital, ED, and SNF services or 30-day rehospitalization rates compared those of with usual care patients.

The Interventions to Reduce Acute Care Transfers (INTERACT) model is a nursing home quality improvement intervention providing tools and strategies to assist nursing home staff in early identification, assessment, and communication regarding changes in resident condition. The Discharge of Elderly from the Emergency Department (DEED) program uses comprehensive geriatric assessment performed by a nurse for patients ≥75 years old who are discharged from the ED to home.

Policy Approaches

Successful strategies and processes from transitional care models form the basis of many of the new models of care encouraged by CMS. Increased emphasis is placed on patient-specific goals, quality, safety, and the avoidance of cost shifting to other components of the health care system. Key stakeholders may be reluctant to invest in prevention of rehospitalizations if they perceive other stakeholders (ie, not the ones making the investments) will reap the benefits. Programs are needed that align the incentives of all stakeholders involved. To this end, the federal government has implemented programs to improve care transitions nationally. The Community-based Care Transitions Program (CCTP) was created by Section 3026 of the Affordable Care Act and was in effect between 2012–2017. Designed to allow for testing of care models, the goals of the CCTP are to improve transitions of Medicare beneficiaries from the inpatient hospital setting to other care settings, to improve quality of care, to reduce rehospitalizations for high-risk beneficiaries, and to document measurable savings to the Medicare program.

In addition to the CCTP, CMS announced new payment codes in 2013 that incentivize ambulatory care providers to participate in transitional care management. Providers can bill under these codes for transitional care management services they perform to assist with care transitions in the first 30 days of discharge from an inpatient hospital setting. Transitions from the hospital to SNFs are the focus of the Protecting Access to Medicare Act (PAMA) of 2014. The PAMA legislation includes language regarding rehospitalization penalties for SNFs starting in 2018.

DISCHARGE DESTINATIONS AND CARE VENUES

When determining a discharge destination, the clinician should match the services available with the needs of the older adult. Home-health care works well for older adults requiring only intermittent skilled services (nursing, physical therapy, or speech therapy), and older adults with one of these needs may also receive assistance (under Medicare) from occupational therapy, medical social work, and/or home-health aides. Medicare requires that older adults receiving home-health care be homebound. Under Medicare, older adults appropriate for SNFs must also have a need for a skilled service, such as a requirement for intravenous therapy, artificial nutrition and hydration, complex wound care, ostomy care, or rehabilitation. Medicare covers all or part of skilled-nursing care for up to 100 days after a qualifying hospital stay, but coverage stops earlier if an older adult's treatment goals are met or if the older adult "plateaus" and no longer demonstrates improvement. Older adults with substantial rehabilitation needs (more than just physical therapy, occupational therapy, or speech therapy) and considerable rehabilitation potential may be appropriate for transfer to an acute rehabilitation unit, but many older adults are deemed ineligible because of an inability to participate in 3 hours per day of intense therapy. Long-term acute care, also known as "chronic hospitalization," is appropriate for the rare hospital patient who requires prolonged, hospital-level care. Long-term acute care facilities provide care for patients requiring long-term mechanical ventilation, multiple intravenous medications, parenteral nutrition, or complex wound care, along with a need for frequent clinician monitoring.

CMS require hospitals to provide discharge planning services for hospitalized patients. Nurses or social workers trained in development of discharge evaluations provide discharge planning services and are required to provide options for SNFs or home-health services after hospital discharge.

THE DISCHARGE MEDICATION REGIMEN

A critical activity near the time of hospital (or other facility) discharge is the preparation of the discharge medication list. This list should include an indication for each medication, stop dates (eg, for antibiotics) or tapering schedules (eg, for systemic corticosteroids) as appropriate, and clear behavioral triggers for as-needed psychiatric medications. Medications added during the hospital stay (such as analgesics, proton-pump inhibitors, or laxatives with as-needed orders) can be tapered or discontinued at this time. Finally, the discharge regimen should be formally reconciled with the preadmission regimen by the discharge team. The discharge medication regimen should also be reviewed by the receiving provider, who may need to further reconcile it with other lists that the patient may have (including but not limited to the home medication list, the medication list kept by the pharmacy, and the medication list kept by the outpatient clinic).

COMMUNICATING WITH THE PATIENT, CAREGIVERS, AND RECEIVING TEAM

The following items should be communicated to older adults (or their caregivers) who are being discharged directly home: follow-up appointments, warning symptoms or signs to watch for with instructions on whom to contact, clinical disciplines (eg, nursing, physical therapy) contracted for provision of services in the home, and the reconciled medication list. Older adults being discharged to other care venues should be oriented with respect to the nature of the new institution, the identity of a new provider (if known), and the expected frequency of provider visits. Tools are available to assist older adults and caregivers with assessing care preferences, clarifying discharge instructions, reconciling medication inaccuracies, and facilitating communication across care sites at discharge (eg, see www.caretransitions.org [accessed Feb 2019]).

If the provider at the receiving institution differs from the hospital clinician, then clear and prompt communication is essential. Some items of information (such as critical but pending study results, nuances of goals of care, or family dynamics) call for direct communication between sending and receiving clinicians. Otherwise, a brief and prompt discharge summary containing the following will suffice: summary of hospital course with the care provided and important test results; a list of problems and diagnoses; baseline physical functional status; baseline cognitive status; physical and cognitive status at discharge; reconciled medication list; allergies; tests results still outstanding; follow-up appointments; and information related to goals, preferences, and advance directives.

THREE STEPS TO IMPROVE CARE TRANSITIONS

Creating a strategy to improve care transitions consists of three essential steps. The first step is setting expectations for both the sending and receiving provider teams. The National Transitions of Care Coalition recommends shifting from the concept of "discharge" to that of "transfer with continuous management."

The second step to creating a strategy to improve care transitions involves tailoring communication strategies to the type of information being communicated and to the type of care transition. Written communication (electronic or paper) is best for information that must be a part of the medical record or used as a reference by the older adult, caregiver, or clinical provider. Written communication can be used for information transfer of discharge summaries, notification of patient admission or discharge, and other nonurgent issues. Verbal communication (phone or in person) is best for situations of urgency or uncertainty, new diagnoses of serious illnesses, difficult social situations, and when preparing patients for their next care transition.

The third step to creating a strategy to improve care transitions focuses on specific processes or outcomes as targets for improvement, using established quality improvement methods. It is important to begin by choosing one or two measures to focus on to track progress, and then expand further once initial goals are achieved.

RESOURCES

- Lindquist LA, Miller RK, Saltsman WS, et al. SGIM-AMDA-AGS Consensus Best Practice Recommendations for Transitioning Patients' Healthcare from Skilled Nursing Facilities to the Community. *J Gen Intern Med*. 2017;32(2):199–203.

- Pauly MV, Hirschman KB, Hanlon AL, et al. Cost impact of the transitional care model for hospitalized cognitively impaired older adults. *J Comp Eff Res*. 2018;7(9):913–922.

- Rennke S, Nguyen OK, Shoeb MH, et al. Hospital-initiated transitional care interventions as a patient safety strategy: a systematic review. *Ann Intern Med*. 2013;158(5 Pt 2):433–440.

CHAPTER 21—REHABILITATION

KEY POINTS

- The World Health Organization conceptual model of functioning and disability provides a useful framework for geriatric rehabilitation by taking into account the complex interactions of body functions and structures, health conditions, individual activities and participation in life situations, and environmental and personal factors.

- As rehabilitation treatments require active patient participation and long-term self-management, the patient and family are core members of the rehabilitation team.

- Optimal rehabilitation outcomes depend on comprehensive assessment of the patient, coordinated interprofessional team management, multifaceted interventions, and access to appropriate and high-quality care.

Rehabilitation is a critical component of geriatric health care because of the high incidence of disabling conditions in the older adult population. Although these conditions drastically influence quality of life, they often improve with treatment. Chronic disease almost always underlies disability in older adults; for example, stroke occurs most often in people with other vascular diseases, and hip fractures occur most often in people with osteoporosis and gait disorders. Disability also worsens in progressive chronic diseases (eg, osteoarthritis, Parkinson disease, or amyotrophic lateral sclerosis) or in the context of deconditioning from inactivity during acute illness. To provide the best functional recovery possible, those providing geriatric rehabilitation must do the following:

- Use systematic approaches to assess the causes of disability

- Be familiar with the advantages and disadvantages of all potential sites of care

- Understand the role of interprofessional teams and care plans

- Adapt care to comorbidities and disabilities

- Be familiar with the basic requirements for rehabilitation of common geriatric conditions

CONCEPTUAL MODEL FOR GERIATRIC REHABILITATION

Geriatric rehabilitation services can be organized around a conceptual model of disability for assessing the status and needs of the patient, matching treatments with specific conditions, and evaluating rehabilitation outcomes. The World Health Organization (WHO) *International Classification of Functioning, Disability, and Health* (ICF) provides a useful framework for measuring health and disability. For an ICF guide and a discussion of the ICF model of disability, see the WHO website (www.who.int/classifications/icf/en/ [accessed Feb 2019]). The ICF has two main domains: "health conditions" and "contextual factors." Disability and functioning are viewed as outcomes of interactions between health conditions (diseases, disorders, injuries) and contextual factors, which includes both environmental and personal. Environmental factors range from a person's most immediate environment, like furniture in the room, to the more general environment, such as access to public transportation. Personal factors include a person's age, race, gender, educational background, personality, fitness, and lifestyle.

In the WHO model, interventions can be designed to modify a person's impairments, limitations in activities, and restrictions in participation. For example, a treatment plan can be developed to improve a person's muscle strength (impairment level), but the significance of this intervention is a result of its effect on his or her physical mobility (activity) and ultimately his or her ability to return to social or physical roles (participation). The effects of gains in strength and physical mobility on participation can be modified by the person's motivation or social support. For example, if patients improve in strength and balance but their family and friends continue to "do everything for them" and do not encourage independent function, they may remain dependent. The physical environment is another powerful modifier. Even the person who achieves improved function cannot return to prior work or household roles if physical barriers to access in the community are not removed or adapted by means such as ramps or modified bathrooms. In summary, the interaction of disease and disability is particularly complex in older adults; the ICF model is useful for structuring their comprehensive rehabilitation care.

SITES OF REHABILITATION CARE

Rehabilitation services for older adults are available and reimbursed through Medicare on a time-limited basis. Physical, occupational, and speech therapy services are offered in inpatient, outpatient, and community-based sites. Inpatient rehabilitation care may be provided in Medicare-certified freestanding rehabilitation centers, units attached to acute hospitals, or in skilled-nursing facilities. The escalating expenditures for Medicare's

Table 21.1—Rehabilitation Sites of Care and Level of Care Requirements

Rehabilitation Sites	Level of Care Requirements	Expected Intensity of Services	Payment Source
Inpatient			
Freestanding rehabilitation hospital or rehabilitation unit attached to acute hospital	24-hour availability of a physician with training or experience in rehabilitation 24-hour nursing care Intense level of rehabilitation services Interprofessional team to deliver coordinated program of care as evidenced by weekly team conferences Reasonable expectation of improvement	An interprofessional team approach is required and in most cases, this calls for 3 hours of therapy 5 days/week of at least two therapies; this can include physical, occupational, or speech therapy in any combination.	Medicare Part A Days 1–60: full coverage Days 61–90: partial coverage but daily co-payment >90 days: daily co-payment for up to 60 lifetime reserve days More than lifetime reserve days: no coverage
Medicare skilled-nursing facility or transitional care unit	Physician supervision, with access 24 hours/day on emergency basis 24-hour nursing care Less intense therapy needs Interprofessional team coordination ideally will occur Maintenance of function without progress can be goal of care	Daily therapy (5 days/week) 1 hour/day or more, as tolerated by patient; ADL assistance and/or skilled-nursing care	Medicare Part A Days 1–20: full coverage Days 21–100: partial coverage with co-insurance >100 days: no coverage
Outpatient			
Home health	Face-to-face physician visit within 90 days to establish need and order; physician certifies need and plan of care every 60 days Skilled need required for homebound patient, including either intermittent skilled nursing, physical, occupational, or speech therapy	Intermittent nursing or therapy provided in home; can be no more than 7 days/week or 8 hours/day; patient must have support system to meet needs of living at home	Medicare Part A
Clinic (hospital-based or independent)	Physician orders Skilled need required; rehabilitation services to include physical, occupational, or speech therapy and reviews plan periodically	Intermittent physical, occupational, or speech therapy provided; patient must be able to get to therapy visits	Medicare Part B There are annual caps on coverage, but these can be waived if medically necessary.

SOURCE: www.cms.hhs.gov (accessed Feb 2019)

postacute benefits from $2.5 billion in 1986 to more than $30 billion in 1996 led to the Balanced Budget Act (BBA) of 1997, which mandated prospective payment systems rather than fee-for-service reimbursement. To receive Medicare Part A coverage for inpatient rehabilitation, a patient must have a qualifying hospital stay of at least 3 consecutive midnights for a related illness or injury with an expectation of discharge to the community. Typically reimbursed through Medicare Part B, outpatient and community-based rehabilitation can be provided in hospital-based or independent clinics, day hospital settings, or the home environment. The patient's eligibility, type of services provided, and costs vary across sites of care. For a summary of the sites of rehabilitation, Medicare requirements and payment sources, and the expected intensity of the rehabilitation services, see Table 21.1.

Sites of Care: Coverage and Services

Medicare Part A covers intensive inpatient rehabilitation for patients who have complex needs requiring an interprofessional team approach, including multiple therapies under the Inpatient Rehabilitation Facility (IRF) Prospective Payment System. In most cases, the patient must be able to tolerate a minimum of 3 hours of multiple rehabilitation therapy services per day at least 5 days per week or 15 hours per week. A Medicare-classified inpatient rehabilitation hospital or rehabilitation unit in an acute care hospital must demonstrate that at least a certain percentage of patients have at least 1 of 13 conditions: stroke, spinal cord injury, congenital deformity, amputation, major multiple trauma, hip fracture, brain injury, neurologic disorders (eg, multiple sclerosis, Parkinson disease), burns, three arthritis conditions for which appropriate aggressive and sustained outpatient therapy has failed, joint replacement for both knees or hips when the surgery immediately precedes admission, a BMI ≥50 kg/m^2, or age ≥85 years. Patients must have close medical supervision by a physician with specialized training or experience in rehabilitation and have 24-hour rehabilitation nursing care needs. In collaboration with the patient, an individualized treatment plan is developed and managed by an interprofessional team of skilled nurses and therapists. Medicare prospective payment reimbursement is based on case-mix groups using information in the patient assessment instrument

Table 21.2—Functional Status and Disease-Specific Assessment Instruments

Instrument	Purpose/Description
Functional Independence Measure (FIM) (https://www.sralab.org/rehabilitation-measures/fimr-instrument-fim-fimr-trademark-uniform-data-system-fro-medical)	■ Measures assistance required for self-care, transfers, locomotion, sphincter control, social cognition, and communication. ■ An 18-item ordinal scale with scores ranging from 0 (total assist) to 7 (complete independence); the possible total score ranges from 18 (the lowest) to 126 (highest), obtained by adding points for each item.
Barthel ADL Index (https://www.sralab.org/rehabilitation-measures/barthel-index)	■ Used to establish degree of independence with regard to ADLs. ■ A 10-item ordinal scale; scores vary depending on the item in question. Bathing and grooming are scored either 0 (dependent/needs help) or 5 (independent); scores for feeding, dressing, bowels, bladder, toilet use, and stairs range from 0 (dependent/unable) to 10 (independent); scores for transfers and mobility on level surfaces range for 0 (unable) to 15 (independent); the possible total score ranges for 0 (the lowest) to 100 (the highest), obtained by adding points for each item.
Activity Measure for Post Acute Care (AM-PAC) (https://www.sralab.org/rehabilitation-measures/activity-measure-post-acute-care)	■ Measures patient's activity limitations in the domains of cognition, self-care, and mobility. ■ Various versions available, including a computer-adapted test; inpatient short form includes 5–8 items per domain and outpatient short form consists of 15–18 items per domain.
Stroke Impact Scale (https://www.sralab.org/rehabilitation-measures/stroke-impact-scale)	■ An 8-domain, 59-item scale that measures the aspects of stroke recovery important to patients and caregivers, as well as stroke experts. ■ Includes measures of physical domain such as strength, mobility, ADLs, and hand function, as well as the domains of memory, emotion, communication, and social participation.
Harris Hip Questionnaire (www.orthopaedicscore.com/scorepages/harris_hip_score.html)	■ Asks questions regarding pain and function, including ambulation distance, presence of a limp, ability with tasks such as public transportation or stairs, and need for an assistive device. ■ Hip deformity and range of hip motion are also included.

NOTE: Above websites accessed Feb 2019.

(IRF-PAI) including admission and discharge scores from the Functional Independence Measure (Table 21.2).

A patient with multiple ongoing medical issues who is unable to tolerate 3 hours of therapy per day may need to be transferred to transitional or long-term acute care before rehabilitation. This is a less intensive alternative to IRF, Medicare Part A covers daily, skilled therapy and skilled-nursing services provided in a certified skilled-nursing facility or unit for 20 days in full and up to 80 additional days with coinsurance. An established rate in addition to a per diem prospective payment covers routine, ancillary, and capital costs with some exceptions. Payments for each admission are case-mix adjusted by use of a resource utilization classification system (RUG IV) that is based on data from scheduled patient assessments (the Minimum Data Set 3.0) and relative weights developed from staff time data. Physical, occupational, and speech therapies are available as well as dietary, pharmaceutical, dental, and medical social services. Physicians must supervise patient care and be available 24 hours per day on an emergency basis. In this setting, maintenance of function without progress may be the goal of care. A legal decision (Jimmo v. Sebelius, 2013) clarifies that the skilled services may include maintenance therapy in addition to those interventions to prevent or slow further deterioration.

For those patients who require skilled-nursing care and home-health aide services on an intermittent or part-time basis, defined as <8 hours per day and 28 or fewer hours per week for all required services, Medicare provides home-health benefits. Physical, occupational, and speech therapies as well as medical social work are available through Medicare-participating home health agencies. Patients must also be homebound, either 1) need the aid of an assistive device (such as a walker or wheelchair), use of special transportation, or the assistance of another person to leave their home; or 2) have a condition such that leaving the home is medically contraindicated. Patients must be unable to leave home or considerable effort is required to do so. However, patients can leave home for medical treatments or for short, infrequent nonmedical reasons, including attendance at religious services. Home-health services must follow an established plan of care that is prescribed and recertified every 60 days by a physician. Initial certification for home health requires a documented face-to-face visit by the physician, or nonphysician practitioner, within 90 days before the start of home-health care or within 30 days after the start of care. There is no prior hospitalization requirement or limit on the number of visits a person may receive. The plan of care is based on a comprehensive assessment from the Outcome and Assessment Information Set (OASIS). Medicare provides care in 60-day episodes. Therapy coverage is based on assessment of the patient's function and need for skilled care; reassessment is completed every 30 days. Home-health care reimbursement is also under a prospective payment system with an initial and final payment. A case-mix methodology adjusts the national 60-day episode payment rate based on characteristics of the patient and resource needs using relevant data from OASIS.

Medicare Part B covers outpatient physical, occupational, and speech therapies, available through independent and hospital-based clinics. Unlike the inpatient and home-health rehabilitation reimbursement, payment is based on the Current Procedural Terminology (CPT) codes that reflect the therapy evaluation and/or treatment provided. To assist in Medicare reform, legislation now requires a claims-based system to collect outcome data on the provision of outpatient therapy services to Medicare B beneficiaries. The current, projected goal, and discharge functional status of the beneficiary are reported using non-payable G-codes and complexity/severity modifiers. The functional data on mobility, self-care, and cognition must be collected using an outcomes assessment such as the Boston University Activity Measure for Post-Acute Care (Table 21.2).

Sites of Care: Outcomes

The effect of site of care on rehabilitation outcomes is not well established. A study of outcomes among patients with stroke and hip fracture examined rates of discharge to home and recovery of function that were based on use of inpatient or nursing rehabilitation services. When controlling for case-mix differences, the researchers found that stroke but not hip fracture patients were more likely to be discharged home and to recover activities of daily living (ADLs) if treated in an inpatient rehabilitation setting (SOE=B). In another cohort study, patients admitted for hip fracture to inpatient facilities had better 12-week functional outcomes than did patients undergoing rehabilitation at skilled-nursing facilities (SOE=B). This type of observational study is vulnerable to bias, despite adjusting the analyses, because the prognosis for recovery may influence discharge site; patients with a poor prognosis are more likely to go to the nursing home, whereas those with a better prognosis go to inpatient or home-health settings.

Each site of care has advantages and disadvantages from the patient's perspective. Inpatient care is the most intense but may not be endurable for frail older patients, because it usually requires 3 hours per day of active (and fatiguing) therapy. Skilled nursing offers 24-hour care for those who cannot care for themselves or do not have a full-time caregiver. Alternatively, patients often prefer to return to their own homes but may not have the care support they need. Participation in day hospitals or outpatient clinics requires transportation, which can be costly and time consuming.

TEAMS AND ROLES

A team approach is necessary to meet the complex rehabilitation needs of older adults. The interprofessional rehabilitation team often includes practitioners from nursing, physical therapy, occupational therapy, speech language therapy, social work/case management, psychology, nutrition services, prosthetics/orthotics, and pharmacy. Medical professionals on team can consist of a nurse, nurse practitioner, physician assistant, and/or physician (Table 21.3). Each health care professional evaluates the patient, identifies goals, and then provides discipline-specific interventions to address the patient's issues in collaboration with other members of the team. The patient's health-related outcome is the sum of the effort of each discipline. According to Medicare regulations, the interdisciplinary team must be able to document participation by professionals with specialized training and experience in rehabilitation from the following disciplines: physician, registered nurse, social worker or case manager (or both), and licensed or certified therapist from each discipline involved in treating the patient. One of the therapy disciplines must be either physical or occupational therapy. Documentation of the interprofessional team meetings, which are held every 7 days, must include the name and professional designation of each team member in attendance. Health care professionals complete comprehensive evaluations on the patient; however, the patient goals and the intervention plan are determined by the entire team, including the patient and his or her family. The patient and family are core members of the rehabilitation team, and their expectations and preferences must be integrated into the care plan. In collaboration, the team members should pool their skills, experience, and knowledge to work toward the patient's goals to achieve the best outcome. Team building and continual efforts to improve team function are important issues for geriatric rehabilitation service providers to achieve positive patient outcomes.

IMPACT OF COMORBID CONDITIONS

In older patients, comorbid diseases and conditions can interrupt or delay treatment and often require the care plan to be modified. Many of the illnesses that can interfere with rehabilitation of older adults are predictable and potentially preventable. A systematic approach to assessment, prevention, and management of comorbid conditions can improve the patient's chance of receiving maximal benefit from rehabilitation services.

Table 21.3—Roles of Core Health Care Providers on Rehabilitation Team

Provider	Primary Role on Rehabilitation Team
Case manager	Assists patient and family in coordinating services to meet recovery needs and transition toward discharge to home
Dietitian	Assesses nutritional status Recommends dietary changes to maximize nutrition
Nurse	Provides ongoing assessment of signs and symptoms of illness, medical conditions, and affect Educates patient and family Evaluates self-care skills
Nurse's aide	Facilitates participation in ADLs (bathing, dressing and mobility) Takes vital sign measurements
Occupational therapist	Assesses ADL and IADL abilities Screens visual perception and cognition Provides home assessment Provides self-care skills training; makes recommendations and provides training in use of assistive technology Fabricates splints and treats upper extremity deficits
Orthotist	Makes and fits braces and other devices to align and/or support limbs
Pharmacist	Conducts thorough medication review Detects therapeutic incompatibilities Reduces or eliminates unnecessary medication use
Physical therapist	Assesses joint range of motion and muscle strength Assesses gait and mobility Provides appropriate assistive devices Instructs in exercise training to increase range of motion, strength, endurance, balance, coordination, and gait Treats with physical modalities (heat, cold, ultrasound, massage, electrical stimulation) Assesses environmental barriers in planned discharge environment
Physician, physician assistant, nurse practitioner	Certifies rehabilitation need (physician only) Supervises patient treatment Treats medical comorbidities Educates patient and family Contributes to postadmission assessment
Prosthetist	Makes and fits prosthetic limbs
Psychologist	Provides clinical and counseling services to patient and family
Social worker	Evaluates family and home-care factors Assesses psychosocial factors Provides counseling
Speech therapist	Assesses all aspects of communication Assesses swallowing disorders Treats communication deficits Recommends changes in diet and positioning to treat dysphagia

Older adults with reduced mobility are at high risk of skin breakdown, which can interfere with recovery and require extensive treatment. Immobility or altered weight bearing can precipitate pressure injuries that heal poorly. Clinicians should monitor pressure and weight-bearing areas and be prepared to modify footwear, wheelchairs, and bedding as needed. Because thromboembolic events are also common with reduced mobility, their prevention should be a routine part of care. Length of time for prophylaxis and medication recommendations varies depending on the medical condition.

Incontinence is prevalent among older adults; causes include detrusor overactivity, obstruction, neurogenic bladder, immobility, and cognitive deficits. Indwelling catheters increase the risk of infection and are rarely appropriate in the nonacute setting. A structured approach to the assessment and treatment of bladder problems should be a basic component of any rehabilitation service.

The risk of pneumonia is increased by inactivity and disordered swallowing, as well as by underlying lung disease. The prevention of aspiration pneumonia involves difficult tradeoffs. Awareness of aspiration has been markedly increased by routine radiologic screening, but the clinical relevance of modest aspiration detected radiologically is unknown. Conservative measures such as changing food consistency with liquid thickeners and cohesive food substances and elevating head position while eating can help alleviate the problem. Sometimes aspiration risk is addressed by discontinuing all oral feeding and placing an enteral feeding tube. This approach eliminates the fundamental human pleasure of eating and may not be successful, because oral secretions or refluxed gastric contents can still be aspirated. Bleeding in the upper GI tract can occur during rehabilitation as a consequence of stress or medications and may not be preceded by typical symptoms.

Anemia is common in older adults and has been associated with adverse outcomes, including functional impairment, decreased muscle strength, and poorer quality of life. Although there is some evidence for improved exercise tolerance in older adults with end-stage kidney disease and congestive heart failure who are given erythropoiesis-stimulating agents, definitive studies are lacking.

Mental functioning is critical for rehabilitation, which requires the ability to follow commands and to learn. Because older adults who have been acutely ill are at increased risk of delirium, clinicians should assess mental status and screen for easily reversible causes in older rehabilitation patients. Depression is endemic in newly disabled individuals and can manifest as low motivation; formal screens for depression and early intervention are essential. Seizures can develop after stroke, and spasticity can develop during stroke recovery. Interventions for spasticity such as physical therapy or muscle relaxants have offered only modest benefit (SOE=B). Studies have shown botulinum toxin to be effective in decreasing muscle tone and increasing range of motion (SOE=A). However, these improvements have not consistently translated into improved function (SOE=B).

Certain comorbid conditions common in older adults, including diabetes mellitus, heart disease, peripheral vascular disease, musculoskeletal disorders, sensory impairments, and dementia, require ongoing adaptations in rehabilitation. Activity level is a powerful factor in glucose metabolism; diabetic patients are therefore likely to experience changes in glucose levels and medication requirements during rehabilitation. Increased caloric intake during recovery can also affect medication needs. Therapy personnel should know how to assess diabetic control, use a glucometer, and intervene for hypoglycemia. Most abnormal gaits increase the energy requirements of walking; an abnormal gait in a patient with coronary artery disease can cause coronary symptoms to worsen. Patients with poor cardiac output may have extreme exercise limitations. Medication adjustments for heart diseases may be necessary but can cause adverse events of their own, such as orthostatic hypotension. Patients with one vascular disease often have others; peripheral vascular disease is common, often associated with insensitive or painful feet and a high risk of skin breakdown. Treatment of painful peripheral neuropathy can foster increased activity and avoid pressure injury. Musculoskeletal status should be monitored to avoid overuse syndromes involving increased demand on vulnerable joints. For those with vision or hearing impairment, corrections must be provided and teaching approaches adapted accordingly. In patients with dementia, rehabilitation progress is still possible, but carryover may be decreased and the need for supervision and cueing may be increased.

ELEMENTS OF A COMPREHENSIVE ASSESSMENT

Comprehensive assessment of rehabilitation patients is necessary for appropriate clinical management and evaluation of outcomes. The treatment plan should be guided by results of the initial assessment. The primary components of any assessment include patient demographics, social support, place of residence before illness, medical comorbidities, severity of current illness, and the patient's prior functional status. The rehabilitation stay is an ideal time for medication review and reconciliation, as patients transition from the hospital to the rehabilitation setting and ultimately to the community.

Impairments such as deficits in range of motion and flexibility, strength, sensory functions, balance, cognition, and depression should always be assessed. In conditions such as stroke, swallowing and language function should be evaluated. The patient's functional status is assessed with standardized measures of ADLs (eg, the Barthel ADL Index [Table 21.2]) and measures of IADLs. The patient's participation or quality of life is assessed with generic measures such as the SF-36 Health Survey (available at www.rand.org/health/surveys_tools/mos/36-item-short-form.html [accessed Feb 2019]) or disease-specific measures such as the Stroke Impact Scale or Harris Hip Questionnaire (Table 21.2).

APPROACHES FOR DIAGNOSIS-SPECIFIC REHABILITATION

Stroke

Stroke is a major cause of mortality and morbidity in the United States, particularly among adults ≥55 years old. Acute stroke occurs in nearly 800,000 people each year (statistics available at www.cdc.gov/dhdsp/data_statistics/fact_sheets/fs_stroke.htm [accessed Feb

2019)] And, 80% or more are likely to survive, many with residual neurologic difficulties, including hemiplegia, dysphagia, aphasia, and visual perceptual and cognitive impairments. These impairments impact participation in daily life activities. Stroke-related deficits are severe in approximately one-third of the survivors, increasing the potential for additional musculoskeletal and neurologic complications such as heterotopic ossification and seizures. As stroke survival continues to increase, the need for early and comprehensive stroke rehabilitation will increase to prevent complications and long-term sequelae. Rehabilitation programs must address a broad range of stroke-related functional disabilities, including those in basic ADLs and IADLs, as well as those impacting participation in work, leisure, and social relationships.

Rehabilitation

The overall goals of rehabilitation for older stroke patients include improving participation and regaining function through remediation or adaptation for specific impairments to reach the highest level of performance. Specific objectives include the following:

- Preventing or recognizing and managing comorbid illness and medical complications
- Preventing recurrent stroke and other vascular conditions such as myocardial infarction
- Assessing each patient comprehensively, using standardized assessments
- Matching the patient's needs to the program capabilities
- Training the patient to maximize independence in ADLs and IADLs
- Facilitating the patient's and family's psychosocial coping and adaptation
- Assisting the patient in reintegrating into the community

Rehabilitation for older adults with stroke is complex because of the variability of causes, symptoms, severity, and recovery. Stroke patients present with varying symptoms, depending on the site and size of the brain lesions. The most common type of neurologic deficit is hemiparesis, but other deficits can include sensory impairment, aphasia, dysarthria, cognitive impairment, motor incoordination, hemianopsia, visual-perceptual deficits, depression, dysphagia, and bowel and bladder incontinence. The degree of initial recovery and the time needed to reach maximal recovery is affected by the number of deficits. For example, individuals who have hemiparesis, hemianopsia, and sensory deficits are less likely to ambulate independently and require a longer time to regain skills than do those with only hemiparesis.

Stroke patients usually experience some degree of recovery. This recovery is most dramatic in the first 30 days but may continue more gradually for months. Stroke severity, which is based on degree of neurologic impairment and size of infarct on CT or MRI, is probably the most important factor to affect short and long-term outcomes. In the Framingham study, improvement in motor function and self-care slowed 3 months after stroke but continued at a reduced pace throughout the first year. In a study of locomotor training after stroke, participants demonstrated functional improvements up to 1 year later, even when training was begun 6 months after the stroke had occurred (SOE=B). Language and visual-spatial function was recovered over 12 months, but cognitive function improved during only the first 3 months.

Management

Guidelines for rehabilitation after stroke have been updated by a team sponsored by the Department of Veterans Affairs and the Department of Defense (available at www.healthquality.va.gov/guidelines/Rehab/stroke [accessed Feb 2019]). The guidelines offer algorithms for initial assessment and rehabilitation referral, followed by management in inpatient or community settings. The guidelines emphasize that clinical outcomes are better when patients with acute stroke are treated in a setting that provides coordinated, interdisciplinary stroke-related evaluation and services (SOE=A). Studies have confirmed that adherence to guidelines promotes better outcomes. Coordinated care reduces 1-year mortality, improves functional independence, and increases satisfaction with care (SOE=A). Stroke severity should be systematically assessed, using the NIH Stroke Scale (www.strokecenter.org/wp-content/uploads/2011/08/NIH_Stroke_Scale.pdf [accessed Feb 2019]).

Benefits of rehabilitation after stroke are not restricted to any particular subgroup of patients. Recent research reviews have demonstrated the complexity of racial disparities and rehabilitation outcomes indicating the need for further inquiry. Two studies investigating motor functioning after post-stroke inpatient rehabilitation found no significant differences in outcomes. Interestingly, there were differences between racial groups in the amount and type of therapy interventions received (SOE=B). In one study, urban-dwelling black stroke patients were more likely to be discharged to an inpatient rehabilitation facility, possibly because of the greater number and severity of stroke cases in this population. Non-Hispanic whites who undergo rehabilitation for a stroke tend to be older, and less likely to have had a hemorrhagic stroke or have Medicaid. In general, therapy should be started early, but later supplementary interventions can also be beneficial. The A Very Early Rehabilitation Trial (AVERT Phase 2) study showed that mobilization within the first

24 hours after stroke and at regular intervals thereafter was safe, with patients in the intervention group being more likely to be discharged home. There are several philosophical approaches to physical rehabilitation after strokes that are based on neurophysiologic, motor learning, or orthopedic principles. In a Cochrane review, a mixed approach was significantly more effective than no treatment or placebo (sham treatment) control for improving functional independence (standardized mean difference 0.78; confidence intervals 95%, 0.58–0.97), and this effect persisted beyond the intervention period. There is no convincing evidence that any one specific technique is superior to another.

Constraint-induced movement therapy discourages use of the unaffected extremity and encourages active use of the hemiparetic extremity, with a goal of improved motor recovery. In a systematic review, constraint-induced movement therapy produced statistically significant and clinically relevant improvements in arm motor function that persisted for at least 1 year (SOE=A). Treadmill walking with partial body-weight support using a harness connected to an overhead system can improve gait velocity and walking endurance significantly. Although this method did not increase the chances of walking independently compared with other physiotherapy interventions, the improvements in walking endurance were sustained among those patients who could walk at the beginning of therapy. There is evidence that mirror therapy improves recovery of arm function (SOE=B). This therapy uses visual imagery by encouraging the patient to exercise both extremities symmetrically while viewing the reflection of only the unaffected limb in a mirror. It is thought that the patient experiences proprioceptive input to the affected side through the visual input. Newer therapeutic interventions for regaining motor function are in development, including use of robotics to provide high-intensity repetitive and task-specific treatments. One systematic review found improvements in ADLs, and arm function but not arm muscle strength using robot-assisted training. The use of virtual reality for upper limb rehabilitation has also been evaluated in a systematic review that included 5 randomized controlled trials. Results showed improved motor impairment but no significant differences in motor function between the control and intervention groups (SOE=A).

Speech and language therapy are often provided for stroke patients with aphasia. However, there is no universally accepted treatment. Although a Cochrane report states that the evidence does not support a finding of either clear effect or lack of effect, the Veterans Affairs guidelines support "good" evidence for follow-up evaluation and treatment by a speech language professional for long-term residual communication difficulties. Dysphagia (or swallowing disorders) is common after stroke, affecting up to 30% of patients. The most commonly used test to diagnose dysphagia is videofluoroscopy, which allows speech therapy professionals to observe and analyze the swallowing process and to assess for aspiration. Patients who aspirate are treated using rehabilitation exercises, changes in food consistency, and changes in posture to reduce the likelihood of aspiration. Transcranial magnetic stimulation to improve muscle function has shown promise. The guidelines also support "good" evidence for cognitive retraining for attention or visual-spatial perceptual deficits and compensatory training for short-term memory deficits. The same guidelines find "good" evidence for medication treatment for depression and emotional lability. In several studies, depression was a consistent factor adversely influencing rehabilitation outcomes. Spasticity can develop gradually after stroke and can inhibit function and interfere with hygiene. Most interventions, including surgery and medications like baclofen, have been disappointing.

Prevention

Patients who have had a stroke are at high risk of recurrence: up to 7%–10% annually. The rehabilitation phase is an appropriate time to ensure that assessment and treatment for stroke prevention has occurred. Assessments for significant carotid stenosis and for atrial fibrillation should be completed. Indications for carotid endarterectomy and anticoagulation with warfarin, dabigatran, or rivaroxaban should be reviewed. Antiplatelet medications such as aspirin alone or in combination with extended-release dipyridamole or clopidogrel should be considered in many patients. Treatment with ACE inhibitors[OL] and statins[OL] has also demonstrated reduced risk of stroke. Other risk factors to be targeted for preventing stroke recurrence include hypertension and smoking (SOE=A).

In summary, the evidence for specific interventions for stroke rehabilitation is weak. The collective benefits of well-organized interprofessional care, including secondary prevention, are well established.

Hip Fracture

Each year in the United States, about 300,000 older adults fracture a hip, with >90% of these fractures being the result of a fall. The risk of fracture is higher in women, whites, nursing-home residents, and in people with dementia. Mortality is about 5% during the initial hospitalization but nears 25% in the year after fracture. About 75% of survivors return to their prior level of function, but their overall mobility is more limited; up to half still require an assistive device. About half of patients will have an initial decline requiring transient long-term care, and about 25% will still be in long-term care 1 year later.

Rehabilitation

Rehabilitation after hip fracture includes pain management, mobilization, and prevention of complications, such as delirium and thromboembolic events. The most important factors influencing recovery appear to be how soon mobilization is started and how frequently therapy is provided. Delay in mobilization is often driven by surgical recommendation, with proper healing of the fracture taking precedence over mobility. Partial weight bearing is difficult for many older adults to achieve. Prolonged inactivity is clearly associated with poorer functional outcomes, and early weight bearing is associated with low rates of surgical failure (SOE=A). Accelerated rehabilitation with rapid mobilization, coordinated planning, early discharge, and community follow-up has been associated with a 17% reduction in costs and no detriment to rates of recovery (SOE=B). Intensity of service clearly affects outcome, because those who receive physical therapy more than once a day during initial rehabilitation are more likely to be discharged directly to home than those who receive physical therapy once a day or less (SOE=A).

Management

Medical management includes interventions to relieve pain and restore bone alignment to allow fracture healing and prepare the older adult to return to his or her prior level of functioning. For medically stable patients, surgical repair is recommended 24–72 hours after fracture. This early repair has been associated with a reduction in 1-year mortality, as well as with a lower incidence of complications such as pressure injury and delirium. For medically unstable patients, delaying surgery is warranted to allow sufficient improvement to tolerate the procedure. The surgical approach is determined by the location of the fracture, the presence or absence of displacement, and the patient's prefracture mobility. One-third of hip fractures occur at the femoral neck, and the other two-thirds are intertrochanteric, occurring lateral to the femoral neck. Prefracture mobility is used as a guide to determine the goal of surgical treatment and to allow the risks and benefits of each surgical procedure to be considered. There is evidence that comanagement by geriatricians and orthopedic surgeons can result in improved outcomes, including lower than predicted length of stay, low complication rates, low mortality, and reduced cost (SOE=B). To be successful, comanagement must be interdisciplinary with shared decision making, equal responsibility for the patient, and daily communication.

Femoral neck fractures, which include subcapital, transcervical, and basilar fracture locations, are more common in older adults, particularly women. A femoral neck fracture without any displacement and intact blood supply can be surgically corrected with simple screws. However, femoral neck fractures with any degree of displacement and/or poor circulation are at increased risk of nonunion or avascular necrosis and, therefore, are usually treated with a prosthetic femoral head (hemiarthroplasty). Patients with significant underlying bony acetabular disease and a displaced femoral neck fracture may benefit from complete hip arthroplasty. Patients are usually allowed to bear weight immediately after repair of a femoral neck fracture, regardless of type of surgical procedure. However, those undergoing a total hip arthroplasty are required to adhere to total hip precautions.

For intertrochanteric fractures, the treatment of choice is open reduction and internal fixation with a compression screw or similar device. Displaced or comminuted intertrochanteric fractures commonly remain unstable, even after surgical fixation; therefore, full weight bearing is often not allowed for up to 6 weeks or until the stability of the fracture is assured. Factors that influence recovery should be assessed, including prior mobility and functional status, comorbid conditions, cognitive status, social support, type of injury, and repair and pain status. Mobility performance can be systematically assessed with numerous instruments, including the Harris Hip Questionnaire, which was developed specifically for hip fracture (Table 21.2).

Prevention

Older adults who have had a hip fracture often have other comorbidities, such as osteoporosis and balance problems, that place them at risk of additional fractures resulting from falls. Efforts to diagnose and treat osteoporosis, improve balance, and reduce injury risk are a key part of treatment planning during rehabilitation. The use of hip protectors for fracture prevention in community-dwelling older adults has been extensively studied with mostly negative results (SOE=B). However, studies conducted in nursing or residential care settings found a small reduction in hip fracture risk with the use of hip protectors (SOE=B).

Total Hip and Knee Arthroplasty

In the United States, joint arthroplasty is the most common elective surgical procedure performed; approximately one million are done annually. The primary indications for joint replacement are progressive pain and limitation of mobility despite conservative care. Plain radiographs are the usual method for determining the severity of joint damage at both the hip and knee. Loss of cartilage is shown by joint-space narrowing, and often osteophyte formation is also present. The most common diagnosis associated with the need for hip and knee joint replacement is osteoarthrosis, followed by rheumatoid arthritis.

The long-term results of joint replacement have generally been excellent and include significant pain relief, increased motion, and improved function. Continued success rates in the 90% range are seen 10–15 years after joint replacement. The most common reason for failure of the hip or knee replacement is loosening of the implant. Joint infection is another major concern, affecting 0.2%–1.1% of total hip and 1%–2% of total knee replacements. Deep infections often necessitate removal of the implant and long-term treatment with antibiotics until there is no sign of infection, followed by ultimate replacement with a new implant.

There are various types of hip prostheses and surgical approaches for the total hip arthroplasty; the prosthetic and approach used are determined by the surgeon and based on the condition of the joint and integrity of the bone. Depending on the approach used, the patient must adhere to certain hip precautions, ie, prevention of specific movements by the affected leg for approximately 6 weeks to ensure healing and prevent dislocation. When the anterolateral surgical approach is used, the patient must avoid external rotation, adduction, and extension of the operated leg. When the posterolateral approach is used, the patient should not internally rotate or adduct the leg and not flex the hip beyond 90 degrees. Many surgeons use a minimally invasive technique for total hip arthroplasty that involves 2-inch incisions (versus the traditional 10-inch) and no detachment of muscle. Because tissue trauma is less, recovery is often quicker.

Various types of prosthetic knees are also available and, like hip prostheses, the type used depends on the joint damage. Typically, patients can begin bearing weight on the operated leg by the first day or two after surgery. However, rotation or torsion at the knee should be avoided for up to 3 months. Surgeons have also applied the concept of minimal incisions to the total knee replacement surgery and with significantly more success, including achieving greater knee flexion. This surgery, in experienced hands, decreases blood loss and length of stay (SOE=A).

Rehabilitation

Rehabilitation focuses on strengthening especially the abductors, which are weakened by the surgical approach, as well as on progressive range-of-motion and gait training. After total knee replacement, recovery of range of motion is the key to return of function. Postoperative swelling is common and interferes with regaining motion. However, thigh-high compression stockings and possibly cryotherapy can be used to manage swelling.

Management

Anticoagulation to prevent thromboembolism and good pain control are the major goals during the immediate postoperative period for both hip and knee arthroplasty. Patients who have undergone a major orthopedic procedure such as total hip or knee arthroplasty are at particularly high risk of both symptomatic and asymptomatic venous thromboembolism. Current guidelines for prevention of venous thromboembolism after total hip arthroplasty recommend a minimum of 10–14 days of antithrombotic prophylaxis (SOE=A). Pain in the initial postoperative period is often controlled with opioids administered orally, intravenously, or by patient-controlled analgesia pumps. For both hip and knee arthroplasty, early mobilization is the standard of care, and weight bearing often begins on the first postoperative day. Patients at low risk can often be discharged from the acute care hospital within 5 days. For those at high risk, defined as being >70 years old or having 2 or more comorbid conditions, early inpatient rehabilitation improves functional outcomes and decreases total length of stay (SOE=B). Age alone should not be used as a criterion for eligibility for joint replacement—excellent results can be achieved even in patients >80 years old who are in good health with stable chronic conditions. In a large retrospective study of patients receiving inpatient medical rehabilitation after hip arthroplasty, non-Hispanic whites and women had the greatest functional improvement from admission to discharge. Asians had the lowest mean change in function scores. Being of nonwhite ethnicity and being male were associated with higher odds of being discharged to home (SOE=B).

Prevention

To decrease the risk of dislocation after total hip arthroplasty, rehabilitation patients are taught to complete their daily activities while adhering to hip precautions through the use of adaptive equipment and assistive devices. To prevent excessive hip flexion during toileting, a raised toilet seat is recommended for the first few months after surgery. If the patient uses a tub/shower combination at home, a tub bench is beneficial for safety in entering and exiting while maintaining hip precautions.

Amputation

Approximately 121,000 people undergo leg amputation each year in the United States. Most of these people have systemic vascular disease, with or without diabetes mellitus. Those with diabetes often have other end-organ disease, such as blindness, chronic kidney disease, and peripheral neuropathy. Mortality in this group approaches 50% at 2 years and 70% at 5 years. For up to one-fifth of patients, amputation of the other leg is needed within the first 2 years after the initial amputation. Most dysvascular amputees have such a burden of comorbid disease that the prosthesis is largely used for limited mobility, such as transfers and ambulation within the home.

The level of amputation and surgical approach depends on the status of the extremity; the surgery may be to remove devitalized tissue or may include reconstruction of the residual limb or stump. Common amputation levels include above or below the knee, as well as hip disarticulations.

Rehabilitation

Rehabilitation starts in the preoperative stage, when the patient begins with strength and flexibility exercises and is educated about the recovery process, including prosthetic preparation and training. Amputation surgery generally aims to preserve the knee, because the energy requirement for walking is much lower for the below-the-knee amputee than for the above-the-knee amputee. This decision must be weighed against risks of poor wound healing with more distal amputation.

Postoperative rehabilitation includes efforts at early mobilization, prevention of contractures, wound healing, edema control, shaping of the stump, and psychosocial support. Patients are educated on maintaining intact skin integrity through wound care, compression wrapping, desensitization, and skin inspection to prepare the residual limb for the prosthesis. Poor wound healing delays rehabilitation in about 25% of cases. Prostheses vary in weight, socket type, style of foot, and suspensions. The older amputee benefits from a prosthesis that is lightweight, stable, and easy to use. Prosthetic rehabilitation involves progressive ambulation, education about prosthesis and stump care, and stump injury monitoring.

Lastly, phantom limb pain is common after amputation, with an estimated incidence of 60%–80%; pain management influences progress with rehabilitation. Treatment remains difficult, and clear evidence-based guidelines are lacking. A Cochrane review that included 14 studies with a primary outcome being change in pain intensity described available evidence. Most of the studies were limited by their small sample sizes. The results for gabapentin[OL] were conflicting, but combined results favored the treatment group compared with controls (SOE=B). Morphine and the N-methyl D-aspartate (NMDA) receptor antagonist ketamine[OL], demonstrated favorable short-term analgesic efficacy compared with placebo (SOE=B). Memantine[OL] and amitriptyline[OL] were not effective in the small number of studies with limited sample sizes. Based on one small study, botulinum toxin A[OL] (versus lidocaine/methylprednisolone) did not decrease phantom limb pain (SOE=C).

Management

Key factors to assess include the patient's prior functional status, stability of comorbid conditions, cognition, arm use, and condition of the stump and the other leg. Successful prosthetic ambulation is associated with independent prior ambulation, ability to bear weight on the contralateral leg, stable medical status, and ability to follow directions. Blindness and chronic kidney disease do not necessarily preclude rehabilitation.

Prevention

Focusing on medical management of the underlying disease process that led to the amputation is important.

APPROACHES FOR COMMONLY ENCOUNTERED REHABILITATION ISSUES

Cardiac Rehabilitation

Cardiac rehabilitation (CR) programs typically include an individualized, medically supervised exercise program combined with an interdisciplinary focus on psychosocial, nutritional, and heart disease risk factor reductions. CR programs have been shown to improve exercise capacity, physical function, and quality of life, and to reduce mortality. In a Cochrane review and meta-analysis of 63 randomized clinical trials including over 14,000 patients with coronary heart disease, CR was associated with an absolute risk reduction from 10.4% to 7.6% from cardiovascular disease mortality. In a study of more than 600,000 Medicare beneficiaries who had been hospitalized for coronary conditions or revascularization procedures and were eligible for cardiac rehabilitation, 1- to 5-year mortality rates were reduced for those who attended rehabilitation (21%) compared to those who did not (34%) ($P<.001$). In addition, a dose effect was demonstrated with better attendance being correlated with reduced risk of myocardial infarction (SOE=A). CR is effective in reducing symptoms of anxiety. In one study of 104 younger (<55 years) and 260 older (>70 years) adults with coronary heart disease, the prevalence of anxiety fell by 61% in the young adults and by 32% in the older ones after formal CR. Unfortunately, <30% of eligible patients are referred to CR and only 40%–60% actually complete the prescribed course of treatment. There are a number of barriers to utilization of CR, including low physician referral and lack of personal resources, making attendance difficult. Low rates of referral by primary care physicians has been attributed to lack of familiarity with CR site locations, lack of standardized referral forms, and inconvenience. The national Million Hearts initiative, which seeks to prevent 1 million cardiovascular disease events over 5 years, has a goal of achieving >70% participation in CR through increased referrals and enrollment and more flexible delivery of CR services. Medicare provides for up to 36 sessions after myocardial infarction, percutaneous revascularization, heart valve, coronary artery bypass surgery, and stable heart failure.

Pulmonary Rehabilitation

Pulmonary rehabilitation (PR) has been defined as "a comprehensive intervention based on a thorough patient assessment followed by patient-tailored therapies which include, but are not limited to, exercise training, education, and behavior change, designed to improve the physical and emotional condition of people with chronic respiratory disease and to promote the long-term adherence to health-enhancing behaviors." PR is most successful when delivered by an interprofessional team. Traditionally, PR has been provided to stable patients with moderate to severe chronic obstructive pulmonary disease (COPD). However, more recent studies have shown that rehabilitation in the peri-exacerbation period can reduce hospital admissions. PR has also been shown to be as effective with equivalent benefits in patients with non-COPD respiratory disease. There is little guidance regarding who should be referred for PR. However, a practical approach that has been suggested is to refer any patient with functional status limitations or persistent respiratory symptoms despite otherwise optimal therapy.

The main aim of endurance exercise training is to improve aerobic capacity and thereby enhance ability to perform activities of daily living. This improvement is attributed, in part, to reduced ventilatory requirements for a given task and improved peak aerobic capacity. In addition, there is evidence of improvements in lower limb muscles, specifically increases in muscle fiber capillarization and mitochondrial density and oxidative capacity of muscle fibers. There is strong evidence for improvements in health-related quality of life and reductions in fatigue and dyspnea with PR (SOE=A). The effect on mortality is less robust. One systematic review found in the control group, 29 of 100 people had mortality over 107 weeks compared with 10 of 100 in the active treatment group. Thus, the number needed to treat for benefit was 6 (95% CI 5–30) over 107 weeks. Treadmill walking and stationary cycle ergometry are the most common forms of exercise in PR and have been shown to improve exercise performance and muscle function (SOE=A). In addition, a number of other types of exercise training have also been explored and may be beneficial, although the evidence is less robust. These include ground walking exercise, Nordic walking exercise training, resistance exercise, aquatic exercise, and tai chi.

Shoulder Rehabilitation

Shoulder disorders, more common in older men than older women, contribute to disability and impact quality of life. Shoulder pain, secondary to rotator cuff tendonitis or tears, proximal humeral fractures from falling on an outstretched arm, or glenohumeral osteoarthritis, inhibits use of the affected extremity with eventual loss of active range of motion and strength, even adhesive capsulitis. Because of the limitations, especially if the dominant extremity is involved, older adults will have difficulties with ADLs, such as putting on a coat and combing their hair, as well as in IADLs involving reaching overhead. Whenever possible, conservative, nonoperative medical management is the preferred approach with a referral to outpatient occupational and/or physical therapy to decrease pain and improve function. Therapists will complete a comprehensive evaluation of the upper extremity using palpation, provocative testing, goniometry, and manual muscle testing. Functional use of the involved extremity may be determined using a standardized assessment such as the Disabilities of the Arm, Shoulder, and Hand Outcome Measure (available at www.dash.iwh.on.ca/about-dash [accessed Feb 2019]). This assessment is a self-report questionnaire used to measure changes in symptoms and function throughout the recovery process.

Typical rehabilitation for shoulder soft-tissue injuries includes pain control and range of motion and strengthening exercises to increase use of the affected extremity during ADLs and IADLs. Occupational therapy includes instructing the patient in alternative methods for grooming, bathing, dressing, and homemaking to compensate for limitations, protect the shoulder, and maximize participation. Both occupational and physical therapy can address physical symptoms. Ice and heat may be applied initially to the area to control pain. Ultrasound, low-level laser therapy, and transcutaneous electrical nerve stimulation (TENS) are physical agent modalities often used to increase energy in the body to reduce pain and promote function. However, an updated Cochrane review that included 47 trials of 2,388 participants found low-level evidence to support pulsed ultrasound and low-level laser therapy as having benefits over placebo. The benefits of TENS beyond placebo remain uncertain. The severity of the injury determines the progression of therapeutic exercises. Patients with significant pain should begin with Codman pendulum exercises allowing gravity to assist with distraction at the glenohumeral joint, enabling passive shoulder motion focused on the muscles of the rotator cuff. As pain-free passive motion increases, patients can move on to active stretching exercises focused on the posterior deltoid, infraspinatus, and teres minor muscles. Isotonic or isometric exercises can be used to strengthen the muscles and often include graded resistive bands. Patient education should focus on proper posture and prevention of further shoulder injury.

Little evidence exists to support standardized medical management of proximal humeral fractures; therefore, conservative treatment is preferred for older adults secondary to their increased risk of complications after surgery. Initially, a sling, with or without a swathe, immobilizes the shoulder. Severity of the fracture, symptoms, and mobility status will determine whether therapy is provided in the outpatient setting or through home-health care services. Occupational therapy provides ADL training in one-handed techniques and adaptive equipment use for eating, grooming, bathing, and dressing. Therapy should start with Codman pendulum exercises and instructing the patient in a home exercise program to maintain joint motion and strength in the elbow, wrist, and hand as the fracture heals. Approximately 1 week after fracture, therapy can begin with active assisted shoulder flexion, abduction, and rotation. Isometric exercises to strengthen the rotator cuff muscles can begin after 3 weeks. Depending on the quality of the healing, strengthening exercises can often begin after 6 weeks.

Older adults not responding to conservative treatment for shoulder osteoarthritis or rheumatoid arthritis, or those with rotator cuff tear arthropathy or severe fractures of the humerus, may require a shoulder arthroplasty. There are various types of arthroplasty surgeries; treatment protocols after surgery that allow passive and active motion and strengthening exercises differ based on the location and type of arthroplasty and the preference of the surgeon. Day one after surgery, the affected extremity is immobilized in a sling and the patient instructed not to extend the shoulder beyond neutral or contract the muscles. Therapy will include passive shoulder forward flexion and external rotation to the patient's tolerance and instructing the patient in Codman pendulum exercises. Frequently icing the area helps reduce inflammation. After discharge from the hospital, patients can continue rehabilitation in the home or outpatient setting depending on their status and needs. Similar to that for a proximal humeral fracture, occupational therapy provides training in one-handed techniques and adaptive equipment to maximize independence in ADLs. Therapeutic exercise aims to gradually increase passive range of motion of the shoulder and strengthen the elbow, wrist, and hand. Shoulder exercises should progress to active range of motion and isometric exercises as the patient recovers. Typically, moderate strengthening exercises begin 6 weeks after surgery.

Rehabilitation services are discontinued when the patient has returned to completing daily activities, has pain-free active motion, and has maximized muscle strength.

MOBILITY AIDS, ORTHOTICS, ADAPTIVE METHODS, AND ENVIRONMENTAL MODIFICATIONS

Assistive devices, orthotics, adaptive methods, and environmental modifications are effective for maximizing function in older adults with disabilities. It is important to identify the underlying cause(s) of a disability before prescribing a device or modification, because medical or surgical treatment for a specific disease or impairment may be more effective or enhance the usefulness of these approaches. Although many of the items considered durable medical equipment are 80% reimbursed for Medicare B beneficiaries if medically necessary and prescribed by a physician, the equipment must be accessed through a Medicare-enrolled and accredited Durable Medical Equipment, Prosthetic, Orthotic, and Supplies supplier.

An estimated 6.8 million Americans use assistive technology devices to enhance mobility. Unfortunately, many older adults who might benefit from the use of mobility aids do not or will not use them. There may be racial/ethnic influences in willingness to use mobility aids. Focus group studies with community-dwelling older adults of white, non-Hispanic black, and Hispanic backgrounds showed that for all groups, perceived benefits of mobility devices in maintaining independence and control produced positive attitudes. However, the association of use of mobility aids with aging and physical decline contributed to stigmatizing attitudes. Black and Hispanic participants expressed apprehension about using unsafe or inappropriate secondhand equipment, heightened concerns about mobility-aid users becoming the subject of negative biases, and a preference for fashionable mobility aids. Hispanic participants expressed a preference for human assistance. Participants of all groups perceived clinicians as influencing their decision to use mobility aids.

Mobility Aids

Canes typically support 15%–20% of the body weight and are used in the hand contralateral to the affected knee or hip. A straight cane has a single tip, while a quad cane has four tips. As the number of tips increases, the degree of support also increases, but the cane becomes heavier and more awkward to use. The handle of the cane may be curved or have a pistol grip; the pistol grip offers more support. Canes can be made of a variety of materials, but most are made of wood or lightweight aluminum. The length of the cane is important for stability. Some canes are adjustable, but wooden canes must be cut to size. One of two methods can be used to evaluate the proper cane length: measuring the distance from the distal wrist crease to the ground when the patient is standing erect, and measuring the distance from the greater trochanter to the ground. Straight canes are often prescribed for patients with a single joint problem, such as osteoarthritis of the knee. The cane decreases the weight bearing through the joint, thereby decreasing pain and improving ambulation. A cane can also be helpful for patients with decreased lower extremity proprioception. Proprioceptors in the hand relay vital information to the brain about where the cane and the ground are in relation to the person. A different version of the single point cane has a small, triangular base with three small feet and a pivot point just proximal to the base. The benefits of this cane include that it stands on its own and has a slightly larger base of support. The pivot mechanism allows all 3 feet to be on the floor without altering a patient's gait pattern. Quad canes are used when a patient requires a more stable platform on which to bear weight, such as after a stroke with resultant hemiparesis. When using a quad cane, it is important that all four tips are placed on the ground simultaneously, to assure the cane is stable before weight bearing (Table 21.4).

Crutches, axillary or forearm, are usually used to provide bilateral support. Axillary crutches are seldom recommended for older adults because greater arm strength and coordination are required for use. In addition, there is a risk of brachial plexus injury if the crutches are used incorrectly. Forearm crutches are more functional because a cuff secures the crutch on the patient's arm, allowing use of the hand to manipulate objects. A single crutch can be used instead of a cane if additional unilateral support is needed.

A walker is prescribed when a cane does not offer sufficient stability. A walker can completely support one leg but cannot support full body weight. Walker types include pick-up and wheeled walkers. Walkers should be adjusted so that the user maintains an erect posture and is not required to lean forward to reach the walker. The pick-up walker is lifted and moved forward by the user, who then advances before lifting the walker again; the result is a slow, staggering gait. It requires strength to repeatedly pick up the walker and cognitive ability to learn the necessary coordination. It may be the mobility device of choice when offloading one limb and maximal stability is preferred, such as after a hip fracture in a patient with a tenuous fixation in which non-weight bearing is needed to allow the bone to heal. A wheeled walker allows for a smoother, coordinated, and faster gait and takes advantage of compensated gait patterns; it is more likely to be correctly used by those with cognitive impairment. The most commonly used type is the two-wheeled walker, which brakes automatically with increased downward pressure. Patients with Parkinson disease often do well with a wheeled walker because once they start walking, they do not have to stop and start as is required with a pick-up walker. The two-wheeled walker is also easier to stop, because patients need only to lean on the device to engage the brakes.

A "rollator" is a four-wheeled walker with hand brakes, which can be locked when the patient is transferring. This type also has a platform seat for resting and a basket for carrying objects. Because of the use of the hand brakes, the rollator requires greater skill and safety awareness. It is preferred for outdoor use, because the wheels are larger and move easier over sidewalks and slightly rough terrain. The rollator is often prescribed for patients with cardiac or pulmonary conditions and deconditioning. The ability to lean on the device increases the distance patients can travel because it decreases energy expenditure, and patients can sit to rest when fatigued.

Patients who cannot safely use or who are unable to ambulate with an assistive device require a wheelchair. A wheelchair must be fitted according to the patient's body build, weight, disability, and prognosis. Incorrect fit can result in poor posture, joint deformity, reduced mobility, pressure injury, circulatory compromise, and discomfort. The Rehabilitation Engineering and Assistive Technology Society of North America Wheelchair Service Guide provide detailed information for determining the most appropriate wheelchair for the patient (www.resna.org/knowledge-center/position-papers-and-provision-guides [accessed Feb 2019]). Several factors are associated with use of a prescribed wheelchair, including age, gender, health, characteristics of the device (eg, type, size), and environmental facilitators and barriers. Often the prescribed devices do not meet the needs of the older adult. In one study, 61% of the older adults reported having difficulty with manual wheelchair propulsion. Important considerations in the evaluation for a wheelchair are cognitive status and functional ability to use the device. Manual wheelchairs are frequently used in the nursing-home setting to allow ease of mobility, either through self- or staff propulsion. The most significant factor associated with manual wheelchair use was not living at home.

The demand for power mobility devices (PMDs), including power wheelchairs and scooters, has increased substantially in recent years. CMS provides a detailed explanation of requirements for physician prescribing of power mobility devices www.cms.gov/Outreach-and-Education/Medicare-Learning-Network-MLN/MLNProducts/downloads/

Table 21.4—Commonly Prescribed Mobility Aids

Assistive Device	Characteristics	Prescribed Conditions
Straight cane	Provide unilateral support Assist with balance and proprioception Reduce weight bearing on opposite leg	Osteoarthritis of knee or hip Peripheral neuropathy
Quad cane	Provides unilateral support More stable than straight cane Allows greater weight bearing on device	Stroke with hemiparesis
Stationary "pick-up" walker	Provides bilateral support Must be lifted and advanced, requiring strength and coordination Very stable and allows non-weight bearing movement	Hip fracture in which non-weight bearing needed Unilateral amputation, before prosthesis
Two-wheeled walker	Less stable than stationary walker but easier to advance Allows for smoother, faster gait	Deconditioning Parkinson disease Total joint replacement
Rollator (four-wheeled walker with seat and brakes)	Less stable but allows for smoother, faster gait Requires more coordination and safety awareness (because of brakes) Good for outside walking because of large wheels Has seat for resting	Cardiopulmonary disease Peripheral neuropathy with balance difficulty
Manual wheelchair	Requires use of arms and some cardiopulmonary endurance Often used in nursing homes and by caregivers for ease of patient mobility Easy to transport	Nonambulatory patient with cognitive impairment Low-level spinal cord injury
Power wheelchair	Allows mobility for those with limited ambulatory ability Controls do not require intact upper extremities Need cognitive ability to operate safely May need home modifications	Neurologic diseases (eg, high-level spinal cord injury, multiple sclerosis, amyotrophic lateral sclerosis) Multiple limb amputations
Scooter	Similar benefits to power wheelchair, except need to operate with upper extremities May be more acceptable to patient than power wheelchair	Cardiopulmonary disease

PMD_DocCvg_FactSheet_ICN905063.pdf [accessed Feb 2019]. The Medicare Fee-For-Service Prior Authorization of PMD demonstration requires prior authorization for PMDs for people with Medicare who reside in certain states. Motorized wheelchairs can be used by mentally alert individuals with bilateral arm weakness or other neurologic disorders that limit arm use. Power wheelchairs can be controlled using a joystick or an alternative control device like a sip-and-puff switch or head control. Examples of patients who might do well with a power wheelchair include those with spinal cord injuries, multiple sclerosis, or amyotrophic lateral sclerosis. Motorized scooters offer less trunk support than motorized wheelchairs but are more acceptable to some people. Patients are more likely to use scooters rather than power wheelchairs if they have a primary diagnosis of cardiovascular and pulmonary disease and if they are living at home. Motorized scooters and wheelchairs increase patients' mobility, but there is a risk of deconditioning because patients might otherwise push a wheelchair or ambulate. The use of a wheelchair or scooter commonly requires home modifications, including ramps and widened doorways. Cars may need to be adapted with lifts.

Orthoses, Adaptive Methods, and Environmental Modifications

Obtaining a physical or occupational therapy evaluation early in the hospitalization is important to assess for equipment needs, including mobility aids and adaptive equipment. This assessment is critical to providing older adults with the correct equipment to maximize their independent function.

Orthoses are exoskeletons designed to assist, resist, align, and control function. Typically, orthoses applied to the extremities use 3 points of pressure to support the structure, limit or increase joint motion, and modify soft tissue. Orthoses can be custom fabricated, custom fit, or prefabricated. They are named by using the letters for the primary and secondary joints that the device involves in its structure, and they are classified by their action—static or dynamic. Thus, an AFO is a static ankle and foot orthotic device used to support weak calf or pretibial muscles (eg, for a stroke patient with leg weakness). A thumb carpometacarpal immobilization splint provides stability for intrinsic muscle weakness and pain in older adults, typically women, with carpometacarpal joint osteoarthritis.

Adaptations and use of equipment may be necessary for older adults with limitations in range of motion, strength, coordination, and endurance to improve or maintain their level of function. Occupational therapy provides training in adaptive equipment and compensatory strategies to maximize independence. Clothing that is easy to clean and tops that fit over the head with little effort or that fasten in the front and allow for freedom of movement are helpful. Hook-and-loop tape is usually easier to use than buttons and can be sewn on to replace buttons and zippers. When buttons are necessary, if they are sewn on with elastic thread, the need to manipulate them can be eliminated. A button hook is a device to assist with closure of button-down shirts, sweaters, and coats. Older adults with limitations in their hip range of motion benefit from use of a reacher or dressing stick, as an extension to their upper extremity, to put on underwear and pants. Putting on shoes and socks is particularly difficult for older adults with decreased flexibility. Longer, looser socks (eg, tubular socks) are easier to put on. For those who find it difficult to reach the feet to put on socks and shoes, a sock aid and long-handled shoehorn may be useful. Elastic shoelaces eliminate the need for tying and untying. Raised toilet seats, height-adjustable shower chairs, and transfer tub benches are available to assist those with lower-extremity weakness, poor balance, or limited endurance. These are also useful for older adults with arthritis of the hips or knees, because they reduce biomechanical stress on the joint. Long-handled bath brushes, hand-held shower heads, and "soap on a rope" can be helpful for older adults with extremity weakness, decreased balance, and limited endurance. Use of energy conservation and work simplification techniques during ADL and IADL tasks enable older adults, particularly those with progressive conditions, to maximize their endurance to participate in their desired leisure and social activities. For example, sitting down to dry off after a shower or while dusting the furniture reduces the typical amount of energy used, reserving it for more desirable activities.

Environmental modifications can have a major impact on the older adult's ability to function independently or with minimal assistance at home (SOE=A). A variety of assistive devices, such as reachers, door knob extenders, and plug pullers, can reduce the difficulty of performing daily tasks, protect joints, and have a significant impact on a person's quality of life. Installation of automatic lighting in hallways and stairwells can contribute to reducing fall risk. The bathroom is a common place for falls. Any older adult with impaired balance or leg weakness should have grab bars installed near the toilet and tub or shower.

RESOURCES

- Hankey GJ. Stroke. *Lancet*. 2017;389(10069):641–654.

- National Institute for Health and Care Excellence Guidelines. Venous thromboembolism in over 16s: reducing the risk of hospital-acquired deep vein thrombosis or pulmonary embolism. https://www.nice.org.uk/guidance/ng89

- Schopfer DW, Forman DE. Cardiac rehabilitation in older adults. *Can J Cardiol*. 2016;32:1088–1096.

CHAPTER 22—NURSING-HOME CARE

KEY POINTS

- Nursing-home regulations, originally driven by the Omnibus Budget Reconciliation Act of 1987, require a periodic comprehensive assessment of all nursing-home residents, set minimum staffing requirements, and foster residents' rights by limiting the use of restraints and psychoactive medications.

- The care of nursing-home residents has become more complex over the past several years, commensurate with an increasing level of medical acuity in an environment constrained by limited resources.

- Dementia is the most common condition in the nursing home.

Nursing homes have evolved dramatically over the past several years, responding to a variety of government and market-driven forces. Highly regulated institutions for people who often have severe physical and mental disabilities, nursing homes, more than ever, present the clinician with a set of unique and complex care issues, many of which are best understood in the context of population needs, government policy, and reimbursement and staffing patterns.

THE NURSING-HOME POPULATION

Currently, more than 1.4 million Americans reside in certified nursing facilities. Relatively speaking, this is a small portion of Americans who are >65 years old (2.6%); 15% of nursing-home residents are <65 years old, and <1% are ≤30 years old. The typical nursing-home resident is a non-Hispanic, white, unmarried (usually widowed) woman >85 years old with limited social supports.

In the last 20 years, the proportion of the nursing-home population that is <65 years old has increased (8%–15%), as has the population of residents >85 years old (38%–43%). The numbers of Hispanic, Asian, and black Americans living in nursing homes have also increased. Although some of this increase is explained by increasing numbers of these populations in American demographics, the rate of increase of minority populations in nursing homes has exceeded changing population demographics, suggesting that nursing-home use is increasing by these populations. Some cultural groups, particularly Hispanic and Asian Americans may be reluctant to consider nursing-home placement because of concerns about the lack of staff on all shifts who speak the same language, as well as the perception that the nursing home will not be able to serve familiar foods or follow other cultural traditions. As their older parent-caregivers are lost, older adults with intellectual and/or developmental disabilities constitute another unique population that is requiring nursing-home level care in higher numbers. These individuals often require specialized care that many nursing homes may have difficulty providing.

Functional disability is prevalent in nursing-home residents. A quarter of long-stay nursing-home residents require supervision or hands-on assistance in 5 ADLs (ie, eating, dressing, bathing, transferring, and toileting). Not surprisingly, most residents have communication problems, with frequent difficulty both in being understood and in understanding others. Currently, few residents (8.8%) walk without assistance or supervision, and most (65.8%) can be described as "chairfast," reflecting reliance on a chair for mobility and an inability to take steps without extensive or constant weight-bearing support.

Over two-thirds of long-stay residents in skilled-nursing facilities have multiple medical conditions. Special treatments are often required; in 2015, more than 20% of residents received injections, 15% received respiratory therapies (respirators/ventilators, oxygen, inhalation therapy, and other treatments), and almost 5% received tube feedings.

Dementia is the most commonly condition in nursing homes. The prevalence of cognitive impairment is reflected in the fact that about 80% of nursing-home residents are felt by nursing home staff to be impaired in their ability to make daily decisions, and two-thirds have orientation difficulties or memory problems, or both. Comorbid physical and mental diagnoses in this population are common; approximately 30% of nursing-home residents have psychological diagnoses with depression diagnosed in 20%–25%. More than 60% of residents are treated with psychoactive medications. Additionally, behavioral issues, such as verbal and social inappropriateness, wandering, and resistance to care, are seen in one-third of nursing-home residents.

NURSING-HOME AVAILABILITY

According to CMS data, there are currently 15,640 certified nursing homes in the United States with 1.65 million beds and 2.4 million discharges (ie, to home, hospital, or secondary to death). Of these facilities, 68.4% are proprietary (ie, for profit), with voluntary nonprofit (23.8%) and government nursing homes (7.1%) accounting for the remainder. Nursing-home care is provided to eligible veterans in 132 Veterans Affairs Community Living Centers. The U.S. Department of Veterans Affairs also recognizes 161 State Veterans Homes, which are owned, operated, and funded by all 50 states and Puerto Rico to provide long-term care services to veterans. In some states, nonveteran spouses and parents may also be eligible for care in a State Veterans Home. Nationally, nursing homes operate an average of 109 beds, but facility size varies greatly by state. Most commonly, nursing facilities have between 100–199 beds (44.1%), with a minority having >200 beds. A little more than half of all nursing homes are part of a chain, and about 5% are hospital-based. Nursing homes vary with respect to what ancillary services are available. Many facilities offer on-site mobile radiography services and infusion service.

Most admissions to nursing facilities come from acute hospitals, followed by private residences and other nursing homes. Not surprisingly, assisted-living facilities are becoming a greater source of older adults admitted to nursing facilities of total admissions. Assisted-living facilities do not operate under the oversight of a single national regulatory or licensure agency. In general, assisted-living facilities have greater heterogeneity than nursing homes in services offered and are most commonly paid for with out-of-pocket funds. Assisted-living facilities accommodate a population of older adults that significantly overlaps that found in nursing homes, particularly regarding their underlying physical and psychological deficits. Although the social model of care still predominates in most assisted-living facilities, rising medical acuity and resident complexity is demanding more substantive medical involvement.

Risk of nursing-home admission is high with 1 of every 3 adults >65 years old requiring a nursing-home admission in their lifetime. The risk of nursing-home admission rises steeply with age. Interestingly, the occupancy rates in nursing homes nationally have declined over the past several years and now stand at 82%. This decline has generally been attributed to the availability of other community-based long-term care options.

Postacute care is increasingly being offered in nursing-home settings, a response to the higher-care needs of older adults in conjunction with shorter hospital stays and the presence of a Medicare payment stream. Although the types of postacute services and programs vary significantly from one locale to another (eg, dialysis, orthopedic, ventilator, postoperative, rehabilitative, wound care), they remain distinct from the standard nursing-home services by integrating the features of acute medical, long-term care nursing, and rehabilitative settings.

The average length of stay for Medicare beneficiaries in a nursing facility is 26.8 days. On any given day, residents with a length of stay of <3 months comprise about 20% of the total nursing-home population.

Among all nursing-home residents, about 25% have a length of stay >3 years.

This continuum spanning subacute and long-term care in nursing homes contributes to the development of 2 populations of residents. Many short-stay residents are admitted for rehabilitation, targeting restoration of the functional ability and endurance that will allow them to return to community-based living settings. Others enter nursing homes for end of life or hospice type care.

In contrast, many of those who ultimately become long-stay residents present to nursing homes for ongoing supportive care of progressive, chronic illnesses.

FINANCING

Across all payers, nursing-home expenditures total more than $140 billion dollars. In 2012, the national median daily rate for a private room in a nursing home was $267, or $97,455 annually. Public health programs primarily finance this cost; Medicaid and Medicare account for 62% and 14% of nursing-home care payments, respectively. With the high annual costs, those paying for nursing-home care out-of-pocket often deplete their personal funds and turn to public funding. Although purchase of long-term care insurance has been increasing, these policies generally pay for only a small fraction of nursing-home care. Medicare funding for nursing-home costs is available for certain limited conditions for beneficiaries who require skilled-nursing or rehabilitation services, following a qualifying hospital stay. A qualifying hospital stay is a hospital stay of at least 3 days before entering a nursing home.

As part of the Balanced Budget Act of 1997, Medicare payments to nursing homes are based on an individual's functional needs and potential for rehabilitation. This prospective payment system, also called PPS, requires careful documentation of functional gains, particularly by rehabilitation therapists.

Supplemental increases in reimbursement are made to offset costs of caring for those with HIV/AIDS. Despite the high cost of nursing-home care, resources remain constrained. In general, psychiatric conditions are undervalued with respect to reimbursement in long-term care. Residents with active psychiatric illness often require increased care and staff time, but mechanisms do not exist for increased reimbursement for those efforts. Shortages of psychiatric specialists trained in nursing-home care, combined with relatively low reimbursement rates for care in nursing homes, add to the challenge of providing optimal mental health care in this setting. Many are exploring telemedicine as one potential means to increase access to urgent and consultative medical care in the nursing home.

STAFFING PATTERNS

Resident care and evaluation in the nursing home largely depend on nurses and nursing assistants. Nursing facilities are required to provide nurse staffing sufficient to provide the care outlined in its care plans. According to federal guidelines, every nursing home must have the following on staff: a licensed nurse who acts as charge nurse on each shift; a registered nurse who is on duty at least 8 consecutive hours, 7 days a week; and a registered nurse who is designated as the director of nursing. Studies have reported the correlation between the provision of quality care to total nursing hours and the ratio of professional nurses (ie, registered nurses) to nonprofessional nursing staff. Current federal regulations do not mandate specific nurse-to-resident staffing ratios. It has been estimated that 9 of 10 nursing homes are inadequately staffed, and nearly $8 billion dollars would be needed to bring staffing to adequate levels.

Recruiting and retaining staff, particularly nursing assistants who constitute the bulk of the nursing-home workforce, also continues to be difficult. Yearly turnover rates of approximately 50% for direct care staff of nursing facilities, including 50% of nurse assistants and registered nurses and 35% of licensed practical nurses, have been reported. Stability of staff has been associated with better quality of care. Turnover rates have been associated with increased rates of hospitalization for nursing-home residents and have been linked to the organizational culture within the nursing facility.

Staffing issues are also pertinent to the medical providers who practice in nursing homes. Many providers avoid nursing-home practice because of perceptions of excessive regulations, paperwork, limited reimbursement, and aversion to the long-term care environment. Use of the nursing home as an academic training site can offer important exposure to this practice opportunity and professional role models and may help to stimulate interest among trainees.

THE INTERFACE OF ACUTE CARE AND THE NURSING HOME

Nursing-home residents account for >2.2 million emergency department visits annually in the United States, or 1.6 emergency department visits for every nursing-home resident. Although most nursing-home residents who were hospitalized were hospitalized once (63.8%), many experienced multiple transfers.

Unfortunately, suboptimal information transfer often complicates transitions between acute- and long-term care settings. Higher nurse staffing ratios are associated with lower readmission rates.

Five conditions account for most (78%) of these rehospitalizations: congestive heart failure, respiratory infection, urinary tract infection, sepsis, and electrolyte imbalances. Polypharmacy and a lack of thorough medication reconciliation have also been found to contribute to higher readmission rates. Reduction of hospital readmission from skilled-nursing facilities is the focus of recently enacted value-based purchasing program for skilled-nursing facilities.

Interventions to Reduce Acute Care Transfers (INTERACT) is a quality improvement program that seeks to improve the identification, evaluation, and management of acute change of conditions in nursing-home residents. Through a focus on advance care planning, structured communication between providers, and the use of care pathways, acute hospital admissions have been reduced.

REGULATIONS

CMS pays Medicare claims and interprets legislation into written regulations for skilled-nursing facilities. CMS interprets federal statutes and also writes regulations for Medicaid that are administered by each state's Medicaid program. Federal regulations, including those pertaining to long-term care, are compiled in the *Code of Federal Regulations*. Each federal regulation is given a tag number, often called "F-tags." To qualify for federal reimbursement under Medicare and Medicaid, facilities must comply with these CMS regulations.

Nursing-home regulations target many residents' rights issues, including setting limits on restraint use and regulating use of psychoactive medications. These regulations have had notable impact on quality of care including significant decreases in the use of restraints in nursing homes, increases in registered nurse staffing, and the establishment of training requirements for certified nursing assistants.

OBRA also mandates comprehensive periodic assessments of all nursing-home residents. This is accomplished by the Minimum Data Set (MDS), which surveys a host of clinical issues thought to directly relate to the quality of resident care and thus considered pertinent to effective care planning. A resident's medical regimen must be consistent with the assessment compiled in the MDS. CMS also uses the MDS for individual facilities to compile nursing-facility quality measures data, which are reported publicly on the CMS website and used for payment (www.medicare.gov/NHcompare/Home.asp). Measures include outcomes data such as prevalence of pain, pressure injury, weight loss, and depression, as well as rates of vaccination, restraint use, and urinary tract infection. Included in the measures of nursing-home quality publicly reported by CMS is the 5-star quality rating for nursing homes. This rating was developed to help consumers, families, and caregivers make comparisons about nursing homes and areas of strength or concern. The 5-star rating is based on three sources of data: the facility's health inspection survey results, staffing levels, and 13 MDS-based quality measures and 3 quality measures drawn from MDS- and

Medicare claims-based data. Nursing-home ratings take into account a variety of measures that are thought to reflect the facility's practice such as the percentages of residents who are prescribed antipsychotic drugs, who have indwelling catheters inserted and left in their bladder, or who experience falls with major injury. In 2016, five new quality measures were introduced into the star rating methodology, including a focus on hospital readmissions and prevention of avoidable declines in resident function.

Adherence to regulations is assessed by mandatory site visit surveys. These surveys are mandated every 15 months but occur on average every 12 months. During traditional nursing-home surveys, facility procedures and records are reviewed, and quality of care and quality of life for residents are observed.

Failure to meet regulatory standards for care is cited in a "deficiency." Penalties imposed for deficiencies depend on the nature and severity of the deficiency and can range from implementation of a corrective action plan to monetary fines, limits on facility admissions, or even facility closure. Each deficiency is rated according to a standard matrix of scope and severity. Severity refers to the level of harm to the resident or residents involved, from no harm or minimal potential for harm to immediate jeopardy to health or safety. Scope of a deficiency may be isolated, a pattern, or widespread in nature. Inspections can also occur at any time in between mandated surveys as a result of a complaint received by the state. In 2015, the mean number of deficiencies received by nursing homes during regulatory visits was 8.6, with 21% of facilities cited for deficiencies relating to actual harm or immediate jeopardy of residents.

The facility must ensure that the resident optimally improves or deteriorates only within the limits of that resident's right to refuse treatments and within the influence of their illnesses and normal aging. When a resident declines (or does not improve), a survey team may investigate whether the decline was avoidable. Documentation of a resident's reasonable prognosis and the risks versus reasonable expected benefits of treatments has an important role in care planning in the nursing home, particularly given current regulatory and liability influences.

OBRA requires that a state agency must screen and preapprove the admission of individuals with intellectual disability or serious mental illness to a nursing facility (F285). This screening is done to ensure that the facility can provide appropriate programs and services to meet the individual's needs.

Medical Director

The quality of medical practice in the nursing home is, in many ways, determined by the medical director. CMS requires that every skilled-nursing facility designate a licensed physician to serve as medical director (F501). The medical director has many roles that differ from the roles of the attending physician and other providers and include coordination of medical care that meets current standards for care in the nursing home. Integral to the medical director's role is providing guidance in development and implementation of resident-care policies. The medical director must ensure compliance with all relevant state and federal guidelines and work with the nursing-home administrator and director of nursing to foster effective team care and continuing staff education.

Medication Oversight

Additional regulations require medication review at regular intervals and that each resident's medication regimen includes no unnecessary drugs. Clinical documentation must demonstrate the indication for all drugs, especially psychoactive medications. Unnecessary medications are those given without indication, at excessive dosages, for excessive duration, without adequate monitoring, or when there has been a significant adverse event. Residents without a history of antipsychotic drug use should not be treated with antipsychotic medication unless the drug is required to treat a specific diagnosed condition (eg, schizophrenia, Huntington disease, psychosis) that is documented in the medical record. For those residents receiving psychoactive medications, gradual dosage reductions and behavioral interventions are mandated unless a clinical contraindication exists and is documented in the medical record.

A thorough evaluation of medication regimens, done monthly by a pharmacist, is also required. This monthly medication review is intended to minimize adverse events and unnecessary medication use and to ensure proper medication monitoring. A facility must ensure that the medication error rate is <5% and that no significant medication errors occur. No errors should occur that cause a resident discomfort or jeopardize his or her health and safety. Care in assisted-living facilities is not subject to the same regulations that guide care in nursing homes.

Quality

The 2010 Affordable Care Act included a provision that requires all nursing homes certified by CMS to establish Quality Assurance and Performance Improvement (QAPI) programs. Effective in November 2017, the addition of performance improvement to the traditional quality assurance required in nursing homes significantly expands the level and scope of facility activities not only to correct defects but also to proactively prevent problems and optimize performance throughout all levels of the organization. Recent regulatory requirements for nursing facilities have also focused on preventing abuse of older adults and promoting person-centered care, improved care planning, and infection control including antibiotic stewardship.

MEDICAL CARE

The care of nursing-home residents has become more complex over the past several years, commensurate with an increasing level of medical acuity in an environment continually constrained by lack of adequate resources. Comprehensive, ongoing assessment within an interdisciplinary framework works to restore function, when possible, and to enhance quality of life.

Clinical challenges abound in the nursing home, created, in part, by the atypical and subtle presentation of illness so characteristic of residents with profound physical and psychologic frailty. In addition, limited access to biotechnology, frequent dependence on nurses and nurse assistants for resident evaluation, and the high prevalence of cognitive impairment in a setting of intense regulatory oversight all complicate the medical decision-making process. Families of nursing-home residents remain an integral part of the overall care plan and may benefit from specific educational and psychosocial supports. Ethical and legal concerns are also very common, particularly those regarding end-of-life, feeding, hydration, and resident rights issues. Finally, the heterogeneity among nursing-home residents demands an individualized, thoughtful, and reasoned approach to each individual.

Problems in nursing homes that commonly require unique diagnostic and treatment strategies include infections, falls, malnutrition, dehydration, incontinence, and behavioral disturbances. For example, determining the risks and benefits of tube feedings for frail nursing-home residents must be predicated not only on underlying illness but also on the resident's and family's value system, the resources available in the nursing facility, and staff acceptance of the intervention. Many of the problems commonly seen in the nursing home result when multiple comorbidities interact with a host of environmental factors, all of which may be only partially remediable. Unfortunately, expectations of family, as well as regulations, often do not account for these complexities and commonly engender "risk-averse" behavior that may be counter to autonomy and optimal quality of life.

Over the last 40 years, many have advocated for culture change in nursing-home care from institutional, provider-centered models to person-centered models that are driven by choice and self-determination of older adults and their caregivers. Transformed nursing-home culture includes resident direction of activities; a homelike atmosphere; close relationships between staff, residents, and families; empowered staff members who are trained to respond to residents' needs; and collaborative decision making with residents and families about care. Several culture-change initiatives, including the Eden Alternative, the Wellspring Model, and the Green House Model, have been described. In the Green House Model, 6 to 10 older adults reside in small non-institutional homes set in residential neighborhoods. Care in these homes is provided by empowered direct-care staff who manage all care and meal preparation. Close relationships between staff and residents are developed in each of the models. Evidence to date suggests these models improve resident quality of life and employee satisfaction, while preserving or improving quality of care; however, additional research regarding the benefits and costs of culture change is needed.

SPECIAL-CARE UNITS

Special-care units, although conceptually attractive, have not consistently been shown to enhance quality of care apart from the involvement of individual professionals. Some nursing facilities have formed distinct nursing-home units specifically designed and staffed for populations of residents with specific care needs or diagnoses. Examples might include dementia care, respiratory care, and dialysis care. However, specific consultation services in the nursing home may improve care practices and condition-specific resident outcomes, such as reduction of falls (SOE=A).

ADVANCE CARE PLANNING

Understanding each nursing-home resident's preference for care in the context of his or her underlying value system will undoubtedly improve overall quality. This can be challenging in the nursing-home setting given that the number of nursing-home residents who do not have medical decision-making capacity has been noted to be as high as 44%. Early advance care planning may be invaluable for nursing-homes residents and those at risk of nursing-home placement. According to the CDC, 65% of nursing-home residents have at least one advance care directive on record. Living wills and do-not-resuscitate orders are the most common advance directives, in place for 18% and 56%, respectively, of all nursing-home residents.

Durable power of attorney for health care documentation is present for 26% of nursing-home residents at admission and for 39% after 1 year of residence. Less than 5% of nursing-home residents have "do-not-hospitalize" orders, which document that the resident is not to be hospitalized even after developing a condition that is generally treated in the hospital. Although ongoing discussion of care preferences appears to be present in the nursing home, there likely remain ongoing opportunities for improved understanding of nursing-home resident preferences for care. A recent study found almost one-third of older adults receive care in a skilled-nursing facility in the last 6 months of life under the Medicare post-hospitalization benefit, and 1 in 11 older adults will die while enrolled in the skilled-nursing facility benefit. Although use of formal hospice programs to augment end-of-life care for long-term residents in nursing homes has increased in recent years, many have called for providing additional palliative care services to care for the diverse population receiving care in nursing-home settings. When ethical dilemmas arise in nursing-home care, institutional ethics committees can provide important guidance. The multidisciplinary nature of these committees ensures a spectrum of opinion and insight critical for nursing-home residents.

RESOURCES

- Lindquist LA, Miller RK, Saltsman WS, et al. SGIM-AMDA-AGS Consensus Best Practice Recommendations for Transitioning Patients' Healthcare from Skilled Nursing Facilities to the Community. *J Gen Intern Med*. 2017;32(2):199–203.

- Martin-Misener R, Donald F, Wickson-Griffiths A, et al. A mixed methods study of the work patterns of full-time nurse practitioners in nursing homes. *J Clin Nurs*. 2015;24(9-10):1327–1337.

- Unroe KT, Nazir A, Holtz LR, et al. The Optimizing Patient Transfers, Impacting Medical Quality, and Improving Symptoms: Transforming Institutional Care approach: preliminary data from the implementation of a Centers for Medicare and Medicaid Services nursing facility demonstration project. *J Am Geriatr Soc*. 2015;63(1):165–169.

CHAPTER 23—COMMUNITY-BASED CARE

KEY POINTS

- Home and community-based supports and services play an important role in helping to keep people living in their homes longer. Many of these services depend on funding from Medicare and Medicaid benefits.

- Community-based services that do not require a change of residence may be used as an alternative to hospitalization or institutionalization. The availability of such services varies depending on location, financial reimbursements, and state policies.

- Health care providers should be familiar with the types of community-based care services available in their own communities to help advise patients and their families about care options.

HOME CARE

Home care services are provided by home health care agencies, home care aide organizations, and hospices. Some of these organizations are Medicare certified, which allows providers to bill Medicare directly for reimbursement. Agencies that are not Medicare or Medicaid certified are reimbursed largely from out-of-pocket payments from the clients who are served.

In 2013, close to 5 million patients received services from home health agencies, and 1.3 million individuals received services from hospices, predominantly in the home setting. For many of these people, home care has the potential to improve quality of life and avoid unnecessary hospitalization or institutionalization.

Under a cost-based reimbursement system, home care grew rapidly in the 1980s and 1990s. This growth coincided with the initiation of the prospective payment system (diagnostic-related groups (DRGs) for hospitals. This shift resulted in shorter hospital stays and an increased need for home services. New technologies created the possibility of providing therapies in the home that were previously available only in hospitals or nursing homes. Because of an increase in costs, Congress placed limits of Medicare spending as mandated in the Balanced Budget Act of 1997, which led to development of a prospective payment system for home-services. By the end of 2001, the number of Medicare-certified home care agencies had declined by 30.4%, many as a result of financial pressures. However, with implementation of a prospective payment system, the financial stability has allowed growth of Medicare-certified agencies to well over 10,000 agencies nationally. The Outcome and Assessment Information Set (OASIS) is a tool that classifies patients into home health–related groups (HHRGs). The OASIS instrument is completed by the home care agency and tracks several domains of the patient's functional status and medical needs. Like the DRGs, the HHRGs provide the basis for agency reimbursement and are based on severity of the patient's illness, disabilities, and nursing needs. This includes a payment adjustment based on location in the United States. The instrument is also intended to provide a means of uniformly measuring quality of care across all home care agencies. The OASIS assessment and the International Classification of Disease (ICD) codes must be accurate to ensure that reimbursement matches the needs of the patient being served. Like other sectors of the health care system, home care agencies are charged with developing cost-effective, high-quality care despite diminishing reimbursement.

Medicare coverage of home health services require that a patient meets the criteria for being homebound and have a need for a skilled service provided by a licensed nurse or rehabilitation professional. To be considered homebound, a patient's condition makes leaving home a "considerable and taxing effort." For example, leaving home may require extensive assistance such as using a wheelchair or walker, needing special transportation, or getting help from another person. The patient may still be able to leave the home for nonmedical reasons as long as these occurrences are "infrequent and short in duration" such as for attending a religious service or special family event.

Home care services paid under Medicare must be provided by a Medicare-certified home health agency. To compare quality measures of agencies, one may use the Home Health Compare tool available at Medicare.gov (www.medicare.gov/homehealthcompare).

Team Approach to Home Care

Home care involves an interprofessional team that typically is composed of nurses, rehabilitation professionals (speech, physical, occupational, and respiratory), social workers, personal care aides, home medical equipment suppliers, and informal caregivers. Physicians certify and recertify the plan of care and the need for individual therapy services for Medicare-covered home health services. To certify a patient's eligibility for the home health benefit, the physician must document that he or she, or an allowed non-physician practitioner, has had a face-to-face encounter with the patient. This requirement is designed to ensure that the physician has current knowledge of the patient's condition to inform the home care orders. The documentation requirements for billing allow activities over multiple days in a month to be combined. Reimbursement can vary in different parts of the country by as much as 20% based on a Medicare adjustment called "Geographical Practices Cost Indices."

Nurse practitioners cannot certify home care services under Medicare, but they are authorized by law to provide both primary care and registered nurse services in the home. Reimbursement for these services depends on the type of care provided. If the nurse practitioner provides a service described by a Current Procedural Terminology (CPT) code made necessary by an ICD diagnosis to a homebound patient, then it is billable to Medicare Part B as a medical service. It does not require a physician's order and could be billed directly using the nurse practitioner's provider number. Nursing services provided by the nurse practitioner working as an employee of a certified home care agency or house call program are billable under Medicare Part A. In such a case, the nurse practitioner bills for these services using the home care agency's Medicare provider number.

Home care teams can vary widely in terms of structure and organization, as well as visit frequency per discipline. Team organization and effective communication has been cited as a key factor in driving quality in home health care. Home health aides or personal care attendants are often the cornerstones in the provision of home care, providing the bulk of hands-on care to assist patients/clients in ADLs. Clinical assessments, case management, and care coordination is most frequently performed by a nurse in home care. Of note, a home visit from a physician is not required for the patient to receive home care services.

House Calls

Physicians, nurse practitioners, and physician assistants may provide house calls on an intermittent basis when a clinical need arises, or house calls may be an integrated component of a clinical practice that focuses on house calls or home-based primary care. House calls can add an important dimension to the primary provider's knowledge of the patient's circumstances, function, and environment. Home evaluation can identify additional problems not readily apparent in office-based assessment. Unlike with home health services under a Medicare-certified agency, a patient does not need to be considered homebound in order to receive a home visit from a primary care provider. There are a variety of reasons for which a patient may have difficulty receiving care in an office-based setting, such as cognitive impairment, limited mobility, or exacerbations in chronic health conditions. House calls have the additional benefit of reducing the burden for patients who lack access to transportation or have functional limitations. Some clinical practices are shifting from an office-based to a house calls practice.

The house call involves a direct face-to-face visit with the patient at his or her residence. There are no specific restrictions on the number of home visits, as long as the clinician can support in the progress note that the encounter was reasonable and necessary. The documentation must justify the medical necessity such as addressing a new health condition, acute change in clinical status, exacerbation of a chronic condition, or assessing the response to a specific therapy or plan of care. For house calls to be financially feasible for clinicians, thorough documentation is key to receiving reimbursement. As is the case with other outpatient visits, the provider's progress note must identify historical data, physical examination findings, diagnostic test results, assessment of an active diagnosis, and a therapeutic plan. Evaluations of the patient's function, caregiver issues, and the medical plan of care are also critical elements of the documentation. There are specific CPT codes for house calls and domiciliary care. When visits are prolonged, time codes can sometimes be used to justify an enhanced reimbursement, such as for goals of care discussions and advance care planning.

Medical care in the home may be provided as part of an ongoing office-based program, as an extension of hospitalization through a postacute care program, or as a free standing clinical entity. Current regulations allow house calls to be provided by physicians, nurse practitioners, and physician assistants. Their services are often delivered as part of an interprofessional team.

Independence at Home Demonstration

Home-based primary care has been proposed as a way to improve the overall quality of health care, reduce costs for vulnerable patients, and support quality of life. The Independence at Home Demonstration was authorized under the Affordable Care Act, beginning in 2012, enrolling >10,000 home-limited Medicare beneficiaries with multiple chronic conditions. The demonstration project provided longitudinal primary care and care coordination services by teams of provider groups led by physicians or nurse practitioners. Care coordination is designed to be comprehensive, informed by assessments, and involves both social service and medical needs. Clinical groups participating in the demonstration who meet the savings target of 5% are eligible for varying levels of shared savings to reinvest in programs. The demonstration has continued to show ongoing high quality of care, with cost savings of more than $25 million dollars in its first year and more than $10 million dollars in the second year.

Patient Assessment

Homebound patients generally have significant functional impairment. Comprehensive geriatric assessment is particularly valuable in this setting to evaluate a patient's functional and cognitive baseline, monitor the course of illness, and evaluate the effects of intervention. However, assessment in the home has some important differences from office-based assessment.

During a home visit, the patient's daily environment can be assessed for safety in the context of the patient's unique needs. Performance-based functional assessment can focus on the practical aspects of performing ADLs by directly observing bathing, dressing, and transferring. Challenges and safety issues can be identified, and the assessor can evaluate the caregiver's abilities to support the patient's needs. The caregiver's needs for counseling, training, support, and education can also be identified and addressed.

Environmental modifications can be recommended to improve function. For example, modifications of the bathtub, a hand-held shower, a shower seat, grab bars, and a bedside commode can improve the patient's quality of life and functioning. Barriers to wheelchairs and walkers (eg, door sills) can be identified and removed. Chair lifts and outdoor ramps can help patients circumvent stairs. Occupational therapy consultation can be particularly useful in identifying other personal care needs and assistive devices for performing ADLs such as dressing, eating, and housekeeping chores. Numerous home safety checklists are available online to help a reviewer assess the home. Additional technological additions to improve home safety, including personal emergency response systems (in which a person pushes a button for emergency assistance), can help aid the homebound patient.

Limitations of Home Care

Many older adults would prefer to remain in their own homes, but situations arise that may make institutional care a more appropriate choice than in-home care. For example, caregivers in the home may not be available or able to safely or adequately meet the needs of the patient. Unstable medical conditions that require frequent laboratory testing, respiratory interventions, IV medications, or frequent dressing changing, may make institutional care a better choice than home care. Additionally, the features of the home setting may make mobility and completion of ADLs unsafe. Another consideration is the substantial cost of home care beyond what is covered by a patient's insurance. Out-of-pocket expenses for additional private-pay services may be prohibitive, making a nursing facility a more feasible option for patients and their families.

Liability and Legal Issues

As in other areas in the practice of medicine, clinicians are potentially liable for adverse outcomes in home care. It is important to maintain accurate and thorough documentation of the patient's needs, conditions, assessments, and care plans. If the patient is receiving home care agency services, clinicians must ensure that the patient meets the defined Medicare criteria for being homebound. Inaccurate certificates of medical necessity for home care could lead to charges of Medicare fraud. All home care forms should be carefully reviewed before they are signed.

When providing home care, a provider must be sensitive to potential conflicts of interest. Federal legislation prohibits physicians from receiving financial benefit, compensation, or rebate for referring a patient to a home care provider. Further, physicians may not refer patients to home care companies in which the physician or the physician's family has a substantial financial interest. Providers should seek legal advice for any question of a potential conflict of interest.

Ethics and Decisions about Institutionalization

Two ethical themes arise commonly in home care. The first is the balance between patient autonomy and maintaining safety. The second involves issues surrounding mistreatment and neglect of older adults. Respect for patient autonomy often means that the patient remains in his or her home as a result of the patient's (or surrogate decision maker's) choice. An assessment of the patient's capacity to make decisions should be conducted if in question. Conflict arises when a patient's medical care or safety cannot be adequately maintained in the home, yet the patient chooses to continue remaining in the home. It is difficult to balance respect for patient autonomy with prevention of medical neglect. In some situations when the patient has a terminal prognosis, a hospice referral can help provide additional services in the home and supports for both the patient and family. In cases when there is a neglectful or abusive situation, local Adult Protective Services should be notified.

COMMUNITY-BASED SERVICES: AGING SERVICES NETWORK

While quality medical care is vital to caring for older adults at home, often the key to maintaining independence and addressing the challenges of aging and disability is the appropriate use of non-medical community-based supports and services. These services are provided throughout the United States by Area Agencies on Aging (AAAs), which were initiated under the Older Americans Act (AOA) in 1965 and provide a scope of services that continues to expand. The aging services network consists of publicly funded and subcontracted public and private organizations and agencies that implement an array of non-medical community-based services coordinated at state and local levels. These services include elder abuse prevention and intervention, home meal services, transportation, respite care, health insurance counseling, legal assistance, chronic disease self-management, and home modifications. AAAs, under AOA funding, provide the Expanded In-home Services for the Elderly Program, which provides person-centered case management and service coordination. AAAs were also instrumental in supporting the development of Aging and Disability Resource Centers, which provides a "single point of entry" for information and referral for long-term care supports and services. Other aging services network programs specifically support caregivers, focus on care transitions, and assist older adults struggling to make payments for rent or utilities. This diverse array of supports and services are crucial for the independence of older adults in their local communities and require a close integration of medical and social aspects of care. The National Association of Area Agencies on Aging provides information on the national scope of services and legislative initiatives related to the aging service network (www.n4a.org/).

COMMUNITY-BASED SERVICES NOT REQUIRING A CHANGE IN RESIDENCE

Adult Day Care

Adult day care is a community-based option that provides a wide range of social and support services in a congregate setting. Adult day care has become increasingly common with >280,000 participants enrolled in adult day services at centers nationally. Providers of adult day care may offer a variety of services, ranging from simple nonskilled custodial care to more advanced skilled services. The availability of a registered nurse allows for onsite health services, clinical assessment and monitoring, and assistance with medication management. Adult day care is also used commonly for patients with dementia who need supervision and assistance with their ADLs while the primary caregiver is at work or tending to other responsibilities. Adult day care may be used on a regular basis or temporarily as a form of respite for the primary caregiver. In general, custodial adult day care is not covered by Medicare, although some costs may be covered by Medicaid or other insurers.

Day Hospitals

Day hospitals provide a broad range of skilled nursing care services, including parenteral antibiotic treatment, chemotherapy, and intensive rehabilitation. They may also be referred to as partial hospitalization programs. Most programs are housed in chronic care hospitals or rehabilitation centers. This arrangement allows for the provider to take advantage of in-house professional expertise and resources, while allowing the patient to return to his or her home or alternative living site after day treatments are complete. Services are covered under Medicare, with similar requirements to those surrounding home health care.

Day hospitals are most often used for 2 groups of patients: those needing multidisciplinary rehabilitation and those with psychiatric illnesses. A systematic review of day hospital care found no significant differences between day hospitals and alternative sources of care with respect to death, disability, or use of health services. Among those receiving care in a day hospital, there was a trend toward less functional decline and less hospital and institutional care.

The Program of All-inclusive Care for the Elderly (PACE)

PACE is a capitated model of care that provides comprehensive care services to frail, community-dwelling older adults by a single organization. The program provides all inpatient, outpatient, and long-term care services to frail older adults. Participants in the PACE program must be age ≥55 years old to meet state-defined requirements regarding their need for a nursing-home level of care. Most will qualify for Medicaid and Medicare, so called "dually eligible"; pooling funds from Medicaid and Medicare allows for comprehensive care to be planned and coordinated by the PACE interdisciplinary team. Without Medicaid and Medicare coverage, out-of-pocket expenses are high. Few private insurance programs provide a PACE program as part of their policies. The average PACE enrollee is 80 years old and has an average of 8 medical conditions and 3 ADL limitations. Half of PACE participants have dementia. As of 2015, there are 114 PACE programs operating in 32 states.

The goal of the PACE program is to keep the participant in the community for as long as is medically, socially, and financially feasible. The system, designed to be seamless, uses an interprofessional team of health care providers who know the patients and their caregivers well. The team provides care across the spectrum of hospital, home, alternative living situations, and institutional care. The team consists of a physician (often a geriatrician), nurse practitioner or physician assistant, clinic and home health nurses, social workers, physical, occupational, and speech therapists, pharmacists, dieticians, and transportation workers. The hub of care is the PACE center, which provides adult day health care. Other care and services may include, but are not limited to, respite care, transportation, prescription drug coverage, audiology, dentistry, optometry, and podiatry. Hospital and nursing-home care may remain an option when necessary. The interprofessional team aims to provide assistance for the complex social needs as well as the medical needs of the participant.

The National PACE Association (NPA) studies and disseminates information on who PACE serves and the experiences of individuals enrolled in PACE. NPA leads the effort to determine how the model should evolve in response to the rapid changes in the health care system. (www.npaonline.org)

In 1997, legislation was passed that changed the status of PACE from a demonstration program to a permanent provider under Medicare. PACE is an optional program under state Medicaid. There are more than 3 million dually eligible and nursing home–certifiable older adults in the United States that might benefit from PACE, but only a small fraction have enrolled. The growth of PACE has generally been slower than expected. Barriers to growth have included large start-up costs, insufficient supply of physicians, and the reluctance of patients to leave their primary care physician. NPA and CMS are evaluating modifications to the PACE model that would allow for community physician involvement as primary care providers (rather than using a PACE-paid, staff health maintenance organization model). This change in the model may result in more significant growth of PACE, because it could allow patients to keep their primary care physicians. The PACE Innovation Act, which was passed in 2016, allows the development of pilot programs using the PACE model to serve patients <55 years old who have chronic illness or disability and are at risk of nursing-home placement.

Managed Long-Term Care Programs

Managed long-term care programs are state-developed systems that aim to streamline the delivery of long-term services to people with chronic illnesses or disability who wish to stay in their homes and communities. These services, such as home care or adult day care, are provided through managed long-term care plans. These programs often include patients with Medicare and Medicaid and those who are eligible for both ("dually eligible"). Some of these programs have been referred to as "PACE without walls" and provide funding to test new models of care that build on the successful PACE model. States are partnering with entities such as home care agencies, nursing homes, hospitals, and integrated delivery systems to develop these programs. These programs provide financing through various capitated per member, per month payments. The aim of the managed long-term care programs is to provide safe and cost-effective care.

Home Hospital

The home hospital focuses on providing more complex care at home to older adults who would have been hospitalized for an acute care need. Patients receiving home hospital care have access to nurses and physicians on a regular basis and for episodic care through an on-call system that allows problems to be addressed promptly. Such programs have been successfully implemented in nations with single-payer health systems. Studies conducted outside of the United States suggest that care is comparable for selected patients and that patient satisfaction is higher. The Veterans Administration Program at Home is a research-based home hospital program run by physicians and nurses with the goal of preventing hospitalization or reducing the length of hospital stays. This program has demonstrated that complications such as falls and confusion are lower for patients in the home hospital program than those who remain in hospital.

In-Home Technology

A wide array of technologies have been developed that can assist patients with ADLs and provide valuable information to caregivers. Devices such as personal emergency response systems, usually worn on the wrist or around the neck, can alert care providers that help is needed. Newer technologies can provide help in administering and tracking medications, monitoring and transmitting vital signs, and connecting patients to care providers through audio and visual telemedicine screens. Homes can be equipped with fully automated systems to adjust heating and lighting, to allow doors to be opened and closed with remote devices and to monitor activity throughout the home. Home robotics are under development that assist in ADLs or IADLs, including meal preparation and service. Computers and smartphones can also be used to connect patients through social networks to combat isolation and loneliness. The rapid development and interconnectivity of these tools will likely become increasingly important in the safe and efficacious delivery of home care services.

Telemedicine

Telemedicine is a rapidly growing modality of providing in-home health care services. Telemedicine can improve access to medical services that may not be readily available otherwise, such as in rural communities.

Table 23.1—Types of Long-Term Care Services

Adult day care	Structured day programs for older and disabled individuals permitting family caregivers time to pursue personal and employment opportunities while those receiving care remain in the home setting.
Respite care	Temporary in-home assistance or placement in an alternative care setting of a disabled individual, usually for a period of days to weeks to allow a rest period for family caregivers. Other respite models may include in-home respite volunteers to help relieve caregivers, day respite programs by faith-based or other community organizations, and up to 5 days of facility-based respite care under Medicare hospice. The goal with respite is that the patient is eventually returned to the home setting.
Assisted living	Residence that provides a variety of services designated to facilitate continued residence in the community for older and disabled persons. Assistance may include meals, administration of medication, homemaker services, transportation, health reminders, and personal care.
Board and care	Board and care homes offer a group living situation for older adults and people with disabilities who generally are mobile (either able to ambulate or self-propel in a wheelchair) but need help with meal preparation, medication monitoring, and personal care. It is a type of an assisted-living environment, but nursing and medical care is usually not provided.
Nursing home/ long-term care	Residence for individuals whose functional disabilities or illnesses preclude a higher level of nursing care due to ADL dependence. Some patients may also have skilled nursing needs, such as wound management, acute rehabilitation, and intravenous antibiotics.

A wide variety of technology and services are broadly included in the telemedicine category. Commonly used technologies include videoconferencing connections, usually through a web-connected camera or tablet computer, allowing a clinician to speak with and observe a patient to conduct a "virtual home visit." More advanced models use trained technicians on-site with a patient and incorporate higher resolution cameras and additional equipment (eg, stethoscope and otoscope attachments), while the off-site clinician can conduct a clinical assessment remotely. Some telemedicine services also include clinical monitoring (telehealth), mobile laboratory/phlebotomy, radiography, and home nursing components, and as such begin to resemble a hospital-at-home type service. Telemedicine psychiatric services, including longitudinal medication management and treatment of depression, have been successfully implemented across many areas of the country. Current obstacles to the wider implementation of telemedicine include unclear or variable regulations across states (including licensing requirements across state lines), as well as marked variation in reimbursement for such services. A number of health care companies and insurers are now adopting telemedicine services as supplemental benefits, which can include urgent care visits and other medical consultations with health care providers. These services have varying levels of insurance coverage, copayment, and out-of-pocket costs to patients.

COMMUNITY-BASED SERVICES REQUIRING A CHANGE OF RESIDENCE

For a comparison of types of long-term care services, see Table 23.1.

Senior Villages and Senior Cohousing

Senior villages and cohousing are intentional communities where residents tend to be more independent, healthy, and active than in other forms of senior housing. These are typically not associated with provision of medical supervision or health care services.

Assisted-Living Facilities

Assisted-living facilities continue to grow in number as the U.S. population ages. They may be categorized or marketed under different titles (such as personal care homes, residential care homes, domiciliary care, and sheltered care) and are housing increasingly frail and medically complex individuals. The average length of stay for persons in an assisted-living facility is 2 years, and the most common reason for discharge is the need for nursing home care.

Assisted-living residences are characterized by some level of coordination or provision of personal care services, social activities, health-related services, and supervision in a home-like atmosphere that maximizes autonomy and privacy. Additional individual services may be provided at additional cost to the resident.

Assisted-living facilities may provide private or shared rooms or apartments. They may provide housekeeping, meals, and assistance with ADLs. Facilities vary with regard to whether they will accept residents with cognitive impairment or dementia. Many assisted-living facilities do not have a registered nurse on staff. State licensing requirements vary in terms of medication administration by facility personnel. Depending on the requirements, medication administration and management can be directed by staff with varying levels of training requirements or licensure.

Table 23.2—Examples of Skilled Versus Nonskilled Nursing Needs

Skilled	Nonskilled
Acute rehabilitation	Dementia/cognitive impairment
Complex wound care	Functional dependence
Intravenous antibiotics	Incontinence
Titrating oxygen and insulin requirements	Lack of a caregiver

In states where regulations do not require skilled care (see Table 23.2) in assisted-living facilities, home health skilled care is often provided as an external or independent service to the individual patient at the facility. In this context, the boundary between assisted-living and skilled-nursing facilities often becomes blurred.

Costs for assisted-living residences vary greatly, depending on the size of the unit, services provided, and location. The national median monthly cost for assisted-living facilities is more than $3,500 per month or in excess of $42,000 annually. Assisted living is covered in a growing number of long-term care insurance policies, but only a small minority of older Americans possess long-term insurance. Assisted living is not covered by Medicare, but certain services are paid under Supplementary Security Income and Social Services Block Grant programs. Some states reimburse or plan to reimburse for assisted-living services through Medicaid. In addition, states have the option to pay for certain assisted-living services under their Medicaid plans or to petition the Department of Health and Human Services for a waiver.

Group Homes

Group homes (including domiciliary care, single room occupancy residences, board-and-care homes, and some congregate living arrangements) are houses or apartments in which 2 or more unrelated people live together. Group homes vary in types of residents they serve, such as those with chronic mental illness or dementia. Residents share common living spaces but have their own bedrooms. Advantages of this arrangement include a lower cost of living and peer socialization. Independence and functional status are supported through the interdependence and relationships of the residents, although staff are present and assist residents to varying degrees. Resident-to-staff ratios may be higher than in other supported-living environments. Most group homes are run as for-profit businesses, and some states require licensing.

Adult Foster Care

Foster care homes generally provide room, board, and some assistance with ADLs by the sponsoring family or by paid caregivers, who customarily live on the premises. Perhaps the longest experience with adult foster care is in the state of Oregon, where it is used as an alternative to long-term care and institutionalization. Adult foster care has the advantages of maintaining frail older adults in a more home-like environment. Regulations for foster care vary by state, and some states require licensing. Some states provide coverage of adult foster care through their Medicaid programs.

Sheltered Housing

Sheltered housing is funded though the Older Americans Act and is offered as an option for housing subsidized through Section 8, Housing and Urban Development programs for seniors and disabled residents. Often, these arrangements are sheltered homes offering personal care assistance, housekeeping services, and meals. Programs may be supplemented by social work services and activities coordinators. Charges to clients are based on a sliding scale, which may cost up to 30% of income.

Continuing Care Retirement Communities

Continuing care retirement communities (CCRC) possess a variety of living options with the expectation that a resident will transition to those offering additional supports as needed over time. Such communities may include houses, condominiums, apartments, assisted living, home care, and skilled-nursing home care. Three financial models are common in such communities: the all-inclusive model, which provides total health care coverage, including long-term care; fee-for-service models, which match payments to the level of care; and the modified coverage model, which covers long-term care to a predetermined maximum. CCRCs often require an entry fee that may or may not be refundable, plus a variable monthly fee to pay for rent and supportive services. Funding for care in such communities is largely private (out-of-pocket or one-time investment), although some facilities have Medicare- or Medicaid-funded beds for skilled care.

RESOURCES

- Han K, Trinkoff AM, Storr CL, et al. Variation across U.S. assisted living facilities: admissions, resident care needs, and staffing. *J Nurs Scholarsh.* 2017;49(1):24–32.

- Medicaid Community-Based Long-Term Services & Supports (https://www.medicaid.gov/medicaid/ltss) (accessed Feb 2019).

- O'Conno M, Hanlon A, Mauer E, et al. Identifying distinct risk profiles to predict adverse events among community-dwelling older adults. *Geriatr Nurs*. 2017;38(6):510–519.

- Thoma-Lurken T, Bleijlevens MH, Lexis MA, et al. Facilitating aging in place: a qualitative study of practical problems preventing people with dementia from living at home. *Geriatr Nurs*. 2018;9(1):29–38.

CHAPTER 24—OUTPATIENT CARE SYSTEMS

KEY POINTS

- A person-centered geriatric approach to care can improve the quality of care and outcomes for older adults and is often provided in a team milieu in accordance with best geriatric medical practice.

- Broad dissemination of effective models of outpatient care for older adults must integrate person-centered geriatric care with particular payment models (eg, fee-for-service, capitation, patient-centered medical homes, accountable care organizations), requiring a broad understanding of existing payment methodologies, practice workflow, and initiatives to improve competencies in the clinical geriatrics workforce.

- Chronic care management codes provide an opportunity to provide coordinated person-centered geriatric care in the fee-for-service environment.

Describing geriatrics as a "metadiscipline" captures the unique approach of outpatient care systems for older adults. Traditional outpatient care, based on the classic internal medicine approach of diagnosis, treatment, and cure, does not deliver the recommended standard of care to older adults for preventive services, chronic disease management, and geriatric syndromes. Ageism continues to have a negative impact on the delivery of health care to older adults, and traditional care approaches are associated with racial and ethnic disparities in preventive and chronic care. A more proactive, person-centered approach based on the core principles of geriatric medicine, including a focus on function and quality of life, is needed to improve the overall quality of geriatric care. To this end, several innovative outpatient care systems have been developed over the past few decades. This chapter focuses on the value of the geriatric approach to care, insofar as it can be delivered in traditional primary care settings as well as through a variety of system-based approaches. Some approaches integrate geriatrics into primary care, whereas others involve geriatrics as a primary care specialty. Consultative geriatrics that is not integrated into a care model has not been proved to work. Hence, geriatrics must be a "metadiscipline" informing all care delivered to older adults.

The traditional fee-for-service payment model has been questioned in regard to the care of older adults, insofar as the incentives for procedurally oriented care often outweigh a more person-centered cognitive approach. Fragmentation of care has also been shown to detract from the type of care needed in a complex population with multiple chronic diseases. This has led to a variety of new models of primary care aimed at improving the quality and outcomes of care for older adults. Many of these models share concepts from the patient-centered medical home (PCMH) model of practice (www.medicalhomeinfo.org/downloads/pdfs/JointStatement.pdf) (Table 24.1). The PCMH model builds on a strong evidence base showing that higher-quality care and lower costs can be achieved through greater emphasis on primary care. However, there has not been evidence that a PCMH model works with older adults without clinicians who are competent in, and models that support, the geriatric approach to care.

The accountable care organization (ACO) is another model for delivery-system reform that can be synergistic with the PCMH model. An ACO aims to manage the full continuum of care and to be accountable for the overall quality of care and costs for a defined population. An ACO is a provider-led organization and may take on many forms, including large integrated delivery systems, physician-hospital organizations, and independent practice associations. ACOs typically receive fee-for-service payment and if specified quality performance metrics are met, share in any cost savings achieved relative to a risk-adjusted projected spending target for their patient population. ACOs need a strong primary care foundation to succeed and, in turn, can provide important infrastructure beyond the primary care practice to facilitate the full realization of the PCMH model. Evidence of success by ACOs in the care of older adults is limited in the absence of a geriatric approach to care. However, there are market-based examples of geriatric practices providing the backbone to a successful ACO or other systems. Payment reform such as that proposed for PCMH and ACOs may offer a means for implementing the system approaches to outpatient geriatric care discussed below. However, for such programs to be successful, geriatric competencies must be instilled in the clinical workforce.

GERIATRICS IN PRIMARY CARE

Person-Centered Geriatric Approach to Care

Person-centered care is an important element in a variety of care models. The very basis of person-centered care is true knowledge of the individual. This requires an effort on the part of the clinician to know the person beyond the traditional set of medically oriented questions. At the heart of this approach is knowledge of the person's goals based on his or her preferences. Person-centered care has been defined by an AGS expert panel (Table 24.2).

Table 24.1—Joint Principles of the Patient-Centered Medical Home

- Each patient has an ongoing relationship with a personal physician.
- A physician-directed medical practice includes a team of individuals who collectively take responsibility for care.
- The practice adopts a "whole-person orientation" and provides or arranges for all the patient's health care needs.
- Care is coordinated across all elements of the complex health care system.
- Clinicians engage in continuous quality improvement, and patients participate in decision making.
- Access to care is enhanced.
- Payment recognizes the added value provided to patients who have a patient-centered medical home (eg, via enhanced fee-for-service, care management fee, and/or shared savings).

Table 24.2—American Geriatrics Society Expert Panel Definition of Person-Centered Care

- An individualized, goal-oriented care plan based on the person's preferences.
- Ongoing review of the person's goals and care plan.
- Care supported by an interprofessional team in which the person is an integral team member.
- One primary or lead point of contact on the health care team.
- Active coordination between all health care and supportive service providers.
- Continual information sharing and integrated communication.
- Education and training for providers and, when appropriate, the person and those important to the person.
- Performance measurement and quality improvement using feedback from the person and caregivers.

Table 24.3—Key Elements of Geriatric Approach to Care

- Focus on function.
- Focus on managing chronic diseases.
- Identify and manage psychological and social aspects of care.
- Respect patient dignity and autonomy.
- Respect cultural and spiritual beliefs.
- Be sensitive to the patient's financial condition.
- Promote wellness.
- Listen and communicate effectively.
- Take a patient-centered approach to care and customer approach to service.
- Maintain a realistic attitude of optimism and hope.
- Use a team approach to care.

Person-centered care is not sufficient to improve care for older adults if it is not accompanied by core geriatric medical principles, which are incorporated in successful models of care. A philosophy of care was developed by a group of geriatricians in the 1990s that describes the key elements of the geriatric approach (Table 24.3)

Many of the other chapters in this syllabus convey the body of evidence that demonstrate clear differences in how health care professionals should approach the care of older adults. It is critical that this knowledge be integrated with the aforementioned philosophy of care to provide for person-centered geriatric care. Many models of care have failed to demonstrate successful outcomes, no doubt because these key elements have been missing.

Enhanced Primary Care

Guided Care was designed to improve the quality of life and efficiency of resource use for older adults with multiple morbidities. Consistent with the PCMH approach, Guided Care aimed to enhance primary care by infusing the operating principles of 7 chronic care innovations: disease management, self-management, case management, lifestyle modification, transitional care, caregiver education and support, and geriatric evaluation and management. A specially trained registered nurse works with assigned primary care physicians (PCPs) and office staff to provide the intervention to a panel of the practice's older patients at highest risk of requiring abundant health care services. Results showed that Guided Care reduced the use of home-health care but had little effect on the use of other health services at 32 months. Interestingly, in the same trial and among the subgroup of Kaiser-Permanente patients, Guided Care reduced skilled-nursing facility admissions and days and also showed a trend toward reduced hospital admissions and emergency department visits. There is no consistently defined geriatric approach to care at the center of this model, likely limiting its potential effectiveness. However, similar principles have worked successfully in the GRACE and PACE models discussed below.

The Geriatric Resources for Assessment and Care of Elders (GRACE) model of primary care, now referred to as GRACE Team Care™, also includes each of the PCMH principles and could be described as an intensive "medical home" or complex care management program for high-risk older patients. GRACE provides patients with home-based comprehensive geriatric assessment and long-term care management by a nurse practitioner and social worker (GRACE support team) who collaborate with the office-based PCP and a geriatrics interprofessional team, including a geriatrician, pharmacist, and mental health liaison. Individualized care planning during weekly team meetings is guided by 12 care protocols for common geriatric conditions (eg, "difficulty walking/falls," "cognitive impairment," "depression"). Three protocols are used in all patients: "medication management," "health maintenance," and "advance care planning." The nurse practitioner and social worker (employees of the primary care practice) review and prioritize the care plan with the patient's PCP, assure the plan is consistent with the patient's goals and preferences, and then implement it in collaboration with the PCP. The GRACE support team provides ongoing home-based care management, including coordination and continuity of care among all health care professionals and sites of care, facilitated by an electronic medical record and a Web-based care management tracking system. By definition, the GRACE model follows a geriatric approach to care.

The GRACE model was developed specifically to improve the quality of care of a mixed-race population of older adults who are poor (many dually eligible for Medicare and Medicaid), have multiple comorbid conditions, and receive primary care in community-based health centers affiliated with an urban safety net health care system. Low-income older adults enrolled in a randomized controlled trial of the GRACE intervention received better quality of care for geriatric conditions (eg, falls and depression) and general health processes (eg, preventive care and advance directives) targeted, had improvements in health-related quality-of-life measures, and made fewer emergency department visits over 2 years (all compared with usual care). In addition, hospital admissions were significantly reduced in the second year among GRACE patients identified at baseline as being at high risk of future hospitalization (SOE=A). Cost analysis of the GRACE intervention revealed that in the high-risk group, increases in chronic and preventive care costs were offset by reductions in acute care costs such that the intervention was cost neutral in the first 2 years. Two-year costs were higher in the low-risk group. The intervention reduced costs in the high-risk group during the post-intervention, or third, year because of continued lower hospital costs for GRACE patients than for those who received usual care.

Replication of the GRACE model has been successful in Medicare managed-care and Department of Veterans Affairs health care settings and demonstrated consistent improvements in quality of care and reductions in hospital utilization (http://graceteamcare.indiana.edu [accessed Feb 2019]). The GRACE model has been applied within a home visitation program, as a care transition intervention, and as a model for integrated medical and social services in older adults enrolled in the Medicaid Home and Community-Based Services waiver. Other successful models of enhanced primary care demonstrating reduced acute care utilization have also involved an interprofessional team that provides ongoing care management (usually including home visitation) in support of and integrated with the PCP (SOE=A).

Incorporating the above models and approaches, the Department of Veterans Affairs Boston Healthcare System has brought the PCMH concept one step further. The Geriatrics in Primary Care model embeds geriatric services directly into primary care. An on-site consulting geriatrician and geriatric nurse care manager work directly in the primary care setting. Preliminary data have been positive, suggesting "care defragmentation," with a significant reduction in subspecialty clinic use.

Disease Management

Disease management programs focus health care delivery around a single disease with the goal of optimizing patient care for that condition. The most effective disease management programs are those that are integrated with the patient's PCP or specialty physician, or both. Single disease specific programs have limited utility in frail older adults with multiple chronic conditions. Successful disease management programs that demonstrated utility in older adults have generally had geriatricians involved in the care delivery model. One notable heart failure program that was nurse-directed and multidisciplinary (geriatrician, cardiologist, nurse, dietitian, and social worker) reduced readmission rates and costs in hospitalized older adults with heart failure (SOE=A). Key components included comprehensive education of the patient and family, a prescribed diet, social-service consultation and planning for an early discharge, medication review, and intensive follow-up.

In the disease management program for late-life depression called Improving Mood—Promoting Access to Collaborative Treatment (IMPACT), patients had access to a depression care manager (a specially trained nurse or psychologist), supervised by a psychiatrist and a primary care liaison physician, who offered education, care management, and support of antidepressant drug therapy prescribed by the patient's PCP or a brief psychotherapy for depression. In a large multicenter clinical trial, depressed patients who received the IMPACT intervention were more likely than patients who received usual care to be given guideline-concordant depression care and to recover from depression (SOE=A).

A collaborative care model developed for older adults with Alzheimer disease has demonstrated improvements in the quality of care and in behavioral and psychological symptoms of dementia among primary-care patients (SOE=A). In this program, known as the Aging Brain Care Medical Home, an advanced practice nurse supported by an interprofessional team (psychologist, neuropsychologist, geriatrician, and geriatric psychiatrist) served as the care manager working with the patient's family caregiver and PCP. The team used standard protocols to initiate treatment and to identify, monitor, and treat behavioral and psychological symptoms of dementia with an emphasis on non-pharmacologic approaches to management.

Outpatient Consultation

Comprehensive geriatric assessment (CGA) is a process intended to determine a patient's medical, psychosocial, and functional capabilities and limitations, with the goal of developing an overall plan for treatment and long-term follow-up. In many ways, it has been the gold standard for a person-centered geriatric approach to care. Because traditional CGA typically requires highly trained teams of geriatricians, geriatric nurse clinicians, physical and occupational therapists, geriatric psychiatrists, and social workers, it is expensive and time consuming. Success generally requires the geriatric team to take over the direct care of the patient, thus becoming a de facto primary care geriatric model. An extended period of intensive team involvement with ongoing care is essential to ensure the efficacy of the intervention. When the geriatric team assumes a purely consultative role (ie, without a role in implementing the recommendations), CGA is unlikely to be successful in improving patient outcomes (SOE=A). However, CGA coupled with an intervention designed to improve PCP and patient adherence to recommendations has demonstrated improved outcomes. In a randomized controlled trial, CGA coupled with adherence strategies was associated with less decline in physical functioning, less fatigue, and better social functioning among community-dwelling older adults with at least 1 of 4 conditions (functional impairment, falls, urinary incontinence, or depressive symptoms [SOE=A]). In this care model, patients undergo an in-depth, standardized assessment from a social worker, a geriatrics nurse practitioner/geriatrician team, and a physical therapist (when indicated by falls or impaired mobility), after which the evaluation team holds a short interprofessional case conference to form the recommendations for care. The adherence intervention includes the geriatrician contacting the patient's PCP to convey the recommendations and also sending a letter describing the recommendations, a copy of the dictated consultation, and full-text references specific to the patient's conditions. In addition, the patient receives a written list of recommendations at the time of the CGA and is subsequently mailed a copy of the dictated consultation and list of recommendations, as well as a "How to Talk to Your Doctor" booklet. Approximately 2 weeks later, a health educator telephones the patient to review the team's recommendations and to help prepare the patient for discussion of the proposed recommendations with the PCP.

A more intensive outpatient consultation model is short-term geriatric evaluation and management (GEM). In GEM, a geriatrics interprofessional team diagnoses *and treats* problems, including adjusting medications, providing counseling and health education, and making referrals to other health professionals and community services. In addition, monitoring and coordination of care between visits is provided through regular telephone calls. In one trial, community-dwelling adults ≥70 years old and found to be at high risk of hospital admission by mailed screening questionnaire underwent CGA followed by interprofessional primary care by the GEM team (geriatrician, geriatrics nurse practitioner, nurse, and social worker) for an average of 6 months before being discharged and returned to the care of their original PCP. This GEM model prevented functional decline, improved patients' satisfaction with their health care, and lessened caregiver burden. Other trials of GEM have shown similar positive results (SOE=A). However, fully implementing the above GEM model was more expensive than usual care. Other GEM trials have produced varying results on costs, with some costing more than usual care, some costing the same, and some costing less.

Forms of CGA may also be attempted in the home setting. Accumulating evidence suggests that preventive home visitation programs, based on CGA with extended follow-up of patients at lower risk of death, can reduce functional decline and nursing-home placement (SOE=A).

GERIATRIC SPECIALTY CARE

Senior Health Clinic

The senior health clinic (SHC) care model is a specialized ambulatory clinical service center for older adults providing primary care using an interprofessional team approach to developing and implementing a plan of care. In the 1990s, this model was cost-reimbursed by Medicare and generally existed as outpatient departments of hospitals. Cost-reimbursement was discontinued by OBRA 1997, and many of these clinics closed their doors. SHCs today depend on traditional reimbursement models, although those that function as outpatient hospital departments have some nuanced reimbursement structure. SHC providers generally have competency in geriatrics, and care is provided and/or coordinated throughout the continuum of care, including hospital, skilled-nursing facility, assisted living, and home care. Team members work with patients, families, and caregivers, and link patients with needed community-based services and information. The chronic care model offers an organized framework to provide the comprehensive resources and processes needed to deliver evidence-based primary care within an integrated health care system that supports the interactions between the informed, activated (ie, engaged) patient and a prepared, proactive team. Patients new to the SHC are screened for risk status, and a comprehensive geriatric-focused evaluation is completed.

The core interprofessional clinical practice team consists of a geriatrician, nurse practitioner, and social worker or geriatric nurse specialist. An extended team may include other professionals, such as a pharmacist, physical therapist, dietitian, and home-health nurse. Provider teams share a common medical record and meet regularly to review complex care plans and discuss new or anticipated patient issues. When SHC patients are admitted to the hospital or skilled-nursing facility, care is delivered directly and/or coordinated by providers from the SHC.

Studies in community settings and Veterans Affairs medical centers have demonstrated that geriatric patients cared for in the SHC model have improved mental health status and better maintained health-related quality of life over time than patients in traditional care (SOE=A). Financially, SHCs may be a cost center when viewed in isolation, with lack of attention given to appropriate coding, billing, and collections. However, these clinics can be considered revenue generators when viewed from the perspective of an integrated health system because of the associated "downstream" fee-for-service revenues generated from hospital inpatient, hospital outpatient, and professional fees (SOE=B). There also exist financially viable private practice groups who provide this type of care in a fee-for-service environment. The key to financial success for these practices is strict adherence to and understanding of the applicable coding and billing requirements. The broad uptake of the SHC model has been limited by health system administrators who consider the clinic in isolation as a cost center, private practitioners who dramatically under-code, and the limited number of specialty-trained geriatrics health care professionals available to staff such clinics. However, under a capitated/risk sharing environment or one of the newer payment models (PCMH or ACO), the SHC model has the potential to thrive by focusing on high-risk Medicare beneficiaries and delivering higher-quality care at lower costs from reduced need for expensive services such as emergency department visits and hospitalizations. One example of such a model is the Independence at Home program, which has demonstrated success in a high-risk population of older adults (SOE=B).

Chronic Care Management

The CMS has identified care management for Medicare beneficiaries as a service that CMS is willing to reimburse. Geriatricians have long believed in the value of care management in the context of a geriatric approach to care. There are now billing codes that PCPs can use in the outpatient, assisted-living, home and nursing-home setting. These chronic care management (CCM) services can be billed by a physician or non-physician practitioner (physician assistant, nurse practitioner, clinical nurse specialist, certified nurse-midwife, and his or her clinical staff, per calendar month, for patients with two or more chronic conditions expected to last at least 12 months or until the death of the patient, and that place the patient at significant risk of death, acute exacerbation/decompensation, or functional decline. Only 1 practitioner can bill CCM per service period (month).

CCM requires the following services be available:

- Use of a certified electronic health record
- Continuity of care with designated care team member
- Comprehensive care management and care planning
- Transitional care management
- Coordination with home and community-based clinical service providers
- 24/7 access to address urgent needs
- Enhanced communication (eg, email)

Verbal consent by the patient, or responsible party, must be documented in the medical record to provide these services.

As of 2017, there are two types of CCM codes. The first is the regular CCM code, and the second is a complex CCM code. The difference between the codes is the amount of clinical staff time, the extent of care planning, and the complexity of the problems addressed by the billing practitioner. The regular CCM code is meant to be for a patient only requiring about 20 minutes per month of care management services. The complex CCM codes are billed for an initial hour of time over the course of a month but additional time in increments of 30 minutes can also be billed.

The CCM codes allow PCPs to bill for services that they or their staff have performed in the past without any compensation. Combined with better attention to appropriate coding and billing, the CCM codes could potentially allow PCPs to more effectively deliver care to older adults while maintaining financial viability.

Program of All-inclusive Care for the Elderly (PACE)

PACE is a capitated model of care that provides comprehensive care services to frail community-dwelling older adults by a single organization. The PACE model follows a person-centered geriatric approach to care. It is essentially a primary care model for a specifically defined geriatric population. The program provides all inpatient, outpatient, and long-term care services to its enrolled population. Participants in the PACE program must be ≥55 years old and meet state-defined requirements regarding their need for nursing-home level of care. Most will also qualify for Medicare and Medicaid; pooling funds from Medicare and Medicaid allows for comprehensive care to be planned and coordinated by the PACE interprofessional team. Without Medicare and Medicaid coverage, out-of-pocket expenses are high. Few private insurance plans provide a PACE benefit as part of their policies. The average PACE enrollee is 80 years old and has an average of 8 medical conditions and 3 ADL limitations; half of PACE participants have dementia.

The goal of the PACE program is to keep the participant in the community for as long as is medically, socially, and financially feasible. The system, designed to be seamless, uses an interprofessional team of health care providers who know the patients and caregivers well and who provide care across the spectrum of hospital, home, alternative living situations, and institutional care. This team includes a physician (often a geriatrician), nurse practitioner, clinic and home-health nurses, social workers, physical therapist, pharmacist, dietician, and transportation workers. The hub of care is the PACE center, which provides adult day health care. Other care includes respite, transportation, medication coverage, rehabilitation (including maintenance physical and occupational therapy), hearing aids, eyeglasses, and a variety of other benefits. The program, at the discretion of the interprofessional team, has the flexibility to pay for nonmedical costs in unusual circumstances (eg, paying a person's electric or gas bill). Care by the interprofessional team provides for the complex social needs as well as the medical needs of the participant. PACE has been described as one of the few truly integrated systems of care in the United States. Although the effectiveness of PACE has not been directly tested by a randomized controlled trial, research has shown that PACE provides high-quality care, albeit with significant site-to-site variation (SOE=B).

In 1997, legislation was passed that changed the status of PACE from a demonstration program to a permanent provider under Medicare. PACE is an optional program under state Medicaid. There are more than 3 million dually eligible and nursing home–certifiable older adults in the United States who might benefit from PACE, but only a small fraction have enrolled. The growth of PACE has been slower than expected. Barriers to growth have included large start-up costs, insufficient supply of physicians, and reluctance of patients to leave their PCP. The National PACE Association and CMS are continuing to evaluate modifications to the PACE model that would allow for community physician involvement as PCPs (rather than using a PACE-paid, staff health-maintenance organization model). PACE has also been looking at ways of moving "upstream" to capture patients before to the level of frailty that makes them eligible for nursing-home care. These changes in the model may result in more significant growth of PACE.

PATIENT SELECTION FOR OUTPATIENT INTERVENTIONS

Patient selection for intensive outpatient interventions is one of the major challenges facing health care organizations that serve older adults. Three complementary approaches have been used to identify high-risk older adults: referral by clinicians, screening by mail or telephone, and analysis of administrative data (predictive modeling). The ideal system for identifying high-risk individuals would rely on multiple sources of information. Clinicians in primary care settings are perhaps well-positioned to identify some high-risk older adults, especially when provided with objective criteria on which to base referral. However, they may lack the time, skills, and incentives to do so. Surveys can be administered systematically by mail or telephone to a defined population of older adults. The Probability of Repeated Admission Questionnaire (Pra) has been used extensively in managed-care settings to identify high-risk older adults upon enrollment. A risk score is calculated based on age, sex, perceived health, availability of an informal caregiver, heart disease, diabetes, and frequency of physician visits and hospitalizations. A score above a certain threshold indicates that the member is at high risk of hospital admission and use of other health-related services during the coming year. The Pra has been found to be valid in many different populations of community-dwelling older adults, including Medicaid, fee-for-service, and managed-care patients (SOE=B). Because of the associated expenses and limited survey response rates, an administrative proxy has been developed as a close substitute to the Pra.

The Vulnerable Elders Survey-13 (VES-13), another risk screening instrument, is a 13-item questionnaire that produces a vulnerability score from 0 to 10 based on age, self-reported health, physical function (ability to stoop, crouch, kneel, walk modest distances, etc), and self-care function (selected basic and instrumental ADLs). Patients with a VES-13 score of ≥3 are at four times the risk of functional decline or death over the next 2 years, compared with those whose scores are <3, and are therefore defined as vulnerable (SOE=B).

There is a growing body of literature related to the concept of frailty and its predictive value. The Frailty Index or Modified Frailty Index (mFI) has demonstrated to have a direct correlation not only to mortality but also to surgical complications. How this type of information can be used in relation to developing improved care plans and approaches to care for this population remains to be seen. There have been predictive modeling approaches that use administrative data for identifying high-risk older adults. These are usually proprietary (and therefore not described in the peer-reviewed literature). They typically analyze health insurance enrollment records and claims data, producing predictions based on age, gender, diagnoses, prior use of health services and associated costs, and pharmacy data. There are also programs that use the Minimum Data Set data in nursing-home residents and correlate this information to frailty.

RESOURCES

- The American Geriatrics Society Expert Panel on Person-Centered Care. Person-centered care: a definition and essential elements. *J Am Geriatr Soc*. 2016;64:15–18.

- Meunier MJ, Brant JM, Audet S, et al. Life after PACE (Program of All-Inclusive Care for the Elderly): A retrospective/prospective, qualitative analysis of the impact of closing a nurse practitioner centered PACE site. *J Am Assoc Nurse Pract*. 2016;28(11):596–603.

- Schubert CC, Dolejs J, May J. Grace Team Care Model. In: Wasserman MR, Riopelle JF, eds. *Primary Care for Older Adults, Models and Challenges*. NY: Springer International Publishing. 2017;1324.

CHAPTER 25—FRAILTY

KEY POINTS

- Frailty occurs in 7%–10% of community-dwelling older adults.

- Frailty is a clinical syndrome of dysregulation of energetics and multiple physiologic systems. Its definable clinical manifestations become apparent when physiologic dysregulation reaches a critical threshold.

- Physical frailty and frailty result from a common pathway of intrinsic physiological alterations. "Index" frailty, by contrast, is characterized by an accumulation of unrelated comorbidities.

- The validated frailty syndrome is manifested when ≥3 or more of 5 phenotypic components are present: weakness, slowed walking speed, low physical activity, low energy or exhaustion, and weight loss.

- Stressors such as hospitalization, surgery, illness, or environmental extremes are less tolerated by frail older adults.

- Frail patients are at high risk of adverse clinical outcomes, including falls, fractures, hospitalization, complications of chemotherapy or surgery, hemodialysis, disability and dependency, and mortality. The most effective preventive approaches appear to be maintaining muscle mass and strength (through walking and resistance exercise) and consuming a Mediterranean diet. Dietary protein supplementation may also be beneficial.

THE CONCEPT OF FRAILTY

The care of frail older adults is a central focus of geriatric medicine. Frail older adults are a subset of the older population at high risk from stressors such as extremes of heat and cold, acute infection or injury, or hospitalization or surgery. In the face of such stressors, frail older adults are more likely to experience delayed recovery from illness, to fall, to develop greater functional impairment (including becoming disabled or dependent), and/or to die. As a group, frail older adults are at high risk of needing hospitalization, and they risk worse outcomes, including dependency, once hospitalized.

Frailty is clinically observed to be a chronic, progressive condition with a spectrum of severity. The most severely frail older adults appear to be in an irreversible, pre-death phase with high risk of mortality over 6–12 months. Those in earlier phases may respond to treatment, which may prevent or ameliorate the clinical manifestations of frailty. The late phase may be an indication for palliative care approaches.

Frailty may, in some individuals, result from intrinsic aging processes, ie, *primary frailty*. In *secondary frailty*, the same phenotype and vulnerability exist in tandem with, and occur as a result of, one or more chronic diseases associated with inflammation and wasting, such as cancer, heart failure, COPD, and HIV/AIDS. The similarity of presentation of primary and secondary frailty suggests that, clinically, frailty is a physiologic entity unto itself that can be triggered by disparate causes but that, ultimately, represents a final common physiological pathway that accelerates vulnerability to adverse health outcomes.

Frailty and Associated Vulnerability: Clinical Implications of Frailty

Frailty is associated with heightened likelihood of adverse outcomes, and this vulnerability is more likely to become manifest in the face of stressors. All frailty theories suggest that, regardless of the causes, frail older adults have decreased reserves to compensate for, or recover from, stressors. Aggregate loss of physiologic function is the process thought to increase the risk of and underlie the vulnerability to adverse outcomes. An emerging research agenda is focused on developing approaches that can identify older adults with this vulnerable physiologic status before phenotypic frailty becomes clinically apparent.

Frailty as a Clinical Syndrome

Beyond the consensus that frailty is a physiologic state of heighted vulnerability, there are 2 major conceptual categories of frailty in common use. These include physical or syndromic frailty, described in this chapter, and index frailty, which is defined by a collection of comorbidities or "deficits." In these conceptual frameworks, index frailty results from accumulation of a number of often unrelated diseases, impairments, and other health conditions in an individual. This state of multimorbidity is associated with increased risk of both mortality and disability; the number of conditions predicts this vulnerability. In this approach, a large number of prevalent conditions marks an individual as frail.

The most common clinical conceptualization of frailty (the so-called *phenotypic* construct used in this chapter, also termed physical frailty and syndromic frailty) arises from distinct dysregulation of physiologic processes that results in a vulnerability to adverse health outcomes and mortality, especially in the face of stressors. These two definitions and measures of

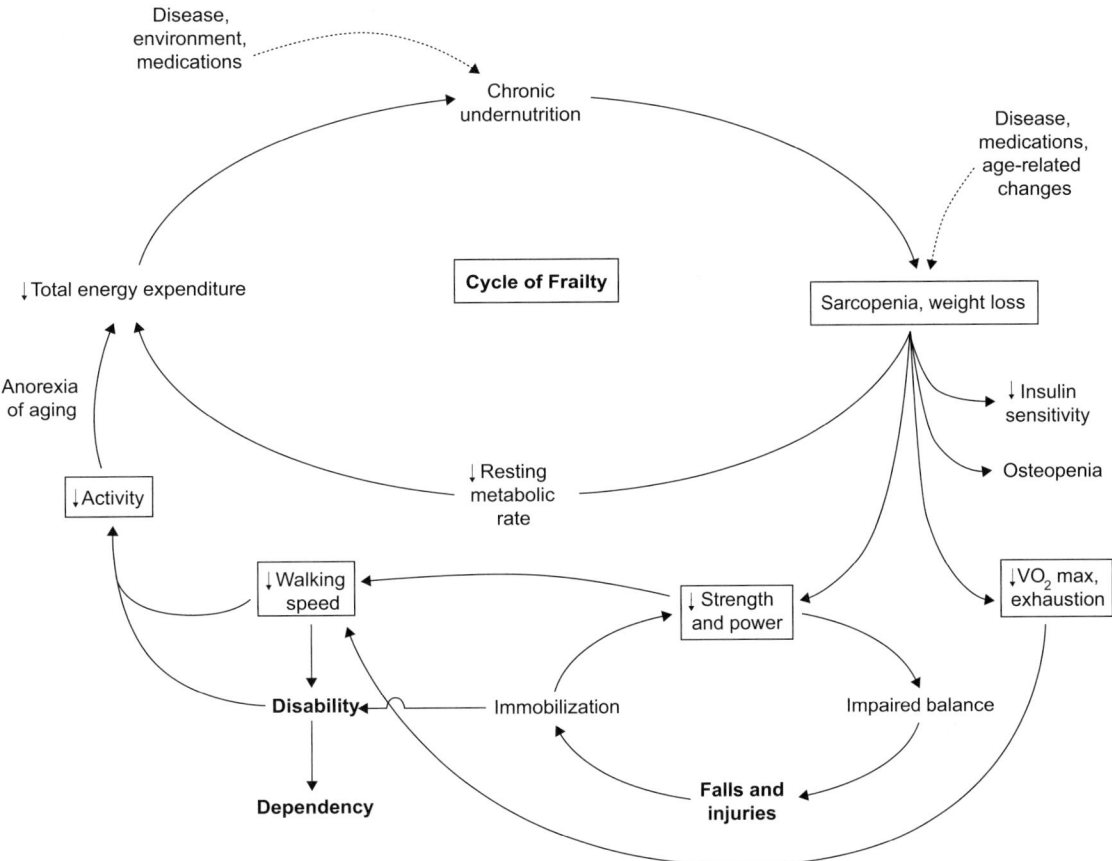

Figure 25.1—The Cycle of Frailty

SOURCE: Fried LP, Tangen CM, Walston J, et al. Frailty in older adults: evidence for a phenotype. *J Gerontol A Biol Sci Med Sci.* 2001;56(3):M146–156. Reprinted with permission by Oxford University Press.

frailty identify populations that overlap to a modest degree (SOE=A).

A phenotype has been developed and validated that links all aspects identified as clinical presentations of frailty (strength, balance, motor processing, nutrition, endurance, physical activity, mobility; note that cognition is excluded), based on the hypothesis that the clinical presentation of frailty results from dysregulated metabolic processes related to energy production, leading to the following:

- Decreased muscle mass, or sarcopenia, with resulting loss of strength
- Slowed motor performance (such as walking speed)
- Decreased physical activity
- Worsened exercise tolerance (or low energy or fatigue or exhaustion)
- Inadequate nutritional intake (even when physical activity is low)

The latter three result in further sarcopenia and, when nutritional intake is inadequate, weight loss as well (Figure 25.1). Research has shown this construct is consistent with the definition of a clinical syndrome, and that it is chronic and progressive, with early stages generally predicting progression to more severe frailty. Progression is not inexorable, however, because some afflicted individuals may show improvement. Early stages of frailty are likely most amenable to intervention. The first manifestations of frailty tend to be weakness, slowed walking speed, and/or decreased physical activity.

Observations to date support the concept of frailty as a clinical syndrome, the manifestations of which become apparent when physiologic dysregulation reaches a critical threshold. It has recognizable causes at the level of both altered physiology and potentially altered genetic, cellular, and molecular processes.

In this model, physical frailty is distinguished from disability, although clinically an individual may display both. In disability, a person has a physical or mental impairment that substantially limits one or more major life activity. In frailty, the presence of the criteria described above identify an individual who has reduced ability and reserve for adapting to stress, whatever their functional state. So, a functionally normal person could be frail but at high risk of decline and even disability after a stressor, while an individual who is disabled from an accidental injury may have intact physiologic compensatory mechanisms and thus not be frail.

Many patients present for medical attention without the full syndromic definition of frailty, and clinicians caring for older adults should be adept at constructing a differential diagnosis for such individuals. Evaluation for weight loss, depression, medication effects, occult malignancies, endocrine abnormalities, and neurologic decline should be considered.

EVIDENCE AS TO CAUSE

Primary Frailty

Sarcopenia, or loss of lean body mass, is a central manifestation of physical frailty and a key predictor of the other clinical manifestations. Predictors of loss of muscle mass and strength with aging include decreased anabolic factors such as testosterone and IGF-1, diminished physical activity, reduced nutritional intake (including protein, energy, vitamin D, and other micronutrients), and older age itself.

Although the fundamental underlying cause of frailty is still unknown, the intermediate process appears to entail the dysregulation of a critical number of physiologic systems. In addition to sarcopenia, systemic abnormalities include a pro-inflammatory state (indicated by increased IL-6 and C-reactive protein), decreased immune function, anemia, glucose intolerance, increased insulin resistance, low levels of DHEA-S and IGF-1, increased cortisol, low testosterone, decreased heart rate variability, and nutritional derangements (low levels of certain vitamins and carotenoids, reduced intake of protein and energy). The number of abnormal systems is a stronger predictor of frailty than dysfunction in any one system, and there is evidence that abnormal physiological systems synergistically interact to increase frailty risk. There is no evidence to date that intervention on any one system modifies frailty risk.

In frail older adults, dysfunction in a physiologic system may not be apparent at rest but is unmasked by a stressor. For example, in a resting state, levels of blood glucose and insulin may be in normal ranges but after a glucose tolerance test, levels are increased and return to baseline is delayed in those who are frail compared with those who are not.

Secondary Frailty

A variety of primary diseases independently predict development of the frailty phenotype, potentially through inflammation and/or their effect on cardiopulmonary function and inactivity. Such diseases include immune disorders (eg, HIV/AIDS), heart failure, COPD, and chronic infections (eg, cytomegalovirus, HIV, tuberculosis). Data on HIV-positive men indicate that HIV infection, even in the absence of clinical AIDS, is associated with rates of a frailty-like presentation that would be found in HIV-negative men who are 10 years older. Additionally, frailty in association with HIV/AIDS predicts a lower response to therapy and a worse prognosis than HIV infection alone. Similarly, there is early evidence that frailty is a risk factor for intolerance of some cancer chemotherapies and worse outcomes after kidney transplantation.

ASSESSMENT OF FRAILTY

To date, frailty assessment has not been fully integrated into clinical practice, in part because of a lack of clear evidence as to how best to manage frail patients once they are identified. Despite this, it is abundantly clear that frail older adults are at much higher risk of adverse outcomes in the face of clinical interventions and, therefore, may well benefit from closer observation in stressful clinical situations. Although the benefits of screening for frailty have not been conclusively demonstrated, an international consensus conference has recommended that adults at least 70 years old be screened. The presence of frailty can be determined by use of several established methods. The approach chosen may differ depending on the setting and goal. In the clinical setting, assessing older adults for frailty is appropriate to identify those at risk of adverse medical or surgical outcomes and to gauge the severity of risks, find those who may benefit from prevention or treatment, track change in status over time, or determine eligibility for palliative care for those at end stage.

Frailty can be assessed in several different ways:

- For frailty as a clinical syndrome with a distinct phenotypic presentation, determining the number of criteria present (out of 5) offers a standardized approach to diagnosis and stage of severity.

- Some rapid screening/assessment tests have been developed and validated, such as the interview-based FRAIL scale. These may be sensitive in clinical settings but should be followed up using more specific evaluations for the syndrome of frailty.

- For frailty as a clinical composite or "gestalt," an instrument providing a clinical global impression of change in frailty has been validated. Called the Clinical Global Impression of Change in Physical Frailty (CGIC-PF), it draws on clinical judgment and incorporates intrinsic domains (mobility, balance, strength, endurance, nutrition, neuromotor performance) as well as outcome/consequence domains (medical complexity, healthcare use, appearance, self-perceived health, ADLs, emotional status, and social status).

- Walking speed predicts mortality and mobility disability. It, along with grip strength, is an early manifestation of frailty, and can serve as a marker in screening (SOE=A).

The cumulative number of symptoms, signs, illnesses, and disabilities present is useful to characterize aggregate morbidity burden, and those present can be combined into an index of accumulated deficits, which predicts risk of mortality.

PREVAILING MANAGEMENT STRATEGIES

Comprehensive geriatric assessment and management is a clinical care model designed to optimize outcomes for frail older adults, particularly preservation of their independence. This team-based, multidisciplinary approach results in positive effects on polypharmacy, falls, functional status, and nursing-home admission, and reduces mortality. The assessment should include accurate screening for frailty, including assessment of gait speed, combined with ongoing, expert geriatric care. The focus of care should be 1) to exclude any modifiable precipitating causes of frailty, particularly those that are treatable or environmental; 2) to improve the clinical manifestations of frailty, especially low physical activity, strength, exercise tolerance, and nutrition; and 3) to minimize the consequences of the vulnerability of frail older adults, by directing attention to environmental risks, extent of social support, falls prevention, and the risks from stressors such as acute illness or injury, hospitalization, or surgery. Frail adults subject to such stressors should be provided support for a potentially prolonged recovery. Resistance, or strengthening, exercise, with added nutritional support, particularly protein-calorie supplementation, appears to be a key management approach for frailty and for its prevention (SOE=C). This can be supplemented by walking for exercise and balance training.

The approach that many older adults use to adapt to age-related psychosocial losses and behaviors can also be applied to challenges in physical health and frailty. In the face of diminished resources or reserves, older adults must carefully choose their goals, focus on optimizing the abilities needed to reach their goals, and then compensate for any diminished competencies by increased reliance on other functions or by replacement. Such compensations could include services such as "meals on wheels" or supportive residential environments that offer personal care or meals if needed. Clinical management needs to include such approaches for care of frail older adults, as well as more standard medical approaches, as described above. Further, implementing systematic approaches to decrease the stress of environments such as hospitals, surgical centers, and rehabilitation facilities may be effective as well. For severe frailty, palliative care or hospice may be appropriate, depending on severity and patient preferences.

POTENTIAL APPROACHES FOR PREVENTION OF FRAILTY

Points of Vulnerability and Precipitants

Exposure to any of a variety of stressors appears to put frail older adults at risk of adverse outcomes and may precipitate clinically apparent frailty in those already at risk. Immobility is one key precipitant, causing frailty to develop or worsen, as well as accelerating the onset of adverse outcomes such as dependency. This holds regardless of whether immobility results from pain, illness, or in the context of hospitalization or surgery. Depression may be another precipitant, given its association with decreased activity, energy, and nutritional intake, as well as with inflammation and social isolation. (Depression also appears to be an outcome of frailty as well as a precipitant.) Overall, attention should be paid to minimizing these precipitants or the stress associated with them, through systematic screening, case finding, and quality improvement approaches. Evidence supporting the benefit of such efforts in the context of frailty is limited.

Potential Pharmacologic Treatments

Although vitamin D deficiency has been associated with physical frailty, no large-scale study has demonstrated a significant treatment effect on frailty with vitamin D repletion. Similarly, replacing deficiencies of any one hormone or repleting defects in other systems as a sole intervention has not been demonstrated to prevent or ameliorate frailty. Theoretically, this is understandable, given that the number of deficits in multiple physiologic systems most strongly predicts frailty, rather than the presence of any one deficit alone. This suggests that improving only one system (eg, immune, hormonal, musculoskeletal) may not be clinically effective, and future effective drug treatments will likely be those that target multiple systems simultaneously. The prototype of such approaches, along with comprehensive geriatric assessment and management, has decreased polypharmacy and related adverse medication events in frail older adults (SOE=A).

Behavioral Approaches to Prevention or Treatment

Maintaining physical activity and muscle mass is critical in older adults at risk of frailty. Evidence is substantial that resistance, or strengthening, exercise is effective in increasing muscle mass, strength, and walking speed in frail older adults, such as nursing-home residents (SOE=A). Other forms of exercise, including stretching, Tai Chi, and aerobic exercise, are also helpful. Prevention of immobility is critical. Overall, exercise has proven beneficial physiologic effects on sarcopenia, inflammation, and other systems associated with frailty, making maintenance of physical activity as well as strength a cornerstone of prevention, "prehabilitation," and treatment. Importantly, randomized controlled trials of exercise interventions have demonstrated increased gait speed and reduced functional limitations. It remains to be determined if they can prevent or ameliorate frailty and disability.

Consumption of a Mediterranean diet lowered the risk of becoming frail over 6 years in community-dwelling adults ≥65 years old. More broadly, attention to preventing nutritional inadequacy is important, including supplementation of protein, calories, and micronutrients. In many studies, nutritional supplementation appears to be effective only when added to exercise.

FRAILTY AND PALLIATIVE CARE

Frailty predicts functional decline and onset and progression of dependency at the end of life. Severe frailty, with 4 or 5 syndrome characteristics, and metabolic abnormalities of low cholesterol and albumin predict particularly high short-term mortality rates in frail older adults (SOE=B); these characteristics can be considered to mark a pre-death phase of severe frailty. Clinical case series document a poor response to treatment in those with end-stage frailty, and the adoption of palliative approaches for such patients may be appropriate.

RESOURCES

- Buta B, Choudhury PP, Xue QL, et al. The association of vitamin D deficiency and incident frailty in older women: the role of cardiometabolic diseases. *J Am Geriatr Soc.* 2017;65(3):619–624.

- Cesari M, Vellas B, Hsu F-C, et al. A physical activity intervention to treat the frailty syndrome in older persons—Results from the LIFE-P Study. *J Gerontol A Biol Sci Med Sci.* 2015;70(2):216–222.

- Chang SF, Wen GM. Association of frail index and quality of life among community-dwelling older adults. *J Clin Nurs.* 2016;5(15):2305–2316.

- Uchmanoqicz I, Jankowska-Polanska B, Wleklik M, et al. Frailty syndrome: Nursing interventions. *SAGE Open Nursing.* 2018;4(7).

CHAPTER 26—VISUAL LOSS AND OTHER EYE CONDITIONS

Key Points

- Visual loss, defined as visual acuity worse than 20/40, increases exponentially with age and affects 20%–30% of the population ≥75 years old. Blindness, defined as visual acuity of 20/200 or worse, affects 2% of the population ≥75 years old. Those ≥65 years old make up 12% of the total U.S. population but 50% of the blind population.

- Cataracts and refractive error are common reasons for visual loss.

- Age-related macular degeneration (ARMD) is a common cause of visual loss in individuals >65 years old. ARMD can be categorized as nonexudative or exudative, and both forms can cause severe vision loss. Antioxidant multivitamins can slow the progression of nonexudative ARMD to exudative ARMD.

- Glaucoma is common, and increased intraocular pressure is no longer required to meet diagnostic criteria. Screening for glaucoma should be done every 1–2 years after age 50 and more often in high-risk individuals.

- Control of blood glucose and blood pressure in type 2 diabetes can delay the onset and slow the progression of diabetic retinopathy. Glycemic and blood pressure control needs to be sustained to achieve significant benefit.

- Chronic eye disease and visual loss can have a significant impact on the quality of life of older adults.

The American Academy of Ophthalmology recommends a comprehensive eye examination every 1–2 years for adults ≥65 years old. Prophylactic and therapeutic ocular management can effectively alter the course of various conditions that cause visual loss. About one-third of all new cases of blindness can be avoided with effective use of available ophthalmologic services. Older adults with eye complaints frequently first seek care from their primary care provider. Common complaints include red eye, ocular swelling or discomfort, blurred or sudden loss of vision, diplopia, and floaters. "Has your vision changed?" is a key question that helps determine whether a patient can be treated by the primary care provider as opposed to needing a referral to an ophthalmologist. For this reason, it is vitally important to check visual acuity in each eye separately with the patient's current corrective aid (eg, eyeglasses) in place for any eye complaint.

Common Eye Conditions

Many changes common with aging involve the eyes and surrounding structures (Table 26.1). Consequences of these changes range from cosmetic concerns to discomfort and disease predisposition. Lid abnormalities are a common problem for older adults. Because of the gradual loss of elasticity and tensile strength that occurs with age, secondary degenerative changes can develop. Blepharochalasis (drooping of the brow) and blepharoptosis (drooping of the eyelid) can cause cosmetic deformity and, if severe, can cause visual loss. Lid ectropion or entropion (ie, eversion and inversion of the lid margins, respectively) can disrupt the ocular surface and cause discomfort. These conditions can be addressed by various surgical procedures. Ocular lubricant ointments (those without antibiotics) can be recommended to minimize discomfort from exposure of the globe. Older adults can also develop squamous cell and basal cell carcinomas of the eyelids. Ulcerations or chronic irritation, especially if associated with loss of eyelashes, should be evaluated by an ophthalmologist. In addition, older adults frequently develop nasolacrimal tear duct obstruction that prevents tears from exiting into the nose, which causes chronic epiphora leading to blurry vision. Patients can be offered surgery if the epiphora is highly symptomatic.

Significant vision loss can be indicated by the presence of a relative afferent pupillary defect, which can be assessed using a "swinging flashlight test." While in a dark room, the patient is asked to stare into the distance. A bright flashlight is then placed in front of one eye to check the pupillary light reflex; the other eye should also constrict because of the consensual light reflex. The flashlight is then quickly swung over to the second eye. If this eye dilates, there is an afferent pupillary defect (ie, the second eye is not detecting the light as the first eye detects it).

For serious eye conditions requiring immediate attention by an ophthalmologist, see Table 26.2. All of the listed conditions are usually associated with a decrease in vision that can be profound but masked by good vision in the other eye. The symptoms of a retinal detachment include new floaters in one eye along with photopsias (the perception of flashes of light), distorted peripheral vision, or decreased vision. Ocular pain and hyperemia do not accompany a retinal detachment; the

Table 26.1—Common Aging Changes of the Eye and Consequences

Change	Finding	Functional Consequence
Eyelids		
Laxity of eyelid tendons	Entropion (turning in of lid) Ectropion (turning out of lid) Ptosis (drooping of lid)	Eyelashes rub and irritate eye, chronic tearing, drying of eye; ptosis blocks visual axis, particularly when looking down to read
Atrophy of periorbital fat	Sunken eyes	Cosmetic
Tear ducts		
Stenosis of nasolacrimal duct	Chronic tearing	Blurred vision
Reduced production of tears	Reduced tears	Dry eye, irritation
Cornea		
Lipid deposition in cornea	Arcus senilis (white ring in peripheral cornea)	Cosmetic
Sclera		
Calcium deposition among scleral fibers	Ovoid zone of grayish translucency on sclera	Cosmetic, sometimes confused for a pigmented tumor
Lens		
Lens thickening	Anterior chamber shallowing	Predisposes to an acute attack of angle-closure glaucoma
Changes in lens proteins	Cataracts	Blurred vision
Pupils		
Unknown etiology	Pupil size shrinks	Difficulty in dim light, glare
Intraocular drainage		
Thickening of basement membranes in trabecular meshwork	Increased intraocular pressure	Glaucoma
Vitreous		
Liquefaction	Posterior vitreous detachment	Floaters and retinal tears
Retina		
Decreased phagocytotic activity of cells	Accumulation of drusen	Macular degeneration

Table 26.2—Common Signs and Symptoms of Eye Conditions Requiring Immediate Referral to an Ophthalmologist

Condition	Symptoms and Signs
Retinal detachment	Flashes, floaters, decreased vision, "curtain over vision"
Acute angle-closure glaucoma	Eye pain or headache, ocular hyperemia, dilated pupil, decreased vision, nausea, vomiting
Ischemic optic neuropathy	Sudden painless loss of vision (complete or partial) in one eye
Central or branch artery occlusion; giant cell arteritis	Sudden painless loss of vision in one eye or in superior/inferior hemifield in case of branch occlusion; if from giant cell arteritis, review of symptoms may reveal accompanying jaw claudication, headache, transient diplopia, etc. Artery occlusion requires stroke protocol evaluation within 2 weeks of event.
Central or branch retinal vein occlusion	Sudden painless blurring of vision or loss of vision; in central occlusion, vision loss is diffuse; in branch occlusion, loss is either superior or inferior
Scleritis	Eye redness, severe pain and/or tenderness, decreased vision
Posterior uveitis	Floaters, decreased vision
Corneal ulcers	Eye redness, pain, decreased vision, corneal infiltrate
Anterior uveitis	Photophobia, eye redness, decreased vision
Herpes zoster ophthalmicus	Eye redness, pain, burning, rash, decreased vision, light sensitivity

only signs a primary care provider may detect are a relative afferent pupillary defect, decreased vision, or a monocular visual field deficit. Signs and symptoms of acute angle-closure glaucoma include an injected eye with fixed, dilated pupil and cloudy cornea; the patient is often in severe pain, nauseated, and/or vomiting. Acute angle closure can be precipitated by sympathomimetic and anticholinergic drugs. In ischemic optic neuropathy, vision in one eye is lost suddenly, usually in the upper or lower hemifield (this can be detected on visual field testing by confrontation). Giant cell arteritis must be excluded quickly in patients

Table 26.3—Treatment of Eye Conditions Commonly Seen by Primary Care Providers

Condition	Treatment and/or Cause
Red eye	
Subconjunctival hemorrhage	Supportive treatment with artificial tears
Dry eye	Artificial tears, cyclosporine 0.2% eye drops
Blepharitis	Lid scrubs, ophthalmic antibiotic ointment qhs, oral doxycycline
Lid malposition/exposure	Ocular lubricant, refer for surgical repair
Allergic conjunctivitis	Cold compresses, allergen avoidance, topical/systemic antihistamines
Viral conjunctivitis	Supportive treatment with artificial tears; refer to ophthalmologist if vision significantly affected
Chalazion	Warm compresses, may refer for excision
Herpes simplex keratitis	Trifluridine eye drops, refer to ophthalmologist
Herpes zoster ophthalmicus	Tear drops, refer to ophthalmologist
Angle-closure glaucoma	Pilocarpine 2% ophthalmic solution, refer to ophthalmologist immediately
Floaters, flashes	Refer to ophthalmologist immediately; may be retinal detachment or vitreous hemorrhage
Sudden decrease in vision	Refer to ophthalmologist immediately; may be secondary to a number of vision-threatening problems
Diplopia	
Monocular	Refractive error, cataract
Binocular	Microvascular infarct to cranial nerve, giant cell arteritis, compressive tumor

with ischemic optic neuropathy to prevent bilateral blindness. Diplopia and central retinal artery occlusion can also be the result of giant cell arteritis. Retinal vein occlusions, which are usually found in patients with systemic hypertension, diabetes, and/or hyperlipidemia, present as sudden, painless vision loss diffusely (if central) or in one hemifield (if only one branch vein is involved). Funduscopic examination may reveal prominent retinal hemorrhages and cotton wool patches. Bacterial keratitis usually presents with pain and a corneal infiltrate. Scleritis is frequently associated with significant autoimmune disease; symptoms include boring pain, decreased vision, and a red eye. Posterior uveitis presents with decreased vision and floaters.

RED EYE

Red eye is an extremely common eye complaint, the cause of which may be benign or malignant (Table 26.3). Hyperemia of the eye can accompany any inflammation or infection. Causes of red eye that require referral include corneal ulcers (which are usually accompanied by a visible white infiltrate on the cornea), anterior and posterior uveitis, herpes simplex and herpes zoster ophthalmicus, scleritis, angle-closure glaucoma, ocular surface tumors, and postoperative infections. The reason for referral is to prevent permanent vision loss, which can be the end point of any of these conditions. Although it is sometimes difficult to differentiate one cause from another without a slit lamp examination, signs and symptoms that should prompt referral are decreased vision, severe pain, photophobia, recent intraocular surgery, or even distant surgery (especially if glaucoma surgery).

Relatively benign causes of red eye include blepharitis or inflammation of the Meibomian glands in the eyelids, dry eye, allergic conjunctivitis, corneal exposure due to lid malposition, viral conjunctivitis, and subconjunctival hemorrhages. Blepharitis and dry eye often present together because blepharitis affects the integrity of the tear film, which then evaporates more readily. Tears serve several important functions, including corneal lubrication, debris clearance, and immune protection. Tear production decreases with age, and older adults are prone to develop keratitis sicca, characterized by redness, foreign body sensation, and reflex tearing. Patients may complain of severe eye discomfort and blurred vision, which usually improves with blinking or eye rubbing because these two maneuvers spread the remaining tear film over the cornea. Dry eye can be especially problematic in older women, in whom hormonal changes are thought to play a role. Keratitis sicca can also be associated with autoimmune disease; conditions such as Sjögren syndrome should be excluded. Management of dry eye includes tear replacement with artificial tears during the day (preservative-free tears if being used more than four times daily) and a lubricant ointment at bedtime. Topical cyclosporine A (0.2%) eye drops can be used for more severe cases of dry eye to combat the underlying ocular inflammation that affects tear production; however, caution is warranted in patients with a history of ocular herpetic infections. If there is a severe tear deficiency, an ophthalmologist can place punctal plugs to retain what tears are made. Treatment for accompanying blepharitis includes lid hygiene,

Table 26.4—Adverse Events of Selected Eye Drops for Glaucoma

Class	Adverse Events
Aqueous suppressants	
α-Agonists (eg, brimonidine)	Allergic dermatoconjunctivitis, dry mouth/nose, mental status changes occasionally
β-Blockers (eg, timolol)	Bradycardia, dyspnea, asthma, heart failure exacerbations, impotence, exercise intolerance, hypoglycemia masking
Carbonic anhydrase inhibitors (eg, dorzolamide)	Blurry vision, stinging, bad taste in mouth, allergic dermatoconjunctivitis
Aqueous outflow facilitators	
Miotics (eg, pilocarpine)	Brow ache, blurriness, detached retina, small pupils
Prostaglandins (eg, latanoprost)	Hyperemia, increased length and thickness and darkness of eyelashes, increased iris and eyelid pigmentation, orbital fat atrophy, cystoid macular edema, exacerbation of herpetic eye disease
Rho kinase inhibitors (eg, netardusil)	Hyperemia

consisting of gentle scrubbing of the lash bases with nontearing baby shampoo twice daily or OTC eyelid cleansing pads and applying topical antibiotic ointment to the eyelids nightly. Oral doxycycline can also be a useful adjunct, especially when blepharitis is associated with acne rosacea. If symptoms continue despite these conservative measures, referral is warranted.

Subconjunctival hemorrhages are very common and, despite being benign, elicit worried responses from patients. Patients may be on anticoagulant medications, and minor trauma, such as eye rubbing, can cause a small conjunctival blood vessel to leak blood in the subconjunctival space.

Herpes zoster ophthalmicus, or shingles, is a painful reactivation of varicella zoster virus that not uncommonly affects older adults. Dermatomal distribution of weeping vesicles affecting the ophthalmic branch of the trigeminal nerve is the classic presentation. Ocular involvement can be signaled by lesions on the tip of the nose (Hutchinson sign) and can include dendritic keratopathy or uveitis. Oral antiviral therapy can shorten the course of disease. Trifluridine eye drops are indicated for herpes simplex dendriform corneal ulcers (not for herpes zoster). Postherpetic neuralgia can be quite debilitating; systemic medications (narcotics, tricyclic antidepressants[OL], gabapentin, pregabalin) can reduce pain.

Viral conjunctivitis (or pink eye) is associated with severe tearing, mucous discharge, and matting of the eyelids, especially in the morning. Symptoms include eye irritation and blurred vision. Viral conjunctivitis is distinguished from bacterial conjunctivitis by history and, because it is highly contagious, patients frequently report either an upper respiratory tract infection or recent contact with someone suffering from a red eye. Viral conjunctivitis is treated conservatively with warm compresses and artificial tears; topical antibiotics are not indicated. If it is accompanied by severely reduced vision, the patient should be referred for an ophthalmologic examination, because corneal infiltrates can (rarely) develop, requiring steroid eye drops. Viral conjunctivitis is extremely contagious (by contact), and patient education is necessary to limit spread of the infection to the other eye or to contacts (including office staff).

Allergic conjunctivitis is a common benign condition; its hallmark is ocular pruritus. Management of allergic conjunctivitis includes cool compresses, systemic antihistamines, topical antihistamines or decongestants, and ophthalmic corticosteroids (if severe) for limited periods of time.

OPHTHALMIC CORTICOSTEROIDS

The use of ophthalmic corticosteroids merits comment. Ophthalmic steroid drops or ointment can have serious potential adverse events, including risks of ocular hypertension and glaucoma development (which can be asymptomatic for a long period of time), secondary infections, cataract formation, and corneal thinning if used in undiagnosed infections. Prescriptions for any steroid-containing eye medication should never be refilled without ophthalmic evaluation. Ocular hypertension that can lead to glaucoma can develop within 2–3 weeks with daily use of topical steroids in susceptible individuals (those with glaucoma, either diagnosed or undiagnosed, or with a family history of glaucoma). Low-potency steroids given for 7–10 days will not be problematic for the vast majority of patients, but patients and caregivers should be warned of the risks of prolonged and unmonitored use of steroids in and around the eyes.

REFRACTIVE ERROR AND CATARACTS

The leading causes of visual loss worldwide are refractive error and cataracts, for which eyeglasses and surgical cataract extraction, respectively, are mainstays of treatment.

Refractive error can be categorized as emmetropia (neutral refraction), ametropia, or presbyopia. Three forms of ametropia exist: myopia (nearsightedness), hyperopia (farsightedness), and astigmatism (distorted vision). Although contact lens wear and laser refractive surgery are available for myopic and hyperopic refractive errors, these forms of refractive treatment are not favored by older people. Corneal refractive surgery, such as LASIK, is not the best remedy for refractive problems in older adults who usually have some degree of cataracts. Removal of the cataract and replacement with an artificial intraocular lens, the power of which can be chosen to eliminate refractive error, is a better option in older adults. Toric intraocular lenses can correct astigmatism, and multifocal lenses can decrease the need for eyeglasses after surgery. After the age of approximately 40, emmetropic individuals begin to develop progressive presbyopia, loss of ability to focus on near objects that is caused by gradual hardening of the lens and decreased muscular effectiveness of the ciliary body. Reading glasses can be obtained OTC, or bifocal eyeglasses can be prescribed.

Approximately 20% of adults ≥65 years old and 50% of adults ≥75 years old have cataracts, a lens opacity that reduces vision. Cataracts are associated with decreased visual acuity that is not correctable by glasses, glare symptoms, changes in color perception, and decreased contrast sensitivity. The most important risk factor is increased age; other risk factors include decreased vitamin intake, light (ultraviolet B) exposure, smoking, alcohol use, long-term corticosteroid use, and diabetes mellitus.

Cataract extraction is one of the most successful surgeries in medicine (90% of patients achieve vision of 20/40 or better). Approximately 3 million cataract procedures are performed each year in the United States. The benefits of cataract surgery include not only improved vision but also a decreased rate of falls and improved vision-related quality of life (SOE=A).

Indications for cataract surgery are a decrease in vision that affects ability to perform activities of daily living. Cataract extraction is safe and can be completed in <30 min under local or topical anesthesia. The surgery involves the use of ultrasound energy and vacuum aspiration to simultaneously break down and remove the lens (phacoemulsification). An artificial implant (intraocular lens) is placed in the residual lens capsule, which is the only remnant of the native lens retained. A secondary laser procedure (capsulotomy) may be necessary to ablate subsequent capsular opacification that can develop in ≥15% of patients. Reasons for not attaining visual acuity of 20/40 or better include diseases of the retina and optic nerve that limit best correctable vision.

AGE-RELATED MACULAR DEGENERATION (ARMD)

ARMD is the most common cause of irreversible blindness in older adults throughout the developed world. It is a multifactorial disease involving age-related changes and multiple genes and environmental interactions. Currently, there is no role for genetic screening as a clinical tool, because it is not yet clear how to use this information. The percentage of patients who harbor these gene mutations and who will subsequently develop disease is unknown. Other risk factors include smoking and hypertension. Exposure to ultraviolet light is a debated risk factor. Researchers are currently exploring links between ARMD and Alzheimer disease. The two diseases share the accumulation of amyloid beta within brain plaques and drusen, respectively, which may contribute to angiogenesis.

ARMD is classified into two forms: nonexudative and exudative, also called dry and wet. The nonexudative form is much more common and is characterized by deposits of drusen, submacular yellow lipoprotein aggregates composed of metabolic by-products. Although drusen do not typically cause vision loss, they may be harbingers of the exudative form of the disease. The presence of larger, more numerous drusen confers a greater risk of development of CNV. The 2001 Age-Related Eye Disease Study (AREDS) found that the risk of CNV development could be decreased by 25% (absolute risk reduction [ARR] of 8% for progression to advanced ARMD, and 6% for loss of vision of 3 lines or more) when patients with high-risk drusen were treated with high-dose oral multivitamin therapy (SOE=A).

Patients with the nonexudative form of ARMD should be examined periodically by an ophthalmologist for development of early signs of CNV. CNV in exudative ARMD is characterized by the presence of a subretinal gray-green membrane, which may be associated with subretinal fluid and/or blood. The development of exudative ARMD is typically associated with sudden vision loss or distortion of vision and requires urgent evaluation because delay in treatment can lead to severe, irreversible central vision loss. The natural history of CNV is progressive subfoveal leakage with eventual fibrotic scarring and central blindness.

Angiogenesis inhibition has proved to be a major breakthrough in treatment of CNV. Inhibitors of vascular endothelial growth factor (VEGF) approved by the FDA for treatment of exudative ARMD include ranibizumab and aflibercept. Bevacizumab, also an anti-VEGF medication, is currently not approved by the FDA for intraocular use but is widely used off-label for exudative ARMD, mainly because of its lower cost. In a multicenter, prospective randomized clinical trial, visual acuity improved by approximately 2 lines in patients with CNV treated with ranibizumab compared with those given sham treatments. Serial intravitreal injections of anti-VEGF medications are now the gold standard of care for all subtypes of exudative ARMD (according to data from the pivotal ANCHOR and MARINA trials). In 2012, the Comparison of AMD Treatments Trial (CATT), sponsored by the National Institutes of Health, published results from a 2-year multicenter randomized controlled trial that compared ranibizumab and bevacizumab, injected either monthly or as needed, for exudative ARMD in which the primary outcome measure was visual improvement. Visual improvement was similar in both groups. Serious adverse events (primarily hospitalizations) occurred at a 24% rate for patients receiving bevacizumab and a 19% rate for patients receiving ranibizumab. However, the number of deaths, heart attacks, and strokes were low and similar for both drugs during the study.

DIABETIC RETINOPATHY

Duration of disease, control of blood glucose, and control of blood pressure are the most important variables in the development and progression of diabetic retinopathy. After 10 years, 70% of those with type 2 diabetes have some form of retinopathy, and nearly 10% show proliferative disease. The Diabetic Control and Complications Trial demonstrated that tight control of blood glucose in individuals with type 1 diabetes resulted in a long-lasting decrease in the rate of development and progression of diabetic retinopathy. The United Kingdom Prospective Diabetes Study (UKPDS) validated these results in an older population with type 2 diabetes.

More recent data from the ACCORD and ADVANCE studies have raised the question of whether intensive glycemic control is of enough benefit to outweigh the risks of hypoglycemia. The ACCORD study was terminated early because of excessive mortality in the intensive control group (relative risk increase 20%, absolute risk increase 1.0%, number needed to harm 100) and showed no significant benefit with respect to macro- or microvascular disease. The ADVANCE study showed reductions in microvascular disease; however, the significant benefits were in reductions of albuminuria rather than retinopathy. The results of these studies prompted significant controversy in both the lay press and the medical literature and led the American Diabetes Association, the American Heart Association, and the American College of Cardiology to issue a revised position statement in 2009 about the value of intensive control in type 2 diabetes mellitus. In this statement, the recommended hemoglobin A_{1c} target remains 7.5%–7.9%; however, it notes that targets should be individualized and that patients with limited remaining life expectancy, those with longstanding diabetes mellitus, and those with preexisting vascular disease are less likely to benefit from intensive control. Many older patients fall into the latter categories; thus, the benefits of intensive control need to be very carefully weighed against the potential for harm. The risk of hypoglycemia is significantly greater in those who are frail, demented, or otherwise unable to comply with medical regimens.

Other systemic risk factors, including kidney disease and increased serum cholesterol, can also influence the course of diabetic retinopathy and should be optimized. ACE inhibitors decrease progressive nephropathy in diabetic patients and may have similar benefits on the retina.

Patients with type 2 diabetes require baseline ophthalmologic screening at diagnosis and annually thereafter. Subsequent follow-up depends on the grade of retinopathy. Nonproliferative diabetic retinopathy, the earliest stage of retinopathy, can first be manifested by retinal microaneurysms. Intraretinal hemorrhages and exudates, with or without associated macular edema, can ensue. The preproliferative stage of diabetic retinopathy is characterized by progressive ischemia with increasing hemorrhages, venous caliber changes or intraretinal microvascular abnormalities or both, and capillary nonperfusion on fluorescein angiography. About 40% of patients with preproliferative retinopathy develop proliferative diabetic retinopathy within 1–2 years, characterized by neovascularization or new blood vessel growth of the retina or disc, or both.

Visual loss in patients with diabetes can occur as a result of macular nonperfusion or macular edema. In 1985, the Early Treatment Diabetic Retinopathy Study demonstrated the benefit of focal or grid laser photocoagulation in stabilizing and improving vision in diabetic patients with clinically significant macular edema. More recently in 2013, the Study of Ranibizumab Injection in Subjects with Clinically Significant Macular Edema with Central Involvement Secondary to Diabetes Mellitus (RIDE and RISE trials) established anti-VEGF injections as the gold standard treatment for diabetic macular edema. Compared with laser therapy, monthly intravitreal injections of ranibizumab were associated with significantly greater visual gains, greater anatomic reduction of macular edema, reduced rate of progression of retinopathy and even improved grade of retinopathy. Intravitreal injection of a slow-releasing steroid (dexamethasone) implant has also been FDA approved for treatment of diabetic macular edema. Steroid injection should be used with caution because it increases the risk of cataracts and glaucoma.

Neovascularization in proliferative diabetic retinopathy is the most important cause of severe vision loss or blindness in diabetic patients. Neovascularization can result in both vitreous hemorrhage and retinal detachment. Proliferative diabetic retinopathy is amenable to treatment by panretinal laser photocoagulation to inhibit the growth stimulus for neovascularization. In the Diabetic Retinopathy Study, incidence of severe visual loss in patients treated with panretinal photocoagulation was 11%, but the incidence in those who did not receive laser during a 2-year follow-up was 26% (ARR=15%, NNT=6–7). Intravitreal anti-VEGF injections are also used in proliferative retinopathy to expedite regression of neovascularization. Pars plana vitrectomy, membrane peeling, and endolaser are surgical methods of addressing nonclearing vitreous hemorrhage or tractional retinal detachment.

GLAUCOMA

Glaucoma is the second most common cause of irreversible blindness worldwide and the most common cause of blindness in black Americans. It affects more than 2.25 million Americans ≥40 years old and results in >3 million office visits each year. The financial burden is considerable because of the prevalence and chronicity of glaucoma and the debilitation that results.

The definition of glaucoma has evolved considerably, and it is now defined as characteristic optic nerve head damage and visual field loss. Increased intraocular pressure (IOP) is no longer considered an absolute criterion, although it is a very important risk factor. There are many different types of glaucoma, of which primary open-angle glaucoma (POAG) is the most common. Adults >50 years old should be screened for glaucoma every 1–2 years. Older adults with a family history of glaucoma, black ethnicity, or other risk factors may need more frequent screening.

POAG is a chronic disease most commonly affecting older adults. Its development is probably multifactorial and polygenic. In POAG, the "clogged" drain of the eye impairs passage of aqueous humor out of the angle. Slow aqueous drainage leads to chronically increased IOP. This is in contrast to acute angle-closure glaucoma, in which the eye's drain is suddenly blocked off, IOP increases precipitously, and the patient has considerable redness and pain with acute vision loss. Pain may be so severe as to cause headache, nausea, and vomiting. Emergent ophthalmologic referral is required to reverse the angle closure and decrease IOP through the use of aqueous suppressants, miotics, and laser iridotomy. Conversely, the increase in IOP in POAG is slow and much less severe. Individuals with POAG are initially asymptomatic and can suffer substantial field loss (insidiously tending toward tunnel vision) before consulting an ophthalmologist, which underscores the importance of regular ophthalmologic screening of older adults.

The management of POAG is approached by the ophthalmologist in a stepwise manner. A variety of IOP-lowering medications, both local and systemic, are available. Mechanisms of action include decreased aqueous production or increased aqueous outflow. Various eye drop formulations are available, and all have some adverse effects (Table 26.4). In the face of visual field progression despite maximal medications, intolerance of medications, or inability to comply with eye drop administration (eg, because of problems such as rheumatoid arthritis or dementia), laser trabeculoplasty (application of laser energy to the trabecular meshwork) can be effective in lowering IOP in approximately 50% of patients for 3–5 years after treatment. Intraocular surgery involves the creation of a fistula to allow an alternative route of aqueous egress (trabeculectomy). Adjunctive antimetabolite use with 5-fluorouracil[OL] or mitomycin-C[OL] has increased the success of this procedure in those patients at high risk of surgical failure because of fibrosis and scarring of the filtration site. Alternative surgeries for glaucoma include aqueous shunts. These devices, made of silicone, shunt fluid from the anterior chamber to the subconjunctival space. Newer mini shunts, which are frequently implanted at the time of cataract surgery, are made of different materials that shunt aqueous fluid to different spaces (into Schlemm's canal or the space between the choroid and sclera). Cryotherapy or laser procedures to destroy the ciliary body (cyclocryoablation or cyclophotocoagulation) can be used when the prognosis for vision in the eye is poor.

The strength of evidence is high in support of treating ocular hypertension to prevent the onset of glaucoma and of treating prevalent glaucoma to slow down progression of disease. Based on a meta-analysis of the literature, 12 ocular hypertensive patients need to be treated to prevent 1 patient from developing visual field defects or optic nerve changes consistent with glaucoma (SOE=A). From a meta-analysis of literature on treatment of established glaucoma patients, the NNT to prevent 1 glaucoma patient from progressive vision damage within 5 years of treatment is 7. The ARR is 14.2%.

ANTERIOR ISCHEMIC OPTIC NEUROPATHY

Anterior ischemic optic neuropathy can result in acute vision or field loss. Microvascular occlusion of the blood supply to the optic nerve can be attributed to atherosclerotic vascular disease or inflammation in the setting of giant cell (temporal) arteritis. The nonarteritic form typically affects patients with vasculopathic risk factors such as diabetes mellitus and hypertension; the arteritic form tends to occur in older adults with a history of myalgias, headaches, and weight loss. An increased Westergren erythrocyte sedimentation rate and a positive temporal artery biopsy are diagnostic of arteritis, and systemic corticosteroid treatment is crucial to avoid visual loss in the other eye.

CHARLES BONNET SYNDROME

Between 10% and 13% of patients with significant vision loss (bilateral acuity worse than 20/60) experience visual hallucinations, a condition known as Charles Bonnet syndrome. Hallucinations may be elementary shapes, or, more commonly, they are complex and highly organized with patients seeing small children, multiple animals, or a vivid scene as from a movie. Patients with this syndrome have a clear sensorium and are aware that the visions are not real. It has been suggested that this syndrome is an analogue of the phantom limb syndrome. Underlying conditions include age-related macular degeneration, glaucoma, diabetic retinopathy, and cerebral infarction. If the cause of vision loss is known and there is no homonymous visual field defect present, neuroimaging is not necessary.

The best treatment for Charles Bonnet syndrome is education, reassurance, and support. Patients should be informed that the hallucinations are a sign of eye disease, not mental illness. An occasional patient has partial insight or loses insight and becomes very distressed by this symptom. When this distress is significant or leads to dangerous behavior, a cautious trial of low dosages of a second-generation antipsychotic medication can be considered.

LOW-VISION REHABILITATION

Despite considerable advancements in the medical treatment of ocular conditions, many patients, especially those with the wet form of ARMD, can sustain permanent visual loss that impedes independent functioning. Visual training and the provision of visual aids are indispensable services for those with low vision (visual acuity <20/60).

Various low-vision aids are available to improve the ability to see both near and far. The fine detail required for reading is the most common indication for visual aids. Improved lighting is a simple modification that can enhance visualization of print. Selection of reading material using bold, enlarged fonts and accentuated black-on-white contrast can be helpful. Magnification is commonly used through various devices such as high-plus spectacles, hand-held magnifiers, stand magnifiers, and closed-circuit television to enhance reading ability. Distance magnification can be achieved with the use of telescopic devices that are hand-held for spot viewing or spectacle mounted for continual viewing. Talking devices, which are computers used to create voice synthesis such as those used at stoplights, or Braille can be especially helpful for those who have completely lost vision. Downloadable smart phone apps that provide magnification, money recognition, and dictation functions are also available.

> ### CHOOSING WISELY® RECOMMENDATIONS
>
> **Visual Loss**
>
> - Do not perform preoperative medical tests for eye surgery without specific indications.
>
> - Most cases of acute conjunctivitis have a viral etiology. Do not treat viral infections with antibiotics; if diagnosis is uncertain, patients may be followed closely for resolution.
>
> **Diabetes Mellitus**
>
> - Avoid using medications to achieve hemoglobin A_{1c} <7.5% in most adults ≥65 years old; moderate control is generally better.

RESOURCES

- Jacobs L. Could links between our senses and cognitive health explain parts of how we age? Experts like the sound of that, according to new AGS report. *Geriatr Nurs*. 2018;39(5):613–615.

- Jonas JB, Aung T, Bourne RR, et al. Glaucoma. *Lancet*. 2017;390(10108):2183–2193.

- Shekhawat NS, Stock MV, Baze EF, et al. Impact of first eye versus second eye cataract surgery on visual function and quality of life. *Ophthalmology*. 2017;124(10):1496–1503.

CHAPTER 27—HEARING LOSS

KEY POINTS

- Hearing loss is among the most common chronic diseases among older adults: 10% of adults 65–75 years old and 25% of those >75 years old have hearing loss.

- Treatment of hearing loss and attention to communication strategies can improve quality of life for individuals who have difficulty with hearing.

- Important issues when considering hearing aids for an older adult with hearing loss include the nature and degree of hearing loss, the person's ability to manipulate the aid and adapt to its use, and the person's social support and financial resources.

Hearing loss is the fourth most common chronic disease among older adults. Hearing loss is often assumed to be benign, but it has profound effects on quality of life. The psychological effects of hearing loss include family discord, social isolation, loss of self-esteem, anger, and depression. Epidemiologic studies suggest an association between hearing loss and cognitive impairment, and between hearing loss and reduced mobility. Hearing loss can also affect an older adult's interaction with clinicians, making history taking and patient education difficult. Treatment of hearing loss and attention to communication strategies can improve quality of life by facilitating interaction with family, friends, and caregivers. Studies indicate that use of a hearing aid can relieve symptoms of depression that are associated with hearing loss.

NORMAL HEARING AND AGE-RELATED CHANGES IN THE AUDITORY SYSTEM

The normal ear is an efficient transducer of sound energy into nerve impulses. Sound energy is transmitted through the external ear to the tympanic membrane and the auditory ossicles. The malleus, incus, and stapes in series transmit vibrations to the oval window of the cochlea. Fluid waves within the cochlea stimulate the outer hair cells of the scala tympani. These cells stimulate the inner hair cells, which generate impulses that are sent via cochlear neurons to the cochlear nuclei and then to auditory pathways elsewhere in the brain.

Age-related changes in the auditory system can interfere with its function. The walls of the external ear canal become thin. Cerumen becomes drier and more tenacious, increasing the likelihood of cerumen impaction, which in turn leads to conductive hearing loss (CHL). The tympanic membrane becomes thicker and appears duller in older adults than in younger people. The ossicular joints undergo degenerative changes, but this generally does not interfere with sound transmission to the cochlea. Cochlear changes include loss of sensory hair cells and fibrocytes in the organ of Corti, stiffening of the basilar membrane, calcification of auditory structures, and cochlear neuronal loss. Changes in the stria vascularis include thickening of capillaries, decreased production of endolymph, and decreased Na^+/K^+-ATPase activity. These degenerative changes occur to varying degrees in different individuals. It is currently not possible to fully correlate the degree of hearing loss with histologic changes in the aging ear.

Changes in central auditory processing also occur with aging. In one study, when competing speech stimuli were presented to each ear, the right ear had a 5%–10% advantage over the left ear in younger people (the effect of right- and left-handedness was not assessed; all the participants were right-handed). In adults 80–89 years old, this difference increased to >40%. This difference may be related to a loss of efficiency of transfer of auditory information from one side of the brain to the other through the corpus callosum.

EPIDEMIOLOGY

Hearing loss can result from dysfunction of the auditory system at any point from the external ear to the brain. This loss can be described in terms of the loss of ability to hear pure tones across the range of audio frequencies important for understanding speech, but in practical terms, difficulty in understanding spoken language and perceiving environmental sounds significantly affects quality of life. The prevalence of hearing loss increases with age. Hearing loss is present in 10% of adults 65–75 years old and in 25% of those >75 years old. In nursing homes, estimates of prevalence vary from 50% to 100%, depending on the criteria used to define hearing loss.

In addition to age, male sex is a risk factor for hearing loss. Loss of hearing in the higher audio frequencies is associated with noise exposure; higher levels of education are associated with a lower prevalence of hearing loss. Black race is associated with a lower risk of age-associated hearing loss. The association of hearing loss with cardiovascular risk factors is less clear, with results differing among studies.

Hearing loss can be caused by pathology in the external ear canal, the middle ear, the inner ear, the auditory nerve, central auditory pathways, or a combination of these.

CHL is caused by disease in the external ear, such as cerumen impaction or a foreign body in the canal, or by middle-ear pathology, such as otosclerosis, cholesteatoma, tympanic membrane perforation, or middle-ear effusion.

Sensorineural hearing loss (SNHL) is most often caused by cochlear disease. Excessive noise is the most common factor in cochlear damage. Hearing loss is less common among people in quiet rural environments than among those in industrialized communities. Other causes of SNHL include ototoxic medications, genotype, vascular disease, and rarely, occupational and environmental chemical exposures. Smokers have higher rates of hearing loss than nonsmokers. Autoimmune disease and auditory nerve tumors are rare causes of SNHL. Neuronal loss can affect the brain stem and cortical ascending auditory pathways. The resulting deficits in central auditory processing can affect perception of sound and the ability to understand speech. These deficits are not apparent on a simple audiogram.

PRESBYCUSIS

Most hearing loss in older adults is categorized as presbycusis (literally, "older hearing"). Presbycusis is a sensorineural, usually symmetrical hearing loss. It is usually due to cochlear pathology but may have central components. Many people with presbycusis can be helped by amplification, especially if speech discrimination is preserved. The typical audiogram in presbycusis slopes from normal or mild SNHL at the low frequencies to severe or worse hearing loss at the high frequencies, and is symmetrical and bilateral. For an example of such an audiogram. Because of the increased hearing loss in the high frequencies where consonant sounds are perceived, speech discrimination may be poorer than the pure tone average might suggest. Early amplification, before the brain loses some ability to adapt to the auditory input, is of great importance in presbycusis.

Sensory presbycusis is attributed to a loss of sensory hair cells in the basal end of the cochlea. It results in a steeply sloping audiogram, with greater loss of hearing acuity at higher frequencies. It is often slowly progressive, beginning with the higher frequencies. Loss of auditory acuity can begin when people are in their twenties but may not become clinically evident until later decades. People with this type of hearing loss often have trouble hearing in the presence of background noise but are able to hear adequately in quiet settings.

Strial presbycusis typically begins between the ages of 20 and 60 years old and is characterized by mild to moderate hearing loss in most frequencies. People with strial presbycusis usually have good speech discrimination and do well with amplification.

Neural presbycusis is caused by a cochlear neuronal loss of ≥50%. Despite preserved pure-tone thresholds, which are not affected until >90% of cochlear neurons have been lost, individuals with neural presbycusis show very poor speech discrimination. Successful use of amplification is difficult for this form of presbycusis.

Cochlear or sensory hearing loss refers to changes in the cochlear microstructures, including hair cell or supporting cell loss or damage, stiffness of the basilar membrane, or strial or spiral ligament atrophy. With primarily cochlear presbycusis, most patients benefit from appropriately fit hearing aids. If they do not, consideration should be given to cochlear implantation.

Most presbycusis is probably a mixture of the forms described above. The shape of the audiogram and speech discrimination scores depend on the extent of injury to various components of the cochlea.

CLINICAL PRESENTATION AND DETECTION OF HEARING LOSS

Patients with hearing loss commonly do not to bring it to medical attention. Partly because of the slowly progressive nature of hearing loss, many older adults are unaware of their hearing deficit. They may also be unaware of advances in hearing instrument technology that can help people who did not benefit from older devices. In some cases, the perceived stigma of wearing a hearing aid causes the patient to deny the problem. The hearing loss may be brought to medical attention by family members, who complain that the patient does not hear them or plays the television or radio too loudly. Clinicians may notice that the patient does not respond when spoken to by someone out of the patient's field of view, or seems to misunderstand questions. Hearing loss can also be interpreted as cognitive impairment. Caregivers and clinicians may not recognize the presence of hearing loss or may assume it is a benign component of aging.

Tinnitus, or "ringing in the ears," can be an early sign of hearing loss. The etiologies of tinnitus are legion, but the possibility of medication-induced tinnitus should always be considered. Individuals with tinnitus or buzzing should be evaluated by an otolaryngologist. Medical treatment for tinnitus is often unsuccessful, but hearing aids for those with hearing loss, or the use of devices that provide background white noise, may be useful to reduce the impact of tinnitus.

Fitting hearing aids early in the course of hearing loss can help the person adjust to their use (SOE=B), and treatment can reduce psychological morbidity related to hearing loss (SOE=A). Hearing aid use may reduce the frequency of behavioral problems in older adults who have both hearing loss and dementia. Robust evidence that treatment of hearing loss can prevent or reduce cognitive decline is lacking.

Hearing loss assessments can include questionnaires, testing with speech or pure tones, or a combination of these assessments. The best screening tool is to ask the patient and/or family members the following questions: "Do you notice that you are having trouble hearing or understanding other people?" "Have family/friends complained that your television volume is too loud?" "Do you have any difficulty following conversations in restaurants or other noisy settings?" "How often do you do things with friends? Is it less than you'd like because you're having trouble hearing what's going on?"

Clinicians should ask each patient about hearing loss. If the patient denies it, questions like those above should be asked (eg, complaints about television volume). The HHIE–Screening Version is a 10-item questionnaire that asks about difficulty with communication in various settings. It can be useful to determine the impact that hearing loss has on a patient's daily activities. A 512-Hz tuning fork allows for a quick, inexpensive screen to distinguish SNHL from CHL or mixed hearing loss (MHL). The two common tests conducted using tuning forks are the Weber and Rinne tests. In primary care settings, the finger rub test, whisper test, and simply asking about hearing loss are easily and rapidly performed, and also have reasonable sensitivity and specificity.

For the Weber test, the fork is vibrated on the knee or elbow (not on a metal or wood surface) and placed on the midline of the face at the forehead, bridge of nose, or on the upper incisors if they are not artificial. Patients are asked where they hear the sound. A normal response is "everywhere" or "in both ears" or "in the center of my face." Patients with SNHL may give a normal response or may indicate that they cannot hear the sound. Patients with CHL or MHL will usually localize the sound to the hearing-impaired ear. For the Rinne test, the fork is vibrated as above. It is placed first on the mastoid bone, and that sound is indicated to the patient as sound #1. The fork is then placed close to (but not touching) the external auditory meatus, and that sound is indicated to the patient as sound #2. The patient is asked which sound is louder. Normal is that air conduction (sound 2) is louder than bone conduction (sound 1). The test should be done on each ear, and results recorded accordingly.

A handheld otoscope with a tone generator can be used by primary care providers to assess for the presence of hearing loss at selected frequencies (0.5, 1, 2, and 4 kHz) and two loudness levels (25 and 40 dB hearing loss). This device should be used in a quiet environment. When set at 40 dB hearing loss, testing at 1 and 2 kHz has a sensitivity of 94% and a specificity of 82%–90% for detecting hearing loss. A similar device costs $660–$900 with accessories; the cost of using it would not be directly reimbursable by third-party payors. Smart phone apps are available that use pure-tone testing; online hearing tests may also be helpful for identifying hearing loss.

When hearing loss is detected by history and/or screening test, referral for complete audiometric evaluation is recommended. If there is asymmetric SNHL or CHL or MHL, referral to an otolaryngologist is necessary.

EVALUATION OF SUSPECTED HEARING LOSS

The clinician should exclude causes of hearing loss that are readily treatable or that warrant referral to an otolaryngologist before signing medical clearance forms for hearing aids (see Table 27.1). The ear canals should be examined with an otoscope to exclude the presence of obstruction or effusion before referral for audiologic testing. Medications should be reviewed for their potential contribution to hearing loss. Furosemide and salicylates can cause reversible hearing loss. Other medications, such as aminoglycosides and vancomycin, can cause irreversible SNHL and should be used only with caution.

Cerumen impaction can cause a clinically significant hearing loss, as much as 40 dB. If the patient has a history of tympanic membrane surgery or perforation, referral to an otolaryngologist for removal of the impaction is advisable. Otherwise, cerumen can be removed by manual extraction in cooperative patients. Cerumenolytics alone, used for several days, are effective about 40% of the time in treating cerumen impaction. Alternatively, cerumenolytics or saline can be applied to soften the wax 15–30 min before irrigating the ear with warm water. If irrigation fails, using a cerumenolytic for several days may clear the impaction or soften it enough that repeat irrigation is successful. It is important for the clinician to ascertain that there is no history of ear surgery (including tubes), tympanic membrane perforation, or other ongoing chronic otitis before offering irrigation as a means of cerumen removal. If the impaction remains, the patient should be referred to an otolaryngologist.

A subset of patients (Table 27.1) with hearing loss should be referred for otolaryngological evaluation. An asymmetrical hearing loss demands thorough investigation. Auditory nerve tumors are rare, but tumors of the posterior pharynx can obstruct the eustachian tube, causing a middle-ear effusion with CHL.

Audiologists assess hearing to determine the presence and type of hearing loss. A comprehensive audiologic assessment consists of pure-tone thresholds for both air and bone conduction, speech-recognition thresholds, speech discrimination, and middle-ear function. This information, along with the medical

Table 27.1—Indications for Medical Evaluation of Hearing Loss

- Unilateral or asymmetrical hearing loss*
- Sudden or recent onset hearing loss (within the last 90 days)*
- Suspected or visualized tympanic membrane perforation*
- Acute or chronic dizziness
- Air-bone gap ≥15 dB at 500, 1000, and 2000 Hz*
- Visible congenital or traumatic ear deformity*
- Pain or discomfort in the ear
- Active drainage from the ear within the previous 90 days
- Visible deformity of the outer ear
- Cerumen impaction or foreign body in the ear canal
- Cerumen impaction with history of tympanic membrane surgery or perforation*

*Indication for referral to an otolaryngologist. Other problems may be addressed by a primary care practitioner.

evaluation, is used to determine appropriate treatment. Audiologists recommend and fit hearing aids and provide auditory rehabilitation. Medicare will pay for an audiologic examination if it is ordered by a physician.

TREATMENT

Some causes of hearing loss are amenable to medical or surgical treatment. Paget disease of the bone can affect the middle ear, causing CHL, or the inner ear, leading to SNHL. Bisphosphonate therapy rarely restores hearing in these patients, although it may stabilize hearing loss (SOE=C). Otosclerosis or tympanosclerosis may be correctable with surgery (SOE=C). Otosclerosis may respond to bisphosphonate therapy (SOE=C). Sudden hearing loss may be autoimmune in nature and sometimes responds to corticosteroids (SOE=B) or immunosuppressive therapy (SOE=C). Most older adults with hearing loss are treated with communication strategies or amplification, or both. Hearing aids often improve ability to understand speech, particularly soft speech and conversational loud speech (SOE=B). Almost all hearing aids currently sold use digital sound processing to limit noise to comfortable levels and to reduce feedback, and have dual microphones for reduction of background noise. Some have automatic volume control.

Surgical treatment of SNHL may include implantation of prosthetic devices (see bone-anchored hearing aids and cochlear implants, below).

Strategies to Enhance Communication

Individuals with hearing loss should be encouraged to let others know about their hearing loss and to suggest strategies that will help them communicate more easily (Table 27.2). In addition to using these strategies, clinicians should provide options for patients with hearing loss, such as sign language interpreters, the use of writing materials (eg, pen and paper, dry-erase board, or computer screen), or assistive devices. Office and hospital staff should be alerted to a patient's hearing loss. Background noise from the environment can interfere with hearing and should be reduced as much as possible.

Lipreading and looking at facial expressions can be useful adjuncts to listening but require thoughtfulness on the part of the speaker. When speaking to a person with hearing loss who lip-reads, it is important to face him or her and to obtain the person's attention before speaking; a gentle touch on the hand or arm will usually suffice. Each word should be spoken clearly and distinctly. Shouting not only distorts lip movements so they are harder to read but also can make the speaker sound angry. It is best to speak in complete sentences; single words are hard to lip-read because the listener often needs cues from context to identify meaning. It is helpful to make certain the person knows the topic of conversation. The language used should be appropriate for the listener's educational level. Unlike deaf persons who have usually had hearing loss all or most of their lives, most older adults with hearing loss do not know sign language. Sometimes, amplification and lipreading are not enough. Gestures can aid communication even with cognitively impaired individuals.

For patients with hearing loss, it can also be helpful to write words down. For those with both hearing loss and visual impairment, large printing with a marker pen or a laptop computer screen with magnified print may be necessary. These patients may benefit from correction of the visual problem, if possible (eg, cataract removal or use of eyeglasses). In any case, providing written instructions generally improves understanding and retention of important information.

The clinician should be alert to misunderstandings, which are common. If a reply does not make sense, repeating the idea of what was said using different words can help, as can asking the patient to express what he or she heard.

Assistive Listening Devices

For some people with hearing loss, a personal amplifier may be more useful than hearing aids. These pocket-sized devices are considerably less expensive than hearing aids and are harder to misplace. Headphones stay on the head better than earbuds and provide sound to both ears. The volume and microphone placement of the amplifier should be adjusted to find the best combination for a given user. At least one or two of these devices should be available in every health care facility; these devices are not personalized and so can be used by different people. If a portable amplification device is not available, one approach is to place a stethoscope into the patient's ears and have the examiner talk into the bell. It is important that the examiner *not* cover his or her own mouth with the bell, because this impedes lipreading on the part of the patient. This is an easily implemented, low-tech, and often effective way to improve communication with patients who have hearing loss. Additionally, it makes patients more aware of the degree of communicative disability they are experiencing from hearing loss.

Adaptive equipment can facilitate telephone use. State agencies may provide amplified telephones, vibrating and flashing ringer alert devices, and text telephones (TTY) or captioned telephones to people with hearing loss. This equipment can also be purchased from retailers of assistive devices. Text telephones can be contacted through telecommunications relay services by dialing 711, then the number. A communications assistant transcribes the caller's voice into text that is displayed for the listener. Captioned telephones and Web-based captioning services allow the user to hear the caller's voice and then to read a transcription of the caller's voice during the call.

Many other assistive devices are available. Television listening devices can spare others from overly loud volume levels. FM loop systems can be used for groups of people with FM receivers or telecoil switches in their hearing aids. Wireless FM transmitters and receivers are also available for indoor or outdoor use. Infrared group-listening devices are primarily useful indoors. Vibrating and flashing devices such as alarm clocks and timers, smoke alarms, doorbell alerts, and motion sensors can improve quality of life and safety for people with hearing loss. These items can be purchased through the agencies mentioned above, or from catalog retailers of assistive listening devices.

Electronic communication such as text messaging and e-mail can be helpful for patients and caregivers with hearing loss. However, measures to protect patient confidentiality must be considered when using these mediums.

Hearing Aids

Hearing aids are the most common form of amplification. Many factors need to be considered in deciding whether to fit an individual with a hearing aid. In addition to the nature and degree of hearing loss, the person's motivation and ability to adapt to use of the aid and to physically manipulate the aid (Table 27.3), the degree of social support, and the ability to afford the aid (Table 27.4) must be considered. Although hearing aids can be purchased from numerous sources, including over the Internet, working with an audiologist or other individual who has master's level training in audiology

Table 27.2—Strategies to Improve Communication with People Who Have Hearing Loss

- Ask the listener what the best way is to communicate with him or her.
- Obtain the listener's attention before speaking.
- Eliminate background noise as much as possible.
- Be sure the listener can see the speaker's lips:
    Speak face-to-face in the same room.
    Do not obscure the lips with hands or other objects.
    Make certain that light shines directly on the speaker's face, not from behind the speaker.
- Speak slowly and clearly, but avoid shouting.
- Speak toward the better ear, if applicable.
- Change phrasing if the listener does not understand at first.
- Spell words out, use gestures, or write them down.
- Have the listener repeat back what he or she heard.

is advisable because of his or her expertise in fitting and adjusting hearing aids.

Not everyone benefits from a hearing aid. The pattern of sensorineural damage can be such that speech discrimination is poor even with amplification. Some individuals are unable to tolerate the presence of a hearing aid in the ear. It is important to be sure that the aid can be returned during an initial trial period, usually 30 days, without having to pay the full cost of the aid. It is equally important not to give up on a hearing aid too soon, because an audiologist often can adjust it to improve comfort and sound quality. The audiologist should provide counseling for optimal use of the aid. In general, two hearing aids are more beneficial than one. The first aid provides the most gain; the second one helps with speech discrimination and with localizing the source of sounds. However, the presence of asymmetrical hearing loss or significant difficulty in understanding competing speech stimuli may mean that use of a single hearing aid is more appropriate.

Many different styles of hearing aids are available (Table 27.3). Behind-the-ear aids hang behind the ear and are connected directly to an earmold. The earmold is usually custom made to fit each ear. Some behind-the-ear aids can be connected to assistive listening devices via a "boot," which fits over the end of the aid to provide direct audio input. Some models of hearing aids can be used with Bluetooth devices, including mobile telephones, remote microphones, and computers. Body aids are worn on the belt or in a pocket or harness, and they are connected to a custom-made earmold by a wire; these are rarely used. All-in-the-ear aids and canal aids usually have cases that are custom fit to the user.

Table 27.3—Advantages and Disadvantages of Styles of Hearing Aids

Style	Degree of Hearing Loss	Advantages	Disadvantages
Completely in the canal (CIC)	Mild to moderate	Almost invisible Less occlusion of ear canal allows more natural sound Easier to use with headphones and telephone	Dexterity may be a problem. Small size may limit available features. May cost more than canal or in-the-ear aids Shorter battery life
Canal	Mild to moderate	More cosmetic than larger aids Telecoil* available in some models May be able to use with headphones	Dexterity may be a problem. Small size may limit available features.
In the ear	Mild to severe	Ease of handling Comfortable fit Available options: telecoil, directional microphone More power than CIC or canal aid	More conspicuous than CIC or canal aid May be difficult to use with headphones
Behind the ear	Mild to profound	Greatest power Available options: telecoil, direct audio input, directional microphone, wireless connectivity with mobile telephones and other devices Earmold can be changed separately	More conspicuous May be more difficult to insert than in-the-ear aids Difficult to use with headphones
Body aid	Severe to profound	Greatest separation of microphone from receiver reduces feedback	Most conspicuous Body-level microphone is subject to noise from clothing. Microphone is on chest or at waist, but speech is usually directed at ear level.
Bone conduction aid	Mild to severe	Bypasses middle ear; used if ear canal is unable to tolerate aid or earmold, or for unilateral hearing loss	Receiver of traditional aid causes pressure on the scalp, which can be uncomfortable; does not correct sensorineural loss. Being replaced by bone-anchored hearing aids

*A telecoil is the small copper coil that serves as the hearing loop wireless receiver and that enables the hearing aid user to use a phone (conventional or cellular) without feedback.

The smaller hearing aids may have remote controls. Selection of aid style for each individual depends on the degree of hearing loss, available features, and the person's dexterity and motivation.

The telecoil is an induction coupling coil built into the hearing aid that detects the magnetic field produced by hearing aid–compatible telephones. The telecoil is used to listen to the telephone with less distraction from noise in the same room. It can also be used with many assistive listening devices. The amount of coupling, and therefore the volume of the signal, depends on the angle of the telecoil with respect to the magnetic field. Users may need to experiment to find the right angle. Strongly magnetic devices such as computer monitors often produce interference, which also depends on the angle and the distance of the telecoil from the device. These drawbacks aside, the telecoil is a useful feature and can be added to hearing aids at relatively low cost. Individuals with moderate to severe hearing loss should be encouraged to consider purchasing an aid with a telecoil.

Analog hearing aids were first type available and are more affordable than digital aids but are rarely sold now. Digital technology has allowed improved sound quality, reduced size, and increased ability to customize the amplification of the aid to the needs of the user. Programmable aids are adjusted for each individual while he or she is wearing the aid. Often, 2 or more programs are available within a single aid. Using a computer, the audiologist makes adjustments to gain, response in different frequency ranges, and loudness balance for each program. One program may be most useful in the presence of background noise, whereas another works better in a quiet environment, and a third works with a telecoil. Patients with Ménière disease can have their aids reprogrammed to accommodate fluctuating hearing loss. Many hearing aids automatically adjust the volume to increase amplification of soft sounds while avoiding uncomfortable loudness, reducing the need for the user to manipulate the aid. This can be helpful for first-time users, although experienced users may require time to adjust to this feature. Hearing aids may have an automatic telecoil feature that switches to the telecoil program when a hearing-aid compatible telephone is brought close to the ear.

Background noise is a significant problem for hearing-aid users. Traditional hearing aids amplify sound indiscriminately, so that background noise,

Table 27.4—Approximate Costs of Assistive Listening Devices and Hearing Aids

Type of Technology	Cost	Comments
Assistive listening devices (eg, personal amplifiers, telephone amplifiers, television listening devices)	$100 and up	Useful for specific situations (see text for details)
Hearing aids		
	One aid/two aids	
Digital, economy	$1,200/$2,200	Economy aids process signals more slowly and have fewer programs. Telecoils are available on request. Background noise suppression may be switched on manually. Economy aids may be very appropriate for persons with a quiet lifestyle.
Digital, value	$1,500/$2,800	Multiple programs, telecoil
Digital, mid-range	$2,100/$4,000	Multiple programs, telecoil, Bluetooth input
Digital, premium	$2,800/$5,400	Multiple features available, including multiple programs, telecoil, Bluetooth input, and more rapid signal processing

NOTE: Assistive listening devices and hearing aids are not covered by Medicare. Features of hearing aids in a given price range vary by manufacturer.

eg, papers rustling or water running, can be very distracting. For new hearing-aid users, this problem can be addressed by having the audiologist gradually increase the gain of the hearing aid as the listener adjusts to being able to hear environmental sounds over the course of weeks. However, background noise in the presence of speech is a problem even for experienced hearing-aid users. The use of multiple microphones in the hearing aid, combined with digital signal processing, can decrease the effects of background noise. This can significantly improve the user's ability to understand speech and increase satisfaction with the aid. Most hearing aids now include noise reduction and feedback suppression.

Unfortunately, the cost of hearing aids is often a significant barrier to their use and can affect the patient's (purchaser's) choice of features (Table 27.4). The current cost of a digital hearing aid to the patient ranges from $1,200 to $4,000 per device, or $2,200 to >$7,000 for a pair, depending on the number and types of features desired, including Bluetooth and other capabilities. Analog hearing aids are less expensive but provide poorer sound quality and are being phased out by manufacturers. Very low-end amplifiers called personal sound amplification products can be useful in mild to moderate hearing loss and are significantly more affordable. They are inappropriate, however, for any hearing loss of a greater degree. Typically, the cost of the aid includes follow-up visits to the hearing-aid dispenser for the first 2–3 years after purchase, although some audiologists may unbundle the follow-up visits from the original fitting and purchase. Patients should be vigilant when contemplating the cost of these devices. Hearing aids can be expected to last 3–5 years, although they may last longer with good care.

Although hearing aid(s) are covered by Medicaid when it is the primary insurance in most states, the amount of reimbursement often does not cover aids with advanced features. Hearing aids are not covered by Medicare or by many private health insurance carriers, and often the coverage is limited even in the private arena. Federal programs such as the Department of Veterans Affairs pay for hearing aids if the recipient is eligible for services. Some charitable organizations assist in providing hearing aids to low-income persons.

In the United States, legislation (the Over-the-Counter Hearing Aid Act of 2017) now allows the FDA to regulate the sale of OTC personal sound amplification systems, which resemble hearing aids. Many types of devices are available, with ability to improve speech comprehension varying widely. Some devices are comparable to a hearing aid, some distort sound and can make comprehension worse, and some are loud enough to damage hearing. These devices are sold directly to consumers without a requirement for evaluation by an audiologist or hearing aid dispenser.

Caring for Hearing Aids

Hearing aids should be stored with the battery compartment door open; this may be the only way to turn the hearing aid off. They should be wiped with a dry cloth daily (earmolds of behind-the-ear aids should be cleaned according to manufacturer's instructions). Cerumen may plug the sound outlet of a hearing aid, and the manufacturer's instructions should be consulted before trying to clean it.

Patients may need assistance to insert the hearing aid. First, it should be noted whether the hearing aid goes into the right ear (the aid may be marked with red)

Table 27.5—Characteristics of Older Candidates for Cochlear Implants

- Severe to profound sensorineural hearing loss in both ears
- Functional auditory nerve
- Short duration of severe hearing loss
- Good speech, language, and communication skills
- Not benefiting enough from other kinds of hearing aids
- No medical contraindication to surgery (eg, active infection, inability to tolerate general anesthesia)
- Realistic expectations about results
- Appropriate support services available for aural rehabilitation after cochlear implant
- Adequate motivation and cognition to participate in aural rehabilitation

or the left ear (marked with blue). The battery door faces the outside of the ear. If there is a vent or a removal string, these are usually at the bottom. The following instructions apply to all except behind-the-ear aids:

The aid should first be turned on to be sure it is working. If so, a high-pitched squeal or vibration (feedback) should be heard; if no noise is heard when the volume is set at maximum, the battery should be replaced. The hearing aid should be oriented right side up, with the canal portion of the aid or earmold facing toward the canal. The wide, flat portion of an in-the-ear aid or earmold should be posterior. This part of the aid may need to be rotated so that it fits into the external ear, and the helix lifted gently to ease this part in. If there is feedback, the aid may be gently pushed to seat it more firmly into the ear. Turning the volume down may also reduce feedback.

Patients with dementia may inadvertently remove and dispose of an aid. To reduce this risk, it can be helpful to order a loop attached to the hearing aid case; a piece of fishing line can be attached to the loop and the other end of the line pinned to the patient's clothing to catch the aid when the patient removes it. In long-term care institutions, a system for collecting the aids each night and placing them in the patients' ears each morning may facilitate use of the aids, while also reducing the number that are lost.

Osseointegrated Implants

People with unilateral hearing loss, inability to tolerate an earmold or hearing aid in the canal, or CHL/MHL may consider an osseointegrated implant. An osseointegrated implant has a small titanium screw post that is surgically implanted in the skull behind and above the ear. This can connect, either via an implanted magnet or a percutaneous abutment, to an external speech processor. Osseointegrated implants are replacing bone conduction aids.

Cochlear Implants

For patients with severe to profound hearing loss who gain little or no benefit from hearing aids yet who are motivated to participate in the hearing world, cochlear implants can provide useful hearing (Table 27.5). A cochlear implant is an electronic device that bypasses the function of damaged or absent cochlear hair cells by providing electrical stimulation to cochlear nerve fibers. A receiver-stimulator and an intracochlear electrode array are surgically implanted. A headset is worn behind the ear. The headset microphone transmits signals to the speech processor, which filters and digitizes the sound into coded signals. The coded signals are sent to the cochlear implant, which then stimulates auditory nerve fibers in the cochlea, from which nerve signals are sent to the brain. Candidate patients must be able to tolerate general anesthesia and to participate in extensive pre-implant testing and post-implant training. Meningitis is a rare complication of cochlear implants.

The cochlear implant procedure is covered by most Medicare carriers and, with appropriate prior authorization, commercial insurance companies. Outcomes of cochlear implantation in the >65 age group are as good as in younger post-lingually hearing-impaired adults. Implantation criteria have changed from profound bilateral hearing loss to moderately severe to severe or worse hearing loss with speech discrimination as good as 60% in the ear to be implanted. Single-sided implants are also approved, in the case of a unilateral severe to profound hearing loss with normal or near-normal hearing in the other ear. Quality-of-life outcomes are excellent in the young-old and in the older-old (>75) population. This has to do with restoration of the ability to participate in the auditory world socially, with family, and at work. Cochlear implants do not restore normal hearing; however, postimplant hearing thresholds are almost always in the mild hearing loss range or better. The initial "robotic" sound is quickly manipulated by the brain to sound near normal, and patients do not report mechanical sounds any longer, fairly early on in their hearing experience with cochlear implants. Users should expect not only awareness of environmental sounds but also excellent closed-set speech discrimination, and most patients enjoy very good to excellent open-set speech discrimination. Many individuals with cochlear implants can use the telephone effectively, and a significant number enjoy music.

Currently, the first large cohort of individuals to receive cochlear implants in the United States will be ≥50 years old, with many of the adults who received implants in the late 1980s and early 1990s now in their 70s and 80s. All of the manufacturers, in working with cochlear implant surgical and audiology teams, have committed to life-long implant hearing care. Therefore, any new upgrade to the external processor portion of the implant can be retrofitted to even the oldest generation of internal implant. There is no reason for explantation and reimplantation other than for trauma or other very unusual circumstance that may have caused damage to the internal device. Medicare and commercial insurance carriers cover an external speech processor "upgrade" every 5 years, allowing patients to continue to take advantage of newer and more powerful and natural-sounding speech processing strategies no matter how long ago they were implanted.

RESOURCES

- Olson A, McKeich M. Assessment and intervention for patients with hearing loss in hospice. *J Hosp Palliat Nurs*. 2017;19(1):97–103.

- Reed NS, Betz J, Kendig N, et al. Personal sound amplification products vs a conventional hearing aid for speech understanding in noise. *JAMA*. 2017:318(1):89–90.

- Strawbridge WJ, Wallhagen MI. Simple tests compare well with a hand-held audiometer for hearing loss screening in primary care. *J Am Geriatr Soc*. 2017;65(10):2282–2284.

CHAPTER 28—DIZZINESS

KEY POINTS

- The classification of dizziness into vertigo, presyncope, dysequilibrium, mixed, or others may be useful in guiding patient evaluation; however, precise classification is often difficult, and multiple causes of the same symptoms are common.

- Dizziness is associated with increased fear of falling, functional disability, and depressive symptoms.

- Multiple factors can contribute to chronic dizziness.

- Expensive tests like electronystagmography, rotational chair testing, posturography, and neuroimaging, such as CT or MRI, are not routinely needed in the evaluation of dizziness.

- Multifactorial interventions can help in ameliorating chronic dizziness.

Dizziness ranks among the most common symptoms presented by older adults to primary care providers. The various and often nonspecific terms—lightheadedness, giddiness, wooziness, vertigo, spinning, floating, and imbalance—that patients typically use to describe dizziness add to the diagnostic and management challenge. Dizziness that continues >1–2 months is considered chronic. The prevalence of dizziness in adults ≥65 years old ranges from 4% to 30%. The wide prevalence range is related to differences in age, symptoms, and sample population among the various studies. The prevalence of dizziness is lower between the age of 65 and 69 years and increases as people get older. Dizziness is more common in women than in men.

Acute dizziness, which is independent of age, usually results from a disorder of one system. The causes, evaluation, and interventions are similar to those of chronic dizziness. The most common causes of acute dizziness are acute vestibular neuritis, cerebrovascular ischemia, and cardiovascular disorders resulting in hypotension. The approach to management in older adults is similar to that in younger patients.

Chronic dizziness is much more common in older adults than in younger adults, has a larger variety of contributing causes, and requires additional skill and patience to evaluate and manage successfully. This chapter focuses on chronic dizziness in older adults, which is commonly associated with increasing fear of falling, depressive symptoms, fall risk, and general functional disability.

CLASSIFICATION

Dizziness has been classified into 4 types of sensations: vertigo, presyncope, dysequilibrium, and other. A fifth type—mixed—results from a combination of two or more of the above and is the most common type of dizziness reported by older adults (Table 28.1).

Vertigo

Vertigo is an often episodic spinning or rotational sensation; objective vertigo ("the room is spinning") versus subjective vertigo ("I am spinning") results from disturbances in the vestibular system. The most common causes of vertigo are benign paroxysmal positional vertigo (BPPV) and Ménière disease. BPPV, an inner ear disorder, is characterized by sudden onset, seconds-long bouts of vertigo precipitated by certain changes in head position (rolling over in bed, gazing up or down). BPPV probably results from changes in endolymphatic pressure during head movements, resulting from dislodged otoconia in the semicircular canal. Ménière disease, an idiopathic inner ear disorder, is characterized by episodic vertigo, tinnitus, fluctuating hearing loss, and a sensation of fullness in the inner ear. Other causes of vertigo include idiopathic recurrent vestibulopathy and central vestibular lesions such as cerebrovascular disease and acoustic neuroma. Absence of spinning sensation does not exclude vestibular diseases, because patients with vestibular problems can describe dizziness as an imbalance, dysequilibrium, or other sensation. Patients with cervical dizziness secondary to cervical arthritis can also present with vertigo.

Presyncope

Presyncope, a feeling of faintness or lightheadedness, usually results from a cardiovascular problem causing brain hypoperfusion through postural hypotension. There is no specific definition of postural hypotension in older adults, but it is commonly defined as a drop in systolic arterial blood pressure of at least 20 mmHg and/or a drop in diastolic blood pressure of 10 mmHg after standing up from a supine position. However, older adults commonly describe dizziness on standing from a supine position without any orthostatic changes in blood pressure. Another common condition, postprandial hypotension, is defined as a decrease in systolic blood pressure of ≥20 mmHg in a sitting or standing posture within 1–2 hours of eating a meal.

Table 28.1—Classification of Dizziness

Type	Common Causes or Coexisting Conditions	Diagnostic Features	Treatment
Vertigo	Benign paroxysmal positional vertigo	History of episodic vertigo; rotational nystagmus; Dix-Hallpike maneuver confirms diagnosis	Epley maneuver is treatment of choice
	Meniere disease	Episodic vertigo lasting for a few hours; tinnitus; fluctuating hearing loss; sensation of fullness in ears; audiogram reveals sensorineural hearing loss (at low more than high frequencies)	Salt restriction, diuretics; vestibular suppressants may be helpful during acute attacks; in severe cases, may need surgical interventions, including endolymphatic decompression, vestibular nerve resection, and labyrinthectomy
	Ototoxic medications, eg, aminoglycosides, diuretics, NSAIDs	Presence of nystagmus, bedside vestibular function tests (eg, head thrust test can be abnormal)	Discontinue, substitute, or reduce dosage of offending medication
Presyncope	Cerebral ischemia secondary to orthostatic hypotension, cardiac causes, dehydration, medications, vasovagal attack, autonomic dysfunction secondary to diabetes, parkinsonism	Near fainting/lightheadedness when getting up from lying down or sitting position; orthostatic changes in blood pressure; investigations relevant to predisposing diseases	Treatment of specific cause, eg, proper hydration; dosage adjustment or removal of offending medications; slow rising from sitting or lying down position; graduated support stockings; physical therapy and/or occupational therapy; medications (eg, fludrocortisone, midodrine) as needed
	Postprandial hypotension	Near fainting/lightheadedness when getting up from lying down or sitting position; orthostatic hypotension usually within 45–60 min of eating	Frequent small meals; avoid exertion after meals; slow rising from sitting position; avoid antihypertensive drugs with or near meal time
Dysequilibrium	Vertebrobasilar ischemia and/or cerebellar infarcts/hemorrhages	History of dizziness usually associated with slurred speech; visual changes; one-sided weakness and/or gait ataxia; truncal ataxia; CT or MRI or magnetic resonance angiography scan may be helpful	Low-dose aspirin, clopidogrel, or extended-release dipyridamole/aspirin; rehabilitation
	Cerebellopontine angle tumor, eg, acoustic neuroma	History of vertigo or dysequilibrium, unilateral hearing loss, tinnitus; audiometry reveals sensorineural hearing loss more for higher frequencies; MRI is diagnostic	Surgery
	Parkinson disease	Bradykinesia; muscular rigidity; tremor; orthostatic hypotension	Drug therapy; rehabilitation therapy
	Peripheral neuropathy secondary to diabetes; vitamin B_{12} deficiency; idiopathic, etc	Decreased vibration or position sense; gait abnormality; hyperglycemia; low vitamin B_{12} level	Treatment of the underlying disease
	Cervical spine degenerative arthritis, spondylosis	Limitation of range of motion of neck; decreased vibratory or joint position sense; signs of radiculopathy or myelopathy; cervical spine radiologic abnormalities	Cervical or vestibular rehabilitation; cervical collar; surgery if needed
Other	Anxiety, depression, or psychosomatic disorders	Usually continual nonspecific dizziness; fatigue; poor appetite; sleep problems; somatic complaints; positive results on anxiety or depression screening scales	Psychotherapy and/or antidepressant therapy
Mixed	Medications: antianxiety drugs, antidepressants, anticonvulsants, antipsychotics, antihypertensives, anticholinergics	History of fatigue; dizziness often vague and can be continual, postural, or associated with confusion	Discontinue, substitute, or reduce dosage of offending medication
	Combination of any of the above causes	Combination of any of the above features	Multifactorial intervention

Dysequilibrium

Dysequilibrium, a feeling of imbalance or unsteadiness on standing or walking, usually results from visual or proprioceptive system abnormalities, with or without vestibular system involvement. Common contributing conditions include vision problems (eg, refractory errors, cataracts, macular degeneration), musculoskeletal disorders (eg, arthritis, muscle weakness, deconditioning after prolonged illness), proprioceptive disorders (eg, neuropathies), and gait disorders (eg, cerebrovascular stroke, Parkinson disease, cerebellar disorders).

Other Forms of Dizziness

Other forms of dizziness include a vague feeling other than vertigo, presyncope, or dysequilibrium. The patient may describe "floating," "lightheadedness," "wooziness," "spaciness," "whirling," or other nonspecific sensations. Patients with psychogenic dizziness commonly report anxiety or depressive symptoms. The psychiatric symptoms can primarily cause or contribute to the dizziness complaint in older adults.

Mixed Dizziness

Mixed dizziness, a combination of two or more of the above types, is the most common type of dizziness reported by older adults. It most likely results from combinations of diseases affecting the vestibular, CNS, visual, or proprioceptive systems. Systemic disorders like anemia, heart failure, diabetes mellitus, and hypothyroidism can contribute to instability or dizziness by affecting the sensory, central, or effector components. Although less commonly reported, carotid sinus hypersensitivity or carotid sinus syndrome can also cause dizziness. Patients with dementia often get fixated on being dizzy or unsteady.

Many medications can contribute to chronic dizziness through various mechanisms. Important classes of medications to consider in the dizziness evaluation include anxiolytics, antidepressants, antihistaminics, antihypertensives, aminoglycosides, anticholinergics, antipsychotics, and NSAIDs.

Research data indicate that chronic dizziness often has a multifactorial etiology. Chronic dizziness is associated with risk factors such as angina, myocardial infarction, stroke, arthritis, diabetes, syncope, anxiety, depressive symptoms, impaired hearing, and the use of medications in several classes. In a study of a large community sample and in another study in which patients attended a geriatric clinic, the complaint of chronic dizziness was associated with factors such as anxiety, depressive symptoms, postural hypotension, use of ≥5 medications, and impaired gait and balance (SOE=B). Complaints of chronic dizziness were more common in patients who had >5 of these risk factors than in those having <2 of these risk factors. Similar to delirium and falls, chronic dizziness can be thought of as a geriatric syndrome that prompts a multifactorial assessment and intervention strategy, which is likely more effective at alleviating symptoms than a standard disease-oriented approach.

EVALUATION

History

The clinical history begins with helping patients to describe their symptoms as precisely as possible, which is potentially daunting for those with multiple sensations. Patients should be encouraged to use their own words to distill the symptoms into specific sensations such as spinning, imbalance or unsteadiness, or fainting. Documenting the frequency and duration of dizziness, and whether changing head position exacerbates the dizziness, is important. Establishing whether symptoms peak at any specific time of day, such as after meals or first thing in the morning, is also useful. Patients should be asked about associated symptoms such as hearing loss, ear fullness, diplopia, dysarthria, and tinnitus. Patients with Meniere disease complain of recurrent dizziness associated with ear fullness and/or tinnitus along with fluctuating hearing loss. Patients with acoustic neuroma complain of hearing loss and tinnitus but not of ear fullness. Patients with Meniere disease, CNS diseases, and BPPV complain of recurrent dizziness, whereas patients with psychogenic and central dizziness usually complain of continual dizziness. Inquiring about precipitating factors such as after eating meals (postprandial hypotension), looking down or rolling over in bed (vestibular conditions), or standing from supine position (orthostatic hypotension) can suggest interventions, as well as corroborate timing of symptoms. Any evaluation must include a critical review of medications, including OTC medications. It is also important to elicit the impact on the patient's quality of life.

Physical Examination

The physical examination should begin with measurements of orthostatic changes in blood pressure. Nystagmus should be evaluated; horizontal or rotatory nystagmus usually indicates a peripheral vestibular lesion, whereas vertical nystagmus is seen in central lesions. Hearing and vision tests should be done, and the cranial nerves examined if vertebrobasilar ischemia or infarction is suspected. The "Timed Up and Go" test can be performed to look for gait and balance problems.

The following provocative tests of the vestibular system can be done at the bedside:

Dix-Hallpike maneuver: This is a useful test for diagnosis of BPPV. Ask the patient to sit on the examination table with the head rotated 30–45 degrees to one side. Instruct the patient to fix his or her vision on the examiner's forehead. The examiner holds the patient's head firmly in the same position, and moves the patient from a seated to a supine position with the head hanging below the edge of the table and the chin pointing slightly upward. The examiner notes the direction, latency, and duration of the nystagmus, if present. A demonstration of the Dix-Hallpike maneuver can be viewed at https://youtu.be/8RYB2QlO1N4 (accessed Feb 2019). The diagnostic criteria for BPPV include 1) paroxysmal vertigo along with a rotatory nystagmus, 2) latency for 1–2 seconds between completion of the maneuver and onset of vertigo and nystagmus, and 3) fatigability (decrease in the intensity of the vertigo and nystagmus with repeated testing).

Side-lying test: This is an alternative to the Dix-Hallpike maneuver for diagnosis of BPPV in patients with limited range of motion of the cervical spine, or when hyperextension of the neck is contraindicated. Ask the patient to sit sideways on the examination table such that there will be sufficient space for the patient to lie on his or her side and be fully supported by the table. The patient begins with the head rotated 45 degrees away from the side being tested. The examiner holds the head firmly in the same position while the patient moves from supine to lying on the side being tested, with the head fully on the table. The examiner notes the direction, latency, and duration of the nystagmus, if present.

Head-thrust test: Ask the patient to fixate on the examiner's nose. The examiner then rotates the head rapidly about 10 degrees to the left or right. In patients with a vestibular deficit, the eyes move away from the target along with the head, followed by a corrective saccade back to the target, whereas normal eyes remain fixed on the target without a saccade.

Diagnostic Testing

A small battery of laboratory tests, including hematocrit, glucose, electrolytes, BUN, vitamin B_{12}, folic acid, and thyrotropin, should be performed on all patients with chronic dizziness. An ECG should be done if a cardiac cause is suspected, and a Holter and event monitor only if suspicion of arrhythmia is strong. Tilt-table testing should be done only for select patients with postural hypotension or syncope. Audiometry assists in the evaluation of patients with tinnitus or hearing loss and helps differentiate between acoustic neuroma and Meniere disease.

Suspected vestibular disorders can be evaluated with vestibular function tests such as electronystagmography, and rotational testing. Electronystagmography helps in detecting unilateral vestibular dysfunction, whereas rotational chair testing helps in identifying bilateral vestibular loss. These tests should be used selectively, based on initial assessment.

Likewise, neuroimaging is not needed in all patients with dizziness. MRI provides better resolution than CT for posterior fossa lesions. However, in a community-based study of adults ≥65 years old, the similar prevalence of MRI abnormalities in the dizzy and nondizzy group led to the conclusion that routine MRI will not identify a specific cause of dizziness in most patients (SOE=B).

MANAGEMENT

Given the multifactorial nature of dizziness, it has been suggested that dizziness may be a geriatric syndrome. Therefore, a multifaceted approach to interventions can help treat chronic dizziness and reduce the impact on day-to-day functioning. Treatment of coincident symptoms from depression, anxiety, hearing loss, and vision loss can help reduce the disability arising from dizziness. Dizziness from medication responds to dosage adjustment or to withdrawal of the offending medication.

Vestibular suppressants, including antihistamines (eg, meclizine), provide effective symptomatic relief of vertigo but generally do not provide benefit in management of chronic dizziness or dysequilibrium. In general, meclizine should be used with caution because of its anticholinergic properties and potential adverse events in older adults. Long-term use should be avoided, because it suppresses central and vestibular adaptation and can thus eventually worsen or exacerbate dizziness. Similarly, long-term use of benzodiazepines should be avoided because they can cause memory impairment, increase the risk of falling, diminish vestibular compensation, and lead to dependence and addiction.

Vestibular rehabilitation therapy (VRT) can help suppress symptoms in patients with peripheral and central vestibular causes of dizziness. VRT includes different exercises such as vestibulo-ocular reflex adaptation exercises and habituation exercises. Vestibulo-ocular reflex adaptation exercises help the CNS to adapt to a change or loss in input of the vestibular system. Habituation exercises include a combination of exercises designed to provoke dizziness; the movements are repeated until they can no longer be tolerated. Initially, the exercises can worsen the dizziness, but over time (weeks to months) movement-related dizziness improves, likely because of central adaptation. VRT has been shown to improve dizziness as well as quality of life (SOE=B).

The canalith repositioning procedure, introduced by Semont as well as Epley, can provide quick relief for those patients with BPPV, and a video demonstration is available at https://youtu.be/jBzID5nVQjk (accessed Feb 2019). Other repositioning procedures include Li's maneuvers, which consist of 3 different sets of movements developed to manage BPPV of posterior, anterior, and horizontal semicircular canals.

A small subset of patients require surgical intervention. Surgical excision remains the treatment of choice for cerebellopontine angle tumors. Surgery should be reserved for disabling unilateral peripheral disease that is unresponsive to medical therapy. Surgical procedures are ablative or nonablative. Surgeons select ablative procedures, including transmastoid labyrinthectomy and partial vestibular neurectomy, for uncontrolled Meniere disease. Nonablative procedures, such as posterior canal occlusion, provide benefit to those patients whose BPPV remains refractory to repeated attempts of canalith repositioning procedures.

RESOURCES

- Avanecean D, Calliste D, Contreras T, et al. Effectiveness of patient-centered interventions on falls in the acute care setting compared to usual care: a systematic review. *JBI Database System Rev Implement Rep*. 2017;15(12):3006–3048.

- Bhattacharyya N, Gubbels SP, Schwartz SR, et al. Clinical Practice Guideline: Benign Paroxysmal Positional Vertigo (Update). *Otolaryngol Head Neck Surg*. 2017;156(3 suppl):S1–S47.

- McDonnell MN, Hillier SL. Vestibular rehabilitation for unilateral peripheral vestibular dysfunction. *Cochrane Database Syst Rev*. 2015;1:CD005397.

CHAPTER 29—SYNCOPE

KEY POINTS

- Syncope is a symptom, not a disease, that can be caused by many different conditions.

- In older adults, the cause of syncope is often multifactorial. The prognosis is generally determined by underlying cardiac and comorbid illnesses. If the cause of syncope is not determined, the prognosis is likely similar to that of other patients of the same age and comorbidity burden.

- Bradycardia is the single most common cardiac cause of syncope in older adults.

- Although many diagnostic procedures are available to search for the cause of syncope, most are expensive and have a low yield unless findings from the history or physical examination suggest a particular cause.

- Treatment of syncope often requires addressing multiple potential causes in geriatric patients, including polypharmacy, frailty, orthostasis, bradycardia, and tachyarrhythmias.

Syncope is a symptom complex composed of a sudden and transient loss of consciousness resulting from a temporary interruption of global cerebral perfusion. It is a common reason for evaluation in both outpatient clinics and emergency departments, and a common symptom resulting in hospital admission. Annually it accounts for approximately 1%–3% of emergency department visits and 2%–6% of hospital admissions. Incidence of syncope increases with age; incidence doubles in those ≥70 years old, and the rate among those ≥80 years old is three to four times that seen among younger people. Approximately 80% of patients hospitalized for syncope are ≥65 years old.

Syncope is a clinically important condition that is challenging to evaluate. Its potential causes range from those that are benign and self-limiting to those that are life threatening. In older adults, the cause of syncope can often be multifactorial, adding to the diagnostic difficulty. Additionally, limited recall of details surrounding the event may make it difficult to determine whether syncope truly occurred. Because syncope encompasses a wide range of potential causes, its diagnostic evaluation can be complex and expensive.

NATURAL HISTORY: DIAGNOSIS AND PROGNOSIS

Causes of syncope in older adults are often multifactorial. Decreases in cardiac output or peripheral vascular resistance, or both, resulting in decreased systemic blood pressure and cerebral perfusion are common mechanisms of syncope. In addition, adverse effects of drugs must be considered, particularly in older adults taking multiple medications. Common causes of syncope in older adults include the following:

- Orthostatic or postprandial hypotension, affected by:

  □ Decreased intravascular volume due to blood loss or dehydration

  □ Alterations in the peripheral vasculature due to arterial vasodilation or increased venous pooling

- Cardiac rhythm disturbances

- Reflex, or neurally mediated, syncope (syncope from autonomic-mediated vasodilation and/or bradycardia), including vasovagal syncope or carotid sinus hypersensitivity

- Medication related

While localized atherosclerotic diseases, such as vertebral basilar insufficiency and subclavian steal, can result in syncope, these causes are uncommon.

Epileptic seizure, a common cause of transient loss of consciousness, is no longer categorized as a cause of syncope, because seizure is not mediated by a decrease in cerebral perfusion. Nevertheless, differentiation of seizure from syncope as a cause of transient loss of consciousness is clinically relevant, because both conditions are common and have overlapping clinical features in the older population. For clinical characteristics differentiating cardiac syncope due to arrhythmia, vasovagal syncope, and seizure, see Table 29.1.

The prognosis of syncope depends on the underlying cause. Patients with syncope from cardiac causes have the worst prognosis; their 1-year mortality is 18%–33%, with deaths chiefly due to underlying cardiac disease, not syncope. Patients with syncope due to noncardiac causes have a 1-year mortality of approximately 6%. Neurally mediated or vasovagal syncope, which has a benign prognosis in the young, is more common in older adults than previously thought. It is responsible for approximately 20%–30% of syncopal events in patients >65 years old (SOE=A). Vasovagal syncope may have a worse prognosis in older adults than in younger individuals, because it may be associated with comorbid

Table 29.1—Distinguishing Characteristics of Seizure and Syncope Due to Arrhythmia and Vasovagal Syncope[a]

Phase	Sign/Symptom	Seizure	Cardiac Syncope Due to Arrhythmia	Vasovagal Syncope
Before	Position	Any	Any	**Upright; aborted by lying flat**
	Warning/prodrome	None	**<5 seconds**	**Seconds to minutes**
	Precipitant	Usually absent	Absent	**Present**
	Palpitations	Absent	Sometimes	Absent
	Nausea/diaphoresis	Rare	Absent	**Common**
	Visual changes	None	None	**Common**
During	Tone	**Rigid**	Flaccid	Motionless, relaxed
	Pulse	**Rapid**	Absent or faint	Slow, faint
	Color	Pale or normal	Blue, ashen	Pale
	Incontinence	**Common**	Rare	Very rare
	Eye findings	**Tonic eye deviation**	Variable pupils	Dilated, reactive pupils
	Oral frothing	**Common**	Absent	Absent
After	Type of recovery	Slow, incomplete	**Rapid, complete**	Fatigue common
	Mental status	**Disorientation**	No retrograde amnesia	No retrograde amnesia
	Nausea/diaphoresis	Rare	Absent	**Common**
	Focal neurologic findings	**Common**	Absent	Absent

[a] Characteristics most distinctive in determining the cause of syncope are highlighted in bold.

illnesses that can increase overall mortality (SOE=B). In approximately 10%–20% of syncopal patients, no cause can be found. The prognosis for these patients is no worse or better than that of the general population (SOE=C).

PATHOPHYSIOLOGY

The integrity of a number of control mechanisms is crucial for maintaining adequate perfusion of the brain and cerebral oxygen delivery after sudden changes in blood pressure. These mechanisms include carotid and aortic baroreceptors, sympathetic renal stimulation of the renin-angiotensin system, and arteriolar autoregulation.

In aging, many of these reflex mechanisms are less responsive. For example, the arterial baroreceptor reflex and cardiac response to β-adrenergic stimulation (cardiac acceleration and increased contractility) decrease with advancing age. In addition, comorbid conditions such as diabetes mellitus and Parkinson disease affect postural reflexes. Medications such as α-blockers, β-blockers, calcium channel blockers, ACE inhibitors, and tricyclic antidepressants can also impair postural reflexes. Because the ability to increase heart rate in response to sympathetic stimulation is decreased in older adults, maintaining blood volume and vasoconstriction become more important in maintaining postural blood pressure. Thus, older adults can be particularly sensitive to the effects of dehydration, diuretics, and vasodilator medications. These three factors—age-related decline in adaptive reflexes, comorbid conditions, and medications—are all likely to have a role in older patients presenting with syncope, and can be addressed by increasing caution with postural change, physical counter-pressure maneuvers (eg, leg crossing) and compression stockings to increase venous return, adequate hydration, and simplification of the patient's medication regimen to eliminate medications that are no longer needed.

EVALUATION

History

The medical history should be informed by a witness to the event if possible. This history, in combination with a physical examination, plays a key role in the initial evaluation. Key elements to obtain from the history include the following:

- Did the patient suffer a true syncopal event, as opposed to dizziness (dysequilibrium) or falls?

- Was there a precipitant? Could the patient's activities around the time of the event have triggered it?

  □ Syncope associated with activities such as eating, urinating, coughing, and experiencing emotional stress suggests reflex syncope.

  □ Syncope occurring while sitting or supine without prodrome suggests a profound hemodynamic disturbance and should raise a concern about a significant cardiac arrhythmia.

- ☐ Syncope occurring during physical exertion should raise the possibility of myocardial ischemia or aortic stenosis.
- ☐ Syncope after turning motions of the head should raise the possibility of carotid sinus hypersensitivity.

■ Were there prodromal symptoms before the event?

■ Chest pain, palpitations, or shortness of breath suggests a cardiac or pulmonary cause.

- ☐ Nausea, diaphoresis, and vomiting can be associated with vasovagal syncope.

- ☐ Sudden onset of syncope with no prodrome or <5 sec of warning is characteristic of syncope due to a cardiac arrhythmia and should be evaluated as such. However, in older adults, vasovagal syncope can present with short or no prodrome. Thus, if the initial evaluation for arrhythmia in an older adult with syncope without a prodrome is unrevealing, a vasovagal mechanism should also be considered.

■ What medications are being used? Timing and dosage of medications that can cause bradycardia or hypotension should be reviewed. Many commonly used medications can increase the propensity for ventricular arrhythmias by prolonging the QT interval (for a full current list, see www.qtdrugs.org).

■ What did witnesses observe?

- ☐ Patients with cardiac causes of syncope are generally flaccid in tone and motionless while unconscious, unless the event lasts for >15 sec, when myoclonic jerks and truncal extension can be seen.

- ☐ Increased body motion, tone, and head turning to one side with loss of consciousness are more common with seizure activity.

■ Are there significant comorbid conditions? A history of coronary artery disease or its associated symptoms is particularly important. Approximately 5% of myocardial infarctions present as syncope. Sustained ventricular tachycardia resulting in syncope is most common in patients with prior myocardial infarction. Patients with diabetes mellitus are at increased risk of coronary atherosclerosis, as well as autonomic dysfunction predisposing to syncope.

For a summary of the characteristics of three common causes of loss of consciousness, see Table 29.1. A scoring system has been useful in distinguishing cardiac from noncardiac syncope (Table 29.2). The probability of cardiac syncope increases with higher scores; notably, scores ≥3 are associated with 95% sensitivity and 61% specificity. Mortality was 17%–21% in those with a score ≥3, and 2%–3% in those with a score <3 after 600 days of follow-up (SOE=B). The available risk scores have all been developed and validated in patient populations with a mean age of 52–59 years; there are no risk scores specifically validated for older adults.

Physical Examination

A physical examination should focus on cardiovascular and neurologic areas of concern raised by the history. Blood pressure should be measured in both arms; blood pressure and pulse should be measured in both supine and standing positions after 1 min and 3 min of standing. Although any definition of postural hypotension is arbitrary, a decrease in systolic blood pressure of >20 mmHg is the definition used most frequently (SOE=C).

The carotid pulse should be assessed for the delayed upstroke characteristic of significant aortic stenosis. A carotid bruit should be noted as a relative contraindication to carotid sinus massage, as are recent myocardial infarction and stroke. Even in the absence of contraindications, carotid sinus massage should be performed only under continuous ECG monitoring in a setting where resuscitation equipment is available.

Physical examination of the patient with syncope should include cardiac examination for evidence of murmurs characteristic of valvular abnormalities or extra heart sounds suggestive of cardiomyopathy. Fecal examination for occult blood and neurologic examination for focal deficits are also important. Potentially informative aspects of the neurologic examination, particularly in patients in whom it is unclear whether true syncope occurred, include assessment of cognitive function, visual acuity, coordination, and gait.

Diagnostic Testing

Several clinical characteristics and diagnostic approaches are particularly important for evaluation of syncope in older adults (Table 29.3).

Electrocardiogram (ECG)

An ECG is indicated for all patients presenting with syncope. Although an ECG establishes a diagnosis in only 5% of those with syncope, abnormalities on an ECG can provide clues for further cardiovascular evaluation. A normal ECG is associated with a more favorable prognosis. Specific abnormalities that indicate underlying cardiac conditions include conduction abnormalities, AV block, preexcitation, evidence of left or right ventricular hypertrophy, Q waves indicative of prior myocardial infarction, ST segment abnormalities, and QT prolongation.

Table 29.2—Evaluation of Guidelines in Syncope Study (EGSYS) Score: Predictors of Cardiac Syncope

Variable	Score[a]
Palpitations preceding syncope	4
Heart disease or abnormal ECG	3
Syncope during effort	3
Syncope while supine	2
Precipitating or predisposing factors, or both[b]	−1
Autonomic prodromes (nausea/vomiting)	−1

[a] Scores ≥3 are associated with higher rates of cardiac syncope and higher mortality.
[b] Warm or crowded place, prolonged orthostasis, fear, pain, or emotional distress

SOURCE: Data from Del Rosso A, Ungar A, Maggi R, et al. Clinical predictors of cardiac syncope at initial evaluation in patients referred urgently to a general hospital: the EGSYS score. *Heart.* 2008;94(12):1620–1626.

Ambulatory Electrocardiographic Monitoring

An ambulatory ECG recording can establish or exclude many causes of syncope if the patient experiences syncopal or presyncopal symptoms during the recording. Unfortunately, the occurrence of symptoms during ambulatory ECG monitoring is relatively infrequent in most patients with syncope that remains unexplained after a history, physical examination, and ECG. A multitude of monitoring devices has been developed, including 24-hour Holter monitors, external loop recorders, patches for longer-term monitoring or telemetry, and smartphone-based patient-initiated recording applications. The monitoring device should be chosen based on the frequency of the patient's symptoms and their capability to activate the recording mechanism (SOE=C). The diagnostic yield increases with the length of time monitored, from 1%–2% for Holter monitors to 25% in external loop recorders.

Implantable Loop Recorders

Implantable loop recorders (ILRs) are implanted subcutaneously in the prepectoral region under local anesthesia. The devices have a battery life of up to 36 months and a solid-state loop memory that stores ECG recordings, when activated either by the patient or a bystander, usually after a syncopal episode or are automatically activated in the case of occurrence of predefined arrhythmias. Current guidelines recommend that use of an ILR can be considered early in patients when an arrhythmic cause of syncope is suspected but not sufficiently proved (SOE=B).

Echocardiography and Exercise Stress Testing

In the absence of features suggestive of heart disease by history, physical examination, or ECG, two-dimensional echocardiography has a low yield (SOE=C). It is most useful in confirming a specific diagnosis suspected by other assessment. Occult coronary artery disease is also prevalent among older adults, and stress testing is often used for screening. In some patients, particularly those in whom the history, physical examination, or ECG suggest structural cardiac abnormalities and ischemia, it is efficient to perform stress echocardiography as a single procedure.

Tilt-Table Testing

Head-up tilt-table testing results in pooling of blood in the legs and, in susceptible individuals, can trigger syncope mediated by vasovagal mechanisms or it can confirm postural hypotension. Tilt-table testing is useful for patients suspected of having vasovagal syncope and those with unexplained syncope who are not suspected of having a cardiac cause. Responses to tilt testing performed for evaluation of syncope tend to differ by age among adults without significant structural heart disease. Those ≥65 years old tend to have far higher rates of symptoms due to pure vasodilatation without significant change in heart rate than individuals ≤35 years old. In contrast, individuals ≤35 years old tend to have more profound cardioinhibitory responses, characterized by profound bradycardia or asystole induced by tilt testing, than those ≥65 years old. The different patterns of responses induced by tilt studies between younger and older adults suggest that different mechanisms for vasovagal syncope predominate at different ages. An exaggerated autonomic response is common in younger people, whereas attenuated autonomic responses become predominant with advancing age.

Electrophysiologic Study (EPS)

The diagnostic efficacy of EPS to determine the cause of syncope greatly depends on patient selection and the degree of suspicion of an arrhythmic substrate for syncope. The development of effective noninvasive methods for prolonged rhythm monitoring has decreased the importance of EPS as a diagnostic test. Nevertheless, this test is still useful for diagnosis in suspected intermittent bradycardia, tachyarrhythmia, or in patients with bundle-branch block (suggestive of impending high-grade AV block). EPS is not recommended for patients with normal ECGs or without a history of heart disease or symptoms of palpitations.

Neurologic Testing

Extensive neurologic testing is generally not required in syncope evaluation. Neurologic testing, including imaging of the head by CT or MRI and electroencephalographic recording, is appropriate in situations when focal neurologic signs or symptoms are present or when the history suggests seizure during the evaluation of loss of consciousness. Also, neuroimaging may be required to evaluate trauma

Table 29.3—Diagnostic Evaluation of Older Adults with Syncope

Evaluation	Finding	Comments
Orthostatic vital signs	Systolic blood pressure drop of >20 mmHg on standing	Maintain adequate hydration. Consider reducing antihypertensive therapy. Repeat measurements to identify situations that precipitate orthostasis (eg, postprandial hypotension).
Gait evaluation	Gait unsteadiness Failure of heart rate to increase	Increased risk of falls Chronotropic incompetence preventing appropriate increase in heart rate
Carotid sinus massage	Reproducible symptoms	Contraindicated in patients with carotid bruits, recent stroke Patients with transient asystole and carotid sinus syncope may benefit from pacemaker placement.
Laboratory testing	Hyperglycemia Electrolyte disturbance Anemia Occult heme in feces Increased creatinine	Correctable pathophysiologic states that either precipitate syncope or result in a state of altered consciousness that can be confused with syncope
Resting ECG	Arrhythmias, Q waves, prolonged QT_c	Increased likelihood of cardiac causes of syncope, including arrhythmias
Echocardiogram	Aortic stenosis, left ventricular outflow tract obstruction	Treatable causes of cardiac syncope are identified.
Ambulatory (24-hour) blood pressure monitor	Diurnal variation in blood pressure	Can identify patterns in variation in blood pressure, in particular, supine hypertension and postprandial hypotension
Holter monitor	Arrhythmias Chronotropic incompetence	Likelihood of identifying cause of syncope is low.
Implantable loop recorder	Arrhythmias	Ultimately demonstrates whether or not infrequent syncope is arrhythmic in origin
Head-up tilt table testing	Reproduces vasovagal syncope	Adequate usefulness in older adults Reproduces vasovagal syncope
Electrophysiologic study	Inducible ventricular tachyarrhythmias	Limited utility
Validated depression assessment	Syncope is more common in depressed patients	Identification of another treatable risk factor for syncope
Autonomic neurologic testing	Autonomic nervous system dysfunction	Diagnoses primary syndromes of autonomic dysfunction and demonstrates extent of dysfunction with targets for therapeutic intervention.
Electroencephalogram	Epileptiform activity	Diagnostic for seizure

Note: Not every test is required; the history and physical examination are used to determine appropriate testing. In all patients, an assessment of orthostatic vital signs, gait, laboratory tests, and ECG are reasonable.

that occurred during the loss of consciousness. Autonomic evaluation should be considered when symptoms and signs of autonomic insufficiency are present.

TREATMENT

The goals of treatment for syncope, particularly in older adults, are to improve quality of life and prevent physical injuries. Effectiveness of therapy depends on whether a cause of syncope can be clearly established.

Polypharmacy is increasingly identified as a risk of syncope because of the actual number of medications and risk of interaction and adverse effects, and potentially because of the number of comorbid conditions requiring complex pharmacotherapy. Before any new medication is added, the medication list must be reviewed for potential culprits (in particular, α-antagonists, clonidine, vasodilators, and excessive diuretics). Discontinuing or reducing antihypertensive medications has been shown to reduce syncope recurrence (SOE=B). Shifting once-daily antihypertensive medications to evening administration may reduce daytime orthostatic symptoms.

Reflex Syncope and Postural Hypotension

Nonpharmacologic measures with physical counter-pressure maneuvers such as leg crossing, arm tensing, hand grip, and buttock clenching are able to induce a significant blood pressure increase during the phase of impending reflex syncope so that the patient can avoid or delay losing consciousness in most cases (SOE=B). These measures in conjunction with conventional therapies have been shown to reduce recurrence by 39% (SOE=A). However, effectiveness of these physical counter-pressure maneuvers in older adults has not been confirmed. Compression stockings and abdominal binders can be helpful in some patients with postural hypotension. Small, frequent meals can be effective in patients with postprandial hypotension.

Medical Management

The baroreceptor reflex plays a key role in blood pressure homeostasis. Drugs that mimic sympathetic activity such as α-agonists, including midodrine, have been used to increase vasoconstriction and reduce syncope recurrence (SOE=B). However, use of an α-agonist is limited by supine hypertension, particularly in older adults with decreased vascular compliance. In men, α-agonists may exacerbate lower urinary tract symptoms due to prostatic hyperplasia. The use of an α-agonist requires careful titration of the drug dosage and close monitoring of blood pressure response and symptoms.

β-Blockers may be useful in older patients with vasovagal syncope, based on age-specific analysis of randomized controlled trials. However, β-blockers in the general population appear to have no significant effect on reduction in syncope.

Pyridostigmine[OL], an acetylcholinesterase inhibitor, facilitates transmission of cholinergic neuronal impulses and increases standing blood pressure by increasing peripheral resistance. Supine blood pressure may increase, but it is generally not significantly affected. Common adverse events include abdominal cramps, diarrhea from increased peristalsis, and urinary urgency (SOE=C). The use of pyridostigmine in syncopal patients with orthostatic hypotension and autonomic failure should be closely supervised. Data in older adults is limited, so pyridostigmine should be used cautiously in this population because the adverse effects may not be tolerated well.

Volume expansion with added salt (liberalize diet) or fludrocortisone, or both, to increase renal sodium retention and intravascular volume can be effective in patients with persistent postural hypotension (SOE=C).

Role of Pacemakers

Beyond the discontinuation of culprit medications, pharmacologic treatment has little place in the long-term treatment of bradycardia associated with syncope. Atropine or isoproterenol is indicated only in emergencies and temporary situations before cardiac pacing can be introduced. The mainstay of treatment for sinus node dysfunction or high-grade AV block is a pacemaker. Permanent pacing is clearly indicated when syncope or near syncope is correlated with bradycardia, regardless of the site of block. Although the recommendation to avoid pacemaker placement but rather discontinue medications causing bradycardia in patients taking them makes sense, often these medications are treatment for a significant cardiac condition (ie, β-blockers) or dementia (acetylcholinesterase inhibitors). Acetylcholinesterase inhibitors are associated with a significant risk of bradycardia, and bradycardic patients have a significant risk of syncope. Recommendations for when it is appropriate or necessary to discontinue acetylcholinesterase inhibitors are needed because it is difficult to weigh the risk of worsening cognitive status against the improvement in bradycardia if these medications are discontinued. Pacemaker therapy is not recommended in patients with unexplained syncope or falls without documentation of bradycardia (SOE=A).

The role of pacemaker therapy in patients with reflex syncope remains to be defined. In older adults with recurrent syncope of a vasovagal nature, pacemaker placement can be considered when a cardioinhibitory response is documented during monitoring (SOE=B). Pacemaker therapy is effective in preventing recurrent syncope in patients with carotid sinus syndrome (SOE=B).

PUBLIC REPORTING

Syncope while driving is uncommon; however, many states have laws restricting driving after a syncopal event. It is important that clinicians be familiar with local driving regulations pertaining to syncope. Finding a balance between protecting the patient and public safety and maintaining the patient's independence is especially relevant in older adults after experiencing syncope.

CHOOSING WISELY® RECOMMENDATIONS

Syncope

- Do not perform cardiac imaging (particularly echocardiography) routinely unless cardiac disease is suggested by history, physical examination findings, or an abnormal ECG.
- Do not perform imaging of the carotid arteries for simple syncope without other neurologic symptoms.
- In the evaluation of simple syncope and a normal neurologic examination, do not obtain brain imaging studies (CT or MRI).

RESOURCES

- De Ruiter SC, Wold JFH, Germans T, et al. Multiple causes of syncope in the elderly: diagnostic outcomes of a Dutch multidisciplinary syncope pathway. *Europace*. 2018;20(5):867–872.

- Hamdon MH, Walsh KE, Brignole M, et al. Outreach syncope clinic managed by a nurse practitioner: Outcome and cost effectiveness. *J Telemed Telecare*. 2018;24(8):566–571.

- Shen W-K, Sheldon RS, Benditt DG, et al. 2017 ACC/AHA/HRS Guideline for the Evaluation and Management of Patients with Syncope. *Heart Rhythm*. 2017;14(8):e155–e217.

CHAPTER 30—NUTRITION AND WEIGHT

KEY POINTS

- Aging is associated with changes in body composition such that well-standardized nutrient requirements for younger or middle-aged adults cannot be generalized to older adults.

- The Mini-Nutritional Assessment–Short Form is a brief and simple instrument useful for nutritional screening in geriatric patients.

- Identification of the presence of undernutrition or obesity can be facilitated by determining a person's BMI.

- In the presence of inflammation, neither albumin nor prealbumin is an accurate indicator of malnutrition.

- Lean body mass (muscle mass) is inversely associated with mortality risk in older adults.

- Many medications cause anorexia or can reduce nutrient availability in older adults.

- Therapeutic diets should be avoided unless their clinical value is certain.

- Appetite stimulants have not been demonstrated to improve long-term survival and may cause serious adverse effects.

- Cultural competence extends to understanding the many factors influencing nutrition and health behaviors in the increasingly heterogeneous population of older adults.

Malnutrition in older adults spans the spectrum from under- to overnutrition. Nutritional problems accompany many chronic disease processes of older adults. Moreover, age-related changes in physiology, metabolism, and function can alter the older adult's nutritional requirements. Better understanding among clinicians of the aging process and of nutritional screening, assessment, and interventions could potentially improve the health and independence of older adults.

AGE-RELATED CHANGES

Body Composition

Aging is associated with notable changes in body composition. Bone mass, lean mass, and water content all decrease, while fat mass generally increases. The volume of distribution of many medications changes as a result of these shifts in body composition, and creatinine-based determinations can overestimate renal clearance in older adults. The increase in total body fat is commonly accompanied by greater intra-abdominal fat stores. The consequence of these changes in body composition is that well-standardized nutrient requirements for younger or middle-aged adults cannot be generalized to older adults. The aging process also affects organ functions, although the degree of change observed is highly variable among individuals. Decline in organ functions can affect nutritional assessment and intervention.

Energy Requirements

The reduced demand for energy (calories) and lower basal metabolic rate in older adults reflects loss of lean body mass, including muscle mass. The resting energy expenditure is the principal contributor to total energy expenditure; energy expenditure in relation to physical activity is the most variable component. The Harris-Benedict or similar equations can be used to predict basal energy expenditure. In any determination of energy needs for older adults, care must be taken to avoid overfeeding while still meeting basal requirements.

Macronutrient Needs

MyPlate (www.choosemyplate.gov [accessed Feb 2019]), a modified food guide pyramid for older adults based on the 2010 U.S. Department of Agriculture food guidelines, is a USDA initiative with helpful, culturally sensitive advice; it has replaced the formerly used Food Pyramid. This pictorial recommendation depicts easy-to-understand examples to balance energy, avoid oversized food and meal portions, encourage lower-fat dairy and low-sodium food choices, and make half the plate fruits and vegetables and half of all grains whole grains.

The Food and Nutrition Board of the Institute of Medicine of the National Academies (formerly National Academy of Sciences) has released macronutrient guidelines that recommend a prudent diet, with 20%–35% of energy as fat, and reduced intakes of cholesterol, saturated fatty acids, and trans-fatty acids. Carbohydrates should constitute 45%–65% of total energy; complex carbohydrates are the preferred fiber source. More specifically, the recommended daily fiber intake for those ≥60 years old is 30 g for men and 21 g for women. Protein intake is recommended at 0.8 g/kg/day at approximately 10%–35% of total energy. With stress or injury, protein requirements are typically estimated at 1.5 g/kg/d, but underlying renal or hepatic insufficiency may warrant protein restriction (SOE=C).

Micronutrient Needs

The Dietary Reference Intakes (DRIs) is a set of reference values used to plan and assess the nutrient intakes of healthy people. Included among the DRIs is the recommended dietary allowance (RDA), which is defined as the average daily nutrient intake level estimated to meet the requirements of 97%–98% of the healthy individuals in a group. For the RDAs for vitamins and elements for the group >70 years old, see data from the Standing Committee on the Scientific Evaluation of Dietary Reference Intakes, Food and Nutrition Board, Institute of Medicine, Dietary Reference Intakes (available at www.ncbi.nlm.nih.gov/books/NBK56068/ [accessed Feb 2019]).The Food and Nutrition Board has also updated the RDAs with population-weighted estimated average requirements, defined as the average daily nutrient intake level estimated to meet the requirements of half of the healthy individuals in a group, based on updated census data. This information may be helpful for individualized recommendations to avoid over-nutrification (http://books.nap.edu/openbook.php?record_id=11537&page=R1 [accessed Feb 2019]).

Fluid Needs

Dehydration is the most common fluid or electrolyte disturbance in older adults. Normal aging is associated with a decreased perception of thirst, impaired response to changes in serum osmolality, and reduced ability to concentrate urine after fluid deprivation. A decline in fluid intake can also result from disease states that reduce mental or physical ability to recognize or express thirst, or that result in decreased access to water. In general, fluid needs of older adults can be met with 30 mL/kg/d or 1 mL/kcal ingested. Fluid needs may increase during episodes of fever or infection, as well as with diuretic or laxative therapy. Common signs of dehydration are decreased urine output, confusion, constipation, and mucosal dryness, although none of these signs is sensitive or specific.

NUTRITION SCREENING AND ASSESSMENT

Anthropometrics

Anthropometrics refers to the study of human body measurements on a comparative basis. Anthropometric measurements are often used for assessing nutritional status of older adults. An involuntary weight loss of 10 pounds in the preceding 6 months is a useful indicator of morbidity in all geriatric populations; this degree of weight loss is predictive of functional limitations, health care charges, and the need for hospitalization (SOE=B).

The Minimum Data Set (MDS-3) used by Medicare-certified nursing homes defines significant weight loss as ≥5% of body weight in the past month or ≥10% in the past 6 months. BMI, calculated by weight in kg/(height in meters)^2, is a useful measure of body size and indirect measure of body fat that does not require use of a reference table of ideal heights and weights. For National Institutes of Health guidelines regarding body size classification based on BMI, see https://www.cdc.gov/healthyweight/assessing/bmi/adult_bmi/index.html (accessed Feb 2019). The risk threshold for low BMI is set at 18.5 kg/m^2 but should be interpreted in the context of the individual's lifelong weight history. Other anthropometric tools include skinfold and circumference measurements, but these have had limited practical application because of the difficulty of achieving acceptable reliability among those taking the measurements.

Nutritional Intake

Generally, inadequate nutritional intake has been defined as average or usual intake of servings of food groups, nutrients, or energy below a threshold level of the RDI. Poor intake is often an indication of illness. The limited reliability of accurately assessing dietary intake measures is well known, so thresholds of 25%–50% below the RDI have generally been selected as an indicator of inadequate intake. In one study, energy intake was reduced (<50% of calculated maintenance energy requirements) in 21% of hospitalized older adults. This subset of patients had higher rates of in-hospital mortality and 90-day mortality than did those with energy intakes above the threshold. Surveys of nutritional status conducted among long-term institutionalized older adults suggest that 5%–18% of nursing-home residents have energy intakes below their recommended energy requirements. However, evidence is lacking to support any benefits of nutritional supplementation in this population (SOE=B).

Energy intakes of men and women 65–98 years old have been estimated in a nationwide food consumption survey; 37%–40% of the men and women studied had energy intakes lower than two-thirds of the RDIs, and many participants reported skipping at least one meal every day. However, estimated intakes obtained from consumption surveys may be unreliable, because some studies suggest that older adults under-report energy intakes by 20%–30%.

Problems with obtaining food commonly contribute to inadequate nutritional intakes among older adults. It is important to ascertain whether limitations in resources, transportation, or functionality may limit access to food or the ability to prepare and/or consume food.

Laboratory Tests: Albumin, Prealbumin, Cholesterol

Serum albumin has been recognized as a risk indicator for morbidity and mortality. Hypoalbuminemia lacks specificity and sensitivity as an indicator of malnutrition; however, it can be associated with injury, disease, or inflammatory conditions. As a negative acute-phase reactant, albumin is subject to cytokine-mediated decline in synthesis and to increased degradation and transcapillary leakage. Longitudinal studies of serum albumin levels suggest that a modest decline with aging may be independent of disease. The prognostic value of hypoalbuminemia may be largely because of its use as a proxy measure for injury, disease, or inflammation. In the hospital setting, hypoalbuminemia has been associated with increased length of stay, complications, readmissions, and mortality (SOE=B). In the community setting, hypoalbuminemia has been associated with functional limitations, sarcopenia, increased health care use, and mortality (SOE=B).

Serum prealbumin is another protein marker of nutritional status with clinical significance. Prealbumin has a considerably shorter half-life (48 hours) than albumin (18–20 days) and may more adequately reflect short-term changes in protein status. In the absence of an inflammatory state, prealbumin appears to have limitations similar to those of albumin as a diagnostic tool for nutritional status assessment. In the presence of inflammation, neither albumin nor prealbumin is an accurate indicator of malnutrition. However, prealbumin can be used to assess the effectiveness of nutritional interventions or as an indicator of recovery (SOE=B). Because of a shorter half-life and a smaller serum pool than albumin, prealbumin can be used to detect small changes in nutritional status over a shorter time period if inflammation is not present.

Serum cholesterol concentration has also been linked to nutritional status. Low cholesterol levels (<160 mg/dL) are often detected in individuals with an underlying serious disease such as malignancy. Poor clinical outcomes have been reported among hospitalized and institutionalized older adults with hypocholesterolemia. In a study of community-dwelling older adults, nutrient intakes were not different in those in the lowest quartile of serum cholesterol levels from other quartiles. It appears likely that acquired hypocholesterolemia is a nonspecific feature of poor health status that is independent of nutrient and/or energy intakes, and that it may be a marker of pro-inflammatory conditions. Of interest is the observation that community-dwelling older adults with both hypoalbuminemia and hypocholesterolemia have higher rates of mortality and adverse functional outcomes than those with hypoalbuminemia or hypocholesterolemia alone (SOE=B).

Table 30.1—Drug-Nutrient Interactions

Drug	Reduced Nutrient Availability
Alcohol	Zinc, vitamins A, B_1, B_2, B_6, B_{12}, folate
Antacids	Vitamin B_{12}, folate, iron
Antibiotics, broad-spectrum	Vitamin K
Colchicine	Vitamin B_{12}
Digoxin	Zinc
Diuretics	Zinc, magnesium, vitamin B_6, potassium, copper
Isoniazid	Vitamin B_6, niacin
Levodopa	Vitamin B_6
Laxatives	Calcium, vitamins A, B_2, B_{12}, D, E, K
Lipid-binding resins	Vitamins A, D, E, K
Metformin	Vitamin B_{12}
Mineral oil	Vitamins A, D, E, K
Phenytoin	Vitamin D, folate
Proton-pump inhibitors	Calcium, iron, magnesium, vitamins B_{12}, C
Salicylates	Vitamin C, folate
Trimethoprim	Folate

Drug-Nutrient Interactions

Medications can modify the nutrient needs and metabolism of older adults. Certain medications, such as digoxin and phenytoin, even at therapeutic levels, can cause anorexia in older adults. Additional agents that have anorexia as a major potential adverse effect include cholinesterase inhibitors, SSRIs, calcium channel blockers (eg, dihydropyridines), H_2-receptor antagonists, proton-pump inhibitors, opioid and nonsteroidal analgesics, furosemide, potassium supplements, ipratropium bromide, and theophylline. Many medications are known to interfere with taste and smell, and others can reduce the availability of specific nutrients (Table 30.1). Some medications can reduce intake by causing inattention, dysphagia, dysgeusia, or xerostomia. Medications that precipitate constipation can also reduce appetite.

Multi-Item Tools for Nutrition Screening

The nutritional status of older adults can be influenced by a variety of factors (Table 30.2). The lack of single assessment measures that are valid indicators of comprehensive nutritional status has prompted the development of multi-item tools. Older adults in acute- or chronic-care facilities have been extensively studied to identify indicators and predictors of nutritional status. In contrast, substantially fewer studies have been conducted in community-dwelling adults. Nutritional screening

Table 30.2—Risk Factors for Poor Nutritional Status

- Alcohol or substance abuse
- Cognitive dysfunction
- Decreased exercise
- Depression, poor mental health
- Functional limitations
- Inadequate funds
- Limited education
- Limited mobility, transportation
- Medical problems, chronic diseases
- Medications
- Poor dentition
- Restricted diet, poor eating habits
- Social isolation

tools for older adults have been widely disseminated and yet their effectiveness in identifying undernourished individuals whose problems are amenable to intervention has not been demonstrated.

The Nutrition Screening Initiative (a collaborative effort of the American Dietetic Association, the American Academy of Family Physicians, and the National Council on Aging, Inc.) developed 3 interdisciplinary tools to screen for nutrition risk and help evaluate the nutritional status of older adults. The DETERMINE checklist (https://nutritionandaging.org/wp-content/uploads/2017/01/DetermineNutritionChecklist.pdf [accessed Feb 2019]) was created to raise public awareness about the importance of nutrition to the health of older adults. This self-report questionnaire is composed of 10 items and is intended to identify risk but not to diagnose malnutrition. The Level I screen, intended for use by health care professionals, incorporates additional assessment items regarding dietary habits, functional status, living environment, and weight change, as well as measures of height and weight. The Level II screen, for use by more highly trained medical and nutrition professionals and suggested for use in the diagnosis of malnutrition, contains all the items from Level I with additional biochemical and anthropometric measures, as well as a more detailed evaluation of depression and mental status.

The Mini-Nutritional Assessment (MNA®) tool was developed to evaluate the risk of malnutrition among frail older adults and to identify those who may benefit from early intervention (SOE=B). This assessment tool requires administration by a trained professional and consists of 18 items, including questions about BMI, mid-arm and calf circumferences, weight loss, living environment, medication use, dietary habits, clinical

Table 30.3—Mini Nutritional Assessment*

Screening

A. Decline in food intake over past 3 months due to loss of appetite, digestive problems, or chewing or swallowing difficulties
   0 = severe decrease in food intake
   1 = moderate decrease in food intake
   2 = no decrease in food intake

B. Weight loss during past 3 months
   0 = >3 kg (6.6 lbs)
   1 = does not know
   2 = 1–3 kg (2.2–6.6 lbs)
   3 = no weight loss

C. Mobility
   0 = bed/chair bound
   1 = able to get out of bed/chair but does not go out
   2 = goes out

D. Psychological stressor acute disease in past 3 months
   0 = yes
   2 = no

E. Neuropsychological problems
   0 = severe dementia or depression
   1 = mild dementia
   2 = no psychological problems

F1. BMI (kg/m^2)
   0 = <19
   1 = 19 to <21
   2 = 21 to <23
   3 = ≥23

Note: If BMI is not available, replace question F1 with question F2. If question F1 is completed, do not answer question F2.

F2. Calf circumference (cm)
   0 = <31
   1 = ≥31

Scoring (maximum 14 points)
12–14 points: normal nutritional status
8–11 points: at risk of malnutrition
0–7 points: malnourished

*For more information, see www.mna-elderly.com.

global assessment, and self-perception of health and nutrition status. The MNA may be incorporated into the electronic medical record, and it is also available as a downloadable phone/tablet application. A shortened screening version that contains only 6 items (Table 30.3), the short form Mini-Nutritional Assessment, is also available as a self-assessment interactive tool for patients and caregivers at (https://www.allacronyms.com/SNAQ/Simplified_Nutritional_Assessment_Questionnaire [accessed Feb 2019]). Another nutritional assessment tool, the Simplified Nutrition Assessment Questionnaire (www.slu.edu/readstory/newslink/6349 [accessed Feb 2019]) can be answered by patients through the mail or while sitting in a waiting room; it has a sensitivity and specificity of 88.2% and 83.5%, respectively, for identifying those at risk of at least 5% weight loss within 6 months. Despite the effectiveness of these tools to identify nutritionally at-risk older individuals, no data exist to demonstrate that these tools positively impact patient outcomes.

NUTRITION SYNDROMES

Involuntary Weight Loss

Involuntary weight loss and low body weight can have potentially serious clinical implications. Clinically important weight loss is commonly defined as loss of 10 lbs (4.5 kg) or >5% of usual body weight over a period of 6–12 months. Weight loss >10% of body weight often represents protein/energy under-nutrition, and 20% loss is associated with impaired physiologic function, including cell-mediated and humoral immunity. A BMI <17 kg/m² is consistent with under-nutrition. Excess loss of lean body mass results in skeletal muscle wasting, loss of visceral protein, and associated nutrient deficiencies, and is associated with poor wound healing, infections, pressure injury, depressed functional ability, and mortality. Involuntary weight loss is present in approximately >50% of nursing-home residents and in 25%–50% of hospitalized and 13% of ambulatory, outpatient, community-dwelling, and home-bound older adults.

Etiologies of involuntary weight loss are approximately 50% organ related, 20% neoplastic, 20% idiopathic that includes sarcopenia associated with aging, and 10% psychosocial conditions (Table 30.4). Detailed testing for involuntary weight loss should be guided by the patient's clinical condition. In evaluating involuntary weight loss, the following strategy is recommended: careful documentation of body weight over time; detailed history, including medical, dietary, and psychosocial elements; a physical examination; focused additional testing based on the history, physical, and limited standard laboratory profile; institution of treatment of underlying cause(s); and appropriate follow-up to assess response to management. Without symptoms, or examination or laboratory findings that might direct radiographic studies, there is no proven utility to all-body imaging.

Nutritional therapy should include dietary education, removing dietary restrictions for chronic conditions, nutritional supplements given between meals and supervised by a dietitian, and a multivitamin/multimineral supplement to prevent micronutrient deficiencies (SOE=C). Unfortunately, the clinical benefits of full replacement nutrition are difficult to document, and avoidance of severe nutritional compromise is of critical importance.

Obesity

The growing prevalence of obesity in America extends to older adults in their 60s and 70s. According to

Table 30.4—Etiologies of Involuntary Weight Loss

Organ-related (50%)
  Congestive heart failure
  COPD
  Chronic kidney disease
  Chronic infection
  Inflammatory states
  GI conditions
  Medications
  Neurodegenerative
    Dementia
    Parkinson's disease

Neoplasm (20%)

Idiopathic (20%)
  Frailty

Psychosocial (10%)
  Depression
  Isolation
  Economic
  Environmental

National Health and Nutrition Examination Surveys, the prevalence of obesity (BMI ≥30 kg/m²) has climbed from 14% to 35% between 1976 and 2010. Trends were similar for all ages, both genders, and all racial or ethnic groups.

Excess body weight and modest weight gain (≥5 kg) in middle age can be associated with medical comorbidities in later life that include hypertension, diabetes mellitus, cardiovascular disease, obstructive sleep apnea, and osteoarthritis. The relationship between BMI and all-cause mortality is a U-shaped curve, with the risk of death rising at both extremes of BMI. Adverse outcomes associated with obesity include impaired functional status, increased use of health care resources, and increased mortality (SOE=B). A BMI ≥35 kg/m² is associated with increased risk of functional decline among older adults. Of interest, poor diet quality and micronutrient deficiencies are relatively common among obese older adults, especially obese older women living alone. However, in older individuals, higher BMI may have a protective effect with mortality rates lowest for individuals with BMIs of 27–29 kg/m². This relationship persists even when BMI is controlled for lean body mass. The interplay between obesity and sarcopenia, termed sarcopenic obesity, is defined as a combination of low muscle mass and strength and high fat mass especially visceral fat, however, the importance and clinical usefulness of sarcopenic obestty requires further research. Many homebound older adults are also obese. The National Institutes of Health has suggested: "Age alone should not preclude weight loss treatment for older adults. A careful evaluation of potential risks and benefits in the individual patient should guide management." The focus must be on achieving a more healthful weight to promote improved health, function, and quality of life. A combination of prudent diet, behavior modification, and physical activity, including exercise, may be appropriate for selected patients. For frail, obese older adults, the emphasis may better be placed on preservation of strength and flexibility and maintaining weight rather than on weight reduction.

NUTRITIONAL INTERVENTIONS

Oral Nutrition and Nutritional Supplements

Preventing undernutrition is much easier than treating it. Food intake can be enhanced by catering to food preferences as much as possible and by avoiding therapeutic diets unless their clinical value is certain. Patients should be prepared for meals with appropriate hand and mouth care, and they should be comfortably situated for eating. Assistance should be provided for those who need help. Placing two or more patients together for meals can increase sociability and food intake. Foods should be of appropriate consistency, prepared with attention to color, texture, temperature, and arrangement. The use of herbs, spices, and hot foods helps to compensate for loss of the sense of taste and smell often accompanying older age and to avoid the excessive use of salt and sugar. Hard-to-open individual packages should be avoided. Adequate time should be given for leisurely meals. Title IIIC of the Older Americans Act has provided for congregate and home-delivered meals for older adults, regardless of economic status. This service is available in most parts of the country, albeit with a waiting list in many locations. Adequate access to nutritious and appetizing food should be assured for patients of various cultural backgrounds and in all settings.

Nutritional supplements containing protein and energy (calories) have been widely used in an effort to enhance caloric and nutrient intake, especially when patients eat only small amounts of food. The use of such supplements may decrease food intake, but overall nutritional intake usually increases owing to the nutrient quality and density of the supplements (SOE=C). Standard supplements contain macro- and micronutrients. Many different oral formulations are available in both liquid and solid bar forms. They can be chosen based on patient preferences, chewing ability, or product cost. Oral formulas can also be selected based on their caloric density, osmolality, protein, fiber, or lactose content. Most formulas provide 1–1.5 calories/mL, and many are lactose- and/or gluten-free. Supplementation with energy and protein produces a small but consistent weight gain in older adults. Mortality may be reduced in older adults who are hospitalized and undernourished. There may also be a beneficial effect on complications, which needs to be confirmed. However, there is no evidence of improvement in functional benefit or reduction in length of hospital stay with supplements. In addition, current evidence does not support routine supplementation for homebound older adults or for well-nourished older patients in any setting.

Interest is also growing in the use of micronutrient supplements in health promotion to ensure adequate dietary intake of essential nutrients. Many vitamin and mineral supplements are commonly available in supermarkets and drugstores and are generally safe except for excessive intake of some, such as vitamins A and D, and iron. Vitamin D deficiency occurs in 30% of individuals >70 years old and is associated with impaired calcium absorption and reduced physical activity level. The U.S. Preventive Services Task Force concluded that the current evidence is insufficient for balancing the benefits and harms of screening for vitamin D deficiency in asymptomatic adults because 1) there is a lack of consensus on the cut-off level for defining vitamin D deficiency, and 2) the sensitivity and specificity of the many tests to measure serum total 25-hydroxyvitamin D [25(OH)D] levels are unknown. Furthermore, there is lack of clarity as to whether current laboratory reference ranges are appropriate for all ethnic groups. For example, while the prevalence rates of vitamin D deficiency are higher among black individuals than white individuals, the risk of fracture in black persons is half that seen in white persons. Screening for vitamin D deficiency with measurement of 25(OH)D levels may be appropriate in older patients at risk of vitamin D deficiency (ie, weight loss, malnutrition), because repletion is associated with improved bone healing and response to bisphosphonates (SOE=B). A daily intake of 800–1,000 IU of vitamin D is sufficient to meet the needs of 97.5% of the adult population >70 years old according to the Institute of Medicine. Supplements of vitamin D up to 4,000 IU daily are considered safe in nonfrail older adults.

Supplemental folic acid, vitamin B_6, and vitamin B_{12} can lower homocysteine levels. However, evidence to date from randomized controlled trials with folic acid or vitamin B_6 supplementation is poor and has not demonstrated reduced risk of coronary artery disease or prevention of cognitive decline. Insufficient evidence also exists to determine whether immune function can be improved by protein, vitamin E, zinc, or other micronutrient supplementation (SOE=C). Whether the effects of antioxidants are beneficial is also controversial. Although it has previously been suggested that antioxidants can help in preventing age-related cataracts and macular degeneration, evidence indicates that they may have little or no effect. Although naturally occurring dietary antioxidants can reduce risk of cardiovascular disease and mortality, supplementation with specific antioxidants, namely β-carotene, vitamin A, and vitamin E, can increase mortality in some settings (SOE=C). In addition, vitamin E supplementation has not been shown to slow progression of Alzheimer disease or prevent cardiovascular disease, but it may be associated with higher risk of hemorrhagic stroke. Further, among individuals with diabetes or vascular disease, supplementation with vitamin E can increase risk of heart failure (SOE=C).

Because approximately 60% of older adults take self-prescribed dietary supplements, it is imperative that the clinician obtain information about the patient's use of all supplements. The appropriateness and safety of each supplement should be evaluated, because patients are often unaware of potential risks and adverse events of many OTC supplements, and solid evidence in favor of purported benefits of these supplements is currently lacking.

Drug Treatment for Undernutrition Syndromes

A number of agents have been suggested to promote appetite or to serve as anabolic aids. Although some studies involving selected patient populations (eg, AIDS, certain cancers) suggest limited efficacy, there are no reports demonstrating improvement in long-term survival, and some agents may cause serious adverse effects, particularly among older adults (SOE=C). Appetite stimulants include mirtazapine[OL], an α_2-antagonist antidepressant that antagonizes the 5-HT3 receptor, possibly stimulating appetite by that mechanism, but proof of this effect is limited (SOE=C). Dosing is 7.5–30 mg po at bedtime. Caution is required for dosages of 15–30 mg/d because of hepatic or renal insufficiency and more noradrenergic and serotonin effects, some of which may counteract the appetite stimulatory effects. Cyproheptadine[OL], a serotonin and histamine antagonist, can also enhance appetite (SOE=C), but there is the potential for confusion in older adults. It is given at a dose of 2–4 mg po with meals. Megestrol[OL] is a progestin that stimulates appetite and is given daily at 320–800 mg po in two equal doses. Appetite and weight usually improve with megestrol acetate; however, this weight gain is primarily fat, and clinical benefits have not been demonstrated (SOE=A). In addition, megestrol acetate in nursing-home populations can be associated with a higher risk of deep-vein thrombosis, fluid retention, edema, and exacerbation of congestive heart failure. There is a strong AGS Beers Criteria® warning to avoid prescribing this agent. Finally, megestrol acetate taken during rehabilitation may negate the benefits of exercise on strength and function. Dronabinol[OL], a cannabinoid, can stimulate appetite at 2.5 mg twice daily before lunch and dinner (maximum 20 mg/d), but it is associated with somnolence and dysphoria in older adults.

Cytokine-modulating agents are experimental in the treatment of undernutrition syndromes, even though anticytokines have been breakthrough treatments for selected forms of disease-related cachexia. Approaches include anti–tumor necrosis factor, consisting of antibodies that can inhibit cytokine-mediated inflammation, and n-3 fatty acids and antioxidants, which can modulate cytokine production.

Anabolic agents include human growth hormone[OL] (HGH), which induces preferential usage of carbohydrates and fats while preserving proteins and increasing muscle mass. However, increased muscle strength and functional capacity depend mostly on exercise rehabilitation. HGH is contraindicated in cancer states. Hyperglycemia and fluid retention can be seen, and no studies have demonstrated significant functional benefits of HGH. Oxandrolone is an anabolic steroid that increases muscle protein synthesis; it is given orally at 2.5–20 mg/d in divided doses. Anabolic agents can increase muscle mass, but questions remain concerning long-term safety and cost that currently mitigate endorsement (SOE=B). Likewise, although muscle mass has consistently improved with anabolic agents, significant improvements in strength and function, or a reduction in fractures have not been demonstrated.

CULTURALLY APPROPRIATE NUTRITIONAL CARE

Cultural factors dramatically influence health behaviors and outcomes. In the United States, minority older adult (>65 years old) populations are projected to increase from 21% of the population in 2012 to 28% by 2030. During that same time period, the older Hispanic population is expected to increase from 7.3% to 11%; older African-Americans from 8.8% to 10.7%; and older American Indians, Eskimos, Asians, and Pacific Islanders from 4.5% to 5.9% . The United States will continue to be characterized as an increasingly diverse population. In addition to genetics and nutrition intake, nutritional status of older adults could be affected by socioeconomic factors, such as education and income level and environmental factors, such as proximity to stores and transportation that can affect food variety and availability. Ethnic and religious customs are 2 of many factors that influence food preferences. Cultural variation is additionally influenced by regionalism and within-culture diversity. Nutrition and aging are connected inseparably, because eating patterns affect progress of many chronic and degenerative diseases associated with aging. In turn, disease progression, health status, and ultimately quality of life may be adversely affected by a number of cultural and ethnic factors associated either directly or indirectly with nutrition and aging.

For example, some Latino groups believe in disease as destiny (ie, fatalism) and often fear adverse effects of medications given to treat disease. Some patients expect the healer to cure the ailment, with difficulty comprehending the concept of chronic illness. This can greatly compromise the care of certain conditions such as diabetes. The hot and cold theory of disease traditionally held by Latino cultures is a continuing influence of ancient Greek and Arabic humoral pathology, which maintained that the four body "humors" regulated health and disease: blood, phlegm, and black and yellow bile, each characterized as warm or cold, wet or dry. Although disagreement exists within Latino populations, warm illnesses (kidney ailments, rashes, dysentery) are produced by the body, and cold illnesses (pain, paralysis, stomachache) are produced by outside influences. Warm illnesses are treated by avoiding cold foods (vegetables, dairy products, tropical fruits), and cold illnesses by avoiding warm foods (lamb, beef, grains, temperate fruits).

Multicultural nutrition counseling competencies are critical in managing nutritional health and chronic illness for diverse populations. It is important for clinicians to be aware of how cultural background and experiences and attitudes, values, and biases influence nutrition counseling and to be advised to acquire cultural knowledge and sensitivity for appropriate nutrition intervention and materials. Many culturally appropriate nutrition education materials are available in English and other languages, including My Plate for Older Adults, a USDA product also available in Spanish (http://hnrca.tufts.edu/myplate/ [accessed Feb 2019]). Oldways® (http://oldwayspt.org [accessed Feb 2019]), a nonprofit organization that promotes healthy eating based on regional diets, has developed consumer-friendly pyramids that display prudent food choices in a culturally sensitive manner. These pyramids include Mediterranean, Latino, Asian, African-American, and vegetarian and vegan alternatives to the USDA My Plate for Older Adults and reflect consistency with eating patterns of healthy populations around the world.

LEGAL AND ETHICAL ISSUES

In the nursing home, unacceptable weight loss, as defined by the Omnibus Budget Reconciliation Act of 1987, is any loss ≥5% in the past month or ≥10% in the past 6 months. Sections of the Minimum Data Set related to nutritional status include those assessing cognitive function, mood and behavior, physical function, health condition, oral and nutritional status, dental status, skin condition, and special treatments and procedures, including restorative care for eating and swallowing. Care Area Assessments (formerly called Resident Assessment Protocols) ensure prompt identification of problems focused on by the MDS. The MDS uses intake of <75% of food provided as the threshold to trigger nutrition assessment. Legal and clinical standards of care dictate the following:

- Acceptable parameters of nutritional status such as body weight and protein levels should be maintained; unless the resident's clinical condition demonstrates that this is not possible.

- A resident should receive a therapeutic diet when there is a problem.

Food and fluids should always be offered to all patients; however, the decision to start or to discontinue artificial nutrition or hydration must be considered very carefully. Competent adults may choose to forgo artificial feeding, just as they have the right to decline any invasive procedure. Some adults have advance directives executed at a time when the individual was competent that prohibit the use of feeding tubes. These should be honored unless there is compelling evidence that the individual would have changed his or her mind in the current situation. Older adults without decision-making capacity and without advance directives pose a greater challenge. The decision to start or to discontinue artificial feeding should be considered carefully with the surrogate, taking into account the risks and burdens of such an action, the risks and burdens of alternative actions, and the evidence to support likely benefits of the various actions. To date, evidence does not support the use of feeding tubes in patients with end-stage cancer, dementia, or COPD.

After total cessation of nutrition, depending on underlying conditions, several weeks may ensue before death, and some patients who consume very little may survive much longer. In this setting, palliative care, including emotional support, is extremely important and complex.

CHOOSING WISELY® RECOMMENDATIONS

Feeding and Swallowing

- Do not recommend percutaneous feeding tubes in patients with advanced dementia; instead offer oral assisted feeding.

- Avoid using prescription appetite stimulants or high-calorie supplements for treatment of anorexia or cachexia in older adults; instead, optimize social supports, provide feeding assistance, and clarify patient goals and expectations.

RESOURCES

- The National Academies of Science, Engineering, and Medicine. www.nationalacademies.org/hmd/Reports.aspx?filters=inmeta:iom_topic=Food%20and%20Nutrition (accessed Feb 2019).

- Wright W, Zelman K. Maximizing your "nutrition minute": Bridging nutritional gaps across the life span. *J Am Assoc Nurse Pract*. 2018;30(3):160–177.

- Yannakoulia M, Ntanasi E, Anastasiou CA, et al. Frailty and nutrition: from epidemiological and clinical evidence to potential mechanisms. *Metabolism*. 2017;68:64–76.

CHAPTER 31—SWALLOWING AND FEEDING

KEY POINTS

- Most healthy people aspirate regularly without any important clinical consequences.

- With aging, chewing becomes less efficient, and swallowing is slowed for most healthy older adults.

- Dementia is the most common cause of oral dysphagia.

- Aspiration pneumonitis results when gastric contents, usually sterile, are misdirected into the lungs. This condition is not treated with antibiotics.

- Aspiration pneumonia is believed to occur when contaminated oral secretions arrive in the lungs in a high enough inoculum to overcome host defenses.

- Many studies identify feeding tubes as major risk factors for aspiration of both oral and gastric contents.

- Given the absence of data linking interventions resultant from swallowing studies with clinical outcomes, the assessment of swallowing function is controversial. Performing swallowing studies in delirious patients is nonsensical.

Swallowing is a complex event affected by both normal aging and diseases that are common in older adults. Treatment of eating and feeding problems depends on identified cause(s) and contributing factors. Many medications contribute to feeding problems at a variety of levels.

SWALLOWING IN HEALTH AND DISEASE

Swallowing and Aging

Swallowing can be divided into 3 phases on the basis of anatomy. First is the preparatory or oral phase, which includes the complex activities of mastication and propelling the food bolus to the back of the mouth toward the pharynx. This stage is under voluntary control and requires attention, praxis, and coordination. The second or pharyngeal phase is involuntary and involves initiation of the swallow reflex with propulsion of the food bolus past the laryngeal vestibule and into the esophagus. Execution of the oral and pharyngeal phases of swallowing requires the complex coordination of 5 cranial nerves and a large number of small muscles in the head and neck, with regulation from cortical input to the medullary swallow center, all in the appropriate sequence, usually within 1 second. The third stage of swallowing is the esophageal phase, during which food is propelled down the esophagus by the action of skeletal muscle proximally and smooth muscle distally; this phase is regulated by its own intrinsic innervation.

Normal aging is associated with several changes in eating. With advanced age, taste sensation decreases but not taste discrimination (older adults may be able to distinguish sweet from salty but may need to add more salt to food to taste it sufficiently). Olfactory function declines with advancing age, further impairing taste sensation. Loss of teeth greatly reduces chewing efficiency (ie, chewing is needed for a longer period of time and with more chewing strokes to achieve the same level of food maceration), which is only partly ameliorated with dental prostheses. Sarcopenia, or age-related loss of lean muscle mass, can contribute to loss in chewing efficiency and to pharyngeal muscle weakness demonstrated on videofluoroscopic deglutition examination (VDE) of asymptomatic older adults. Whether aging alone contributes to esophageal dysmotility (so-called presbyesophagus) remains a subject of debate. Esophageal function is probably well preserved, except perhaps in very advanced age. In total, these changes with age result in a prolonged duration of each swallow.

Dysphagia

Dysphagia, or difficulty swallowing, can occur when a disease affects any level of swallowing function. Dysphagia is usually classified as oral, pharyngeal, or esophageal. In oral dysphagia, there is difficulty with the voluntary transfer of food from the mouth to the pharynx. This might be diagnosed, for example, when scrambled eggs are discovered in the cheeks of a patient with dementia shortly before lunch. The most common cause of oral dysphagia is dementia.

In pharyngeal dysphagia, there is a problem with reflexive transfer of the food bolus from the pharynx to initiate the involuntary esophageal phase of swallowing while simultaneously protecting the airway from misdirection of food. The affected person or a caregiver may notice coughing, choking, or nasal regurgitation while eating and localize the symptoms to the throat. The most common cause of pharyngeal dysphagia is stroke, but any disease that impairs the swallowing center in the brain stem or the cranial nerves involved (eg, Parkinson disease, CNS tumor), the oropharyngeal striated muscle (eg, myasthenia gravis, amyotrophic lateral sclerosis), or the local structures involved (eg, retropharyngeal abscess, tumor) can lead to pharyngeal dysphagia. Management of both oral and pharyngeal dysphagia involves treating the underlying disorder and devising an individualized, often labor-intensive, feeding program.

In esophageal dysphagia, the patient has the sensation that food has gotten "stuck" after a swallow. Dysphagia for both solids and liquids suggests an esophageal motility disorder (eg, achalasia, scleroderma), whereas progressive dysphagia for solids suggests a mechanical obstruction (eg, cancer, esophageal ring, stricture from mucosal irritation). None of these diseases is unique to the geriatric population, although older adults tend to take more medications and are therefore more likely to experience medication-induced esophagitis (which manifests initially as odynophagia, followed by dysphagia). Medications most commonly causing esophagitis in older adults are potassium, NSAIDs, oral bisphosphonates, and tetracycline-related antibiotics. Indirectly, medications that promote candidal esophagitis, such as prednisone or immunosuppressants, also contribute to esophageal dysphagia usually with odynophagia.

Aspiration

The misdirection of oral or gastric contents into the airway is termed *aspiration*. However, controversy persists over the definition of *aspiration pneumonia*. Aspiration pneumonia is believed to occur when bacteria arrive in the lungs from the pharynx in a large enough inoculum to overcome host defenses. In the case of more virulent organisms, defenses can be overwhelmed by smaller inocula, and when host defenses are weak, smaller inocula may also be problematic. Pneumococcal pneumonia arises from aspiration of *Pneumococcus* from a colonized oropharynx and is usually not considered an aspiration pneumonia, highlighting how inexactly the nomenclature is applied. Aspiration of gastric contents, or Mendelson syndrome, usually results in a chemical pneumonitis; the usefulness of antibiotics in this situation is questionable. Most often, after a period that can include fever, tachypnea, hypoxemia, and rales that last <24 hours, local host defense mechanisms clear the lung of the offending aspirate, without serious clinical effect unless the volume of aspirate is large or recurrent aspiration leads to pulmonary scarring. Many healthy individuals episodically aspirate without any important clinical consequences.

Aspiration of contaminated oral or of gastric contents is not prevented by placement of a feeding tube. In fact, tube feeding is universally cited as a risk factor for major aspiration, and some patients who have never previously aspirated begin to do so after a feeding tube has been placed.

Assessment of Oropharyngeal Dysphagia

Several tools can be used to assess swallowing function when oropharyngeal dysphagia is suspected clinically. The most common are the full bedside evaluation (of which there are many variations), the VDE (a variant of the modified barium swallow), and nasopharyngeal laryngoscopy performed by an otolaryngologist. There is considerable controversy regarding the relative efficacy of these tools.

VDE is usually performed by a speech-language pathologist who videotapes the patient swallowing barium-impregnated foods of several consistencies while maintaining various head positions. This can permit identification of the food consistency or compensatory mechanisms that minimize fluoroscopic evidence of aspiration. Depending on the results of the VDE, the therapist may recommend swallow therapy or diet modifications, or both. Swallow therapy may be compensatory (eg, turn head toward weaker side while swallowing), indirect (eg, exercises to improve the strength of the involved muscles), or direct (ie, exercises to perform while swallowing, such as swallowing multiple times per bolus). Dietary recommendations generally consist of altering bolus size or consistency of food or fluid, or of restricting foods of certain consistencies. Unfortunately, there is insufficient evidence to support any clinical benefit in altering dietary consistency (SOE=D).

FEEDING

Tube Feeding Versus Hand Feeding

When an older adult experiences difficulty eating, the two main therapeutic approaches are careful feeding by tube or hand. Tube feeding is an invasive intervention associated with its own risks; hand feeding requires extraordinary patience and is labor intensive. Data about either approach are limited, and randomized comparisons have not been done.

The number of percutaneous endoscopic gastrostomy feeding tubes placed in patients ≥65 years old had been growing at an astonishing rate. Low procedure-related complication rates are often cited; however, long-term studies reveal substantial mortality among tube-fed patients. Despite the popularity of feeding tubes, studies have not demonstrated improved survival, reduced incidence of pneumonia or other infections, improved symptoms or function, or reduced pressure injury with the use of feeding tubes of any type in patients with dementia who have eating difficulties, and the American Geriatrics Society lists the practice of feeding tube placement in patients with dementia as one of the Choosing Wisely practices that patients and physicians should question. Median survival after placement of a feeding tube is well under a year, but it is unknown whether this results from tube feeding or if the need for tube feeding is a marker that death is near.

Complications described with feeding tubes are numerous and include an increased risk of aspiration pneumonia, metabolic disturbances, diarrhea, and local cellulitis. Monitoring for these complications should be meticulous. Patients in nursing homes fed by tube have less contact time with nursing and support staff than those who are hand fed. Although paradoxically likely a marker of poorer quality of care in a nursing home, feeding by tube is reimbursed at a higher rate than the more labor-intensive hand-feeding approach. Tube feedings may interfere with absorption of some medications, eg, levodopa/carbidopa and phenytoin. Time-released medications cannot be crushed for administration through the tube.

Overall, there is a lack of evidence that feeding tubes are of benefit to most older adults. The American Geriatrics Society has issued a helpful position statement regarding the use of feeding tubes (see Resources).

Contraindications to gastrostomy include the inability to pass an endoscope into the stomach, uncorrectable coagulopathy, massive ascites, peritonitis, and bowel obstruction. After successful placement of a gastrostomy, the stoma is not epithelialized for up to a month but the tube may be used right away with tube feedings of commercially available canned nutritional supplements as slow gravity boluses for gastrostomy tubes over 30–60 minutes or as a continuous infusion. The feeding tube should be flushed with water before and after each feeding or at least 4 times a day in cases of continuous feeding.

For many older adults, a viable, albeit time-intensive alternative to tube feeding is careful hand feeding. With age, chewing and swallowing become slower; this is compounded significantly when cognitive impairment and apraxia exist. Aspiration may be reduced by feeding the person in an upright posture, but not all older adults are capable of maintaining this position. Feeding one or two individuals by hand requires impressive patience, made easier when combined with a genuine commitment to each person's well-being. Nursing-home staff are often harried, poorly reimbursed, infrequently appreciated, and do not remain in the job long enough to develop deeply caring relationships with the residents. Although evidence does not support improved safety of tube feeding over hand feeding, many nursing home administrators—and often other providers and family members—perceive this to be the case. As noted previously, financial incentives also favor the use of expensive, burdensome, and likely less compassionate feeding tubes in this setting. While the use of feeding tubes in older adults is declining, these barriers to more substantial reductions remain challenging.

Approaches to Nondysphagia Feeding Problems

Not all feeding problems are related to dysphagia, and many contributing factors are quite amenable to therapy. Oral hygiene is often neglected but when addressed, through meticulous mouth care and properly fitting dental prostheses, can result in substantial improvements in eating. Other approaches to consider in older adults who demonstrate eating or feeding problems are evaluating for depression or metabolic disorders, eliminating unduly restrictive diets, considering individual food preferences, considering the environment in which the person eats to improve socialization and reduce disruptive stimuli, determining the need for personal assistance with feeding, and reducing or eliminating medications that can cause inattention, xerostomia, movement disorders, or anorexia. Small studies have documented improved clinical outcomes in nursing-home residents with the use of flavor enhancers, increased food variety, and attention to the meal ambiance.

CHOOSING WISELY® RECOMMENDATIONS

Swallowing and Feeding

- Do not recommend percutaneous feeding tubes in patients with advanced dementia; instead offer oral assisted feeding.
- Avoid using prescription appetite stimulants or high-calorie supplements for treatment of anorexia or cachexia in older adults; instead, optimize social supports, provide feeding assistance, and clarify patient goals and expectations.

RESOURCES

- American Geriatrics Society. Feeding tubes in advanced dementia position statement. *J Am Geriatr Soc.* 2014;62(8):1590–1593.

- Batchelor-Murphy M, McConnell E, Amelia E, et al. Experimental comparison of efficacy for three handfeeding techniques in dementia. *J Am Geriatr Soc.* 2017;65(4):e89–e94.

- Sura L, Madhavan A, Carnaby G, et al. Dysphagia in the elderly: management and nutritional considerations. *Clin Interv Aging.* 2012;7:287–298.

CHAPTER 32—URINARY INCONTINENCE

KEY POINTS

- The prevalence of urinary incontinence (UI) increases with age and ADL dependence, affecting 15%–30% of all adults ≥65 years old and 60%–70% of long-term care residents.

- The etiology of UI in older adults is usually multifactorial and may include medical conditions, functional and cognitive impairment, and medications, with or without concomitant lower urinary tract dysfunction. Therefore, assessment of comorbidity, medications, and function are essential components of evaluation.

- Even in frailer older adults, UI is manageable through a stepped approach that starts with addressing comorbidity, impairments, and medications, followed by lifestyle interventions, behavioral therapy, medications, minimally invasive, and surgical interventions as appropriate.

Urinary incontinence (UI) is the involuntary leakage of any amount of urine. In younger people, the etiology of UI often can be attributed after evaluation to a specific pathophysiology in the lower urinary tract (LUT) and/or pelvic floor. In older adults, however, the cause of UI can be comorbid conditions, medications, or functional and cognitive impairments, either alone or in combination with LUT dysfunction. Thus, UI is a classic geriatric syndrome, common in older adults with multiple chronic conditions, in which multiple risk factors interact with one another and other modulating factors to produce a clinical phenotype, ie, urine leakage.

There are 4 main types of types of UI symptoms in older adults:

- Urge UI—leakage associated with urgency, a compelling and often sudden need to void that is difficult to forestall.

- Stress UI—leakage associated with coughing, sneezing, laughing, or physical activity.

- Mixed UI—leakage occurs with both urgency and activity.

- UI associated with incomplete bladder emptying—leakage occurs in the setting of an increased postvoid residual (PVR) due to either bladder outlet obstruction (eg, by an enlarged prostate) or an impairment in bladder contractility.

There is no consensus on a clinically important definition of increased PVR. Some suggest a cut-off of 200 mL, others suggest a lower volume (100–150 mL) cut-off.

UI may be accompanied by other lower urinary tract symptoms (LUTS), including frequency, nocturia (awakening to void >1 time during sleep), slow urine stream, hesitancy, sense of incomplete emptying, and intermittent stream. "Overactive bladder" refers to a symptom complex of urgency, with or without urge UI, often accompanied with frequency and nocturia. UI, LUTS, and "overactive bladder" are all nonspecific terms and may be due to a range of lower urinary tract pathophysiology as well as comorbid conditions and medications.

UI caused or exacerbated by comorbid conditions and medications or impaired mobility has been called "transient UI" and "functional UI." These terms do not acknowledge the underlying LUT dysfunction.

PREVALENCE AND IMPACT

UI increases with age and affects women more than men (ratio 2:1) until age 80, after which men and women are equally affected. The prevalence is 15%–30% in community-dwelling adults ≥65 years old, and 60%–70% in long-term care settings. In most studies, overall rates of UI are higher in white women than in black, Hispanic, and Asian women, and stress UI is more common in white and Hispanic women than in black women. Racial and ethnic differences among older men are less clear. The few longitudinal studies in older women suggest annual UI incidence rates of 5%–11% in the community and 22% in long-term care, with remission rates that nearly match incidence. Estimating the prevalence of the different types of UI is difficult because of wide variability in source populations and definitions. In general, young-old women are most likely to have mixed UI and old-old women more likely to have more urge UI. Young-old men are most likely to have more mixed UI (stress-predominant) because of the prevalence of prostatectomy, and old-old men more likely to have more urge UI. UI due to impaired bladder emptying is the least prevalent type in both women and men (<10%).

UI significantly impairs quality of life, including emotional well-being, social function, and general health. Older adults with UI may maintain social activities but do so with an increased burden of coping, embarrassment, and poor self-perception. Morbidity from UI includes dermatitis and cellulitis, pressure injury, urinary tract infections, falls with fractures, sleep deprivation, social withdrawal, depression, and sexual dysfunction. UI is not associated with increased mortality. UI increases caregiving time and burden, which may be why it remains a significant factor in families' decision to place a loved one in long-term care placement. Out-of-pocket costs per year for women (for pads and medical complications) are

Table 32.1—Medications That Can Cause or Worsen Urinary Incontinence

Medication	Effect on Continence
Alcohol	Polyuria, frequency, sedation, delirium, immobility
α-Adrenergic agonists	Outlet obstruction (men)
α-Adrenergic blockers	Stress incontinence (women)
ACE inhibitors	Stress incontinence from associated cough
Anticholinergics	Impaired emptying, retention, delirium, sedation, constipation, fecal impaction
Antipsychotics	Anticholinergic effects plus rigidity, sedation, and immobility
Calcium channel blockers	Impaired detrusor contractility, dihydropyridine agents cause nocturnal polyuria from pedal edema
Cholinesterase inhibitors	Urinary incontinence, potential interactions with anticholinergics
Estrogen (oral)	Stress and mixed leakage in women
GABAergic agents (eg, gabapentin, pregabalin)	Sedation, dizziness; edema causing nocturnal polyuria
Loop diuretics	Polyuria, frequency
Narcotic analgesics	Urinary retention, fecal impaction, sedation, delirium
NSAIDs	Edema causing nocturnal polyuria
Sedative hypnotics	Sedation, delirium, immobility
SGLT2 inhibitors	Polyuria, frequency
Thiazolidinediones	Pedal edema causing nocturnal polyuria
Tricyclic antidepressants	Anticholinergic effects, sedation

up to $900 a year. Estimated annual costs related to UI in older adults total more than $26 billion.

RISK FACTORS AND ASSOCIATED COMORBID CONDITIONS

Other than age, the evidence-based risk factors for UI in older adults include obesity (best demonstrated in young-old women), functional impairment, dementia, medications (Table 32.1), diabetes, and environmental barriers to toilet access. The association of vaginal delivery and parity with UI attenuates with age. These data pertain primarily to white women; much less is known about UI risk factors in other racial and ethnic populations. In men, the best studied risk factors are benign and malignant prostate disease and their treatment, but there are few data on other risk factors.

Especially in older adults, continence depends not only on LUT function but also on the ability to toilet, which requires sufficient physical function (mobility and manual dexterity), cognition, motivation, and available toilets.

Medications (Table 32.1) and medical conditions can cause or worsen UI via multiple pathways that include direct and indirect effects on LUT function, toileting, and/or urine output. For example, incontinence in people with diabetes can occur from direct neurologic effects (with detrusor overactivity [DO] being far more common than underactivity [cystopathy]), disease complications (eg, constipation, glycosuria, impaired ambulation from peripheral vascular disease), and complications from treatment (eg, thioglitazone- and gabapentin-associated edema causing nocturia).

Not every older adult with a comorbid condition or taking a medication that is associated with UI will develop UI, and the presence of such factors in an individual person with UI does not imply that they are causative. The best example of this is the relationship between UI and dementia. Although older adults with dementia may have impairment in central inhibitory pathways that control urgency, impaired functional status and mobility are at least as strong or stronger predictors of UI than cognitive status. Older adults with advanced dementia may remain continent if they can transfer and ambulate with minimal to moderate assistance. Furthermore, older adults with dementia may have other types of LUT dysfunction and symptoms than urge UI: one-third of nursing-home residents with UI have stress UI or bladder outlet obstructions on urodynamic testing.

PATHOPHYSIOLOGY

Age-Related LUT Changes

A number of age-related physiologic changes in LUT function predispose older adults to UI. In both

Table 32.2—Medications Used to Treat Urge-Predominant UI

Agent	Formulation	Dosage
Darifenacin		7.5–15 mg/d
Fesoterodine		4–8 mg/d
Mirabegron		25–50 mg/d
Oxybutynin	Immediate release	2.5–5 mg q6–12h
	Extended release	5–20 mg/d
	Topical patch	3.9 mg/24 hr applied twice weekly to abdomen, thighs, or buttocks
	Topical gel (3% gel or 10% sachet)	Daily
Solifenacin		5–10 mg/d
Tolterodine	Immediate release	1–2 mg q12h
	Extended release	2–4 mg/d
Trospium	Immediate release	20 mg q12h or q24h
	Extended release	60 mg/d in am

genders, bladder contractility decreases, uninhibited bladder contractions are more prevalent, diurnal urine output occurs later in the day, and sphincteric striated muscle attenuates, while bladder capacity decreases and PVR increases (both modestly and without clear clinical significance). In women, urethral closure pressure decreases, and vaginal mucosal atrophy is prevalent. Benign prostatic hyperplasia and prostate hypertrophy increase in men. Why some older adults with age-related LUT changes develop UI and others do not remains unclear; differences in LUT function and other compensatory mechanisms may play a role.

LUT Pathophysiology in UI

Specific UI symptoms and LUT pathophysiology overlap substantially. However, some general associations (with caveats) are possible:

- **Urge UI with DO:** Up to 40% of continent healthy older adults demonstrate DO on urodynamic testing, suggesting that urge UI requires not only DO but also impaired compensatory mechanisms. Research now emphasizes the roles of afferent stimulation from the bladder urothelium and impaired CNS control of urgency in DO and overactive bladder. DO may be idiopathic, age-related, secondary to lesions in cerebral and spinal inhibitory pathways, due to bladder outlet obstruction, or (less commonly) result from local bladder irritation (eg, infection, stones, tumor).

- **Stress UI and impaired urethral sphincter support and/or closure:** Stress UI can result from 1) damage to pelvic floor supports (levator ani, connective tissues), such that they fail to provide firm resistance and compress the urethra with any increase in intra-abdominal pressures; or 2) failure of the proximal urethra and its sphincter components to remain closed during bladder filling (usually due to surgical damage or severe atrophy or, in rare cases, subsacral spinal cord injury). DO can cause apparent "stress" UI when a cough triggers an uninhibited detrusor contraction. In such cases, leakage usually occurs after and not coincident with the cough, is large in volume, and difficult to stop.

- **Mixed UI with both DO and impaired sphincter support/function:** Mixed UI occurs when the mechanisms of urge and stress UI are both present. The contribution of the different mechanism can vary, such that some mixed UI is urge-predominant and some stress-predominant.

- **UI with impaired bladder emptying due to bladder obstruction and/or detrusor underactivity:** The most common cause of obstruction in men is prostate hyperplasia causing prostate enlargement, and in women urethral surgical scarring or a large cystocele/prolapse that kinks the urethra. Detrusor underactivity can be caused by intrinsic bladder smooth muscle damage (eg, from ischemia, scarring, fibrosis), peripheral neuropathy (diabetes mellitus, vitamin B_{12} deficiency, alcoholism), or damage to the spinal cord and spinal bladder efferent nerves by disc herniation, spinal stenosis, tumor, or degenerative neurologic disease. Neurologic diseases affecting the spinal cord (eg, multiple sclerosis, spinal cord injury) can cause detrusor underactivity and/or neurally mediated obstruction, depending on the exact level and extent of spinal cord involvement.

- **Nocturia:** This is a nonspecific symptom, even in older men, and providers should consider causes other than urge UI and prostate disease.

EVALUATION

Similar to other geriatric syndromes, UI requires multifactorial evaluation with a focus on multimorbidity, function, and medications as contributing factors. Evaluation and management of UI in nursing-home residents are discussed separately below.

Screening

All older patients, especially women, should be asked at least yearly about UI, because 50% of affected individuals do not voluntarily report their symptoms to a health care provider.

Screening questions

- Do you have any problems with bladder control?
- Do you have problems making it to the bathroom on time?
- Do you ever leak urine?

Follow up positive screen with questions to determine the type of UI (SOE=B)

Do you leak urine most often:

- When you are performing some physical activity, such as coughing, sneezing, lifting, or exercising? (stress)
- When you have the urge or feeling that you need to empty your bladder but cannot get to the toilet fast enough? (urge)
- With both physical activity and a sense of urgency? (mixed)
- Without physical activity and without sense of urgency? (other)

History

The history should include UI onset, frequency, volume; timing, and exacerbating and ameliorating factors, including any new medical problems or medications; other LUT symptoms; amount and types of fluid intake; past treatments and results; and pad use. Review of systems should include fecal incontinence and depression (both SOE=B), because both are common in older adults with UI. Screening for sleep apnea should be considered in patients with nocturia with nocturnal polyuria (see below).

UI may be the herald symptom of neurologic disease and cancer. "Red flag" symptoms that require prompt evaluation and referral are abrupt onset of UI, pelvic pain (constant, worsened, or improved with voiding), hematuria, and association with new neurologic symptoms.

Providers should ask patients (and/or caregivers) about UI-associated bother and impact on quality of life, starting with simple questions (eg, "What bothers you most about your leakage?" or "How does leakage affect your daily life?"), followed by more specific probes, as appropriate, regarding impact on ADLs and IADLs, social role, emotional and interpersonal relations, sexual function and relations, self-concept, general health perception, and financial burden.

Physical Examination

The initial general examination should include cognition and functional status, if not recently assessed, and focus on presence and severity of comorbid conditions that may be associated with UI (SOE=D). Abdominal palpation is insensitive and nonspecific for bladder distention. Digital rectal examination can check for masses, fecal loading, and prostate nodules or firmness, but it cannot accurately determine prostate size. Neurologic evaluation is especially important in patients with known neurologic disease, new-onset or sudden worsening of UI, or motor and sensory symptoms. Tests for integrity of the sacral cord (the origin of the pelvic and pudendal nerves innervating the LUT) are perineal sensation, anal "wink" (lightly scratch the perianal area and look for [or palpate during a digital rectal examination] anal sphincter contraction), and bulbocavernosus reflex (lightly touch the clitoris or glans and look for or palpate for anal contraction same as with anal wink). A basic pelvic examination in women should include checking for labial and vaginal lesions and marked pelvic organ prolapse (eg, large uterine prolapse, cystocele extending to or through the introitus). Uncircumcised men should be checked for phimosis, paraphimosis, and balanitis.

A clinical stress test can corroborate stress UI symptoms. The patient should have a full bladder and is instructed to relax the perineum and buttocks, while the examiner is positioned to observe or catch any leakage when the patient gives a single vigorous cough. Clinical stress testing is highly sensitive (most helpful when negative) but less specific (SOE=B). Sensitivity is highest when the patient is standing. It is insensitive if the patient cannot cooperate, is inhibited, or the bladder volume is low.

Additional Testing

The only recommended test for all patients is urinalysis to look for hematuria (and glycosuria in diabetic patients) (SOE=D). If a woman does not have an acute onset of UI, dysuria, fever, or other signs of urinary tract infection, then any pyuria and bacteriuria represent asymptomatic bacteriuria. Asymptomatic bacteriuria is not associated with UI and should not be treated with antibiotics.

Bladder diaries (also called frequency-volume charts) can help to determine whether urine volume contributes to UI frequency and especially nocturia and can assist in evaluation of UI frequency, timing, and circumstances. Typically, a diary entails recording the time and volume of all continent voids and UI episodes for 2–3 days, including day and evening.

PVR measurement is not routinely needed in evaluation of UI (SOE=B), because the cut-off for an "increased" PVR is not standardized, the overall prevalence of high PVR (eg, >200 mL) is low, and there is insufficient evidence that routine PVR measurement affects outcomes. Even older men with LUT symptoms and/or known prostate disease do not require routine PVR testing. PVR measurement may be considered in patients with prior urinary retention, longstanding diabetes, recurrent urinary tract infections, severe constipation, complex neurologic disease, higher than routine risk for prostate enlargement (eg, men with known increased PSA) and in women with marked pelvic organ prolapse or who have had prior surgery for UI (SOE=C). PVR can be measured in the office with ultrasonography or catheterization.

Routine urodynamic testing is not necessary or desirable; it should be considered only if the cause of UI is unclear and knowing it would change management (eg, determine whether a man with severe urge UI also has bladder outlet obstruction), or when empiric treatment has failed and the patient would consider invasive or surgical therapy.

TREATMENT AND MANAGEMENT

As with all geriatric practice, it is important to establish the goals of care for incontinence management from the patient and/or caregivers. For example, desired outcomes may range from complete continence, control sufficient to prevent large volume leakage with tolerance of small volume, to skin integrity and comfort. Patients and caregivers may have different tolerance for or perceptions of the bother, invasiveness, burden of treatment, and desired outcome of treatment.

Treatment should proceed stepwise, from correcting contributory factors and lifestyle modification, to behavioral therapy, medications, and then minimally invasive procedures and surgery as appropriate and consistent with the goals of care. Not all steps will be needed or appropriate for all patients, and some patients may want to proceed directly to specific therapy (eg, women with severe stress UI desiring surgery). Some treatments are effective for several UI symptoms (see below). Management should focus on relieving the aspect of UI that is most bothersome for the patient; for example, treatment that only decreases daytime UI episodes may not be sufficient for those most bothered by the timing of UI, nocturia, or leakage with exercise.

Clinicians should be able to conduct an initial evaluation and begin stepped treatment for most older patients with UI. However, patients presenting with pelvic pain, hematuria, recurrent symptomatic urinary tract infections, pelvic mass, previous pelvic irradiation, prior pelvic or LUT surgery, significantly increased PVR, significant pelvic organ prolapse, or suspected fistula should be referred for specialty management, if appropriate for goals of care.

Lifestyle Modification

Weight loss significantly reduces stress incontinence in obese, young-old women (SOE=A). Other lifestyle interventions lack confirmatory evidence but may be helpful (SOE=D): avoiding extremes of fluid intake, caffeinated beverages, and alcohol; minimizing evening intake in those with nocturia; and quitting smoking (to decrease coughing) in patients with stress UI.

Behavioral Therapies

Bladder training and pelvic muscle exercises (PMEs) are effective for urge, mixed, and stress UI, and are often used in combination (SOE=A).

Bladder training uses two principles: frequent voluntary voiding to keep bladder volume low, and urgency suppression using CNS and pelvic mechanisms.

- The initial voiding frequency can be every 2 hours or based on the smallest voiding interval on bladder diary.

- To decrease or suppress a strong urge, patients should not walk to or focus on getting to the bathroom but instead stand still or sit down, do several pelvic muscle contractions, and concentrate on making the urgency decrease by taking a deep breath and letting it out slowly, or visualizing the urgency as a wave that peaks and then falls. Once patients feel more in control (the urgency can still be present), they should walk to the bathroom and void.

As patients progress, they can increase the time between scheduled voids by approximately 30-minute intervals, until they reach a comfortable level balancing voiding frequency and continence. Successful bladder training usually takes several weeks, and patients need reassurance to proceed despite any initial failure.

PMEs strengthen the muscular components of urethral support and are effective for urge, mixed, and stress UI. PMEs also are effective for prevention and treatment of UI after prostatectomy. PMEs are based on similar strategies to other muscle strength training: correct isolation of the target muscle(s), high intensity contraction, and low repetitions. Patient instruction and motivation are necessary, although simple instruction booklets alone have moderate benefit (SOE=A). Instructions for PMEs are available online (www.acog.org/Patients/FAQs/Pelvic-Support-Problems).

For patients with moderate to severe cognitive impairment, the only behavioral treatment with proven efficacy is prompted voiding (SOE=B). A caregiver monitors the patient and encourages him or her to report any need to void; prompts the patient to toilet on a regular schedule during the day (usually every 2–3 hours); leads the patient to the bathroom; and gives the patient positive feedback when he or she toilets. Patients most likely to improve are able to state their name, transfer with a minimum of one assist, void ≤4 times during daytime hours, and are able to accept and follow the prompt to toilet at least 75% of the time with an initial 3-day trial. Toileting routines without prompting, such as habit training (based on a patient's usual voiding schedule without prompting) and scheduled voiding (using a set schedule) are not effective.

Medications

Medications are used to treat urge UI or urge-predominant mixed UI insufficiently responsive to behavioral therapy. There are currently no approved medications for stress UI.

Antimuscarinic agents are moderately effective for urge UI, overactive bladder, and mixed incontinence (SOE=A). They work by decreasing basal excretion of acetylcholine from the urothelium and thus increasing bladder capacity; they do not ablate uninhibited contractions. Data are conflicting whether combined antimuscarinic and behavioral therapy is better than either alone for reducing UI; the combination is significantly better for improving quality of life (SOE=A). In stepped therapy, behavioral therapy is usually continued when medications are added. Antimuscarinics are safe and effective in men with urgency and urge UI associated with benign prostatic hyperplasia who have a PVR <200 mL (SOE=A). Antimuscarinics are contraindicated for patients with narrow-angle glaucoma (not open-angle), impaired gastric emptying, and urinary retention. It is not necessary to routinely monitor PVR with antimuscarinic treatment. However, PVR should be checked if UI increases with antimuscarinic treatment, because a significant PVR reduces the functional capacity of the bladder, making voiding and UI more frequent.

There are 6 antimuscarinics with established efficacy (Table 32.2). Based on systematic reviews, the 6 antimuscarinic agents have similar efficacy in reducing urge UI frequency (best data are in women, ARR for continence 0.9–0.13, NNT 8–11; ARR for clinically important improvement 0.08–0.18, NNT 6–13) but differ in adverse events, metabolism, drug interactions, and dosing requirements. Only fesoterodine has been evaluated in a community-based population of vulnerable older adults; efficacy and tolerability were similar to those observed in trials of younger and healthy old adults (SOE=A). Comparative effectiveness trials are limited and industry supported.

Anticholinergic adverse events can limit tolerability and safety of these medications. The major concern is cognitive impairment. Although antimuscarinics as a class are associated with cognitive impairment, the risk, prevalence, type, and magnitude of cognitive changes from specific antimuscarinic UI medications in individual patients or patient groups are not clear. Short-term (4 week) use of extended-release oxybutynin (5 mg/d) did not increase delirium in frail nursing-home patients (SOE=A). A systematic review found low-moderate evidence for impairment of divided attention and reaction time, but overall the effects were inconsistent. Evidence is insufficient that one drug is "safer" for all patients, for those with mild cognitive impairment, or for those with moderate-severe dementia. What is clear is that antimuscarinics should not be combined with cholinesterase inhibitors because of lack of efficacy and risk of increased functional and possibly cognitive impairment.

Other important anticholinergic adverse effects include dry mouth with increased risk of dental caries, and constipation, with similar rates across antimuscarinics except for dosages of oxybutynin ≥10 mg/d, which is highest.

All antimuscarinics except trospium are metabolized by cytochrome P-450 pathways and can interact with drugs that induce CYP2D6 (eg, fluoxetine) or are metabolized by CYP3A4 (eg, erythromycin, ketoconazole). Fesoterodine is a prodrug that is metabolized to tolterodine by nonspecific peripheral esterases. Trospium is renally cleared and should be given once daily in patients with renal insufficiency; it should be taken on an empty stomach. Other antimuscarinics that should be considered for dose adjustment in chronic renal disease are tolterodine, fesoterodine, and solifenacin. Therefore, choice of agent for a particular patient should depend on potential adverse events to be avoided, possible drug-drug and drug-disease interactions, dosing frequency, titration range, and cost. A lack of response to one agent does not preclude response to another.

Mirabegron (25–50 mg/d) is a β3-adrenergic agonist that facilitates detrusor relaxation and increases bladder capacity, with similar moderate efficacy as the antimuscarinics (SOE=A). To date, it has not been shown to have cognitive adverse effects, but it can raise blood pressure. Important drug-drug interactions can occur with digoxin, metoprolol, venlafaxine, desipramine, and dextromethorphan.

There is insufficient evidence for the efficacy of propantheline, dicyclomine, imipramine, hyoscyamine, calcium channel blockers, NSAIDs, and flavoxate. Vasopressin (DDAVP) should not be used for nocturia in older adults because of the risk of hyponatremia (SOE=A).

The serotonin–norepinephrine uptake inhibitor antidepressant duloxetine decreases stress UI but is not FDA approved for this indication. Oral estrogen, alone or in combination with progestins, increases UI (SOE=A). There is insufficient evidence whether vaginal topical estrogen improves UI (cream, vaginal tablet, or slow-release ring), but it is helpful for uncomfortable vaginal atrophy and may decrease recurrent urinary tract infections.

Minimally Invasive Procedures

These procedures are used primarily for refractory urge UI. Sacral nerve neuromodulation has some effect for both urge UI refractory to drug treatment and urinary retention (idiopathic and neurogenic). The mechanism of action is unknown. The procedure involves percutaneous implantation of a trial electrode at the S3 sacral root, which is connected to an external stimulator. Patients responding to the trial have a permanent lead with a pacemaker-like energy source implanted. Posterior tibial nerve stimulation is a less invasive form of neuromodulation with a variably defined response rate of 60%–81% in small short-term trials (SOE=C). Patients will likely not experience a response until completing about 6 weekly treatments.

Intravesical injection of botulinum toxin is effective for refractory urge UI (SOE=A). Optimal dosing for specific patient groups is uncertain, and patients must be willing to do self-catheterization because of the risk of urinary retention.

Pessaries may benefit women with stress and urge UI exacerbated by bladder or uterine prolapse.

Surgery

Surgery provides the highest cure rates for stress UI in women (SOE=A). The most commonly used procedures are colposuspension (Burch operation), and midurethral and bladder neck slings (synthetic mesh or autologous fascia placed transvaginally). Older women have similar improvement with midurethral slings as middle-aged women, but older women have more persistent postoperative urgency (SOE=A). Periurethral injection of a bulking agent is a short-term (≤1 year) alternative and usually requires a series of injections; previously widely used, collagen is no longer commercially produced.

Artificial sphincters are used for refractory stress UI from sphincter damage, typically after radical prostatectomy. A cuff is placed internally around the urethra, and its inflation controlled by the patient squeezing a reservoir device placed in the scrotum. They are moderately effective (SOE=B) but require manual dexterity and intact cognition; an alert bracelet should be considered, because catheter insertion through a closed artificial sphincter can cause significant damage. Revision rates can be high (up to 40%).

Supportive Care

Pads and protective garments should be chosen based on patient gender, type of UI, and volume of leakage. For example, an absorbent sheath may be sufficient for a man with mild UI after prostatectomy. In some states, Medicaid may cover the cost of pads; Medicare and private insurance do not. Medical supply companies and patient advocacy groups publish illustrated catalogs to guide product selection. Because these products are often expensive, some patients may not change pads frequently enough.

EVALUATION AND MANAGEMENT OF UI IN NURSING-HOME RESIDENTS

The CMS *Guidance for Surveyors for Long Term Facilities* sets the nursing-home compliance standards, known as the F-tag 315, for evaluation and management of UI and urinary catheters. The 2006 revision of F-tag 315 changed the focus from documentation of toileting plans to an increased emphasis on screening, the process and documentation of UI assessment, and reevaluation. The Minimum Data Set requires that residents are screened for UI at admissions and quarterly, and with any change in cognition, function, or urinary tract function. F-tag 315 guidance suggests an evaluation essentially equivalent to that described above. Instead of bladder diaries, toileting patterns and UI episodes are monitored over several days. Although evaluation is largely a nursing responsibility, provider input is especially important given the F-tag 315 emphasis on physical examination, evaluation of medications and comorbidity as a cause of UI, and differential diagnosis.

Nearly all studies of UI treatment in long-term care involve behavioral therapy. Evidence is moderate that prompted voiding is effective in reducing daytime UI (SOE=B), but treatment is rarely continued long term. Interventions that combine prompted voiding with bedside exercise improve both incontinence and physical function (SOE=B). Long-term care residents who do not respond should be managed with "check and change." The revised F-tag 315 supports this targeted approach and the role of patient and family preferences in evaluation and treatment. Unfortunately, many nursing homes practice only scheduled toileting without prompting, which is ineffective. Quality improvement efforts focused on staff organization and systems may ultimately be necessary to reduce UI in long-term care.

The only randomized studies of antimuscarinic efficacy in nursing-home residents used oxybutynin. A 4-week randomized controlled trial found no difference between extended-release oxybutynin given at 5 mg/d and placebo. Consequently, antimuscarinics are infrequently prescribed, despite evidence that patients may prefer medications over behavioral therapy and "check and change." It is reasonable to consider an antimuscarinic trial for residents with urge UI who respond to prompted voiding but still have bothersome incontinence.

It is important to remember that up to a third of nursing-home residents with UI have an underlying bladder outlet problem (stress incontinence or bladder outlet obstruction) and may be candidates for alternative medical or surgical treatment.

CATHETERS AND CATHETER CARE

Indwelling catheters cause significant morbidity, including polymicrobial bacteriuria (universal by 30 days), febrile episodes (1 per 100 patient days), nephrolithiasis, bladder stones, epididymitis, chronic renal inflammation and pyelonephritis, and meatal damage. Condom catheters, often assumed to be less morbid than indwelling catheters, also cause bacteriuria, infection, penile cellulitis and necrosis, and even urinary retention and hydronephrosis if the condom twists or its external band is too tight. Indwelling catheters should be used only for short-term decompression of acute urinary retention, chronic retention that cannot be managed medically or surgically, protection of wounds that may be contaminated by urine, and for comfort in terminally ill or severely impaired patients who cannot tolerate garment changes with informed preference for catheter management despite risks. Inappropriate and/or poorly documented indications for catheter use are a major focus in the revised F-tag 315 guidance for nursing homes. The guidance states that catheters should primarily be used for short-term decompression of acute retention but also allows for the indications above.

All patients with acute retention should have decompression with an indwelling catheter while being evaluated and treated for potentially remediable causes, such as medications that impair detrusor contractility or increase urethral tone, outlet obstruction, and constipation. Duration of catheterization before voiding trial should depend on time course for reversing underlying cause. A voiding trial without catheter should follow decompression. To do so, the catheter should be removed (never clamped), the patient adequately hydrated, and a PVR checked after the first void or bladder volume checked if there is no void after about 6 hours. Studies have not confirmed any benefit of bethanechol chloride for patients with retention (SOE=B).

Intermittent clean catheterization is an effective alternative to an indwelling catheter for willing and able patients and/or caregivers. Strict sterility is not necessary, although good hand washing and regular decontamination of the catheters is needed. Specialized stiff and smooth short catheters are available for use. Bacteriuria can be minimized by a frequency of catheterization that keeps bladder volume <400 mL. Sterile intermittent catheterization is preferred for frailer patients and those in institutionalized settings.

Bacteriuria is universal in catheterized patients and should not be treated unless there are clear symptoms of cystitis or pyelonephritis, eg fever. Routine cultures should not be done because of changing flora and difficulty in differentiating colonization from active infection. In symptomatic patients, urine for culture is best obtained by removing the old catheter and urine obtained from a newly placed catheter. Institutionalized patients with catheters should be kept in separate rooms to decrease cross-infection. Topical meatal antimicrobials, catheters with antimicrobial coating, collection bag disinfectants, and antimicrobial irrigation are not effective in preventing catheter-associated urinary tract infection. Use of antibiotics for anything other than symptomatic infection induces resistant organisms and secondary infections (such as with *Clostridium difficile*) and should be avoided. Prophylactic antibiotics are recommended only in high-risk patients (eg, those with prosthetic heart valves) during short-term catheterization. For patients with chronic obstruction, suprapubic catheters may be preferable to avoid meatal and penile trauma.

Catheters do not need to be changed routinely as long as monitoring is adequate and catheter blockage does not develop. Risk factors for blockage include alkaline urine, female gender, poor mobility, calciuria, proteinuria, copious mucin, *Proteus* colonization, and bladder stones. Changing the catheter every 7–10 days may decrease blockage in such patients. If patients cannot be monitored, changing catheters every 30 days is reasonable (SOE=D). Possible causes of persistent leakage around the catheter are large Foley balloon, detrusor overactivity, bacteriuria, constipation or impaction, and improper catheter positioning. These can be addressed by trials of partial deflation of the balloon, smaller catheter, treatment of constipation, use of an anticholinergic, or treatment with pyridium.

Catheters coated with silver alloys reduce asymptomatic bacteriuria in hospitalized patients requiring short-term urethral catheterization, but their use in reducing symptomatic bacteriuria is less certain. Data are scant whether silver alloy catheters reduce asymptomatic or symptomatic bacteriuria in other settings (such as long-term care or home care) or with longer-term catheterization.

> **CHOOSING WISELY® RECOMMENDATIONS**
>
> *Urinary Incontinence*
>
> - Do not order creatinine or upper tract imaging if only lower urinary tract symptoms are present.

RESOURCES

- Madhuvrata P, Cody JD, Ellis G, et al. Which anticholinergic drug for overactive bladder symptoms in adults. *Cochrane Database Syst Rev.* 2012;1:CD005429.

- Moss MC, Rezan T, Karaman UR, et al. Treatment of concomitant OAB and BPH. *Curr Urol Rep.* 2017;18(1):1–7.

- Talley KM, Wyman JF, Shamliyan TA. State of the science: conservative interventions for urinary incontinence in frail community-dwelling older adults. *Nurs Outlook.* 2011;59(4):215–220, 220.e1.

CHAPTER 33—PRESSURE INJURIES AND WOUND CARE

KEY POINTS

- Empiric evidence to guide the treatment of pressure injuries is limited. This requires clinicians to focus on critical components of management, including wound examination, documentation, and diagnosis, as well as understanding and implementing basic principles of wound care.

- Pressure injuries are only one type of chronic wound seen in older adults. However, because of their association with the perception of quality, pressure injuries have become an important concern in regulatory, reimbursement, and risk-management arenas.

- Pressure injuries have severe consequences, including increased length of stay, increased chance of readmission within 30 days of hospital discharge, prolonged rehabilitation, pain, disfigurement, infection, loss of limb, and death.

- Risk assessment and risk factor intervention are key to pressure injury prevention. It is now accepted that nonmodifiable risk factors in many patients can lead to pressure injuries even when appropriate interventions are implemented.Many wounds have reduced or no chance of healing. For these wounds, palliative care principles may curtail suffering, improve quality of life, and decrease health care costs. When wounds are considered palliative, caregivers must reconsider expensive advanced wound care modalities and surgical procedures such as sharp debridements.

Pressure injuries are a common chronic wound in the geriatric population. Care of pressure injuries is interdisciplinary and involves nursing, nutrition, rehabilitation, and surgical subspecialties. Pressure injuries cause pain and are associated with a decreased quality of life, longer hospital stay, increased chance of readmission within 30 days after hospital discharge, increased chance of admission to a long-term care facility, and increased risk of death. Infectious complications include cellulitis, abscess, sepsis, pyarthrosis, and osteomyelitis. Pressure injuries often require surgical procedures ranging from sharp debridements to myocutaneous flaps, amputations, and ostomies for fecal diversion. According to the Agency for Healthcare Research and Quality, pressure injuries cost $9.1 to $11.6 billion per year, with the cost of individual patient care ranging from $20,900 to $151,700 per pressure ulcer. A vexing variety of treatments is available with few studies to prove efficacy of one over the other. The standard of care for pressure injuries is evolving, and all primary care providers need to be aware of prevention strategies, documentation standards, and treatment choices. These choices include a palliative care approach, which can avoid unnecessary and futile procedures, improve quality of life, and curtail health care costs.

Pressure injuries affect from 1.3 to 3 million adults in the United States, and their incidence and prevalence vary greatly depending on stage, setting, and how data are collected. In acute care, one study showed incidence ranging from 7% to 9% per year. Higher rates are consistently reported in older populations. Hospital prevalence rates range from 11.9% to 15.8%. In long-term care, prevalence ranges from 8.5% to 32.2%. In one study, up to 54.7% of terminally ill nursing-home residents had pressure injuries. The increase in pressure injury prevalence that occurred in the 20th century was largely a result of modern public health measures and advances in medical technology that resulted in longer life expectancy and greater numbers of people living with multiple chronic illnesses.

Pressure injuries are a designated quality measure in hospitals, long-term care, and home-care settings. As a result of their association with quality of care, pressure injuries have become a major risk management issue, and, according to the Agency for Healthcare Research and Quality, >17,000 lawsuits related to pressure injuries are filed annually. Pressure injury data for skilled-nursing facilities is currently published by CMS on the Nursing Home Compare Web site, but as yet there is no federal mandate for publication of pressure injury statistics for hospitals and home care. In addition, pressure injuries have been spotlighted in value-based purchasing and pay-for-performance initiatives. For example, in 2008 the CMS introduced a policy to decline payment to hospitals for certain hospital-acquired conditions that include stage 3 or 4 pressure injuries. These factors have resulted in an evolving standard of care that designates physicians as key players. Many hospitals and long-term care facilities require orders for wound care products, dressings, and devices to obtain Medicare reimbursement. Because pressure injuries are an identified geriatric syndrome, geriatrics providers with proper training can play a pivotal role in improving quality of care for this condition.

It has become increasingly recognized that many pressure injuries are unavoidable. Patients at severe risk with immobility and multiple chronic conditions, and patients who are dying, can develop pressure injuries even when standards of care for prevention are met. A pressure injury is therefore not necessarily indicative of poor quality care but rather may be a marker for disease severity or impending death. An expert panel (SCALE Panel 2009) assembled consensus statements about skin changes at life's end that support the concept of unavoidable pressure injuries in patients who are actively dying. An extensive literature review and consensus study summarizing factors that lead to unavoidable pressure injuries was published. A key concept for understanding unavoidable pressure injuries is the nonmodifiable risk factor for which effective interventions cannot be implemented. The National Pressure Ulcer Advisory Panel (NPUAP) defines an unavoidable pressure injury as one that develops despite the provider having 1) evaluated the individual's clinical condition and pressure injury risk factors; 2) defined and implemented interventions consistent with individual needs, goals, and recognized standards of practice; and 3) monitored and evaluated the impact of the interventions, revising the approaches as appropriate.

The skin is the largest organ of the body, and the concept of "skin failure" has been advanced to account for unavoidable pressure injuries in patients who are dying and other situations such as multiple organ system failure. Unlike other organ systems such as kidney, liver, and lung, there is currently no laboratory marker identifying skin failure. Although the concept of skin failure makes sense, universal agreement on its definition or clinical application has not yet been achieved.

CHRONIC WOUND HEALING

Normal wound healing is a complex but orderly sequence of biologic events that includes hemostasis, inflammation, proliferation, and remodeling. Neutrophils are involved in the inflammatory phase, phagocytizing debris and microorganisms and providing a first line of defense. Macrophages play an important role in phagocytosis, debriding damaged tissue with proteases, creating granulation tissue, laying down extracellular matrix, and secreting chemotactic and growth factors. Granulation tissue consists of new blood vessels, fibroblasts, endothelial cells, myofibroblasts, and extracellular matrix. Fibroblasts produce collagen that increases the strength of the wound, plus other critical substances such as elastin, fibronectin, glycosaminoglycans, and proteases. Myofibroblasts, descended from fibroblasts, assist in contraction. Keratinocytes are the main cells responsible for epithelialization, the process of migrating across a bed of granulation tissue. Because of the disruption in normal anatomy and disorganization of new collagen, the tensile strength of a healed wound is only 50%–80% of that of undamaged skin.

Pressure injuries are one of a diverse group of lesions classified as chronic wounds (see Table 33.1). Chronic wounds share in common prolonged healing time and interference with normal wound healing that renders them stalled in the inflammatory and proliferative phases. The surface of a chronic wound often harbors an "antihealing environment" with elements that include biofilm, exudate that contains pro-inflammatory cytokines such as matrix metalloproteases and tumor necrosis factor alpha (TNF-α), and lack of pro-regenerative agents such as transforming growth factor (TGF-β), platelet-derived growth factor, and vascular endothelial growth factor.

Conditions leading to chronic wounds include repetitive trauma, decreased vascular perfusion, poor nutrition, poor oxygenation from anemia, diabetes or pulmonary disease, edema that interferes with nutrient delivery, pharmacologic barriers such as corticosteroids and immunosuppressants, incontinence, and biofilms. A biofilm is a community of microorganisms that secretes a mucilaginous extracellular coating that protects them from antibiotics and inhibits healing. These factors have greater impact on older adults, because they add to the processes of aging that include reduced fibroblasts, macrophages, and mast cells; loss of extracellular matrix components such as collagen and glycosaminoglycans; decreased amount and morphology of elastin; altered surface pH; reduced sebum secretion with decreased pilosebaceous units; and flattening of the dermal-epidermal junction.

PRESSURE INJURY DEFINITION AND CLASSIFICATION

A pressure injury is defined as localized damage to the skin and/or underlying tissue, usually over a bony prominence that results from pressure, or pressure in combination with shear. The current staging system defined by NPUAP is used only for pressure injuries (see Table 33.1). Staging of pressure injuries is determined by visible depth. If the base of the wound cannot be seen, the wound is determined as "unstageable." A wound is designated a deep tissue pressure injury (DTPI) when the skin is intact and a purple bruise-like area is present in an area subjected to pressure. A DTPI can dissipate leaving intact skin, or it can evolve into a wound of varying severity. Stage 1 and DTPI can be difficult to assess in persons with dark skin, and examinations should be performed with adequate lighting and include palpation for detection of induration or warmth.

The heel, the second most common site for pressure injuries after the sacrum, has unique anatomic features that warrant special consideration when evaluating an ulcer. These include thick skin, very little subcutaneous

Table 33.1—National Pressure Ulcer Advisory Board Staging Criteria for Pressure Ulcers

Stage 1 Nonblanchable erythema	Intact skin with nonblanchable redness of a localized area, usually over a bony prominence. Darkly pigmented skin may not have visible blanching; its color may differ from the surrounding area. The area may be painful, firm, soft, or warmer or cooler than adjacent tissue. May be difficult to detect in those with dark skin tones. May indicate "at risk" patients.
Stage 2 Partial thickness	Partial-thickness loss of skin presenting as a shallow open ulcer with a red pink wound bed, without slough. May also present as an intact or open/ruptured blister filled with serum or serosanguineous fluid. Presents as a shiny or dry shallow ulcer without slough or bruising (the latter indicates deep-tissue injury). This category should not be used to describe skin tears, tape burns, incontinence-associated dermatitis, maceration, or excoriation.
Stage 3 Full-thickness tissue loss	Full-thickness tissue loss; subcutaneous fat is visible, but bone, tendon, or muscle are not exposed/visible or directly palpable. Slough may be present but does not obscure the depth of tissue loss. May include undermining and tunneling. The depth of a Stage 3 pressure ulcer varies by anatomical location. The bridge of the nose, ear, occiput, and malleolus do not have (adipose) subcutaneous tissue, and Stage 3 ulcers can be shallow. In contrast, areas of significant adiposity can develop extremely deep Stage 3 pressure ulcers.
Stage 4 Full-thickness tissue loss	Full-thickness tissue loss with exposed/visible bone, tendon, or muscle that is directly palpable. Slough or eschar may be present. Often includes undermining and tunneling. The depth of a Stage 4 pressure ulcer varies by anatomical location. The bridge of the nose, ear, occiput, and malleolus do not have (adipose) subcutaneous tissue, and these ulcers can be shallow. Stage 4 ulcers can extend into muscle and/or supporting structures (eg, fascia, tendon or joint capsule) making osteomyelitis or osteitis likely to develop.
Unstageable Full-thickness skin or tissue loss, depth unknown	Full-thickness tissue loss in which actual depth of the ulcer is completely obscured by slough (yellow, tan, gray, green, or brown) and/or eschar (tan, brown, or black) in the wound bed. Until enough slough and/or eschar are removed to expose the base of the wound, the true depth cannot be determined; but it will be either a Stage 3 or 4. Stable (dry, adherent, intact without erythema or fluctuance) eschar on the heels serves as "the body's natural (biological) cover" and should not be removed.
Deep tissue pressure injury, depth unknown	Purple or maroon localized area of discolored intact skin or blood-filled blister due to damage of underlying soft tissue from pressure and/or shear. May be preceded by tissue that is painful, firm, mushy, boggy, and warmer or cooler than adjacent tissue. May be difficult to detect in those with dark skin tones. Evolution may include a thin blister over a dark wound bed. The wound may further evolve and become covered by thin eschar. Evolution may be rapid, exposing additional layers of tissue even with optimal treatment.

© National Pressure Ulcer Advisory Panel, 2016
SOURCE: Adapted with permission of the National Pressure Ulcer Advisory Panel, 2018. The permission granted through this process cannot be transferred to others or used for other purposes than expressed above and approved by the NPUAP. ©NPUAP

tissue and muscle, and vascular perfusion delivered around the large calcaneus bone that underlies the rear portion of the foot. The foot is also susceptible to circulatory impairment because of atheromatous disease of the leg, microvascular disease from diabetes mellitus, and decreased sensation from peripheral neuropathy of any etiology. Pressure injuries of the heels often present as blisters. A clear blister over a bony prominence is considered a stage 2 pressure injury, whereas a blood-filled blister is considered a DTPI.

Definitions and nomenclature for pressure injuries was recently modified by the NPUAP. The recommendation to change the term "pressure ulcer" to "pressure injury" has garnered controversy. Concerns include potential unintended consequences upon increased litigation risk as well as the burden of modifying CPT codes. For practical purposes, "pressure ulcer" and "pressure injury" are synonymous.

PRESSURE INJURY ASSESSMENT AND DOCUMENTATION

Pressure injuries must be detected early, because these wounds can usually heal quickly if discovered in early stages and treated properly. Alternatively, wounds can deteriorate quickly, particularly in patients with severe immobility in conjunction with multisystemic disease. As a result, timely examination and documentation is an important component of management. Consistent and complete documentation is required for coding and reimbursement, public reporting, risk management, and accurate transmittal of information as patients traverse the health care continuum. Providers should take the time to perform the examination rather than rely on others for the information. Proper wound evaluation can be time consuming, particularly in patients with multiple wounds. It often involves obtaining assistance with lifting or turning an immobile patient who may be in pain, and removing and replacing dressings. However, timely and thorough examination is mandatory for all patients with pressure injuries and will bring dividends in accurate documentation and improved decision making.

Wound documentation includes diagnosis, stage, location, length, width, depth, presence of odor and/or drainage, presence of undermining and tunneling, as well as characteristics of the wound bed, margin, and surrounding skin. Supplemental information can include warmth, capillary refill, and presence of pulses, edema, anasarca, and lymphedema. Measurement is an important component of wound assessment, particularly for determining the effectiveness of clinical interventions. Measurement involves head-to-toe length, width, and depth and should be both consistent and accurate. The simplest method uses a centimeter ruler to measure length and width, and a cotton-tipped swab to measure depth, tunneling, and undermining. Wound clinics and skilled-nursing facilities usually have structured documentation sheets with entry points for diagnosis, length, width, and depth, along with diagrams to designate location and undermining, as well as treatment in progress and response to treatment. If such structured documents are unavailable, it is advisable to describe the wound with as much detail as possible in narrative form.

Documentation of wound progression is an important component of management and should be ongoing, systematic, and consistent. Wounds should be formally assessed at least weekly, with descriptors that include measurements, nature of the wound bed and periwound area, pressure redistribution modalities, treatments in progress, and response to healing. Some authorities recommend a validated healing scale such as the Pressure Sore Status Tool or the Pressure Ulcer Scale for Healing. No single standard exists that mandates the type and extent of information to include in a wound assessment, but the more descriptors the better. Patients with pressure injuries frequently undergo transitions between locations within the health care continuum, and wounds should be thoroughly documented on both admission and discharge from hospitals and long-term care facilities. Similarly, initial home care visits should include thorough skin inspection. Reverse staging is not a recognized standard, because it does not accurately characterize the anatomic and physiologic process that occurs during healing.

Photographs can be valuable adjuncts to wound documentation; however, their implementation in a medical record must be consistent and within a formal policy and procedure guideline. Photographs must be of reasonable quality and accompanied by a label within the visual field that contains a patient identifier (name, initials, or medical record number), location of the wound, and date. Haphazard use of photographs or poor photographic technique can create discontinuities in documentation with risk-management implications. Providers who use personal cell phones to take photographs are committing potential HIPAA violations.

PRESSURE INJURY PREVENTION

The standard of care for pressure injury prevention includes risk assessment followed by appropriate pressure redistribution interventions if the patient is deemed at risk.

Risk Assessment

There are many recognized risk factors for pressure injuries, and several validated instruments that quantify risk are available. The most widely used tool is the Braden Scale (www.in.gov/isdh/files/Braden_Scale.pdf), which combines sensory perception, moisture, activity, mobility, and friction and shear. This scale has been validated in home, skilled-nursing facilities, and hospital settings but not in ICUs. However, other studies have noted that risk assessment tools can be weak predictors of which patients are more likely to develop pressure injuries (SOE=B). Current scales also do not contain information related to organ system failure or physiologic factors such as hypoxia and hypotension, which may also engender increased pressure injury risk. Therefore, clinical judgment should be relied on to determine "at risk" status in addition to the formalized risk assessment scale.

Risk factors for pressure injuries can be classified as either extrinsic, intrinsic, or both. Immobility is a major risk factor that results from causes that are both external and internal to the patient. Nutritional compromise is a known risk factor for pressure injuries, and patients >75 years old with malnutrition and weight loss are 3.8 times more likely to develop pressure injuries.

Medical devices are increasingly recognized as causes of pressure ulceration. These include external devices such as tubing and orthopedic splints, casts, limb immobilizers, abdominal binders, and CPAP masks. Care plans for patients with external orthopedic devices should always include periodic skin assessment. Pressure injuries can develop over internally placed medical devices such as implantable neurostimulators and pain-control pumps that create new pressure points under the skin.

Skin assessment is an important component of prevention and should be done at least once per day for patients considered at risk in any setting. Areas of skin exposed to chronic moisture, over bony prominences, or under medical devices require special attention to detect early signs of impairment. Inspection of skin over bony prominences and under medical devices should be a routine part of the physician assessment, particularly on admission to the hospital or nursing home. Routine nursing care should include skin assessment, and skin should be cleansed with efforts to minimize both dryness and excessive moisture.

Moisture-associated skin damage (MASD) that occurs from perspiration, urine, diarrhea, fistulas, or wound exudate increases susceptibility to pressure injuries, and is a common occurrence in patients with constant loose stools from tube feeding or *Clostridium difficile* colitis. MASD involves more than simple maceration of skin, and contributors include mechanical factors such as friction, chemical irritants, and microbes, including bacteria and fungi. Strategies to avoid or treat MASD include moisture barrier creams, absorbable undergarments, continence care, and fecal and urinary diversion devices. Fungal infections require early diagnosis, because they can lead to impaired skin integrity if untreated. The diagnosis of fungal infection is sometimes missed because of the similarity in appearance to MASD, but close inspection of the border of redness and inflammation can reveal telltale satellite lesions characteristic of *Candida albicans*.

Prevention Strategies

There are many strategies for minimizing pressure, friction, and shear. Positioning devices such as pillows and foam wedges can help keep pressure off bony prominences, and lifting devices and draw sheets can minimize friction. Shear is a mechanical force that occurs when skin is pulled parallel to the body and is commonly caused by sitting up in bed. Backrest elevation of 30–45 degrees is associated with reduced risk of ventilator-associated pneumonia and aspiration related to tube feeding; however, sustained backrest elevation of >30 degrees is associated with increased pressure and shear to the lower back and buttocks. There is no current consensus as to how to balance the risks of pressure ulceration with minimizing the risks of ventilator-associated pneumonia and aspiration.

The industry standard for turning and positioning is every 2 hours, but there is minimal research to support this schedule (SOE=C). In addition, this standard was developed before the advent of advanced mattress and continence care technology. Research challenges the need for every-2-hour repositioning for patients using high-density foam mattresses (SOE=B). Patients who sit for long periods of time in chairs should be assessed for proper posture and alignment and provided with pressure relief schedules and cushioning. Strategies for preventing heel wounds include local skin care, cushioning, and lifting the heels off the mattress by placing a pillow under the legs when supine, also called "floating the heels" (SOE=B).

NPUAP defines "support surface" as a specialized device designed for management of tissue loads, microclimate, and/or other therapeutic needs. There are a large variety of support surface technologies and features. Mattress overlays go between the mattress and the patient and are more commonly used in rehabilitation facilities and home environments. A mattress replacement is a device placed in the bed frame that generally uses the low air-loss (LAL) technology; such a support surface provides a flow of air for managing skin microclimate, including heat and humidity.

Surfaces designed to prevent pressure injuries are defined by "immersion" and "envelopment." Immersion refers to the depth that a mechanical load sinks, and envelopment is the characteristic that takes the shape of the applied load. The combination of immersion and envelopment gives the protective effect against pressure injuries. An alternating pressure air mattress does not use these characteristics, but rather "force redistribution" by taking a load from one place to another and allowing reperfusion of the previously loaded area, thereby preventing pressure injuries. Other advanced features of the specialized bed include pulsations for pulmonary toilet, multizoned surfaces, and lateral rotation. The evidence to guide surface choices is conflicting regarding efficacy at preventing pressure injuries, and efforts are underway by the NPUAP to standardize testing and measure outcomes objectively.

PRINCIPLES OF PRESSURE INJURY TREATMENT

A holistic, patient-centered approach to pressure injury treatment involves assessing the overall health status of the patient, addressing psychosocial needs, treating underlying comorbidities, assessing and correcting causes of tissue damage, and assessing and monitoring the wound. It is essential to understand the patient's functional and cognitive status, home environment, family support, and other factors such as the presence of depression. Wound assessment entails examination and description as discussed above, along with proper documentation. If the wound is an alteration in skin or tissue integrity over a bony prominence, it is most likely a pressure injury and staged in accordance with NPUAP criteria. Local malignancy must be considered in any chronic wound with consideration of biopsy, and all wounds should be assessed for infection (discussed below). Elements of pressure injury treatment involve offloading and pressure redistribution strategies, removing debris and necrotic tissue, and addressing moisture balance. Finally, the clinician must address pain, acknowledge advance directives, and be able to recognize wounds appropriate for a palliative approach and alter the plan accordingly.

Laboratory tests provide important information regarding the patient's health and ability to heal. Anemia contributes to decreased oxygen delivery to vulnerable or healing tissue. Nutritional status as reflected in serum albumin and prealbumin levels can impair wound healing, but these laboratory tests are unreliable in the presence of inflammation and are losing their status as nutritional indicators. Increases in WBC count, erythrocyte sedimentation rate, or C-reactive protein may indicate ongoing infection or inflammation. The clinician must be aware of endocrinopathies such as hypothyroidism and poorly controlled diabetes mellitus. For wounds of the lower extremity, tests such as ankle-brachial index (ABI), pulse volume recording, and Doppler ultrasound can assist in evaluating arterial supply. ABI loses diagnostic value when arteries are noncompressible because of advanced atherosclerotic disease.

Numerous wound products are available, and the lack of controlled clinical trials and reliable measures of efficacy can make choosing an appropriate treatment bewildering. The lack of research is partially attributable to the FDA classification of most wound care products as medical devices (as opposed to pharmaceuticals), which exempts manufacturers from the requirement to demonstrate efficacy. As for all chronic wounds, correction of underlying factors leading to the chronic ulcer formation is more important than choice of topical dressing. With little evidence-based support for individual treatments, choices are often made based on product availability, insurance coverage, personal preference, cost considerations, expert opinion, and intrinsic rationale for product type. Table 33.2 presents some commonly used treatment modalities along with rationale for each (SOE=C).

Wound bed preparation has emerged as a useful tool to conceptually organize the array of wound products in a manner that achieves maximal benefit for chronic wounds such as pressure injuries. Wound bed preparation focuses on critical components of management, including moisture and exudate, bacterial balance, and debridement. The foundation of this concept is an orderly approach to accelerate endogenous healing and facilitate the effectiveness of therapeutic measures. The goal is to reestablish the balance of growth factors, cytokines, proteases, and their natural inhibitors as found in acute wounds, thereby stimulating the healing process.

Moisture balance is an important component of wound healing, because a moist environment promotes autolytic debridement and encourages matrix formation. Alternatively, excess moisture inhibits wound healing through maceration that impairs both the wound bed and periwound area. Several products promote moist wound healing such as hydrocolloids, hydrogels, and other bio-occlusives. The exudate of chronic wounds contains heightened proteolytic activity, matrix metalloproteases, and macromolecules that inhibit growth factors, and products such as foams, hydrofibers, and alginates provide absorptive capabilities. Collagen-containing products inactivate harmful cytokines and factors that inhibit healing.

Bacterial balance in the wound bed is facilitated by cleansing, topical antibiotics, disinfectants, and debridement. Debridement removes necrotic tissue and bacteria, providing a clean surface that promotes healing. Debridement can be achieved by several ways, and selection should be individualized in accordance with goals of care and degree of necrosis. Autolytic debridement uses moisture-retentive topical dressings to take advantage of endogenous enzymes present in the wound, whereas enzymatic debridement uses a commercially produced enzyme to digest debris and dead tissue. Mechanical debridement methods include hydrotherapy (whirlpool), irrigation (pulsed lavage), and scraping the wound base and periwound area with a blunt instrument. Wet-to-dry or wet-to-moist gauze dressings are discouraged because of their nonselective nature in removing both debris and healthy granulation tissue.

Management of eschar depends on whether the tissue is stable or unstable. The term stable eschar is used to describe leathery or dry tissue, whereas unstable describes tissue that is undergoing a softening process caused by bacteria or developing infection. Sharp or excisional debridement includes the use of a scalpel, curette, or scissors, and requires written informed consent regardless of the location of care delivery. Other methods of debridement are available using ultrasonic or laser technology. Sharp debridement is best handled by an experienced clinician. Options for sharp debridement include scoring of the eschar with application of topical enzymatic debriding agents and use of a curette, scalpel, or scissors to remove eschar. Depending on the extent of the eschar, considerations include local or general anesthesia. Timing of debridement is a matter of clinical judgment as to whether the eschar is stable or unstable, and serial debridements are often needed. Pain management and control of bleeding are important components of mechanical and sharp debridement. Some clinicians advocate maggot debridement therapy, also called biological or larval therapy, which involves application of sterilized larvae of the *Lucilia sericata* fly directly in the wound. The fly larvae digest bacteria, secrete proteinases that degrade necrotic tissue, and stimulate granulation.

NPWT is the application of suction to a wound bed to facilitate healing. The wound is packed with foam and sealed with adhesive membrane, and a vacuum device delivers controlled negative pressure while

Table 33.2—Common Wound Treatment Modalities

Type	Content	Rationale	Best Use
Gauze	Cotton, polyester, or other fabrics	Versatile, can be absorptive or protective, primary or secondary dressing	Secondary dressing, wet to moist, or wet to dry, or as a protective to the wound and surrounding skin. *Note:* wet to dry is not recommended.
Hydrocolloid	Adhesive pad with moisture-activated, gel-forming material; gelatin and pectin	Moisture retention	Superficial, clean pressure ulcers with no necrosis or infection
Semipermeable films	Transparent polymer with acrylic adhesive	Moisture retention	Superficial, clean pressure ulcers with no necrosis or infection
Hydrogel	Water in a delivery vehicle such as glycerin or cross-linked polymer sheets	Promote moist wound healing and autolytic debridement	Dry wounds; wounds with some necrosis
Foam	Polyurethane with or without adhesive borders	Absorb exudate, cushioning, secondary dressing	Control of exudate, protect the wound
Alginate	Seaweed derivative; can be in different forms, including sheet or rope, and combined with other materials such as silver or charcoal	Absorptive dressing	Control of exudate
Collagen	Animal-derived collagen formulated into gel, powder, paste, or sheet	Deactivates matrix metalloproteases that inhibit wound healing	Partial- or full-thickness wounds with minimal necrosis
Silver-containing dressings	Silver can be impregnated into multiple types of dressings	Silver has broad-spectrum antimicrobial activity	Wounds requiring control of bacterial balance
Enzymatic debriding agent	Enzyme in a petrolatum vehicle	Selected degradation of denatured collagen	Wounds with necrosis and slough
Cadexomer iodine dressing	Iodophor in a polysaccharide polymer	Absorbent, antimicrobial	Wounds with slough, infected wounds
Silicone dressings	Inert silicone polymer; sometimes has pores that allow passage of exudate	Contact layer that can be removed without causing trauma to wound or surrounding skin	When a nonadherent dressing is required, protects the wound and surrounding skin
Activated charcoal	Combined with silver or other vehicles	Control odor	Palliative wounds with odor
Honey	Medicinal grade honey can be used as a gel or impregnated into other dressing types	Antimicrobial properties, anti-inflammatory	Autolytic debriding agent on noninfected wounds
Topical antiseptics	Includes hydrogen peroxide, Dakin solution (hypochlorite), povidone-iodine	Reduce bacterial burden of wounds	Can be cytotoxic to healing wounds; for limited use in heavily contaminated or nonhealable wounds
Petrolatum-impregnated gauze	Woven mesh; medical petrolatum and 3% bismuth tribromophenate	Bacteriostatic, nonadherent, retains moisture	Use with larger wounds with minimal necrosis and slough

collecting exudate and debris into a collection chamber or absorptive pad. Since its introduction in the 1980s, NPWT has become a multimillion dollar industry despite limited evidence in controlled clinical trials for efficacy. NPWT has been used in treatment of all types of wounds, including open abdominal incisions, dehisced surgical wounds, burns, preparation for skin grafts, traumatic wounds, venous stasis ulcers, diabetic foot ulcers, and pressure injuries.

The mechanism by which NPWT promotes healing is not known but may include removal of excess fluid, improved circulation, reduced bacterial load, and the mechanical effect of negative pressure. The FDA has issued a safety communication regarding complications of NPWT, including pain, retention of foreign bodies from the dressing, bleeding, infection, death, and complications stemming from power outages. NPWT should not be used over necrotic or infected wounds and is not a substitute for good nursing care to keep a wound clean. Patients should be carefully selected for NPWT and educated regarding its use and risks. NPWT initiation should be cautiously considered for a wound that is not expected to heal; if no observable improvement is seen after 2 weeks, NPWT should be discontinued.

Most experts agree that nutrition is an important component of pressure injury management. Carbohydrates and fats supply energy to cells, and protein is used in anabolic repair, whereas many vitamins and trace elements are essential for healing. Nutritional recommendations should be individualized in response to clinical conditions and goals of care. In general, the caloric requirement for wound healing is 30–35 Kcal/kg/day (SOE=B). Protein is required for wound healing, but the exact amount is not established. The current recommendation for protein is 1–1.5 g/kg/day, but more may be required depending on clinical condition. When determining nutritional needs, it is important to consider other factors such as preexisting protein-calorie nutrition and comorbidities. There is some evidence that 8 weeks of supplementation with an oral nutritional formula enriched with arginine, zinc, and antioxidants improves pressure ulcer healing (SOE=B).

Caution is advised when delegating wound care decisions to consultants, particularly with regard to procedures and ancillary treatment such as NPWT. Long-term care facilities that outsource wound care must ensure that treatment decisions remain part of the interdisciplinary team approach. Many types of providers practice wound care, including general surgeons; plastic and vascular surgeons; emergency physicians; dermatologists; physicians from nonsurgical specialties; podiatrists; advanced practice nurses; wound, ostomy, and continence nurses; physician assistants; and physical therapists. Wound care practitioners may not have had training in geriatrics or palliative care and may lack knowledge or skill with decision making in light of advance directives and end-of-life issues. The wound care consultant should be integrated into an overall and reasonable plan, particularly for patients in whom palliative principles apply. Wound care takes teamwork and communication, and weaknesses in the system have adverse consequences in terms of unnecessary procedures, pain, increased health care costs, risk-management, and quality of patient-centered care.

INFECTIOUS ASPECTS OF PRESSURE INJURIES

Localized infection or cellulitis occurs when microorganisms replicate and produce large enough numbers to elicit host response and cause injury. Local infectious complications of pressure injuries include cellulitis, abscess, osteomyelitis, and pyarthrosis. Pressure injuries can be the starting point for necrotizing fasciitis, a rapidly progressive infection that spreads along fascial planes within subcutaneous tissue. Systemic infections resulting from pressure injuries include sepsis and hematogenous seeding of distant structures, causing further problems such as endocarditis, infected prosthetic joints, and bacterial meningitis.

Identification and treatment of infection are critical to healing a pressure ulcer; however, there is little consensus on definition of wound infection in a chronic wound. Signs and symptoms include fever, increased drainage, pain, warmth, edema, erythema, slough, odor, cessation of healing, or worsening of the wound. Many of these may not be present in older patients, people with diabetes, or patients with malnutrition or immunocompromise. Diagnosis is based on clinical evaluation of local and systemic symptoms in concert with laboratory studies. Increased WBC count may be found when the infection is acute but is an unreliable indicator of chronic infection.

Because all wound surfaces are contaminated, swab cultures are best reserved for wounds with purulent drainage in the setting of high suspicion for infection. One reliable technique involves rotating a swab over a 1-cm^2 area with enough pressure to express fluid from the wound (SOE=B). Tissue biopsy culture method includes removing a piece of the wound with a scalpel or curette, but this is painful and unavailable in many settings.

Treatment of infected wounds involves managing underlying conditions, including diabetes, anemia, poor nutritional status, cardiopulmonary disease, and any cause of edema. All wounds should be protected from contamination with urine and feces. Wound cleansers include water, saline, commercial cleansers, and irrigation devices, but these do not remove deeper bacteria. Bioburden can be managed by removing devitalized tissue with debridement, which can be autolytic, enzymatic, mechanical, or surgical. Antiseptics such as povidone-iodine, betadine, peroxide, and Dakin solution are generally discouraged because they harm living tissue, but they can be useful in heavily contaminated wounds when used in limited fashion.

Wound infections can be treated locally, systemically, or both, depending on the clinical situation. Local treatments include dressings containing antimicrobial compounds such as gentian violet, methylene blue, silver, and cadexomer iodine. Topical antibiotics include mupiricin, neomycin, polymixin B, and bacitracin. Multiple topical antifungals are available, including the imidazole, triazole, and thiazole compounds. Systemic treatment depends on the suspected organisms and clinical setting, and bone infection requires 6 weeks of intravenous therapy. Aggressive treatment and hospitalization should be guided by goals of care and advance directives in conjunction with education of the patient and family.

DIFFERENTIAL DIAGNOSIS OF LOWER EXTREMITY WOUNDS

Ulcers of the foot and leg generally result from multiple etiologies. The most common causes of lower extremity ulcers are venous insufficiency, arterial insufficiency, neuropathic disease, and pressure injury. The most common cause is chronic venous insufficiency. These wounds are generally not painful and are seen most often above the medial or lateral malleolus and occur in beds of chronic venous insufficiency evidenced by edema and hemosiderin staining of the lower extremities.

Arterial wounds are painful and are seen in distal portions of the foot, generally in the presence of chronic atherosclerotic disease evidenced by pale, shiny, and cool skin; loss of skin appendages such as hair and sweat glands; decreased pedal pulses; and poor capillary refill. The presence of peripheral arterial disease (PAD) increases the risk of pressure injury. The ABI is unreliable in the geriatric population for assessment of arterial wounds, because hardening of the arteries falsely increases the result. Other noninvasive tests are recommended such as pulse-volume recordings, toe pressure, and Doppler ultrasound. Suspected PAD requires assessment by a vascular surgeon, and endovascular procedures can increase circulation and assist in healing.

Diabetic foot ulcers usually occur in the setting of longstanding diabetes mellitus and peripheral neuropathy. They result from various factors, including mechanical changes in the bony architecture of the foot, atherosclerotic PAD, loss of sensation, and disease of the microcirculation. Infected diabetic wounds often present atypically, and all diabetic foot ulcers require evaluation by a vascular surgeon and/or podiatrist.

Miscellaneous causes of leg ulceration in older adults include trauma, malignancy such as basal or squamous cell carcinoma, pyoderma gangrenosum, and vasculitis.

PALLIATIVE CARE FOR CHRONIC WOUNDS

Skin integrity compromise impacts up to one-fourth of patients at life's end. Fifty percent of these cases are pressure injuries, 20% are ischemic wounds related to PAD, and the remainder are related to malignancy, venous insufficiency, lymphedema, diabetes, skin tears, surgery, radiotherapy, and other causes. A palliative approach can reduce suffering, improve quality of life, and decrease health care costs by eliminating expensive and/or painful procedures and treatments. Palliative care for chronic wounds should be considered when it becomes clear that there is little or no realistic chance of healing within the patient's lifetime and when the burdens of operative procedures or advanced treatment options outweigh the benefits. The decision to designate a wound as palliative arises when the wound is unresponsive to therapy and the process of achieving healing is inconsistent with overall goals of care. Some wounds that are designated as palliative can show signs of healing, but this should not alter the palliative plan. Because of the difficulty of studying this population, evidence-based guidelines are limited and the strength of evidence for existing guidelines is generally level C. For a mnemonic that summarizes the palliative care approach to wounds, see Table 33.3.

Table 33.3—Palliative Care of Wounds: the Mnemonic "SPECIAL"

S	= Stabilize the wound
P	= Prevent new wounds
E	= Eliminate odor
C	= Control pain
I	= Infection prophylaxis
A	= Absorbent wound dressings
L	= Lessen or reduce dressing changes

SOURCE: Alvarez OM, Kalinski C, Nusbaum J, et al. Incorporating wound healing strategies to improve palliation (symptom management) in patients with chronic wounds. *J Pall Med.* 2007;10(5):1161–1189e.

Factors leading to designating a wound as palliative include unmodifiable risk factors or medical conditions such as poor nutrition, inadequate perfusion, multisystem organ failure, immunocompromise, irreversible anasarca, a terminal prognosis that prevents the normal healing process, and the presence of artificial life support. NPWT, hyperbaric oxygen, and other ancillary treatments are generally used when the goal is healing. The decision to consider a palliative approach is made in consultation with the patient, family, and wound specialist with honest and open dialogue regarding prognosis for healing and the burdens, benefits, adverse effects, and potential complications of more aggressive cure-oriented procedures.

A palliative approach to wounds involves providing counseling and emotional support for the patient and family, preventing further skin deterioration and infection, promoting comfort, and optimizing pain management and other symptoms such as odor and bleeding. The timing of dressings and repositioning can be modified to decrease pain associated with physical manipulation of the patient and the wound. Topical pain treatments include viscous lidocaine gel and dressings that deliver locally applied ibuprofen and opiates. An FDA advisory warns that topical skin-numbing products may have cardiopulmonary adverse effects when absorbed into the bloodstream, so caution is advised. Wound odor can be minimized with charcoal- or chlorophyll-containing dressings, or metronidazole gel[OL]. Dressings such as alginates and absorptive foam can manage excess drainage and protect the periwound areas from MASD.

RESOURCES

- Edsberg LE, Black JM, Goldberg M, et al. Revised National Pressure Ulcer Advisory Panel Pressure Injury Staging System: Revised Pressure Injury Staging System. *J Wound Ostomy Continence Nurs*. 2016;43(6):585–597.

- National Pressure Ulcer Advisory Panel. Prevention and Treatment of Pressure Ulcers: Clinical Practice Guideline. Washington, DC: NPUAP; 2014.

- Westby M, Dumville JC, Soares MO, et al. Dressings and topical agents for treating pressure ulcers. *Cochrane Database Syst Rev*. 2017 Jun 22;6:CD011947.

- Woo KY, Krasner DL, Kennedy B, et al. Palliative wound care management strategies for palliative patients and their circles of care. *Adv Skin Wound Care*. 2015;28(3):130–140.

CHAPTER 34—GAIT IMPAIRMENT

KEY POINTS

- Gait disorders are common in older adults and are a predictor of functional decline.

- The cause of gait impairment in older adults is usually multifactorial; therefore, a full assessment must include consideration of a number of different causes, as determined from a detailed physical examination and a functional performance evaluation.

- Various interventions, ranging from medical to surgical to exercise, can reduce the degree of impairment, although some residual impairment is often present.

EPIDEMIOLOGY

Limitations in walking increase with age. At least 20% of noninstitutionalized older adults admit to difficulty with walking or require the assistance of another person or special equipment to walk. In some samples of noninstitutionalized older adults ≥85 years old, the prevalence of walking limitations can be over 50%. Age-related gait changes such as slowed speed are most apparent after age 75 or 80, but most gait disorders appear in connection with underlying diseases, particularly as disease severity increases. For example, advanced age (>85 years old); three or more chronic conditions at baseline; and the occurrence of stroke, hip fracture, or cancer predict catastrophic loss of walking ability (SOE=B).

Determining that a gait is disordered is difficult, because there are no clearly accepted general standards of normal gait for older adults. Some believe that slowed gait speed suggests a disorder; others believe that deviations in smoothness, symmetry, and synchrony of movement patterns suggest a disorder. Regardless, a slowed and aesthetically abnormal gait can nevertheless provide an older adult with a safe, independent gait pattern. Attributing a gait disorder to one specific disease in older adults is particularly difficult, because similar gait abnormalities are common to many diseases.

Longitudinal observational studies suggest that certain gait-related mobility disorders progress with age and that this progression is associated with disability, morbidity and mortality. Community-dwelling older adults with gait disorders, particularly neurologically abnormal gaits, are at higher risk of institutionalization and death (SOE=B).

CONDITIONS THAT CONTRIBUTE TO GAIT IMPAIRMENT

Impaired gait may not be an inevitable consequence of aging but rather a reflection of the increased prevalence and severity of age-associated diseases. These diseases, both neurologic and non-neurologic, are the major contributors to impaired gait. (For a glossary of gait abnormalities, see Table 34.1.)

Patients in primary care report that pain, stiffness, dizziness, numbness, weakness, and sensations of abnormal movement are the most common causes of their walking difficulties. The most common conditions seen in primary care that are thought to contribute to gait disorders are degenerative joint disease, acquired musculoskeletal deformities, intermittent claudication, impairments after orthopedic surgery and stroke, and postural hypotension. Usually, more than one contributing condition is found. In a group of community-dwelling adults >88 years old, joint pain was by far the most common contributor, followed by multiple causes such as stroke and visual loss. Factors such as dementia and fear of falling also contribute to gait disorders. The disorders found in a neurologic referral population include frontal gait disorders (usually related to normal-pressure hydrocephalus [NPH] and cerebrovascular processes), sensory disorders (also involving vestibular and visual function), myelopathy, previously undiagnosed Parkinson disease or parkinsonian syndromes, and cerebellar disease. Known conditions causing severe gait impairment, such as hemiplegia and severe hip or knee disease, are commonly not mentioned in these neurologic referral populations. Thus, many gait disorders, particularly those that are classical and discrete (eg, those related to stroke and osteoarthritis) and those that are mild or may relate to irreversible disease (eg, vascular dementia), are presumably diagnosed in primary care and treated without a referral to a neurologist. Other less common contributors to gait disorders include metabolic disorders (related to renal or hepatic disease), CNS tumors or subdural hematoma, depression, and psychotropic medications. Case reports also document reversible gait disorders due to clinically overt hypo- or hyperthyroidism and B_{12} and folate deficiency.

Factors associated with slowed gait speed are also considered contributors to gait disorders. These factors are commonly disease associated (eg, cardiopulmonary or musculoskeletal disease) and include decreased leg strength, vision, aerobic function, standing balance,

Table 34.1—Glossary of Gait Abnormalities

Term	Description
Antalgic gait	Pain-induced limp with shortened stance phase of gait on painful side
Circumduction	Outward swing of leg in semicircle from the hip
Equinovarus	Excessive plantar flexion and inversion of the ankle
Festination	Acceleration of gait
Foot drop	Loss of ankle dorsiflexion secondary to weakness of ankle dorsiflexors
Foot slap	Early, frequent audible foot–floor contact with steppage gait compensation
Freezing of gait	Sudden, short duration diminution or cessation of walking usually associated with shift in attention or movement circumstance or direction
Genu recurvatum	Hyperextension of knee
Propulsion	Tendency to fall forward
Retropulsion	Tendency to fall backward
Scissoring	Hip adduction such that the knees cross in front of each other with each step
Shuffling	Not lifting feet off ground when walking
Steppage gait	Exaggerated hip flexion, knee flexion, and foot lifting, usually accompanied by foot drop
Trendelenburg gait	Hip abductor weakness causes contralateral pelvis to drop, which may be compensated by trunk lean to affected side
Turn en bloc	Moving the whole body while turning

and physical activity, as well as joint impairment, previous falls, and fear of falling. Longitudinal data suggest that multiple organ system changes contribute to age-related changes in gait speed, but no single system is primarily associated with this decline. Combining factors can result in an effect greater than the sum of the single impairments (as when combining balance and strength impairments). Furthermore, the effect of improved strength and aerobic capacity on gait speed may be nonlinear; that is, for very impaired individuals, small improvements in strength or aerobic capacity yield relatively larger gains in gait speed, whereas these small improvements yield little gait speed change in healthy older adults.

Although older adults can maintain a relatively normal gait pattern well into their 80s, some slowing occurs, and decreased stride length thus becomes a common feature in descriptions of gait disorders of older adults. Some authors have proposed the emergence of an age-related gait disorder without accompanying clinical abnormalities, ie, essential "senile" gait disorder. This gait pattern is described as broad-based with small steps, diminished arm swing, stooped posture, flexion of the hips and knees, uncertainty and stiffness in turning, occasional difficulty initiating steps, and a tendency toward falling. These and other nonspecific findings (eg, the inability to perform tandem gait) are similar to gait patterns found in a number of other diseases, and yet the clinical abnormalities are insufficient to make a specific diagnosis. This "disorder" may be a precursor to an as-yet-undiagnosed disease (eg, related to subtle extrapyramidal symptoms) and is likely to be a manifestation of concurrent, progressive cognitive impairment (eg, Alzheimer disease or vascular dementia). Thus, "senile" gait disorder may reflect a number of potential diseases and is generally not useful in labeling gait disorders in older adults.

Subclinical as well as clinically evident cerebrovascular disease is increasingly recognized as a major contributor to causes of gait disorders (SOE=B). Individuals without a dementia diagnosis and with clinically abnormal gait (particularly unsteady, frontal, or hemiparetic gait) followed for approximately 7 years were found to be at higher risk of developing non-Alzheimer, particularly vascular, dementia. Of note, those with abnormal gait at baseline may not have met criteria for dementia but already had abnormalities in neuropsychologic function, such as in visual-perceptual processing and language skills. Gait disorders with no apparent cause (also termed "idiopathic" or "senile" gait disorder) are associated with a higher mortality rate, primarily from cardiovascular causes (SOE=B). These cardiovascular causes are likely linked to concomitant, possibly undetected, cerebrovascular disease.

ASSESSMENT

Gait disorders can be assessed and categorized according to the sensorimotor levels that are affected.

Disorders that are the result of pathology of the low sensorimotor level can be divided into peripheral sensory and peripheral motor dysfunction, including myopathic or neuropathic disorders that cause weakness and musculoskeletal diseases. These disorders are generally distal to the CNS. With peripheral sensory impairment, unsteady and tentative gait is commonly caused by vestibular disorders, peripheral neuropathy, posterior column (proprioceptive) deficits, or visual impairment. With peripheral motor impairment, a number of classical gait patterns emerge. Examples of these patterns include Trendelenburg gait (ie, hip abductor weakness causes the contralateral pelvis to drop, which may be compensated by trunk lean to the affected side), antalgic gait (weight bearing is avoided and stance shortens on one side because of pain), and foot drop (due to ankle dorsiflexor weakness and characterized by a frequently audible foot-floor contact with steppage gait compensation, ie, excessive hip flexion). These gait impairments are the result of body segment and joint deformities, pain, and focal myopathic and neuropathic weakness. In general, if the gait disorder is limited to this low sensorimotor level (ie, the CNS is intact), the person can adapt well to the gait disorder, compensating with an assistive device or learning to negotiate the environment safely.

At the middle sensorimotor level, the execution of centrally selected postural and locomotor responses is faulty, and the sensory and motor modulation of gait is disrupted. Gait may be initiated normally, but stepping patterns are abnormal. Diseases causing spasticity (eg, those related to myelopathy, B_{12} deficiency, and stroke), parkinsonism (idiopathic as well as medication induced), and cerebellar disease (eg, alcohol induced) are examples of those that cause this type of impairment. Gait abnormalities appear when the spasticity is sufficient to cause leg circumduction and fixed deformities (eg, equinovarus), when the Parkinson disease produces shuffling steps and reduced arm swing, and when the cerebellar ataxia increases trunk sway sufficiently to require a broad base of gait support. Freezing of gait is found commonly in parkinsonian syndromes.

At the high or central level, gait impairments become more nonspecific. Lesions in the frontal lobe account for most gait abnormalities at this level. The severity of the frontal-related disorders runs a spectrum from difficulty with initiation of gait to frontal dysequilibrium, in which unsupported stance is not possible. Cerebrovascular insults to the cortex, as well as to the basal ganglia and their interconnections, may contribute to difficulty with initiation of gait and to apraxia.

Dementia and depression are also thought to contribute to an abnormal gait at the high or central level. With increasing severity of the dementia, particularly in patients with Alzheimer disease, frontal-related symptoms also increase. Gait impairments in this category have been given a number of overlapping descriptions, including *gait apraxia*, *marche a petits pas*, and *arteriosclerotic parkinsonism*.

More than one disease or impairment is likely to contribute to a gait disorder; one example is the longstanding diabetic patient with peripheral neuropathy and a recent stroke who is now very fearful of falling. Certain disorders can actually involve multiple parts of the nervous system, such as Parkinson disease affecting cortical and subcortical structures. Drug and metabolic causes (eg, from sedatives, tranquilizers, and anticonvulsants) can involve both central and peripheral nervous systems (eg, phenothiazines can cause central sedation and extrapyramidal effects).

History and Physical Examination

A careful medical history can help elucidate the multiple factors contributing to gait impairments in older adults. A brief systemic evaluation for evidence of subacute metabolic disease (eg, thyroid disorders), acute cardiopulmonary disorders (eg, myocardial infarction), or other acute illness (eg, sepsis) is warranted because an acute gait disorder may be the presenting feature of acute systemic decompensation in older adults. The physical examination should include an attempt to identify motion-related factors, eg, by provoking both vestibular and orthostatic responses. A focused examination, based on symptoms, should include the Dix-Hallpike test to test for vestibular dysfunction, postural blood pressure measurements to exclude orthostatic hypotension, and vision screening at least for acuity. In addition, the neck, spine, extremities, and feet should be evaluated for pain, deformities, and limitations in range of motion, particularly regarding subtle hip or knee contractures. Leg-length discrepancies such as can occur with a hip prosthesis and either as an antecedent or subsequent to lower back pain can be measured simply as the distance from the anterior superior iliac spine to the medial malleolus. A formal neurologic assessment is critical and should include assessment of strength and tone, sensation (including proprioception), coordination (including cerebellar function), station, and gait. The Romberg test screens for simple postural control and whether the proprioceptive and vestibular systems are functional. Some investigators have proposed that one-legged stance time <5 seconds is a risk factor for injurious falls, although even relatively healthy adults ≥70 years old can have difficulty with one-legged stance. Given the importance of cognition as a risk factor, assessing cognitive function is also indicated.

Laboratory and Imaging Assessments

Depending on the history and physical examination, further laboratory and diagnostic imaging evaluation may be warranted. A CBC, serum chemistries, and other metabolic studies may be useful when systemic disease is suspected. Head or spine imaging, including radiography, CT, or MRI, are not indicated unless history and physical examination identifies neurologic abnormalities, either preceding or of recent onset, that are related to the gait disorder. In a recent review of multiple imaging modalities, a number of pathologies (white matter, hippocampal volume, ventricular enlargement, and amyloid and tau aggregation) were associated with poor gait performance, with grey matter atrophy having the most consistent link (SOE=A). Other pathologies associated with poor gait performance included white matter atrophy, hippocampal volume decline, ventricular enlargement, and amyloid and tau aggregation. Gait disruption was also associated with both under- and overactivation of neuronal activity. Beause of substantial methodologic heterogeneity for measuring both neuropathology and gait, a meta-analysis was not possible.

Performance-Based Functional Assessment

A number of timed and semiquantitative balance and gait scales have been proposed as a means to detect and quantify abnormalities and to direct interventions. Fall risk, for example, can be increased with more abnormal gait and balance scale scores, such as with the Berg Balance Scale or the Performance-Oriented Mobility Assessment. Perhaps the simplest battery in the clinical setting is the "Timed Up and Go" (TUG), a timed sequence of rising from a chair, walking 3 meters, turning, and returning to sit in the chair. One study suggests a TUG score of ≥12 seconds as an indicator of fall risk. Other investigators have found limitations in TUG in the presence of cognitive impairment and difficulty in completing the test because of immobility, safety concerns, or refusal. Another functional approach that can be useful clinically is the Functional Ambulation Classification scale, which rates the use of assistive devices, the degree of human assistance (either manual or verbal), the distance the person can walk, and the types of surfaces the person can negotiate.

Comfortable gait speed and related endurance measures (such as the 6-minute walk) are powerful predictors of a number of important outcomes, such as falls, disability, hospitalization, institutionalization, and mortality (SOE=B). Another endurance measure, the 400-meter walk, has been increasingly used in research settings and considered a marker of major mobility disability that was responsive to a physical activity intervention. Gait speed is faster in individuals who are taller, who have a lower disease burden, and who are more active and less functionally disabled. Usual gait speed is frequently tested from a standing start over a distance of 4 meters. Although speeds between 0.6 and 0.8 m/s are associated with poor outcomes, a speed of 0.6 m/s has been proposed as the cut point for dismobility, given the rapid rise in disability and poor health outcomes below this speed. As expected, in clinical settings, gait speed is slowest in the acute hospital versus in subacute or outpatient settings (0.46, 0.53, and 0.74 m/s respectively, in a review). Speeds of >1.0 m/s and perhaps 1.2 m/s are associated with better functional outcomes and increased life expectancy. Several studies have found age- and disease-associated deficits in the ability to walk and perform a simultaneous cognitive task ("dual tasking," such as talking while walking), and also linked these deficits with increased fall risk (SOE=B), and include gait speed changes as well as gait variability. However, dual task changes in gait speed as well as variability may be equivalent to single task changes in discriminating fallers from non-fallers even when considering those who walk more slowly or who are cognitively impaired. The dual task effect may thus be most clinically useful in very high-risk groups who require extensive attentional resources to maintain safe gait. Although slower gait speed can predict decreased cognition in healthy older adults, the opposite is true as well, namely that decreased cognitive function, in multiple domains including executive function, is associated with slower speed.

INTERVENTIONS TO REDUCE GAIT DISORDERS

Even if a condition can be diagnosed on evaluation, many conditions causing a gait disorder are, at best, only partially treatable. The patient is often left with at least some residual disability. However, other functional outcomes such as reduction in weight-bearing pain may be equally important in justifying treatment. Functional improvement becomes the treatment goal. Comorbidity, disease severity, and overall health status tend to strongly influence treatment outcome.

Achievement of premorbid gait patterns may be unrealistic, but improvement in measures such as gait speed is reasonable as long as gait remains safe. Recent studies have estimated the extent to which a change in gait performance, such as usual gait speed, is clinically meaningful. For example, in cohorts that include mobility-impaired individuals, estimates range from 0.05 m/s to 0.10 m/s for small and substantial change, respectively. Exercise interventions in more physically impaired older adults may have lower meaningful differences (eg, 0.07 m/s in one review). However, using a cut-off of even 0.10 m/s may not coincide with perceived change in mobility in certain patient populations, such as in patients with a previous hip fracture. The most striking changes in gait speed occur with strength or combined training (including aerobic exercise), especially with higher intensity or dosage. An innovative program using goal-oriented, progressively more difficult stepping and walking patterns to promote the timing and coordination of stepping in subclinically gait-impaired older adults may be more effective than treadmill walking training (SOE=B). Task-specific training may also improve dual-task performance, but the same training in impaired populations may also improve single-task performance. Finally, recent trials using exercise or combined exercise–cognitive training may improve dual task performance (mainly gait speed), but the results are mixed and the mechanism for improvement (eg, applying a different cognitive response strategy) is not clear.

Modest improvement with residual disability is also the result of surgical treatment for compressive cervical myelopathy, lumbar stenosis, and NPH. Few controlled prospective studies and no well-controlled randomized studies address the outcome of surgical versus nonsurgical treatment for these 3 conditions. A number of problems plague the available series: outcomes such as pain and walking disability are not reported separately, the source of the outcome rating is not clearly identified or blinded, the criteria for classifying outcomes differ, the outcomes may be subjective and subject to interpretation, the follow-up intervals are variable, the participants who are reported in follow-up may be a highly select group, the selection factors for conservative versus surgical treatment between studies differ or are unspecified, and there is publication bias (only positive results are published). Many of the surgical series include all ages, although the mean age is usually >60 years old. A few studies document equivalent surgical outcomes with conservative, nonsurgical treatment.

With regard to lumbar stenosis procedures, many older adults have reduced pain after laminectomies and lumbar fusion surgery, although they have continued residual disability and if there is improvement in walking ability, the improvement may wane long term (SOE=B). Nonoperative treatment (with a variety of interventions, including oral anti-inflammatory medications, heating modalities, exercise, mobilizations, and epidural injections) can also result in modest improvements such as in walking tolerance (SOE=B). A randomized trial found that physical therapy yielded similar effects to those of surgical decompression (no gait data shown). However, methodologic differences, such as a large percentage of physical therapy patients crossing over to surgery, undermine the outcome, and similar to results of other studies, long-term benefits of surgery diminish after 24 months. Part of the problem in determining long-term gait outcomes of surgery for lumbar stenosis is other comorbidity, such as cardiovascular or musculoskeletal disease, that influences mobility. Regarding cervical stenosis, studies involving postoperative gait outcomes in older adults are limited, but in one nonrandomized study, walking speed improved significantly in most of the postcervical myelopathy decompression patients whose mean age was 60 years old (SOE=B).

Outcomes for hip and knee replacement surgery for osteoarthritis are better, although some of the same study methodologic problems exist. Multidisciplinary rehabilitation (versus more limited rehabilitation) after hip or knee replacement results in improved global functioning beyond walking measures (SOE=A). Other advances include "total body preoperative exercise," ie, "prehabilitation," which may have positive effects on length of stay and possibly postoperative function, as noted in a review that included primarily orthopedic surgeries. Despite rehabilitation after joint replacement, some residual weakness, stiffness, and slowed/altered gait and balance may remain. Simple function may be maintained after knee replacement, such as maintaining the ability to safely clear an obstacle, but usually at the expense of additional compensation by the ipsilateral hip and foot. Other than pain relief, sizable gains in gait speed and joint motion occur, although residual walking disability continues for a number of reasons, including residual pathology on the operated side and symptoms on the nonoperated side. Controlled trials of specific exercise programs offered at least 2 months after total knee replacement (such as aquatic or general exercise) generally show retention of strength but varying retention of walking speed gains at 1-year follow-up. In patients undergoing total hip replacement for osteoarthritis versus patients with osteoarthritis who received medical therapy, self-reported walking-related function at 6 months was improved (SOE=B). Nevertheless, in a review of hip replacements, reduction in strength output continues compared with controls and the nonoperated hip, with reductions in walking speed at long term (eg, 2 year) follow-up.

Finally, the use of orthoses and other mobility aids can help reduce gait disorders (SOE=C). Although there are few data supporting their use, lifts (either internal or external) to correct for limb length inequality can be used in a conservative, gradually progressive manner. Other ankle braces, shoe inserts, shoe body and sole modifications, and their subsequent adjustments are part of standard care for foot and ankle weakness, deformities, and pain but are beyond the scope of this chapter. In general, well-fitting walking shoes with low heels, relatively thin firm soles, and if feasible, high, fixed heel collar support are recommended to maximize balance and improve gait. Mobility aids such as canes and walkers reduce load on a painful joint and increase stability. Note that light touch of any firm surface like walls or "furniture surfing" provide feedback and assist with balance.

RESOURCES

- Plummer P, Zukowski LA, Giuliani C, et al. Effects of physical exercise interventions on gait-related dual-task interference in older adults: a systematic review and meta-analysis. *Gerontology*. 2015;62(1):94–117.

- Taylor JL, Parker LJ, Szanton SL, et al. The association of pain, race and slow gait speed in older adults. *Geriatr Nurs*. 2018;39(5):580–583.

- Wennberg AM, Savica R, Mielke MM. Association between various brain pathologies and gait disturbance. *Dement Geriatr Cogn Disord*. 2017;43(3-4):128–143.

CHAPTER 35—FALLS

KEY POINTS

- Falls are not only common events that threaten the independence of older adults, but also the leading cause of death from injury in this age group.

- Falls are generally multifactorial in origin, with complex interactions among intrinsic risk factors (age-related declines, chronic disease, medications), challenges to postural control (environment, changing position, routine activities), and mediating factors (risk-taking behaviors, situational hazards, acute illness).

- Older adults with even a single fall should have a gait and balance evaluation.

- For older adults with two or more falls in the past 12 months, or with gait or balance abnormalities, a multifactorial falls risk assessment should be pursued.

- Important components of a fall history include the activity of the patient at the time of the fall, the occurrence of prodromal symptoms (lightheadedness, imbalance, and dizziness), and the location of the fall.

- Interventions shown to be effective in reducing falls include medication review, exercise programs that include muscle strengthening and balance training, vitamin D supplementation, use of appropriate footwear, and multifactorial interventions including home hazards assessment for those at high risk of falls.

A fall is one of the most common events threatening the independence of older adults. A fall is considered to have occurred when a person comes to rest inadvertently on the ground or lower level. Most of the literature on falls in older adults does not include falls associated with loss of consciousness (eg, syncope, seizure) or with overwhelming trauma, because most falls are not associated with syncope or trauma.

PREVALENCE AND MORBIDITY

Every second of every day, an older person in the United States will fall. According to a CDC report, one of three adults ≥65 years old reports falling in the previous year. The incidence of falls is more frequent with advancing age and among nursing-home residents, such that one-half of individuals >80 years old or nursing-home residents will fall each year. Among those with a history of a fall in the previous year, the annual incidence of falls is close to 60%. Almost one-third of those who fall need to restrict their activities for a day as a result of the fall or need medical attention related to the fall. Most falls result in minor soft-tissue injury, whereas 5%–10% of falls result in fracture or a more serious soft-tissue injury or head trauma. Women and nursing-home residents are more likely to experience a nonfatal fall-related injury than men. Even among those who do not experience physical injury, falls are associated with subsequent declines in functional status, greater likelihood of nursing-home placement, increased use of medical services, and development of a fear of falling. Of those older adults who fall, only half are able to get up without help, thus experiencing the "long lie." Long lies are associated with lasting declines in functional status. Fall-related injuries are not a common cause of death in older adults; however, complications resulting from falls are the leading cause of death from injury in adults ≥65 years old. The death rate attributable to falls increases with age, with white men ≥85 years old having the highest death rate (>180 deaths per 100,000 population).

The true cost of falls in healthcare dollars is difficult to ascertain. Because many falls result in injury, use of emergency department facilities among those who fall is common. In 2014, 2.8 million nonfatal falls were treated in emergency rooms, with 27% of these visits resulting in hospitalization. Thus, the direct cost of medical visits for falls and services/therapies for fall-related injuries is substantial. Indirect costs from fall-related injuries, such as hip fractures, can also be considerable.

CAUSES AND RISK FACTORS

Falls, incontinence, delirium, and other geriatric syndromes result from the accumulated effects of multiple impairments. In older adults, falls rarely have a single cause. Rather, there is often a complex interaction among intrinsic risk factors (age-related physiologic changes, chronic disease, medications), challenges to postural control (environment, changing positions, routine activities), and mediating factors (risk-taking behaviors, acute illness, or situational hazards, such as unfamiliar staff or high patient-to-staff ratios in hospitals and long-term care facilities).

In multiple prospective cohort studies, several risk factors have been consistently associated with falls, including older age, cognitive impairment, female gender, past fall history, arthritis, foot disorders, balance problems, hypovitaminosis D, psychotropic medication use, pain, Parkinson disease, and stroke (SOE=B). These studies differed significantly in the types of risk factors evaluated, the types of population studied (eg,

Table 35.1—Medication Classes Associated with an Increased Risk of Falls in Older Adults

Amiodarone
Antidepressants (SSRIs, TCAs, others)
First-generation antihistamines or anticholinergic drugs
Other antihypertensives
Antimuscarinic incontinence agents
Antipsychotics, first- and second-generation
Benzodiazepines
Non-benzodiazepine hypnotics
α-Blockers
Dementia medications, acetylcholinesterase inhibitors*
Insulin
Opioids
Muscle relaxants
Parkinson drugs

* Associated with increased risk of syncope

past fall history was sometimes an entry criterion), and the outcome (one fall, two or more falls, rate of falls, injurious falls). The differences in risk factors found across the studies highlight the multifactorial nature of falls and suggest the importance of unique mediating factors unaccounted for in these studies. In general, the risk of falling increases with the number of risk factors, although as many as 10% of falls occur in individuals with no identifiable risk factor for falls. Also, risk factors for indoor and outdoor falls differ: indoor falls tend to occur among older, frail adults with mobility disorders, whereas outdoor falls occur in younger, healthier persons.

Successful prevention of falls begins with knowledge of the age-related changes that increase the risk of falls. With aging, there are declines in the visual, proprioceptive, and vestibular systems. For example, visual changes with aging include reduced visual acuity, depth perception, contrast sensitivity, and dark adaptation. The proprioceptive system loses sensitivity in the legs. The vestibular system has a loss of labyrinthine hair cells, vestibular ganglion cells, and nerve fibers.

Despite these age-related changes in sensory systems, quantifying the age-related changes in postural control that are independent of disease is difficult. When postural stability is tested in young and older people with no apparent musculoskeletal or neurologic impairment, there are measurable age-related differences in sway with perturbations of stance, such as changing the support surface, changing body position, changing the visual input, or moving the support surface horizontally or rotationally. This occurs because these perturbations of stance stress the redundancy of the sensory systems in their ability to maintain postural control. This is borne out by the observation that gait speed deteriorates when individuals are presented with a dual task ("walking while talking"). In addition, there may be other age-related changes in the CNS that affect postural control, including the loss of neurons and dendrites, and the depletion of neurotransmitters, such as dopamine, within the basal ganglia.

Some of the most striking postural control differences between young and old people relate to the order or grouping of muscle activation patterns: in response to perturbations of the support surface, older adults tend to activate the proximal muscles, such as the quadriceps, before the more distal muscles, such as the tibialis anterior. This strategy may not be an efficient way to maintain postural stability. Similarly, in older adults, there may be greater co-contraction of antagonistic muscles, and the onset of the muscle activation and associated joint torque may be delayed. Finally, the ability to recover balance after a postural disturbance may be compromised by an age-related decline in the ability to rapidly develop joint torque by using muscles of the leg. All these mechanisms potentially impair maintenance of upright posture.

Another important physiologic contributor to the maintenance of upright posture is regulation of systemic blood pressure. With advancing age, baroreflex sensitivity declines, which manifests as an inability to increase heart rate in response to common stresses (such as changing posture, eating a meal, or suffering an acute illness) and results in subsequent hypotension. Because many older adults have a resting cerebral perfusion that is compromised by vascular disease, even slight reductions in blood pressure can result in cerebral ischemic symptoms and subsequent falls. Finally, with aging, the amount of total body water is reduced, which places older adults at increased risk of dehydration with acute illness, diuretic use, or hot weather. Because basal and stimulated renin and aldosterone levels progressively decrease with aging, dehydrating stresses can lead to orthostatic hypotension and falls.

A number of age-related chronic conditions deserve special mention because of their association with fall risk. Parkinson disease increases the risk of falls through several mechanisms, including the rigidity of leg musculature, the inability to correct sway trajectory because of the slowness in beginning movement, hypotensive effects of medication, and in some cases, cognitive impairment. Strokes can result in an increased risk of falls secondary to visuospatial defects, impaired peripheral sensation, cerebellar dysfunction, muscle weakness, and residual dizziness. Knee osteoarthritis can affect mobility, the ability to step over objects and maneuver, and balance due to a tendency to avoid complete weight bearing on a painful joint. Chronic pain has been associated with an increased risk of falls possibly due to changes in gait and muscle strength or because pain can act as a cognitive distractor.

One of the most modifiable risk factors for falls that has been repeatedly demonstrated in observational studies is medication use (Table 35.1). Individual classes of psychotropic medications, such as the benzodiazepines, other sedatives, antidepressants, and antipsychotic medications, have been associated with an increased risk of falls and hip fracture. There appears to be no difference in the risk of falling with the use of older antidepressants or antipsychotics compared with the newer SSRIs or atypical antipsychotics. Similarly, there is no protection with respect to risk of falls and fracture by choosing a nonbenzodiazepine hypnotic ("Z-drug") to treat insomnia versus using a benzodiazepine. As might be expected, the risk of falls increases in older adults taking more than one psychotropic medication, and among older adults taking more than 3 or 4 medications of any type.

Other classes of medications affect falls risk as well. Conflicting data exist with respect to the role of antihypertensive medications and falls risk, but these medications likely increase falls risk in persons with a history of falls. Given their favorable effect on bone density, long-term use of thiazides is associated with a decreased risk of hip and pelvic fracture than use of other antihypertensives. Meta-analyses have demonstrated an increased risk of falls among those taking digoxin, diuretics, type 1A antiarrhythmic agents, and NSAIDs. Acetylcholinesterase inhibitors, which are used to treat dementia, have been associated with an increased risk of syncope. Diabetic medications can also be associated with falls risk during periods of hypoglycemia.

Older adults may be particularly vulnerable to falls in the days to weeks after a new medication is started or the dosage of an existing medication is increased. An increased risk of falling has been observed after a new prescription or dosage increase of a non-SSRI antidepressant, benzodiazepine, antihypertensive, or diuretic medication. Older adults are more vulnerable to hip fractures after a new prescription for a nonbenzodiazepine hypnotic, diuretic, or antihypertensive medication. Providers should alert older patients and their caregivers to the increased risk of falls after a new prescription of these medications in an effort to avoid injury.

The relative importance of environmental and mediating factors on the risk of falling has not been well quantified. Most intervention studies have focused on improving the risk-factor profile of the individual or have combined individual interventions with environmental manipulation, making it difficult to isolate the contributions of the environmental factors. Nevertheless, attention to safety hazards in the home environment appears to be worthwhile in those at high risk of falls.

CLINICAL GUIDELINES

The CDC has published an Algorithm for Falls Risk Assessment and Interventions (Figure 35.1) For older adults presenting with a fall, or an adult who is worried about falling or feels unsteady while standing or walking, it is recommended that gait, strength, and balance be evaluated. Further, if the older adult has had two or more falls, or a fall with injury, a multifactorial falls risk assessment should be pursued.

For older adults who have no history of falling, providers should still ask about falls and use traditional geriatric assessment to target major risk factors. For a summary of the recommendations of the expert panel on falls prevention assembled by the American Geriatrics Society (AGS) and the British Geriatrics Society (BGS), see http://bit.ly/2rJPkM3 (accessed Feb 2019).

DIAGNOSTIC APPROACH

History and Physical Examination

Many falls never come to clinical attention for a variety of reasons: the patient may never mention the event, there is no injury at the time of the fall, the clinician may neglect to ask the patient about a history of falls, or the patient or clinician may make the invalid assumption that falls are an inevitable part of the aging process. The treatment of injuries resulting from falls commonly fails to include an investigation of the cause of the fall.

In the clinical evaluation of noninstitutionalized older adults who are not being seen specifically as the result of a fall, it is still important to include an assessment of fall risk in the history and physical examination. The most important point in the history is asking whether there has been a previous fall, because this is a strong risk factor for future falls. Older adults presenting with a single fall should be evaluated for gait and balance problems. Older adults with two or more falls in the past 12 months or with gait or balance abnormalities should undergo a multifactorial falls risk assessment; evaluation of recurrent indoor falls is most likely to uncover multiple risk factors.

For patients presenting with a fall, important components of the history include the activity at the time of the fall, the occurrence of prodromal symptoms (lightheadedness, imbalance, dizziness), and the location and time of the fall. Loss of consciousness is rare, but it should raise important considerations, such as orthostatic hypotension or cardiac or neurologic disease.

Information on previous falls should be collected to identify patterns that may help determine strategies to reduce future falls. A complete medication history should focus on newly added medications or recent dosage changes, as well as the use of antihypertensives, diuretics, and psychotropic medications because of their association with falls and their common use in older adults.

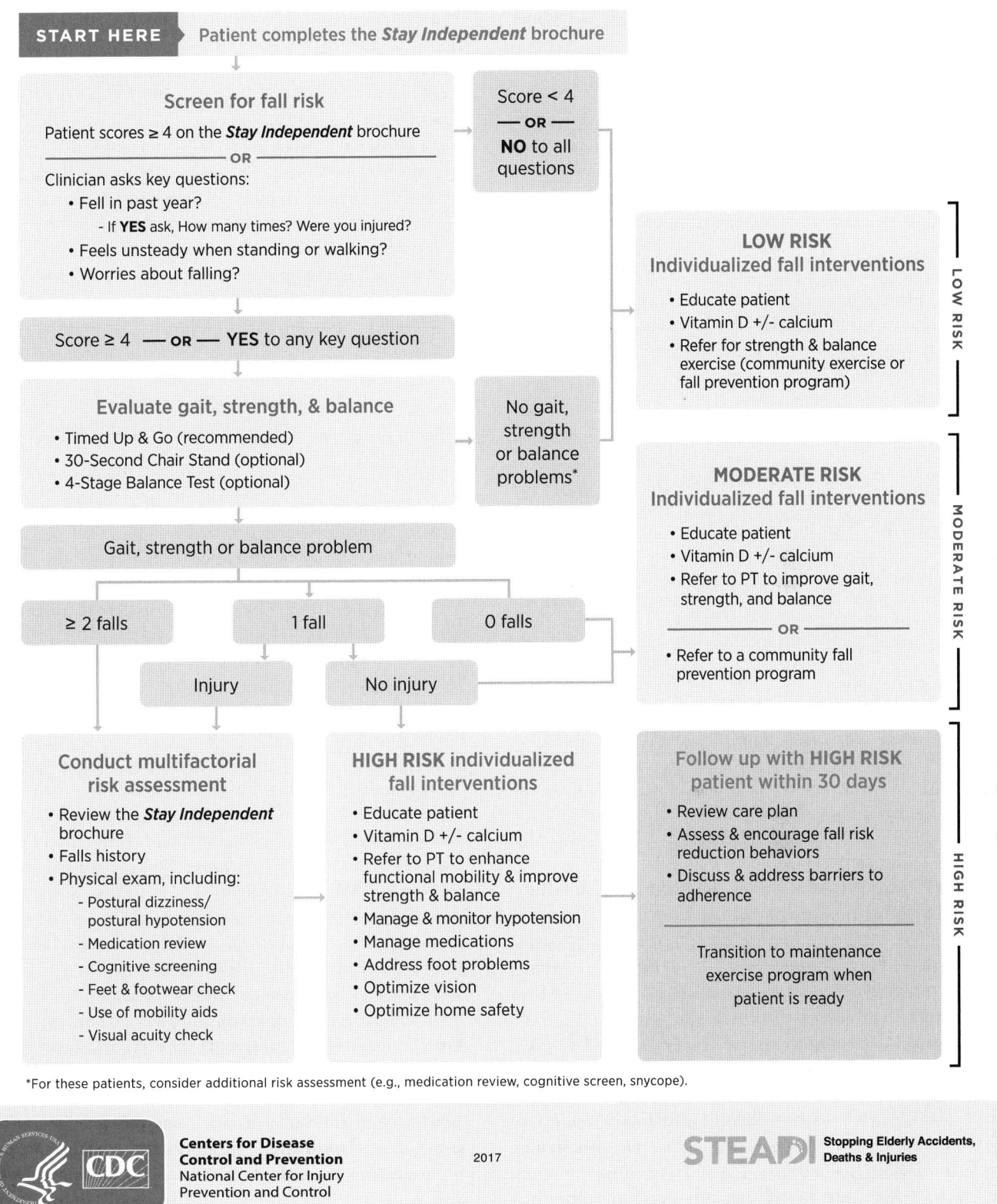

Figure 35.1—Fall Risk Screening, Assessment, and Intervention

EDITORIAL NOTE: Recent systematic reviews of vitamin D and calcium supplementation in community-dwelling older adults do not support routine use in persons who are not frail, at high risk of falls, or who have normal 25(OH)D serum concentrations.

SOURCE: Centers for Disease Control and Prevention. STEADI: Stopping Elderly Accidents, Deaths, and Injuries

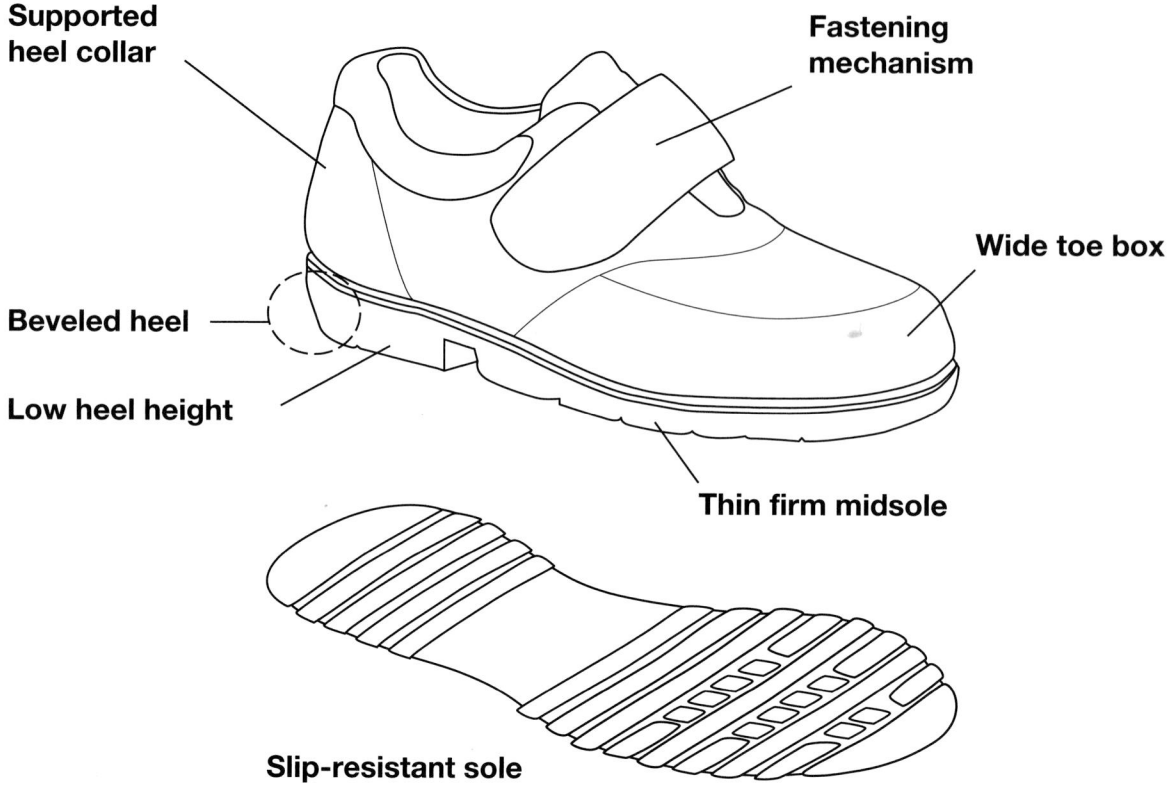

Figure 35.2—Characteristics of shoes recommended for older adults

In addition to inquiring about the circumstances surrounding the fall, the clinician should attempt to identify any potential contributing environmental factors. Information on lighting, floor coverings, door thresholds, railings, and furniture can add important clues. Footwear can also be an important factor (Figure 35.2). In one small study that evaluated the effect of various shoe types on balance in older men, shoes with thin, hard soles produced the best results, even though they were perceived as less comfortable than thick, soft, mid-soled shoes, such as running shoes. In another nested case control study of men and women, athletic shoes were associated with the lowest risk of falls, and shoes with increased heel height and decreased surface area between the sole and the floor were associated with a higher risk of falls.

When performing a physical examination on an older adult with a fall, the provider should focus on risk factors, including gait assessment. Probably the most important part of the physical examination is an assessment of integrated musculoskeletal function, which can be accomplished by performing one or more of the following tests of postural stability. The most commonly used test of integrated strength and balance is the Up and Go test, which can be performed with or without timing. It consists of observation of an individual standing up from a chair, walking across a room (about 3 meters), turning around, walking back, and sitting down without using the arms. This test can grade muscle weakness, balance problems, and gait abnormalities using a scale of 1–5, with 5 indicating severe abnormalities. The need to use arms to stand may indicate hip extensor weakness. This test may be timed, with inability to complete the test within 12 seconds suggesting an increased risk of falls. The 30-second chair stand is another integrative test of balance and strength. Patients are asked to cross their arms over their chest while seated in a chair. It should be noted if the patient needs to use his or her arms to arise from the chair. The provider records how many times the patient can fully stand and sit in 30 seconds. For patients 75–79 years old, <11 stands in men and <10 stands in women is considered abnormal and represents an increased fall risk. The 4-stage balance test is a third integrative test whereby patients are asked to stand for at least 10 seconds in the following positions: feet adjacent, semitandem stance, tandem stance, and on one foot. Patients unable to perform the semi-tandem test for 10 seconds are at increased risk of falling. The functional reach test, Berg Balance Test, and Performance-Oriented Mobility Assessment are infrequently used in clinical settings, but they are used in research studies as other integrated measures of neuromuscular support. Impaired performance on these tests has been demonstrated to predict falls in older adults

A number of screening tools for risk of falls have been developed for use in the acute hospital setting,

Table 35.2—Evidence-Based Interventions for Lowering Fall Risk by Site of Care

Home
Muscle strengthening or balance training prescribed by clinician (SOE=A)
Tai Chi (SOE=B)
Home-hazard assessment prescribed for those with history of falls (SOE=A)
Multidisciplinary, multifactorial health and environmental risk-factor screening or intervention for: (SOE=A) <ul><li>unselected community-dwelling older adults</li><li>older adults with a history of falling</li><li>older adults selected because of known risk factors</li></ul>
Withdrawal of psychotropic medications (SOE=B)
Vitamin D supplementation at ≥800 IU/d in persons with vitamin D deficiency (SOE=A) <ul><li>First cataract surgery, when indicated (SOE=B)</li></ul>

Hospital
Many risk assessments have reasonable sensitivity and specificity to be of potential value in targeting high-risk patients. Multifactorial interventions that target an individual's greatest risk factors for falls, including a plan that uses health information technology, has been effective in reducing falls (SOE=B).

Nursing Home
No proven interventions have been reported other than vitamin D supplementation.
Reasonable to assume all nursing-home residents are at high risk of falls and to target resident's most important individual risk factors, using an interprofessional team (SOE=C).
Vitamin D supplementation at ≥1,000 IU/d for residents independent in transfers at risk of falls (SOE=A)
Exercise programs may reduce risk of falls (SOE=C).

NOTE: MDS = minimum data set

including the Morse Fall Scale and the St. Thomas's Risk Assessment Tool (STRATIFY). The Morse Fall Scale, one of the more commonly used scales, comprises 6 items: history of falling in the past 3 months, presence of any secondary diagnosis, use of an ambulatory aid, receipt of intravenous therapy, abnormal gait, and impaired mental status. Scores range from 0 to 125, with higher numbers indicating a greater risk of falls. A cutpoint of >45 is often used to identify patients at high risk of falls.

Although these screening tools perform relatively well in predicting falls, a systematic review and meta-analysis of prospective studies suggests that they are comparable with nursing clinical judgment when predicting falls in the hospital setting. Screening tools are likely to be even less useful in the nursing-home setting, where most residents have multiple risk factors for falls. For this reason, all nursing-home residents that can transfer or ambulate should be considered at high risk of falls, prompting a consideration of modifiable, individual risk factors.

Laboratory and Diagnostic Tests

There is no standard diagnostic evaluation of a person with a history of falls or a high risk of falling. Laboratory tests for hemoglobin, BUN, creatinine, or glucose concentrations can help to exclude anemia, dehydration, or hyperglycemia with hyperosmolar dehydration as the cause of falling. There is no proven value of routinely performing Holter monitoring of individuals who have fallen. Because data demonstrate that carotid sinus hypersensitivity contributes to falls and even hip fracture, some have advocated performing carotid sinus massage with continuous heart rate and phasic blood pressure measurement in older adults with unexplained falls. Similarly, the decision to perform echocardiography, brain imaging, or radiographic studies of the spine should be driven by the findings of the history and physical examination. Echocardiography should be reserved for those with cardiac conditions believed to contribute to the maintenance of blood flow to the brain. Spine radiographs or MRI can be useful in patients with gait disorders, abnormalities on neurologic examination, leg spasticity, or hyperreflexia to exclude cervical spondylosis or lumbar stenosis as a cause of falls.

TREATMENT AND PREVENTION

The evaluation and management of falls in older adults may differ according to the clinical setting. For example, in the home, the fall may be reported by the patient or family, or in response to clinician query. In the hospital or nursing home, staff may directly witness a fall, or find the patient on the floor. For evidence-based approaches to the management of falls, see Table 35.2.

Multiple studies of preventive interventions have been conducted, including programs to improve strength or balance, educational programs, optimization of medications, and environmental modifications in homes or institutions. Some interventions have targeted single risk factors; others have attempted to address multiple factors by either targeting patient-specific risk factors (multifactorial intervention) or by offering the interventions to an entire population (multicomponent intervention).

A Cochrane collaboration systematic review of interventions to reduce the incidence of falling in older adults has been performed. Because of the large numbers of fall intervention trials and because interventions may be more effective in certain settings, systematic reviews of fall prevention interventions were divided into 2 groups: those among community-dwelling adults and those among institutionalized adults. The 2012 update of the Cochrane systematic review of fall interventions among community-dwelling adults included 159 individual trials. The results of this review demonstrated that the following falls prevention interventions are likely to be beneficial in the community setting: medication review; home hazards assessment by health care professionals in older adults at high risk of falling; Tai Chi; multiple-component interventions (strength, balance, or gait training) or home-based exercises; vitamin D supplementation in patients with vitamin D deficiency; an antislip shoe device to be worn in icy conditions; pacemaker placement in patients with carotid sinus hypersensitivity; first cataract surgery; and multifactorial, multidisciplinary interventions.

In 2011, the AGS and the BGS updated clinical practice guidelines for the prevention of falls in older adults. These guidelines advocate for interventions tailored to major falls risk factors, coupled with an appropriate exercise program. All older adults in the community at risk of falling should be offered an exercise program incorporating balance, gait, and strength training. Flexibility and endurance training should also be offered but not as sole components of the program. Interventions should include an education component tailored to the individual's cognitive ability and language. The interventions most commonly identified and that are considered to be efficacious in preventing falls in community dwellers include the following:

- **Modify the home environment:** When included as part of a multifactorial intervention, home environment assessments with environmental modification performed by a health care professional reduced the risk of falling among older adults who have fallen or are at high risk of falling because of visual impairment (2 trials; 491 participants; relative risk [RR] 0.56; CI 95%, 0.42–0.76) (SOE=A). Home environment assessment and intervention performed by a health care professional should be included in a multifactorial assessment and intervention for older adults who have fallen or who have risk factors for falling.

- **Discontinue or minimize psychoactive medications:** In one study of 93 community-dwelling adults, a gradual taper of psychotropic medications was associated with a decreased rate of falls (relative hazard 0.34; CI 95%, 0.16–0.74) (SOE=B).

- **Discontinue or minimize other medications:** A prescribing modification program for primary care physicians that included a medication review checklist, education and feedback from a pharmacist, and financial incentives significantly reduced the risk of falling (1 cluster randomized trial; 20 providers and 849 participants; RR 0.61; 95% 0.41–0.91) (SOE=B). There was no effect of medication reviews led by pharmacy on the risk of falls (2 trials; 445 participants; RR 1.03; CI 95%, 0.81–1.31). Multifactorial interventions that have been successful in preventing falls often include a review of medications.

- **Manage postural hypotension:** The sensation of dizziness is strongly associated with an increased risk of falls; thus, assessment and treatment of postural hypotension should be included as components of multifactorial interventions to prevent falls in older adults. Achieving better control of systolic blood pressure has been associated with a decrease in postural changes in blood pressure. It is unclear whether this might also translate into a decreased risk of falls. Although no trial to date has addressed whether a single intervention to reduce orthostasis results in decreased falls, multifactorial interventions that include fluid optimization, medication review and reduction, and behavioral changes have shown a modest effect in reducing the risk of falls among community-dwelling adults (SOE=C).

- **Manage foot problems and footwear:** One trial comparing multifaceted podiatry intervention including foot and ankle exercises with standard care in people with disabling foot pain significantly reduced the rate of falls (305 participants; relative attributable risk (RAR) 0.64; CI 95%, 0.45-0.91) but not the risk of falls (SOE=B). Footwear associated with higher heels and decreased surface area has been associated with an increased risk of falls (SOE=C). Clinicians should advise their patients to wear walking shoes with high contact surface area. Although nonslip soles are generally recommended, they should be avoided in those with a shuffling gait. In older adults with disabling foot pain, falls may be reduced by a multifaceted intervention, including customized insoles, attention to shoe wear, foot and ankle exercises, and falls prevention education.

- **Prescribe exercise, particularly balance, strength, and gait training:** The 2012 Cochrane review of fall interventions included 59 trials that tested the efficacy of exercise as an isolated intervention to prevent falls in the community setting. Exercise classes incorporating more than one type of exercise (eg, gait training, balance, strengthening) were effective in reducing the risk of falls (22 trials; 5,333 participants; RR 0.85; CI

95%, 0.76–0.96) (SOE=A). Multiple-component home-based exercise was also effective in reducing the risk of falls (6 trials; 714 participants; RR 0.78; CI 95%, 0.64–0.94). In a separate meta-analysis, home-based and group exercises reduced the rate of injurious falls in community dwellers (10 trials; 2,922 participants; RAR 0.63; CI 95%, 0.51–0.77) (SOE=A). Tai Chi, which combines both strengthening and balance measures, is effective in reducing the risk of falls among community-dwelling adults (6 trials; 1,625 participants; RR 0.71; CI 95%, 0.57–0.87) (SOE=A).

The AGS/BGS recommendations state "Exercise programs should consider the functional status and comorbidities of the older person, and they should be prescribed by qualified health professionals or fitness instructors, whenever possible. The exercise program should include regular review, progression and adjustment of the exercise prescription as appropriate." For homebound older adults, programs such as the Otago Exercise Program that include in-home physical therapy and requires fewer one-on-one sessions over the course of a year, have been shown to reduce the rate of falls (SOE=A).

- **Treat vision impairment:** There is insufficient evidence to recommend for or against the inclusion of vision interventions within multifactorial fall prevention interventions. However, first cataract surgery results in a decreased rate of falls (1 trial; 306 participants; RR 0.66; CI 95%, 0.45–0.95) (SOE=B). Second cataract surgery showed no benefit in reducing the rate of falls or number of fallers. Although routine eye screening with correction of visual defects is considered good medical practice, one trial with an intervention to treat vision problems resulted in a significant increase in the risk of falls (616 participants; RR 1.54; CI 95%, 1.24–1.91). In another trial of 597 participants, regular wearers of multifocal glasses who routinely participated in outdoor activities experienced a reduced rate of falls when given single lens glasses (SOE=B). However, there was a significant increase in outside falls in intervention group participants who infrequently participated in outside activity. The AGS/BGS recommends cautioning older adults with multifocal lenses to be more attentive to falling while walking, particularly on stairs (SOE=C).

- **Manage heart rate and rhythm abnormalities:** One trial demonstrated a reduction in the rate of falls among older adults with carotid sinus hypersensitivity treated with a pacemaker (175 participants; weighted mean difference −5.20; CI 95%, −9.40 to −1.00) (SOE=B). In contrast, a small randomized cross-over trial of 34 participants with carotid sinus hypersensitivity and a history of falls found no benefit in preventing falls when their pacemaker was switched to the on mode as compared with the off mode (RR of falling when pacemaker was off: 0.82, CI 95%, 0.62–1.10) (SOE=B).

Additionally, several multifactorial interventions in which participants received more than one intervention targeting their major risk factors were effective in reducing the rate of falls (19 trials; 9,503 participants; RR 0.76; CI 95%, 0.67–0.86) (SOE=A). Because these trials were conducted in different populations and used different interventions, it is unclear which combinations of interventions are the most effective.

The health professional or team conducting the fall risk assessment should directly implement interventions or assure that the interventions are carried out by other qualified health care professionals. It is also reasonable to educate cognitively intact older adults at risk of falls on home hazards, proper footwear choices, and the importance of regular exercise. In one trial of 1,206 hospitalized older adults, intensive falls education as provided by a physiotherapist in combination with written and video materials on falls reduced the risk of falls as compared with usual care in cognitively intact persons (RR 0.51; CI 95%, 0.28–0.94) (SOE=B). However, results from a meta-analysis do not demonstrate that education reduces falls risk or fall-related injuries (4 trials; 2,555 participants; RR 0.88; CI 95%, 0.75–1.03). Thus, education alone should not be provided as a single intervention to prevent falls.

A number of interventions have not been effective for fall prevention, including group-delivered exercise interventions (SOE=B), nutritional supplementation (SOE=C), isolated modification of home hazards (SOE=B), cognitive-behavioral approach (SOE=B), and hormone therapy (SOE=C). Fall prevention programs in nursing-home settings have been largely unsuccessful in reducing the number of fallers, although they may reduce the number of recurrent fallers. Interventions that include medication reduction show some promise in preventing falls in this setting (SOE=B). Multifactorial interventions were successful in reducing falls in the hospital setting and, when delivered by an interprofessional team, were successful in reducing falls in the nursing-home setting. Among 8 trials of exercise in the acute hospital and rehabilitation settings, there was no clear effect of exercise on the risk of falls (1,887 participants; RR 1.07; CI 95%, 0.94–1.23). A multicenter randomized controlled trial of more than 10,000 acutely hospitalized adults found that a fall prevention tool kit using individual patient

Table 35.3—Preventing Falls: Selected Risk Factors and Suggested Interventions

Factors	Suggested Interventions
General Risk	Offer exercise program to include combination of resistance (strength) training, gait, balance, and coordination training: ■ tailor to individual capabilities ■ start with low intensity and graduate slowly in those with limited mobility not accustomed to physical activity ■ prescribed by qualified health care provider ■ regular review and progression Education and information, cognitive-behavioral intervention to decrease fear of falling and activity avoidance Recommend daily supplementation of vitamin D_3 (1,000 IU) to older adults with vitamin D deficiency and to those residing in long-term care facilities. After supplementation, vitamin D levels may be appropriate for select patients at risk of vitamin D deficiency with the goal of achieving a 25-hydroxy vitamin D level of 30 ng/mL.
Medication-Related Factors	
Use of benzodiazepines, sedative-hypnotics, antidepressants, antipsychotics, and antihypertensive medications	Consider whether medication is really needed. If medication is needed, reduce dosage as possible. Address sleep problems with nonpharmacologic interventions. Educate regarding appropriate use of medications and monitoring for adverse events.
Recent change in dosage or number of prescription medications, *or* use of ≥4 prescription medications, *or* use of other medications associated with fall risk	Review medication profile and reduce number and dosage of all medications, as possible. Counsel patients at risk of falls with new prescription or dosage increase. Monitor response to medication changes.
Mobility-Related Factors	
Presence of environmental hazards (eg, improper bed height, cluttered walking surfaces, lack of railings, poor lighting)	Improve lighting, especially at night. Remove floor hazards (eg, loose carpeting in home or carpeted flooring in nursing home). Replace existing furniture with safer furniture (eg, correct height, more stable). Install support structures, especially in bathroom (eg, railings, grab bars, elevated toilet seats). Use nonslip bath mats.
Impaired gait, balance, or transfer skills	Refer to physical therapy for comprehensive evaluation, rehabilitation, and training in use of assistive devices. Provide gait training. Prescribe balance and strengthening exercises. If able to perform tandem stance, refer for Tai Chi, dance, or yoga. Provide training in transfer skills. Prescribe appropriate assistive devices. Recommend appropriate footwear (eg, good fit, nonslip, low heel height, large surface contact area).
Impaired leg or arm strength or range of motion, or proprioception	Strengthening exercises (eg, use of resistive rubber bands, putty) Resistance training 2–3 times/week, 3 sets of 10 repetitions with full range of motion, then increase resistance Tai Chi Refer to physical therapy or occupational therapy
Medical Factors	
Parkinson disease, osteoarthritis, depressive symptoms, impaired cognition, carotid sinus hypersensitivity, other conditions associated with increased falls	Optimize medical therapy. Monitor for disease progression and impact on mobility and impairments. Determine need for assistive devices. Use bedside commode if frequent nighttime urination. Cardiac pacing in patients with carotid sinus hypersensitivity who experience falls due to syncope

Table 35.3—Preventing Falls: Selected Risk Factors and Suggested Interventions (continued)

Factors	Suggested Interventions
Postural hypotension:	Review medications potentially contributing and adjust dosing or switch to less hypotensive agents; avoid vasodilators and diuretics if possible. Educate on activities to decrease effect (eg, slow rising, ankle pumps, hand clenching, elevation of head of bed) and to slow rising from recumbent or seated position, grab bars by toilet and bath. Prescribe pressure stockings (eg, Jobst). Optimize hydration. Liberalize salt intake, if appropriate. Recommend caffeinated coffee (1 cup) or caffeine 100 mg with meals for postprandial hypotension. Consider medication to increase blood pressure (if hypertension, heart failure, and hypokalemia not serious): ▪ midodrine 2.5–10 mg given 3 times/day 4 hr apart ▪ fludrocortisone 0.1 mg q8–24h
Visual impairment	Cataract extraction (first but not second cataract removal found to reduce falls, but second cataract extraction still useful for improvement in vision) Increase awareness and vigilance when wearing multifocal lenses while walking, particularly up stairs.

SOURCE: Adapted with permission from Reuben DB, Herr KA, Pacala JT, et al. *Geriatrics At Your Fingertips*, 20th ed. New York: American Geriatrics Society; 2018:124–125.

characteristics as ascertained from health information technology reduced the absolute rate of falls by 1.16 falls/1,000 bed days (CI 95%, 0.17–2.16). Vitamin D supplementation has been demonstrated in the nursing-home setting to reduce the rate of falls (5 trials; 4,603 participants; RAR 0.63; CI 95%, 0.46–0.86) but not the risk of falling (6 trials; 5,186 participants; RR 0.99; CI 95%, 0.90–1.08) (SOE=A).

The AGS/BGS makes the following recommendations regarding interventions to prevent falls in the nursing-home setting: Multifactorial/multicomponent interventions should be considered in long-term care to reduce falls. Exercise programs should be considered to reduce falls in older adults living in long-term care settings with caution regarding risk of injury in frail persons. Limited data exist on falls prevention in the assisted-living setting. These individuals often resemble nursing-home residents, and thus, it is reasonable to approach falls prevention in the assisted-living setting using a similar multidomain approach.

A practical approach for clinicians who are treating older adults, including nursing-home residents, at risk of falls targets risk factors in 3 major domains: medications, mobility, and medical conditions (Table 35.3).

Considerations for Recurrent Fallers

A small number of older adults will fall repeatedly despite interventions. These patients generally have non-modifiable risk factors that place them at particularly high risk, including Parkinson disease and dementia. For these patients, every attempt should be made to reduce modifiable risk factors, including reducing medications associated with falls, treating pain, and assessing environmental hazards. As with all fallers, it is important to get a history of the events surrounding the fall to exclude syncope, seizures, and other less common medical conditions. These patients frequently seek medical attention as a result of the falls, and often times medical providers suggest moving to a nursing home or environment with more intense supervision. Patients who are able to understand the risks and alternatives and express their choice to remain independent have the right to do so. In these instances, a direct discussion of goals of care with or without a palliative care consult may be helpful (SOE=C).

RESOURCES

- Francis-Coad J, Etherton-Beer, C, Bulsara C, et al. Evaluating the impact of a falls prevention community of practice in a residential aged care setting: a realist approach. *BMC Health Serv Res.* 2018;18:21.

- Guirguis-Blake JM, Michael YL, Perdue LA, et al. Interventions to prevent falls in older adults: updated evidence report and systematic review for the US Preventive Services Task Force, *JAMA.* 2018;319(16):1705–1716.

- Vlaeyen E, Coussement J, Leysens G, et al. Characteristics and effectiveness of fall prevention programs in nursing homes: a systematic review and meta-analysis of randomized controlled trials. *J Am Geriatr Soc.* 2015;63(2):211–221.

CHAPTER 36—OSTEOPOROSIS

KEY POINTS

- Osteoporosis is a common metabolic bone disorder affecting older adults that is preventable and treatable. The resultant fractures can lead to chronic pain, decreased mobility, loss of independence and function, and increased mortality.

- Bone mineral density (BMD) measurement establishes the diagnosis of osteoporosis (T-score ≤–2.5). Osteoporosis can also be defined clinically in at-risk people who sustain a fragility or low-trauma fracture.

- Secondary osteoporosis should be excluded in men and women with osteoporosis. Common causes of secondary osteoporosis include glucocorticoid use, hyperparathyroidism, hypogonadism, hyperthyroidism, hypercalciuria, and vitamin D deficiency.

- Screening for osteoporosis is recommended for all postmenopausal women ≥65 years old and both women and men ≥50 years old with risk factors for osteoporosis. FRAX is a free online clinical tool for estimating the 10-year probability of osteoporotic fracture based on a patient's clinical risk factors and femoral neck BMD.

- Prevention of osteoporosis includes adequate calcium and vitamin D intake, weight-bearing exercise, and reduction of known risk factors for osteoporosis.

- Bisphosphonates are first-line pharmacologic therapy for osteoporosis. Other pharmacologic therapies to consider include denosumab, teriparatide, and abaloparatide.

Osteoporosis, the most common metabolic bone disease, is a major cause of morbidity, loss of independence, and mortality in older adults. It is a systemic skeletal disorder defined by decreased bone strength, density, and quality with an increasing risk of fractures. Osteoporosis is a silent disease that requires astute clinical monitoring for risk factors and active screening. Once osteoporosis is diagnosed, multiple treatment options for reducing risk of fractures are available.

Although strong evidence exists for fracture prevention with appropriate treatment, prescription of osteoporosis medications has been declining. In fact, use of the first-line treatment for osteoporosis, bisphosphonates, has declined by 50% from 2008 to 2012. Declining use of osteoporosis treatments is primarily driven by concerns over rare medication adverse effects, despite the known reduction in fracture risk with treatment. It is imperative for clinicians to be well versed in identification and safe treatment of osteoporosis to reduce the morbidity and mortality associated with this disease.

OSTEOPOROSIS DEFINITION

Osteoporosis is defined by a bone mineral density (BMD) measurement ≤2.5 standard deviations below the young normal adult reference (T-score ≤–2.5), or a minimal trauma fracture of the spine, proximal humerus, hip, and/or forearm in a patient with osteopenia (T-score between –1 and –2.5). For the WHO standardized criteria for BMD measurements of the spine, hip, or forearm, see Table 36.1. A low-trauma fracture is defined as any nonpathologic fracture that occurs from a fall from standing height or less. While still controversial, there is also a call by organizations like the National Osteoporosis Foundation (NOF) and the European and Canadian counterparts to incorporate risk assessment tools like the FRAX score in the categorization of osteoporosis.

EPIDEMIOLOGY AND IMPACT

In 2010, NOF estimated that approximately 10.2 million Americans have osteoporosis by bone density criteria. An additional 43.4 million adults ≥50 years old were found to have low bone density, increasing their risk of fractures. Osteoporosis affects people of all ethnic backgrounds. While less prevalent than in the estimated 7.7 million white and Asian American adults, osteoporosis is found in 600,000 Mexican Americans and 500,000 non-Hispanic blacks ≥50 years old.

Osteoporosis is the most common cause of fracture in older adults. In 2005, osteoporosis caused >2 million fractures in the United States; this number is expected to rise to >3 million by the year 2025. One in two postmenopausal women and up to one in five men >50 years old will have an osteoporotic-related fracture in their remaining lifetime. Mortality risk is estimated to increase 20% in older adults in the year after a hip fracture, with the rate of death in men nearly double that in women (SOE=B). Vertebral and pelvic fractures have also been linked with increased mortality, generally from associated comorbidities. Based on several meta-analyses, the increased mortality risk persists for at least 10 years after the hip-fracture event. Hip fractures are also associated with 2.5-fold increased risk of future fractures. Hip fracture rates in black Americans, Japanese Americans, Hispanics, and Native Americans

Table 36.1—WHO Bone Mineral Density Definitions

Classification	Bone Mineral Density (BMD)	T-score
Normal	Within one SD[a] of reference mean[b]	≥–1.0
Osteopenia (low bone mass)	More than 1 but less than 2.5 SD below reference mean	Between –1.0 and –2.5
Osteoporosis	2.5 or more SD below reference mean	≤–2.5
Severe osteoporosis	Below 2.5 SD of reference mean in the presence of one or more fragility fractures	<–2.5

[a] Standard deviation
[b] For young, normal adult

occur at lower frequencies than in white Americans, with the rate of hip fractures in Mexican Americans higher than that of other Hispanic groups.

Osteoporotic fractures can lead to permanent declines in functional status, independence, and quality of life. In patients who were previously ambulatory, approximately 40% regained their previous level of functioning after hip fracture and 20% required long-term nursing-home care. Pain, kyphosis, height loss, and other changes in body habitus can develop from vertebral fractures. Patients may be unable to bathe, dress, or walk independently. The economic costs associated with osteoporotic-related fractures are substantial. In 2005, the total direct health care costs were estimated at $19 billion. By 2025, this number is expected to rise to $25.3 billion. Thus, because of the substantial social and economic costs associated with osteoporotic fractures in older adults, reduction of this burden is widely seen as a health care policy imperative.

BONE REMODELING AND BONE LOSS IN AGING

Bone is a dynamic tissue that undergoes active remodeling (also called bone turnover), a coupled process of bone resorption followed by bone formation occurring throughout adult life. Bone remodeling maintains both skeletal strength (through repair of microfractures) and systemic calcium homeostasis.

Bone mass changes over the life span of an individual. In women, bone mass increases rapidly from puberty until approximately the mid-20s to mid-30s, when bone mass peaks. Once women reach peak bone mass, bone loss occurs very slowly until the onset of menopause. After menopause, the rate of bone loss is accelerated for 8–10 years. Bone loss continues in later life, albeit at a slower rate of 1%–2% per year; however, some older women may lose bone density at a higher rate. Data suggest that reducing bone loss and skeletal turnover will decrease fracture risk.

Like women, men also lose bone with age, starting slowly in their late 20s to early 30s. However, the pattern of bone loss between sexes is different. Cortical bone, which forms the hardened exterior of the bones and provides most of the support and resistance to compression, undergoes accelerated decline in women at around age 50; this occurs later in men, around age 75, and correlates with the increase in vertebral fractures from osteoporosis. This difference in cortical bone thinning between women and men is predominantly mediated by reduction in sex hormones with age and menopause.

RISK FACTORS FOR OSTEOPOROSIS

Intrinsic

The pathogenesis of osteoporosis in men and women is complex, encompassing factors that affect the level of peak bone mass, the rate of bone resorption, and the rate of bone formation. A multitude of factors, including genetic, endocrine, nutrition, skeleton loading, disease states, and medication combine to affect the risk of developing osteoporosis.

Genetics

Heritable traits account for 75%–80% of a person's peak bone mass. Epidemiologic studies demonstrated possible linkage of low birth size, late menarche, and low childhood height and weight to increased risk of osteoporosis. Genetic factors can also contribute to an increased risk of coronary artery disease, hypertension, and type II diabetes, all of which correlate with greater likelihood of osteoporosis. Furthermore, sex and genetic traits affect levels of sex hormones and sensitivity to hormonal and nutritional factors. Genetic variations are rarely the direct cause of osteoporosis but increase a person's susceptibility to osteoporosis through intrinsic and extrinsic pathways.

Sex Hormones

After menopause, the natural decline of estrogen levels is associated with increased risk of osteoporosis and fracture (SOE=A). Increased resorption appears to be the major factor for bone loss in estrogen deficiency. Evidence also suggests a role of estrogen deficiency in reducing bone formation over time.

Estrogen has both direct and indirect effects on osteoclasts, the cells that are responsible for bone resorption and bone loss. It acts through multiple

Table 36.2—Risk Factors for Osteoporosis

- Age (postmenopausal women, men >70 years old)
- Female sex
- Low body weight (BMI <20 kg/m^2)
- 10% decrease in weight (from usual adult body weight)
- Physical inactivity
- Glucocorticoids
- Previous fragility fracture as adult
- White or Asian race
- Current smoking
- Low dietary calcium
- Alcohol intake ≥3 drinks a day

pathways to decrease the expression of human receptor activator of nuclear factor kappa-B ligand (RANKL), the major cytokine that promotes development and differentiation of osteoclasts to mature forms. Estrogen also has direct effects on cells of hematopoietic lineage, including osteoclast precursors, mature osteoclasts, and lymphocytes.

In men, bioavailable testosterone and estrogen decrease with aging mainly due to an increase in sex hormone–binding globulin levels. Approximately half of men >70 years old have bioavailable testosterone levels below the normal reference range of young adults. Several studies demonstrated that late-onset hypogonadism plays a role in osteoporosis in men; however, estrogen has shown a stronger correlation with bone metabolism than testosterone.

Skeleton Loading

Weight-bearing bones require a level of stress from gravity while walking and dynamic strain of muscular contractions to maintain BMD. The importance of bone loading is most evident in space flight, where astronauts have been shown to lose 3% of vertebral bone mass within 15 days of weightlessness. Similar effects on weight-bearing bones are seen in studies evaluating prolonged bedrest. Exercise that stresses or mechanically loads bones, including strength training, aerobics, walking, and Tai Chi, reduce BMD loss in the spine and hip in postmenopausal women based on a Cochrane review (SOE=B).

Calcium and Vitamin D Deficiency

Calcium deficiency and disruption of calcium homeostasis is another mechanism for bone loss in older adults. With age, intestinal absorption of calcium declines. Vitamin D plays a vital role in regulating calcium homeostenosis. Vitamin D production is lowered in aging skin, and decreased exposure to sunlight reduces the conversion of 7-dehydrocholesterol to cholecalciferol (vitamin D$_3$) by ultraviolet light. Older black Americans are at particular risk of vitamin D deficiency as they age.

The hormonally active form of vitamin D is 1,25(OH)$_2$D$_3$, or calcitriol. It is necessary for optimal intestinal absorption of calcium and phosphorus, and it also exerts a tonic inhibitory effect on parathyroid hormone (PTH) synthesis. Vitamin D deficiency not only contributes to accelerated bone loss and increasing fragility but also appears to promote muscle weakness that can increase risk of falls.

Decreased serum concentration of calcium and 1,25(OH)$_2$D$_3$ lead to increased levels of PTH. When levels are chronically increased, PTH becomes a stimulator of bone resorption. Trials involving older adults at high risk of calcium and vitamin D deficiency show that supplementation of both can reverse secondary hyperparathyroidism (SOE=A), increase bone mass (SOE=B), and decrease bone resorption (SOE=A) and fracture rates (SOE=B).

Extrinsic Factors

Smoking increases risk of fractures in both current and former smokers. The risk of fractures is moderated more by the amount of nicotine smoked and how recently one quit smoking than by the duration of tobacco use. Also, chronic heavy alcohol use decreases bone turnover and bone formation. Drinking ≥3 drinks per day early and/or later in life increase bone loss and fracture risk (SOE=A). Nutrition, exercise, and use of certain medications can further modulate a person's risk of fractures.

PREDICTION AND DIAGNOSIS OF FRACTURES

Osteoporosis is a preventable disease; however, because bone loss is silent, it is often not diagnosed until a fracture occurs. The NOF recommends clinical assessment of osteoporosis risk factors for all postmenopausal women and men ≥50 years old. The diagnosis of osteoporosis should be considered in any older adult with a fracture.

Evaluation of Risk Factors

Clinical evaluation begins with a thorough history to identify risk factors that may lead to increased bone fragility. Risk factors for osteoporosis and osteoporotic fracture have been identified (Table 36.2) and can be used to determine who should be placed on preventive or therapeutic regimens. Obtaining a thorough history of fractures and the setting in which the fractures occurred is important. Fracture from osteoporosis is the greatest risk factor for future fractures. WHO has developed a 10-year fracture risk model (FRAX) (www.shef.ac.uk/FRAX [accessed Feb 2019]) that can be used

Table 36.3—Causes of Secondary Osteoporosis

Endocrine	■ Hypogonadism
	■ Hyperthyroidism
	■ Hypercortisolism (Cushing syndrome)
	■ Hyperparathyroidism
	■ Diabetes mellitus (insulin dependent)
GI disorders/ nutrition/ malabsorption	■ Celiac disease
	■ Inflammatory bowel disease
	■ Gastric resection or gastric bypass
	■ Vitamin D deficiency
	■ Alcoholism
	■ Chronic liver disease
Hematologic disease	■ Multiple myeloma
	■ Leukemia
	■ Lymphoma
	■ Thalassemia
Medications	■ Glucocorticoids
	■ Proton-pump inhibitors
	■ Gonadotropin releasing-hormone agonists
	■ Androgen deprivation therapy
	■ Aromatase inhibitors
	■ Thiazolidinediones
	■ Canagliflozin and other SGLT-2 inhibitors
	■ Anticonvulsants
	■ SSRIs
	■ Cancer chemotherapeutic agents
	■ Methotrexate
	■ Heparin
	■ Excess thyroid hormone replacement
Other	■ Idiopathic hypercalciuria
	■ Solid organ transplantation
	■ Immobilization

clinically, independent of BMD, to identify adults at high risk of fracture. Given that falls are a major cause of osteoporosis-related fractures, a fall risk evaluation should be conducted.

Secondary Causes

Excluding other causes that lead to fractures or low bone mass is important in evaluating women and men with osteoporosis. For the major secondary causes of osteoporosis, see Table 36.3. Certain laboratory tests should be considered for all older adults with a new diagnosis of osteoporosis; additional specific tests are recommended for adults in which there is clinical suspicion of secondary causes (Table 36.4).

Idiopathic hypercalciuria, found in approximately 10% of the general population, is an important secondary cause of osteoporosis. It is diagnosed by a 24-hour urinary calcium excretion >4 mg/kg and can be treated with a thiazide-type diuretic. Primary

Table 36.4—Recommended Initial Laboratory Testing in Those with Osteoporosis*

Initial recommended testing
- Fasting comprehensive metabolic panel, including electrolytes, creatinine, calcium, serum phosphorus, liver enzymes, total protein, albumin, and alkaline phosphatase
- Complete blood count
- 25-hydroxy vitamin D
- 24-hour urine collection for calcium and creatinine
- Parathyroid hormone
- Thyrotropin-stimulating hormone

Consider in select patients
- Serum protein electrophoresis (suspect multiple myeloma)
- Urine protein electrophoresis (suspect multiple myeloma)
- Tissue transglutaminase antibodies (suspect celiac disease)
- Urine free cortisol (suspect Cushing syndrome)
- Testosterone in men (suspect hypogonadism)

*Modified from National Osteoporosis Foundation and American College of Endocrinology Clinical Practice Guidelines

hyperparathyroidism is a common cause of secondary osteoporosis in women, with an incidence in older women as high as 1:500. An observational study suggested preservation of BMD in women who undergo parathyroidectomy. Secondary causes of osteoporosis are commonly found in men, with only 40% of cases having no identifiable secondary cause on laboratory testing (SOE=B). The most commonly reported secondary causes of osteoporosis in men include hypogonadism, medications, and excessive alcohol use.

Medication use is an important secondary cause for osteoporosis, with glucocorticoids being the most common culprit in men and women. An estimated 2.5% of people 70–79 years old take an oral glucocorticoid. Glucocorticoid-induced osteoporosis is caused by an early increase in bone resorption. Prolonged exposure reduces osteoblastogenesis, resulting in low bone turnover and decreased bone formation. Fracture risk increases rapidly in the first 3–6 months and continues to progress during the duration of glucocorticoid use. Increased fracture risk may be present with daily dosages as low as 2.5–7.5 mg/d (prednisone or equivalent). The risk of fracture positively correlates with increasing glucocorticoid dosages and duration, partially independent of BMD. Stopping glucocorticoids is associated with a decrease in fracture risk, although it is unclear if the risk ever returns to the preexposure level. Limited evidence suggests that large doses of high-potency inhaled steroids can also result in bone loss. The best strategy for older adults who require long-term glucocorticoid therapy is to maximize bone health by a variety of interventions, including using the lowest possible dosage of glucocorticoids, ensuring adequate intake of calcium and vitamin D, serial monitoring of BMD, and starting prescription osteoporosis therapy if appropriate (see treatment, below). Other medications that adversely affect BMD are listed in Table 36.3. When evaluating patients for osteoporosis, clinicians should also remember to review medications that increase risk of falls.

Physical Examination

The physical examination is directed toward detecting signs of fracture as well as potential secondary causes. Key elements include height, weight, posture, mobility, nutritional status, and overall build. Vertebral fractures are suggested by thoracic kyphosis, although this finding is not diagnostic. Wall-to-occiput distance >0 cm and ribs-pelvis distance ≤2 fingerbreadths suggests a spinal thoracic or lumbar fracture. Height loss >4 cm in women and >6 cm in men from peak young adult height or prospective height loss of 2 cm in women and 3 cm in men is also suggestive of previous vertebral fracture.

Bone Mineral Density Measurement

BMD measurement establishes the diagnosis of osteoporosis and is a potent predictor of fracture risk. The relative risk of fracture is 10 times greater in women whose BMD is in the lowest quartile versus those whose BMD is in the highest quartile (SOE=A).

BMD of the hip, spine, wrist, or calcaneus can be measured by a variety of techniques. The preferred method is central DEXA, which measures BMD of the proximal femur and lumbar spine. Femoral neck BMD is the best predictor of hip and other osteoporotic fractures. Other methods (not currently recommended in the United States although used globally) of measuring BMD include quantitative CT, ultrasonography of the calcaneus, single radiographic absorptiometry of the calcaneus, peripheral DEXA, and radiographic absorptiometry.

BMD measurements are typically expressed as a Z or a T-score. Z-scores represent the relationship between a patient's BMD to the expected BMD for the patient's age and sex, while a T-score compares the BMD to "young normal" adults of the same sex. The lowest T-score from the lumbar spine, femoral neck, or total proximal femur is used to make the overall diagnosis. Forearm BMD from the distal third of the radius can be used for diagnosis, specifically if the hip or spine imaging cannot be interpreted, the patient has a history of hyperparathyroidism, or the patient weighs >300 pounds. For every 1-unit decrease in T-score, fracture risk at the spine and hip approximately doubles. For example, if a woman has a T-score of −2, her risk of fracture is 4 times that of a woman with normal bone density for her age (controlled for height and weight).

Osteoporosis Screening Guidelines

Based on U.S. Preventive Services Task Force guidelines, there is insufficient evidence to recommend screening in men (SOE=C). However, the NOF recommends screening all men ≥70 years old regardless of risk factors (SOE=C). Per the NOF, DEXA is also recommended in men and women 50–69 years old with diseases or medications known to increase risk of osteoporosis and in those with a history of fracture after age 50. Although information relating BMD to fracture risk are derived mostly from studies of women, data also suggest that similar associations may be valid for men. Men tend to fracture at a higher BMD than women, but most fractures occur in men with a T-score less than −2.5, just like women. There is limited information to determine the frequency of screening or the age to stop screening for osteoporosis. In the Study of Osteoporotic Fractures, no additional benefit was achieved from repeat BMD testing at an interval of 15 years for healthy, older postmenopausal women with normal BMD or mild osteopenia. Post-hoc analyses of the Framingham Osteoporosis study suggest no benefit of a screening interval of <4 years in older men and women (mean age 75).

Interpretation of BMD involves evaluating the quality of the DEXA as well as the T-scores. Several considerations are important when evaluating BMD of the spine over time. BMD of lumbar vertebrae L1–L4 should be measured when making a decision about therapy. Vertebral, arterial, or lymph node calcification as well as any scoliosis can falsely increase BMD of the anterior-posterior spine DEXA. Thus, a woman with osteoporosis of the spine can have a DEXA T-score that is higher than −2.5. Usually, these changes can be seen on the DEXA report if the picture of the scan is included in the report. Proximal femoral neck BMD is preferred because it is more likely to be free of osteoarthritic changes and is most associated with fracture risk. Proximal femur is based on the lower measure of the total hip or femoral neck. Another important issue of DEXA testing is measurement variability. It is critical to scan a patient on the same DEXA machine, given that unaccountable differences between machines can substantially impair the ability to detect statistically different changes in BMD over time. In addition, patient positioning should be consistent on repeated measurements. The International Society of Clinical Densitometry offers guidelines and standardized training courses for technicians and clinicians acquiring and interpreting the results.

Table 36.5—Components of FRAX Risk Score Calculator

Component	Comments
Race	In USA: black, Hispanic, white, Asian-American
Age	Model evaluated for patients between 40 and 90 years old
Sex	
Weight and height	
Previous fracture	Specifically, a spontaneous or traumatic fracture in an adult that would not have resulted in a fracture in a healthy individual
Parent fractured hip	History of hip fracture in either mother or father
Currently smoking	
Glucocorticoid use	Currently using oral glucocorticoids or previous exposure to oral glucocorticoids for >3 months at a dose equivalent to prednisone ≥5 mg/d
Rheumatoid arthritis diagnosis	
Secondary osteoporosis	Diagnosed with a disorder strongly associated with osteoporosis, including insulin-dependent diabetes, osteogenesis imperfecta in adults, untreated long-standing hyperthyroidism, hypogonadism, premature menopause (<45 years old), chronic malnutrition, malabsorption, and chronic liver disease
Alcohol use	Drinks ≥3 units of alcohol daily
BMD	Need to know the DXA scanning equipment and femoral neck BMD NOTE: BMD is not required to calculate FRAX risk score.

FRAX

The WHO fracture risk assessment tool (FRAX) has been the most widely adopted method to incorporate clinical risk factors and BMD. FRAX is a free online clinical tool (www.shef.ac.uk/FRAX [accessed Feb 2019]) that estimates the 10-year probability of fracture at the hip or major osteoporotic fracture (hip, spine, proximal humerus, or distal forearm). It is used for both women and men from different geographic settings. For components of the FRAX risk score, see Table 36.5. FRAX was developed through WHO after analyzing 12 population-based cohorts of nearly 60,000 men and women with approximately 250,000 person-years of observation; this data was then externally validated in another 11 cohorts comprising 230,000 men and women with >1.2 million person-years of observation. It is most useful for patients who have a low hip BMD, because fracture risk may be underestimated if BMD is low at the spine but relatively preserved at the hip. It has not been validated in patients who have or are currently taking medications for osteoporosis or for individuals <40 years old or >90 years old. FRAX score also does not take into account fall risk. Currently in the United States, the FRAX algorithm is validated for four ethnicities (white, black, Hispanic, and Asian).

Vertebral Fracture Assessment

Vertebral fracture assessment (VFA) is a technology used for diagnosis of vertebral fractures that can be performed as part of a routine DEXA measurement. Vertebral fractures are highly associated with future fracture risk and morbidity (SOE=A), but they are often not clinically apparent and can be present in patients with T-scores greater than −2.5. In addition, under-reporting of radiographic vertebral fractures by radiologists is well established. Treatment of patients with vertebral fractures, including those with T-scores greater than −2.5, reduces further fracture risk (SOE=A). For diagnosing vertebral fractures, VFA has lower resolution than CT and spine radiographs but has the advantage of less radiation, lower cost, convenience (at time of BMD), and comparable sensitivity and specificity to spine radiographs. VFA can therefore be a useful adjunct to BMD testing, particularly when results can influence clinical decision making. Risk stratification of patients at risk of fracture, who otherwise might not be considered for pharmacologic therapy, is an important benefit of this technology. Repeat measurements should only be done for patients with recent height loss, new back pain, postural changes, or on evaluation for a medication "holiday." The International Society of Clinical Densitometry published a position statement in 2015 on indications for VFA (Table 36.6).

Biochemical Markers of Bone Turnover

Serum and urine biochemical markers can estimate the rate of bone turnover (remodeling) and provide additional information to assist the clinician. A number of markers have been developed that reflect collagen breakdown, bone resorption, and or bone formation. A decrease in the level of these markers from baseline after 3–6 months of therapy may indicate a therapeutic

Table 36.6—Indications for Vertebral Fracture Assessment from The International Society of Clinical Densitometry 2015 Position Statement

T-score is < −1.0 and one or more of the following is present:
- Women ≥70 years old or men ≥80 years old
- Historical height loss >4 cm (>1.5 inches)
- Self-reported but undocumented prior vertebral fracture
- Glucocorticoid therapy equivalent to ≥5 mg of prednisone or equivalent per day for ≥3 months

response. However, the use of markers in clinical practice is controversial because of high within-patient variability and gaps in understanding the magnitude of biochemical marker reduction necessary to prevent bone loss or, more importantly, fractures. Therefore, routine measurement is not recommended.

PREVENTION AND TREATMENT

Whom to Treat

Treatment should be offered to all postmenopausal women and men ≥50 years old who meet the criteria for osteoporosis by DEXA or have a history of hip, vertebral, or prior fragility fracture. However, recommendations for treatment of adults with osteopenia (defined as a T score of −1.0 to −2.5) and a high fracture risk remains uncertain. The NOF recommends considering treatment in patients with osteopenia who have a 10-year probability of hip fracture ≥3% or major osteoporotic fracture ≥20%, as calculated by FRAX-US algorithm (SOE=C). In patients in whom treatment is being considered, secondary causes should be evaluated and excluded as appropriate. All patients should be counseled on osteoporosis risk and receive falls prevention counseling.

There is no identified age cutoff for initiating pharmacologic treatment. Studies show a reduction in risk of fractures after 6–12-months of treatment in the oldest-old. Thus, treatment should be considered in any patient with >1 year of remaining life expectancy. In addition, no clear guidelines exist for when to start pharmacologic treatment after a fragility fracture. Preliminary evaluation of secondary causes and patient education on osteoporosis should begin as soon as possible. The general consensus is to start pharmacologic therapy 14 days after acute fracture. A decision to start therapy should focus on patient preferences, fracture risk profile, harm, benefit, and cost of medications.

The Role of Exercise

Weight-bearing and muscle strengthening exercises are an important component of osteoporosis treatment and prevention; however, exercise alone is insufficient to prevent the rapid bone loss associated with estrogen deficiency in early menopause. Regular exercise is positively associated with BMD, and starting an exercise program even late in life can help to preserve BMD (SOE=A). Studies support use of resistance strength training in helping maintain femoral neck BMD as well as improve muscle mass, strength, and balance in postmenopausal women (SOE=B).

Weight-bearing exercise, such as walking, can be recommended for all adults. Older adults should be encouraged to start slowly and gradually increase the amount of time as well as the number of days spent walking.

Calcium and Vitamin D

Current recommendations for calcium intake in postmenopausal women >50 years old is elemental calcium at 1,200 mg/d. For men 51–70 years old, the recommendation for calcium is 1,000 mg/d, increasing to 1,200 mg/d after the age of 70. The upper intake level for all groups is 2,000 mg/d. The average dietary intake of calcium for postmenopausal women in the United States is 500–700 mg/d; thus, most require some form of additional dairy or calcium supplementation to ensure adequate intake. For information on the amount of calcium in selected foods, see Table 36.7. Common calcium supplements are carbonate or citrate, and absorption of either supplement is best in dosages ≤600 mg at a time. Calcium carbonate is best absorbed with food, while calcium citrate can be absorbed efficiently without food. Calcium carbonate also has a higher risk of bloating and constipation than calcium citrate. Calcium supplementation <2,500 mg/d is considered safe from a cardiovascular standpoint based on joint guidelines of NOF and the American Society for Preventive Cardiology (SOE=A).

The recommended requirement of vitamin D is 600 IU/d for women and men 51–70 years old, and 800 IU/d for women and men >70 years old. Research in frail older adults has shown an increased risk of falls with daily vitamin D_3 intake between 3,000 and 4,000 IU. All patients should limit vitamin D intake to <4,000 IU/d. Dietary sources of vitamin D include liver, egg yolks, saltwater fish, and vitamin D–fortified food.

There is disagreement on vitamin D monitoring and target 25-hydroxy vitamin D concentration goals. Current laboratory tests lack sufficient standardization, and guidelines differ on the importance of increasing supplementation to achieve a target vitamin D level. Vitamin D insufficiency has been commonly defined as 25-hydroxy vitamin D between 21 and 29 ng/mL and vitamin D deficiency as a level ≤20 ng/mL. The American Geriatrics Society 2014 consensus statement continues to emphasize treating to a target serum

Table 36.7—Calcium-Containing Foods

Food	Serving Size	Calcium (mg) per serving
Dairy Products		
Milk	1 cup	290–300
Yogurt	1 cup	240–400
Swiss cheese	1 ounce (1 slice)	250–270
American cheese	1 ounce (1 slice)	165–200
Ice cream	½ cup	90–100
Cottage cheese	½ cup	80–100
Parmesan cheese	1 tablespoon	70
Powdered nonfat milk	1 teaspoon	50
Other		
Sardines in oil with bones	3 ounces	370
Calcium-fortified orange juice	1 cup	300
Canned salmon with bones	3 ounces	170–210
Broccoli	1 cup	160–180
Tofu (soybean curd)	4 ounces	145–155
Turnip greens	½ cup, cooked	100–125
Kale	½ cup, cooked	90–100
Cornbread	2 ½-inch square	80–90
Egg	1 medium	55
Other fortified foods (eg, bread, cereal, fruit juices)	1 serving	Varies; read label

concentration of 25-hydroxy vitamin D of ≥30 ng/mL (75 nmol/L).

Studies involving postmenopausal women question the benefit of routine supplementation when there is an absence of risk factors for osteoporosis and the patient has adequate dietary intake of calcium and vitamin D. Vitamin D supplementation alone has not been shown to be beneficial in osteoporosis prevention in community-dwelling older adults (SOE=A). The greatest benefit for dual supplementation in reducing fracture risk is in homebound or institutionalized older adults who often have low calcium intake and vitamin D deficiency (SOE=A).

Pharmacologic Options

For dosing and special considerations for medications used to prevent and treat osteoporosis, see Table 36.8. Combination therapy is not recommended.

Bisphosphonates

Bisphosphonates decrease bone resorption and bone remodeling, leading to increase in BMD. Bisphosphonate treatments can be provided by oral or IV dosing. Oral bisphosphonates include alendronate, risedronate, and ibandronate. Alendronate and risedronate are approved for osteoporosis prevention in both men and women. Both medications increase BMD and decrease fractures at the spine and hip in postmenopausal women with osteoporosis (SOE=A). Ibandronate, which can be taken orally on a monthly basis or intravenously every 3 months, is approved for osteoporosis prevention and treatment in postmenopausal women. Ibandronate is used less frequently, because it has only shown efficacy in preventing vertebral fractures (SOE=A). In post-hoc analyses of the Fracture Intervention Trials, alendronate decreased the relative risk of hip, symptomatic vertebral, and wrist fractures in postmenopausal women up to age 85. Risedronate has been shown to decrease the relative risk of new vertebral fractures in women >80 years old with osteoporosis. Alendronate and risedronate are also approved to treat glucocorticoid-induced osteoporosis.

Zoledronic acid is an IV bisphosphonate approved for osteoporosis prevention and treatment in postmenopausal women, and for patients after osteoporotic hip fracture. It is also indicated as treatment for osteoporosis in men and for prevention of osteoporosis in men and women who are expected to receive ≥12 months of glucocorticoid therapy. Zoledronic acid has also been proved to reduce all-cause mortality when given to patients after surgical hip-fracture repair (SOE=A). Post-hoc analyses have shown a risk reduction for new clinical fracture in women ≥75 years old with treatment.

The major adverse events of oral bisphosphonates are GI symptoms, which can include abdominal pain, dyspepsia, esophagitis, nausea, vomiting, and diarrhea. Musculoskeletal pain can also rarely occur. Esophagitis, particularly erosive esophagitis, is seen most commonly in patients who do not take the medication properly, including not remaining upright

Table 36.8—Prescription Medications Used to Prevent and Treat Osteoporosis

Medication	Dosage	FDA Indication	Medication Adverse Effects/Risks	Usage/ Contraindication
Bisphosphonates				
Alendronate	Treatment: 70 mg/wk po; Prevention: 35 mg/wk po	PMO prevention; PMO, male, and GIOP treatment	Upper GI symptoms; musculoskeletal pain; esophagitis; acute-phase response Rare: ONJ, atypical femur fractures	Take oral bisphosphonates on an empty stomach with limited water. Need to sit up and wait at least 30 minutes before any oral intake. *Contraindication:* GFR≤30 mL/min
Risedronate	35 mg/wk or 150 mg/mo po	PMO prevention; PMO, male, and GIOP treatment		
Ibandronate	150 mg/mo or 3 mg IV or po every 3 mo (treatment only)	PMO prevention; PMO treatment	Musculoskeletal pain; Zoledronic acid has increased acute-phase response; hypocalcemia Rare: ONJ, atypical femur fractures	Use only for vertebral fractures. *Contraindication:* GFR ≤30 mL/min
Zoledronic acid	Treatment: 5 mg/yr IV; Prevention: 5 mg every 2 yr	PMO and GIOP prevention; PMO, male, and GIOP treatment		Tylenol premedication limits acute-phase reaction. *Contraindication:* GFR ≤35 mL/min
RANKL inhibitor				
Denosumab	60 mg SC every 6 months	PMO, male treatment	Eczema; injection site reaction; hypocalcemia; increased infection risk (especially of skin); Rare: ONJ, atypical femur fractures	Transition patient to other osteoporosis medication on completion of treatment to maintain BMD gain.
Parathyroid hormone				
Teriparatide	20 mcg/d SC	PMO, male, and GIOP treatment	Potential increase of osteosarcoma based on animal studies; hypocalcemia; nausea; vomiting; injection site reaction; fatigue	Do not use for >2 years; black box warning for patients with high risk of osteosarcoma.
Abaloparatide	80 mcg/d SC	PMO treatment		
Selective estrogen-receptor modulators and Estrogen				
Raloxifene	60 mg/d po	PMO prevention and treatment	Increased risk of venous thromboembolism; fatal stroke; flu-like symptoms; hot flashes; leg cramps; peripheral edema	Mainly used for patients in need of breast cancer prevention or treatment.
Estrogen/ bazedoxifene	0.45 mg/20 mg po	PMO prevention	Increased risk of venous thromboembolism; fatal stroke; flu-like symptoms; hot flashes; leg cramps; peripheral edema	Prescribe lowest effective dose for shortest duration of time.
Estrogen	Regimens vary	PMO prevention	Increased risk of venous thromboembolism, cardiac disease, breast cancer	Prescribe lowest effective dose for shortest duration of time.
Calcitonin				
Calcitonin	200 IU intranasally once daily; 100 IU SC every other day	PMO treatment in women ≥5 years postmenopause	Hypocalcemia, nausea, vomiting, allergic reaction, possible increased risk of cancer	Do not use as first-line treatment because of risk of malignancy and limited efficacy.

NOTE: PMO = postmenopausal osteoporosis, GIOP = glucocorticoid-induced osteoporosis, ONJ = osteonecrosis of the jaw

for 30 minutes after administration. Because absorption of oral bisphosphonates is poor, it is important to inform patients to limit intake to water only for at least 30 minutes after ingestion. Zoledronic acid and rarely alendronate and risedronate have been associated with an acute-phase response (fever, myalgias, arthralgias, and headache) as soon as 6 hours and lasting up to 72 hours after infusion or oral ingestion.

Bisphosphonate use is rarely associated with osteonecrosis of the jaw, a necrotic area of bone more commonly found in the mandible than the maxilla. Most reported cases have been in patients receiving parenteral bisphosphonates for malignant bone disorders who have undergone dental procedures such as tooth extraction. There are rare reports of patients contracting osteonecrosis of the jaw on long-term conventional oral bisphosphonates for osteoporosis. Long-term use of bisphosphonates has also been associated with atypical fractures, such as subtrochanteric and diaphyseal femur fractures. Cohort studies have shown an increased risk of subtrochanteric and femoral shaft fractures with ≥5 years of bisphosphonate use as well as a drug-dose effect. Overall, the absolute risk of osteonecrosis of the jaw and atypical femoral fractures is very low (1:10,000 person-years of use) and is outweighed by the benefits of bisphosphonate use in the vast majority of patients.

Patients taking bisphosphonates are encouraged to report new groin or thigh pain to their health care providers. When such pain is reported, radiographs of both femurs should be obtained, which can identify those who may be at risk of these atypical fractures. Further studies such as MRI or whole-body scan may be warranted in certain circumstances given the low sensitivity of plain radiographs in detecting stress fractures. Evidence is conflicting for an association between bisphosphonates and esophageal cancer. No clear association with atrial fibrillation and bisphosphonates exists.

The optimal duration of treatment with bisphosphonates is unclear; however, the effects of bisphosphonates may extend for months to years after treatment is stopped. In the FLEX study, patients who took alendronate for 10 years had less decline in their BMD at the hip and spine than those who stopped the drug after 5 years. Risk of clinical (symptomatic) vertebral fractures, but not total fractures or hip fractures, was higher in those who stopped alendronate after 5 years (SOE=A). This data suggest that alendronate can be discontinued after 5 years of treatment in patients at low risk of future fracture (eg, no new fractures on therapy, T-score greater than −2.5, and T-score that has increased while on therapy). The American Association of Clinical Endocrinologists guidelines recommend a "drug holiday" of 1–2 years. After 10 years of therapy, those at highest risk of fracture should be offered a drug holiday with consideration of possible interval treatment with another agent. In the long-term care population, expert opinion recommends discontinuation of bisphosphonates when a person is no longer ambulatory or has a remaining life expectancy of <2 years. An FDA review of the clinical studies that explored the long-term benefit of bisphosphonates concluded that patients at low risk of fracture may be good candidates to discontinue treatment after 3–5 years, while those at increased risk may continue to benefit from continued bisphosphonate treatment. However, further research is needed to better understand an individual's risk of fracture after stopping bisphosphonate therapy and when and whether to resume therapy in the future.

RANKL Inhibitor

Denosumab is a human monoclonal antibody that binds and neutralizes RANKL, a critical mediator of bone resorption by cells of osteoclast lineage. This leads to decrease in bone turnover and increase in BMD. Denosumab is FDA approved for postmenopausal women at high risk of fracture, women receiving adjuvant aromatase inhibitors therapy for breast cancer, and men on androgen deprivation therapy for nonmetastatic prostate cancer. A patient's risk of a vertebral fracture returns to the pretreatment level shortly after medication discontinuation (SOE=B). Because of this finding, it is recommended to transition patients to other antiresorptive treatment after discontinuing denosumab.

Denosumab is administered through subcutaneous injections every 6 months. Unlike bisphosphonate treatment, renal insufficiency is not a contraindication for medication use. The most statistically significant adverse events associated with denosumab include eczema, an injection site reaction, hypocalcemia, and increased risk of infections, especially of the skin. There are case reports of osteonecrosis of the jaw with denosumab use, as well as atypical femoral fractures. Because of the risk of hypocalcemia, NOF guidelines recommend evaluating and repleting calcium before starting treatment. Furthermore, monitoring serum calcium, phosphorus, magnesium, and for signs of infection should be a regular part of follow-up care while a patient is on denosumab.

Parathyroid Hormone Analogues

Teriparatide is a 1-34 human PTH anabolic agent approved for treatment of men with primary or hypogonadal osteoporosis, glucocorticoid-induced osteoporosis, and in postmenopausal women with osteoporosis. A newer medication, abaloparatide, is a synthetic analogue of PTHrp and is currently indicated for use only in postmenopausal women with osteoporosis. These anabolic agents increase bone formation by stimulating osteoblast activity through intermittent spikes of PTH or PTHrp. In a comparison 18-month study with teriparatide, abaloparatide, and placebo, both anabolic agents demonstrated a significant reduction in nonvertebral and vertebral fractures and in increased BMD. However, the study showed no statistical difference in fracture rates between the abaloparatide and teriparatide groups.

Both medications are injected subcutaneously on a daily basis and are typically reserved for those with severe osteoporosis and a higher prevalent fracture burden (SOE=A). Cost and parenteral administration also limit their use. Risk from PTH analogue medication includes potential increased incidence of osteosarcoma (seen in rat studies). This finding led to a "black box" warning and contraindication of use for patients with Paget disease, history of skeletal irradiation, and a higher baseline risk of osteosarcoma. Hypercalcemia can also occur, but most observed cases were mild and treated with reduction in calcium supplementation. Other adverse effects include nausea, vomiting, injection site reactions, and fatigue. If fatigue becomes a concern, some clinicians suggest injecting the medication before bedtime.

These drugs should be prescribed for no more than 2 years because of the plateau of benefit over time and concern over increased risk of osteosarcoma. The BMD benefits of the medication decline after discontinuation, so it is recommended to transition patients to an antiresorptive agent to maintain BMD gains. The impact of this strategy on fracture risk is still not completely understood.

Selective Estrogen-Receptor Modulators
The selective estrogen-receptor modulators (SERMs) act as estrogen agonists in bone and cardiac tissue, and as estrogen antagonists in breast and uterine tissue. SERM medications are mainly used for the treatment and prevention of estrogen receptor–positive breast cancer. Of the SERM medications, only raloxifene is approved for treatment and prevention of osteoporosis in postmenopausal women. Raloxifene reduces incident vertebral fractures; however, it has not been shown to decrease nonvertebral fractures. A combination of estrogen/bazedoxifene is approved only for prevention of postmenopausal osteoporosis in women with a uterus. As with all estrogen-containing products, the FDA recommends limited duration of use. Adverse events of both medications include increased risk of venous thromboembolism, fatal stroke, flu-like symptoms, hot flashes, leg cramps, and peripheral edema (SOE=A). Because of the risk profile, raloxifene is recommended for postmenopausal women with osteoporosis and in need of breast cancer prevention or treatment.

Estrogen
Estrogen replacement therapy is approved by the FDA solely for osteoporosis prevention in women who are at significant risk of osteoporosis and in whom nonestrogen medications have been deemed inappropriate. In the Women's Health Initiative (WHI) trial, hormone therapy reduced hip fracture rates by 34% and total osteoporotic fractures by 24%. However, hormone therapy also increased the risk of breast cancer, heart disease, and venous thromboembolism. Given the WHI findings, USPSTF guidelines advise against the routine use of estrogen plus progesterone for prevention of chronic conditions in postmenopausal women. If used, estrogen and hormonal therapy should be prescribed at the lowest effective dose for the shortest duration of time. When stopping treatment, rapid bone loss can occur and other treatments for BMD preservation should be initiated.

Calcitonin
The FDA recommends calcitonin as a second-line therapy in women with osteoporosis who are >5 years after menopause. Calcitonin inhibits bone resorption through decrease in osteoclast activity. Although the medicine is available as a subcutaneous injection, it is most commonly prescribed as a nasal spray. Conflicting evidence exists for fracture reduction with calcitonin, and there is insufficient data for calcitonin effectiveness in the first few years after menopause. Calcitonin has also shown some benefit for acute pain relief within 10 days after an osteoporotic fracture (SOE=C); however, this is not an FDA-indicated use. Safety and efficacy data are available for up to 5 years of treatment. Adverse effects include hypocalcemia, nausea, vomiting, allergic reaction, and possible increased risk of cancer. Medication should be frequently reevaluated because of the adverse effect profile and limited efficacy of use.

Monitoring
Patients receiving treatment for osteoporosis commonly undergo serial BMD measurements at least every 2 years to assess effectiveness, an interval currently covered by Medicare. This interval is not a universal recommendation, as evidence is insufficient to support modifying treatment based on BMD response. Because of the limited evidence, as of 2017 the American College of Physicians no longer recommends BMD monitoring after initiation of treatment. Proponents of measuring BMD report that benefits of monitoring include identification of patients with poor adherence, secondary cause of bone loss, and possible evidence of treatment failure. Adherence to treatment should be assessed at each visit for all patients, especially those on oral bisphosphonates. Patients on bisphosphonates who experience GI adverse events are 50% more likely to discontinue their medication, and poor adherence is associated with increased risk of fractures (SOE=A).

VERTEBRAL FRACTURE MANAGEMENT

Vertebral compression fractures are often asymptomatic and diagnosed incidentally by spinal radiographs. They most commonly occur in the thoracolumbar transition zone or midthoracic region. In affected individuals, height may decrease, kyphosis may increase, or clothes may no longer fit properly over time. Many older adults have chronic back pain caused by changes in the spine that develop with degenerative osteoarthritis or vertebral compression; distinguishing the source of the pain can be difficult. On a practical level, pain should be treated if it interferes with ADLs and quality of life, regardless of cause. However, identifying vertebral fractures is important so that future fractures can be prevented.

In the case of symptomatic vertebral compression fractures, adequate pain control is essential. The pain usually lasts 2–4 weeks and can be quite debilitating. In addition to medication, physical therapy is an important part of osteoporosis treatment programs to manage acute and chronic pain and to provide patient education. A physical therapist can provide postural exercises, alternative interventions for pain reduction, and information on changes in body mechanics that can help prevent future falls. Back braces may help to decrease pain and disability after a fracture. Support groups for patients with osteoporosis can also be helpful.

Vertebroplasty and Kyphoplasty

Vertebroplasty and kyphoplasty are minimally invasive surgical approaches for management of painful vertebral compression fractures. In vertebroplasty, the cement is injected directly into the vertebral body, with the goal of alleviating pain and preventing further bone compression. Kyphoplasty uses an inflated balloon inserted through a fluoroscopically placed needle to elevate the fracture and fill the cavity with cement. The goal is to improve pain while reducing loss of height and decreasing kyphosis. The American Academy of Orthopedic Surgeons states that kyphoplasty is an option for pain control in neurologically intact individuals (SOE=C). However, the Academy recommends against vertebroplasty based on 2 randomized trials showing no significant differences in pain reduction between vertebroplasty and sham procedure (SOE=A). Both procedures, although minimally invasive, carry complications.

CHOOSING WISELY® RECOMMENDATIONS

Osteoporosis

- Do not routinely repeat BMD more than once every 2 years.
- Do not perform population based screening for vitamin D deficiency

RESOURCES

- American Geriatrics Society Workgroup on vitamin D supplementation for older adults. Recommendations abstracted from the American Geriatrics Society Consensus Statement on Vitamin D for Prevention of Falls and Their Consequences. *J Am Geriatr Soc.* 2014;62(1):147–152.

- Prah A, Richards E, Griggs R, et al. Enhancing osteoporosis efforts through lifestyle modifications and goal setting techniques. *J Nurse Pract.* 2017;(13)8:552–561.

CHAPTER 37—DEMENTIA

KEY POINTS

- Alzheimer disease is the most common form of degenerative dementia seen in late life.

- Cholinesterase inhibitors and N-methyl-d-aspartate receptor antagonists can produce modest improvements in measures of cognition and ADLs in some patients with Alzheimer dementia.

- Behavioral and psychological symptoms in dementia should be primarily managed with a combination of psychosocial and environmental modifications.

With the publication of the *Diagnostic and Statistical Manual of Mental Disorders, Fifth Edition (DSM-5)*, the major neurocognitive disorder (NCD) category encompassed various disorders that cause significant decline in one or more cognitive domains severe enough to result in functional decline. The *DSM-5* further defined mild NCD as cognitive decline beyond that associated with normal aging but without significant functional decline. By seeing cognitive decline on a continuum, the *DSM-5* hoped to provide an opportunity for early detection and potential treatment of cognitive decline before it becomes more debilitating. For purposes of maintaining consistency with the clinical identification of these disorders in current practice, the term "dementia" will be used when referencing the various disorders.

Of those who suffer from dementia, most have Alzheimer disease (AD), which affects an estimated 5.5 million people in the United States. Millions of caregivers and relatives are challenged as they cope with the patient's progressive and irreversible decline in cognition, functioning, and behavior. Both caregivers and patients can misinterpret the initial symptoms of dementia as normal age-related cognitive losses; clinicians as well may not recognize early signs or can misdiagnose them. However, dementia and aging are not synonymous. Cognitive aging is the gradual decline in certain cognitive abilities that parallels a number of common decreases in physiological function that occur in conjunction with normal developmental processes. These cognitive declines typically are not significant enough to cause impairment in functional abilities. In contrast, the cognitive disorders go beyond what may be considered normal aging and are typically progressive to the point of loss of social and/or occupational functional abilities. These progressive forms of cognitive deterioration are caused by a variety of neurodegenerative conditions and dementing diseases.

Early and accurate diagnosis of dementia and its cause can minimize use of costly medical resources and give patients and their relatives time to anticipate future medical, financial, and legal needs (SOE=B). Sustained reversal of the progressive cognitive decline of dementia is not currently possible, but psychosocial and pharmacologic treatments can improve overall quality of life, permit the institution of safety measures, and provide caregiver support and training.

EPIDEMIOLOGY AND SOCIETAL IMPACT

Dementia is typically a disease of later life, generally beginning after 65 years of age. AD is the most common type of dementia, accounting for approximately two-thirds of all cases and affecting 6%–8% of those ≥65 years old. The disease prevalence doubles every 5 years after age 60; an estimated 45% or more of those who are ≥85 years old have AD. Vascular dementia is thought to cause an estimated 15%–20% of cases and often coexists with AD pathology, ie, so-called "mixed dementia." In recent years, dementia associated with Lewy bodies has received increased attention and is now thought to be the second most common cause of dementia. Frontotemporal dementia is less common and typically has a younger age of onset than seen in other dementias. Neurodegenerative diseases such as Huntington disease, Parkinson disease, or other causes such as head injury and alcoholism account for other dementia syndromes.

Dementia has significant social and economic implications in terms of direct medical costs, direct social costs, and the costs of informal care. According to the World Health Organization, in 2015, the total global societal cost of dementia was estimated to be $818 billion (USD), equivalent to 1.1% of the global gross domestic product. This was a sharp increase from 2010, during which time global costs were estimated to be $604 billion. Medicare, Medicaid, and private insurance pay much of the direct cost, but families caring for patients with dementia bear the greatest burden of expense. In 2016, the Alzheimer's Association reported family caregivers provided an estimated 18.2 billion hours of care, estimated to cost more than $230 billion dollars in the United States alone.

In addition to the financial costs, the emotional toll is immense for both patients and their families. Nearly half of primary caregivers of patients with dementia experience psychologic distress, particularly depression, and have more physical health issues.

ETIOLOGY

Research into the pathophysiologic mechanisms of dementia has rapidly evolved over the last several decades. For each type of dementia, a putative protein or set of proteins has been implicated in the cause and progression of the neurodegenerative process. Whether it is the amyloid plaques/oligomers or tau neurofibrillary tangles (or both) associated with AD, the tau or ubiquitin proteins of frontotemporal dementia, or the cytoplasmic α-synuclein inclusion bodies of Lewy body dementia and Parkinson dementia, it is the accumulation of these proteins or protein aggregates within the brain that appears to set off a cascade of events that directly affect neuronal function and ultimately cell death in a disease-specific pattern. Efforts continue to better understand the genetics and environmental influences on these mechanisms, which appear to be well underway, possibly even up to 30 years, before any pathology is clinically identifiable.

RISK FACTORS AND PREVENTION

The two greatest risk factors for AD are age and family history. Studies that account for death from other causes suggest that by 90 years of age, nearly half of those with first-degree relatives (eg, parents, siblings) with AD develop the disease themselves. Rare forms of familial AD are caused by mutations in one of three genes—amyloid precursor protein (APP), presenilin 1 (PS1), or presenilin 2 (PS2)—and account for approximately 1% of individuals with AD. These individuals usually have a pattern of illness in the family called autosomal dominant, which describes many family members, who are closely related to each other, with AD before age 60. Most commonly, AD begins late in life, and for many such late-onset cases, the apolipoprotein E gene (APOE) on chromosome 19 influences risk. The APOE gene has three alleles: epsilon (ε) 2, 3, and 4. Epsilon 4 (ε4) is the risk-conferring allele; it does not cause AD directly. Epsilon 2 (ε2) is considered a protective allele, and epsilon 3 (ε3) is neutral. Individuals with two APOE ε4 alleles have increased lifetime risk, as compared with those in the general population. Those carrying one APOE ε4 allele are still at increased risk. Using APOE genotyping as a prognostic test for asymptomatic older adults is not currently recommended. Merely a risk factor, the ε4 allele cannot accurately predict whether or not a person will develop AD. Genome-wide association studies have identified genes in addition to APOE that confer risk of AD. These additional risk genes include triggering receptor expressed on myeloid cells 2 (TREM2), bridging integrator 1 (BIN1), ATP-binding cassette subfamily A member 7 (ABCA7), clusterin (CLU), and phosphatidylinositol-binding clathrin assembly protein (PICALM). Genetic testing is not clinically available for these genes. Other types of dementia have genetic etiologies. Huntington disease is caused by mutations in the Huntington gene. A proportion of frontotemporal dementia with or without amyotrophic lateral sclerosis is also genetic in origin and may be caused by mutations in select genes. Any evaluation should include a thorough family history and referral to a genetics counselor if indicated.

Prevention of dementia, especially AD, is an active area of research. The general premise behind most of the research is understanding risk and protective factors thought to have an impact on cognitive function. Potential factors that have been identified can be classified according to lifestyle and physical environmental factors (smoking, alcohol, diet, physical activity, education, cognitive and social activity) and vascular risk factors (hypertension, hyperlipidemia, diabetes, obesity, vascular insults, neuronal damage). An additional area of increased interest includes head trauma, which is thought to disrupt neuronal synapses and predispose to β-amyloid formation. Various research projects have examined how to mitigate the risks and exploit the protective factors to prevent cognitive decline. Research in healthy older adults has found encouraging although inconclusive evidence to support interventions that can slow cognitive aging or prevent or slow clinical dementia. Data suggest that cognitive training and increased physical activity can delay or slow cognitive decline. Blood pressure management in patients with hypertension is thought to be able to prevent, delay, or slow dementia.

Several randomized controlled trials are beginning to test multicomponent interventions that target several of these risk factors together. Reviews suggest that interventions, including diet, exercise, cognitive training, and vascular risk monitoring, could improve or maintain cognitive functioning in at-risk individuals. For both risk and protective factors for dementia, see Table 37.1.

ASSESSMENT

In general, the diagnosis of dementia is a clinical one, and laboratory assessment and imaging are used to identify uncommon treatable causes and common treatable comorbid conditions and, when used in the setting of specialty care clinics, can help further differentiate atypical presentations.

Most cases of dementia can be diagnosed in the primary care setting on the basis of a complete history, physical examination, and cognitive testing. Although cognitive screening of all geriatric patients is not recommended by the U.S. Preventive Task Force, it is prudent for primary care providers (PCPs) to ask patients about changes in memory or cognition and to perform a cognitive evaluation of appropriate patients. Indeed, early-stage or mild dementia is often undetected until an adverse event, such as medication errors or behavioral disturbances, flags its presence. Subjective complaints from the patient or family member should be heeded and followed by a cognitive assessment and potentially a dementia evaluation. Of note, early signs of cognitive decline may be subtle, eg, missing appointments, misplacing things frequently, increasing difficulty in managing complex tasks such as finances or paying bills, or giving up a hobby or interest that may have become too challenging.

Various medical, neurologic, and psychiatric conditions can affect memory and cognition, so PCPs must approach evaluation of the subjective complaint of memory loss with a broad differential before attributing symptoms to dementia. Potential causes of cognitive changes include depression, delirium, hypothyroidism, vitamin B_{12} deficiency, sleep impairment, or adverse effects of medication. According to the American Academy of Neurology, laboratory evaluation for memory loss should include a CBC, glucose, thyroid function test, electrolytes, BUN/creatinine, serum B_{12}, and liver function test. Of note, the American Academy of Neurology does not recommend the routine evaluation of those with suspected dementia by syphilis serology, EEG, lumbar puncture, positron emission tomography (PET), or APOE genotyping.

The informant interview and office-based clinical assessment are the most important diagnostic tools for dementia. Both the patient and a reliable informant (if available) should be interviewed to obtain information on the patient's past and current cognitive state, medical and medication history, functional abilities, and psychosocial concerns, including behavioral changes and living arrangements. For a helpful mnemonic for obtaining a complete but concise cognitive history, see Table 37.2. Determination of onset, nature, and course of symptoms can help differentiate dementia from benign age-associated memory impairment as well as other clinical syndromes such as delirium and depression. Note that functional decline should be judged against previous performance and may require the provider to probe specific tasks (eg, driving, bill payments, medication management) given the common denial or minimization of symptoms by patients or even family members. The presence of behavioral changes such as hallucinations and delusions should be asked about specifically, as well as adequacy of caregiver support.

Cognitive Evaluation

Several consensus guidelines are available for the clinical diagnosis and treatment of most types of dementia. Common quantified screening tests of cognitive function

Table 37.1—Protective Factors and Risk Factors for Alzheimer Disease

Probable Protective Factors	Risk Factors
Blood pressure control	Age
Physical activity	Family history
Cognitive training	APOE4 allele
Education	Down syndrome
	Head trauma
	Fewer years of formal education
	Cardiovascular risk factors (hypertension, hypercholesterolemia, diabetes, obesity)

Table 37.2—NW-CALMS Mnemonic for Obtaining a Cognitive History

Nature	Forgetting appointments, driving problems, misplacing things, getting lost, missed bill payments, personality change
When	Days, months, years, decades
Course	Abrupt, stepwise, slowly progressive, fluctuating, after new medications
ADLs/IADLs	Functional impairment
Life situation	Bereavement, home safety
Mood	Depression (anorexia, insomnia, anhedonia)
Status of health	Acute illness (delirium), thyroid problems, electrolyte abnormalities, etc

include the Mini-Cog Assessment Instrument for Dementia, the St. Louis University Mental Status, and the Montreal Cognitive Assessment (MoCA) (Table 37.3). These are screening tools only with general score cut-offs regarding cognitive functioning and should not be used to diagnose dementia. Diagnosis of dementia is a clinical diagnosis taking into account multiple factors with cognitive screening being only one.

Cognitive performance is influenced by number of years of formal education. Affected patients with more years of education may have normal cognitive test scores, whereas patients with less education may have low scores and no decline in function. This must be considered, especially in patients with more subtle deficits or subjective complaints. In addition, in tests that are most sensitive to language performance, cultural differences can lead to an overdiagnosis of dementia in minority patients. One way to improve the accuracy of assessment is to perform serial evaluations (using a medical interpreter if needed), which allow determination of decline in an individual that is consistent with a neurodegenerative process. In addition, measuring changes in everyday memory function by evaluating a person's performance of ADLs and IADLs, either by direct observation or by

Table 37.3—Screening Instruments for the Evaluation of Cognition

Instrument Name	Time of Administration (minutes)	Number of Items (score)	Domains Assessed	Website (accessed Feb 2019)
Mini-Cog	3	2 (5)	Visuospatial, executive function, recall	https://mini-cog.com
St. Louis University Mental Status (SLUMS) Examination	7–10	11 (30)	Orientation, recall, calculation, naming, attention, executive function	http://medschool.slu.edu/agingsuccessfully/pdfsurveys/slumsexam_05.pdf
Montreal Cognitive Assessment (MoCA)	7–10	12 (30)	Orientation, recall, attention, naming, repetition, verbal fluency, abstraction, executive function, visuospatial	www.mocatest.org
Folstein Mini–Mental Status Examination (MMSE)	10–15	19 (30)	Orientation, registration, attention, recall, naming, repetition, 3-step command, language, visuospatial	www.minimental.com (for purchase)
Functional Activities Questionnaire	5	10 (30)	Informant based, executive functioning, ADLs, attention, concentration, memory, home safety	https://www.healthcare.uiowa.edu/familymedicine/fpinfo/Docs/functional-activities-assessment-tool.pdf

obtaining information from a reliable informant may be helpful. Cognitive and functional assessments should be conducted in the patient's native language, if at all possible. (In the face of cognitive decline, patients with dementia commonly retain the greatest fluency in their native language.)

Functional Status Evaluation

Through questioning of patient and reliable informants, practitioners can determine if there has been any change in performance of ADLs/IADLs. However, it is important to know baseline level of functioning and to be able to differentiate functional decline secondary to cognitive impairment from other causes of functional impairment (eg, stroke with residual weakness that prevents independence with ADLs or IADLs). Any changes are best determined by comparing present with previous performance, because functional decline and multiple cognitive deficits support the diagnosis. For cases in which there is incongruence between functional status and assessment performance (eg, MoCA score of 13 with full independence in ADLs and IADLs), further neuropsychological testing could be warranted.

Neuroimaging

Neuroimaging is often obtained during the evaluation of cognitive impairment, although it is not required to reach a diagnosis of dementia. Most clinicians in the primary care setting utilize a CT scan of the brain without contrast to exclude any overt pathology. It provides a general view of brain anatomy and can detect generalized atrophy, space-occupying lesions, previous large territory infarcts, and subdural hematoma and stroke. MRI of the brain without contrast is more specific and can provide information on cerebral brain volume, specific areas of atrophy (ie, hippocampal in AD), white matter changes, and smaller infarcts (ie, vascular dementia, mixed dementia). Further evaluation for abnormal metabolism/activity is typically reserved for differentiating between types of dementia and not used for routine diagnosis. To differentiate between Alzheimer disease and frontotemporal dementia, a PET scan or FDG-PET scan can be used to increase diagnostic accuracy that can impact management. PET identifies areas of reduced brain activity. FDG-PET directly measures brain metabolism by measuring glucose uptake by parts of the brain (decreased uptake in temporal and parietal areas in AD, decreased uptake in frontal and temporal areas in frontotemporal dementia). Brain imaging studies may be especially useful in the following situations:

- Age at onset <65 years
- Symptoms begin suddenly or progress rapidly
- Evidence of focal or asymmetrical neurologic deficits

- Clinical picture suggests normal-pressure hydrocephalus (eg, onset has occurred within 1 year, gait disorder or unexplained incontinence is present)
- History of a recent fall or other head trauma

Diagnosis Reporting

According to the Alzheimer's Association, fewer than half of people with AD or their caregivers have been told of their diagnosis by their health care provider. Clinician, patient, and system-based factors contribute to the lack of disclosure. Conveying the diagnosis can be associated with a sense of distress but has not been definitively associated with increased risk of suicide. Although age is a risk factor for suicide, further research is needed to clarify if suicide in patients with dementia is a result of the dementia or unrecognized psychiatric symptoms. However, knowing the diagnosis facilitates a conversation about issues that go along with the disease.

DIFFERENTIATING BETWEEN DEMENTIA, DEPRESSION, AND DELIRIUM

Older patients with depression may present with a syndrome of cognitive impairment resembling dementia that subsides after remission of depression. Therefore, it is necessary to screen for depression and treat if present, because it may be a reversible cause of the cognitive impairment (previously described as pseudodementia). Patients with primary depression can demonstrate decreased motivation during the cognitive examination and express cognitive complaints that exceed objectively measured deficits. Moreover, patients with primary depression usually have intact language and motor skills, whereas patients with primary dementia may show impairment in these domains. Patients with primary dementia commonly experience symptoms of depression, and such patients may minimize cognitive losses. Depression and dementia can coexist; in fact, dementia with depressed mood is fairly common and can respond to antidepressants. As many as half of older adults who present with severe depression and signs of cognitive loss become progressively demented within 5 years.

Delirium and dementia are in some ways similar; both are characterized by global cognitive impairment. Delirium, however, is defined as an acute alteration of consciousness, characterized by inattentiveness which can often present as memory loss. Delirium typically has a reversible cause (eg, infection) but even after identifying and addressing the cause, delirium can persist for days, weeks, or months before resolving completely. Delirium can present in hyperactive, hypoactive, and mixed forms. Recognition is critical, because there is an increased risk of morbidity and mortality with delayed diagnosis and treatment. Patients with underlying dementia are at increased risk of delirium, so it is important for patients to be screened for cognitive impairment once delirium has resolved.

SUBTYPES OF DEMENTIA

For an overview of diagnostic features of the most common dementias, see Table 37.4.

Common to all types of dementia, cognitive impairment eventually has a profound effect on the patient's daily life. Difficulties in planning meals, managing finances or medications, using a telephone, and driving without getting lost are not uncommon. Such functional impairments may first alert others that a problem is emerging. Numerous functions are maintained in patients with dementia of mild to moderate severity, including such ADLs as eating, bathing, and grooming, and the behaviors of many patients remain socially appropriate during the early disease stages.

Behavior and mood changes eventually become commonplace, including personality changes, apathy, irritability, anxiety, or depression. During the middle and late stages of the disease, delusions, hallucinations, aggression, resistance to care, and wandering may develop. These behaviors are extremely troubling to caregivers and often result in family distress and long-term care placement. Although the course of dementia is variable, the progression of dementia often follows a sequential clinical and functional pattern of decline (Table 37.5).

Alzheimer Disease

Clinically, AD is characterized by gradual onset and progressive decline in cognitive functioning; motor and sensory functions are spared until middle and late stages. Memory impairment is often a core symptom of any dementia, but in AD it is typically *the* core feature present in the earliest stages. Typically, AD patients demonstrate difficulty learning and retaining new information with impairment most prominent in short-term memory. In later disease stages, their ability to access older, more distant memories also become impaired. Aphasia, apraxia, disorientation, visuospatial dysfunction, impaired judgment, and executive dysfunction are also often present in the moderate to late stages. Neurologic examination is usually nonfocal in earlier stages, although impairments in gait, coordination, and other vital motor functions such as swallowing appear in the later stages. The "probability" of AD is amplified by the presence of risk factors such as age over 65 years, history of head trauma, and family history of AD in a first-degree relative.

Table 37.4—Diagnostic Features and Treatment of Dementia Syndromes

Syndrome	Onset	Cognitive Domains, Symptoms	Motor Symptoms	Progression	Neuropathology	Pharmacologic Treatment of Cognition
Alzheimer disease	Gradual onset, primarily memory loss	Memory, language, visuospatial	Rare early, apraxia later	Gradual (over 8–10 years)	Cortical atrophy, hippocampal atrophy, tau protein	ChI for mild to severe (SOE=A); memantine for moderate to severe stages
Vascular dementia	May be sudden or stepwise	Depends on location of ischemia	Correlates with ischemia	Gradual or stepwise with further ischemia	Ischemic, hemorrhagic, or hypoxic lesions	Consider ChI for memory deficit only (SOE=C); risk-factor modifiers
Lewy body dementia	Gradual, typically patient presents with visual hallucinations, REM sleep behaviors	Memory, visuospatial, hallucinations, fluctuating symptoms	Parkinsonism	Gradual but faster than Alzheimer disease	Lewy bodies, possible global atrophy	ChI (SOE=B); ± carbidopa/levodopa for movement
Parkinson disease dementia	Typically has Parkinson disease for many years before onset	Memory, visuospatial, hallucinations, fluctuating symptoms	Parkinsonism	Progressive	Lewy bodies, possible global atrophy	Carbidopa/levodopa for movement ± ChI
Frontotemporal dementia	Gradual, age <60 years	Executive, disinhibition, apathy, language, ± memory	None	Gradual but faster than Alzheimer disease	Atrophy in frontal and temporal lobes	Not recommended per current evidence

Vascular Dementia

Vascular dementia refers to cognitive deficits most often associated with vascular damage in the brain, either micro or macro in nature. It is sometimes associated with focal neurologic deficits that accompany cognitive loss, and the cognitive and neurologic impairments should correlate anatomically with the areas of ischemia, although the often diffuse nature of vascular disease may make this correlation difficult to identify. This is especially true in the case of small-vessel ischemic disease, which can be found in up to 50% of the cases of vascular dementia. Small-vessel ischemic disease involves white-matter damage and subcortical vessel damage, which in contrast to large-vessel disease, can present with more subtle neurologic signs, ie, pronator drift, gait instability, slowing of motor performance, and/or a neuropsychologic profile consistent with a dysexecutive syndrome of slow information processing and inattention. These changes are often seen as focal or diffuse white-matter changes on MRI (T2-weighted hyperintensities) and, as a function of volume, are often associated with worsening cognitive function. Parsing the differences between AD and vascular dementia can be challenging, especially given the relatively high rate of "mixed" etiology found in AD. The temporal association of cardiovascular events, genetic predispositions, and/or neuroimaging data increase the probability of a diagnosis of vascular dementia.

Dementia (or NCD) with Lewy Bodies

For a diagnosis of dementia with Lewy bodies, both dementia and at least one of the following core features must be present: recurrent and detailed visual hallucinations, parkinsonian signs, and fluctuations in levels of alertness or attention. Additional suggestive features may include autonomic dysfunction, sleep disorder, severe neuroleptic sensitivity, and psychiatric misidentification syndromes. The diagnosis may overlap with AD and the dementia associated with Parkinson disease but having at least 2 core features raises the probability of dementia with Lewy bodies. Poor visuospatial abilities are also often out of proportion to other cognitive deficits. Symptoms of dementia with Lewy bodies may overlap with Parkinson disease dementia. If the motor symptoms of Parkinson disease have been present for ≥1 year before cognitive symptoms are seen, the diagnosis is more consistent with Parkinson disease dementia. If parkinsonian symptoms are present at the same time as cognitive symptoms, a diagnosis of dementia with Lewy bodies should be considered.

Frontotemporal Dementia

Frontotemporal dementia (FTD) is a disease often seen in patients with onset of cognitive symptoms at a younger

Table 37.5—The General Progression of Dementia

Stage 1: No cognitive impairment
Unimpaired individuals experience no memory problems, and none is evident to a health care professional during a medical interview.

Stage 2: Very mild cognitive decline
Individuals at this stage feel as if they have memory lapses, especially in forgetting familiar words or names or the location of keys, eyeglasses, or other everyday objects. However, these problems are not evident during a medical examination or apparent to friends, family, or coworkers.

Stage 3: Mild cognitive decline
Early-stage Alzheimer disease can be diagnosed in some, but not all, individuals with these symptoms.

Friends, family, or coworkers begin to notice deficiencies. Problems with memory or concentration may be measurable in clinical testing or discernible during a detailed medical interview. Common difficulties include the following:
- Word- or name-finding problems noticeable to family or close associates
- Decreased ability to remember names when introduced to new people
- Performance issues in social or work settings noticeable to family, friends, or coworkers
- Reading a passage and retaining little material
- Losing or misplacing a valuable object
- Decline in ability to plan or organize

Stage 4: Moderate cognitive decline (mild or early-stage Alzheimer disease)
At this stage, a careful medical interview detects clear-cut deficiencies in the following areas:
- Decreased knowledge of recent occasions or current events
- Impaired ability to perform challenging mental arithmetic, eg, to count backward from 100 by 7s
- Decreased ability to perform complex tasks, such as marketing, planning dinner for guests, or paying bills and managing finances
- Reduced memory of personal history

The affected individual may seem subdued and withdrawn, especially in socially or mentally challenging situations.

Stage 5: Moderately severe cognitive decline (moderate or mid-stage Alzheimer disease)
Major gaps in memory and deficits in cognitive function emerge. Some assistance with day-to-day activities becomes essential. At this stage, individuals may:
- Be unable during a medical interview to recall such important information as their current address, their telephone number, or the name of the college or high school from which they graduated
- Become confused about where they are or about the date, day of the week, or season
- Have trouble with less challenging mental arithmetic, eg, counting backward from 40 by 4s or from 20 by 2s
- Need help choosing proper clothing for the season or occasion
- Usually retain substantial knowledge about themselves and know their own name and the names of their spouse or children
- Usually require no assistance with eating or using the toilet

Stage 6: Severe cognitive decline (moderately severe or mid-stage Alzheimer disease)
Memory difficulties continue to worsen, significant personality changes may emerge, and affected individuals need extensive help with customary daily activities. At this stage, individuals may:
- Lose most awareness of recent experiences, events, and surroundings
- Recollect their personal history imperfectly, although they generally recall their name
- Occasionally forget the name of their spouse or primary caregiver but generally can distinguish familiar from unfamiliar faces
- Need help getting dressed properly; without supervision, may make errors such as putting pajamas over daytime clothes or shoes on wrong feet
- Experience disruption of their normal sleep-wake cycle
- Need help with handling details of toileting (flushing toilet, wiping, and disposing of tissue properly)
- Have increasing episodes of urinary or fecal incontinence
- Experience significant personality changes and behavioral symptoms, including suspiciousness and delusions (eg, believing that their caregiver is an impostor); hallucinations (seeing or hearing things that are not really there); or compulsive, repetitive behaviors such as hand wringing or tissue shredding
- Tend to wander and become lost

Stage 7: Very severe cognitive decline (severe or late-stage Alzheimer disease)
This is the final stage of the disease when individuals lose the ability to respond to their environment, to speak, and ultimately to control movement.
- Frequently lose the ability for recognizable speech, although words or phrases may occasionally be uttered
- Need help with eating and toileting, and there is general urinary incontinence
- Lose the ability to walk without assistance, then the ability to sit without support, smile, and to hold up head; reflexes become abnormal, muscles grow rigid, and swallowing is impaired

SOURCE: Excerpted from www.alz.org/AboutAD/Stages.asp and reproduced with permission of the Alzheimer's Association. © 2011 Alzheimer's Association. All rights reserved. This is an official publication of the Alzheimer's Association but may be distributed by unaffiliated organizations and individuals. Such distribution does not constitute an endorsement of these parties or their activities by the Alzheimer's Association.

age (<65 years old). FTD is divided into 3 subtypes: 1) behavioral variant FTD is characterized by prominent behavioral issues such as disinhibition, hyperorality, lack of social awareness, and impulsivity; 2) semantic dementia manifests as impaired comprehension with generally fluent speech; and 3) progressive nonfluent aphasia presents with impairment in speech production. These symptoms of FTD appear relatively early in the course of the disease. Memory deficits are often not as pronounced in these patients in the early stages as they are in patients with other dementias. It is important to recognize the difference between FTD and AD with "frontal" symptoms. The latter refers to social disinhibition and behavioral impulsivity that can be seen with moderate to late-stage AD. In these patients, the behavioral problems occur much later in the course of illness, after a cognitive problem is already clearly evident. In contrast, patients with FTD display social disinhibition or language impairments before prominent memory decline. The probability of FTD is increased by evidence of disproportionate frontal and/or temporal lobe involvement from neuroimaging (eg, FDG-PET).

TREATMENT AND MANAGEMENT

Geriatric care providers should be able to manage dementia-related cognitive, behavioral, and psychosocial issues. Consultation from behavioral neurologists, neuropsychologists, psychiatrists, and other specialties (eg, social work) can be requested in certain cases in which the presentation is atypical and/or the behavioral and psychosocial challenges are not responsive to interventions. The primary treatment goals for patients with dementia are to enhance quality of life and maximize functional performance by improving or stabilizing cognition, mood, and behavior. Both pharmacologic and nonpharmacologic treatments are available, and the latter should be emphasized. Available pharmacologic treatments show only modest effects on cognition, and providers should educate patients and caregivers to have realistic expectations. Any acute change requires an evaluation for undiagnosed medical problems, pain, depression, infection, metabolic disturbance, or delirium. Other factors that can contribute to behavioral symptoms include interpersonal or emotional issues. Addressing such issues, treating underlying medical conditions, providing reassurance, and attending to the possible need for changes in the patient's environment and care interactions can reduce agitation. The use of pharmacologic treatments for behavioral problems is recommended only after nonpharmacologic interventions prove ineffective, or when there is an emergent need such as extreme patient distress or risk of physical violence.

Nonpharmacologic Treatment

Cognitive Training

Memory retraining and cognitive stimulation have been proposed as possible techniques to perhaps improve cognitive function. A 2012 Cochrane review of randomized controlled trials (RCTs) of cognitive stimulation for dementia showed evidence of benefit in persons with mild to moderate dementia. Studies in this review were limited by variable quality of study design, small sample sizes, and limited details of randomization methodology. A 2017 meta-analysis of RCTs found a small to moderate benefit of cognitive stimulation.

Supportive Therapy

Emotion-oriented psychotherapy, such as "pleasant events" and "reminiscence" therapy, and stimulation-oriented treatment, including art and other expressive recreational or social therapies, such as exercise or dance, are examples of psychosocial treatments that can minimize depressive symptoms and reduce behavioral symptoms. These interventions can be provided by professionals or informal caregivers who have been specifically trained. Support groups can provide meaningful assistance and education for both patients and caregivers. Early-onset dementia groups are especially helpful for patients with mild deficits and insight. Research has begun to demonstrate benefits of caregiver education and support in reducing behavioral symptoms and improving quality of life among patients and caregivers with dementia (SOE=C).

Other Therapies

There are some data supporting physical exercise as having effects on functional performance, cognitive function, and behavioral symptoms. A recent Cochrane review reported evidence on ADL performance and cognition, as well as promising data on caregiver burden associated with exercise programs. Physical activity should be encouraged as part of the treatment plan for any patient with dementia. Early research also suggests a role for occupational therapy in providing caregiver education strategies and environmental modification.

Family and Caregiver Education and Support

Many caregivers experience high levels of stress that place them at risk of physical and mental health problems. These include poor health maintenance practices (eg, lack of exercise, increased smoking and alcohol consumption, poor sleep), more physical health conditions (eg, cardiovascular conditions, lower immunity, diabetes), reduced sense of well-being, stress, anxiety, and depression. Perceived burden from the caregiver role is a strong predictor of premature institutionalization of the care recipient. Thus, education of family and caregivers about diagnosis, clinical course, treatment options, and management strategies is critical. Recent research has focused on developing a framework to analyze behaviors and develop individualized strategies for use by caregivers. Several of these studies have demonstrated efficacy on reducing caregiver burden, especially around behavioral symptoms.

Relatives are often helpful sources of information about cognitive and behavioral changes, and generally they take the primary responsibility for implementing and monitoring treatment. Often, they are also responsible for medical and legal assistance. However, early identification of dementia can allow the affected individual to participate in treatment decisions and future planning. Subjects to pursue with family members include medical and legal advance directives (also called advance care plans in some contexts). It is often best for a trusted relative to co-sign important financial transactions and attend to paying bills.

Community programs such as enrollment in adult daycare centers or respite programs can provide support to family caregivers, allowing the individual with dementia to remain at home longer. Patients also benefit from these programs through opportunities for socialization and structured activities. Although most care for dementia patients is provided in the home, some may need alternative living situations such as assisted living, board-and-care, or nursing home care. Discussion about long-term care placement options should be started early to provide the individual or family members time to complete arrangements and begin to adjust emotionally. In the late stages of dementia, palliative care teams may be consulted to assist in developing goals of care around symptom management and may provide support in planning for this very unpredictable prognosis. Hospice can be an alternative for end-stage dementia patients who wish to remain at home and have comfort as the goal for care.

Environmental Modification

Patients with dementia can be extremely sensitive to their environment; in general, a moderate level of stimulation is best. When they experience overstimulation, confusion or agitation can increase, whereas too little stimulation can cause boredom and withdrawal. As deficits change over time, this balance must be reevaluated, and activities adjusted regularly. Familiar surroundings maximize existing cognitive functions, and predictability through daily routines is often reassuring. Other helpful orientation and memory measures in early stages include conspicuous displays of clocks, calendars, and to-do lists. Links to the outside world through newspapers, radio, and television can benefit some mildly impaired patients.

Adaptive strategies for more impaired individuals can involve providing visual clues to assist patients (eg, picture of a toilet for the bathroom, or of food for the dining room) or to distract patients from exposure to unsafe situations (eg, STOP sign on door, covering elevator buttons). Attention to a simple and compassionate communication style can reduce behavioral symptoms in the patient and burden for the caregiver. Strategies such as using simple sentences, phrasing commands in a positive fashion, avoiding slang and pronouns, and speaking in a calm tone of voice can enhance communication.

Attention to Safety

In early stages, safety concerns include difficulty with IADLs such as finances, transportation, and medication management. However, the need for supervision usually increases as the disease progresses to the moderate stage and the person becomes more forgetful and judgement becomes impaired. Interventions should balance allowing as much independence as possible while ensuring safety, focusing initially on environmental strategies. Door locks or electronic guards prevent unsafe wandering, and many families benefit from registering with Safe Return through the Alzheimer's Association (www.alz.org). Medical-alert bracelets can assist in locating lost patients. Emerging technologies include watches and other devices that incorporate a global positioning system to monitor the individual's location.

Cognitive impairment affects driving skills, and the visuospatial and planning disabilities of even mildly demented patients can make them unsafe drivers. Discussions about driving are best started early in treatment. Patients with advanced dementia definitely should not drive, but clinicians disagree about whether mildly demented patients should drive. Referral for an independent driving assessment is recommended if there is any concern regarding safety. Certainly, when a patient has a history of traffic accidents or significant spatial and executive dysfunction, driving abilities should be carefully scrutinized.

Pharmacologic Treatment

All current FDA-approved medications for Alzheimer disease and other dementias are symptomatic; none has been shown to halt cognitive and functional decline. The magnitude of cognitive enhancement with these medications is generally modest, and it is important for clinicians to inform patients and families to set realistic expectations. Many older patients take medications that can affect cognition, and thus a medication review for adverse reactions and interactions is warranted. Medications with anticholinergic effects are a particular problem for patients with dementia, because they can worsen cognitive impairment and lead to delirium.

Psychoactive medications such as sedative/hypnotics and benzodiazepines can worsen cognition and cause CNS sedation. Any nonessential medications with CNS adverse events should be considered for dose reduction or discontinuation. When starting a new medication, it is generally best to start with low dosages and increase gradually ("start low and go slow") with the goal of identifying the lowest effective dosage. Before starting any treatment, a thorough medical examination should be conducted to identify and treat any underlying medical conditions that might impair cognition.

Cholinesterase Inhibitors (ChIs)

Three ChIs are approved by the FDA for treatment of AD: donepezil, rivastigmine, and galantamine. By slowing the breakdown of the neurotransmitter acetylcholine, which is associated with memory, these medications are thought to facilitate memory function.

In clinical trials, these medications demonstrated a modest delay in cognitive decline compared with placebo in patients with AD. Onset of behavioral problems and decline in ADLs is modestly delayed compared with treatment with placebo (SOE=A). In a Cochrane review of 10 randomized, double-blind, placebo-controlled trials, treatment for 6 months resulted in less decline of cognitive function on average -2.7 points (95% confidence interval, -3.0 to -2.3, $P<.00001$) on the 70-point Alzheimer's Disease Assessment Scale-Cognitive Subscale; there was also small improvement on measures of ADLs and behavior. Despite statistically significant findings of efficacy in research settings, clinical experience with these drugs has been less positive.

Results of studies of patients with dementing disorders other than AD are also becoming available. Some studies suggest that ChIs may be helpful in managing attention and behavioral disturbances (eg, hallucinations) associated with dementia with Lewy bodies (SOE=B), and one ChI, rivastigmine, is approved by the FDA for mild to moderate dementia in Parkinson disease. There appears to be no role for ChIs in treating frontotemporal dementia, and in fact, evidence suggests they may worsen agitation (SOE=B). Because effects are modest in all disorders, patients and families should be counseled to have realistic expectations, and discontinuation of medication should be considered after a reasonable time period if decline continues at the rate expected without treatment. Clinical evaluation after 3–6 months of therapy is suggested to assess response. In the case of long-term therapy with initial positive responses to treatment but continued advancement of cognitive decline, the question of discontinuation effect on cognition ultimately arises. If cognitive decline persists despite maximal treatment with ChIs, the clinician should discuss the risks and benefits of therapy with the patient and caregivers. Tapering the medication over time may be considered.

All three ChIs can be dosed once daily, either in oral form (donepezil and galantamine) or as a 24-hour patch (rivastigmine). Dosing adjustments should follow a slow titration curve to maximize the tolerable dosage while avoiding adverse events, such as nausea, diarrhea, insomnia, headaches, dizziness, orthostasis, and nightmares. However, a lower initial dosage and/or an even slower titration curve can help further mitigate adverse events if they occur, especially GI adverse events. High dose ChI (donepezil 23 mg/d or rivastigmine patch to 13.3 mg/24 hours) is FDA approved for severe dementia based on modest incremental cognitive benefit over lower doses but is unlikely to affect overall global functioning. It should only be used very selectively in patients in whom a modest enhancement of cognition will justify the observed increase in cholinergic adverse events (SOE=A). The most serious adverse event associated with ChIs is bradycardia. Because of limited direct comparisons, there is currently no evidence for any difference in efficacy among the ChIs.

Memantine

Memantine, an N-methyl-d-aspartate antagonist, has been used worldwide for many years. It is thought to have neuroprotective effects by reducing glutamate-mediated excitotoxicity. A Cochrane review of two 6-month studies showed minimal beneficial effects of memantine on measures of cognition, ADLs, and behavior (SOE=A). Memantine is approved by the FDA for treatment of moderate to severe AD. Research has not supported use in earlier stages of AD, and trials have yet to establish efficacy in other dementias. A Cochrane review and a meta-analysis of memantine in vascular dementia found limited effect on cognition and no evidence to recommend widespread use (SOE=A). The recommended dosage of memantine in management of Alzheimer-type dementia starts at 5 mg/d po, which may then be increased on a weekly basis in 5-mg increments to a target dosage of 20 mg/d dosed as 10 mg q12h after a 4-week titration period. For the extended-release formulation, the starting dosage of 7 mg/d can be increased to the maximal dosage of 28 mg/d over 3 weeks. The most common adverse events are constipation, dizziness, and headache. Memantine has been used safely as a single agent and in conjunction with ChIs for moderate to severe AD (SOE=B). Overall, as with ChIs, clinical experience with memantine has typically been disappointing.

Other Cognitive Enhancers

Ongoing studies are assessing a variety of other agents in AD, including antioxidants and *Ginkgo biloba* extract. In a trial including >300 patients with moderately severe AD, treatment with vitamin E (α-tocopherol) or the selective monoamine oxidase B inhibitor selegiline (approved for treatment of Parkinson disease) lowered rates of functional decline but was not associated with evidence of cognitive improvement. However, this study involved patients with moderate to severe dementia, so effects on cognition earlier in the illness remain unknown. Results from a randomized, placebo-controlled trial of vitamin E and donepezil in MCI showed some short-term benefit from donepezil in delaying conversion to AD but no effect of vitamin E.

Extract from the leaf of the *Ginkgo* tree has been promoted primarily in Europe for peripheral vascular disease as well as for "cerebral insufficiency." Other studies in Europe and the United States have explored its use in AD. However, a recent large, multicenter, randomized, double-blind, placebo-controlled trial in normal individuals and individuals with MCI did not show any slowing of cognitive decline in either population over a median follow-up of 6.1 years.

Nutrient-based interventions have failed to show any consistent, clinical benefit in improving cognition or function. Trials of antioxidants, B vitamins, omega-3 fatty acids, and medium-chain triglycerides have all been negative. There are also medical foods, approved by the FDA, that have been suggested to have some benefit with cognitive disorders. However, because these foods do not undergo the same rigorous evaluation process as drugs, more testing and extensive RCT studies are needed to provide clearer information on potential benefits.

Many patients also use OTC preparations for cognitive enhancement. A complete review of medications should always include questions about use of OTC medications.

Antidepressants

Antidepressant drug treatment is generally considered for AD patients with depressive symptoms, including depressed mood, appetite loss, insomnia, fatigue, irritability, and agitation. Of note, depression in persons with dementia may manifest as agitation, combativeness, and/or apathy that may be misattributed to the progression of dementia. A trial of high-dose citalopram demonstrated significant improvements in behaviors but also resulted in worsened cognition and QT prolongation. In addition, patients with dementia are at risk of falls, and the use of SSRIs and SNRIs can possibly exacerbate these risks, especially those with greater anticholinergic tone (eg, paroxetine).

Psychoactive Medications

Behavioral and psychologic symptoms of dementia such as paranoia, agitation, and irritability are best managed by nonpharmacologic strategies, such as distraction, redirection, physical activity, and reducing overstimulation. However, when medications are required, target symptoms should be identified, and therapy selected accordingly. The 2016 American Psychiatric Association practice guidelines in the use of antipsychotics in persons with dementia provides an evidence-based review that can help guide clinicians and caregivers. There is some limited evidence that first- and second-generation antipsychotics help control these symptoms, but recent trials have revealed that all antipsychotics increase the risk of "all-cause" mortality in the setting of dementia (SOE=A). Therefore, these medications must be used cautiously to manage delusions, hallucinations, and paranoia as well as some of the irritability associated with dementia. To help mitigate these risks, frequent attempts to taper off each medication should be undertaken (SOE=A). Medications such as carbamazepine[OL] and valproic acid[OL] are possible alternatives for managing irritability and agitation, but again both have limited evidence for effectiveness in dementia and can also be associated with increased mortality risk (SOE=B). The use of benzodiazepines and medications with anticholinergic effects should be avoided. Finally, antidepressants with sedating effects such as mirtazapine and trazodone can be considered in management of insomnia.

Other Resources

Most PCPs successfully treat and manage most patients with dementia, but referral to a specialist is sometimes necessary, especially for diagnosis of atypical presentations or uncontrolled behavioral symptoms. When the presentation or history is atypical or complex, particularly when the onset begins before age 60, consultation with a specialist in treating dementia patients (eg, geriatrician, geriatric psychiatrist, behavioral neurologist) can be helpful in establishing diagnosis, treatment, and prognosis. Geriatric specialists with psychology or psychiatry training can assist with behavioral management, particularly when patients are agitated, psychotic, or violent. They are also helpful when patients have concurrent major depressive disorder or when individual or family therapy is indicated for patients or caregivers.

A behavioral neurologist can be helpful for patients with early-onset/familial dementias, parkinsonism, focal neurologic signs, unusually rapid progression, or abnormal neuroimaging findings such as masses or ventricular dilatation suggesting possible normal pressure hydrocephalus. Neuropsychologic consultation can clarify diagnostically complex cases such as discrepancy between subjective memory complaints and performance in objective cognitive testing or in persons with low or high literacy levels.

Clinical psychologists can provide support and/or psychotherapy for caregivers suffering from stress or strain. Social workers can provide counseling and contact with community resources. Physical therapists can provide guidance on physical and group activity, and occupational therapists can assess the patient's functional level and suggest approaches to maximize functioning. Nurses can make management suggestions and guide behavior management, feeding, and other care issues. Pharmacists can perform medication reviews to minimize adverse drug events and can assist caregivers with practical advice on administration of medications to patients with dementia. Wills, conservatorships, estate planning, and other legal matters are best addressed with the assistance of an attorney, preferably one who specializes in elder law. Because dementia is a progressive disease, patients with early dementia should be offered an opportunity to plan for future incapacity and illness by having frank but sensitive discussion about goals of care.

Community support can be informal, in which neighbors or friends help out, or formal, through home-care or family service agencies, the aging or mental health networks, or adult daycare centers. Available specialized services include adult daycare and respite care, home-health agencies that can provide skilled nursing, help lines of the Alzheimer's Association, and outreach services offered by Area Agencies on Aging and Councils on Aging, which are mandated and funded under the federal Older Americans Act. Food services for the homebound are available from Meals-on-Wheels, and many senior citizens' centers, church and community groups, and hospitals offer transportation options. Clinicians who deliver care for persons with dementia need to have some familiarity with available community-based services for both patients and family caregivers. Referral to the local Alzheimer's Association chapter is a good starting point.

Choosing Wisely® Recommendations

Dementia

- Do not order APOE genetic testing as a predictive test for Alzheimer disease.

- Do not prescribe cholinesterase inhibitors for dementia without periodic assessment for perceived cognitive benefits and adverse GI effects.

- Do not routinely use antipsychotics as first choice to treat behavioral and psychological symptoms of dementia.

- Do not recommend percutaneous feeding tubes in patients with advanced dementia; instead offer oral assisted feeding.

RESOURCES

- Reus VI, Fochtmann LJ, Eyler AE, et.al. The American Psychiatric Association Practice Guideline on the Use of Antipsychotics to treat Agitation or Psychosis in Patients with Dementia. *Am J Psychiatry.* 2016;173(5):543–546.

- Scott J, Mayo AM. Instruments for detection and screening of cognitive impairment for older adults in primary care settings: A review. *Geriatr Nurs.* 2018;39(3):323–329.

- Treatment guidelines from The Medical Letter™ Drugs for Cognitive Loss and Dementia. *Med Lett Drugs Therap.* 2017;59(1530):155–161.

CHAPTER 38—BEHAVIORAL DISTURBANCES IN DEMENTIA

KEY POINTS

- Behavioral disturbances in dementia require evaluation of the specific symptoms, including the comfort of the patient, medical comorbidities, the environment of care, the needs of the caregiver, and the degree of distress of all those involved in the life of the adult with dementia.

- Delirium secondary to an underlying condition such as dehydration, urinary tract infection, or medication toxicity is a common cause of abrupt behavioral disturbances in patients with dementia.

- Nonpharmacologic interventions must be considered the first-line choice for all behavioral disturbances in dementia. These include caregiver education and support, patient-centered use of music, physical activity, support for activities of daily living, and cognitive stimulation programs.

- Pharmacologic treatment of behavioral disturbances in dementia is of limited efficacy and should be used only after environmental and nonpharmacologic interventions have been implemented.

- Increased mortality has been identified with the use of both first-generation antipsychotic agents such as haloperidol and perphenazine, as well as second-generation antipsychotic agents such as risperidone and olanzapine. All antipsychotic agents carry an FDA warning regarding increased all-cause mortality in patients with dementia. The absolute risk of mortality is likely between 1% and 2%.

- Despite these FDA warnings, antipsychotic medications may be needed for treatment of distressing delusions and hallucinations, and antidepressants may be helpful if symptoms of depression are evident. There is limited evidence for use of mood stabilizers for symptoms such as impulsivity and aggression in patients who have a significant behavioral disturbance.

Most dementias are associated with a range of behavioral and psychologic disturbances, with as many as 80%–90% of patients developing at least one distressing symptom over the course of their illness. The development of behavioral disturbances or psychotic symptoms in dementia often precipitates early nursing-home placement and causes significant caregiver burden and distress. These disturbances are potentially treatable, and it is vital that they are anticipated and recognized early. As these symptoms emerge, it is essential to perform a thorough evaluation of contributing factors, identify the target symptoms for treatment, and implement appropriate interventions for the patient and caregiver.

The *Diagnostic and Statistical Manual of Mental Disorders, Fifth Edition (DSM-5)* uses the term *neurocognitive disorders* to classify conditions of acquired cognitive loss but retains the term *dementia* for clinical and practical uses. ICD-10 continues to use the term dementia in its classifications.

Research that compares different treatment strategies for the behavioral and psychologic symptoms of dementia is growing in response to the great need for evidence-based guidelines. Some conclusions can be drawn from randomized controlled trials evaluating medications for the treatment of depression and psychosis, but these results are limited by marginal efficacy and FDA warnings regarding increased mortality among patients with dementia who are treated with antipsychotic agents. Interventions using behavioral treatment modalities have also been studied, with more robust outcomes in the ability to delay the need for nursing-home placement (SOE=A) and to improve quality of life among patients and caregivers (SOE=B). These studies have allowed for recommendations in many areas; however, many aspects of treatment must still draw on case reports and clinical experience.

CLINICAL FEATURES

Common behavioral and psychological symptoms of dementia include anxiety, apathy, depression, sleep disturbance, resistance to care, appetite changes, elation, irritability, disinhibition, wandering, hoarding, verbal disruptions, physical aggression, delusions, and hallucinations. Discrete psychiatric symptoms may develop that take on a variety of characteristics resembling mental disorders such as depression or mania; however, the course and features are more difficult to predict, and treatments are less reliably effective than when these symptoms occur in younger adults without dementia. Depressive symptoms are common and often manifest as sadness, tearfulness, or a lack of interest in previously enjoyed activities. This depressive syndrome can also include a loss of interest in self-care, eating, or interacting with peers.

A propensity for irritability and impulsivity can also occur. If these features become progressive, overt hostility or violence may ensue, and patients may be characterized as "agitated," reflecting a loss of the ability to modulate their behavior in a socially acceptable way. These behaviors may include verbal outbursts, physical aggression, resistance to bathing or other care needs, and restless motor activity such as pacing or rocking. Among the behavioral complications of dementia, the most severe disruptions in caregiving occur when patients develop physical behaviors such as hitting, scratching, or pushing, or when they develop paranoid delusions that lead to hostility and altercations with others. Paranoia may also prompt patients to mistrust food or medications provided by caregivers. This overlapping of symptoms, in which some are associated with a well-described psychiatric disorder but others such as wandering and hoarding are considered atypical, often creates a significant challenge in diagnostic labeling. In this situation, the nonspecific term *agitation* is commonly used to describe the patient, but it is too broad and nonspecific to be clinically useful and may best be accompanied by additional description as to whether the problem is accompanied by irritability, vocal or physical aggression, or motor disturbances. Assessment of disruptive behavior must include a careful description of the nature of the symptom, when it occurs, where it develops, and if any precipitants or antecedents are identified. Treatment cannot be provided without adequate assessment of the behavioral disturbance.

In many cases, behavioral disruption can occur concomitantly with evidence of paranoia or delusional thinking, such as a fixed false belief that caregivers have stolen possessions or money, or are plotting against the patient. When delusions occur, the patient is then characterized as suffering from "psychotic" symptoms. Sensory experiences without stimuli such as hallucinations are another type of psychotic symptom that can accompany episodes of agitated behavior. Depending on the degree of communication deficits in a given patient, the ability to discern the presence of psychosis is variable, and in many cases disruptive behaviors can occur without clear evidence as to whether delusions or other psychoses may be precipitating the disturbance. Antipsychotic medications are commonly used in management of disruptive behaviors, with the presumption that disturbed perceptions may be the underlying problem. There is little evidence to support this presumption, and there is increasing concern over both the lack of efficacy of antipsychotic agents for nonspecific symptoms of disruptive behavior and the risks of adverse events and mortality related to these medications in dementia.

Occasionally, a behavioral syndrome occurs that includes features of hyperactivity, mood lability, disinhibition, and grandiose beliefs that resemble a manic episode associated with bipolar affective disorder. The features of this "manic-like" syndrome are described below, and much like other mood symptoms in dementia, the features in older adults are similar but less predictable than those seen in younger adults; treatment strategies are also more challenging. One key feature of the manic-like syndromes seen in patients with dementia is the tendency to develop additional symptoms outside the typical course of a bipolar manic episode, such as resistance to care, stubbornness, wandering, and hoarding behaviors, as well as a significant degree of fluctuation in symptoms over the course of a single day. Additionally, the manic-like symptoms may not follow an episodic pattern that is typically seen with bipolar disorder.

The complaints from family caregivers and professional caregivers in a nursing home or assisted-living facility often arise from behavioral complications occurring during care, such as resistance to bathing, dressing, feeding, or other routines. Environmental precipitants such as excessive stimuli or a change in the environment (eg, a new roommate, frequent changes in staff and caregivers) can induce behavioral problems. A presenting complaint may relate to internal cues such as pain, hunger, thirst, or other needs that the patient is not able to express. Family members may feel more overwhelmed than professional caregivers and may consequently attribute more overall distress to these episodes. Overt resistance to care is most often seen in later stages of dementia, but behavioral problems can also be a first sign of incipient cognitive decline.

ASSESSMENT AND DIFFERENTIAL DIAGNOSIS

Comprehensive assessment includes a history from both the patient and an informant or other source. The information should include a clear description of the behavior: temporal onset, course, associated circumstances, and its relationship to key environmental factors such as caregiver status and recent stressors. The problem behaviors and symptoms should then be considered in the context of the patient's family and personal, social, and medical history.

Rating scales are available for the behavioral and psychologic symptoms of dementia. Some of these include the Cohen-Mansfield Agitation Inventory (CMAI), the Neuropsychiatric Inventory (NPI), and the Behavioral Pathology in Alzheimer Disease Rating Scale (BEHAVE-AD). These allow the clinician to note and quantify the symptoms based on a caregiver interview.

A differential diagnosis of the disturbance should proceed based on findings of a comprehensive geriatric evaluation. The first step is to decide whether the disturbance is a symptom of a new condition, of a preexisting medical problem, or of an adverse drug event. Disturbances that are new, acute in onset, or evolving rapidly are most often due to a medical condition or medication toxicity. An isolated behavioral disturbance in a patient with dementia can be the *sole* presenting symptom for many acute conditions such as pneumonia, urinary tract infection, gout flare, angina, constipation, electrolyte abnormalities, or poorly controlled diabetes mellitus. Additionally, the need to satisfy basic physical needs, such as hunger, sleepiness, thirst, boredom, or fatigue, which the patient cannot adequately communicate, can precipitate a behavioral disturbance. Sensory limitations in hearing or vision can also contribute to behavioral disruptions. Medication intolerance or toxicity, from either new or existing medications, may present solely with behavioral symptoms. Treatment or stabilization of the medical or physical cause is often sufficient to resolve the disturbance, but older adults with dementia may require several weeks longer to recover from routine medical problems than those who are cognitively intact.

The second step is to consider whether the behavioral disturbance is related to an environmental precipitant. These include disruptions in routine, time change (eg, with daylight savings time or travel across time zones), changes in the caregiving environment, new caregivers, a new roommate, or a life stressor (eg, death of a spouse or family member). Other common environmental precipitants include overstimulation (eg, too much noise, crowded rooms, close contact with too many people, too much time spent out of the familiar environment), understimulation (eg, relative absence of people, spending much time alone, use of television as a companion), and the disruptive behavior of other patients. For many disturbances, correcting an environmental precipitant or removing the stressor commonly improves the symptoms.

It can be useful to consider whether the disturbance results from stress in the patient-caregiver relationship. Caring for patients with dementia is difficult and requires a degree of perseverance of which most caregivers are capable, with guidance and support. Inexperienced caregivers, domineering caregivers, or caregivers who themselves are impaired by medical or psychiatric disturbances can exacerbate or cause a behavioral disturbance. Caregiver burden can be a problem both in community settings and in nursing homes. Assessing the level of stress and burden on the caregiver is an important part of the evaluation of behavioral disturbances. Interventions to improve the patient-caregiver relationship and to provide caregiver education and support are a vital part of treatment of behavioral disturbances in dementia. Providing resources to caregivers such as referral to support groups and respite services is often very helpful.

After medical, environmental, and caregiving causes are excluded, it is often concluded that the behavioral problem is a manifestation of the dementia and may not be amenable to a pharmacologic intervention. Some disturbances that are closely linked to the dementia syndrome take on the form of a *catastrophic reaction*. A catastrophic reaction is an acute behavioral, physical, or verbal reaction to environmental stressors that results from an inability to make routine adjustments in daily life. The reaction might include anger, emotional lability, or aggression when patients are confronted with a deficit, such as the inability to find a word, or confusion about where they are or what they are supposed to do. Catastrophic reactions are best treated by identifying and avoiding their precipitants, by providing structured routines and activities, and by recognizing early signs of the impending disturbance so that the patient can be distracted and supported before reacting.

If the disturbance is not related to an identifiable cause or environmental precipitant, it may be a consequence of the brain deterioration that occurs during the course of dementia. Disturbances with a more insidious onset or that are persistent are more likely to be symptoms of the underlying disease. Epidemiologic and clinical studies suggest that such disturbances fall into three groups: mood symptoms, psychosis, and specific behavior problems that occur without significant specific psychiatric symptoms. The overlap in the symptoms of these groups can make treatment choices difficult. One approach is to decide whether the predominant symptom of a polysymptomatic disturbance is psychosis (delusions or hallucinations), mood symptoms (dysphoria, sadness, irritability, lability), aggression, or behavioral disruption, and then direct treatment toward the most distressing feature.

Behavioral disturbances can occur in all types of dementias, including Alzheimer type, vascular, and mixed. Frontotemporal dementia is a less common type of dementia, often with a younger age of onset, associated with prominent disinhibition, compulsive behaviors, and social impairment due to more advanced frontal lobe degeneration. In severe cases of this dementia, a syndrome of hyperphagia, hyperactivity, and hypersexuality can occur that is related to bilateral temporal lobe atrophy. Another disorder associated with prominent psychiatric symptoms and behavioral disturbances is dementia with Lewy bodies. This form of dementia may be more common than previously thought. It is characterized by cognitive deterioration and parkinsonian features with prominent psychosis characterized by visual hallucinations. Affected older adults often suffer from distressing hallucinations and a fluctuating clinical course. These patients are extremely sensitive to the extrapyramidal adverse events of antipsychotic medications (eg, muscle rigidity and

Table 38.1—Behavioral Interventions for Dementia Care

- Evaluate and treat underlying medical conditions.
- Assess for new medical problems.
- Correct sensory deficits; replace poorly fitting hearing aids, eyeglasses, and dentures.
- Remove offending medications, particularly anticholinergic agents.
- Keep the environment comfortable, calm, and homelike with use of familiar possessions.
- Provide regular daily activities and structure; refer patient to adult daycare programs, if needed.
- Attend to patient's sleep and eating patterns; offer regular snacks and finger foods.
- Install safety measures to prevent accidents.
- Ensure that the caregiver has adequate respite.
- Educate caregivers about practical aspects of dementia care and about behavioral disturbances.
- Teach caregivers the skills of caregiving: communication skills, avoiding confrontational behavior management, techniques of support for activities of daily living, activities for dementia care.
- Simplify bathing and dressing with use of adaptive clothing and assistive devices if needed; offer toileting frequently, and anticipate incontinence as dementia progresses.
- Provide access to experienced professionals and community resources.
- Consult with caregiving professionals, such as geriatric case managers.
- Refer family and patient to local Alzheimer's Association.
- Encourage family caregivers to become "savvy caregivers" by enrolling in a multisession series by the Alzheimer's Association (www.alz.org). This evidence-based training enables caregivers to gain personal knowledge and skills, modify their caregiving outlook, understand the course of Alzheimer's and related disorders, and develop confidence in setting caregiving goals.

tremor) and often cannot tolerate even low dosages of second-generation antipsychotic medications.

TREATMENT APPROACH

The treatment of the psychiatric and behavioral disturbances in dementia is complex and may require several interventions as part of a comprehensive plan of care. Specialists should be consulted in refractory cases. In general, treatment begins with appropriate environmental and caregiver interventions. Caregiver education and support interventions have been useful in reducing distress and delaying the need for nursing home placement (SOE=A). Nonpharmacologic interventions should always be used as a first-line treatment in the management of disruptive, aggressive, or agitated behavior. For a list of key behavioral interventions that might ameliorate behavioral symptoms in patients with dementia, see Table 38.1. Maintaining a daily routine and introducing meaningful activities is vital. Behavioral disturbances in patients with dementia may decrease with the use of music, particularly during meals and bathing, and with light physical exercise or walking (SOE=B). Massage, pet therapy, white noise, videotapes of family, and cognitive stimulation programs may also be helpful. If the disturbances persist despite best efforts, pharmacologic interventions for specific target symptoms are often necessary.

TREATMENTS FOR SPECIFIC DISTURBANCES

The core of treatment is identifying any possible underlying cause of the behavior change, recognizing that multiple causes may exist. Managing pain, dehydration, hunger, and thirst is paramount. Other common culprits are uncomfortable physical positioning or nausea secondary to medication effects. Environmental modifications can improve patient orientation. Good lighting, one-on-one attention, supportive care, and attention to personal needs and wants can be important aspects of treatment. If there is sleep-wake cycle disturbance, efforts should be made to stabilize the sleep cycle by maintaining a consistent routine, using bright lights, or prescribing short-term use of medications.

Mood Disturbances

In patients with dementia who are experiencing mood symptoms, measures similar to those used in other behavioral disturbances should be implemented, ie, the environment should be optimized by reducing adverse stimuli, and physical health should be assessed comprehensively. Recreational programs and activity therapies have shown positive results in improving mood in depressive symptoms in dementia. Criteria for the diagnosis of depression in Alzheimer dementia have been proposed that note common features of irritability and social isolation or withdrawal. The waxing and waning course of mood symptoms in dementia is attributed to the cognitive loss and reduced communication skills related to the dementia. In patients with depression that lasts ≥2 weeks and that results in significant distress or functional impairment, a trial of an antidepressant medication should be strongly considered. Similarly, if depressive symptoms last >2 months after behavioral interventions have been implemented, treatment with antidepressant medications is warranted.

First-line agents are the SSRIs, preferred for their favorable adverse-event profiles. Studies of depression in patients with dementia have demonstrated the efficacy of sertraline and citalopram versus placebo (SOE=B), but other studies using the same medications as well as

Table 38.2—Medications to Treat Depressive Features of Behavioral Disturbances in Dementia

Medication	Dosage (mg/d)	Uses	Precautions
Selective serotonin reuptake inhibitors (SSRIs)			
Citalopram	10–20	Depression, anxiety[OL]	GI upset, nausea, insomnia (common among all SSRIs), risk of QT_c prolongation with doses >20 mg
Escitalopram	5–20	Depression, anxiety	
Fluoxetine	10–40	Depression, anxiety	Long half-life, greater inhibition of the cytochrome P-450 system, give in the morning (most stimulating of the SSRIs)
Paroxetine	10–40	Depression, anxiety	Greater inhibition of cytochrome P-450 system, some anticholinergic effects
Sertraline	25–100	Depression, anxiety	
Vilazodone	10–40	Depression, anxiety	Should be taken with food, dosage adjustment required in severe hepatic impairment, reduce dose to 20 mg if given with CYP3A4 inhibitors
Vortioxetine	5–10	Depression	Nausea, dizziness, fewer sexual adverse events than other SSRIs
Serotonin-norepinephrine reuptake inhibitors (SNRIs)			
Desvenlafaxine	25–50	Depression, fibromyalgia	Nausea, hypertension, dry mouth, headaches, dizziness
Duloxetine	20–60	Depression, diabetic neuropathy	Nausea, dry mouth, dizziness, hypertension
Mirtazapine	7.5–30	Useful for depression with insomnia and weight loss	Sedation, hypotension, potential for neutropenia
Venlafaxine	25–150	Useful in severe depression, anxiety	Hypertension may be a problem, insomnia
Tricyclic antidepressants (TCAs)			
Desipramine	10–100	Useful in severe depression, anxiety; high degree of efficacy	Anticholinergic effects, hypotension, sedation, cardiac arrhythmias (conduction delays)
Nortriptyline	10–75	High efficacy for depression if adverse events are tolerable; therapeutic range 50–150 ng/mL	Anticholinergic effects, hypotension, sedation, cardiac arrhythmias (conduction delays), caution in patients with glaucoma
Other			
Bupropion	75–225	More activating, lack of cardiac effects	Irritability, insomnia
Gabapentin	100–300	Anxiety[OL], insomnia[OL]	Sedation, falls, hypotension
Trazodone	25–150	When sedation is desirable	Sedation, falls, hypotension

paroxetine and fluoxetine have been inconclusive. For the antidepressants most commonly used to treat depressive symptoms in dementia, see Table 38.2. The FDA warns that there is a dose-dependent risk of QT prolongation with citalopram and advises that for patients >60 years old the maximum dose should be 20 mg/d.

The treatment of depression in dementia requires persistence. If a first agent has failed after administration of an adequate therapeutic dose for 8–12 weeks, an alternative agent should be tried. Venlafaxine, bupropion, mirtazapine, and the tricyclic agents desipramine and nortriptyline might be considered. Tricyclics should be avoided if a bundle-branch block or other significant cardiac conduction disturbance is present. For patients who have a partial response to an antidepressant, augmentation strategies can be considered. The addition of a stimulant such as methylphenidate[OL] (2.5–10 mg/d) may be helpful in some cases (SOE=C), but there is some risk of increasing psychotic symptoms if the patient tends to be suspicious or delusional. The addition of stimulants such as methylphenidate to augment bupropion should be avoided, because bupropion already has stimulant effects. If the patient does not improve, the agents should be tapered and discontinued. If a patient continues to be significantly depressed after several antidepressant trials and is in danger because of serious weight loss or suicidal ideas, consideration may be given to electroconvulsive therapy. This is the most efficacious and rapidly effective treatment for severe major depression and has a favorable safety profile even in mild dementia (SOE=B).

Common adverse effects of antidepressants include sedation, insomnia, GI upset, falls, and for

Table 38.3—Mood Stabilizers for Behavioral Disturbances in Dementia with Manic-like Features

Medication	Geriatric Dosage	Adverse Events	Comments
Carbamazepine[OL a,b]	200–1,000 mg/d (therapeutic level 4–12 mcg/mL)	Nausea, fatigue, ataxia, blurred vision, hyponatremia	Poor tolerability in older adults; monitor CBC, liver function tests, electrolytes every 2 weeks for first 2 months, then every 3 months
Lamotrigine[OL b]	25–200 mg/d	Skin rash, rare cases of Stevens-Johnson syndrome, dizziness, sedation, neutropenia, anemia	Increased adverse events and interactions when used with divalproex, slow-dose titration required
Lithium[OL a,b]	150–1,000 mg/d (therapeutic level 0.5–0.8 mEq/L)	Nausea, vomiting, tremor, confusion, leukocytosis	Poor tolerability in older adults; toxicity at low serum concentrations; monitor thyroid and renal function
Divalproex sodium[OL a,b]	250–2,000 mg/d (therapeutic level 50–100 mcg/mL)	Nausea, GI upset, ataxia, sedation, hyponatremia, tremor	Monitor CBC, platelets, liver function tests at baseline and every 6 months; better tolerated than other mood stabilizers in older adults

[a] Approved by FDA for treatment of bipolar disorder
[b] 2009 FDA warning regarding increase in suicidal thoughts and behaviors among all populations treated with anticonvulsant agents, including those used as mood stabilizers

tricyclic agents, cardiac adverse events. The serotonin-norepinephrine reuptake inhibitors venlafaxine, duloxetine, and desvenlafaxine may cause dose-related hypertension. Patients should be monitored for development of serotonin syndrome, a potentially fatal result of multiple or high-dose agents that increase synaptic availability of serotonin.

Manic-like Behavioral Syndromes

Occasionally, mood syndromes may develop in patients with dementia that are characterized by pressured speech, disinhibition, elevated or irritable mood, intrusiveness, hyperactivity, impulsivity, and reduced sleep. These syndromes frequently bear a resemblance to the manic episodes seen in the context of bipolar affective disorder in younger adults, although they are generally considered to be secondary to the dementing disorder. The important distinction in the patient with dementia is the frequent co-occurrence with confusional states and a tendency to have more of a fluctuating mood; the patient's mood may also be irritable or hostile as opposed to euphoric. The appearance of hypersexual behaviors may be seen in this clinical presentation, although sexual disinhibition frequently occurs with dementia as a consequence of reduced frontal-executive functioning and may not necessarily be part of a manic syndrome.

Treatment of manic-like states, emotional lability, disinhibition, or irritability typically begins with the use of mood-stabilizing agents such as divalproex sodium[OL] (Table 38.3). The sustained-release preparation divalproex sodium is commonly recommended (SOE=C). In patients with dementia, a typical starting dosage of divalproex is 125 mg q12h. The dosage should be titrated upward slowly while the patient is monitored for sedation, ataxia, and falls. Serum concentrations in the range of 50–100 mcg/mL have been shown to be effective, but individual variability in dosage and response is great. Because of the potential adverse effects on the liver and platelet counts (thrombocytopenia), transaminase levels and a CBC with platelets should be measured before therapy is started, rechecked with each dosage increase, and repeated at least every 6 months while the patient remains on the medication. Alternatives to divalproex sodium are carbamazepine[OL], lamotrigine[OL], or lithium[OL]. Carbamazepine starting at 100 mg q12h (with monitoring of liver enzymes and CBC) is an acceptable alternative for manic-like states, mood lability, or irritability in dementia. Leukopenia is of concern with carbamazepine, and monitoring the CBC with every dosage increase and at least every 3 months while the patient remains on the medication is needed. Lamotrigine is approved by the FDA for treatment of mania, but no trials have been conducted in older adults. Lithium is valuable as a mood stabilizer, but its use may be a problem in older adults because of enhanced sensitivity to adverse events. Increased lithium concentrations may occur in the context of reduced renal function and dehydration, resulting in ataxia, tremor, GI distress, and confusion.

Delusions and Hallucinations

Delusions (fixed false beliefs) or hallucinations (sensory experiences without stimuli), whether occurring independently or in association with mood syndromes, typically require specific pharmacologic treatment if the patient is disturbed by these experiences, or if the experiences lead to disruptions in the patient's environment that cannot otherwise be controlled. Clinical criteria for the diagnosis of Alzheimer dementia with psychosis specify that the presence of delusions

Table 38.4—Antipsychotic Medications for Treatment of Psychosis (Hallucinations and Delusions) in Dementia

Medication	Dosage (mg/d)	Adverse Events[a]	Formulations	Comments
Aripiprazole[OL]	2–20	Mild sedation, mild hypotension	Tablet, rapidly dissolving tablet, IM injection, liquid concentrate	Give in AM
Asenapine[OL]	5–10	Sedation	Sublingual tablet	Only sublingual use
Brexpiprazole[OL]	0.25–4	Respiratory tract infection, akathisia, weight gain	Tablet	Pharmacologic action similar to that of aripiprazole (partial D_2 dopamine agonist)
Clozapine[OL]	12.5–200	Sedation, hypotension, anticholinergic effects, agranulocytosis	Tablet, rapidly dissolving tablet	Weekly CBCs required; poorly tolerated by older adults; reserved for treatment of refractory cases
Haloperidol[OL]	0.5–3	Extrapyramidal symptoms, sedation	Tablet, liquid, IM injection, long-acting injection	First-generation agent
Iloperidone[OL]	1–12	Sedation, orthostatic hypotension	Tablet	Dosage reduction with use of CYP3A4 and CYP2D6 inhibitors
Lurasidone[OL]	40–80	Sedation	Tablet	Do not exceed 40 mg/d with CYP3A4 inhibitors
Olanzapine[OL]	2.5–15	Sedation, falls, gait disturbance	Tablet, rapidly dissolving tablet, IM injection	Weight gain, hyperglycemia
Paliperidone[OL]	1.5–12	Sedation, fatigue, GI upset, extrapyramidal symptoms	Sustained-release tablet, depot IM long-acting injection	Dosage reduction in renal impairment
Perphenazine[OL]	2–12	Extrapyramidal symptoms, sedation	Tablet	First-generation agent
Pimavanserin[OL]	17–34	Peripheral edema, nausea, constipation, confusion	Tablet	No dosage adjustment required in mild-moderate renal impairment; not advised in hepatic impairment; only approved for hallucinations and delusions associated with Parkinson disease psychosis
Quetiapine[OL]	25–200	Sedation, hypotension	Tablet, sustained-released tablet	Ophthalmologic examination recommended every 6 months
Risperidone[OL]	0.5–2	Sedation, hypotension, extrapyramidal symptoms with dosages >1 mg/d	Tablet, rapidly dissolving tablet, depot IM long-acting injection, liquid concentrate	
Ziprasidone[OL]	40–160	Higher risk of QT_c prolongation	Capsule, IM injection	Risk of increased QT_c prolongation; little published information on use in older adults

[a] All listed medications have warnings about hyperglycemia, cerebrovascular events, and increase in all-cause mortality in patients with dementia.

or hallucinations occur for at least 1 month, at least intermittently, and must cause distress for the patient. For a listing of potentially useful antipsychotic drugs, along with dosing information, see Table 38.4. The second-generation agents risperidone[OL], olanzapine[OL], quetiapine[OL], and aripiprazole[OL] are used more commonly than first-generation agents such as haloperidol[OL]. The first-generation agents are more likely to cause extrapyramidal adverse events, such as parkinsonism and tardive dyskinesia. Sedation, hypotension, and falls are common adverse events with all antipsychotic agents.

As these medications are more widely used, differences in adverse-event profiles are emerging. The FDA has required that warnings regarding diabetes mellitus, hyperglycemia, ketoacidosis, and hyperosmolar states be included as a risk of therapy with all second-generation antipsychotic agents.

Clozapine[OL], the first of the second-generation agents to be introduced, is difficult to use because of the need for weekly CBC monitoring, adverse events of sedation and orthostatic hypotension, and risk of agranulocytosis. Another risk of clozapine relates to the influence of various substances (certain antibiotics, even cigarettes) on its metabolism. Despite these concerns, the drug can still be helpful in treating a small group of patients with psychosis associated with Parkinson dementia or dementia with Lewy bodies who are unable to tolerate the extrapyramidal adverse events of other agents; quetiapine can also be used in this situation. Clinicians must be prepared to monitor for the emergence of adverse effects among all patients treated with antipsychotic agents and to counsel caregivers regarding the possible adverse effects of these medications before treatment is started.

An increased risk of cerebrovascular events in patients with dementia was identified with use of second-generation agents in 2002. All such agents, including risperidone, olanzapine, aripiprazole, quetiapine, clozapine, ziprasidone, and paliperidone must carry this warning. It should be noted that most cerebrovascular events were not fatal.

In 2005, the FDA required that the manufacturers of aripiprazole[OL], olanzapine[OL], quetiapine[OL], risperidone[OL], clozapine[OL], and ziprasidone[OL], and all additional second-generation antipsychotic agents add a "black box" warning to their labeling describing an increased risk of mortality; this was was observed in 17 placebo-controlled studies (SOE=A), in which the rate of death for patients with dementia was approximately 1.6–1.7 times that for patients given placebo. In most cases, the cause of death appeared to be cardiac or infectious (eg, pneumonia). All new second-generation agents, including rapid-release clozapine and paliperidone, must carry this warning. Based on two observational studies, in 2008, the FDA required that all first-generation antipsychotic agents also have a "black box" warning regarding an increase in all-cause mortality among patients with dementia who are treated with these agents (SOE=B). The mechanism of action of the increase in mortality is not understood, and the FDA has stated that it is not indicating that clinicians should never use these agents to treat patients with dementia and psychosis. It is strongly suggested that clinicians discuss the risks and benefits of treatment with these agents with families and caregivers before starting therapy. More information on these warnings is available at www.fda.gov.

Although antipsychotic agents have demonstrated efficacy in large controlled trials in the treatment of dementia with psychosis and aggression, overall positive effects have been relatively modest (SOE=B). Controlled studies of older adult patients have had very high placebo responses. Although 45%–55% of patients improved on antipsychotic medications, the response to placebo ranged from 30% to 50% across studies. Studies of several antipsychotic agents show that risperidone and aripiprazole may be more effective than placebo for symptoms such as anger, aggression, and paranoid ideation when used for ≤12 weeks (SOE=B). However, use of antipsychotic agents did not appear to improve functional status, care needs, or quality of life.

Pimavanserin is an atypical antipsychotic with a unique mechanism of action as a selective inverse agonist of serotonin but no significant interactions with dopamine receptors. In phase 3 clinical trials, pimavanserin showed significant improvement of hallucinations and delusions in Parkinson disease psychosis, which led to its approval for this indication in 2016.

Antipsychotic agents clearly play an important role in the treatment of delusions, hallucinations, and aggression in dementia, but they must be part of a comprehensive treatment plan that includes frequent dosage evaluation, monitoring of adverse effects, and time-limited treatment.

There is some evidence that cholinomimetic agents such as donepezil or galantamine may reduce the onset of psychosis and behavioral disturbances of Alzheimer disease. Studies comparing these agents with placebo in patients with mild to moderate Alzheimer disease have suggested that they may reduce the rate of emergence of behavioral disturbances and psychosis (SOE=B). One area in which cholinesterase inhibitors may be likely to improve psychosis is in the case of dementia with Lewy bodies. Reduced visual hallucinations have been reported with cholinesterase inhibitor treatment (SOE=C). Galantamine[OL] in dosages of 16–24 mg/d may be useful in the treatment of patients with Lewy body dementia, who are uniquely sensitive to the extrapyramidal adverse events of antipsychotic agents. More recent studies including patients with Alzheimer dementia and behavioral disturbances failed to demonstrate that agents such as donepezil or memantine were effective in reducing behavioral and psychologic disturbances once the symptoms were present. Benzodiazepines are generally avoided because of concerns about causing disinhibition with increased agitation in older patients and patients with dementia.

Disturbances of Sleep

Treatment of insomnia and sleep-wake cycle disturbance should begin with improvement of sleep hygiene (Table 38.5). This consists of efforts to get the patient to go to sleep later every day, around 10:00 or 11:00 pm, while keeping the environment calm, comfortable, and conducive to sleep, into the next morning. If the sleep disturbance is associated with depression, suspiciousness, or delusions, those conditions should be treated.

For primary sleep disturbances when good sleep hygiene and increasing daytime activity level are not successful, trazodone^{OL} (25–50 mg at bedtime) or mirtazapine^{OL} (7.5–15 mg at bedtime) can be used (SOE=D). Gabapentin^{OL} is used because of its sedative properties, but there are concerns because of adverse effects of ataxia and confusion (SOE=D). Benzodiazepines or antihistamines, such as diphenhydramine, should be avoided, because they carry a high risk of falls, hip fractures, disinhibition, and cognitive disturbance when prescribed for patients with dementia.

Zolpidem^{OL} and zaleplon^{OL} are short-acting nonbenzodiazepine sedative hypnotics that may be helpful for sleep disturbances in older adults, although there have been no controlled trials for their use in patients with dementia. Use of zolpidem is associated with increased falls and fractures. Zaleplon has also been studied in older patients and appears to have properties similar to those of zolpidem.

Melatonin is available OTC and has been found to be helpful in some older adults with sleep problems. It has a relatively benign adverse-event profile (SOE=C).

Inappropriate Sexual Behavior

Inappropriate sexual behavior includes exposing oneself, touching, or grabbing in a sexually aggressive manner. When evaluating this behavior, it is imperative to first exclude treatable causes such as underlying urinary tract infections or other general medical conditions. Simple solutions like changes in bedding, providing adaptive clothing, following a toileting schedule, and providing comfort measures may reduce the incidence of inappropriate sexual behaviors. If this occurs in association with another recognizable syndrome such as a mania-like state, treatment of the specific syndrome, such as with mood stabilizers, should be undertaken. SSRIs have also been used for sexual behavioral issues in patients with dementia with variable results (SOE=D).

In men with dementia who are dangerously hypersexual or aggressive, clinical case reports have suggested that a trial of an antiandrogen might be attempted to reduce the sexual drive (SOE=D). Patients have been tried on medroxyprogesterone^{OL} starting at 5 mg/d. The dosage should be adjusted to suppress serum testosterone well below normal. If the patient responds well behaviorally, 100–600 mg of depot intramuscular medroxyprogesterone may be given weekly to maintain reduced sexual drive. An alternative treatment to reduce sexual drive is the antiadrogen leuprolide acetate^{OL} (5–10 mg IM every month). Antipsychotic medications are often used empirically, given the seriousness of hypersexual behaviors in institutionalized settings such as nursing homes; however, there are no controlled studies supporting

Table 38.5—Behavioral Management of Insomnia in Patients with Dementia

- Establish a stable routine for going to bed and awakening.
- Advise and educate caregivers regarding the natural fragmented sleep patterns associated with dementia.
- Optimize sleep environment (attention to noise, light, temperature).
- Increase daytime activity, use of regular light exercise and exposure to natural sunlight.
- Reduce or eliminate caffeine, nicotine, alcohol.
- Reduce evening fluid consumption to minimize nocturia.
- Give activating medications (eg, steroids) early in the day.
- Control nighttime pain.
- Limit daytime napping to periods of 20–30 min.
- Use relaxation, stress management, breathing techniques to promote natural sleep.
- Provide a safe environment for the patient to stay awake if unable to sleep.

this use. Presumably, these medications may enhance the cognitive focus of the individual's perceptions by reducing any psychotic thinking that may be contributing to hypersexual behavior. Although study of nonpharmacologic interventions is needed for this problem, it is suggested that behavioral, environmental, and educational domains be considered before medication use. Behavioral modifications may include distraction, or switching to another stimulating activity such as socializing, exercise, or eating. Environmental modifications may include switching the sex of the staff member working directly with the patient and avoiding overstimulating television. Finally, patients, caregivers, and staff should be offered sex-education programs that emphasize the need for healthy sexual expression while minimizing inappropriate sexual conduct.

Intermittent Aggression or Agitation

When disruptive behavior occurs intermittently or episodically, such as once per week or less, behavioral interventions focusing on identifying the antecedents of the behavior and avoiding the triggers are often most useful. Behavior modification using positive reinforcement of desirable behavior has been shown to be helpful, and it also helps encourage the caregiver to focus on times when behavior is not a problem. Caregiver education and support, music therapy, and physical activity appear to show promise in reducing behavioral disturbances (SOE=B). Reminiscence, validation therapy, and environmental modifications (ie, of light, sound, and space) may all help promote positive behavior. Distraction techniques, activity therapies, and aromatherapy also show promise in reducing troublesome behaviors (SOE=C).

The combination agent dextromethorphan-quinidine is being studied for the treatment of generalized agitation in multiple types of dementia. Early studies show promise but are limited.

Physical restraint in any form should be avoided if at all possible. Every attempt should first be made to understand the underlying reason for the aggression and agitation and to address the problem or change the approach to care. If restraining measures are necessary for the safety of the patient or others around them, careful supportive care with frequent monitoring of the patient should be provided. Over time, it is usually possible to reduce or eliminate the amount of restraint.

Choosing Wisely® Recommendations

Behavioral Problems in Dementia

- Do not use antipsychotics as first choice to treat behavioral and psychological symptoms of dementia.

RESOURCES

- De Giorgi R, Series H. Treatment of inappropriate sexual behavior in dementia. *Curr Treat Options Neurol.* 2016;18(9):41.

- Phillips LJ, Birtley NM, Petroski GF, et al. An observational study of antipsychotic medication use among long-stay nursing home residents without qualifying diagnoses. *J Psychiatr Ment Health Nurs.* 2018;25(8):463–474.

- Solmi M, Murru A, Pacchiarotti I, et al. Safety, tolerability, and risks associated with first- and second-generation antipsychotics: a state-of-the-art clinical review. *Ther Clin Risk Manag.* 2017;13:757–777.

CHAPTER 39—DELIRIUM

KEY POINTS

- The *Diagnostic and Statistical Manual of Mental Disorders, Fifth Edition (DSM-5)* criteria characterize delirium as a disorder of attention and awareness that develops acutely and tends to fluctuate.

- The first key step in delirium management is accurate diagnosis; several brief diagnostic assessments are available that operationalize the Confusion Assessment Method diagnostic algorithm after administration of a brief mental status examination that includes testing attention.

- All delirious patients require a thorough evaluation for reversible causes; all correctable contributing factors should be addressed.

- Delirium is associated with numerous poor outcomes, including death, functional decline, nursing home placement, prolonged cognitive decline, and dementia.

- Pharmacologic intervention should be reserved for target symptoms that are a threat to safety or disrupt needed medical care and cannot be adequately managed with nonpharmacologic interventions; low-dose, high-potency antipsychotics are usually the treatment of choice.

- Prevention of delirium is more effective than treatment. Proactive, multifactorial interventions have reduced the incidence, severity, and duration of delirium.

Delirium has been described in the medical literature for more than two thousand years. Despite this, it remains underrecognized and often inappropriately evaluated and managed. Clinicians call delirium by many different names; up to 30 synonyms exist in the peer-reviewed literature. *Acute confusional state* is the most common synonym and the term still preferred today by some specialties, such as neurology. Other common synonyms include *acute mental status change*, *altered mental status*, and *toxic* or *metabolic encephalopathy*.

INCIDENCE AND PROGNOSIS

Delirium is common and associated with substantial morbidity and mortality. Approximately one-third of patients ≥70 years old admitted to a general medical service experience delirium: one-half of these are delirious on admission to the hospital, while the other half develop delirium in the hospital. Among those admitted to ICUs, the prevalence of delirium is much higher, and when rates for delirium are combined with those for stupor and coma, prevalence rates exceed 75%. Ten to fifteen percent of older adults presenting to the emergency department are delirious. In post-acute skilled-nursing facilities, approximately 15% of new admissions meet criteria for delirium. The prevalence of delirium at the end of life is reported to be as high as 85%, while the overall prevalence in the community is reported to be 1%–2%, largely among older patients recently discharged from the hospital.

Although traditionally viewed as a transient phenomenon, delirium, or residual symptoms of delirium (termed "attenuated delirium" in *DSM-5*), may persist for weeks to months in a substantial portion of affected individuals (SOE=A). Risk factors for delirium persistence predominantly relate to preexisting patient factors, such as advanced age, dementia, multiple comorbidities, and functional impairment, but also include severity of delirium and use of restraints.

Delirium is strongly and independently associated with poor patient outcomes (SOE=A). A meta-analysis that included almost 3,000 patients followed for a mean of 22.7 months demonstrated that delirium was independently associated with an increased risk of death (OR 2.0; 95% CI, 1.5–2.5), institutionalization (OR 2.4; 95% CI, 1.8–3.3), and dementia (OR 12.5; 95% CI, 11.9–84.2). Further, rates of mortality, nursing-home placement, functional decline, and dementia are consistently higher in patients with persistent delirium than in patients whose delirium resolves more quickly.

DIAGNOSIS AND DIFFERENTIAL DIAGNOSIS

Underrecognition of delirium is a major problem, with less than half of all cases recognized in routine care. Several systematic reviews have recommended the Confusion Assessment Method (CAM) as the most useful bedside assessment tool for delirium (www.hospitalelderlifeprogram.org). Clinicians can establish the diagnosis of delirium by judging the presence or absence of the 4 CAM diagnostic features: 1) acute change or fluctuating course, 2) inattention, 3) disorganized thinking, and 4) altered level of consciousness. The diagnosis of delirium requires the presence of features 1) and 2), and either 3) or 4). Although the CAM can be completed by using observations from routine care, use of a formal mental status evaluation greatly improves detection and reliability of the assessment. CAM has been modified to CAM-ICU and B-CAM for diagnostic accuracy in a particular setting (eg, ICU, emergency department, general medicine service). 3D-CAM and 4AT have been developed for brevity.

To improve recognition of delirium, medical centers are starting to use these standardized tools to evaluate high-risk patients, such as those in the ICU or who have had major surgery or are very old. Such case finding is particularly important for identifying hypoactive delirium, which might otherwise go unnoticed by the care team. Even shorter "ultra-brief" screening tools, which consist of only 1 or 2 questions and can be completed in <1 minute, may be useful for widespread screening of lower-risk patients. For instance, the 2-item combination of asking patients to recite the months of the year backward and to state the day of the week (either question incorrect is a "positive" screen) achieved 93% sensitivity and 64% specificity for delirium. All such ultra-brief tools are sensitive but not specific, and a positive screen requires further evaluation, such as with one of the diagnostic tools described above, to confirm the presence of delirium.

Despite growing interest in widespread screening for delirium, there is no consensus on how to best implement this strategy. It could be performed by physicians, nurses, or other hospital personnel; if performed by personnel other than the patient's physician or nurse, the results need to be promptly and reliably communicated to the primary care team to allow for timely intervention. Importantly, there is currently no evidence that widespread screening for delirium improves patient outcomes (SOE=D). Improved delirium identification could either improve or worsen patient outcomes, depending on what interventions follow. To improve outcomes, screening needs to be coupled with education on best practices of delirium evaluation and management (see below).

The differential diagnosis of delirium includes dementia, depression, and acute psychiatric syndromes. In many cases, it is not truly a "differential" diagnosis, because these syndromes can coexist and indeed are risk factors for one another. Instead, it is better thought of as a series of independent questions: Does this patient have delirium? Does he or she have dementia? Does he or she have depression? Does the patient have more than one disorder? The most common diagnostic issue is whether a newly presenting confused patient has dementia, delirium, or both. To make this determination, the clinician must ascertain the patient's baseline status. In the absence of prior knowledge or documentation of the patient's baseline cognitive function, information from family members, caregivers, or others who know the patient is essential. An acute change in mental status from baseline is not consistent with dementia and suggests delirium. In addition, a rapidly fluctuating course (over minutes to hours) and an abnormal level of consciousness are also highly suggestive of delirium. Depression can also be confused with hypoactive delirium. Finally, certain acute psychiatric syndromes, such as mania, can present similarly to hyperactive delirium. Hyperactive patients are best initially evaluated and managed as if they have delirium rather than attributing the presentation to psychiatric disease and potentially missing a serious underlying medical disorder.

THE SPECTRUM AND NEUROPATHOPHYSIOLOGY OF DELIRIUM

The classic presentation of delirium is thought to be the extremely agitated patient. However, agitated, hyperactive, or mixed delirium represents only 25% of cases, with the remaining having hypoactive ("quiet") delirium. Evidence suggests that hypoactive delirium is associated with an equal or poorer prognosis than delirium with hyperactive or normal psychomotor features (SOE=B). Potentially, one of the reasons for this poorer prognosis is that hypoactive delirium is less frequently recognized. As described above, special case-finding efforts are necessary to detect hypoactive delirium among high-risk older adults. If agitation is present, behavioral interventions may be necessary (see below), but such measures alone are not adequate treatment for delirium, and, in some cases, they can exacerbate or prolong delirium.

Although delirium is often said to be either present or absent, the number and severity of symptoms vary widely. To more completely describe delirium, several severity scales have been validated and published. One such scale, termed CAM-Severity (or CAM-S), is derived directly from the CAM and has both a long form that uses all 10 CAM delirium features (scored 0–19, 19 worst) and a short form that uses only the 4 CAM diagnostic features (scored 0–7, 7 worst). The CAM-S has excellent predictive validity (incremental beyond diagnosis) for several important clinical and health utilization outcomes. Short-form severity scales have also recently been published for use with the 3D-CAM and CAM-ICU.

Patients who have some delirium features, but do not meet all diagnostic criteria, have subsyndromal delirium, which is renamed "attenuated delirium" in *DSM-5*. Attenuated delirium can occur during onset or recovery from delirium, or in those who never develop full syndromal delirium. The latter entity has been associated with poor outcomes, although not as serious as full delirium. There is a gradient of worsening outcomes over the spectrum of delirium.

Table 39.1—Mnemonic for Reversible Causes of Delirium

Drugs	Any new additions, increased dosages, or interactions Consider OTC drugs and alcohol Consider especially high-risk drugs (Table 39.3)
Electrolyte disturbances	Especially dehydration, sodium imbalance Thyroid abnormalities
Lack of drugs	Withdrawals from chronically used sedatives, including alcohol and sleeping pills Poorly controlled pain (lack of analgesia)
Infection	Especially urinary and respiratory tract infections
Reduced sensory input	Poor vision, poor hearing (lack of glasses, hearing aids in the hospital)
Intracranial	Infection, hemorrhage, stroke, tumor
Urinary, fecal	Urinary retention: "cystocerebral syndrome" Fecal impaction
Myocardial, pulmonary	Myocardial infarction, arrhythmia, exacerbation of heart failure, exacerbation of COPD, hypoxia, hypercarbia

RISK FACTORS

In the absence of a clear neuropathophysiologic basis for delirium, the cornerstone of management of delirium focuses on the assessment and treatment of modifiable risk factors. Several consistent risk factors for delirium have been identified and classified into two groups: baseline factors that predispose patients to delirium, and acute factors that precipitate delirium. Predisposing factors include advanced age, preexisting dementia, preexisting functional impairment in ADLs, and multimorbidity. Male gender, sensory impairment (poor vision and hearing), depressive symptoms, laboratory abnormalities, and history of alcohol abuse have also been reported in some studies. Acute precipitating factors include medications (especially those that are sedating or highly anticholinergic), surgery, uncontrolled pain, low hematocrit level, bed rest, and use of certain indwelling devices and physical restraints. A useful model suggests that delirium develops when the sum of predisposing and precipitating factors crosses a certain threshold. In such a model, the greater the predisposing factors, the fewer precipitating factors are needed for delirium to develop. This would explain why older, frail adults develop delirium in the face of stressors that are much less severe than stressors that can cause delirium in younger, healthy adults. In some frail older adults, particularly those with dementia, even an environmental change (eg, trip to unfamiliar surroundings) may be enough to precipitate delirium. For a mnemonic for reversible risk factors for delirium, see Table 39.1.

DELIRIUM AND DEMENTIA

The links between delirium and dementia are strong and likely bidirectional. Dementia is an established and perhaps the strongest predisposing risk factor for delirium (SOE=A). Recent evidence suggests that individuals with mild cognitive impairment also have an increased risk of delirium after elective surgery (RR=1.9; 95% confidence interval (CI), 1.3–2.7) (SOE=B). Moreover, delirium is emerging as an important risk factor for cognitive decline and dementia. As described above, a meta-analysis demonstrated that nondemented patients who develop delirium are at increased risk of incident dementia over the next 1–5 years (SOE=B). Complementing these studies in nondemented patients is a growing body of literature demonstrating that patients with Alzheimer disease experience accelerated cognitive decline after an episode of delirium (SOE=B).

A growing body of literature provides evidence that delirium may exert a negative long-term impact on cognitive function. One study examined the 1-year cognitive trajectories of older cardiac surgery patients and found that delirium is associated with an acute decline in cognitive function and persistent deficits. Patients who did not develop delirium returned to their preoperative cognitive baseline by 1 month after surgery, whereas those with delirium had not returned to baseline 1 year after surgery. In a second study that measured cognitive function in survivors of an ICU stay 1 year later, 24% of these patients were functioning at or below the level of patients with mild Alzheimer disease. This study was not restricted to older adults, and this level of cognitive dysfunction was seen in all age groups (as young as 18–45 years) and all levels of comorbidity. Finally, a study of older patients without dementia undergoing elective surgery found that delirium was associated with accelerated decline in cognitive function for at least 3 years after surgery, and that the most severe delirium was associated with the fastest long-term decline. Taken together, this evidence suggests that efforts to prevent and treat delirium (see below) may have a significant public health impact by reducing the burden of cognitive impairment among older adults (SOE=B).

POSTOPERATIVE DELIRIUM

Delirium may be the most common complication after surgery in older adults. The incidence is 15% after elective noncardiac surgery and up to 50% after high-risk procedures such as hip fracture repair, aortic aneurysm repair, and coronary artery bypass grafting. In a prospectively validated clinical prediction rule for delirium after elective noncardiac surgery, 7 risk factors were identified preoperatively: advanced age, cognitive impairment, physical functional impairment, history of alcohol abuse, markedly abnormal serum chemistries, intrathoracic surgery, and aortic aneurysm surgery. Patients with none of these risk factors had a 2% risk of delirium, those with 1 or 2 risk factors had a 10% risk, and those with ≥3 risk factors had a 50% risk. A clinical prediction rule for delirium after cardiac surgery has also been validated; 4 risk factors were identified: cognitive impairment, history of stroke or transient ischemic attack, depressive symptoms, and low or high albumin.

In addition to baseline risk factors, intraoperative and postoperative management plays an important role in the development of delirium. Multiple studies demonstrate that the type or route of intraoperative anesthesia, whether general, spinal, epidural, or combined, has little impact on the risk of delirium (SOE=A). However, the total dose of anesthetic agents may play an important role (SOE=B) and efforts to reduce or titrate this dose to the lowest effective amount may reduce delirium. For instance, a randomized trial used Bispectral Index™ monitoring to titrate the dosage of intraoperative sedative medications among hip-fracture patients undergoing surgical repair using spinal anesthesia. Patients in the low-dose arm had a markedly reduced rate of postoperative delirium relative to the high-dose arm (19% versus 40%, $P<.01$).

Postoperative medication management also plays an important role in delirium. Postoperative use of benzodiazepines and certain opioids, especially meperidine, is strongly associated with development of delirium. Although pain medications can cause delirium, adequate pain management is also important, because high levels of postoperative pain have been associated with delirium. Strategies to provide adequate analgesia with minimally effective doses of opioids should be used. These include the use of scheduled rather than as-needed dosing, patient-controlled analgesic pumps, regional analgesia, opioid-sparing analgesics, and nonpharmacologic approaches, such as ice packs. Low postoperative hematocrit level (<30%) has also been associated with postoperative delirium, although transfusions have not been shown to reduce delirium. The AGS recently published delirium management guidelines focused on surgical patients (see below).

Postoperative cognitive dysfunction (POCD) is a phenomenon that has received considerable attention. As opposed to delirium, POCD does not have *DSM-5* or ICD diagnostic criteria. POCD is usually defined by declining performance on serial testing with a neurocognitive battery, although there is no consensus as to the battery that should be used, when it should be administered, or what threshold of decline constitutes POCD. New guidelines have been published, in which POCD is renamed postoperative neurocognitive disorder, to align with the new terminology for dementia. Additionally, these guidelines suggest that cognition not be assessed for at least 1 month after surgery to allow residual symptoms of delirium to clear.

Interestingly, many studies of POCD have not included good measures of delirium, and many studies of postoperative delirium do not measure POCD. Results from the more recent studies that have both measures well integrated suggest that delirium and POCD are associated but do not fully explain each other, ie, some patients with delirium do not go on to develop POCD, and some patients who develop POCD did not have delirium. Ongoing studies will further elucidate the complex relationship between these 2 entities.

EVALUATION

All patients with newly diagnosed delirium require a careful history, physical examination, and targeted laboratory testing. Most treatable causes of delirium lie outside the CNS, and these should be investigated first. Moreover, multiple contributing factors are often present, so the diagnostic evaluation should not be terminated because a single "cause" is identified. For key steps in the evaluation and management of delirium, see Table 39.2.

The history should focus on the time course of the changes in mental status and their association with other symptoms or events (eg, fever, shortness of breath, medication change). Because medications are the most common and treatable cause of delirium, a careful medication history, using the nursing administration sheets in the hospital or a "brown-bag" review in the outpatient setting, is imperative. In the outpatient setting, it is also important to review the patient's use of OTC drugs, herbal or other supplements, and alcohol. The physical examination should include vital signs and oxygen saturation, a careful general medical examination, and a neurologic examination to assess for new focal findings. The emphasis should be on identifying acute medical problems or exacerbations of chronic medical problems that might be contributing to delirium.

Laboratory tests and imaging studies should be selected based on the history and examination findings. Most patients require at least a CBC, electrolytes, and kidney function tests. Urinalysis, urine toxicology

Table 39.2—Management of Delirium

Step	Key Issues	Proposed Treatment
Identify and treat reversible contributors	Medications	Reduce or eliminate offending medications, or substitute less psychoactive medications.
	Infections	Treat common infections: urinary, respiratory, soft tissue.
	Fluid balance disorders	Assess and treat dehydration, heart failure, electrolyte disorders.
	Impaired CNS oxygenation	Treat severe anemia, hypoxia, hypotension.
	Severe pain	Assess and treat; use local measures and scheduled pain regimens that minimize opioids; avoid meperidine.
	Sensory deprivation	Use eyeglasses, hearing aids, portable amplifier.
	Elimination problems	Assess and treat urinary retention and fecal impaction.
Manage distressing or disruptive behaviors	Behavioral interventions	Teach hospital staff appropriate interaction with delirious patients; encourage family visitation.
	Pharmacologic interventions	Only if necessary, use low-dose high-potency antipsychotics (Table 39.5).
Anticipate and prevent or manage complications	Urinary incontinence	Implement scheduled toileting program.
	Immobility and falls	Avoid physical restraints; mobilize with assistance; use physical therapy.
	Pressure injury	Mobilize; reposition immobilized patient frequently and monitor pressure points.
	Sleep disturbance	Implement a nonpharmacologic sleep hygiene program, including a nighttime sleep protocol; avoid sedatives; minimize unnecessary awakenings (for vital signs, etc).
	Feeding disorders	Assist with feeding; use aspiration precautions; provide nutritional supplementation as necessary.
Restore function	Hospital environment	Reduce clutter and noise (especially at night); provide adequate lighting; have familiar objects brought from home.
	Cognitive reconditioning	Have staff reorient patient to time, place, person at least three times daily.
	Ability to perform ADLs	As delirium clears, match performance to ability.
	Family education, support, and participation	Provide education about delirium, its causes and reversibility, how to interact, and family's role in restoring function.
	Discharge	Because delirium can persist, provide for increased ADL support; follow mental status changes as "barometer" of recovery.

for drugs of abuse, blood alcohol level, tests for liver function, serum medication levels, arterial blood gases, as well as chest radiographs, an ECG, and appropriate cultures are helpful in selected situations. Cerebral imaging is often performed but is rarely helpful, except in cases of head trauma or new focal neurologic findings. In the absence of seizure activity or signs of meningitis, electroencephalograms and cerebrospinal fluid analysis rarely yield helpful results.

MANAGEMENT

Delirious hospitalized patients are particularly vulnerable to complications and poor outcomes. Special care is needed and requires an interprofessional effort by clinicians, nurses, family members, and others. A multifactorial approach is the most successful, because many factors contribute to delirium; thus, multiple interventions, even if individually small, can yield marked clinical improvement (Table 39.2). If delirium is not diagnosed and managed properly, costly and life-threatening complications and long-term loss of function can result.

Modifying the risk factors that contribute to delirium is critically important. Some factors, such as age and prior cognitive impairment, cannot be modified. However, some predisposing factors, such as sensory impairment, can be modified through proper use of eyeglasses and hearing aids. Newly admitted older adults should be screened for cognitive loss, severity of illness, sensory deficits, and markers of dehydration with a goal of addressing correctable risk factors proactively before the onset of delirium.

Medications are the most common reversible causes of delirium. Anticholinergics, H_2-blockers, benzodiazepines, opioids, and antipsychotic medications should be replaced with medications that have no central effects. For example, H_2-blockers can be replaced by antacids or proton-pump inhibitors, and regular dosing of 650 mg of acetaminophen 3 or 4 times daily can reduce or eliminate the need for opioids in many patients (Table 39.3).

The delirious patient is susceptible to a wide range of iatrogenic complications, and careful surveillance is critical. Bowel and bladder function should be monitored closely, but urinary catheters should be avoided unless absolutely required for monitoring fluids or treating urinary retention. Bowel stimulants and fecal softeners can be used to prevent obstipation, particularly in those who are concomitantly using opioids. Complete bed rest should be avoided, because it can lead to increasing disability through disuse of muscles and development of pressure injury and atelectasis in the lungs. Physical exercise and ambulation prevent the deconditioning often associated with hospitalization. Malnutrition can be avoided through use of nutritional supplements and careful attention to intake of food and fluids. Some delirious patients may need assistance for eating. Of note, all the above interventions may also be useful for preventing delirium in high-risk individuals.

Managing Behavior in Delirium

Managing behavioral problems while ensuring both the comfort and safety of the patient can be challenging. Nonpharmacologic behavioral measures provide orientation and a feeling of safety. Orienting items such as clocks, calendars, and even a window view should be made available. Patients should be encouraged to wear their eyeglasses and hearing aids. Physical restraints, which are often justified as a means to reduce the risk of patient self-injury, have actually been associated with increased injury (SOE=B).

Medications used as chemical restraints extract a costly toll in accidents, adverse events, and loss of mobility and should also be avoided if possible. Pharmacologic intervention may be necessary for symptoms such as delusions or hallucinations that are frightening to the patient when verbal comfort and reassurance are not successful. Some delirious patients display behavior that is dangerous to themselves or others and cannot be calmed by a family member or aide. Similar to those for physical restraints, indications for pharmacologic intervention should be clearly identified, documented, and constantly reassessed. The lowest dose of the least toxic agent should be used for the shortest time possible. Daily renewal of orders for physical or chemical restraints is one way of ensuring they are stopped when no longer needed.

The literature on pharmacologic management of delirium is growing rapidly and is best understood keeping several important factors in mind: 1) Except in unusual cases (eg, alcohol withdrawal delirium), antipsychotics have a more favorable risk:benefit ratio than benzodiazepines or other sedatives. 2) All use of antipsychotics for delirium is off-label—there are no FDA-approved drugs indicated for delirium. 3) Many drug treatment and prevention studies were conducted in mixed-age groups in the ICU; it is unclear whether the risk:benefit ratio for use of these drugs will be similar in older hospitalized patients on the general wards. 4) Many studies are not blinded, not placebo controlled, or corporate sponsored, raising concerns about validity. 5) The outcome of some studies is delirium severity; yet, existing delirium severity scales tend to weigh hyperactive symptoms too heavily, so that converting hyperactive delirium to hypoactive delirium (which has worse outcomes, as noted above) is measured as a reduction in severity.

A 2016 meta-analysis summarized the case for use (or non-use) of antipsychotics for the prevention and treatment of delirium. For prevention, the meta-analysis included 7 randomized trials that tested prophylactic administration of low-dose antipsychotics in high-risk surgical patients. The incidence of delirium appeared lower in the intervention than control groups, but there was significant heterogeneity among studies, and the between-group difference was not significant (pooled OR=0.56; 95% CI, 0.23–1.34) (SOE=C). Further, this meta-analysis reported no significant effect of prophylactic antipsychotics on ICU or total hospital length of stay or mortality. For treatment, the meta-analysis included 12 randomized trials that tested administration of antipsychotics in response to delirium in medical, surgical, and ICU patients. These trials found that antipsychotics did not reduce delirium duration or severity, ICU or hospital length of stay, or mortality. In sum, the meta-analysis did not provide compelling evidence supporting the use of antipsychotics for either delirium prevention or treatment (SOE=C). Thus, the decision whether to use antipsychotics must account for the trade-off between amelioration of specific symptoms that cause patient distress or are disruptive to medical care versus risks of antipsychotic-induced complications. Importantly, administration of antipsychotics should never substitute for the other evaluation and management best practices described above.

If treatment with antipsychotics is required, the literature suggests that all of the drugs listed in the Table 39.4 are equally effective. The choice of agent is often made based on adverse effects. Drugs such as haloperidol and risperidone have the least sedation but greatest risk of extrapyramidal side effects, whereas olanzapine and quetiapine are more sedating and have fewer extrapyramidal adverse effects. Regardless of the drug selected, the initial dose should be as low as possible, because there is a wide variability in response. Another dose of the drug can always be administered, but once a dose is administered, it cannot be taken away. For the most part, dosing in delirium (as opposed to in dementia with behavioral disturbances) is on an as-needed basis, although patients with prolonged delirium with behavioral symptoms may need continual scheduled

Table 39.3—Drugs to Reduce or Eliminate in Management of Delirium

Agent	Adverse Events	Possible Substitutes	Comments
Alcohol	CNS sedation and withdrawal	If history of heavy intake, careful monitoring and benzodiazepines for withdrawal symptoms	Alcohol history is imperative
Anticholinergics (oxybutynin, benztropine)	Anticholinergic toxicity	Lower dosage, behavioral management of urinary incontinence	Rare at low dosages
Anticonvulsants (especially primidone, phenobarbital, phenytoin)	CNS sedation and withdrawal	Alternative agent or consider stopping if low risk and no recent history of seizures	Toxic reactions can occur despite "therapeutic" drug concentrations
Antidepressants, especially tertiary amine tricyclic agents (amitriptyline, imipramine, doxepin)	Anticholinergic toxicity	Secondary amine tricyclics (nortriptyline, desipramine), SSRIs, serotonin-norepinephrine reuptake inhibitors	Secondary amines as good as tertiary for adjuvant treatment of chronic pain
Antihistamines (eg, diphenhydramine)	Anticholinergic toxicity	Nonpharmacologic protocol for sleep, pseudoephedrine for colds, nonsedating antihistamines for allergies	Must take OTC medication history Many patients do not realize that compounds ending in "PM" contain diphenhydramine
H_2-blocking agents	Possible anticholinergic toxicity	Lower dosage, antacids or proton-pump inhibitors	Most common with high-dose intravenous infusions
Antiparkinsonian agents (levodopa-carbidopa, dopamine agonists, amantadine)	Dopaminergic toxicity	Lower dosage; adjusted dosing schedule	Usually with advanced disease and high dosages
Antipsychotics, especially low-potency anticholinergic agents and second-generation agents (clozapine)	Anticholinergic toxicity, CNS sedation	No agents or, if necessary, low-dosage high-potency agents	See note for Table 39.5 for warnings about second-generation antipsychotics
Barbiturates	CNS sedation, severe withdrawal syndrome	Gradual discontinuation or benzodiazepine substitution	In most cases, should no longer be prescribed; avoid inadvertent or abrupt discontinuation
Benzodiazepines	CNS sedation, potential for withdrawal	Nonpharmacologic sleep management	Associated with delirium in medical and surgical patients
Nonbenzodiazepine hypnotics (eg, zolpidem)	CNS sedation and withdrawal	Nonpharmacologic sleep protocol	Like other sedatives, can cause delirium
Opioid analgesics (especially meperidine)	Anticholinergic toxicity, CNS sedation, fecal impaction	Local and regional measures and nonpsychoactive pain medications (acetaminophen, NSAIDs) around the clock, reserve opioids for breakthrough and severe pain	Consider risks versus benefits, because uncontrolled pain can also cause delirium Naloxone for severe overdoses Higher risk in patients with renal insufficiency
Almost any medication if time course is appropriate			Consider risks and benefits of all medications in older adults

dosing. As noted above, these drugs should be stopped as soon as possible. In the rare circumstances that they are needed beyond hospital discharge, clear parameters for their discontinuation should be included in the discharge paperwork.

Family Counseling

It is important to stress to family members that delirium is usually not a permanent condition, but rather that it improves over time. Unfortunately, as described above, persistence of delirium is common. Thus, when counseling families, it is important to point out that many cognitive deficits associated with the delirium syndrome can continue, abating weeks and even months after the illness. Advanced age (≥85 years old), preexisting cognitive impairment, and severe illness (ICU stay) are risk factors for slow (or absent) recovery of cognitive function after delirium. Careful monitoring of mental

Table 39.4—Pharmacologic Therapy of Agitated Delirium

Agent	Mechanism of Action	Dosage	Benefits	Adverse Events	Comments
Haloperidol[OL]	Antipsychotic	0.25–0.5 mg po, IM, or IV q4h prn; [a]Max dose 3 mg per 24h	Relatively nonsedating; few hemodynamic effects	EPS, especially if >3 mg/d	Usually agent of choice[a]
Risperidone[OL]	Second-generation antipsychotic	0.25–0.5 mg po q4h prn [a]Max dose 2 mg per 24h	Similar to haloperidol	Might have slightly fewer EPS than haloperidol	Small trials[b]
Olanzapine[OL]	Second-generation antipsychotic	2.5–5 mg po, SL, or IM q12h (cannot be given IV) [a]Max dose 20 mg per 24h	Fewer EPS than haloperidol	More sedating than haloperidol	Small trials[b]; oral formulations less effective for acute management
Quetiapine[OL]	Second-generation antipsychotic	12.4–25 po q12h [a]Max dose 50 mg per 24h	Fewer EPS than haloperidol; can be used in patients with parkinsonism	More sedating than haloperidol; hypotension	Small trials[b]
Ziprasidone	Second-generation antipsychotic	5–10 mg po, IM [a]Max dose 20 mg per 24h	Fewer EPS than haloperidol; moderate sedation	Risk of cardiac arrhythmia, heart failure, agranulocytosis	Small trials[b]; large trial ongoing. Due to risks, used primarily in ICU
Lorazepam[OL]	Benzodiazepine	0.25–0.5 mg po or IV q8h prn for agitation	Use in sedative and alcohol withdrawal; history of neuroleptic malignant syndrome	More paradoxical excitation, respiratory depression than haloperidol	Generally should not be used except for specific indications noted under "benefits"

NOTE: EPS = extrapyramidal symptoms
Use of all these drugs for delirium is off-label. Based on recent meta-analyses, the SOE=C.
[a] Maximum dose per 24 hours is the recommended total cumulative dose threshold to minimize risk of adverse events in frail older adults. Younger patients may be able to tolerate somewhat higher doses.
[b] In a randomized trial comparing haloperidol, chlorpromazine, and lorazepam in the treatment of agitated delirium in young patients with AIDS, all were found to be equally effective in treating symptoms of psychosis, but haloperidol had the fewest adverse events.
[c] Second-generation antipsychotics have been tested primarily in small equivalency trials with haloperidol and recently in small placebo-controlled trials in the ICU. The FDA requires a "black box" warning for all second-generation antipsychotics because of the increased risk of cerebrovascular events, stroke, and mortality in patients with dementia. First-generation antipsychotic agents also have an FDA "black box" warning regarding an increase in all-cause mortality among patients with dementia.

status and providing adequate functional supports during this period are necessary to give the patient the maximal chance of returning to his or her baseline level.

Family members can play an important role in the hospital and postacute setting by providing appropriate orientation, support, and functional assistance. Hospitals are increasingly making provisions for family members to sleep overnight with relatives who are already delirious or at high risk of developing delirium. Although symptoms of delirium may persist, acute exacerbation of cognitive dysfunction is not expected during the convalescent period and therefore likely heralds a new medical problem. Families should be counseled to seek prompt medical attention if a patient's mental status acutely worsens.

Delirium and Care Transitions

Delirium further complicates already challenging care transitions for older adults. First, diagnosis of delirium often requires knowledge of the patient's baseline cognitive function, which can be challenging if documentation is lacking (eg, when a nursing-home resident is transferred to the hospital). Improved documentation of the patient's baseline by the "sending" facility helps to facilitate accurate diagnosis of delirium. Second, the presence of delirium at hospital discharge to a skilled-nursing facility (SNF) is a risk factor for hospital readmission, reduces likelihood of return home within 30 days, and possibly leads to misdiagnosis of dementia. Again, good communication is important, including clear documentation of delirium in the hospital discharge summary and recommendations for management, including discontinuation of antipsychotics if still being used at discharge. Third, the prolonged cognitive and functional disability associated with delirium can make care planning difficult, because affected patients often need increased supports for months after the acute episode. Specialized intervention programs have been developed to facilitate recovery after an episode of delirium. In one 2016 study that targeted delirium superimposed on dementia in the SNF setting, intensive therapy could facilitate cognitive recovery but did not shorten the duration of delirium (SOE=B). Until such models are refined, the best course of action

Table 39.5—Key Recommendations of the AGS Guideline for Postoperative Delirium

Clinical Practice Guideline Summary

Eight *strong* recommendations: benefits clearly outweighed the risks, or the risks clearly outweighed the benefits.
- Multicomponent nonpharmacologic interventions delivered by an interprofessional team should be administered to at-risk older adults to prevent delirium.
- Ongoing educational programs regarding delirium should be provided for health care professionals.
- A medical evaluation should be performed to identify and manage underlying contributors to delirium.
- Pain management (preferably with nonopioid medications) should be optimized to prevent postoperative delirium.
- Medications with high risk of precipitating delirium should be avoided.
- Cholinesterase inhibitors should not be newly prescribed to prevent or treat postoperative delirium.
- Benzodiazepines should not be used as first-line treatment of agitation associated with delirium.
- Antipsychotics and benzodiazepines should be avoided for treatment of hypoactive delirium.

Three *weak* recommendations: current level of evidence or potential risks of the treatment did not support a strong recommendation.
- Multicomponent nonpharmacologic interventions implemented by an interprofessional team may be considered when an older adult is diagnosed with postoperative delirium to improve clinical outcomes.
- The injection of regional anesthetic at the time of surgery and postoperatively to improve pain control with the goal of preventing delirium may be considered.
- The use of antipsychotics (eg, haloperidol, risperidone, olanzapine, quetiapine, or ziprasidone) at the lowest effective dose for the shortest possible duration may be considered to treat delirious patients who are severely agitated or distressed or who are threatening substantial harm to self and/or others.

One "insufficient evidence" recommendation: current level of evidence or potential risks of the treatment did not support either a strong or weak recommendation.
- Use of processed electroencephalographic (EEG) monitors of anesthetic depth during intravenous sedation or general anesthesia may be used to prevent delirium.

Insufficient evidence to recommend either for or against the following:
- Prophylactic use of antipsychotic medications to prevent delirium
- Specialized hospital units for inpatient care of older adults with postoperative delirium

Reproduced with permission from the American Geriatrics Society: AGS Expert Panel on Postoperative Delirium. Clinical Practice Guidelines for Postoperative Delirium in Older Adults. New York: American Geriatrics Society; 2014.

---

is to continue therapy for as long as the patient shows signs of improvement and to not make any permanent decisions about care needs until the patient's status plateaus. Finally, care transitions themselves are likely risk factors for delirium, particularly in highly vulnerable individuals, and should be minimized whenever possible. For instance, it may be preferable to keep a patient in the hospital for a day or two longer to allow direct transition to home, rather than mandating an early discharge to SNF, followed by a second transition to home.

Models of Care

A growing body of literature has focused on prevention and management of delirium. These studies can be best understood along a continuum, ranging from proactive interventions to prevent delirium or to reduce its severity and consequences, to reactive interventions designed to treat delirium after it has developed. The overall trend suggests that the more proactive, the more successful the intervention.

In a landmark 1999 study, a unit-based proactive multifactorial intervention termed HELP (the Hospital Elder Life Program [www.hospitalelderlifeprogram.org]) reduced the incidence of delirium among hospitalized patients ≥70 years old by 40% (matched OR=0.60; 95% CI, 0.39, 0.92; number needed to treat [NNT] =19.6) (SOE=A). Six intervention components were used selectively based on patient-specific risk factors determined at an admission assessment: cognitive impairment, sleep deprivation, immobility, visual impairment, hearing impairment, and dehydration. The HELP model was subsequently demonstrated to be cost-effective for hospitals in medium-risk patients and for the health care system in all patients because of the large savings in postacute care. This model has now been disseminated widely, including in community hospitals and surgical patients.

A 2015 meta-analysis examined the effectiveness of multifactorial nonpharmacologic interventions for delirium, such as HELP. Of the 14 high-quality intervention studies identified, 11 studies demonstrated a significant reduction in delirium incidence (OR=0.47; 95% CI, 0.38, 0.58), and 4 studies demonstrated a significant reduction in in-hospital falls (OR=0.38; 95% CI, 0.25,0.60) (SOE=A). There were also nonsignificant trends toward shorter hospital length of stay and reduced need for postacute nursing home placement. However, in 2018, a single hospital study showed that the intervention group who received HELP had reduced 30-day readmissions (SOE=B).

Finally, several studies have examined treatment of delirium using multifactorial strategies similar to those used for delirium prevention. For the most part, these have not yielded as dramatic benefits as the prevention models (SOE=B), although some have demonstrated improved recognition of delirium, reduction in delirium severity or duration, or faster cognitive recovery in the intervention group. New trials are underway to test treatment interventions.

QUALITY MEASURES AND CONSENSUS GUIDELINES

In 2014, the American Geriatrics Society Section for Enhancing Geriatric Understanding and Expertise among Surgical and Medical Specialists (SEGUE) released guidelines for prevention and management of postoperative delirium (Table 39.5). Although aimed specifically at the surgical setting, many of the recommendations in these guidelines are applicable to other patient populations. The level of evidence supporting various recommendations varies widely, from consistent randomized trials (SOE=A) to a reliance on best clinical practices (SOE=C).

CHOOSING WISELY® RECOMMENDATIONS

Delirium

- Avoid physical restraints to manage behavioral symptoms of hospitalized older adults with delirium.

- Do not use benzodiazepines or other sedative-hypnotics in older adults as first choice for insomnia, agitation, or delirium.

RESOURCES

- Guthrie PF, Rayborn S, Butcher HK. Evidence-Based Practice Guideline: Delirium. *J Gerontol Nurs*. 2018;44(2):14–24.

- Marcantonio ER. Delirium in hospitalized older adults. *N Engl J Med*. 2017;377(15):1456–1466.

- Oh ES, Fong TG, Hsheih TT, et al. Delirium in older persons: advances in diagnosis and treatment. *JAMA*. 2017;318(12):1161–1174.

CHAPTER 40—SLEEP ISSUES

KEY POINTS

- Among older adults, insomnia is common and often present with other comorbid psychiatric and/or medical conditions.

- Compared with younger adults, older adults generally take longer to fall asleep at night and have more nighttime wakefulness and more daytime napping. An earlier bedtime and earlier wake time are also common.

- Older adults, especially older men, have less N3 sleep (the slow-wave, or deeper stage of sleep) than younger adults.

- The appropriate treatment of sleep problems must be guided by knowledge of likely causes and potential contributing factors.

- Several trials, meta-analyses, and guidelines recommend behavioral interventions (eg, cognitive-behavioral therapy for insomnia) as first-line treatment for chronic insomnia in older adults.

Sleep problems are common among older adults, particularly those with other psychiatric and medical conditions. More than two-thirds of older adults with multiple comorbidities have sleep problems. The most common sleep complaints among community-dwelling older adults are difficulty falling asleep, nighttime awakening, early morning awakening, and daytime sleepiness. Many community-dwelling older adults use OTC and/or prescription sleeping medications.

EPIDEMIOLOGY

Epidemiologic studies in older adults have demonstrated an association between sleep complaints and risk factors for sleep disturbance (eg, chronic illness, multiple medical problems, mood disturbance, less physical activity, physical disability) but little association with older age, suggesting that these risk factors, rather than aging per se, account for much of the increase in sleep disturbance with age. However, certain primary sleep disorders do increase in prevalence with age, such as sleep-related breathing disorders (eg, sleep apnea), restless legs syndrome, and certain circadian rhythm sleep disorders.

Insomnia is more common in women than in men at all ages (SOE=A), with a risk ratio in women that increases from young adulthood (risk ratio [RR]=1.28) to older age (RR=1.73). Self-reported sleeping difficulties are more common in older black Americans, particularly women and in those with depression and chronic illness.

Late-life insomnia is generally a chronic problem. Studies often report persistence of insomnia symptoms over (at least) several years, and most hypnotic use occurs among chronic users of these medications. Even among very old women (≥85 years old), there is evidence that the majority report sleeping difficulties, and many regularly use alcohol and/or OTC sleeping agents in an attempt to improve their sleep. Studies in the United States suggest that approximately 5% of older adults use prescription sedative-hypnotics on a daily basis. Insomnia has been reported as a predictor of death and nursing-home placement (particularly in older men). In addition, in several epidemiologic studies, subjective sleep disturbance is associated with worse health-related quality of life in older adults (SOE=B). Evidence also suggests an association between worse sleep (measured subjectively and objectively) and subsequent cognitive decline in older adults.

CHANGES IN SLEEP WITH AGING

In general, older adults have decreased sleep efficiency (time spent asleep divided by total time spent in bed), decreased total sleep time, and increased sleep latency (time to fall asleep) (Table 40.1). Older adults also often report an earlier bedtime and earlier morning awakening, more awakenings and more wakefulness during the night, and more daytime napping. Notable age-related changes in sleep structure as measured by polysomnography include changes in both nonrapid eye movement (NREM, ie, stages N1, N2, and N3) and rapid eye movement (REM) sleep. Most age-related changes in sleep begin in early adulthood and progress throughout life, with notable changes occurring by middle age and a relative plateau in older adults. Older adults, especially older men, have less N3 sleep (the slow-wave, or deeper stage of sleep), whereas the percentage of stage N1 and N2 sleep (the lighter stages of sleep) increases with age. A decrease in REM sleep and an earlier onset of REM sleep in the night (ie, shorter REM latency) have also been reported. In addition, older adults can have an advance in circadian rhythms of sleep and wake (ie, they go to bed earlier, wake up earlier) and a reduced amplitude in (ie, less robust) circadian rhythms.

As suggested above, most age-related changes in sleep occur by age 60, with many sleep parameters remaining relatively stable among people in good health after 60 years of age. In addition, the clinical significance of these age-related changes in sleep is not clear. For example, after a period of sleep deprivation, older adults may actually show less daytime sleepiness, less evidence of decline in performance measures, and a quicker recovery of normal sleep structure than younger people. However, older adults have more sleep disturbance with jet lag and shift work, which may reflect physiologic changes in circadian rhythms with age. In studies comparing good sleepers with poor sleepers, poor sleepers were found to take more medications, make more clinician visits, and have poorer self-ratings of health.

EVALUATION OF SLEEP

Symptoms of sleep disturbance in older adults can be identified with simple screening questions, such as asking whether the person is satisfied with their sleep, whether sleep or fatigue interferes with daytime activities, and whether a bed partner or others complain of unusual behavior during sleep, such as snoring, interrupted breathing, or leg movements. If the patient has a sleep complaint, having them keep a sleep log for 1–2 weeks can be helpful in obtaining a careful description. For example, each morning, the patient can record the time they went to bed the prior night, their estimated total amount of sleep, the number of awakenings, the time of morning awakening, when they got out of bed for the day, and any symptoms that occurred during the night. Any medications or other agents taken for sleep the night before, and time spent napping during the day should also be recorded. The patient's sleep log should be supplemented by information from a bed partner (if available) or from others who may have observed unusual symptoms during the night. Examples of sleep logs and validated sleep questionnaires are available in the literature and online (eg, www.sleepassociation.org/epworth-sleep-scale/ and http://www.opapc.com/uploads/documents/PSQI.pdf). The focused physical examination depends on evidence from the history. For example, reports of painful joints should be followed by a careful examination of the affected areas. Mental status testing should also be considered in patients with sleep disturbance, with a focus on memory and mood problems, particularly depression. The findings of the history and physical examination should guide laboratory and other testing.

Polysomnography is indicated when a sleep-related breathing disorder (sleep apnea) or narcolepsy is suspected, or when there are symptoms of violent or injurious behaviors during sleep (SOE=A). Polysomnography may also be indicated when other unusual behaviors occur during sleep or if periodic limb movement disorder is suspected (SOE=B). Portable sleep monitoring systems for use in the home are available and used primarily when sleep apnea is suspected. Wrist activity monitors (ie, wrist actigraphy) estimate

Table 40.1–Age-Related Changes in Sleep

Sleep Characteristic	Age-Related Change
Total sleep time	Decrease
Sleep latency (time to fall asleep)	Increase or no change
Sleep efficiency (time asleep over time in bed)	Decrease
Daytime napping	Increase
Stages N1 and N2	Increase
Slow-wave sleep (stage N3)	Decrease
Percent rapid eye movement (REM)	Decrease
Awakenings after sleep onset	Increase

sleep versus wakefulness based on wrist movement. Most research using actigraphy as an objective measure of sleep has used validated, research-grade actigraphs. Wrist actigraphy can be used in identifying circadian rhythm disorders (SOE=A) and in nursing-home residents, in whom traditional sleep monitoring can be difficult to obtain (SOE=B).

COMMON SLEEP PROBLEMS

Insomnia

Insomnia disorder is defined by the *Diagnostic and Statistical Manual of Mental Disorders, Fifth Edition (DSM-5)* as a difficulty in initiating or maintaining sleep or waking up too early, which is associated with daytime impairment (such as fatigue, poor concentration, daytime sleepiness, or concerns about sleep). In addition to other features, diagnostic criteria also indicate that the sleep problems must occur at least 3 times per week and (to meet criteria for chronic insomnia) must have been present for at least 3 months. Insomnia diagnostic criteria listed in the *International Classification of Sleep Disorders, 3rd Edition,* are similar. The prevalence of insomnia disorder increases from about 10% in young adulthood to about 30% in those ≥65 years old. However, the prevalence of sleep complaints is even greater than the prevalence of insomnia disorder meeting strict diagnostic criteria. Among older adults in particular, insomnia generally coexists with other conditions, which has been termed comorbid insomnia. Older adults with insomnia are more likely to have medical and/or psychiatric illness than are good sleepers. Risk factors for insomnia include female gender, social isolation, low socioeconomic status, use of multiple medications, and other factors.

Some studies report that an associated psychiatric disorder is present in 30%–60% of patients presenting with insomnia. Depression is strongly associated with insomnia, and many patients with depression also have sleep complaints. Common sleep complaints with depression include early morning awakening, increased sleep latency, and more nighttime wakefulness. Chronic insomnia is a risk factor for development of major depressive disorder in older (and younger) adults, and studies suggest that insomnia symptoms commonly precede the onset of depressive symptoms. In depressed older adults with sleep disturbance, treatment of depression can improve sleep complaints. Conversely, lack of attention to sleep complaints in older depressed adults can make depression less likely to respond to treatment. Sleep disorders in older adults are also associated with increased suicide risk. Anxiety disorder is another psychiatric condition commonly associated with insomnia symptoms, particularly difficulty falling asleep and early awakening. Caregiving is associated with insomnia, and older caregivers report more sleep complaints than do noncaregivers of similar age.

Many medical problems are associated with insomnia in older adults. Epidemiologic studies in older adults suggest a greater prevalence of insomnia in those with conditions such as hypertension, heart disease, arthritis, lung disease, gastroesophageal reflux, stroke, neurodegenerative disorders (eg, dementia, Parkinson disease), and other conditions. Common symptoms of medical illness that can contribute to sleep disturbance (particularly nighttime awakening) include pain, paresthesias, cough, nocturnal dyspnea, gastroesophageal reflux, and nighttime urination. In older adults with sleeping difficulties who describe pain at night, the painful condition should be assessed and managed. Nighttime urination is common in both older men and women and may be associated with insomnia and increased fatigue in the daytime. Reports of nocturia that disrupts sleep should be followed by evaluation for cardiac, renal, or prostatic disease, or diabetes mellitus. Efforts to determine whether the patient has nocturnal polyuria (eg, using a voiding diary) should be considered, and a review of lifestyle habits (eg, evening fluid intake) that may be contributing to the nocturia should be addressed. Multicomponent treatment (eg, lifestyle modifications and behavioral treatment) is first-line therapy for older adults with nocturia and sleep disturbance. In addition, further evaluation for another sleep disorder (eg, sleep apnea) should be considered in patients with disturbed sleep and nocturia who do not respond to these treatments.

Many medications can contribute to insomnia in older adults. Sleep can be impaired by diuretics or stimulating agents (eg, caffeine, sympathomimetics, bronchodilators, activating psychiatric medications) taken near bedtime. Some antidepressants, antiparkinson agents, antihypertensives, and cholinesterase inhibitors can induce nightmares and impair sleep. Required medications that are sedating (eg, sedating antidepressants) should be given at bedtime if possible. Chronic use of sedatives can cause light, fragmented sleep. For some sleeping medications, chronic use can lead to tolerance and the potential for increasing dosages. When chronic use of hypnotics is suddenly stopped, rebound insomnia can occur. Alcohol abuse is associated with lighter sleep of shorter duration. In addition, some older adults try to treat their sleeping difficulties with alcohol. Although nighttime alcohol causes an initial drowsiness, as alcohol is metabolized it impairs sleep later in the night. Finally, sedatives and alcohol can worsen sleep apnea; the use of these respiratory depressants should be avoided in older adults with untreated sleep apnea.

Sleep-Related Breathing Disorders

Sleep-related breathing disorders are characterized by disordered respiration during sleep. In older adults, sleep-disordered breathing is highly prevalent and is associated with heart disease (eg, heart failure, atrial fibrillation), diabetes, stroke, cognitive decline, and other problems. Limited evidence and even fewer guidelines are specific to older adults to guide the diagnosis and treatment of sleep-related breathing disorders, so management recommendations, in general, are based on findings from middle-aged or mixed-aged populations. Evidence suggests that sleep-disordered breathing, including central sleep apnea (CSA), has a higher prevalence in older adults than in younger adults. CSA syndromes are sleep-related breathing disorders in which respiratory effort is absent because of CNS or cardiac dysfunction. Obstructive sleep apnea (OSA) is characterized by an obstruction in the airway resulting in continued breathing effort but inadequate ventilation. Attended (ie, staff present all night), in-laboratory, full-night polysomnography is the gold standard for diagnosis of sleep-disordered breathing (SOE=A). However, portable devices that combine oximetry with additional measures (eg, heart rate, respiratory effort, nasal airflow) are increasingly used for in-home OSA testing. The sensitivity of home testing may be lower than that of laboratory polysomnography (SOE=B). Therefore, negative results from in-home OSA testing may need to be followed by in-laboratory polysomnography to exclude sleep apnea.

In adults, CSA can be a primary disorder or secondary to neurodegenerative disease, stroke, or heart failure. Treatment of CSA associated with heart failure focuses on management of the heart failure. The role of positive-airway pressure (PAP) in treatment of patients with CSA and heart failure has been debated. However, evidence suggests that patients with CSA related to heart failure who are successfully treated with PAP to an apnea-hypopnea index (AHI) <15 have improved transplant-free survival (SOE=B). Nighttime oxygen supplementation can reduce the apnea and oxygen desaturation and has been recommended in CSA patients who are unable to tolerate PAP therapy (SOE=C). Adaptive servo-ventilation (ASV) is a form of ventilation that can normalize breathing patterns in CSA by providing expiratory PAP and dynamic (ie, breath-by-breath) adjustment of inspiratory pressure support and an automatic backup rate. ASV is contraindicated in CSA patients with an ejection fraction ≤45% because of increased cardiovascular mortality (SOE=A).

OSA is common among older adults, but reported prevalence varies considerably. Patients with OSA usually present with excessive daytime sleepiness and may be unaware of their frequent arousals at night. Patients can have morning headache, personality changes, poor memory, confusion, and irritability. A bed partner may report loud snoring, cessation of breathing, and choking sounds during sleep. The classic sleep apnea patient is an obese, sleepy snorer with hypertension. Middle-aged OSA patients are generally obese, but there is less association between obesity and OSA in older age, and many older OSA patients have a normal BMI. Other reported predictors identified in community-dwelling older adults include falling asleep at inappropriate times, male gender, and napping. OSA should be considered in patients with treatment-resistant hypertension. Large neck circumference has also been reported as a marker for sleep apnea in middle-aged adults but may not be a significant predictor for older adults. Alcohol abuse and dependence is an important risk factor for sleep apnea, and sleep-disordered breathing is a significant contributor to sleep disturbance in men >40 years old with a history of alcoholism. Finally, there appears to be an association between sleep apnea, cognitive loss, and dementia (SOE=B). Of note, evidence suggests that OSA patients with mild-moderate dementia can tolerate PAP well, with acceptable adherence to treatment, improvement in OSA parameters, and some evidence of beneficial effects on cognition (SOE=B).

OSA is a treatable condition associated with cardiovascular disease, including hypertension, stroke, myocardial ischemia, arrhythmias, fatal and nonfatal cardiovascular events, and all-cause mortality (SOE=A). PAP therapy may reduce blood pressure in OSA patients with cardiovascular disease or multiple cardiovascular risk factors (SOE=A). OSA is also associated with motor vehicle accidents (SOE=A). The importance of mild degrees of sleep-disordered breathing in older adults is unclear. In one study, no association was found between mild or moderate sleep-disordered breathing and subjective sleep-wake disturbance. The long-term consequences of mild, asymptomatic OSA in older adults are also unclear.

Patients suspected of having OSA should be referred to a sleep laboratory for evaluation and, if the diagnosis is documented, considered for treatment. As mentioned above, portable in-home monitoring devices are available. Although controversial, evidence suggests that home sleep testing followed by use of auto-titrating PAP (autoPAP) treatment in patients diagnosed with OSA (ie, completely home-based diagnosis and treatment of OSA) may be noninferior to (the more costly) in-laboratory polysomnography testing for OSA and PAP titration. PAP therapy reduces sleepiness and improves quality of life in people with moderate and severe OSA (SOE=A). Older adults may tolerate PAP as well as younger adults. Efforts to promote use of devices (eg, variations in mask, humidification) that improve comfort may improve adherence with PAP. Early successful adherence (eg, within the first week of therapy) with PAP may predict long-term adherence with PAP treatment. Behavioral approaches have also been used to improve PAP adherence (SOE=B). Unfortunately, clinicians may not recommend PAP in older adults, perhaps because they assume that the treatment will not be tolerated or successful in this population.

Most OSA patients are treated with continuous PAP (CPAP) therapy. Other mechanical options are available. For example, bi-level PAP (BPAP) devices reduce expiratory pressure compared with CPAP. Evidence suggests that BPAP does not improve efficacy or adherence in treatment of sleep apnea compared with CPAP (SOE=B), but these alternative devices can be appropriate in certain patients. Oral (ie, dental or mouth) appliances are also available, but PAP is more effective in improving OSA. Oral appliances are generally recommended only in patients with mild symptomatic OSA or in those unwilling or unable to tolerate PAP (SOE=B). Several upper airway surgical approaches have also been used, but evidence of effectiveness from large trials is limited. Other novel treatment options for OSA have been considered, but the role of these therapies (particularly in older adults) remains unclear.

Periodic Limb Movements During Sleep and Restless Legs Syndrome

Periodic limb movements during sleep (PLMS) is a condition of repetitive, stereotypical leg movements that generally occur during non-REM sleep. PLMS increases in prevalence with age, but the significance of this is unclear, because some studies have found little relationship between PLMS and sleep disruption. In one study, evidence of PLMS was found in more than one-third of community-dwelling older adults. Some authors have suggested that the high prevalence of PLMS with age is associated with delayed motor and sensory latencies noted on nerve conduction testing. When PLMS is associated with clinical sleep disturbance or a complaint of daytime fatigue that is not better explained by another sleep disorder, this is termed periodic limb movement disorder (PLMD). Polysomnography is required to establish a diagnosis of PLMD.

Restless legs syndrome (RLS) is a condition of an uncontrollable urge to move one's legs at night, usually accompanied by an uncomfortable and unpleasant sensation of the legs that worsens with inactivity and improves with movement. The symptoms occur while the person is awake and can also involve the arms. The diagnosis is based on the patient's description of the symptoms; polysomnography is not required to make the diagnosis. There may be a family history of the condition (particularly in patients with an earlier age onset of RLS) and, in some cases, an underlying medical disorder (eg, anemia, or renal or neurologic disease). RLS is 1.5 times more common in women than in men, and evidence suggests that RLS prevalence increases with age. PLMS occurs in most (80%–90%) patients with RLS, but the presence of PLMS is not specific for RLS. RLS can also be seen in patients with dementia, in which the patient may not be able to adequately describe the symptoms. RLS should be considered in dementia patients who have signs such as rubbing or massaging of legs, increased motor activity (eg, pacing, wandering), and evidence of leg discomfort that occurs in the evening and/or with inactivity and improves with movement. A diagnostic model that combines observation for behavioral indicators plus clinical indicators of RLS has been described and may assist in the recognition of RLS among those with dementia. Many medications can aggravate or induce RLS symptoms, such as antiemetics, antipsychotics, SSRIs, tricyclic antidepressants, and diphenhydramine. These and other medications should be addressed in patients with new or worsening RLS.

If pharmacologic treatment for RLS is indicated (because of severity of symptoms or significant effects on quality of life), dopaminergic agents are the initial agent of choice. An evening dose of a dopamine agonist (eg, pramipexole or ropinirole, about 1–2 hours before bedtime) is effective in treatment of RLS and PLMD (SOE=A). A nighttime dose of carbidopa-levodopa[OL] may also be effective (SOE=A) and can be used for patients who need medication infrequently (ie, for as-needed use). However, some patients describe a shift of their symptoms to daytime hours with successful treatment of symptoms at night; this problem (termed augmentation) appears more frequently with use of carbidopa-levodopa as treatment for RLS. RLS can be associated with iron deficiency, in which case RLS symptoms can improve with iron replacement therapy (SOE=B). Patients with RLS should be screened for iron deficiency, and the cause of identified iron deficiency should also be addressed. Gabapentin[OL] can also be effective (SOE=B), particularly in patients who cannot tolerate dopamine agonists. Benzodiazepines[OL] and opioids[OL] have also been used for RLS but carry greater risk of adverse effects in older adults. Guidelines suggest that there is insufficient evidence to evaluate the use of pharmacologic therapy for patients with PLMD alone (ie, in the absence of coexisting RLS).

Circadian Rhythm Sleep Disorders

Disturbances in circadian rhythms of the sleep-wake cycle may be more common with advanced age. In particular, older adults are more likely to have an advanced sleep phase (ie, fall asleep early and awaken early) rather than a delayed sleep phase (ie, fall asleep late and awaken late), but a delayed sleep phase can be seen in older adults. Some older adults have extremely irregular sleep-wake cycles, including some patients with dementia and nursing-home residents. Some common changes in sleep pattern seen in older adults (such as increased daytime napping and disrupted nighttime sleep) can be due to alterations in circadian rhythms. Dementia is associated with sleep-wake cycle disturbance and frequent nighttime awakenings, nighttime wandering, and nighttime agitation.

A sleep log can help establish the presence of a circadian rhythm sleep disorder (SOE=B). Wrist actigraphy can also be useful for making a diagnosis (particularly in patients who are unable to complete a sleep log) and in monitoring treatment response in patients with a circadian rhythm sleep disorder (SOE=B), including older patients with dementia and nursing-home residents. Polysomnography is not routinely indicated in patients in whom a circadian rhythm sleep disorder is suspected, but referral to a sleep specialist may be indicated when symptoms do not respond to initial management, when the diagnosis is unclear, or when another sleep disorder is suspected (SOE=C). Treatment depends on the particular circadian rhythm sleep disorder. An advanced sleep phase may respond to appropriately timed evening exposure to bright light (SOE=B). A delayed sleep phase may respond to appropriately timed morning bright light and/or evening melatonin (SOE=B). Blind people with a non-24-hour sleep-wake pattern (eg, a free-running rhythm not entrained to the external environment because of lack of light/dark perception) may correct with melatonin given at night (SOE=B). The melatonin dose in these studies has ranged from 0.5 to 10 mg, but lower doses may be most effective. Several weeks or months of treatment with nighttime melatonin may be required to correct the blind person's rhythm, and it is believed that melatonin treatment must be continued indefinitely because the free-running rhythm will return if the melatonin is discontinued. The melatonin receptor agonist, tasimelteon, has been approved by the FDA for this indication (ie, non-24-hour rhythm in blind people [SOE=A])

REM Sleep Behavior Disorder

REM sleep behavior disorder (RBD) is characterized by excessive motor activities associated with dream enactment behavior during sleep and a pathologic absence of the muscle atonia that normally occurs during REM sleep. The presenting symptoms are usually vigorous sleep behaviors associated with vivid dreams, and patients may first present because of injuries (to themselves or their bed partner). The condition can be acute or chronic, and it is much more common in older men (in some case series, >85% of cases are older men). There may be a family predisposition. Transient RBD has been associated with toxic metabolic abnormalities, primarily drug or alcohol withdrawal or intoxication. The chronic form of the disorder can be idiopathic but is increasingly recognized as associated with neurodegenerative disorders such as the synucleinopathies (eg, Parkinson disease, Lewy body dementia, multisystem atrophy) and other conditions. RBD may predate (by many years) the development of Parkinson disease and related disorders. Several psychiatric medications have been associated with RBD, including tricyclic antidepressants, monoamine oxidase inhibitors, fluoxetine, venlafaxine, cholinesterase inhibitors, and other agents. Polysomnography is indicated to establish the diagnosis. Removal of the offending agent is indicated for drug-induced RBD. Clonazepam^{OL} is reported in the literature to be effective for treatment of RBD, with little evidence of tolerance to treatment effect over long periods of treatment, but older adults are at increased risk of adverse events with this agent. Use of nighttime melatonin may be effective as an alternative treatment for RBD in older adults with coexisting neurodegenerative disorders (SOE=C). Environmental safety interventions are also indicated, such as removing dangerous objects from the bedroom, putting cushions on the floor around the bed, protecting windows, and in some cases, putting the mattress on the floor.

CHANGES IN SLEEP WITH DEMENTIA

Meta-analyses suggest that older adults who report sleep disturbances have a higher risk of incident all-cause dementia, Alzheimer disease, and vascular dementia. In addition, poor self-reported sleep in cognitively normal adults is associated with cerebrospinal fluid biomarkers of Alzheimer disease pathology. Older adults with dementia have more sleep disruption and arousals, lower sleep efficiency, a higher percentage of stage N1 sleep, and more sleep fragmentation than older adults without dementia. Circadian rhythm sleep disorders are more common with dementia, resulting in excessive daytime sleeping and nighttime wakefulness. The sleep disturbance seen in older adults with dementia is likely multifactorial, related to changes in brain centers involved in sleep, wakefulness, and circadian rhythms, in addition to comorbidities and adverse effects of medication. Sleep disturbance is also common among older adults with mild cognitive impairment. Cholinesterase inhibitors (often used in treatment of dementia symptoms) can exacerbate insomnia and cause vivid dreams in some patients; changing dose timing to morning hours can help alleviate this problem. Sedative-hypnotic agents have not been adequately tested in patients with dementia and should generally be avoided. As mentioned above, evidence suggests that those with coexisting OSA and mild to moderate dementia can tolerate PAP, with improvement in OSA parameters and beneficial effects on cognition. Results of studies using melatonin for sleep disturbance in dementia have been mixed, but results of one large, randomized controlled trial in patients with Alzheimer disease suggested melatonin was not effective for sleep disturbance in these individuals (SOE=B). Bright light therapy has also been used in dementia patients, with some beneficial effects on sleep and circadian rhythms (SOE=B).

SLEEP DISTURBANCES IN THE HOSPITAL

Sleep deprivation is common among hospitalized older adults, and hospitalization can precipitate insomnia. This insomnia is likely multifactorial in origin and related to illness, medications, change from usual nighttime routines at home, and a sleep-disruptive hospital environment (eg, high noise levels at night). Sleep loss in hospitalized older adults may be associated with worse health outcomes, including increased risk of delirium (SOE=B). There is evidence that untreated OSA is also common among hospitalized patients and may contribute to adverse outcomes, particularly among postoperative, poststroke, and heart failure patients (SOE=B). In one small uncontrolled study, nighttime melatonin levels increased in hospitalized older patients treated with daytime bright-light exposure. Another small study implemented "flexible medication times" that allowed inpatients to sleep longer in the morning; their resulting in-hospital sleeping patterns were more similar to their at-home sleeping patterns. However, adherence with nonpharmacologic interventions can be difficult to achieve in the acute-care hospital. For example, one large clinical trial of nonpharmacologic interventions to prevent delirium in hospitalized older adults reported only a 10% adherence rate for the sleep protocol portion of the intervention. In a large study that tested the feasibility of a nonpharmacologic sleep protocol (consisting of a back rub, warm drink, and relaxation tapes) administered by nurses for hospitalized older adults, the use of sedative-hypnotic medications was successfully reduced; the sleep protocol had a stronger association with improved quality of sleep than the sedative-hypnotic medications.

Sleeping medications are commonly prescribed in hospitalized older adults. Unfortunately, clear guidelines are not available to guide the choice of a sleeping medication for hospitalized older adults. Benzodiazepine-receptor agonists are commonly used for insomnia in this setting, but prescribers should remember to try use of smaller dosages (than those used for younger adults) first, which are likely safer in older adults. Sedating antihistamines (eg, diphenhydramine) should not be used as a sleep aid in hospitalized older adults because of possible complications related to anticholinergic adverse events (eg, delirium, urinary retention, constipation). Melatonin (not FDA approved) has also been used (eg, 1–5 mg at bedtime), with modest evidence for effectiveness (SOE=C).

Sleep apnea is a common comorbidity in hospitalized adults, particularly among those with cardiac illness and stroke. Sleep apnea among stroke patients is associated with worse survival and less functional recovery. Sleep apnea patients should continue their use of PAP when hospitalized, particularly when sedating and narcotic medications are used and in the peri- and postoperative period.

SLEEP IN LONG-TERM CARE SETTINGS

Nursing-home residents often have marked sleep disruption, frequent nighttime awakening, and excessive daytime sleeping. Evidence suggests that sleep disturbance is also common among older adults in assisted-living facilities. Many residents nap on and off throughout the day and wake up frequently during the night. Nursing-home residents may have little or no exposure to outdoor bright light, which likely exacerbates sleep-wake abnormalities. Other common conditions in nursing-home residents that can contribute to sleep disturbance include multiple physical illnesses, the use of psychoactive medications, debility and inactivity, large amounts of time spent in bed during the daytime, increased prevalence of sleep disorders, and environmental factors (eg, nighttime noise, light, and disruptive nursing care). Sleep disturbance in nursing-home residents is associated with decreased functional status, increased agitation and falls, and other adverse consequences (SOE=B). OSA is also common among nursing-home residents, particularly in those with daytime sleepiness and nighttime sleep disturbance, and in those with dementia. As described above, RLS may also occur among nursing-home residents with dementia.

Nonpharmacologic interventions are recommended as the first-line approach to improve sleep disturbance in nursing-home residents. Results of studies involving bright light therapy in the nursing-home setting have been mixed, but there is some evidence for improved nighttime sleep and less daytime sleepiness. In a study of institutionalized residents with dementia and sleep and behavior problems, morning exposure to bright light was associated with better nighttime sleep and less daytime agitation. In another study of ambient bright light therapy (2,500 lux delivered in the morning, evening, or all day) compared with standard lighting among older adults with dementia in a psychiatric hospital and a dementia-specific residential care facility, nighttime sleep increased significantly in participants exposed to morning and all-day light, with the increase most prominent in those with severe or very severe dementia. Daytime exercise and social activity may improve objective measures of nighttime sleep and measures of daytime functioning (SOE=B). A study of residents with dementia and behavioral problems found that social interaction with nurses reduced behavioral problems and sleep-wake rhythm disorders in some residents. Multicomponent behavioral interventions on sleep in the nursing home have had mixed results but may decrease nighttime awakenings and daytime sleeping. (SOE=B). In a small trial, nighttime sleep increased and agitation decreased among nursing-home residents randomized to receive a daytime physical activity program plus nighttime intervention to decrease noise and light disruption. Evidence suggests that sleep disturbance is also common among older adults in assisted-living facilities. In one prospective, observational cohort study, sleep disturbance was common in this population, and subjective and/or objective evidence of sleep disturbance was associated with more symptoms of depression, decline in functional status, and worse health-related quality of life over 6 months of follow-up. A trial that combined an enforced schedule of structured social and physical activity for 2 weeks in a small sample of assisted-living residents found that treated residents had enhanced slow-wave sleep and improved performance in memory-oriented tasks.

MANAGEMENT OF INSOMNIA

Guidelines for all adults in general, and for older adults in particular, uniformly recommend behavioral approaches as first-line therapy for management of insomnia. Sedative-hypnotics have a documented association with falls, hip fracture, and daytime carryover symptoms of sedation in older adults. However, there is also some evidence that untreated insomnia symptoms are associated with increased risk of falls in older adults. A trial of improved sleep habits (eg, sleep hygiene techniques) may improve mild symptoms of insomnia (Table 40.2). However, more intensive behavioral treatment (as described below) is generally indicated for treatment of chronic insomnia, because simple sleep hygiene alone is generally not effective for chronic insomnia. If the person takes daytime naps, it is important to determine whether these are needed rest periods or due to inactivity, boredom, or sedating medications. Patients should be educated that daytime napping will decrease nighttime sleep.

Short-term sedative-hypnotic medication may be appropriate in cases of transient, situational insomnia, particularly during bereavement and other periods of temporary acute stress. If a decision is reached to use a sedative-hypnotic in an older adult, the smallest dosage of the agent with the least risk of adverse events should be chosen and used for the shortest duration possible. Chronic use of sedative-hypnotic agents should generally be avoided if possible because of complications associated with long-term use. Recommendations for management of chronic insomnia in adults of all ages suggest that if initial behavioral therapy is not effective, the decision to use a sedative-hypnotic medication should involve a discussion of risks and benefits with the patient. The chronic use of benzodiazepines can lead to dependence or cognitive impairment. The newer, nonbenzodiazepine hypnotics have been tested in healthy older adults and have less risk of daytime carryover and tolerance to sedative effects, but morning-after effects have been reported, prompting recommendations for lower starting dosages, particularly in women. There has been very little study of these (or other hypnotic) agents in the common situation of older adults with significant comorbidity, where the risks of adverse consequences are likely higher.

Behavioral and Nonpharmacologic Interventions

Extensive evidence has demonstrated that behavioral treatment of insomnia is effective in older adults, including those with insomnia comorbid with other conditions (SOE=A). It is important not to confuse these effective insomnia behavioral interventions with simple sleep hygiene, which (as mentioned above) is generally not effective when used alone for chronic insomnia. For a summary of behavioral insomnia interventions, see Table 40.3. Several systematic reviews and meta-analyses of behavioral interventions for insomnia have been published; the strongest evidence currently supports cognitive-behavioral therapy for insomnia

Table 40.2—Measures to Improve Sleep Hygiene

- Maintain regular rising and bed time.
- Do not go to bed unless sleepy.
- Decrease or eliminate naps, unless necessary rest period.
- Exercise daily but not immediately before bedtime.
- Do not use bed for reading, eating, or watching television.
- Relax mentally before going to sleep; do not use bedtime as worry time.
- If hungry, have a light snack (except with symptoms of gastroesophageal reflux or medical contraindications), but avoid heavy meals at bedtime.
- Limit or eliminate alcohol, caffeine, and nicotine, especially in the evening and before bedtime.
- Wind down before bedtime and maintain a routine period of preparation for bed (eg, washing up, going to the bathroom).
- Control the nighttime environment with comfortable temperature, quiet, and darkness.
- Try a familiar background noise (eg, a fan or other "white noise" machine).
- Wear comfortable bed clothing.
- If unable to fall asleep within 30 minutes, get out of bed and perform soothing activity such as listening to soft music or light reading (but avoid exposure to bright light).
- Get adequate exposure to sunlight or bright light during the day.

(CBTI, which generally combines stimulus control, sleep restriction, and cognitive therapy; additional components may also be provided) (SOE=A). The American College of Physicians recommends that all adult patients receive CBTI as the initial treatment for chronic insomnia disorder. Behavioral interventions for insomnia produce reliable therapeutic benefits, including improved sleep efficiency, decreased nighttime wakefulness, and greater satisfaction with sleep; treatment is also helpful in reducing chronic hypnotic use. In randomized trials of older adults with insomnia that compared cognitive-behavioral therapy with a prescription sedative-hypnotic agent, participants generally reported better improvement in their sleep patterns and more satisfaction with the cognitive-behavioral therapy, and sleep improvements were better sustained over time with behavioral treatment. Evidence suggests that even brief behavioral treatments (eg, 2 in-person sessions plus 2 phone calls; 4 group sessions) are effective in older adults with chronic insomnia (SOE=A). To improve access to these treatments, other formats have been developed and tested for providing cognitive-behavioral therapy for insomnia in older adults, such as online programs and use of nonclinician sleep coaches to provide

Table 40.3—Examples of Nonpharmacologic Interventions to Improve Sleep

Intervention	Goal	Brief Description
Stimulus control	To recondition maladaptive sleep-related behaviors	Patient is instructed to go to bed only when sleepy, not use the bed for eating or watching television, get out of bed if unable to fall asleep, return to bed only when sleepy, get up at the same time each morning, not take naps during the day.
Sleep restriction	To improve sleep efficiency (time asleep over time in bed) by limiting time in bed	Patient first keeps a sleep diary for 1–2 weeks to determine average total daily sleep time, then stays in bed only that amount of time plus about 15 minutes, gets up at same time each morning, takes no naps in the daytime, gradually increases time allowed in bed as sleep efficiency improves.
Cognitive interventions	To change misunderstandings and false beliefs regarding sleep	Patient's dysfunctional beliefs and attitudes about sleep are identified (eg, "I'll sleep better if I spend more time in bed"); patient is helped to correct these maladaptive beliefs and attitudes, including education about changes in sleep that occur with aging.
Relaxation techniques	To recognize and relieve tension and anxiety	In progressive muscle relaxation, patient is taught to tense and relax each muscle group; in electromyographic biofeedback, the patient is given feedback regarding muscle tension and learns techniques to relieve it; meditation or imagery techniques are taught to relieve racing thoughts or anxiety.
Cognitive-behavioral therapy	Combines features of several behavioral interventions	Typically combines stimulus control, sleep restriction, and cognitive interventions, with or without relaxation techniques; often also includes sleep hygiene.
Bright light	To correct circadian rhythm causes of sleeping difficulty (ie, sleep-phase problems)	Patient is exposed to sunlight or a light box. For delayed sleep phase: early morning bright light; for advanced sleep phase: evening bright light; light intensity generally ≥2,000 lux. Appropriate time of day of the light exposure is important. Routine eye examination is recommended before treatment; do not use light boxes with ultraviolet exposure.

the intervention (SOE=A). Additional research demonstrates that in older adults with osteoarthritis pain and insomnia, combined behavioral treatment for both pain and insomnia is effective in improving insomnia (SOE=B).

Several small studies have also tested the effectiveness of exposure to bright light (either natural sunlight or with commercially available light boxes) on the sleep of older adults with insomnia (SOE=B). Variable results have been reported for insomnia, with better results seen for circadian rhythm disorders. As mentioned above, appropriately timed morning bright light may be useful in delayed sleep phase, and evening exposure may be useful in older adults with an advanced sleep phase. Even short durations of bright light may be useful.

There is less evidence to support other nonpharmacologic interventions for insomnia, but some patients may find these methods useful. For example, bathing before sleep may enhance the quality of sleep in older adults, perhaps related to changes in body temperature with bathing. Moderate-intensity exercise also improves sleep in healthy, older adults; however, strenuous exercise performed immediately before bedtime can interfere with sleep. Studies have also suggested beneficial effects on sleep with Tai Chi (SOE=B).

Pharmacotherapy

Pharmacotherapy may be considered in individuals with transient sleep problems, such as problems associated with an acute stressor, or in individuals with chronic insomnia that has not responded to behavioral therapy, after a discussion with the patient about potential risks and benefits. As mentioned above, if a decision is made to use a sedative-hypnotic in an older adult, the smallest dosage of an agent with the least risk of adverse events should be chosen and used for the shortest duration necessary. Short-acting sedative-hypnotic agents are recommended for patients with problems falling asleep, and intermediate-acting agents are recommended for patients with problems staying asleep (Table 40.4). Evidence suggests that use of sedative-hypnotics is increasing in the United States, and new prescription sleep medication use is more likely among older adults with poor mental and physical health.

Benzodiazepines (eg, the intermediate-acting agents estazolam and temazepam) bind nonselectively to the gamma-aminobutyric-acid benzodiazepine (GABA-BZ) receptor subunits. As a class, these agents have potential adverse events, including confusion, rebound insomnia, tolerance (to treatment effects), and withdrawal symptoms on discontinuation. Older adults can be more sensitive to the sedating effects of benzodiazepines, with greater risk of confusion and falls (SOE=B). Long-acting benzodiazepines (eg, flurazepam, quazepam), in particular, should not be used in older adults. Short-acting agents may have less association with falls and hip fractures, presumably because of less daytime carryover, but there is evidence

Table 40.4—Prescription Medications for Insomnia in Older Adults

Class, Medication	Starting Dose (mg)	Usual Dose (mg)	Estimate of Half-Life (hours) in Older Adults	Comments
Intermediate-acting benzodiazepine				
Temazepam	7.5	7.5–15	8.8	Psychomotor impairment, increased risk of falls. Caution suggested because of adverse cognitive and psychomotor effects in older adults. Guidelines recommend avoiding use in older adults.
Short-acting nonbenzodiazepines				
Eszopiclone	1	1–2	6	Increased risk of falls; may be associated with unpleasant taste, headache. Avoid administration with high-fat meal. Evidence for next-day impairment of driving skills prompted lowering of recommended starting dose, especially in women.
Zaleplon	5	5–10	1	Increased risk of falls; occasional adverse effects include headache, dizziness, nausea, abdominal pain, and somnolence.
Zolpidem	2.5–5 (6.25 extended release)	5 (6.25 extended release)	3	Increased risk of falls. Available in extended release, as a dissolvable tablet, and as an oral spray. Complex sleep-related behaviors reported. Evidence for next-day impairment of driving skills prompted FDA warning and lowering of recommended starting dose, especially in women.
Melatonin receptor agonists				
Ramelteon	8	8	2.6	Dizziness, myalgia, headache, other adverse events reported; no significant rebound insomnia or withdrawal with discontinuation.
Tasimelteon	20	20	1.3	Headache, increased ALT, nightmares and abnormal dreams, FDA approved selectively for non-24-hour sleep-wake disorder.
Orexin receptor antagonist				
Suvorexant	5	5–20	8–19	Next-day somnolence and impaired performance (eg, driving); cataplexy-like symptoms also reported.
Sedating antidepressants				
Doxepin	3	3–6	15.3 (doxepin); 31 (metabolite)	Somnolence/sedation, nausea, and upper respiratory tract infection reported; antagonizes central H_1-receptors (antihistamine); active metabolite; should not be taken within 3 hours of a meal.
Mirtazapine[OL]	7.5	7.5–30	31–39	Increased appetite, weight gain, headache, dizziness, daytime carryover; long half-life may limit use in some older patients; lower doses tend to be more sedating than higher doses.
Trazodone[OL]	25–50	25–100	6 ± 2; may be prolonged	Orthostatic effects, increased risk of falls, risk of priapism in men; limited evidence for use in insomnia.

of an association between short-acting agents and falls at night (SOE=B). Agents with rapid elimination in general also result in the most pronounced rebound and withdrawal syndromes after discontinuation. Rebound insomnia after discontinuation of short-acting agents is dose dependent and can be reduced by tapering the dosage before discontinuing the drug.

The nonbenzodiazepine benzodiazepine-receptor agonists (NBRAs [eg, eszopiclone, zolpidem, zaleplon]) are structurally unrelated to benzodiazepines but bind to the GABA-BZ receptor with relative selectivity for sedative and amnestic properties. Evidence suggests that NBRAs are relatively well tolerated in healthy older adults (SOE=B), but evidence is limited in older adults with significant comorbidity. Zolpidem is a nonbenzodiazepine imidazopyridine. In older adults, studies suggest that zolpidem does not result in rebound insomnia, agitation, or anxiety when discontinued. Evidence of next morning impairment in driving ability (that the patient may not be aware of and that may increase risk of motor vehicle accidents) above a threshold blood level of zolpidem has prompted recommendations for use of lower doses of these agents, particularly in women, who clear zolpidem more slowly than men. Zaleplon is a nonbenzodiazepine hypnotic from the pyrazolopyrimidine class, and has also been studied for short-term use in older adults with insomnia. Because of their rapid onset of action, zolpidem and zaleplon should be taken only immediately before bedtime. Eszopiclone is an s-isomer of the cyclopyrrolone zopiclone, and it has a longer duration of action than the other nonbenzodiazepines. Epidemiologic evidence suggests that NRBAs may be associated with an increased age-adjusted risk of falling that is similar to that of the benzodiazepines. Given these and other findings, concerns remain regarding the risks of confusion, falls, and fracture with chronic use of NBRAs in older adults (particularly those who are frail), and caution is warranted even with these agents. The use of benzodiazepines and NRBAs should be limited to ≤6 months, because long-term use is associated with an increased risk of cognitive impairment and dementia.

Orexin receptor antagonists are reported to promote sleep at doses that do not disrupt cognition. Suvorexant is the first dual orexin receptor antagonist approved for treatment of insomnia in the United States. Orexin promotes wakefulness, and suvorexant promotes sleep by blocking orexin neuropeptides from binding to their receptors. Suvorexant may cause next-day somnolence and impaired performance (eg, impaired driving). Cataplexy-like symptoms with leg weakness has also been reported.

The melatonin receptor agonist ramelteon is a selective MT1/MT2 receptor agonist. Ramelteon reduces sleep latency and increases total sleep time in older adults (SOE=B), without evidence of significant rebound or withdrawal effects with discontinuation.

The tricyclic antidepressant doxepin is available in a low-dose formulation (3–6 mg) approved for treatment of insomnia characterized by problems with sleep maintenance (SOE=B). At low dosages, doxepin selectively antagonizes H_1 receptors, which is believed to promote the onset and maintenance of sleep. Low dosages of other sedating antidepressants such as trazodone[OL] or mirtazapine[OL] at bedtime have been used as sleeping aids for many years, but there is limited research evidence to support this practice (SOE=D). Sedating antidepressants have been suggested for use at low dosages as a nighttime aid for sleep in depressed patients receiving another antidepressant at therapeutic dosages during the daytime. Other indications include patients with a history of psychoactive substance use problems, lack of response to other sleeping medications, suspected untreated sleep apnea (in which further respiratory depression with certain other agents is a concern), and fibromyalgia (in which there is some evidence of antidepressant medication treatment effect). However, the adverse effects of sedating antidepressants may limit their usefulness.

Guidelines from the American Academy of Sleep Medicine for the pharmacologic management of insomnia in adults of all ages recommend against use of several agents, primarily because of limited evidence to support effectiveness, including trazodone, tiagabine, diphenhydramine, melatonin, tryptophan, and valerian (SOE=C). Sedating antipsychotics[OL] should not be used in routine management of insomnia in older adults unless the patient has other serious psychiatric illness that warrants treatment with an antipsychotic medication.

Chronic Hypnotic Use

In European studies, a relatively high prevalence of chronic sedative-hypnotic use in older adults (5%–8% in older men, up to 25% in older women) has been reported. There is epidemiologic evidence for increased morbidity and mortality with chronic use of prescription sleeping pills; however, much of this literature is older and predates the availability of newer, nonbenzodiazepine hypnotics, so the relationship between these hypnotics and morbidity/mortality is not clear. In addition, after tolerance to hypnotics develops, long-term use of these agents can actually make sleep quality worse. Data reported from a longitudinal study of older adults in Germany indicated a higher rate of sleep-related complaints in those who took sleeping medications than in those who did not.

Methods to help older chronic hypnotic users reduce or eliminate their use of these agents have been reported (SOE=B). In general, tapering of the hypnotic in chronic users may prevent rebound insomnia and other adverse withdrawal effects. One reported strategy involved decreasing the hypnotic dose by one-half for 2 weeks, followed by full withdrawal, which was effective in eliminating hypnotic use without adverse events on nighttime sleep, depressive symptoms, or daytime sleepiness. In another small controlled trial in which benzodiazepine use was tapered to complete withdrawal over as many as 6 weeks, more success was seen in those participants randomized to receive a nightly dose of 2 mg of controlled-release melatonin rather than placebo. At follow-up 6 months later, nearly 80% of those who successfully discontinued benzodiazepines continued to report good sleep quality. Cognitive-behavioral therapy, when combined with gradual tapering of the hypnotic dose, has also been demonstrated to be effective in reducing or eliminating chronic benzodiazepine use (SOE=B).

Nonprescription Sleeping Agents

Nearly half of older adults report using nonprescription OTC sleeping agents; however, there is little evidence to support this practice. Commonly used nonprescription agents include sedating antihistamines, acetaminophen, alcohol, melatonin, and herbal products. Sedating antihistamines (eg, diphenhydramine) are common ingredients in OTC sleeping agents as well as in combination analgesic-sleeping agents that are marketed for nighttime use. Diphenhydramine has potent anticholinergic effects, and tolerance to its sedating effects develops after several weeks, so it is not recommended for older adults. Individuals with mild nighttime discomfort and mild insomnia may have adequate relief with a simple pain reliever (eg, acetaminophen) at bedtime. Although alcohol causes some initial drowsiness, it can interfere with sleep later in the night and can actually worsen sleeping difficulties. There is some evidence in older adults with insomnia that melatonin administration decreases sleep latency and wake time after sleep onset and increases sleep efficiency (time asleep over time in bed), but results are mixed. In placebo-controlled trials lasting up to 6 months, sustained-release melatonin improved several parameters of sleep quality and was well tolerated in older adults with insomnia, and 2 days of treatment with sustained-release melatonin did not impair psychomotor function, memory recall, and driving skills in older adults. However, current guidelines found insufficient evidence to recommend the use of melatonin in the treatment of chronic insomnia in older adults. Valerian is an herbal product with mild sedative action that has been marketed for insomnia. Its mechanism of action is uncertain, and it contains several potentially active compounds, with risk of adverse events. A systematic review found the existing evidence for efficacy of valerian to be inconclusive (SOE=C). Kava, another herbal product marketed for insomnia, has a significant risk of adverse events, including hepatotoxicity, and is not recommended.

CHOOSING WISELY® RECOMMENDATIONS

Sleep Issues

- Do not use benzodiazepines or other sedative-hypnotics in older adults as first choice for insomnia, agitation, or delirium.

RESOURCES

- Leggett A, Pepin R, Sonnega A, et al. Predictors of new onset sleep medication and treatment among older adults in the United States. *J Gerontol A Biol Sci Med Sci.* 2016;71(7):954–960.

- Qaseem A, Kansagara D, Forciea MA, et al. Management of chronic insomnia disorder in adults: a clinical practice guideline from the American College of Physicians. *Ann Intern Med.* 2016;165(2):125–133.

- Reynolds ME, Cone PH. Managing adult insomnia confidently. *J Nurse Pract.* 2018;4(10):718–724.e1.

- Sawyer AM, King TS, Weaver TE, et al. A tailored intervention for PAP adherence: the SCIP-PA Trial. *Behav Sleep Med.* 2019;17(1):49–69.

CHAPTER 41—DEPRESSION AND OTHER MOOD DISORDERS

KEY POINTS

- Major depressive disorders are rare among physically healthy older adults but depressive symptoms are common among persons with physically debilitating illnesses, adding morbidity and increasing both the costs of care and risk of a major depressive episode.

- Treatment of depression may require up to 12 weeks before remission is complete, but an initial response to medication should be seen within the first 4 weeks.

- In a substantial minority of cases, trials of more than one antidepressant or combination therapy with two antidepressants may be required before remission is achieved.

- Executive cognitive dysfunction is easily assessed and when present predicts poor response to medication, as well as the need for adapted psychotherapy.

- Exercise reduces depressive symptoms and should be prescribed for all depressed older adults who can increase their level of physical activity.

- Bipolar depression in older adults may be more common than previously thought and should be treated with a mood stabilizer rather than an antidepressant.

EPIDEMIOLOGY

Depression is a leading cause of disability-adjusted life years lost across the life span and projected to be a greater factor within a generation. Mood disorders are implicated in 10% of all hospitalizations. However, prevalence studies of community residents demonstrate surprisingly low rates of depressive disorders among those ≥65 years old. Only 1%–2% of women and <1% of men interviewed with standardized instruments met diagnostic criteria for major depressive disorder (SOE=A). Both current and lifetime prevalence rates for older adults are lower than those for middle-aged adults; furthermore, these relatively low rates persist after accounting for possible premature death and institutionalization, both of which can be associated with depression. Similarly, the incidence of first-episode major depressive disorder decreases after age 65. Data demonstrating that older adults are less likely to recognize depression and to endorse depressed mood offer one explanation for the lower prevalence and incidence of depressive syndromes among older community residents.

However, the prevalence of depressive symptoms that do not meet the threshold for a major depressive disorder as defined by the *Diagnostic and Statistical Manual of Mental Disorders, 5th Edition (DSM-5)* is substantial in older adults, with most studies reporting rates in the range of 15%. These subsyndromal states are not inconsequential. "Minor" or "subsyndromal" depression, defined variably as the presence of depressed mood with 2 or 3 additional symptoms of major depressive disorder has been associated with increased use of health services, excess disability, and poor health outcomes, including higher mortality. *DSM-5* uses a more descriptive, precise terminology to capture these depressive states and assigns them the status of "other specified depressive disorder" in recognition of their associated morbidity.

The prevalence rates of both major and subsyndromal depression vary greatly by the setting in which older adults are seen and by methods used to identify cases. Increased rates of depression are found among older adults seen in health care facilities and inpatient settings. Major depressive disorder has been identified in 6%–10% of older adults in primary care clinics and in 12%–20% of nursing-home residents. More varied rates of 11%–45% have been reported among older adults requiring inpatient medical care. The reported prevalence rates of minor depression in outpatient medical settings have varied as well, with reported rates of 8% to >40%. Studies that count symptoms due to physical illness toward a diagnosis of depression can inflate prevalence rates among medical patients because of symptom overlap. In mental health settings, major depressive disorder is the most common diagnosis seen among older patients and accounts for >40% of outpatient caseloads and inpatient psychiatry admissions.

Studies show that risk factors for depression in older ethnic minority patients can differ from those in whites. For example, lack of spirituality was a risk factor for depression in black Americans but not in white Americans. In general, older adults of ethnic minorities exhibit less use of mental health services. Shorter length of residence in the United States as well as personal beliefs influence the use of mental health services among older immigrants and members of ethnic minority groups.

CLINICAL PRESENTATION AND DIAGNOSIS

The Geriatric Syndrome of Late-Life Depression

Although aging does not markedly affect the phenomenology of depression, older adults are more often preoccupied with somatic symptoms and less frequently report depressed mood and guilty preoccupations. Among those who do not acknowledge sustained sadness, a persistent loss of pleasure and interest in previously enjoyable activities (*anhedonia*) for at least 2 weeks is necessary for a diagnosis of major depressive disorder. The phrase "with seasonal pattern" may be added to recurrent major depressive disorder, but depression induced by the shorter day length during winter is uncommon in older adults. Responses to a catastrophic loss such as bereavement, onset of crippling disability or illness, financial collapse, or natural disaster may include profound sadness, preoccupation with the event, impaired concentration, sleep disturbance, and loss of appetite—all consistent with the diagnosis of a depressive disorder. However, grief should be considered an appropriate and even adaptive response, rather than evidence of pathology. Nonetheless, when the response is out of proportion to personal expectations or cultural norms, or when there is a history of depression, clinical judgment may dictate a diagnosis of major depression. When bereavement is associated with prolonged, angry, embittered, nearly paralyzing preoccupation with the lost loved one, *DSM-5* places the condition under "other specified trauma- and stressor-related disorder" as a "persistent complex bereavement disorder." Psychotherapy for complex bereavement more closely resembles that used for post-traumatic stress disorder, but adherence is improved when an SSRI is added to the regimen.

The diagnosis of depression in physically ill older adults is confounded by the overlap among symptoms of major depressive disorder and somatic illness. Patients with advanced physical illness may be preoccupied with thoughts about death or worthlessness because of marked disability, yet not meet criteria for a major depressive episode. The *DSM-5* criteria require that the depressive symptoms are not a direct result of a general medical condition or medication used to treat it. The alternative diagnosis of mood disorder due to a general medical condition should be used for patients with depression that appears to result directly from a specific medical condition (eg, hypothyroidism, pancreatic cancer, end-stage renal disease). In either case, when symptoms are disabling, treatment should be offered.

Screening

Simply screening for the presence of depressed mood and anhedonia identifies most medically ill patients who also meet diagnostic criteria for major depressive disorder. These symptoms are less likely to be confounded by those of a medical illness. When the clinician fears an older adult is minimizing distress or associated disability, it is helpful to obtain further information from involved family members or caregivers. However, without a protocol for treatment initiation and response assessment or referral for mental health services, screening for depressive disorders in primary care or social service settings is ineffective. Informing the primary care clinician of the results of screening without linking to mental health consultation or referral too often leads to subtherapeutic dosages of an antidepressant, inadequate assessment of treatment response, and the patient's abandonment of therapy.

The nine items of the Patient Health Questionnaire (PHQ-9) cover the diagnostic criteria for major depressive disorder, and the initial two questions (the "PHQ-2") can be used for screening. In addition, serial administrations of the PHQ-9 can be used to reliably assess response to treatment.

The PHQ-9 and PHQ-2 are available online in English and Spanish as public access (http://phqscreeners.com). Patients scoring a total of ≥3 on the depressed mood plus anhedonia questions on the PHQ-2 should be assessed with the remaining seven questions of the PHQ-9. Patients scoring 3 on the anhedonia questions alone should also be fully assessed. A complaint of depression need not be present for a diagnosis of major depressive disorder, provided the other symptoms significantly impair function and are not the direct result of somatic illness. For management based on PHQ-9 score, see Table 41.1.

At a score of ≥10, the PHQ-9 has good sensitivity and specificity for major depressive disorder among primary care patients versus a structured diagnostic interview conducted by a mental health professional. People scoring ≥15 and those with suicidal ideation may require psychiatric consultation. A change of 5 points is considered a minimal clinically important difference and evidence of response to treatment (Table 41.2). Remission is best defined as a total score of ≤5. When the score has changed by <5 points despite 4 weeks of treatment at recommended dosages, the medication should either be switched or combined with another antidepressant.

Those who acknowledge thinking they would be "better off dead" or "hurting themselves" (the 9th item of the PHQ-9) should be asked about intent, plan, or method of attempting suicide and the presence of a firearm in the home. Firearms are the leading means

Table 41.1—Indications to Start Antidepressant Therapy Based on Patient Health Questionnaire-9

PHQ-9 Score	Depression Severity	Clinician Response
1–4	None	None
5–9	Mild to moderate	If not currently treated, rescreen in 2 weeks. If currently treated, optimize antidepressant and rescreen in 2 weeks.
10–14	Major depressive disorder	Start antidepressant therapy.
≥15	Major depressive disorder	Start antidepressant therapy; obtain psychiatric consultation if suicidality or psychosis suspected.

For additional information, see http://phqscreeners.com.

of suicide among older adults. Unloading the weapon, placing it in a lock box, or removing it from the premises can be recommended to reduce access. The presence of suicidal thoughts indicates greater severity and the need for referral. When intent or a plan is present, safety trumps confidentiality and emergency interventions may be justified. Older white men exhibit the highest risk.

Another standardized instrument for evaluating depressive symptoms is the 15-item Geriatric Depression Scale (GDS). Although it offers the convenience of a "yes/no" response, and it is virtually free of somatic and sleep queries, it does not query suicidal or death ideation and is not useful for assessing treatment response. The PHQ-9 and the GDS may be reliable when administered to people with mild to moderate dementia; response to treatment with SSRI therapy in dementia with depression may be no better than with placebo (SOE=A).

Emerging evidence suggests that the diagnostic process for older patients should include an assessment of executive cognitive function. When present, executive dysfunction complicating depression predicts poor response to SSRI therapy and may be better addressed with psychotherapy (SOE=A).

Bipolar Disorder

Although the prevalence of bipolar disorder is low, the increasing numbers of older adults means primary care clinicians will encounter more patients with a bipolar disorder, particularly bipolar depression. Bipolar disorders do not "burn out" in old age. Indeed, few patients with bipolar disorder recover full function despite symptom remission. Among those with bipolar disorder, mania is a more frequent cause of hospitalization than depression, but depression accounts for more disability. Late-onset mania is seen equally among men and women. Age has little impact on the symptom profile except for less sexual preoccupation among older adults. Impaired cognitive processing, executive dysfunction, and changes in subcortical brain structures are common, further reducing the chances of return to full function.

The *DSM-5* criteria for bipolar disorder type 1 (mania with or without depression) and type 2 (major depressive disorder without mania but with hypomania) are unchanged with age. The manic episode (prevalence 1 to 4 per 1,000) often presents with confusion, disorientation, distractibility, and irritability rather than with elevated, positive mood. The clinical interview can be characterized by irrelevant content delivered with an argumentative, emotionally intense yet fluent quality. Grossly unrealistic ideas concerning finances, travel, or plans for the future are common. Inflated self-esteem, grandiosity, and contentious claims of certainty in the face of evidence to the contrary are also seen. The unsuspecting examiner may be puzzled or irritated by the difficulty of the clinical interaction until the diagnosis of mania is considered.

Table 41.2—Prescriber Response Guidelines at 4 Weeks Based on the Patient Health Questionnaire-9 and the Sequenced Treatment Alternatives to Relieve Depression (STAR*D) Studies

PHQ-9 Score or Change	Outcome	Prescriber Response
No decrease or increase	Nonresponse	Switch medication
Decrease of 2–4 points	Partial response	Augment medication
Decrease of ≥5 points	Response	Maintain medication
Score <5	Remission	Maintain medication

For additional information, see http://phqscreeners.com.

The presence of psychosis, sleep disturbance, and aggressiveness may lead to the mistaken diagnosis of dementia or depressive disorder rather than mania. Because mania in late life is less frequent than depression or dementia, these patients are often treated with antipsychotics, antidepressants, or benzodiazepines, which provide partial relief. Late-onset mania is more often secondary to or closely associated with other medical disorders, most commonly stroke, dementia, or hyperthyroidism, and also with medications, including antidepressants, steroids, stimulants, and other agents with known CNS effects. A search for treatable components that contribute acutely to the person's disability should be pursued.

Risk factors for cerebrovascular disease, including excessive use of alcohol or tobacco, suboptimal control of hypertension, hyperlipidemia, and other cardiovascular risk factors, should be explored. Careful inquiry of the family may reveal repeated hypomanic episodes that did not seriously impair the individual but in retrospect are clear indications of earlier disease. The difficulty of recognizing the diagnosis, care for contributing conditions, age-related vulnerability to adverse events of medication, and the frequency with which structural brain changes are associated all make treatment more difficult.

Occurring in approximately 0.5% of the U.S. population, bipolar disorder type II is characterized by recurrent major depressive episodes interspersed with periods of hypomania. Because interpersonal difficulties can be minimal, and some symptoms can temporarily increase performance with tasks, past episodes of hypomania may be unrecognized by the patient and family. Major depressive episodes also occur in bipolar disorder I, in which the occurrence of one or more manic episodes is the distinguishing diagnostic feature. There are also mixed states in which criteria for both mania and major depressive disorder are present. As a result, the term "bipolar depression" spans the spectrum of bipolar disorders.

Psychotic Depression

The recognition of psychotic depression has particular relevance for primary care clinicians. Patients with psychotic depression have sustained, fixed, false beliefs (delusions) in association with depressed mood. These delusions are often plausible and focused on physical or medical preoccupations, such as the belief that one's bowels are "blocked with cancer" or "I know there's something there and the doctors are just not telling me." Psychotic depression may be suspected when the irrational belief focuses on somatic symptoms or around fears of a serious physical condition when no medical evidence can be identified to support the belief. Patients with somatic delusions often visit multiple specialists and obtain repeated testing to identify problems that they "know" exist rather than for the purpose of seeking relief from persistent somatic "worries."

TREATMENT

Although mood disorders are eminently treatable, effective treatment remains a goal not easily attained. Only 50% of patients with major depressive disorder fully respond to initial antidepressant treatment (SOE=A). An additional one-third recover when the antidepressant is switched to another agent or is combined with a second antidepressant or psychotherapy. For those who do recover, 40%–60% experience recurrence depending on the severity of the initial episode and persistence of symptoms. Although a substantial number of patients with "subclinical," "subsyndromal," or "minor" depression experience a remission of symptoms without intervention, each category is associated with as much as a 5-fold risk of a subsequent major depressive episode. Poor self-assessed health, apathy, anxiety, executive dysfunction, and perceived lack of social support predict a less benign course. The onset of macular degeneration, stroke, and myocardial infarction are reliable indicators of depression risk, especially in the context of a prior history of mood disorder.

The current approach to mood disorders in late life includes a more aggressive acute phase of treatment to bring about remission of the current episode, continuation of treatment for an additional 6 months after symptom remission to prevent relapse, and maintenance treatment to prevent recurrence. For patients with bipolar disorders or a history of depression complicated by psychosis, suicidality, or recurrent episodes, maintenance treatment should be provided for ≥3 years. However, the duration of maintenance therapy should be based on the frequency and severity of previous episodes and may need to be lifelong. Combined pharmacotherapy with psychotherapy is recommended for all patients with bipolar disorders and recurrent, severe psychotic or suicidal depression (SOE=B).

The First Weeks of Treatment

Substantial data indicate that 4 weeks is adequate to identify those patients who at 12 weeks will be nonresponders or partial responders (SOE=B). The sooner the response occurs, the sooner the remission is likely to be achieved. More severe depression at baseline is associated with slower response; higher self-esteem is associated with rapid response. At 4 weeks, one-third of medicated patients will be nonresponders, one-third will have responded fully, and one-third partially. As treatment duration extends, the response rates for both partial and nonresponders decelerate. The longer the patient remains symptomatic, the greater the indication that either the dosage or the medication should be changed. In addition, partial response predicts a greater likelihood of recurrence of a major episode of depression as opposed to complete response.

Pharmacotherapy of Single or Recurrent Episodes of Major Depression

Currently available antidepressants are thought to work through the enhancement of monoamine function by either blocking the reuptake or stimulating receptors of serotonin, dopamine, or norepinephrine. For a summary of antidepressants and adverse effects in older adults, see Table 41.3. GI distress is the most

Table 41.3—Selected Antidepressants for Older Adults

Drug	Initial Dosage	Final Dosage	Comments/Precautions
SSRIs			
Citalopram	10 mg qam	20 mg qam	Risk of QT_c prolongation in doses >20 mg/d, nausea, tremor, hyponatremia, serotonin syndrome
Escitalopram	10 mg qam	10–20 mg qam	Nausea, tremor, hyponatremia, serotonin syndrome; reduce dosage in renal insufficiency
Sertraline	25 mg qam	100–200 mg qam	Nausea, tremor, hyponatremia, insomnia, serotonin syndrome
Selective Serotonergic and Noradrenergic Reuptake Inhibitors (SSRIs/SNRIs)			
Duloxetine	20–30 mg qam	60 mg qam	Drug interactions (CYP1A2, -2D6 substrate); chronic liver disease, alcoholism, increased serum transaminase; reduce dosage in renal insufficiency
Venlafaxine XR	37.5–75 mg qam	75–225 mg qam	Can increase blood pressure; headache, nausea, vomiting; do not stop abruptly; reduce dosage in renal insufficiency
Vortioxetine	5 mg qam	10-20 mg qam	Nausea; no data available on doses >5 mg in older adults
Tricyclic Antidepressants (TCAs)			
Nortriptyline	10–25 mg qhs	25–100 mg qhs	Glaucoma (avoid if closed-angle), constipation, urinary retention, diabetes; may be fatal in overdose; therapeutic window 50–150 ng/mL serum level
Others			
Aripiprazole	5 mg qam	15 mg qam	Adjunctive treatment with SSRIs and venlafaxine; prolonged half-life, may produce agitation at high dosages because of D_2 dopamine receptor agonist activity
Bupropion	75 mg q12h 150 mg qam	150–300 mg q12h 300 mg extended release qam	Agitation, insomnia, seizures
Methylphenidate	5 mg qam	20 mg q12h	Adjunctive treatment with citalopram; weight loss, insomnia, agitation, hypertension
Mirtazapine	7.5 mg qhs	15–45 mg qhs	Dry mouth, weight gain, sedation, daytime drowsiness, potential for neutropenia; reduce dosage in renal insufficiency

common transient adverse reaction to serotonergic agents. The syndrome of inappropriate antidiuretic hormone (SIADH) is an uncommon, life-threatening adverse reaction to serotonergic agents; it is generally treated with fluid restriction. The even rarer serotonin syndrome is difficult to diagnose and easily overlooked; it requires supportive care and treatment of associated symptoms (Table 41.4).

When psychosis complicates major depressive disorder, the evidence directing choice of pharmacotherapy for older adults is evolving. Electroconvulsive therapy (ECT, discussed further below) is effective for depression complicated by psychosis and is often considered the treatment of choice for patients with severe depression accompanied by suicidal thoughts and for those who do not respond to augmentation therapies (SOE=B). Yet, few patients or their family members will consider ECT without having exhausted other alternatives. In the multisite Study of Pharmacotherapy of Psychotic Depression (STOP-PD), remission was achieved in >60% of the geriatric patients who received a combination of sertraline and olanzapine over 12 weeks. Remission rates with combination therapy were substantially better than with sertraline alone. The average end-of-study daily doses were nearly 150 mg of sertraline and more than 12 mg of olanzapine. Therefore, although ECT remains an effective treatment option for late-life psychotic depression, intensive antipsychotic and antidepressant pharmacotherapy can be an effective initial strategy.

Pharmacotherapy of Mania

For a summary of treatment of bipolar disorders in older adults, see Table 41.5. Expert opinion, guidelines, and the Systematic Treatment Enhancement Program for Bipolar Disorder (STEP-BD) reports agree that anticonvulsants, called mood stabilizers in this context, are preferable for both acute treatment and prevention

Table 41.4—Clinical Signs and Symptoms of Serotonin Syndrome

- Use of medication(s) with serotonergic activity
- Cognitive and behavioral changes: agitation, hyperactivity, worsening confusion, restlessness
- Diaphoresis
- Diarrhea and GI upset
- Fever usually >100.5°F (38°C)
- Hyperreflexia with or without myoclonus
- Incoordination, ataxia, or new onset of falls
- Ocular clonus
- Rhabdomyolysis
- Shivering
- Seizures
- Tremor

of recurrence in late-life bipolar mania (SOE=A). The anticonvulsant divalproex is increasingly considered first choice for treatment and prevention of mania. A therapeutic blood level of 50–100 mcg/mL is considered both safe and efficacious. When the level is subtherapeutic and the patient response inadequate, the dose should be increased. When the level is at or above the upper limit and there is little or no response after 2 weeks, the drug trial should be declared a failure. Partial response accompanied by a blood level within the therapeutic range indicates the need to increase the dosage or add an antipsychotic. Divalproex inhibits hepatic enzymes that metabolize medications frequently used by older adults. Patients taking β-blockers, type 1C antiarrhythmics (eg, flecainide, propafenone), benzodiazepines, or anticoagulants should be monitored more closely until the divalproex dosage has been stabilized. Laboratory tests (including CBC with platelets, AST, ALT, and amylase) should be performed when treatment is started, when the dosage is increased, and at least every 6 months. Dosage reduction is indicated for tremor interfering with self-care, ataxia or unsteady gait, excess sedation, or heart rate <50 beats per minute. Divalproex should be held or discontinued if the following do not remit after dosage reduction or dosage withholding: platelet count <80,000/μL, or AST, ALT, or amylase ≥2-fold above upper limit of normal.

Response to divalproex requires at least a 3-week period, including titration to a therapeutic range. In the interim, individuals whose mania is exhausting or associated with overly aggressive behavior require an antipsychotic or benzodiazepine. A number of second-generation antipsychotics are approved by the FDA for treatment of mania (Table 41.5). Meta-analyses indicate that these second-generation antipsychotics appear to be equally effective (SOE=A) such that the choice of an individual agent is based on the adverse-event profile. However, the available data on the treatment of mania in these studies include few older adults.

Older adults who have had good results with lithium should not be switched to an alternative unless adverse events become disabling. Nonetheless, the use of lithium as initial treatment should be considered cautiously. Structural brain changes that may not be clinically apparent are associated with a higher risk of toxicity. Diabetes insipidus, hyperglycemia, thyroid abnormalities, severe tremor, confusion, heart failure, arrhythmia, and psoriasis are among the more frequent reasons for discontinuing lithium. Manifestations of lithium toxicity include GI complaints, ataxia, slurred speech, delirium, or coma. Toxicity in older adults can occur at plasma concentrations below the therapeutic threshold of 1 mEq/L. Mild tremor and nystagmus without functional consequences frequently accompany lithium treatment and should not be considered signs of toxicity. Dosage reduction is indicated for tremor interfering with self-care or for ataxia or unsteady gait. The onset of diabetes insipidus can also be cause for discontinuing lithium.

Pharmacotherapy of Bipolar Depression

Similar to the case in treatment of mania, there is a relative consensus that mood stabilizers are preferable to antidepressants for acute treatment and prevention of recurrence of late-life bipolar depression (SOE=B). Indeed, antidepressants should be used with caution in bipolar depression because of the risk of a manic reaction or other adverse events, and common lack of efficacy. However, the prescribing pathway for bipolar depression in late life is characterized more by off-label use of medications than by FDA-approved indications. Beyond the initial step of prescribing either lithium or lamotrigine, next steps are dictated by the patient's symptom profile. For episodes of depression in both bipolar types I and II in which the patient's history includes relatively less mania, the antidepressant bupropion is a reasonable addition. However, for instances characterized by mixed symptoms or more frequent episodes of mania, a second-generation antipsychotic or a second mood stabilizer is preferable. Purely based on its adverse-event profile and the likelihood of drug interactions (Table 41.5), lamotrigine would appear to be preferable to lithium, divalproex, and carbamazepine for bipolar depression (SOE=D). Although lamotrigine may be given twice daily, its prolonged half-life, which requires slow titration, suggests once-a-day dosing may be adequate for older adults.

Table 41.5—Medications Used to Stabilize Mood in Mania and Bipolar Depression

Drug	Initial Dosage (mg)	Final Dosage (mg)	Sedative Potential	Precautions	FDA-Approved Indications and Comments
Anticonvulsants					
Carbamazepine	100 q12h 100 qhs (extended release)	500 q12h 800 qhs	Moderate	Delayed onset of action, drug interactions, dizziness, unsteady gait, anemia; CBC and serum chemistries at baseline, then q6mo; enhances cytochrome P450 activity and decreases other drug concentrations	Acute manic and mixed bipolar I episodes; therapeutic concentration 4–12 mcg/mL
Divalproex sodium Extended-release Delayed-release	125–250 q12h 250 qhs 250 qhs	1,000 q12h 1,000 qhs 500 qhs	Moderate	Delayed onset of action, drug interactions, GI upset, tremor, weight gain, edema, thrombocytopenia, sedation; CBC and serum chemistries at baseline, then q6mo; inhibits hepatic enzymes and increases other drug concentrations; hepatotoxicity, pancreatitis; reduce dosage in renal insufficiency	Acute manic and mixed bipolar I episodes; better tolerated than carbamazepine; therapeutic concentration 50–100 mcg/mL
Lamotrigine	25 qhs	100 q12h	Low	Headaches; prolonged half-life, requires slow dose titration; appearance of rash calls for immediate cessation; clearance reduced by valproate	Bipolar I depression to prevent recurrence; does not alter cytochrome P450 activity
Antipsychotics					
Aripiprazole	5 qam	15 qam	Low	Prolonged half-life, may produce agitation at high dosages because of D_2 dopamine receptor agonist activity	Acute manic and mixed bipolar I episodes and for adjunctive treatment of major depressive disorder
Olanzapine	2.5 qhs	15 qhs	Moderate	Slightly anticholinergic as dosage increases, weight gain, metabolic syndrome, diabetes	Acute manic and mixed bipolar I episodes
Quetiapine	25 qhs	800 in divided doses	Moderate	Sedation, weight gain, metabolic syndrome, diabetes, arrhythmia	Acute manic and bipolar I and II depression; sedative; less extrapyramidal symptoms, tardive dyskinesia
Risperidone	0.25 qhs	6 in divided doses	Low	Extrapyramidal symptoms likely at doses >3 mg, weight gain, metabolic syndrome, diabetes	Acute manic and mixed bipolar I episodes
Lithium compounds					
Lithium carbonate Controlled-release	150–300 q24h 225 q24h	600–900 q24h in divided doses 450 q12h	Low	Renal clearance is sole route of elimination; toxicity may appear below therapeutic range; neurotoxicity at low levels including ataxia, myoclonus, confusion; polyuria, polydipsia may be signs of diabetes insipidus; nausea, vomiting are signs of toxicity; risk of hypothyroidism, renal impairment and hypercalcemia	Acute manic episodes: 0.6–1 mEq/L Maintenance therapeutic level: 0.4–0.6 mEq/L

Titration of lamotrigine should be conducted very carefully in patients who may also be taking hepatic cytochrome isoenzyme–inducing medications or valproic acid. In the absence of these, treatment can begin at 25 mg/d for 2 weeks, then 50 mg/d for 2 weeks, then 100 mg/d for 1 week, then 200 mg/d for usual maintenance. As with most anticonvulsants, dosages should be reduced by approximately 50% for patients with moderate liver dysfunction and by approximately 75% for those with more severe dysfunction.

Electroconvulsive Therapy

ECT is highly effective for treatment of major depressive disorder and mania in older adults. ECT is the first-line treatment for patients at serious risk of suicide or life-threatening poor oral intake due to a major depressive disorder (SOE=B). Patients with delusional depression can demonstrate paranoia about their food or caregivers, precluding pharmacologic treatment because of unreliable oral intake. Also, delusional depression is less responsive to standard medication regimens. Therefore, ECT is generally the first-line treatment for these patients and is associated with response rates that approximate 80%.

The cognitive adverse events of ECT are the principal factor limiting its acceptance. Anterograde amnesia or the inability to learn new information can be pronounced initially, particularly during bilateral ECT, but improves rapidly after treatment is completed. Retrograde amnesia is more persistent, and the recall of events that immediately preceded ECT can be lost permanently. Although patients may complain that ECT has had a long-term effect on their memory, longitudinal studies have not demonstrated lasting cognitive effects; furthermore, improved memory, perhaps owing to recovery from depression, has been reported. There are few absolute medical contraindications other than the presence of increased intracranial pressure or unstable angina. Patients with coronary artery disease or cerebrovascular disease can be administered ECT safely by appropriate pharmacologic management of the autonomic responses that can occur during treatment. Nevertheless, a recent myocardial infarction or cerebrovascular event and unstable coronary artery disease increase the risk of complications. Right unilateral treatment produces fewer cognitive adverse events than bilateral treatment but is less effective unless doses markedly exceeding a patient's seizure threshold are used.

The selection of ECT over aggressive pharmacotherapy is generally made by weighing the risk of waiting for medication to work against the burden of hospital treatment, any medical conditions that can complicate general anesthesia, and fears of the patient and family. After a course of ECT, usually administered twice weekly for 4 weeks, pharmacotherapy should be continued. Patients not responding to intensive antidepressant treatment before receiving ECT have lower acute response rates and are more likely to relapse subsequently, even when antidepressant treatment is continued with a new medication. Although maintenance ECT is sometimes used to prevent relapse, the burden that maintenance ECT places on patients and their families may limit its usefulness for long-term management of late-life major depressive disorder. However, some patients who respond uniquely well to ECT can tolerate maintenance ECT performed on an outpatient basis.

Repetitive Transcranial Magnetic Stimulation (rTMS)

rTMS is a newer treatment for depression in which an electrical coil is positioned over the left prefrontal cortex to generate a focal magnetic field. It is considered noninvasive and has also been studied in an array of psychiatric and neurologic conditions. Typically, treatments are delivered daily for 6 weeks or 30 treatments. Dropout rates and adverse reactions are comparable to those of placebo condition with sham rTMS. However, in a meta-analysis of 6 trials comparing ECT to rTMS, ECT showed greater remission rates. Response to rTMS in older adults is not as robust as in younger adults; only one large multisite trial did not show that younger age was a significant predictor of response (SOE=A). rTMS is not covered by either Medicare or Medicaid.

Psychosocial Interventions

Although evidence-based psychosocial interventions are not accessible to all depressed older adults, many components of the interventions have commonsense appeal and can be incorporated into the practices of primary care clinicians. Studies demonstrating the efficacy of psychotherapy for major depressive disorder in older adults have included problem-solving therapy (SOE=B), cognitive-behavioral therapy, and interpersonal psychotherapy. Problem-solving therapy involves working with the patient to identify practical life difficulties that are causing distress and providing guidance to help the patient identify solutions. Therapy is generally conducted in 6 to 8 meetings spaced 1–2 weeks apart. It has been adapted for administration via Skype with symptom reduction and acceptability equivalent to face-to-face, in-home administration (SOE=C). Cognitive and interpersonal psychotherapy are also time-limited but less highly structured. Psychotherapy for minor depression has been promising, with efficacy demonstrated particularly in individuals who have suffered a loss; the goal is prevention of progression to major depressive disorder. Also, caregivers of older adults can develop depressive syndromes that benefit from psychotherapy. Psychosocial interventions can be effective without psychotropic medication. However, psychotherapy combined with an antidepressant has been associated with a longer period of remission after recovery from the acute episode (SOE=A).

Aerobic exercise is also prescribed as a treatment for mild to moderate depression in older adults who can increase their level of physical activity. It incorporates the concept of behavioral activation central to cognitive-behavioral psychotherapy. (Behavioral activation is the behavioral component of cognitive behavioral therapy. It asks patients to identify and engage in stimulating physical, social, and intellectual activities, and reduces depressive symptoms among primary care patients [SOE=B]). Exercise performed with a partner also adds to the perception of social support. Exercise in combination with antidepressants can yield faster, more lasting results than either alone (SOE=A). Encouraging physical activity should be part of the prescription for all depressed older adults and is the cornerstone of behavioral activation.

Treatment of depression through a disease management model using behavioral health managers is being used more often. The behavioral health manager, usually a master's level social worker, psychologist, or nurse, collaborates with the primary care clinician, patient, and family. Even when routine care is enhanced by improved access to psychiatric consultation, the collaborative disease management model proves superior. Most, if not all, of the patient screening, assessment, and follow-up are conducted over the phone by the behavioral health manager. Large-scale, multisite studies have shown greater rates of response and remission as well as lower levels of suicidality with the disease management model than with enhanced routine care (SOE=A).

Several studies have found telephone-based psychotherapy to be effective (SOE=B). It is possible that telemedicine is less disruptive for older adults in that they need not prepare for a therapist visit at home. It is certain that for home-bound adults, particularly in rural areas, psychotherapy via telephone or the Internet may be the only therapy available.

RESOURCES

- Butcher HK, Ingram TN. Evidence-Based Practice Guideline: Secondary Prevention of Late-Life Suicide. *J Gerontol Nurs*. 2018;44(11):20–32.

- Conwell Y. Suicide later in life: challenges and priorities for prevention. *Am J Prev Med*. 2014;47(3S2):S244–S250.

- Kok RM, Reynolds CF III. Management of depression in older adults: a review. *JAMA*. 2017;317(20):2114–2122.

CHAPTER 42—ANXIETY DISORDERS

KEY POINTS

- Late-life anxiety is often seen with other medical illnesses or depression.

- Comorbid medical problems that commonly lead to anxiety include cardiovascular and pulmonary disorders.

- SSRIs, including citalopram and sertraline, are often used as first-line treatment for anxiety in late life.

- Nonpharmacologic therapies, particularly cognitive-behavioral therapy and other types of psychotherapies, are beneficial in older adults.

- Screening for anxiety in older adults is recommended, particularly in primary care and hospital settings.

The term "anxiety disorder" encompasses a spectrum of psychiatric illnesses that includes panic disorder, phobias, and generalized anxiety disorder. Older adults can suffer from the full spectrum of anxiety disorders, which are described in the *Diagnostic and Statistical Manual of Mental Disorders, 5th Edition (DSM-5)*. Older adults can experience a subjective feeling of anxiety that can meet a level of clinical concern that warrants treatment but does not necessarily fulfill the full diagnostic criteria for an anxiety disorder. Although such symptoms merit clinical attention, true anxiety disorders are the focus of this chapter. In addition, obsessive-compulsive disorders, including hoarding, as well as posttraumatic stress disorder will be discussed. These disorders are often associated with significant anxiety symptoms and were classified under the heading of "anxiety disorders" in previous editions of the *DSM*.

Because the published literature on anxiety disorders in older adults is limited, some of the characterizations and treatment strategies described are based on research conducted in younger populations. Such strategies have been modified to take into account the physiologic and psychologic differences between older and younger adults.

Numerous complexities are involved in a proper assessment of anxiety in older adults. Understanding the common issues faced in such an assessment will lead to a more accurate diagnosis and treatment plan. Examples of these complexities include differentiating anxiety disorders from symptoms related to medical conditions or medications, differentiating anxiety disorders from the appropriate ("normal") experience of anxiety associated with the stressors of late life, appropriately attributing the cause of anxiety to an adverse event of medication, and differentiating anxiety from depression. These common challenges are further complicated by the tendency of older adults to resist psychiatric evaluation because of stigma surrounding mental illness or frank denial of illness.

Assessment of anxiety in older adults generally begins with a clinical psychiatric interview to determine the course and nature of symptoms. The interview should include an evaluation of the patient's mental status, including appearance, stated mood, observed affect, and thought process. Consideration of the patient's social context and support systems is particularly relevant in the geriatric population. Assessment of any impairment in functioning related to the anxiety is an important part of the evaluation. A review of all medications, both prescription and OTC, should be done to exclude an alternative medical or pharmacologic explanation for what appears to be an anxiety disorder, or to identify an aggravating condition. Questioning should be done to explore substance use, because use of alcohol or other drugs can exacerbate anxiety symptoms, or may represent an attempt to self-medicate anxiety. Laboratory tests to check for common medical conditions such as renal, thyroid, or hematologic diseases are important. Urine toxicology should be considered in cases in which substance abuse or misuse is suspected.

The Generalized Anxiety Disorder-7 (www.phqscreeners.com) is a 7 item self-report questionnaire that is useful for identifying anxiety disorders in primary care settings. Each item is scored on a scale from 0 to 3, with a score of 5 indicating a likely anxiety disorder and 10 or higher indicative of moderate to severe anxiety.

Clinical anxiety disorders and anxiety as a symptom related to a life stressor are common problems. The ability to recognize and effectively treat anxiety in older adults is important, given the debilitating effects that an unhealthy level of anxiety can have in this vulnerable population.

CLASSES OF ANXIETY DISORDERS

The types of anxiety disorders as currently defined in *DSM-5* are discussed below.

Panic Disorder

Panic disorder is characterized by chronic, repeated, and unexpected panic attacks—spontaneous bouts of overwhelming and irrational fear, terror, or dread when there is no specific cause. During a panic attack, the person experiences a constellation of physical and cognitive symptoms that can include palpitations, sweating, trembling, shortness of breath, the feeling of choking, chest pain or discomfort, nausea or abdominal distress, dizziness or lightheadedness, feelings of derealization (ie, that oneself or others are unreal) or depersonalization (ie, feeling detached from oneself), paresthesias, chills or hot flashes, fear of losing control, "going crazy," or dying. A diagnosis of a true panic attack requires that at least 4 of the somatic symptoms listed above are experienced. Attacks are fairly brief, lasting typically 10–30 minutes. In between panic attacks, individuals with panic *disorder* worry excessively about when and where the next attack may occur and/or significantly change their behavior to avoid having an attack. A clinically significant degree of panic symptoms exists if the history reveals that recurrent and unpredictable panic attacks have occurred for at least 1 month and that time is being spent in worried anticipation of possible recurrence. Agoraphobia may be associated with panic disorder, but is now given a separate diagnosis. In the context of panic disorder, agoraphobia involves the persistent fear of situations that might trigger a panic attack, such as fear of having an attack in the mall or on pubic transportation, and therefore consistently remaining at home.

Individuals who experience one or more panic attacks may not necessarily warrant a diagnosis of panic disorder unless they are worrying about and changing their behavior because of fear of panic attacks. Panic attacks in late life often present with more limited symptoms, often related to one or two organ systems, such as shortness of breath, nausea, and diarrhea; the sensation of palpitations; or dizziness. These limited-symptom panic attacks may be accompanied by feelings of doom, dread, or fear of dying.

The literature suggests that the usual onset of panic disorder is between 15 and 40 years of age and that <1% will have a new-onset panic disorder after age 65, although a Canadian community health survey suggested that almost 25% of older adults with panic disorder in late life had onset after age 55. Panic disorder is considered fairly rare in older adults with a prevalence rate of 0.7% in adults >64 years old. Panic *attacks* in older adults are commonly associated with other psychiatric diagnoses, including major depressive disorder, as well as with medical illnesses, including COPD, hyperthyroidism, arrhythmias, irritable bowel syndrome, and pheochromocytoma.

Agoraphobia

In *DSM-5*, agoraphobia warrants its own diagnosis, separate and distinguishable from panic disorder. It is defined by marked anxiety about ≥2 of the following, including using public transportation, open spaces, enclosed spaces (shops, theaters), being in a crowd, and being outside unaccompanied. This fear is associated with being afraid of panic symptoms or severe embarrassment; the responses to the feared situations are consistent, persistent, and causes significant distress or impairment in social or occupational functioning. It may be associated with panic disorder. It usually begins in teens to mid 20s and is usually persistent. It is associated with significantly increased risk of depression. In older adults, it may be associated with a fear of falling. In one study of older adults with agoraphobia, 11% reported having symptom onset after age 65.

Specific Phobia

A specific phobia is defined as a marked, persistent, excessive, unreasonable fear in the presence of or in anticipation of a particular distinct trigger, such as a specific person, animal, place, object, event, or situation. Examples of simple phobias include fear of snakes, mice, dogs, elevators, flying, or heights. Commonly, the person's anxiety level increases instantly when the feared trigger is encountered. Interestingly, he or she is able to identify this fear as unrealistic and unsupported, even though the cognitive and physiologic responses persist. Specific phobias often involve a great amount of anticipatory anxiety (ie, thoughts of the *possibility* of encountering the feared stimulus), and avoidance behaviors are likely to be reported. The consequence is that the person experiences a variety of personal difficulties as a result of the anxiety. These behaviors interfere with work and daily routines, and they decrease the person's opportunities to experience pleasurable situations (for fear that a trigger might be present). They can also contribute to secondary symptoms, such as frustration, hopelessness, and a sense of lack of control in one's life. The level of anxiety or fear usually varies as a function of both the degree of proximity to the phobic stimuli and the degree to which escape is limited. Specific phobias may be seen with panic disorder, with or without agoraphobia. Among older adults, especially in urban settings, fear of crime seems to be particularly prevalent, and it is important to explore whether this is a realistic fear or a phobia. Phobic disorders tend to be chronic and persist into old age. However, fear of falling is a specific phobia that is increasingly recognized to have an onset in later life. The prevalence of specific phobias in older adults is thought to be 3%–8%.

Social Anxiety Disorder

People with social anxiety disorder (social phobia) suffer from fears that they will behave in a manner that is inept or embarrassing while in a public place or setting. Commonly, the fear is that of trembling, blushing, or sweating profusely in social situations. Other common fears involve giving public speeches, going on dates, or simply socializing with others at a function or party. Similar to specific phobias, social anxiety disorder is often accompanied by a significant degree of anticipatory anxiety or avoidance, or both.

Although systematic studies of social anxiety disorder in older adults are lacking, epidemiologic data indicate that this disorder is chronic and persistent in old age (SOE=A). The 12-month prevalence in older adults is 2%–5%, and social anxiety disorder is more common in women, with some studies suggesting a 2:1 ratio of women to men. One Canadian study suggested that most social anxiety disorder begins in childhood, but onset after age 50 may occur in up to 10% of affected individuals. Common manifestations in old age include the inability to eat food in the presence of strangers, embarrassment concerning physical decline (tremor, vision, hearing) and, especially in men, being unable to urinate in public rest rooms. Despite medical comorbidity, symptoms are out of proportion to actual disability.

Generalized Anxiety Disorder (GAD)

The distinctive symptoms of GAD include excessive anxiety and worry in addition to experiencing other symptoms, such as muscle tension, feeling easily fatigued, difficulty sleeping through the night, difficulty concentrating on a task, and feeling irritable or on edge. These symptoms need to have occurred for at least 6 months and must be accompanied by the sense that one cannot control the feelings of anxiety. In addition, these feelings of intense worry must concern intense worry over more than one activity. The worries are generally out of proportion to the stressors. Many older adults with GAD also have symptoms of depression. The clinician must try to distinguish between the two diagnoses. When these symptoms occur in the context of a major depressive disorder, it is the latter diagnosis that must be assigned, but it is not surprising that >25% of patients with major depressive disorder have symptoms that would qualify them for a diagnosis of GAD. Some studies suggest that GAD may be the most common anxiety disorder in older adults, with prevalence rates between 1.2% and 7.3%. That said, <1% of individuals >74 years old have new-onset GAD. In 2 smaller studies, looking only at older adults with GAD, the age of onset of almost half was over the age of 50. In those studies, disability was associated with increased risk. Thus, it is important to keep GAD in the differential diagnosis, even if there is no lifetime history. Throughout the life span, the prevalence of GAD in women is twice that of men.

Obsessive-Compulsive Disorder (OCD)

OCD involves persistent thoughts (obsessions) and behaviors (compulsions) that are performed in an effort to decrease the anxiety experienced as a result of the obsessions. Obsessions are thoughts or ideas that come to a person's mind, often while completing a specific task or during a particular type of situation, that are generally experienced as intrusive. Compulsions are either clearly excessive or are not connected in any realistic way with the thought/obsession that they are designed to "neutralize." For example, a person may wash his or her hands repeatedly, for hours at a time, after shaking a stranger's hand; the unwanted thought is of possibly having been exposed to a disease. In this example, the act of washing is the compulsion. Other compulsive behaviors include turning lights on and off and checking locks on doors repeatedly. The obsessive-compulsive person may realize that this behavior is excessive but feels intense anxiety if he or she tries to control the compulsion. OCD is chronic and often disabling. Sufferers may spend many hours every day carrying out their compulsions. Depression and other symptoms of anxiety can also be comorbid illnesses in the older population.

In general, the prevalence of OCD is low, the 1-year prevalence being <1%. OCD first appearing in late life is unlikely. More commonly, new symptoms of obsessions may occur along with a depressive syndrome or early dementia. For example, obsessions about paying bills on time can occur in the context of difficulty in estimating time and planning. One study suggested that late onset OCD (>40 years old) was associated more with female gender, a precipitating factor, and fewer sexual and aggressive obsessions.

Hoarding Disorder

Hoarding disorder is now recognized as a clinical disorder characterized in *DSM-5*. It is a late-life disorder that previously was thought to be related to OCD. However, hoarding was minimally responsive to OCD treatments. The key feature of hoarding disorder is the persistent difficulty discarding or parting with possessions regardless of actual value. These collected things may clutter and impede needed living space (eg, preventing the use of a kitchen, bathroom, or bedroom). It often manifests itself with compulsive hoarding and the pathologic collection and storage of objects, often including items that have been collected from garbage cans and dumpsters and that the individual believes have value and meaning. The epidemiology is unclear; some surveys suggest a prevalence of approximately 5%. Unlike that of many psychiatric disorders, the prevalence is thought to be 3 times as common in adults aged 55–94 years old than in younger adults. The differential diagnosis of hoarding includes CNS disorders such as strokes or traumatic brain injury.

Posttraumatic Stress Disorder (PTSD)

The distinctive feature of PTSD is that the person has experienced, either as a witness or a victim, a traumatic event to which he or she has reacted with fear and helplessness. Examples of such events include those that involve actual or threatened death or serious injury, other threats to personal integrity, witnessing an event that involves death or serious injury of another, or even hearing about death or serious injury of a family member or close associate. Commonly observed symptoms include the reexperiencing of the traumatic event, avoidance (both cognitively and behaviorally) of stimuli associated with the event, psychological numbing, and increased physiologic arousal. Reexperiencing can take the form of recurrent, intrusive recollections or images, thoughts, or even physical perceptions of the traumatic event. Such experiences are commonly termed flashbacks. Symptoms of hyperarousal include difficulty falling or staying asleep, hypervigilance, and exaggerated startle response. Nightmares, or recurrent distressing dreams of the traumatic event, are evidence of both hyperarousal and reexperiencing. Disorders often seen with PTSD include depression, panic disorder, and substance-use disorders. Symptoms must be present for at least 1 month and cause clinically significant distress or impairment in social, occupational, or other important areas of functioning. Individuals who experience these symptoms after a recent trauma (from 2 days to 1 month) are diagnosed with acute stress disorder. PTSD must be considered if distress persists for >1 month, and is considered chronic PTSD if the symptoms last for >3 months.

Although <50% of people exposed to a traumatic event go on to develop PTSD, those who experience symptoms of acute stress disorder are at higher risk than those who do not develop acute symptoms (SOE=B). In older adults, PTSD can have a delayed onset, eg, a new presentation of the disorder in a Holocaust survivor. It is postulated that lack of social supports in the context of new stressors in an older adult's life can contribute to such a presentation. PTSD symptoms have been suggested to be associated with increased cardiovascular events, as was seen in a prospective study from 2007.

The *DSM-5* now classifies PTSD in a new category of trauma-and stressor-related disorders.

COMORBIDITY

Depression with Marked Anxiety

Anxiety can be a prominent symptom of depression in many older adults. In fact, anxiety can be the presenting symptom that belies an underlying diagnosis of major depressive disorder. It is commonly believed that the expression of anxiety is more culturally acceptable in this cohort of older adults than the expression of depression. Patients presenting with a chief complaint of anxiety should routinely be evaluated for a major depressive disorder. Patients suffering from a combination of depressive and anxious symptoms can have clinically significant levels of distress despite the fact that they do not meet the full criteria for a diagnosis of either disorder.

Anxiety and Medical Disorders

Comorbid anxiety and medical disorders are commonly present. In many cases, medical illness can mimic an anxiety disorder in its presentation. Medical illness can also exacerbate a concurrent anxiety disorder, or vice versa. Finally, adverse effects of medications can produce or contribute to anxiety symptoms.

Common medical illnesses that can cause or contribute to an anxiety disorder include cardiovascular or pulmonary conditions and hyperthyroidism. Medical illnesses that can be exacerbated by high levels of anxiety include angina pectoris or COPD.

Adverse effects of medications include those commonly encountered with thyroid hormone replacements, antipsychotics, caffeine, and theophylline, and can also be the primary cause of anxiety symptoms. Given the complicated clinical picture that results when anxiety and medical disorders coexist, a thorough assessment, including a clinical history, review of both prescribed and OTC medications and caffeinated beverages as well as herbal supplements (with an eye toward possible interactions), appropriate laboratory tests, and measurement of therapeutic medication concentrations when appropriate, is imperative before treatment begins.

PHARMACOLOGIC MANAGEMENT

Numerous drugs have been used over the years as anxiolytics: alcohol, barbiturates, antihistamines, benzodiazepines, antipsychotic medications, and β-blockers. Evidence to support the use of many of these agents is lacking. Although empirical studies of the use of medications in treating older adults were initially limited, the body of literature to support this practice is increasing, including several randomized controlled trials of the treatment of late-life anxiety disorders (most often GAD). For some disorders, the body of literature supporting the efficacy of these medications is gleaned from use in younger patients, modified by age considerations. For example, a study of time for treatment for an anxiety disorder suggested that, in younger adults, if a patient responds, continuing on medication for a year decreases risk of relapse; this treatment recommendation should be considered with older adults as well. A brief description of the various

Table 42.1—Treatment Strategies for Anxiety Disorders in Late Life

Disorder	First-Line Treatments	Second-Line Treatments or Adjunctive Therapies
Panic disorder, agoraphobia	SSRIs[a], SNRIs[a], CBT[a]	Benzodiazepines[b]
Social anxiety disorder	SSRIs[a] plus CBT[b]	Benzodiazepines[b]
Social anxiety disorder, specific type (eg, public speaking)	β-blockers[OL] plus CBT[b]	Buspirone[b]
Specific phobia (eg, rats, blood)	CBT[b] or PRN benzodiazepines[b]	SSRI[b]
Obsessive-compulsive disorder	SSRIs[a], SNRIs[b], CBT[b]	Clomipramine[b] (adverse effects in older adults)
Posttraumatic stress disorder	SSRIs[b], SNRIs[b]	CBT[b], prazosin[b]
Generalized anxiety disorder	SSRIs[a], SNRIs[a], CBT[a] relaxation training	Benzodiazepines[b]
Anxiety and medical disorders	Identify and treat underlying cause; use SSRIs[a] or SNRIs[a] in primary anxiety disorder.	Benzodiazepines[b]
Depression with severe anxiety	SSRIs[a], SNRIs[a], CBT[a]	Buspirone[b], benzodiazepines[b]

NOTE: SNRIs=serotonin-norepinephrine reuptake inhibitors; CBT=cognitive-behavioral therapy
[a]SOE=A in studies of the geriatric population
[b]SOE=A in studies of the general adult population; insufficient studies in the geriatric population

classes of compounds currently favored as anxiolytics follows. For a summary of the treatment strategies for anxiety disorders in late life, see Table 42.1.

Antidepressants

Antidepressants have proved efficacious in treatment of panic disorder, OCD, GAD, and PTSD in younger patients. Studies have demonstrated that SSRIs, particularly citalopram, are safe and efficacious in specific treatment of late-life anxiety disorders. Given their relatively favorable adverse-event profile, the SSRIs should be considered the medications of choice for these disorders (SOE=A). Further, SSRIs should also be considered treatments of choice for depression with severe anxiety symptoms. Compounds such as venlafaxine and duloxetine (serotonin-norepinephrine reuptake inhibitors) should be considered as alternatives for those patients who do not respond to SSRIs or who experience adverse events.

Benzodiazepines

Over the past several decades, benzodiazepines have been the most commonly prescribed anxiolytics for both younger and older patients, but their use is now discouraged. When needed because symptoms are severe, benzodiazepines with shorter half-lives and without active metabolites, such as lorazepam and oxazepam, are preferable for treating older adults, because they are metabolized by direct conjugation, a process relatively unaffected by aging. However, the use of even short-acting benzodiazepines should be limited to <6 months because long-term use is fraught with complications, such as motor incoordination and falls, cognitive impairment, depression, and the potential for abuse and dependence.

Other Medications

Several studies have suggested that buspirone, an anxiolytic medication with some serotonin-agonist properties, is efficacious for treatment of GAD (SOE=A), although clinical experience is less positive. Buspirone appears to be a safer choice than benzodiazepines for patients taking several other medications or needing treatment for longer periods of time. One drawback of buspirone is the amount of time required to see a clinical response (approximately 4 weeks). At times, concomitant use of a short-acting benzodiazepine in the initial stage of treatment could be useful for some patients. Although antihistamines such as hydroxyzine[OL] and diphenhydramine[OL] are sometimes used to manage mild anxiety in younger patients, the anticholinergic properties of these agents can cause serious problems in older adults, in whom their use is not recommended. Second-generation antipsychotics, such as risperidone[OL], olanzapine[OL], and quetiapine[OL], are not recommended choices for treatment of a nonpsychotic older adult with an anxiety disorder.

PSYCHOLOGIC MANAGEMENT

Although pharmacotherapy is commonly the first-line treatment for late-life anxiety disorders, psychologic treatments are often efficacious, either alone or as adjuncts to medication (SOE=A). The psychotherapeutic remedies that have been most rigorously tested all fall under the rubric of cognitive-behavioral therapy CBT).

Techniques generally fall into 3 categories: 1) relaxation training used with music, visual imagery, aromatherapy, and instruction in relaxation techniques; 2) cognitive restructuring to help the patient identify triggers and stimuli that increase or sustain anxiety, gain more control over the effect of such stimuli, and develop a range of coping strategies and tools; and 3) exposure with response prevention (ie, the individual is exposed to the feared stimuli and prevented from performing a compulsive action), which is used with and particularly effective for OCD. Graded desensitization, which is used in panic and phobias, relies on exposure to gradually more anxiety-producing stimuli, with techniques to manage and tolerate the resultant anxiety. More studies are exploring the use of CBT in older populations and have found it to be as effective as in younger cohorts.

RESOURCES

- Balsamo M, Cataldi F, Carlucci L, et al. Assessment of anxiety in older adults: a review of self-report measures. *Clin Interv Aging*. 2018;13:573–593.

- Bower ES, Wetherell JL, Mon T, et al. Treating anxiety disorders in older adults: current treatments and future directions. *Harv Rev Psychiatry*. 2015;23(5):329–342.

- Kennedy GJ, Ceide ME. Screening older adults for mental disorders. *Clin Geriatr Med*. 2018;34(1):69–79.

CHAPTER 43—SCHIZOPHRENIA SPECTRUM AND OTHER PSYCHOTIC DISORDERS

KEY POINTS

- Hallucinations are perceptions without stimuli that can occur in any sensory modality (ie, visual, auditory, tactile, olfactory, gustatory). In late life, multimodal hallucinations are common.

- Delusions are abnormal false beliefs that in late life are often paranoid or persecutory, such as a belief that one's safety is in jeopardy or that one's belongings are being stolen.

- Psychosis occurring for the first time in late life is often due to dementia or neurologic conditions such as Parkinson disease or stroke, as opposed to a primary psychotic disorder such as schizophrenia.

- Dementia with Lewy bodies is associated with characteristically vivid visual hallucinations, often including people or animals.

- When psychotic symptoms arise in the context of depression, the symptoms are often "mood congruent," such as delusions that one is penniless or that one is already dead.

Psychotic symptoms are defined as either *hallucinations*, ie, perceptions without stimuli, or *delusions*, ie, fixed, false, idiosyncratic ideas. Hallucinations are abnormal perceptions without a physical stimulus that can be in any of the five sensory modalities (auditory, visual, tactile, olfactory, and gustatory). Delusions are false beliefs or ideas that are tightly held by the individual despite any evidence. Delusions can be suspicious (paranoid), grandiose, somatic, self-blaming, or hopeless. This chapter focuses on conditions in which psychotic symptoms are prominent and central to making the diagnosis. It only briefly discusses other disorders, such as dementia, delirium, and the mood disorders, in which psychotic symptoms can occur but the defining features are in the cognitive or mood realms.

Hallucinations and delusions occur in a variety of disorders. Evaluation of an older adult with hallucinations and delusions should begin with evaluation for underlying causes such as delirium, dementia, stroke, Parkinson disease, or substance use disorders. An acute onset of cognitive change with inability to sustain attention and impaired level of awareness and/or arousal suggests delirium. Next, a primary mood disorder should be considered. Only after other causes are excluded should the diagnosis of a schizophrenia spectrum disorder be made. Delirium, most often superimposed on an underlying dementia, is the most common cause of new-onset psychosis in late life.

SCHIZOPHRENIA AND SCHIZOPHRENIA SPECTRUM SYNDROMES

Schizophrenia is defined as a chronic psychiatric disorder characterized by positive symptoms (eg, hallucinations, delusions, and disorganized speech, known as thought disorder) and negative symptoms (eg, social withdrawal and apathy). Mood disorder and cognitive disorder should be excluded before the diagnosis is made. In men, schizophrenia has a modal onset at age 18; onset after age 45 is uncommon. In women, modal age of onset is 28, and 20%–30% of cases begin after age 45. Approximately 85% of older adults with schizophrenia experienced onset of illness in early adult life. However, schizophrenia first comes to clinical attention after patients are 45 years old in 10%–15% of cases. Schizophrenia with onset between the ages of 40 and 60 is called "late-onset schizophrenia," while patients with onset after age 60 are considered to have "very-late-onset schizophrenia-like psychosis."

In older adults, late-onset schizophrenia-like conditions are characterized by onset after age 40, prominent persecutory (paranoid) delusions, and multimodal hallucinations (SOE=C). For example, patients commonly complain that items are being stolen or report that they are being persecuted unjustly. Hallucinations often manifest in complaints, for example, that a neighbor is persistently banging on walls or the roof, that someone is pumping gas under the door, or that electrical sensations are being sent through the walls of the person's home and into his or her body. A schizophrenia-like psychosis can be diagnosed only when cognitive disorder, mood disorder, or other explanatory medical conditions such as delirium or focal brain pathology have been excluded.

The schizophrenia-like psychoses of late life differ from schizophrenia beginning in early life in two ways (SOE=C). First, thought disorder, a sign described as speech in which a series of thoughts are not connected to one another in a logical fashion, is much less common in older adults, comprising only 5% of cases. In early-onset schizophrenia, thought disorder is present in approximately 50% of cases.

Schizoaffective disorder is a chronic mental illness that presents earlier in life and that typically requires ongoing treatment for both psychotic and mood symptoms as patients age.

A second significant difference is the rarity of social deterioration and dilapidation among older adults with late-onset schizophrenia. Thus, personality and social functioning are often better preserved in late-onset cases. However, there is a dearth of long-term follow-up studies, so it is unknown whether social deterioration and personality changes occur after many years of symptoms.

Epidemiology and Clinical Characteristics

Late-onset schizophrenia is more common among women, whereas early-onset schizophrenia is equally common in women and men. The population-based incidence of late-onset schizophrenia is unknown, but the lifetime prevalence of schizophrenia is 1% among both men and women.

Late-onset schizophrenia-like psychoses affect predominantly women, with the female:male ratio ranging from 5:1 to 10:1. Many older adults with late-onset schizophrenia-like psychosis have been married at some time and have been able to hold responsible jobs and work efficiently, but premorbid isolation and "schizoid" (socially detached personality) traits are common.

One condition that may be confused with late-onset schizophrenia is frontotemporal dementia, because it can involve features of socially inappropriate and odd behaviors as well as premorbidly odd or "schizoid" personality features.

Although many individuals with schizophrenia experience fewer hallucinations and delusions as they age, others remain significantly functionally impaired by psychotic symptoms. Moreover, older adults with schizophrenia have an increased risk of suicidal behavior than their peers without mental illness (SOE=C). Some individuals with schizophrenia experience remission of psychotic symptoms with aging, though this clinical remission may be temporary. Indeed, a longitudinal study of community-dwelling people with schizophrenia spectrum disorder found that remission status fluctuates over time. The study further found that remission status was affected by community support and integration, suggesting that social interventions help sustain clinical well-being in these older patients. In addition, individuals with early-onset schizophrenia have more cognitive deficits than patients with late-onset schizophrenia, although these cognitive changes remain relatively stable over time. Neither early-onset nor late-onset schizophrenia is considered a dementing illness, and rapid memory loss should prompt further evaluation for possible comorbid conditions, such as delirium or dementia. Recent studies indicate that older patients with schizophrenia have higher rates of dementia than persons without schizophrenia (SOE=B). They also have significantly higher rates of congestive heart failure, COPD, and hypothyroidism than individuals without schizophrenia, underscoring the importance of comprehensive health care for these older individuals (SOE=C).

Treatment and Management

Nonpharmacologic

Because suspiciousness and paranoid delusions are commonly the most prominent symptoms, the clinician's first task in treating late-onset psychosis is often to establish a trusting therapeutic relationship with the patient. On occasion, the suspicious ideas are conceivable (eg, the claim that the patient is being financially abused by a relative), but usually the delusions are bizarre and improbable. It is rarely effective to confront the patient with the unreality or implausibility of his or her ideas. The patient is more likely to respond positively if the clinician empathizes with the distress that the symptoms cause ("I can see how upset you are by all of this"). If patients ask whether the clinician "believes" them, a response such as, "I don't hear anything like that, but I appreciate the fact that you do" is both honest and empathetic. The symptoms are usually frightening and distressing to patients and can lead to unusual behaviors. For example, patients who develop concerns that their food is being poisoned may exhibit unusual eating habits or food avoidance. Furthermore, suspiciousness can isolate the patient from friends and family. Therefore, encouraging patients to maintain important relationships and seeking their permission to discuss the source of symptoms with close family members or friends can help patients maintain important, supportive relationships.

Pharmacologic

Clinical consensus and descriptive case series suggest that antipsychotic medications are as effective in late-onset schizophrenia as in early-onset cases (SOE=B). Most specialist clinicians recommend second-generation antipsychotic medications, because such agents are less likely to cause tardive dyskinesia (TD), an adverse event for which older age is a predisposing factor. Dosages should be increased at semiweekly or weekly intervals as needed. While dosages are being titrated, patients should be monitored for emergence of extrapyramidal adverse events (eg, parkinsonian tremor, rigidity, dystonia) and other movement disorders. These should be treated by lowering the dosage and switching to an alternative antipsychotic if necessary. Polypharmacy should be avoided by reducing the dosage or switching the antipsychotic medication rather than by adding a medication for extrapyramidal symptoms. Although prescribing anticholinergic medications is generally avoided in older adults, patients with antipsychotic-induced extrapyramidal symptoms whose psychotic symptoms cannot be managed on a lower dose of antipsychotic medication may benefit from concomitant anticholinergic medication. In these instances, a low daily dose of a nonsedating medication such as benztropine (0.5–1 mg/d) or trihexiphenidyl (2–4 mg/d) can be beneficial (SOE=D). Prophylactic use of benztropine or trihexiphenidyl to prevent extrapyramidal symptoms is not recommended. The more common adverse events with quetiapine are sedation and orthostatic hypotension; with risperidone, extrapyramidal symptoms; and with olanzapine, weight gain and sedation (Table 43.1).

No studies are available to guide the duration of treatment. Clinical experience suggests that patients who respond to antipsychotic medications should be continued on the minimal effective dosage for at least 6 months. Patients with early-onset schizophrenia and chronic stable symptoms may be able to tolerate a gradual reduction in dosage of antipsychotic medication. For all patients who relapse on treatment or who relapse when the dosage is lowered, maintenance treatment over a longer term (at least 1–2 years) is recommended (SOE=D). Patients should be monitored for emergence of TD, a syndrome characterized by repetitive involuntary movements of the oral and limb musculature. Rating scales for TD, such as the Abnormal Involuntary Movement Scale (AIMS [www.cqaimh.org/pdf/tool_aims.pdf]) or the Dyskinesia Identification System Condensed User Scale (DISCUS) are clinically useful and easy to administer in the office or institutional setting. If TD develops, the dosage of the antipsychotic medication should be lowered if possible. Depending on the duration of exposure, TD may worsen or appear when the antipsychotic is discontinued or the dosage is lowered, or when switching from one antipsychotic to another. At the time antipsychotic medications are started or as soon as symptoms improve enough so that the patient can understand the risk, the patient should be informed of the risk of TD and the possibility that it can be irreversible.

In April 2017, valbenazine became the first FDA-approved medication to treat tardive dyskinesia. Valbenazine is an inhibitor of vesicular monoamine transporter 2. In phase 3 trials, a dosage of 80 mg/d effectively improved symptoms of tardive dyskinesia after several weeks; improvement was sustained while valbenazine treatment was continued. Adverse effects were mild and included somnolence and possible QT prolongation.

PSYCHOTIC SYMPTOMS ASSOCIATED WITH OTHER NON-SCHIZOPHRENIC DISORDERS

Psychotic symptoms can occur in a number of other disorders in addition to schizophrenia.

Delirium

Hallucinations, particularly visual hallucinations, can be a symptom of delirium, even when it is mild. The onset of delirium is usually acute, and there is generally an identifiable metabolic, pharmacologic, or infectious cause, or a combination of underlying causes. The hallmark feature of delirium is markedly impaired attention and impaired level of awareness. Typically, the mental status examination reveals multiple cognitive impairments and a diminished or waxing and waning level of consciousness with periods of lucidity and alertness alternating with periods of lethargy. Treatment of delirium involves treating the underlying medical condition(s) provoking the delirious state.

Delusional Disorder

Some older adults present with long-standing chronic delusions without hallucinations. When these occur in patients with a normal mood and who do not have cognitive impairment, then a diagnosis of delusional disorder may be made. A recent study found that delusional disorder is more frequent among women but that men experience more severe symptoms. Most commonly, the delusions are persecutory or paranoid in nature, but delusions of jealousy or somatic delusions of bodily dysfunction also occur. Patients with somatic delusions may present to multiple health practitioners and request medical interventions. Management strategies include reassurance, avoidance of unnecessary medical interventions, amelioration of sensory deficits, and sometimes antipsychotic medication.

Mood Disorder

Psychotic symptoms, especially delusions, can be seen in major depressive disorder and in the manic phase of bipolar disorder. These delusions are described as "mood congruent." That is, in patients with depression, the delusional content usually reflects extreme self-deprecation, self-blame, hopelessness, or the conviction of ill health. A patient may complain, for example, that he or she has no blood or that his or her intestines are not working; another patient may believe that he or she has caused a terrible wrong and deserves to be punished (a self-blaming delusion). Some patients become convinced that they are dying and nothing can be done to help them, although there is no physiologic evidence to support their concerns. Other common depressive delusions are the conviction that one has no insurance, no clothing, or no money when this is not true (delusion of poverty). Delusions congruent with mania are grandiose. Examples include the person's belief that he or she is infallible, can do impossible physical or intellectual activities, has skills and abilities that no other human being has, or is a special personage such as Jesus Christ. Treatment of psychotic symptoms in mood disorders includes antipsychotic medication as well as antidepressant or antimanic medications.

Dementia

Patients with dementia experience both hallucinations and delusions. These are usually less complex than the delusions seen in schizophrenia or mood disorder. Common delusions in dementia are the belief that one's belongings have been stolen or moved, or the conviction that one is being persecuted. Delusions that one's spouse is unfaithful (delusions of infidelity) are also common.

Management of psychosis in dementia is particularly challenging, because the use of antipsychotic medication warrants careful consideration of risks and adverse events. Nonpharmacologic interventions, such as redirection and reassurance, should be tried first. However, if the patient is physically aggressive or severely distressed by the psychotic symptoms, then a trial of low-dose antipsychotic medication is warranted (SOE=C). All antipsychotic agents carry an FDA warning regarding increased all-cause mortality in patients with dementia.

Psychotic Disorder Due to Another Medical Condition

It is appropriate to consider this diagnosis when a patient is experiencing hallucinations or delusions that are likely to be a direct result of another medical condition, rather than due to a psychiatric disorder such as schizophrenia or a mood disorder. Patients with Parkinson disease, stroke, and other brain disorders may experience delusions and hallucinations without prominent cognitive impairment or other evidence of psychiatric disorder (SOE=C). Delirium caused by a superimposed condition should be excluded. In patients with Parkinson disease, psychotic symptoms are common and may be secondary to a prescribed dopaminergic agent, although some patients experience visual hallucinations before any medications are started, indicating that the brain disease process itself may have an etiologic role. Education and support should be offered to all patients with these symptoms. Judicious discontinuation or dosage reduction of nonessential antiparkinsonian medications often provides relief from psychotic symptoms. If patients experience significant emotional distress or if the symptoms lead to dangerous or upsetting behavior, cautious use of an antipsychotic medication is appropriate (SOE=B). Use of first-generation antipsychotic medications is usually avoided because of the potential for exacerbating parkinsonian symptoms (SOE=B). For patients with Parkinson disease and concomitant hallucinations or psychosis, quetiapine^{OL} 12.5–75 mg/d may be beneficial. Some patients require clozapine^{OL} 12.5–75 mg/d. However, patients taking clozapine should have a CBC with absolute neutrophil count done once a week for 6 months and then biweekly thereafter because of the risk of granulocytopenia. All patients taking clozapine must be enrolled in a national patient registry to ensure safe administration. Pimavanserin, a 5-HT$_{2A}$ receptor inverse agonist, was approved by the FDA in April 2016 specifically for treatment of psychosis in Parkinson disease. As the only agent with FDA approval for this indication, it is likely to become first-line treatment, although it was somewhat less effective than clozapine in clinical trials (SOE=A) (Table 43.1).

Dementia associated with Lewy bodies is increasingly recognized as an important cause of hallucinations in late life. The clinical scenario typically involves cognitive decline accompanied by motor features of parkinsonism. However, prominent visual hallucinations, which are often vivid and troubling, are a key part of the diagnosis.

Dementia associated with Lewy bodies presents a challenge similar to that of psychosis in Parkinson disease, because the medications in the class approved to treat psychosis (the antipsychotics) worsen the parkinsonian symptoms. At least two placebo-controlled clinical trials and multiple case studies report significant improvement through the use of cholinesterase inhibitors^{OL} (SOE=B). If an antipsychotic medication must be used, then the treatment strategies outlined above are appropriate if there is careful attention to the risk of extrapyramidal adverse events. Nonpharmacologic treatments include redirection, reassurance, and nonconfrontational explanation.

Substance/Medication-Induced Psychotic Disorder

Drugs of abuse, such as alcohol, cannabis, and cocaine, can cause persistent psychotic symptoms after the period of acute intoxication or withdrawal. Alcohol can induce a psychotic disorder marked by persistent auditory hallucinations in individuals who have a moderate or severe alcohol use disorder. Although substance use disorders are less frequent among older patients than in younger individuals, this is an area of growing concern. In addition, many classes of

Table 43.1—Dosing and Adverse Events of Commonly Used Antipsychotic Medications[a] for Psychotic Disorders

Medication	Starting Daily Dosage (mg)	Maximal Daily Dosage (mg)	Adverse Events		
			Extrapyramidal Signs[b]	Drowsiness	Weight Gain
Aripiprazole	2	15	++	+	+
Asenapine	5	10	+	+++	++
Clozapine	12.5	100	+	+++	+++
Haloperidol	0.5	10	+++	++	+
Iloperidone	1	12	+	++	+
Lurasidone	40	80	+	++	+
Olanzapine	2.5	15	+	++	+++
Paliperidone	1.5	12	++	++	+
Perphenazine	4	32	++	++	++
Pimavanserin[c]	34	34	+	++	+
Quetiapine	12.5	300	+	+++	++
Risperidone	0.25	4	++	+	++
Ziprasidone	20	120	+	++	+

NOTE: + = uncommon, ++ = somewhat common, +++ = common
[a] All listed medications have warning about hyperglycemia, cerebrovascular events, and increase in all-cause mortality in patients with dementia.
[b] Rigidity, parkinsonian tremor, dystonia, akathisia
[c] FDA-approved to treat hallucinations/delusions associated with Parkinson disease psychosis only

medications are associated with psychotic adverse events causing hallucinations or delusions. Older adults, especially those with CNS impairments, are particularly vulnerable. In a number of case reports, β-blockers such as metoprolol have been associated with persistent hallucinations and confusional states (SOE=C). In these cases, withdrawal of metoprolol resulted in rapid and complete resolution of psychosis. In addition, psychotic symptoms have been reported related to treatment with other medications such as dopaminergic agents, interferon, cyclosporine, and steroids. Antiarrhythmic agents, antiviral agents, opioids, antineoplastic agents, and other medications such as baclofen have also been associated with psychosis. In these instances, the appropriate therapeutic management is to reduce the dosage of or to discontinue the associated medication.

Charles Bonnet Syndrome

Between 10% and 13% of patients with significant visual loss (bilateral acuity worse than 20/60) experience isolated visual hallucinations. These can take the form of shapes such as diamonds or rectangles but more commonly consist of complex silent hallucinations such as small children, multiple animals, or a vivid scene such as would be seen in a movie. This condition, first described more than 200 years ago, goes by the eponym Charles Bonnet syndrome. The criteria for this syndrome are as follows:

- Silent visual hallucinations
- Partially or fully intact insight (the patient is aware that the perceptions cannot be real but still reports that they appear absolutely real and vivid)
- Visual loss
- Lack of evidence of brain disease or other psychiatric disorder

The best treatment for Charles Bonnet syndrome is education, reassurance, and support. Patients should be informed that the hallucinations are a sign of eye disease, not mental illness. An occasional patient has partial insight or loses insight and becomes very distressed by this symptom. When this distress is significant or leads to dangerous behavior, a cautious trial of low-dosage second-generation antipsychotic medication is occasionally beneficial.

RESOURCES

- Cort E, Meehan J, Reeves S, et al. Very late-onset schizophrenia-like psychosis: a clinical update. *J Psychosoc Nurs Ment Health Serv*. 2018;56(1):37–47.
- Davis MC, Miller BJ, Kalsi JK, et al. Efficient trial design—FDA approval of valbenazine for tardive dyskinesia. *N Engl J Med*. 2017;376(26):2503–2506.
- Reinhardt MM, Cohen CI. Late-life psychosis: diagnosis and treatment. *Curr Psychiatry Rep*. 2015;17(2):1.

CHAPTER 44—PERSONALITY AND SOMATIC SYMPTOM DISORDERS

KEY POINTS

- Personality disorders persist into late life and pose complex challenges in patients across various medical and psychiatric settings.

- Personality disorders can be more difficult to detect in late life because of age-associated changes in symptoms, comorbid psychopathology, and lack of age-adjusted diagnostic instruments.

- The goal of treatment of personality disorders in late life is not to cure the disorder but to decrease the frequency and intensity of symptoms. To this end, both psychotherapeutic and psychopharmacologic strategies are needed.

- Somatic symptom and related disorders represent the presence of prominent physical symptoms or complaints that are associated with significant distress and impairment. The new diagnostic formulation de-emphasizes the previous focus on a lack of established underlying pathology.

- Treatment of somatic symptom and related disorders must attend to the affected individual's distress and belief in the veracity of his or her symptoms. Repeated reassuring clinical visits help to build a therapeutic relationship. Both psychotherapy and pharmacotherapy can be helpful for some individuals.

PERSONALITY DISORDERS

Personality refers to the unique characteristics and qualities that define an individual's ability to form relationships, cope with life stressors, and approach the tasks of daily living. However, when these patterns become debilitating or interfere with interpersonal relationships or overall functioning, the result is referred to as a disorder. Personality disorders are defined in the *Diagnostic and Statistical Manual of Mental Disorders, 5th Edition* (*DSM-5*) by the presence of chronic and pervasive patterns of inflexible and maladaptive inner experiences and behaviors. These patterns lead to significant disruptions in several spheres of function, including cognitive perception and interpretation, affective expression, interpersonal functioning, and impulse control. Individuals with personality disorders are often distinguished by repeated episodes of disruptive or noxious behaviors and, as a result, they often receive pejorative labels, depending on their form. Descriptive terms often applied to those with personality disorders include "difficult," "dramatic," and "strange," to name just a few. Personality disorders can also negatively impact an individual's overall compliance with general medical care in the primary care setting (SOE=B). The developmental roots of personality disorders are believed to lie in childhood and adolescence, but their features can present clinically at any age in adulthood. Personality disorders are influenced by both genetic and environmental factors. A personality disorder cannot be the manifestation of substance use or other mental disorder.

The *DSM-5* describes 10 personality disorders, grouped into 3 broad clusters that are based on common phenomenology; however, they are no longer documented on a separate axis. For late-life features of all 10 personality disorders, see Table 44.1. Depressive and passive-aggressive personality disorders were 2 additional categories that were considered provisional in the previous edition of the *DSM* (*DSM-IV-TR*) but have not been included in *DSM-5* because of a lack of empirical support. Nonetheless, some clinicians continue to see older adults who present with the symptom constellations of these 2 personality disorders. Mixed diagnoses and those that do not fit into any existing category are labeled in *DSM-5* as "other specified personality disorder" and "unspecified personality disorder."

The *DSM-5* classification for personality disorders also includes the category of "personality change due to another medical condition" to represent emergent personality changes resulting from medical compromise. Such personality change has classically been described within the context of an "organic" personality disorder, but this term is no longer used in *DSM* nomenclature. Most often, personality changes with an "organic" source involve impairments in executive functioning, consisting of poor impulse control, poor planning, and greater vulnerability to irritability or agitation. Along these lines, Alzheimer disease and other dementias are often associated with personality changes, including apathy, egocentricity, and impulsivity. Frontal lobe injury can result in a disinhibited impulsive syndrome, or conversely, an apathetic, avolitional syndrome. Frontotemporal dementia has been associated with distinct personality changes, including impulsivity, disinhibition, apathy, and compulsive behaviors such as hoarding. Temporal lobe epilepsy can be associated with personality change, including emotional deepening, verbosity, hypergraphia, hypersexuality, and

Table 44.1—Features of Personality Disorders and Cluster-Specific Management Strategies

Cluster/Disorder	General Features	Features Specific to Older Adults	Cluster-Specific Management Strategies (SOE=D)
Cluster A: Odd or Eccentric Behaviors			
Paranoid	Pervasive suspiciousness of the motives of others, which often leads to irritability and hostility	Increased risk of paranoid psychosis, agitation, and aggression	Always assess for and treat comorbid psychosis.
Schizoid	Disinterest in social relationships, coupled with isolative and sometimes odd behaviors	Poor, strained, or absent relationships with caregivers	Do not force social interactions but offer support and problem-solving assistance in a professional and consistent manner.
Schizotypal	Characteristic appearance, behaviors, and beliefs that are strange, unusual, or inappropriate	Beliefs that can become delusional and lead to conflicts with others; relationships with caregivers can be strained or absent	Do not challenge paranoid ideation; instead, solicit and empathize with emotional responses to inner turmoil and fear of paranoid states.
Cluster B: Dramatic, Emotional, or Erratic Behaviors			
Antisocial	Poor regard for social norms and laws; lack of conscience and empathy for others; frequent reckless and criminal behaviors	Frequent remission of antisocial behaviors with less aggression and impulsivity	Assess for and treat underlying mood lability, depression, anxiety, and substance abuse.
Borderline	Impaired control of emotional expression and impulses associated with unstable interpersonal relations, poor self-identity, and self-injurious behaviors	Persistent emotional lability and unstable relationships but less self-injurious and impulsive behaviors	Adopt a consistent, structured, and predictable approach with strict boundaries to contain disruptive behaviors. Do not personalize belligerent behaviors directed toward staff members; instead, provide opportunities for staff to discuss frustration and negative thoughts and emotions with professional colleagues.
Histrionic	Excessive emotionality and attention-seeking behaviors, sometimes appearing overly seductive or provocative	Behaviors that can become excessively disinhibited and disorganized, appearing hypomanic	Adopt a team approach with all involved clinicians to devise a common plan; avoid staff splits between "supporters" and "detractors" of the patient.
Narcissistic	Pervasive sense of entitlement, grandiosity, and arrogance, coupled with lack of empathy	Can present as hostile, enraged, paranoid, or depressed	Use behavioral contracts and authority figures when necessary to address recurrent disruptive behaviors.
Cluster C: Anxious or Fearful Behaviors			
Avoidant	Excessive sensitivity to rejection and social scrutiny; social demeanor that can be timid and inhibited	Social contacts that can be extremely limited, providing for inadequate support	Assess for and treat underlying anxiety, panic, and depression.
Dependent	Excessive dependence on others to help make decisions and provide support	Comorbid depression is common; clinical appearance often with demanding or clinging behaviors if dependency needs not met	Provide regularly scheduled clinical contacts rather than on an as-needed basis.
Obsessive-compulsive	Pervasive preoccupation with orderliness and cleanliness; a perfectionistic, rigid, and controlling approach that can become more inflexible and indecisive under stress	Obsessive-compulsive traits can become exaggerated in efforts to maintain control over somatic and environmental changes	When possible, provide case managers to solicit the needs of avoidant patients and to provide extra reassurance and attention to the needs of dependent and obsessive-compulsive patients.

NOTE: Descriptions of the clusters and of the disorders in each cluster are based on the *Diagnostic and Statistical Manual of Mental Disorders*. 5th ed. Washington, DC: American Psychiatric Association; 2013.

preoccupation with religious, moral, and cosmic issues. Other disorders found in older adults that are associated with personality disorders include brain tumors, multiple sclerosis, and encephalopathies.

Many older adults with personality disorders can easily become overwhelmed by age-associated losses and stresses, largely because they lack appropriate coping skills and the personal, social, or financial resources to buffer their losses. In particular, admission to a hospital or long-term care setting poses a unique stress on all individuals with personality disorders in late life. The loss of a familiar environment, personal items, privacy, and the control over one's schedule can lead to a sense of disorganization and displacement. Conflict in an institutional setting begins when patients with personality disorders try to cope with the stresses from their new environment by exaggerating their maladaptive behaviors. Dependent individuals may feel helpless and panicked without enough attention to their needs, responding with clinging behaviors and excessive questions or requests for assistance. Paranoid, antisocial, and borderline patients may refuse to cooperate with treatment plans or institutional rules. Individuals with personality change, such as due to head trauma, often have great difficulty accommodating to age-related changes and may respond with characteristic labile or disinhibited moods and behaviors or, conversely, with an overall apathetic demeanor.

Epidemiology

Prevalence rates of late-life personality disorders in the community range from 5% to 13%, which is a slightly lower range than the 10%–20% prevalence estimates for individuals of all ages in the community. Prevalence rates in inpatient settings and with comorbid depression are much higher, ranging from 10% to >50%, depending on the method of diagnosis. The most common personality disorders identified in late life are obsessive-compulsive, paranoid, and schizoid; dependent, borderline, and avoidant personality disorders appear to be less common. Although most research has demonstrated fewer diagnoses in older age groups, it is unclear whether this represents an actual difference in prevalence or merely reflects the fact that it is more difficult to make a diagnosis in late life. Some researchers have suggested that prevalence rates can be influenced by increased mortality among those with antisocial or borderline personality traits that are associated with higher rates of reckless, impulsive, and self-injurious behaviors. Other research exploring the neural substrates of emotion has demonstrated an attenuation of emotional reactivity in late life across a number of physiologic and behavioral parameters. These findings can partially explain the reduced prevalence of the more impulsive and emotionally reactive personality features, such as those associated with borderline personality disorder.

Diagnostic Challenges

Establishing a diagnosis of personality disorder in older adults can be especially challenging, because it requires a detailed, longitudinal psychiatric and psychosocial history. Older patients and their informants are not always able to provide sufficient history, especially when it may span ≥50 years. The history can be distorted by recall bias (the tendency to present more socially desirable traits) or memory impairment. Records often do not provide sufficient information to determine prior personality dynamics. Remote diagnoses from previous decades cannot be easily correlated with current ones, because the diagnostic criteria for personality disorders have changed significantly in the past 50 years. As a result of all of these limitations, clinicians often are unable to make a diagnosis or end up making judgments based on insufficient information.

A further diagnostic challenge for clinicians is the need to isolate lifelong personality characteristics from a multitude of comorbid psychiatric and medical problems. Acute and chronic episodes of major depression, psychosis, and other major psychiatric disorders can considerably distort personality features. Even the current diagnostic nomenclature might serve to handicap late-life diagnosis because it is not age adjusted, and many criteria do not apply in late life. A final barrier to diagnosis can be present if the clinician erroneously considers all older patients to have disruptive personality features as a normal function of age.

Personality disorders are multifactorial, including early developmental life experiences. Determined risk factors include history of sexual abuse, childhood neglect, substance abuse, and chaotic life.

Differential Diagnosis

In clinical settings, it is important to remember that not every older patient with prominent or troubling personality features has a personality disorder. Those who demonstrate rigid and maladaptive personality traits but without the pervasiveness or severity as represented by *DSM-5* criteria are better described as suffering from certain personality traits or an adjustment disorder. An adjustment disorder might best characterize previously healthy and well-adjusted individuals who demonstrate acute changes in personality as a result of severe stresses. For example, physical pain and disability can lead to dependent or avoidant behaviors that resemble those seen in personality disorders but without the pervasive pattern and degree of maladaptiveness. Often, the symptoms of major psychiatric disorders and those of personality disorders overlap considerably, and without longitudinal history it can be difficult to distinguish between them. Diagnosis of a personality disorder becomes more certain when seemingly acute behaviors emerge as enduring and pervasive personality traits. This process depends on the opportunity to observe a person over time and in multiple settings or situations.

Long-Term Course

Personality disorders can follow 1 of 4 possible courses: persist unchanged, evolve into a different form or major psychiatric disorder (eg, depression), improve, or remit. Few disorders have actually been studied over time, and rarely into late life. Several studies have suggested that personality disorders can enter a period of relative quiescence in middle age, with fewer and less intense symptoms and increased adaptation (SOE=C). However, this period may precede their reemergence in late life. Other researchers have proposed that personality disorders characterized by emotional and behavioral lability, including antisocial, borderline, histrionic, narcissistic, and dependent disorders, tend to improve over time, although patients remain vulnerable to depression. Personality disorders characterized by an overcontrol of affect and impulses, including paranoid, schizoid, schizotypal, and obsessive-compulsive personality disorders, are thought either to remain stable or to worsen in late life.

Only antisocial and borderline personality disorders have been looked at longitudinally, and both have shown symptom improvement and even remittance into middle and later life for a significant percentage of patients (SOE=B). At the same time, there can be persistent psychopathology that is not recognized within the context of existing antisocial or borderline diagnostic criteria. In other words, chronic personality dynamics can manifest in new behaviors. For example, those with antisocial personality disorders demonstrate less aggressiveness, violence, and criminal acts as they age but can still have antisocial tendencies expressed through substance abuse, disregard for safety, and noncompliance with institutional rules. Older borderline patients display less impulsivity, self-mutilation, and risk taking but more aging-related symptoms, such as the use of multiple medications and nonadherence with treatment.

Treatment

The treatment of personality disorders in late life is complicated and often has limited success. Given the chronic and pervasive nature of personality disorders, the overall goal of treatment in late life is not to cure the disorder but to decrease the frequency and intensity of disruptive behaviors. The first step should always be to clarify the diagnosis and then to identify recent stressors that may account for the current presentation. The resultant formulation can guide the selection of realistic target symptoms and therapeutic approaches, and allow a treatment team to anticipate future stressors. Treatment of personality disorders in late life uses the same basic approaches as with younger patients, but clinicians must incorporate a much broader understanding of the impact of age-related stressors and comorbid disorders. All forms of psychotherapy have been used to treat personality disorders in older adults, ranging from intensive and long-term insight-oriented approaches to equally intensive but more focused cognitive-behavioral models, such as dialectical behavior therapy or an integrative approach such as schema therapy (SOE=B). In late life, time and intensity of therapy may be more limited and, as a result, treatment must focus more on short-term approaches, with realistic goals focusing on coping skills for daily life and basic interpersonal skills.

In outpatient settings, control over a patient's environment is limited, and clinicians must therefore rely on one-to-one interventions (if the patient is willing to cooperate with treatment). With some patients, it may be necessary to convey a basic formulation of their behaviors, along with suggested approaches, to caregivers and affiliated health care professionals, such as primary care providers, social workers, and visiting nurses. This communication is important when patients are vulnerable to self-harm or likely to cause significant disruptions in other settings when they are not understood and approached in a therapeutic manner. For some therapeutic approaches that can be used with various personality disorders, see Table 44.1.

Long-term care settings allow more opportunities for intervention. A staff meeting or case conference often provides the best forum to discuss disruptive patients and to coordinate a consistent treatment plan. Disruptive behaviors can sometimes be traced to particular activities or staff interactions, which can be adapted as part of an overall treatment strategy. Sometimes, disengagement from patients reduces the intensity of disruptive interactions. In other situations, the continuity of staffing and of daily schedules is critical. In all situations, a treatment plan should be well documented and conveyed to the patient, as well as to all involved staff and caregivers. All plans must provide appropriate limits to ensure the safety of patients and staff. A written contract, signed by all parties, may be needed with nonadherent patients to eliminate ambiguity. Although it is important to involve family members in the treatment plan, clinicians must recognize that patients with personality disorders often have conflictual relationships with them. Attention should also be given to individual staff members who must work with difficult patients. These staff members need opportunities to discuss feelings of anxiety and frustration and to feel acknowledged and supported by administrative and other clinical staff.

Few studies have specifically evaluated pharmacologic strategies for personality disorders in late life, so guidelines are extrapolated from those for younger people. Psychotropic medications can be targeted at a particular personality disorder; specific symptoms or symptom clusters; or comorbid depression, anxiety, or psychosis. Again, the goal is not to cure the disorder but to reduce the frequency and intensity of targeted symptoms. Antidepressant medication can be helpful for the target symptoms of depression and anxiety found in most personality disorders (SOE=B). Mood stabilizers (eg, lithium carbonate[OL], carbamazepine[OL], divalproex sodium[OL], and lamotrigine[OL]) and antipsychotic medications can reduce mood lability and impulsivity in borderline patients, and they can be useful with similar symptoms in antisocial personality disorder (SOE=B). Antianxiety agents are commonly used for transient agitation seen in borderline, antisocial, narcissistic, and paranoid disorders, and they may reduce social anxiety and panic in avoidant and dependent patients (SOE=C). Antidepressants are used commonly to treat impulsive aggression as well as obsessive-compulsive personality symptoms, although efficacy has not been established for treatment of these symptoms (as it has been demonstrated for obsessive-compulsive disorder). Antipsychotic agents can treat the transient psychosis, agitation, and impulsivity seen in dramatic cluster and paranoid disorders, as well as the borderline psychosis and paranoia seen in cluster A disorders (SOE=B).

For personality disorders, psychotropic medications are best used as adjuncts to psychotherapy. In older adults, multiple medications should be avoided in general, and particularly when there is a history of nonadherence, confusion, or impulsivity. Attention must be given to potential interactions with multiple other medications used to treat medical disorders. It is important to obtain and document informed consent (or consent of family members or guardians) for the use of psychotropic medications when there is a history of dementia, recent delirium, paranoia, or conflictual doctor-patient relationships.

Finally, clinicians must recognize that in some cases it is best not to prescribe a psychotropic medication. Such cases include older adults with personality disorders and comorbid substance abuse, chronic nonadherence, or a history of or potential for abusive or self-injurious use of medications. Antisocial and borderline individuals often demonstrate such behaviors. Dependent patients often insist on medications as a means of fostering dependency on the clinician, and obsessive-compulsive patients can perpetuate a maladaptive relationship with the clinician through detailed and controlling discussions of medication management. In each example, medication management is corrupted by dysfunctional interpersonal behaviors that lie at the heart of personality disorders.

SOMATIC SYMPTOM AND RELATED DISORDERS

Somatic symptom and related disorders is the updated terminology in *DSM-5* from the previous category of somatoform disorders. This allows for inclusion of more symptoms that were often encountered usually in primary care medical settings. The revision was aimed at improving relevance in primary care settings. Somatic symptom and related disorders encompass a heterogeneous group of 5 diagnoses that have in common the presence of distressing physical symptoms, as well as abnormal thoughts, feelings, and behaviors in response to these physical symptoms. *DSM-5* does not require that the somatic symptoms be medically unexplained. Instead, somatic symptom disorder can also accompany a diagnosed medical disorder as long as the somatic symptoms are associated with significant emotional distress and impairment. In somatic symptom disorder, the patient must have one or more distressing and/or disruptive somatic symptom(s) that is accompanied by at least one of the following: 1) concerns about the seriousness of the medical symptom that is out of proportion to what is typically experienced, 2) persistent high level of anxiety about the symptom, and/or 3) excessive time and energy focused on the somatic symptom. The clinician can also specify if the somatic symptom disorder occurs with predominant pain.

Illness anxiety disorder is a preoccupation with being susceptible to or having an illness. Patients with illness anxiety disorder tend to have milder somatic symptoms but higher anxiety levels than those with somatic symptom disorder. Symptoms must be persistent for ≥6 months, and patient behaviors can be described as care seeking or care avoidant. Conversion disorder is defined by one or more symptoms of altered voluntary motor and/or sensory function that causes significant social and occupational impairment and is not explained by a neurologic disease. Motor symptoms of conversion disorders may include weakness, paralysis, and abnormal movements (eg, tremor) and gait disorders. Sensory symptoms include changes in vision or hearing, or skin sensations. Psychological factors affecting medical conditions are psychological or behavioral factors that have an adverse effect on a diagnosed medical condition. For example, a patient may exacerbate symptoms of COPD because of anxiety, or a patient may manipulate insulin dosage in an attempt to lose weight. *DSM-5* also includes factitious disorders in this category, which are characterized by false symptoms associated with deception on the part of the patient. Patients with factitious disorder present as ill or injured without any obvious evidence of external reward or reinforcement. Distressing somatic symptoms that do not fit any of the above diagnoses are classified as other or unspecified somatic symptom and related disorders. Specific diagnostic criteria for these 5 conditions can be found in the *DSM-5*.

All of these disorders are especially relevant to geriatric care because affected older adults are seen in all health care settings, and they tend to overuse medical services. Somatic symptom disorders in late life have not been well studied, and existing research has usually focused on select diagnoses, such as hypochondriasis, in limited or biased samples. Research also has looked at somatic symptom reporting rather than at specific diagnoses. Prevalence rates in middle and late life have been found to be <1%. The presence of these disorders has not been found to be strongly associated with age, although there is weak evidence for a slight increase in hypochondriasis with age (SOE=C). However, increased somatic preoccupation and symptoms are associated with depression in late life, and older age of onset for depression may be most predictive. In addition to depression, increased somatic preoccupation is associated with the presence of neuroticism, a personality trait in which a person displays a tendency to experience more negative emotions. Somatic symptom disorders are found more commonly in women and in lower socioeconomic groups. Late onset may suggest associated neurologic illness.

Clinical Characteristics and Causes

Somatic symptom disorders do not represent delusional thinking as is seen in psychotic states, and they are different from psychosomatic disorders, which are characterized by actual disease states with presumed psychological triggers. They also differ from malingering, with its intentional and fully conscious goal of avoiding a specific responsibility such as work. Rather, somatoform disorders represent a complex interaction between mind and brain in which an affected person is unknowingly expressing psychological stress or conflict through the body. It is not surprising, then, that depression and anxiety are associated with increased somatic expressions. In late life, somatic symptom disorders, in particular illness anxiety disorder, can be a way for a person to express anxiety and attempt to cope with accumulating fears and losses. These may include fears of abandonment by family and caregivers, loss of beauty and strength, financial setbacks, loss of independence, loss of social role (eg, through retirement, loss of spouse, occupational disability), and loneliness. The psychological distress and anxiety over such losses can be less threatening and more controllable when shifted to somatic complaints or symptoms. In turn, the resultant state of debility might be reinforced by increased social contacts and support.

Somatic symptom and related disorders, except for factitious disorder, are not caused by intentional, conscious attempts by older adults to present factitious physical symptoms. Individuals with these disorders experience real pain and distress, and they are usually without insight into associated psychological factors. The etiology of somatic symptoms disorder is unclear. There are few theories on this, one of which is increased perceptual disposition that leads to an affected individual to equate these sensations as organic illness. Another theory comes from a psychodynamic approach, which suggests that these disorders result from unconscious conflict in which intolerable impulses or affects are expressed through more tolerable somatic symptoms or complaints. Although psychodynamic explanations can apply across the life span, these conflicts often begin early in life, perhaps accounting for the relatively young age of onset for most somatic symptom disorders. In late life, psychological conflict that results in significant depression and anxiety are, for the most part, the same conflicts that can lead to somatization.

Personality disorders are also associated with severe somatization, with avoidant, paranoid, and obsessive-compulsive being the most common. In addition, the presence of many comorbid medical problems and the use of multiple medications can provide readily available somatic symptoms around which psychological conflict can center. In long-term care, older adults are faced with many overwhelming losses, and their own bodies often serve as the last bastion of control. Somatic preoccupation thus serves as a means of coping with stress, even though it is maladaptive and can result in excessive and unnecessary disability.

For somatic symptom and related disorders and their respective diagnostic features, see Table 44.2.

Treatment

People with somatic symptom disorder do not usually present as such; by definition, they appear to have legitimate somatic complaints. It is only after repeated but fruitless evaluations, multiple and persistent complaints and requests, and sometimes angry and inappropriate reactions to treatment that clinicians begin to suspect a somatic symptom disorder. In some cases, the manner of presentation and symptom complex is more immediately suggestive of a particular somatic symptom disorder. In any event, it is important for the clinician to remember that from the perspective of the patient, the symptoms and complaints are quite real and disturbing. It is never wise to challenge the patient or to suggest that the symptoms are "all in your mind," even after diagnostic evaluation has made it obvious that psychological factors are involved. The typical response to such advice is for the patient to seek additional opinions and medical tests, which in turn can perpetuate a cycle of somatization that never addresses the underlying issues.

Table 44.2—Somatic Symptom and Related Disorders with Diagnostic Features

Somatic Symptom and Related Disorder	Diagnostic Features
Somatic symptom disorder	■ Multiple, current, somatic symptoms that are distressing or result in significant disruption of daily life are typical. ■ Sometimes, only one severe symptom, most commonly pain, is present. ■ Symptoms may be specific (eg, localized pain) or relatively nonspecific (eg, fatigue). ■ Symptoms sometimes represent normal bodily sensations or discomfort that does not generally signify serious disease. ■ Somatic symptoms without an evident medical explanation are not sufficient to make this diagnosis; the individual's suffering is authentic, whether or not it is medically explained.
Illness anxiety disorder	■ Most individuals with hypochondriasis are now classified as having somatic symptom disorder; however, in a minority of cases, the diagnosis of illness anxiety disorder applies instead. ■ Illness anxiety disorder entails a preoccupation with having or acquiring a serious, undiagnosed medical illness. ■ Somatic symptoms are not present or, if present, are only mild in intensity. ■ Preoccupation with the idea that one is sick is accompanied by substantial anxiety about health and disease. ■ Individuals with the disorder often examine themselves repeatedly.
Conversion disorder	■ Alternative names include "functional" or "psychogenic" to describe the symptoms of conversion disorder (functional neurologic symptom disorder). ■ There may be one or more symptoms of various types. ■ Motor symptoms include weakness or paralysis; abnormal movements, such as tremor or dystonic movements; gait abnormalities; and abnormal limb posturing. ■ Sensory symptoms include altered, reduced, or absent skin sensation, vision, or hearing. ■ Episodes of abnormal generalized limb shaking with apparent impaired or loss of consciousness may resemble epileptic seizures (also called psychogenic or nonepileptic seizures). ■ There may be episodes of unresponsiveness resembling syncope or coma. ■ Other symptoms include reduced or absent speech volume (dysphonia/aphonia), altered articulation (dysarthria), a sensation of a lump in the throat (globus), and diplopia.
Psychological factors affecting other medical conditions	■ Essential feature is the presence of one or more clinically significant psychological or behavioral factors that adversely affect a medical condition by increasing the risk of suffering, death, or disability. ■ These factors can adversely affect the medical condition by influencing its course or treatment, by constituting an additional well-established health risk factor, or by influencing the underlying pathophysiology to precipitate or exacerbate symptoms or to necessitate medical attention. ■ This diagnosis should be reserved for situations in which the effect of the psychological factor on the medical condition is evident and the psychological factor has clinically significant effects on the course or outcome of the medical condition.
Factitious disorder	■ Essential feature involves a person producing or faking illness when he or she is not sick and that is associated with the identified deception. ■ Individuals with factitious disorder can also seek treatment for themselves or another after induction of injury or disease. The diagnosis requires demonstrating that the individual is taking surreptitious actions to misrepresent, simulate, or cause signs or symptoms of illness or injury in the absence of obvious external rewards.

Other specified somatic symptom and related disorders	■ This applies to presentations in which symptoms characteristic of a somatic symptom and related disorder that cause clinically significant distress or impairment in social, occupational, or other important areas of functioning predominate but do not meet the full criteria for any of the disorders in the somatic symptom and related disorders diagnostic class.
	■ Examples:
	  ■ Brief somatic symptom disorder: duration of symptoms <6 months
	  ■ Brief illness anxiety disorder: duration of symptoms <6 months
	  ■ Illness anxiety disorder without excessive health-related behaviors: avoids doctors' appointments and hospitals with negative impact on health
	  ■ Pseudocyesis: a false belief of being pregnant associated with objective signs and reported symptoms of pregnancy

Unspecified somatic symptom and related disorders	■ Applies to presentations in which symptoms characteristic of a somatic symptom and related disorder that cause clinically significant distress or impairment in social, occupational, or other important areas of functioning predominate but do not meet the full criteria for any of the disorders in the somatic symptom and related disorders diagnostic class. ■ This category should not be used unless there are decidedly unusual situations in which information is insufficient to make a more specific diagnosis.

NOTE: Descriptions of the somatic symptoms and related disorders with diagnostic features are adapted from the *Diagnostic and Statistical Manual of Mental Disorders*. 5th ed. Washington, DC: American Psychiatric Association; 2013.

Instead, the clinician should attempt to foster an ongoing, supportive, consistent, and professional relationship with the affected patient. Such a relationship serves to provide reassurance as well as to protect the patient from excessive and unnecessary medical visits and procedures. The clinician should focus on responding to individual complaints, perhaps with periodic but regularly scheduled appointments, and to set limits on evaluation and treatment in a firm but empathetic manner. This can be difficult to do when patients become demanding and attempt to consume excessive amounts of time, but the clinician must endeavor to remain professional, without personalizing the situation or feeling that he or she is failing the patient. Overall, the role of the clinician is to focus on reducing symptoms and rehabilitating the patient, and not attempting to force the patient to have insight into the potential psychological nature of his or her symptoms.

It would be hazardous to prematurely diagnose a somatic symptom disorder when there might actually be an underlying medical problem that has eluded diagnosis. For example, disorders such as multiple sclerosis, systemic lupus erythematosus, and acute intermittent porphyria commonly have complex presentations that elude initial diagnostic evaluation. Moreover, many somatic symptom disorders coexist with actual disease states; for example, many individuals with pseudoseizures also have an actual seizure disorder. At the same time, it is important for the clinician to set limits on what he or she can offer and to make appropriate referrals to specialists and mental health clinicians.

The mental health clinician should have an active role in addressing the somatic symptom disorder. Unfortunately, no particular treatment for any specific disorder has been found to have good efficacy, and most disorders tend to be lifelong. As a result, the goal of treatment is not to cure but to control symptoms. The clinician first forms a therapeutic alliance based on empathetic listening and acknowledgment of physical discomfort, without trivializing the somatic complaints. Sometimes an offer to review all available medical records can be a tangible way of conveying one's seriousness to the patient. Underlying anxiety and depression must be identified and treated with psychotherapy and, when necessary, antidepressant or antianxiety medications, or both. Cognitive-behavioral therapy focuses on identifying distorted thought patterns and triggers of anxiety, and then replacing them with more realistic and adaptive strategies. A mental health professional can assist in determining whether cognitive-behavioral therapy may be of benefit. In many cases, however, the supportive nature of regular visits to a primary care provider may be sufficient to meet the needs of individuals with somatic symptom disorders. The goal of treatment is not curative but rather to decrease the distress of the individual and improve their ability to function.

RESOURCES

- Conway CC, Boudreaux M, Oltmanns TF. Dynamic associations between borderline personality disorder and stressful life events over five years in older adults. *Personal Disord.* 2018;9(6):521–529.

- Cruitt PJ, Oltmanns TF. Age-related outcomes associated with personality pathology in later life. *Curr Opin Psychol.* 2018;21:89–93.

- Dixon-Gordon K, Conkey L, Whalen DJ. Recent advances in understanding physical health problems in personality disorders. *Curr Opin Psychol.* 2017;21:1–5.

CHAPTER 45—ADDICTIONS

KEY POINTS

- Alcohol and other substance use disorders can remain undetected when screening questions are omitted during routine medical visits.

- Substance use can be an unrecognized cause of falls, cognitive decline, and medical problems (eg, anemia, increased results of liver function tests, hyponatremia, thrombocytopenia).

- It is important to consider a diagnosis of alcohol or benzodiazepine withdrawal in older adults who develop delirium with hospitalization or facility placement.

- Cognitive impairment from chronic substance use in older adults can improve with sustained abstinence.

- Inappropriate use of prescription drugs, including benzodiazepines and opioids, is often unrecognized and is estimated as the second most common cause of substance use disorders among older adults.

- Substance cessation efforts should persist throughout life, including efforts to minimize chronic use of benzodiazepines, whether illicit or prescribed.

The misuse of alcohol, psychoactive medications, illicit drugs, and nicotine has become a significant public health concern for the growing population of older adults. Substance use disorders among older adults is common, and older adults are particularly vulnerable to the cognitive and physical effects of these substances. Typically, substance use disorders are thought to develop only in those who use substances in large quantities and at regular intervals. Among older adults, however, negative health consequences have been demonstrated at consumption amounts previously thought of as light to moderate. A growing number of effective treatments for these problems lead not only to reduced substance use but also to improved general health. Both the risks and emergence of new treatments underscore the need to identify problems and provide appropriate treatment for older adults suffering from the effects of substance use disorders.

DEFINITIONS OF SUBSTANCE USE DISORDERS

Many older adults are not recognized as having problems related to their substance use, partly because the diagnostic criteria have been difficult to interpret and apply consistently to this population. For instance, many older adults drink at home by themselves; thus, they are less likely than younger drinkers to be arrested, get into arguments, or have employment difficulties. Moreover, because many of the diseases potentially associated with substance use (eg, hypertension, stroke, and peptic ulcer disease) are common disorders in late life, the effects of substance use in older adults who have these other medical disorders can be overlooked. The literature indicates that older adults with alcohol use disorders are identified less often by clinicians and are less often referred for treatment than their younger counterparts.

Given the challenges in applying this terminology to older adults, the *Diagnostic and Statistical Manual of Mental Disorders, 5th Edition (DSM-5)* represents a potential advance, because it no longer uses the terms substance "abuse" and "dependence." The diagnosis of a "substance use disorder" is now based on 11 criteria that encompass the following domains: impaired control, social impairment, risky use, and pharmacologic criteria. Severity is determined by the number of criteria met, from mild (2 or 3), to moderate (4 or 5) or severe (≥6); legal problems are no longer criteria.

Regardless of the diagnostic system, many experts advocate screening to identify those at risk of problem behaviors or who have at-risk or problem use. *At-risk use* is defined as any use of a substance at a quantity or frequency greater than a recommended level. The level of use is often determined empirically based on association with significant disability. For instance, the recommended upper limit of alcohol consumption for older adults has been established as no more than an average of 1 standard drink per day and no more than 2 episodes of binge drinking (>2 drinks for women and >3 drinks for men on any single occasion) during a 3-month period. *Problem substance use* is defined as the consumption of any amount of an abusable substance that results in at least one problem related to this use. For example, the use of benzodiazepines by a patient who has a preexisting unsteady gait would be considered problem use.

On the other end of the spectrum, *abstinence* is defined as no illicit drug or alcohol use in the previous year. Although a large portion of older adults report abstinence, it is important to assess past use patterns. Individuals who have a previous history of substance use problems can require preventive monitoring to determine if any new stresses could exacerbate an old pattern. In addition, a previous history of at-risk drinking or alcohol dependence increases the risk of developing other mental health problems in late life, such as depressive disorders or cognitive problems, and can limit treatment response because of brain damage.

Low-risk or *moderate use* of alcohol is use that falls within the recommended guidelines for consumption and is not associated with problems. Older adults in this category not only consume amounts that fall within recommended drinking guidelines but also are able to reasonably limit their alcohol consumption (ie, they do not drink when driving a motor vehicle or boat, or when using contraindicated medications). However, a change in either physical health or prescription medications can increase even low-risk use to a problem level.

Similarly, *low-risk use* of potentially misused prescription substances, such as opioids or benzodiazepines, is use strictly within the parameters of a clinician's recommendations and is not associated with problem use (ie, taking more than prescribed, supplementing with illicitly procured prescription substances, use resulting in functional impairment or increased morbidity and mortality, etc). A unique challenge for providers of older adults is that benzodiazepines and opioids in particular—even when taken within prescribed guidelines—can cause major health problems, with more recent attention paid to the medical burden of long-term benzodiazepine and opioid use. This is particularly pronounced when opioids and benzodiazepines are co-prescribed.

The most practical method for identifying individuals who could benefit from intervention is to determine the quantity, frequency, and consequences of their substance use. It is important to note that even with stable patterns of use, functional impairment may dramatically increase over time and with advanced age. This method has advantages over formal diagnostic interviews because of its brevity, easily interpretable results, and absence of stigmatizing language, such as "addiction," "alcoholism," or "alcoholic."

MAGNITUDE OF THE PROBLEM

Illicit Drug Use

The most commonly studied substance in older adults is alcohol; however, the prevalence of illicit drug use in older adults has increased dramatically over the last 20 years. The National Survey on Drug Use and Health (NSDUH) reports that nearly 469,000 older adults used an illicit substance in the past month. This does not reflect misuse of prescribed medications, which is the second most common form of substance use in older adults. Nearly 16.2 million adults ≥65 years old drank alcohol in the last month, with 3.4 million reporting binge use. The next most commonly used illicit substance is marijuana (its use is still illegal under federal law), with 132,000 older adults reporting use on an average day in the last month. The NSDUH also reports 43,000 older adults used cocaine on an average day in the last month. These figures are increased from previous studies and may be explained by the population of baby boomers who grew up in the 1960s and 1970s when drug experimentation was accepted and prevalent. For example, in 2012, 19.3% of adults ≥65 years old reported lifetime substance use, versus 47.6% of adults 60–64 years old, which represents the "baby boomer" population.

Prescription Medication Misuse

An increasing problem with the older age group is the misuse or inappropriate use of prescription and OTC medications, with 2.1% of adults aged 50 in the NSDUH reporting nonmedical use of prescription-type drugs, the most commonly used illicit class among those ≥65 years old. This problem includes the misuse of substances such as sedatives, hypnotics, narcotic and non-narcotic analgesics, diet aids, decongestants, and a wide variety of OTC medications. Community surveys have found that 60% of older adults are taking an analgesic, 22% are taking a CNS medication, and 11% are taking a benzodiazepine. Many medications used by older adults have the potential for inducing tolerance, withdrawal syndromes, and harmful medical consequences, such as cognitive changes, kidney disease, falls, and liver disease. A growing body of literature demonstrates a concerning increase in morbidity and mortality associated with misuse of prescription and nonprescription medications, even though this is not considered as a disorder in *DSM-5*.

Of particular concern is the rapid rise in opioid use and misuse, especially in older adults, in whom chronic pain is among the most prevalent complaints. Between 1995 and 2010, opioid prescriptions at office-based visits for older adults in the United States increased nearly 9-fold. The increase in the rate of benzodiazepine prescribing during that time frame was similar. Benzodiazepines are the most commonly prescribed psychotropic medication in developed countries, even among older adults who are particularly vulnerable to adverse effects. The prevalence of benzodiazepine use in adults 51–64 years old is 7.4% and increases to 8.7% for adults 65–80 years old. Rates of use are higher among women and increase with age. Most benzodiazepine prescriptions for older adults are written by primary care providers (9 of 10) to treat anxiety and insomnia. Benzodiazepine prescriptions written by psychiatrists for older adults significantly decrease with age. Although receiving a benzodiazepine prescription does not translate into misuse, the risks in older adults are notable. Despite mounting evidence for adverse effects of benzodiazepines in older adults and recommendations against long-term use in this population, prescribing this class of medications remains common practice. More data are needed to evaluate the specific incidence of misuse in the older adult population versus inappropriate prescribing.

Medication use by all older adults needs to be monitored carefully; prescribing potentially hazardous combinations of medications, medications with a high risk of adverse events, and ineffective or unnecessary medications should be avoided. A practical approach to monitoring psychoactive medications is to reevaluate the older patient's use every 3–6 months. Maintenance treatment should be continued only in those who have specific target symptoms and a documented response to the treatment. Patients who have no response or only a partial response should be reevaluated to consider the appropriate diagnosis and further care. In such cases, consultation with a geriatric mental health professional could be advantageous.

The use of a reversal kit for naloxone overdose should be encouraged among patients with active prescriptions for opioids. Many community-based organizations and pharmacies offer training in its use.

Alcohol Use

Community-based epidemiologic studies define the extent and nature of alcohol use in the older population by reporting percentages of abstainers, heavy drinkers, and daily drinkers. Abstention from alcohol ranges from 31% to 58%, and daily drinking ranges from 10% to 22% in samples of older adults. "Heavy" drinking, defined as a minimum of 12–21 drinks per week, is present in 3%–9% of the older population; alcohol abuse, as defined clinically, is present in approximately 2%–4%.

Longitudinally designed community studies give valuable insight regarding the natural course of drinking patterns in older age groups. Studies that examined longitudinal alcohol use indicate an incidence of heavy drinking of 0.2%–4% in older adults per year. Although older adults are likely to decrease the amount of alcohol consumed on a given day, the frequency or pattern of use changes very little over time.

Cultural and Demographic Factors
The prevalence of alcohol use and alcohol-related problems among older adults is much higher for men than for women. Among younger adults, however, the ratio of male to female drinkers has changed over the past several decades, with the result that more women present for treatment. These changes are likely to continue to be reflected in the next generation of older women. Similar patterns by gender are seen with illicit drug use, except that benzodiazepines are much more commonly used by older women than by older men.

Clinical Settings
Older adults constitute most admissions to acute care facilities and are frequent users of outpatient medical services, including primary care. The prevalence rates for alcohol problems among hospital populations are substantially higher than those among community dwellers. High prevalence rates for problems related to drinking are also becoming more common in retirement communities. Data from a survey of a Veterans Affairs nursing home demonstrated that 35% of patients interviewed had a lifetime diagnosis of alcohol abuse. A significant number of patients seen in outpatient clinics also have active alcohol use disorders. The high prevalence of alcohol-related problems in both hospital and outpatient populations underscores the need for thorough screening of older adults in medical settings.

The epidemiology of substance use suggests that the prevalence of misuse among older adults will likely increase as the baby boomers age. The growing numbers of patients in potential need of treatment will be paired with an ongoing shortage of providers trained in the treatment of older adults with mental health or substance use disorders. This growing public health problem is addressed in the recent Institute of Medicine report *The Mental Health and Substance Use Workforce for Older Adults: In Whose Hands?*

RISKS OF SUBSTANCE USE
Excess Physical Disability

Substance abuse has clear and profound effects on the health and well-being of older adults in all spheres of life. Older adults are particularly prone to the toxic effects of substances on many different organ systems because of both the physiologic changes associated with aging and the changes associated with other illnesses common in late life. The social and economic impact is also tremendous. Substance abuse has adverse effects on self-esteem, coping skills, and interpersonal relationships, which may be compounded by losses that are common in later stages of life.

Levels of alcohol consumption higher than 7 drinks per week, so-called at-risk drinking, have been associated with a number of health problems, including an increased risk of stroke caused by bleeding, impaired driving skills, and an increased rate of injuries such as falls and fractures (SOE=A). The risk of breast cancer in women who consume 3–9 drinks per week is approximately 50% higher than that of women who consume fewer than 3 drinks per week. Of particular importance to older adults are the potential harmful interactions between alcohol and both prescribed and OTC medications, especially psychoactive medications such as benzodiazepines and antidepressants. Alcohol also interferes with the metabolism of many medications, including warfarin.

Older adults who consume more than an average of 4 drinks per day or whose drinking has led to a diagnosis of

Table 45.1—Risk Factors for Substance Use in Older Adults

- More affluent (predictor of increased drinking in older adults)
- White
- "Young old"
- Female gender associated with increase in prescription drug misuse
- Smokers are at increased likelihood of being at-risk drinkers
- History of substance use disorder
- Exposure to drugs of abuse potential (eg, opiates, benzodiazepines)
- Avoidance coping style
- Being divorced/separated/single
- Lack of religious affiliation
- Increased social interaction increases likelihood of drinking, social isolation increases prescription drug misuse
- Involuntary retirement/broadened social network after retirement increases drinking

alcohol dependence are at greatest risk of excess physical disability and physical illness related to drinking. The most common problems associated with alcohol dependence are alcoholic liver disease, COPD, peptic ulcer disease, and psoriasis. Moreover, unexplained multisystem disease should alert the clinician to probe more closely for alcohol use. With smoking, the risks are much clearer, including increased rates of pulmonary disease, especially cancer. Medications such as benzodiazepines are also associated with excess physical disability, increased rates of falls, and driving-related impairment. Research is beginning to demonstrate that the disability associated with these problems is also reversible with reduced substance use (SOE=B).

Over the last several years, more attention has been paid to the burden of prescription opioid and benzodiazepine medications, including within the geriatric population. Benzodiazepine use has been linked to cognitive impairment, falls, and respiratory depression. In addition, overdose deaths with prescribed opioids have increased dramatically in the geriatric population, for whom age-related pharmacokinetic changes that prolong medication effects and the increased occurrence of additional drug interactions that can compound adverse effects, complicate the calculation of an effective and safe dosing regimen. This has led to an increased risk of unintentional overdoses, both lethal and non-lethal, and an increased incidence of the development of dependence and subsequent emergence of use disorders. Although more studies are needed to fully understand the burden of prescription drug misuse, enough evidence has emerged that the FDA, through its Opioid Action Plan and several recent boxed warnings, has recommended strict new guidelines on the long-term prescription of opioids in particular, and of concurrent prescription of opioids with benzodiazepines and other CNS depressants. Additionally, a growing body of evidence suggests that it is safe and, in most cases, preferential to reduce and discontinue long-term treatment with benzodiazepines and/or opioids.

Mental Health Problems

Substance use can be a significant factor in the course and prognosis of nearly all mental health problems of late life. Use of alcohol, benzodiazepines, opioids, and cigarettes has been demonstrated to be related etiologically to mood disturbances, but these substances also complicate the treatment of concurrent mood disorders. Individuals with both alcoholism and depression have a more complicated clinical course of depression with an increased risk of suicide and more social dysfunction than nondepressed individuals with alcoholism. Overall, older adults with alcohol abuse or dependence are nearly 3 times more likely to have a lifetime diagnosis of another mental disorder. Alcoholism has been implicated in mood disorders, suicide, dementia, anxiety disorders, and sleep disturbances. Although benzodiazepines provide dramatic short-term relief of anxiety disorder, long-term use raises concern for paradoxical worsening of anxiety as well as for development of tolerance and withdrawal symptoms, with patients subsequently mistaking relief from physical and psychological withdrawal with continued benzodiazepine administration as relief from the underlying anxiety disorder. A similar challenge exists in the chronic use of benzodiazepines for treatment of insomnia, which is prevalent among older adults. In addition to paradoxical worsening of insomnia symptoms through development of tolerance and withdrawal, benzodiazepines directly disrupt sleep architecture, exacerbating underlying sleep disturbances. In addition, even after benzodiazepines have been discontinued, disturbances to sleep architecture and development of rebound insomnia can persist for months.

The effects of substance use in the geriatric population also play a significant role in development of dementia. As might be expected, patients with alcohol-related dementia who become abstinent do not show a progression in cognitive impairment comparable to that of those with Alzheimer disease. The complex role of alcoholism in the development of Alzheimer disease is not fully understood, but alcoholism does lead independently to a syndrome of dementia. Clinical features supporting the diagnosis of alcohol-related dementia include end-organ damage (eg, liver disease), cognitive stabilization or improvement after abstinence, and evidence of cerebellar atrophy in brain imaging. Further research is needed to understand the potential benefits of long-term abstinence in alcohol-related dementia. Similarly, those with comorbid depression and alcohol use are likely to have better depression outcomes if they become abstinent. Moderate alcohol use has also been demonstrated to have negative effects on the treatment of late-life depression, further underscoring the need for reducing moderate use in the context of chronic health problems in older adults.

Benzodiazepine use in older adults can confound the assessment and treatment of mental health problems, because many of the cognitive, emotional, and behavioral adverse effects of benzodiazepines, whether as part of intoxication or withdrawal, can mimic other illnesses, in particular neurocognitive disorders. Although the greatest risk of cognitive impairment with benzodiazepine use is associated with high dosage and/or chronic use, such impairment in older adults has been seen even at low dosages and short durations of treatment. Some studies have suggested that >10% of patients referred to memory clinics have cognitive impairments that are substance-induced, particularly related to benzodiazepine use.

IDENTIFYING SUBSTANCE USE DISORDERS: RISK FACTORS AND SCREENING

Several risk factors for substance use in older adults should be kept in mind when screening for problematic use (Table 45.1) In addition, although clinical examination remains the most valuable tool for identifying substance use problems, screening instruments can help increase the sensitivity and efficiency of diagnosis. Several instruments have been developed for identifying alcohol use disorders, including self-administered questionnaires and laboratory studies. Self-administered questionnaires provide a rapid, sensitive, and inexpensive method of screening for alcohol problems. Two questionnaires have been developed with these principles in mind: the Michigan Alcoholism Screening Test (MAST)-Geriatric Version and the AUDIT C. Both of these instruments have high sensitivity and specificity for identifying alcohol misuse in middle-aged and older adults. The CAGE is a brief clinician-administered screening test that may be useful to identify problem drinking using a cutoff of 2 as a positive screen, although some suggest ≥1 should be considered positive if the prevalence is high in the population (www.uspreventiveservicestaskforce.org/Home/GetFileByID/838 (accessed Feb 2019).

TREATMENT

Older adults with a substance use problem often need a variety of treatments. Therefore, it is important to have an array of services available that can be tailored to individual needs and that have the flexibility to adapt to changing needs over time. The most important aspect of treating an older adult who is misusing a substance is to engage the individual in the intervention. Older adults engaged in treatment generally have robust improvement, especially compared with younger cohorts. The spectrum of interventions for substance misuse in older adults ranges from prevention and education for those who are abstinent or low-risk users, to minimal advice or brief structured interventions for at-risk or problem users, to formalized substance treatment for individuals who meet criteria for substance use disorders. The array of formal treatment options available includes psychotherapy, education, rehabilitative and residential care, and psychopharmacologic agents.

Assuring that the patient enters a long-term treatment program increases the likelihood of long-term success. The management of patients already maintained on long-term opioid or benzodiazepine treatment presents a particularly difficult challenge to providers treating older adults, with the development of dependence all but assuring significant withdrawal effects. Abrupt discontinuation of preexisting regimens risk rebound symptoms and rupture of therapeutic alliance. However, it should not be assumed that geriatric patients cannot be discontinued from both long-term opioids and long-term benzodiazepines. Complacency with potentially harmful medication regimens that risk the development of use disorders is likewise inappropriate. Alternatives to long-term opioid use, including referral to a pain specialist for nonopioid and possibly even nonpharmacologic interventions is appropriate. Additionally, while specific guidelines and robust data are lacking, office-based treatment for opioid use disorder can also be considered in older adults. Long-term benzodiazepine use should likewise be addressed, with several guidelines emerging over the years for tapering and discontinuing in patients for whom long-term use is causing significant problems.

Brief Interventions

Low-intensity, brief interventions have been suggested as cost-effective and practical techniques that can be used as an initial approach in at-risk and problem drinkers in primary care settings. Studies of brief intervention have been conducted in a wide range of health care settings, from hospitals and primary health care locations to mental health clinics. Two trials of brief alcohol intervention with older adults have been reported. Both studies were randomized trials of brief intervention to reduce hazardous drinking by older adults, and both used advice protocols in primary care settings. These studies showed that older adults can be engaged in brief intervention

Table 45.2—Late-Life Addiction Treatment Research and Strength of Evidence

Indication	Treatment Strategy	SOE	Comments	Limits
Detoxification				
Alcohol	Substitution with benzodiazepine	A	Prevents sequela such as seizures, severe withdrawal symptoms; should be driven by specific plan and measurement of effects	Few specific studies in older adults, who may be at greater risk of idiosyncratic responses
	Gabapentin	C	Effective in several clinical trials	No studies specific to older adults
	Carbamazepine[OL] and other mood-stabilizing medications	D	Small-scale studies have shown promise, but these medications are somewhat more complicated to use.	Very limited evidence base for older adults
Benzodiazepines	Slow tapering	B	Effective in managing withdrawal	Limited evidence base for older adults; long-term outcomes not well correlated with success of detoxification
Opioids	Substitution/taper	B	Effective in managing withdrawal	Limited evidence base for older adults
Treatment Strategies				
Problem and at-risk drinking	Brief interventions	A	Randomized trials have showed efficacy in primary-care settings with less evidence in high-risk settings such as behavioral health, home care, and the emergency room.	Limited effect in those with alcohol dependence; limited dissemination
Alcohol dependence	Psychotherapy	C	Several naturalistic trials demonstrated increased adherence to treatment and generally better outcomes for older adults than for middle-aged adults. Individual therapy such as cognitive-behavioral therapy may be particularly effective.	Randomized trials designed to better understand age-dependent adherence and treatment outcomes are needed.
	Naltrexone	B	Well tolerated and showed some evidence of efficacy in post-hoc analyses	
	Acamprosate	C	Inconsistent evidence base but approved for use	Very limited evidence base for older adults
	Disulfiram	C	Antabuse reaction can be particularly harmful for older adults with preexisting medical problems.	No age-specific studies or studies that have included significant numbers of older adults
	Topiramate	D	Not FDA approved but several positive clinical trials	Can have cognitive effects; not studied in older adults
	Other agents	D	Antidepressants and mood-stabilizing agents are all used clinically but with an inconsistent evidence base.	No age-specific studies or studies that have included significant numbers of older adults
Nicotine dependence	Brief interventions	A	Less than for alcohol but consistent evidence for benefit	Limited evidence specifically for older adults
	Nicotine replacement	B	Strong evidence base for use	Limited evidence specifically for older adults
	Varenicline	B	Several evidence-based studies	Very limited evidence for older adults; case reports of depression and behavior disturbance
Opioid dependence	Methadone, buprenorphine	B	Strong evidence for decrease in use and improved function	Limited evidence base for older adults, many of whom have been on methadone for many years

protocols and that the protocols are acceptable in this population; drinking was substantially reduced among at-risk drinkers receiving the interventions than among a control group.

Detoxification and Stabilization

The assessment of any substance abuser starts with a thorough history, physical examination, and laboratory tests. The patient's potential to suffer acute withdrawal should also be assessed. Severe withdrawal such as that from alcohol use can be life threatening and warrants careful attention. Patients with severe symptoms of dependency or withdrawal potential and patients with significant medical or psychiatric comorbidity can require inpatient hospitalization for acute stabilization before implementing an outpatient management strategy. Detoxification is achieved by placing the patient on the minimal dose that suppresses withdrawal symptoms and then decreasing the dosage by 10% every three half-lives. In general, longer-acting formulations of the drug being abused are preferred to shorter-acting formulations, but many clinicians find that prescribing the specific drug that a patient was abusing makes the process more acceptable to the patient and minimizes the time needed to determine the initial dose.

For patients who are hospitalized for an elective surgery or condition unrelated to the substance problem, remaining vigilant for any evidence of withdrawal is extremely important. Unrecognized alcohol withdrawal can result in serious morbidity and mortality in older adults. Early symptoms include tachycardia, diaphoresis, tremulousness, and hypertension. These symptoms can progress to overt delirium, psychosis, and seizures. Intravenous lorazepam^{OL} is the most expedient intervention in this scenario, followed by oral lorazepam, in tapering dosages.

Outpatient Management

Traditionally, outpatient substance abuse treatment has been reserved for specialized clinics focused on substance abuse. However, it is becoming increasingly apparent that this model is inadequate in addressing the broader public health demand, and there is a need to involve a variety of clinicians and clinical settings to deliver substance abuse treatment. This is particularly important for older adults, who frequently seek medical services but rarely seek specialized addiction services. The traditional addiction clinic is focused on supportive group psychotherapy and encouragement to attend regular self-help group meetings such as Alcoholics Anonymous, Alcoholics Victorious, Rational Recovery, or Narcotics Anonymous. For older adults, peer-specific group activities are considered superior to mixed-age group activities. Outpatient rehabilitation, in addition to focusing on active addiction issues, usually needs to address issues of leisure time and social activity.

Clinicians should be wary of focusing on abstinence as the only positive outcome of treatment and should commend patients for making progress in decreasing use as well as stopping. This can be particularly relevant for misuse of medications such as benzodiazepines, because eliminating use may be more difficult. For benzodiazepines, the risk of adverse events such as falls is greater with higher dosages and with medications that have a longer half-life such as diazepam or clonazepam. Therefore, using medications with a half-life of 6–12 hours reduces the risks for that patient. If benzodiazepines seem to be indicated for an anxiety condition and treatment is started for the first time, shorter-acting agents that do not have active metabolites (eg, lorazepam) are preferred to long-acting preparations. However, for patients already receiving long-acting benzodiazepines (eg, diazepam at ≥50 mg/d), the risk of withdrawal complications is increased, and the dosage should be reduced very gradually. The use of resources such as day programs and senior centers can be beneficial, especially for cognitively impaired patients. Social services, including financial support, are often needed to stabilize the patient in early recovery. Supervised living arrangements, such as halfway houses, group homes, nursing homes, and residing with relatives, should also be considered.

Pharmacotherapy

For alcohol use disorders, the American Psychiatric Association recently released new guidelines for the pharmacologic treatment of alcohol use disorder, recommending the use of naltrexone or acamprosate for adults with moderate to severe use disorders. However, the use of medications to support abstinence in the geriatric population has not been well studied (Table 45.2). Small-scale studies have demonstrated that naltrexone for alcohol abuse is well tolerated and efficacious in older adults. Studies of antidepressants, including the SSRIs, do not support their widespread use as a treatment for alcohol misuse, although they can be effective in treating concurrent depression. Some of the general principles used in treating younger patients should be applied to older patients as well. For example, benzodiazepines are important in treatment of alcohol detoxification, but they have no clinical place in maintaining long-term abstinence because of their potential for abuse and for fostering further alcohol or benzodiazepine abuse. Disulfiram can benefit some well-motivated patients, but cardiac and hepatic disease limits its use by older adults who abuse alcohol.

For opioid use disorders, methadone maintenance and buprenorphine (or buprenorphine with naloxone combination) are approved. Older adults can be started and maintained on methadone or buprenorphine, following the same principles of use as in younger patients. However, given the complexity of treating opioid dependence, systematic training, practice, monitoring, regulation, and evaluation are necessary in a multidisciplinary treatment setting to optimize outcomes. Guidelines for developing treatment programs using buprenorphine are available on the website of the Substance Abuse and Mental Health Services Administration (http://buprenorphine.samhsa.gov [accessed Feb 2019]).

OTHER ADDICTIONS

Nicotine Dependence

In patients with nicotine dependence, multiple attempts to quit with repeated interventions over the life span are typically required. Smoking cessation at any age slows the decline in lung function, and aggressive cessation efforts are appropriate even in very old patients (>85 years). There is significant evidence to demonstrate that brief interventions performed at each office visit will promote smoking cessation (SOE=A). The basic elements of the approach are the "Five A's" from the Agency for Health Care Policy and Research:

- **A**sk patients about nicotine use at every office visit.
- **A**ssess readiness to quit.
- **A**dvise patients to quit.
- **A**ssist patients in the quit attempt with aids such as a local cessation program and pharmacologic agents such as bupropion, nicotine replacement, or varenicline.
- **A**rrange both a quit date and a follow-up visit or contact to discuss the quit attempt.

Establishing abstinence from nicotine follows the same principles as that from other addicting substances. For smoking cessation, it is important to prepare the patient for quitting by discussing management strategies before quitting, setting a quit date, and implementing a monitoring plan for maintaining success. Initially, pharmacologic substitution with either nicotine gum or patch is followed by a gradual decrease in dosage. In several trials, antidepressant medications improved rates of continued abstinence, but only bupropion has been approved for this purpose by the FDA.

Gambling

Gambling in late life is less prevalent than in young adulthood. However, older adults who have engaged in problematic and compulsive gambling behaviors earlier in life often continue this pattern of destructive behavior. Gambling in late life, both recreational and problematic, is associated with a higher prevalence of mental and physical health problems (SOE=B). Many older adults report that gambling is a means of coping with loneliness and boredom, ie, a source of socialization. Regardless, clinicians should be mindful of asking about problematic gambling when taking a history. Such symptoms include preoccupation with gambling, restlessness or irritability when trying to quit, loss of control, need to bet more money with increasing frequency, "chasing" losses, and continuation of gambling despite negative social or occupational consequences. No medications have been helpful in reducing pathologic gambling behaviors. States that allow legalized gaming activities are required to post toll-free telephone numbers to access assistance with problematic gambling. Many 12-step programs are focused on problematic gambling. Older adults who engage in gambling activities should be screened for alcohol, smoking, and other substance use disorders. Dopamine agonists (eg, pramipexole) have been implicated in increasing risk of pathologic gambling. Referrals to community resources and 12-step programs may be useful.

RESOURCES

- American Psychiatric Association Practice Guideline for the Pharmacological Treatment of Patients with Alcohol Use Disorder. *Am J Psychiatry.* 2018;175(1 Suppl):86–90.

- Le Roux C, Tang Y, Drexler K. Alcohol and opioid use disorder in older adults: neglected and treatable illnesses. *Curr Psychiatry Rep.* 2016;18(9):87.

- Maree RD, Marcum ZA, Saghafi E, et al. A systematic review of opioid and benzodiazepine misuse in older adults. *Am J Geriatr Psychiatry.* 2016;24(11):949–963.

CHAPTER 46—INTELLECTUAL AND DEVELOPMENTAL DISABILITIES

KEY POINTS

- Individuals with intellectual disability surviving into adulthood and old age are increasing in numbers.

- Nonadaptive behavioral symptoms, as well as difficulties learning and retaining new skills of coping and adaptation, are significant problems for adults with intellectual disability and, consequently, for their caregivers.

- Medical causes of new behavioral problems should be actively pursued before psychotropic medications are considered.

- Receptive and expressive communication impairments and coexisting cognitive limitations can contribute to diagnostic and treatment difficulties for medical, psychiatric, and behavioral symptoms.

- Physiologic changes related to age as well as to disease states in individuals with intellectual disability can exacerbate or attenuate behaviors.

- Therapeutic interventions for nonadaptive behaviors or psychiatric illnesses that coexist with intellectual disability can include medications and behavioral therapies.

- Individuals with intellectual disability often outlive their family caregivers, and caregiver succession planning is an important part of long-term management.

- The term developmental disability can describe a variety of medical conditions that are not defined by intellectual disability. However, these conditions can contribute to challenging behaviors and impact an individual's quality of life.

Intellectual disability, as used in the *Diagnostic and Statistical Manual of Mental Disorders, Fifth Edition (DSM-5)*, is defined as deficits in intellectual abilities that impact adaptive functioning in three areas: 1) conceptual skills, such as reading, writing, math, reasoning, and knowledge; 2) social and interpersonal skills, such as empathy, communication, and maintaining friendships; and 3) self-management skills, including personal care, recreation, and job skills. Cognitive processes such as attention and memory remain intact. Intellectual disability does not have a specific age requirement; however, the symptoms must occur during the developmental period and result in an inability to meet standards for personal independence. Diagnosis of an intellectual disability is based on the severity of the intellectual impairment and its impact on adaptive function and support needed. While the *DSM-5* no longer considers specific IQ scores in the grading of symptom severity, an IQ of approximately 70 or below based on formal testing is suggestive of an intellectual disability. Intellectual disability replaces the outdated terms of mental retardation and mental handicap.

According to the *DSM-5*, the etiologies of intellectual disability are vast and include prenatal, perinatal, and postnatal causes. Examples of prenatal causes consist of genetic syndromes; brain malformations; and prenatal exposures to alcohol, drugs, or other toxins. Perinatal causes typically involve some type of trauma during labor and delivery, with resulting encephalopathy. Postnatal causes include factors such as hypoxic injury, traumatic brain injury, severe infections, and intoxications or poisoning (eg, lead poisoning).

A demographic issue to remember is that not everyone with a developmental disability has intellectual disability. Developmental disabilities are a group of conditions that cause impairment in physical areas, language, learning, and behavior. Developmental disabilities begin during a child's developmental period, cause impairment in functioning, and remain throughout an individual's life. Some developmental disabilities may not cause an intellectual disability but can contribute to other medical conditions and behavioral/psychiatric symptoms. Examples of developmental disabilities that may not have a corresponding intellectual disability are autism spectrum disorders, cerebral palsy, seizure disorders, and some forms of visual impairment. This chapter primarily focuses on individuals with intellectual disability who may or may not have other comorbid conditions, such as autism spectrum disorders, cerebral palsy, and epilepsy.

PREVALENCE

The number of individuals with intellectual disability surviving into old age is increasing because of improved health care overall, including earlier detection and treatment of some conditions. It is difficult to quantify the prevalence of older adults with intellectual disability because of methodologic considerations and heterogeneity of conditions; however, it is estimated that intellectual disability has a worldwide prevalence of approximately 1%. Prevalence rates vary by age and severity of intellectual disability. Individuals with severe intellectual disability are estimated at 6 per 1,000.

Although the life expectancy of individuals with intellectual disabilities has been increasing, particularly over the past 20 years, it continues to remain lower than that of the general population for individuals with moderate or severe intellectual ability. Life expectancy for individuals with mild intellectual disability is similar to that of the general population. In addition, those who are ≥50 years old are at increased risk of chronic, multiple comorbid medical conditions, such as cardiovascular disease, osteoporosis, and seizure disorders, and are less likely to engage in health promotion activities.

Multimorbidity is associated with advanced age and severe intellectual disability. In a 2014 study in the Netherlands, 80% of individuals with intellectual disability who were ≥50 years old experienced 2 or more chronic medical conditions, and 47% had 4 or more chronic medical conditions.

Published estimates of the number of people of all ages with intellectual disability have ranged from 1% to 2% in the United States, with 2% used in some more recent reports. Regardless of the number, it is expected to double for individuals ≥60 years old by 2030. In general, longevity decreases with severity of intellectual impairment, certain comorbid conditions (eg, seizure disorders, Down syndrome), and the general health of the population and socioeconomic status of the country or culture.

Intellectual Disability and Mental Illness

The literature on older adults with intellectual disability and mental illness (other than dementia) has been relatively sparse over the last few decades. This makes it even more problematic to determine accurate numbers for several reasons: definitions have changed (ie, through various editions of the *DSM* and various versions of the *International Classification of Diseases*), health care has improved, studies have been conducted in different countries or regions, standard methodologies are lacking, and the relative numbers of institutionalized versus community-based individuals have changed.

Several studies conducted over the last decades have had diverse methodologies and research goals; regardless, some common general conclusions have been drawn, one of which is that the prevalence of psychiatric disorders among adults with intellectual disability is much greater than that of age-matched controls (SOE=B). Adults with intellectual disability have similar risk factors (biological, psychological, and social) for mental illnesses as their peers without disability but may have additional risks depending on the cause of their mental disability. Older adults who were raised in institutional settings or who have not benefitted from modern medical care are also at greater risk.

There are many reports of greater than expected rates of certain mental illnesses or behavioral disorders associated with specific physical illnesses or genetic disorders. For example, older adults with autistic spectrum disorders exhibit higher rates of compulsive behaviors requiring psychiatric treatment.

There is general agreement that among all groups of older adults with intellectual disability, behavioral problems are more common, or at least more commonly diagnosed, than are major psychiatric disorders, such as major depressive disorders and psychotic disorders. Some terms, such as "challenging behaviors," are used to describe various behavioral symptoms of autism and fragile X syndrome, whereas other behaviors may have a relationship to brain abnormalities or to impaired acquisition of typically learned social behaviors. Additionally, some behaviors are learned and, in some situations perhaps, chronic nonadaptive behaviors become symptomatic. Learned problematic behaviors are likely to occur from residing in an institutional setting for years.

There is nothing protective against a psychiatric disorder by virtue of having intellectual disability. The cloud of uncertainty is increased perhaps by lack of objective signs and an individual's ability to report their inner feelings. Some of life's stressors that are common for older adults may have a greater impact on those with intellectual disability. Loss of family or friends, income, residence, or vocational status may strain coping strategies as well as overwhelm caregivers or support systems, resulting in an overt decline in level of functioning or a worsening of symptoms.

Major psychiatric disorders are estimated to occur in about 10% of older adults with intellectual disability. Among the most common disorders is dementia. The presence of psychotic disorders increases with age as well. Some disorders are seen at a higher rate than in the general population, such as certain anxiety disorders. Mood disorders also continue into old age, and the management is complex if the individual's ability to participate in certain psychotherapies is limited. Some intellectual disabilities, such as Down syndrome, may increase the likelihood of some disorders such as obsessive-compulsive disorder, which may be three times more prevalent than in the general population. Again, the difference is in the presentation of symptoms in individuals with intellectual disability, and not in the possibility of psychiatric illness.

DIAGNOSTIC AND TREATMENT ISSUES

Clinicians face many diagnostic and treatment challenges when seeing patients with intellectual disability with or without comorbid issues of behavioral symptoms or mental illness. The best treatment requires obtaining a thorough history to arrive at an accurate diagnosis. Unfortunately, all too often the patient's history and his or her subjective reporting are limited or unavailable. The availability of a family member or caregiver who knows the individual well is extremely valuable when making a diagnosis and developing an effective treatment plan.

Barriers to communication can exist for both clinician and patient. Under these circumstances, the clinician should try to be as effective as possible by recognizing the limitations of the patient. For the purposes of this discussion, these limitations are grouped into three broad categories: self-awareness, communication abilities, and diagnostic overshadowing.

For adult and older adult patients with intellectual disability, the clinician needs to estimate the degree to which the patient is aware of his or her problem, condition, or feelings. Barriers to that process of evaluation can come from the organic cause of intellectual disability or from the interviewer by asking questions that are too complex or by using vocabulary beyond the grasp of the patient.

The patient's receptive and expressive abilities need to be considered. These two abilities can be comparable in some individuals with intellectual disability or quite different in others with autism or fragile X syndrome. Differences in these abilities can be characteristic features for some conditions. The goal is to adapt the questions to fit the communication abilities of the patient. Collateral sources of information, including family members or caregivers who can provide adequate descriptions of symptoms and response to treatment, are critically important in both diagnostic and treatment considerations.

An enduring and important concept is that of diagnostic overshadowing, or the idea that the patient's symptoms and behavior are attributed to his or her intellectual disability, leaving comorbid conditions (including both medical and potentially other psychiatric conditions) undiagnosed and untreated. Such overshadowing is a barrier to critical thinking and, therefore, clinicians should guard against it when presented with new or exacerbated symptoms.

PSYCHIATRIC AND BEHAVIORAL DISORDERS

The prevalence of psychiatric disorders among adults with intellectual disability is about 5 times that of age-matched control groups. Depending on the exact population studied and the type of diagnoses included, rates range from 10% to 40%. It is, of course, more complicated, because human aging and pathologic processes are neither simple nor linear. In older adults with intellectual disability, the occurrence and severity of psychiatric disturbances can vary by age and comorbid conditions. For example, in a study of individuals with Down syndrome who subsequently developed Alzheimer disease, these individuals were far more likely to suffer from psychological and behavioral symptoms with more rapid decline in functional status than those who did not develop dementia.

Some symptoms may improve as the individual ages or develops comorbid problems. In adults with Down syndrome, it is not uncommon to have complaints of significant obsessive and compulsive symptoms. This can be the primary focus of concern from young adulthood through the fifth or sixth decade of life or until symptoms of dementia become evident. As the dementia worsens, obsessions and compulsions typically wane, and these symptoms may be less apparent or become of less concern.

It is also true that some behaviors or conditions can worsen with age through various processes. Individuals with intellectual disability experience the same disorders of aging as others but possibly with reduced coping mechanisms. For example, they may be more affected by chronic pain conditions or by vision or hearing loss.

In lower-functioning individuals or in those with expressive communication disorders, a new behavioral concern can be a sentinel sign of a physical disorder. As a general rule, before determining that a new problem behavior should be the focus of a psychotropic medication or intervention, physical causes should be excluded. In particular, new-onset, self-injurious behavior can be an important clue to occult illness. Self-injurious behavior to the ears can be a sign of otitis externa or media. Self-injurious behavior to the eyes can be a clue to vision loss or changes. Delaying attention for a treatable vision condition, eg, presbyopia, can cause permanent loss through self-injury, such as a detached retina or corneal scarring.

Dementias

Individuals with intellectual disability have a higher prevalence of dementias overall than age-matched controls in the general population; this is especially true for dementia associated with Down syndrome

(SOE=A). The challenge is to diagnose the condition correctly given the individual's baseline cognitive impairment and diminished reporting skills. All causes of dementia are possible, but some are more likely than others. The dementia of alcoholism is relatively rare given the lower rates of alcohol dependence (and other substance use disorders) in this particular population. In contrast, chronic traumatic encephalopathy is seen more often than might be expected in this population because of repeated self-injuring blows to the head from coup/contrecoup effects.

It has long been recognized that there is an association and a significantly increased risk of dementia and Down syndrome. Research studies using amyloid imaging agents have added to the postmortem data identifying the association between Alzheimer disease and Down syndrome. Adults with Down syndrome are at increased risk of early onset of Alzheimer disease, with nearly 100% already having developed the characteristic histologic neuropathology of plaques and tangles by age 40. However, it is not typical for individuals with Down syndrome to develop overt dementia at that young an age. Prevalence estimates vary by study, but it is common for at least 50% of adults with Down syndrome who are ≥60 years old to have clinical evidence of dementia (SOE=B).

Most individuals with Down syndrome and dementia die during the sixth decade. In a 2002 survey of nearly 18,000 individuals with Down syndrome compiled by the CDC for the years 1983–1997, the median age of death increased from 25 years of age in 1983 to 60 years of age in 2016. Based on data from death certificates, standardized mortality odds ratios (SMOR) of people with Down syndrome were more likely to show congenital heart defects (SMOR=29.1), dementia (SMOR=21.2), hypothyroidism (SMOR=20.3), or leukemia (SMOR=1.6) than those of people without Down syndrome. Apart from leukemia and testicular cancer, the risk of other malignant diseases was low in those with Down syndrome. Advancing age, presence of dementia, severity of intellectual disability, immobility, and institutional living were found to be significant predictors of mortality among individuals with Down syndrome.

The diagnosis of dementia among individuals with intellectual disability is made according to the same criteria as in the general population. The evaluation includes establishing presence of cognitive and adaptive deterioration; demonstration of deficits on examination (preferably with longitudinal follow-up showing progression of deficits); and exclusion of other possible causes of deterioration, such as medical or environmental factors, or other mental disorders, such as depression or delirium. The Dementia Screening Questionnaire for Individuals with Intellectual Disabilities (DSQIID) is presently the instrument of choice to screen for dementia in those with Down syndrome. The DSQIID requires a knowledgeable informant, has evidence of validity and reliability, and is more sensitive in this population than many commonly used cognitive screening instruments (Mini–Mental Status Exam, Montreal Cognitive Assessment).

Interest has been growing in determining the efficacy of medications such as cholinesterase inhibitors (donepezil, rivastigmine, galantamine) and the glutamate antagonist memantine in individuals with intellectual disability. A randomized trial showed minimal benefit with the use of donepezil[OL] for patients with Down syndrome who developed progressive dementia (SOE=C). Another study did not demonstrate any benefit from use of memantine in a placebo-controlled randomized trial of patients with dementia secondary to Down syndrome (SOE=A). A 2015 Cochrane review assessed the effectiveness of anti-dementia pharmacologic interventions and nutritional supplements for treating cognitive decline in people with Down syndrome found that most studies had methodologic challenges and did not produce consistent results of effectiveness. Risks associated with cholinesterase inhibitors were primarily GI symptoms and syncope.

Adaptive Behavioral Difficulties

Adaptive behaviors are learned social and practical skills concerned with daily functions. Limitations in these skills have a negative impact on people's lives; however, these skill abilities are not fixed in place or easily assigned to a particular level of intellectual disability. In general, the greater the severity of intellectual disability, the more likely the individual will display less adaptive abilities. However, these abilities can be improved over time with behavioral supports.

Adaptive behavior skills can be conceptual, such as in language, reading, and writing; social such as rules, self-esteem, and sense of responsibility; and practical such as job skills, eating, dressing, using the phone, or taking medications. As in any group, aging adults with intellectual disability can lose or become less adept with some adaptive behavior skills, significantly diminishing their quality of life.

Behavioral Disorders

Nonadaptive behaviors are observable phenomena that are counterproductive or disruptive for the individual. Various other terms are sometimes used to describe these acts, including target behaviors (behaviors targeted for extinction) or challenging behaviors. As many as 50%–60% of adults with intellectual disability have nonadaptive behavior (such as withdrawal, self-injury, stereotypy) that is severe or that occurs frequently, and follow-up studies show that these behaviors can persist for years. The proportion decreases with age for various reasons, including worsening overall health status. In Down syndrome, the prevalence of disruptive behaviors tends to be higher, and the incidence of behavioral problems increases with the severity of intellectual disability. Aggression is seen with similar frequency in all age groups and has an extremely variable presentation.

Diagnosis and Treatment

The diagnosis of a mental disorder in an older adult with an intellectual disability is based on the same principles of history and examination that apply in the general population. However, as discussed above, the patient's presentation or reported symptoms can be different, and the perceptions of the clinician and the criteria used pose additional challenges.

Typically, it is difficult for individuals with intellectual disability to report their emotional or physical state because of impaired verbal skills or a limited awareness of their internal state. Often, mental disorders present as behavioral changes; therefore, the reports of family or other caregivers are extremely important. Their interpretation of an individual's behaviors or symptoms, as well as any physical or behavioral responses to therapeutic interventions, can be extremely valuable.

It is important to not over-diagnose and therefore over-treat an individual's presentation. Because insight, judgment, and adaptive or coping skills are limited, individuals may be more likely to "act out," which may be incorrectly perceived as a serious symptom of illness when, in fact, it may be an expression of frustration. Medication may not be called for in a situation in which supportive therapy, a modified caregiver approach, and/or time could lead to resolution. Medication can be used, however, to create a window of opportunity to make behavioral supports or strategies more effective.

Changes in daily routines; staff, residential or vocational settings; or family health should be elicited and considered as precipitating factors for all behavioral changes. The concepts of applied behavioral analysis are important tools to use in determining cause and effect of behavioral symptoms.

Nonadaptive behaviors, such as aggression, can be common in individuals with intellectual disability and can be either a learned or an impulsive response to a stressor. An appropriate treatment or response, as mentioned earlier, might be instructional or behavioral. Preferred behavior programs reward desirable behavior using individualized, positive reinforcement techniques.

Despite appropriate attempts to control physical aggression through behavioral methods, pharmacologic intervention may be necessary for the safety of the patient or those nearby. Very few medications are approved for the most common and challenging behaviors, and prescribing medications off-label is common. Medication management for symptoms of major mental illnesses in older adults with intellectual disability is not much different from that in the general population, keeping in mind the diagnostic caveats already mentioned.

A discussion of the various treatment options for such a diverse patient group is beyond the scope of this chapter. However, medication management is common in certain situations. Autism spectrum disorders probably represent the largest diagnostic group among aging individuals for whom medication management is common and challenging. Self-injurious behaviors are the most common reason medications are considered; these include several potentially life-threatening behaviors that can result in damage to the brain, eyes, and ears, as well as have the potential for systemic infections. Treatment of this diverse population should be symptom driven with clear target behaviors. This may include SSRIs for mood and anxiety, mood stabilizers for impulsivity and aggression, and antipsychotic agents for defined delusions or hallucinations.

There are a few good guidelines when considering pharmacologic interventions. When two medication options exist, a risk-benefit analysis should be done to identify the best choice, ie, the option that poses the least potential for harm with the greatest potential for benefit. Changing only one medication at a time decreases the number of variables. New medications should be started at a low dosage, and results monitored ("start low and go slow"). If possible, dosages of all medications should be tapered and, ultimately, pharmacotherapy discontinued. The use of antipsychotic medications should be avoided if possible, unless the presenting disorder includes distressing psychotic symptoms.

MEDICAL DISORDERS

Adults with intellectual disability have more medical problems than age-matched individuals (approximately 5 medical conditions per person; those with more severe intellectual disability have more problems). Approximately two-thirds of those in a community setting have chronic conditions or major physical disability. It is estimated that 50% of these medical conditions go undetected. Prompt detection and treatment is associated with better survival. Visual or hearing impairments are more common in individuals with intellectual disability; they increase with age and affect approximately 25%.

Life expectancy decreases with increasing severity of intellectual disability and with functional impairments, such as inability to ambulate, lack of feeding skills, and incontinence. The most common causes of death among individuals with intellectual disability are cardiovascular and respiratory disorders, cancer, and dementia (particularly in Down syndrome).

SOCIAL CONDITIONS

At least 80% of adults with intellectual disability live outside institutions and are cared for by aging family members; 20% live in residential programs. It is estimated that about 40% of eligible individuals may not be served by the formal service system. This situation often leads to a crisis when the parent is no longer able to provide adequate care or is unable to manage a behavioral problem. It is estimated that about half of intellectually disabled adults with a behavior problem eventually need a different living arrangement.

Typically, more than half of families have not made plans for the future care of adult relatives with intellectual disability. Individuals in day programs or workshops do not typically have pensions or Social Security benefits to allow retirement. Not surprisingly, the degree of intellectual disability, physical health, and functional skills of the aging individual correlate with the degree of parental stress and burden, although maternal and family characteristics such as education and income are positively correlated with overall life satisfaction and maternal well-being. Aging parents who continued to care for their adult child with intellectual disability at home were noted to be more socially isolated and have worse psychological functioning than parents who lived separately from their adult child. Care, support, and anticipatory guidance should be provided to the individual with disability, family, and caregivers. The Arc (www.thearc.org) is the largest national community-based organization (nearly 700 state and local chapters) that advocates for and serves people with intellectual and development disabilities and their families.

Because individuals with intellectual disability are more likely to outlive their family caregivers, caregiver succession planning becomes important for the clinician to address with the family before a crisis. A variety of alternatives for guardianship of person or property can provide for more flexible decision making, and save some time and money. Options include supported decision making; advance health care directives; appointment of a surrogate decision maker, power of attorney, and representative payee if income is primarily from the government; and establishment of trusts. (Supported decision making is an alternative to the court process of appointing a guardian; it provides the person with an intellectual disability with individual supports and services needed to make informed decisions.) Additionally, some organizations that coordinate care for individuals with intellectual disabilities provide medical and ethical review boards that can give guidance regarding treatment risks and benefits in the absence of a family decision maker. Guardianship of person, property, or both should be considered only if there is no less restrictive alternative and there is a significant need to safeguard the welfare of the individual with intellectual disability. State laws vary; however, information about adult public guardianship frequently can be obtained from state departments of aging and social services. Because guardianship is a legal proceeding in which a petitioner (often a family member or friend) asks the court to find that a person is unable to manage his or her affairs because of a disability, consultation with an attorney is generally necessary.

DEVELOPMENTAL DISABILITIES AND COMORBIDITY

Some developmental disabilities may not cause an intellectual disability but nonetheless can contribute to other morbidities and challenging behaviors, resulting in reduced quality of life. Among these disabilities are cerebral palsy, seizure disorders, and a variety of genetic disorders. Some genetic disorders have significant variability in their impact on cognitive functioning; others once thought to affect only a single generation or gender are now thought to have broader implications, such as fragile X syndrome.

Seizure disorders can negatively impact an individual both directly (if the seizures are uncontrollable) or indirectly (through the medications needed for seizure control). Pre- and postictal states can be times of distinct vulnerability for some individuals. Chronic pain conditions associated with some developmental disabilities, such as the contractures of cerebral palsy, can be a source of medical and psychiatric morbidity. Medical conditions that require frequent hospitalizations or surgeries can carry a great behavioral cost to the individual.

In general, as the degree of cognitive impairment increases, the risk of morbidity due to physical causes increases. For the approximate prevalence and severity of some common conditions found in individuals with developmental disabilities with and without intellectual disability, see Table 46.1.

Table 46.1—Developmental Disabilities and Health Problems

System/Condition	Change with Developmental Disabilities	Management Strategies
Intellectual disability	Two-thirds of patients with developmental disabilities suffer from intellectual disability, many in the mild to moderate range.	Evaluation and referral to specialized services to maximize intellectual and functional potential
Growth retardation	Usually found in individuals with moderate to severe disabilities; it may present as short stature, inability to gain weight, lack of sexual development, or failure to thrive.	Medical evaluation for treatable causes
Sensory and speech impairment	Nearly 90% of individuals have impairments in hearing, vision, and speech. Strabismus is common, as is dysarthric speech.	Regular evaluation of hearing, vision, and speech; correction of deficits
Dental/oral conditions	Poor dentition and oral health are very common.	Oral hygiene and tooth brushing; regular dental visits
Thyroid	Thyroid problems can be a cause or a result of developmental disability.	Regular testing and treatment as indicated
Spinal deformities	Kyphosis, scoliosis, and lordosis are common among individuals with muscle weakness and spasticity.	Monitoring of body habitus; physical therapy
Seizure disorders	Half of individuals may suffer from some type of seizure disorder.	Diagnosis; anticonvulsant medications
Degenerative joint disease	Chronic muscle spasticity and mobility limitations often lead to osteoarthritis and joint disease. Strength and functional status may be prematurely impaired.	Physical therapy, occupational therapy, pain management
Osteopenia and osteoporosis	Lack of weight bearing leads to these chronic conditions in individuals who are unable to ambulate.	Promotion of mobility (physical therapy); adequate calcium and vitamin D supplementation, screening and treatment of osteoporosis
Chronic pain syndromes	Muscle abnormalities and associated spinal deformities often result in chronic pain syndromes. Sensory abnormalities can result in the inability to describe the type, location, and source of the pain.	Regular monitoring of function and behavior to detect possible painful conditions; pain management
Functional decline	Aging individuals with cerebral palsy and other similar conditions often develop fatigue, pain, weakness, and overuse syndromes that result in premature loss of function. This is referred to as *postimpairment syndrome* and often requires a reduction in work hours, increase in assistance or use of adaptive devices, and sometimes nursing-home placement.	Physical therapy, occupational therapy, pain management
Cardiac and pulmonary conditions	Individuals with cerebral palsy and other similar physical disabilities typically require 3–5 times the energy level of unimpaired adults, predisposing to premature conditions of aging, such as hypertension, heart failure, and coronary artery disease.	Monitoring for hypertension, shortness of breath, angina; risk factor management; regular physical activity and healthy diet
GI conditions	Gastroesophageal reflux disease and constipation common; constipation can be chronic and severe.	Monitoring; medications, fiber-rich diet, exercise
Incontinence	Many individuals are incontinent of bowel and bladder from childhood, but others develop these problems with age.	Screening for treatable causes; identifying and addressing functional impairments that can limit toileting; toileting schedules
Depression and mood disorders	Individuals with cerebral palsy are 4 times more likely to develop depression than age-compared other adults. The stress associated with multiple disabilities is a risk factor, as is the premature decline in functional status associated with the disorder.	Regular screening; counseling and/or medications for those diagnosed with mood disorder

RESOURCES

- Axmon A, Björne P, Nylander L, et al. Psychiatric diagnoses in older people with intellectual disability in comparison with the general population: a register study. *Epidemiol Psychiatr Sci.* 2017;23:1–13.

- Livingstone N, Hanratty J, McShane R, et al. Pharmacological interventions for cognitive decline in people with Down syndrome. *Cochrane Database Syst Rev.* 2015 Oct 29;(10):CD011546.

- Schoufour JD, Oppewal A, van der Maarl HJK, et al. Multimorbidity and polypharmacy are independently associated with mortality in older people with intellectual disabilities: a 5-year follow-up from the HA-ID Study. *Am J Intellect Dev Disabil.* 2018;123(1):72–82.

CHAPTER 47—DERMATOLOGY

KEY POINTS

- Photoaging increases the fragility of the skin and decreases the elasticity/tensile strength of the skin.

- Older adults are at risk of xerosis and neurodermatitis, or lichen simplex chronicus.

- Venous insufficiency can cause stasis dermatitis and chronic leg ulcers. Treatment should begin by controlling venous hypertension with compression therapy.

- Ultraviolet (UV) light exposure and age are associated with increased incidence of skin cancers, including squamous cell carcinomas, basal cell carcinomas, and melanomas.

AGING AND PHOTOAGING

The incidence and prevalence of skin disease increase with aging and sun exposure. Dermatologic care of older adults requires an awareness of cutaneous changes of aging and the effects of cumulative UV radiation exposure, as well as knowledge of the common tumors, inflammatory diseases, and infections seen in this population. The skin of older individuals is characterized by several changes, including increased fragility, graying of hairs, and increased wrinkles, particularly at rest. Each of the skin layers changes with aging. In normal young skin, the epidermis interdigitates with the dermis. With time, the epidermis becomes flattened with reduced keratinocyte turnover and melanocyte numbers, contributing in part to the decreased rate of wound healing. In the dermis, the fibroblasts are elongated and collapsed. Types I and III collagen and microfibrils of elastin all decrease, leading to the appearance of laxity and atrophy. Changes in hair include graying, which is caused by changes in follicular melanocytes, and a decrease in scalp hair density secondary to a shortened length of anagen (the growth phase of the hair cycle) and an increased proportion of hairs in telogen (the resting phase). In aging skin, the number of immune antigen-presenting cells, such as Langerhans cells, decrease, which may have consequences for cutaneous immune surveillance.

Aging of skin is a result of both intrinsic and extrinsic factors. The largest contributor is the cumulative exposure to UV light. This leads to the clinical appearance of lentigines, guttate hypomelanosis, poikiloderma (areas of hyperpigmentation, hypopigmentation, and telangiectasia), laxity, yellow hue, and leathery appearance. *Photoaging* refers to the effects of UV exposure on skin. UV light appears to activate signaling pathways that lead to increased matrix metalloproteinase activity and decreased collagen production. In a vicious cycle, the fibroblasts become elongated and collapsed and respond by decreasing collagen production. UV light also causes DNA injury in part via oxidative damage, which likely also contributes to the aging phenotype. Cutaneous malignancies are also more common in photodamaged skin because of photocarcinogenesis and UV light–mediated immunosuppression.

Prevention of photodamage involves using broad-spectrum sunscreens (ie, sunscreens that protect against both UVA and UVB radiation), as well as avoiding direct sunlight and wearing protective clothing, including hats and sunglasses. Although various topical agents claim to decrease photodamage, only topical tretinoin has been shown to increase the thickness of the superficial skin layers, reduce pigmentary changes and roughness, and increase collagen synthesis (SOE=A). Topical and even oral antioxidants (particularly vitamins E and C) have been shown to have some photoprotective and chemoprotective capabilities. In addition, over 70 botanicals, including soy and green tea, are currently found in many cosmaceuticals, but pharmacokinetic, safety, and double-blinded efficacy studies are lacking.

Soft-tissue augmentation and facial volume restoration via injectable fillers composed of hyaluronic acid, calcium hydroxylapatite microspheres, or poly-l-lactic acid, can also reverse the degradation of extracellular matrix, in part by reversing the collapse of fibroblasts. One of the most popular cosmetic procedures is injection of a neurotoxin, botulinum toxin, that relaxes dynamic muscles and thereby reduces furrows and wrinkle lines. Complications of these treatments need to be discussed with patients and include the following: 1) bruising, swelling, injection site reactions, rarely granulomas, and reactivation of herpes with lip injections from filler injections, and 2) headaches or blepharoptosis, or both, with neurotoxins.

INFLAMMATORY AND AUTOIMMUNE SKIN CONDITIONS

Seborrheic Dermatitis

Seborrheic dermatitis (Figure 47.1) is a chronic inflammatory dermatosis characterized by symmetric pink patches with overlying greasy bran-like scaling distributed in the areas where sebaceous glands are found, namely on the scalp, the face, and sometimes the presternal chest and intertriginous areas. On the face,

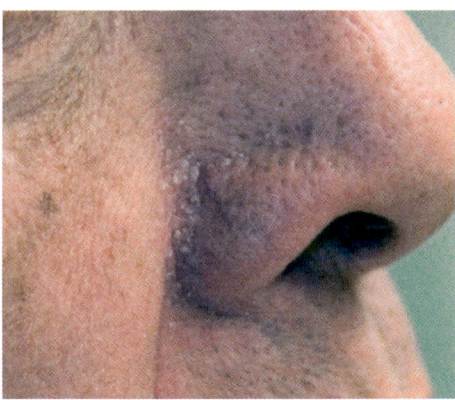

Figure 47.1—Seborrheic dermatitis. Erythema with greasy scaling noted along nasolabial folds.

the lesions are found on the forehead, medial portions of the eyebrows, upper eyelids, nasolabial folds and lateral aspects of the nose, retroauricular areas, and occasionally the occiput and neck. At times, the lesions may be arcuate or petaloid, resembling flower petals. Occasionally, patients have features of both psoriasis and seborrheic dermatitis, particularly in the hairline and eyebrows, and this condition is therefore known as sebopsoriasis.

The pathogenesis of seborrheic dermatitis is unclear but may be related to the yeast colonies that normally colonize the skin, ie, *Malassezia furfur*. Seborrheic dermatitis is more prevalent in patients with Parkinson disease. Extensive and severe eruptions of seborrheic dermatitis often warrant an examination of HIV status. Rebound flares of seborrheic dermatitis can follow tapering of corticosteroid medications.

Although seborrheic dermatitis can be treated, it cannot be cured or eliminated. Treatment can be in the form of creams (face and body) or shampoos (scalp). Medications that target yeast, including selenium sulfide, ketoconazole, and various tar shampoos, are effective. In an acute flare, patients can be treated with mild topical corticosteroids such as hydrocortisone 1%; if treatment is unsuccessful, a trial of topical calcineurin inhibitors (eg cyclosporine, tacrolimus) can be tried. Aggressive topical or systemic therapy should be avoided because of risk of rebound.

Rosacea

Rosacea is a common condition in fair-skinned people. There are 4 subtypes with overlapping prevalence: erythematotelangiectatic rosacea has been reported in 96% of rosacea patients, papulopustular rosacea in 51%, phymatous rosacea in <5%, and ocular rosacea in 14%. In the erythematotelangiectatic subtype, there is persistent erythema of the central convex areas of the face (ie, nose, forehead, cheeks, and chin [Figure 47.2]), with telangiectasias and flushing. In

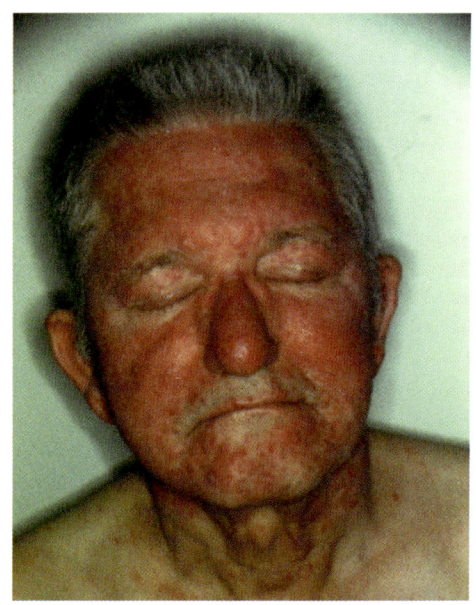

Figure 47.2—Rosacea. Diffuse erythema and erythematous papules and papulopustules are seen on the cheeks, forehead, and chin. The nose shows thickening of the skin and changes consistent with an early rhinophyma.

the papulopustular subtype, there are follicular and nonfollicular papules and pustules in addition to the persistent erythema. In the phymatous subtype, there is sebaceous hyperplasia and thickening of the skin, in part due to recurrent flushing and edema; in some cases, this leads to rhinophyma ("bulbous" or "ruddy" nose). In ocular rosacea, irritation and burning of the eye can present as conjunctival injection, blepharitis, episcleritis, chalazion, or hordeolum. Other variants of rosacea include granulomatous rosacea, periorificial dermatitis, and pyoderma faciale.

Incidence of rosacea peaks in the third and fourth decades, but the disease is seen in young and older adults as well. The cause of acne rosacea is likely multifactorial, including contributions from vasodilatation, *Demodex* mites, and propionobacterium. In addition, thermal stimuli, sunlight exposure, and a number of medications can contribute to rosacea, including oral niacin and topical steroids. Often, seborrheic dermatitis and rosacea are seen together.

The treatment of rosacea depends on the subtype and severity. Topical antibiotics such as benzoyl peroxide, erythromycin[OL], and metronidazole can be used to treat papulopustular rosacea. Oral antibiotics such as tetracyclines (eg, doxycycline, minocycline) and macrolides are used to treat moderate to severe cases. Alternative therapies include topical azelaic acid, topical tretinoin, and oral isotretinoin[OL] for severe cases. For the persistent erythema, nasal decongestants such as oxymetazoline hydrochloride have shown some

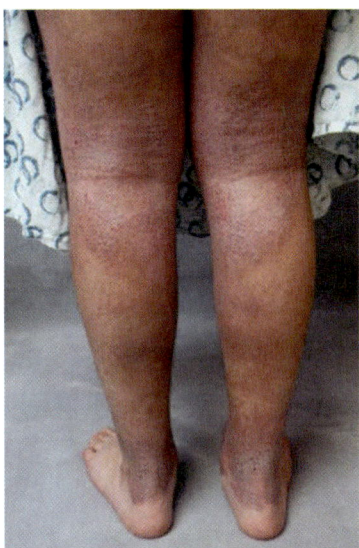

Figure 47.3A—Atopic dermatitis with classic eczematous dermatitis behind the knees.

promise in small case series. For treatment of the telangiectasias, lasers, such as the potassium-titanyl-phosphate laser, intense pulsed light, and the pulsed dye laser, can be used. Rhinophyma can be treated with surgical reduction or electrosurgery.

Xerosis

Dryness of the skin, often a concern for older adults, is due to altered barrier function in the aging epidermis and a reduced ability to retain water. It is exacerbated by environmental factors such as decreased humidity; prolonged exposure to water, which can dilute out natural moisturizing factors; and use of harsh soaps, which can further damage the stratum corneum. During winter, when the heat is turned on, indoor humidity falls and dry skin conditions become more prevalent. Similarly, although summertime often is associated with an increase in ambient humidity outdoors, in many locations, indoor air conditioning can result in a drop in the humidity in home and office environments, causing dryness of the skin. Xerosis is often more pronounced on the legs. Depending on the severity of the dryness, xerosis can present as rough, itchy skin or as scales that give the skin a dry, cracked riverbed appearance known as *eczema craquelé*. Dry skin can precipitate a flare of atopic dermatitis. Classic red, scaling pruritic lesions can be seen in the antecubital or popliteal fossae (Figure 47.3A) or present as coin-shaped eczematous lesions referred to as nummular eczema (Figure 47.3B).

Treatment usually begins with avoiding the exacerbating factors mentioned above. Patients should be advised to take tepid showers and avoid using washcloths, sponges, or brushes to scrub the skin. Moisturizing agents, especially those containing lactic

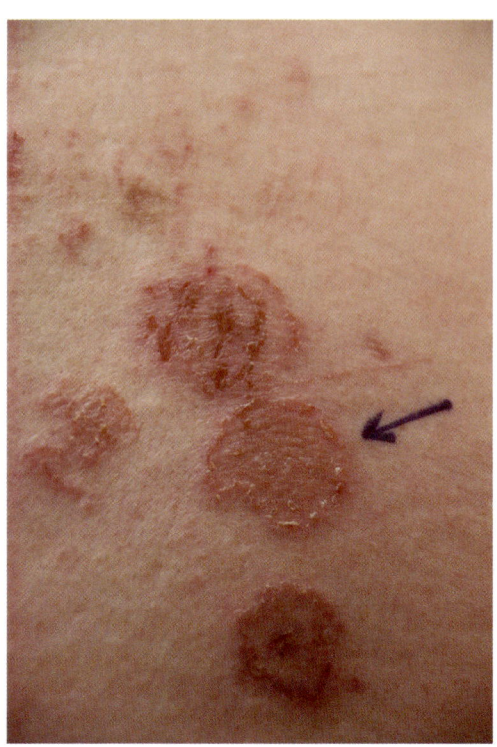

Figure 47.3B—Nummular or coin-shaped eczematous lesions.

acid or α-hydroxy acids, can reduce roughness and scaliness. Moisturizing agents are often most helpful when applied immediately after a bath or shower. Home humidifiers may also be beneficial during seasons when home heating is being used. When irritation or inflammation is prominent, episodic use of mild topical corticosteroids for a short time provides relief.

Neurodermatitis

Neurodermatitis is a nonspecific term used to refer to chronic, pruritic conditions of unclear cause. Another commonly used term is *lichen simplex chronicus* (Figure 47.4). It is most common in adults >60 years old. The lesions show signs of chronic scratching, hyperpigmentation, and lichenification (increased skin markings), along with redness and scaling. Scratching these lesions is often satisfying and leads to a vicious cycle of skin changes and more pruritus. Treatment consists of potent topical corticosteroids (often under occlusion), emollients, and behavior modification. Other causes of pruritus such as irritant or allergic contact dermatitis, drug allergy, or xerosis must be excluded.

Intertrigo

Intertrigo (Figure 47.5) is any infectious or noninfectious inflammatory condition of 2 closely opposed skin surfaces (intertriginous area). It is more common in older adults because of the increased skin folds secondary to

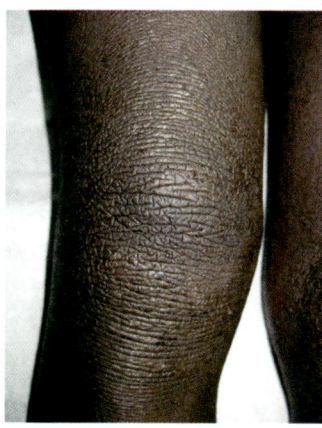

Figure 47.4—Lichen simplex chronicus. Chronic rubbing has caused the skin of this patient to become thickened and lichenified with an exaggeration of skin markings

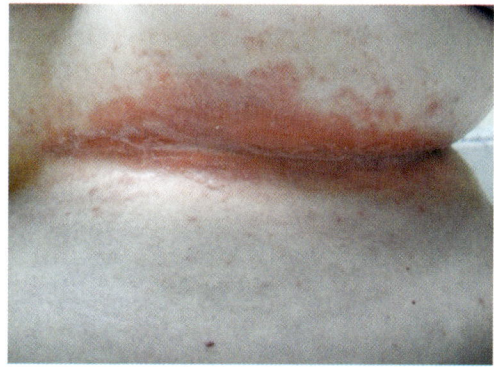

Figure 47.5—Intertrigo. Macerated skin under the breasts of an overweight woman.

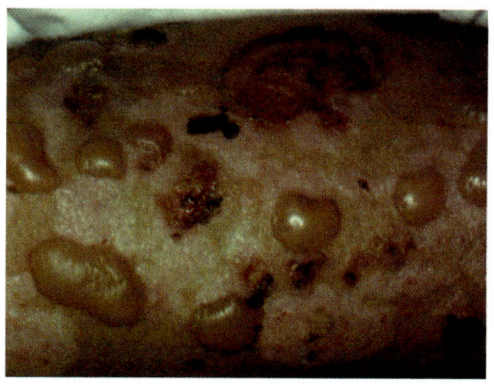

Figure 47.6—Bullous pemphigoid. Tense, fluid-filled, and hemorrhagic bullae on an erythematous base are seen on the trunk and extremities. Some of the bullae have ruptured and left a scab with crusting.

decreased dermal elasticity. Additional contributory factors include decreased mobility, moisture, friction, and poor hygiene. Factors that increase moisture (eg, obesity) or decrease immunity (eg, diabetes or systemic corticosteroids) predispose patients to develop intertrigo. Commonly involved areas, such as the inframammary area, abdominal folds, groin, and axillae, appear erythematous, macerated, moist, and mildly malodorous. Differential diagnosis includes seborrheic dermatitis and inverse psoriasis. Intertrigo often is associated with superficial infection with bacteria or *Candida*. Successful treatment involves decreasing moisture with topical drying agents, such as corn starch and antifungal powder (eg, miconazole or nystatin powder). Physical means of keeping the area dry include bed sheets/handkerchiefs to separate skin folds and frequent airing, or careful use of a hairdryer. If candidal intertrigo is suspected, treatment involves the topical polyene and azole antifungals, such as topical nystatin or ketoconazole. Occasionally, a very mild topical corticosteroid such as 1%–2% hydrocortisone is needed for a short period to reduce inflammation and irritation.

Bullous Pemphigoid

Bullous pemphigoid (Figure 47.6) is the most common autoimmune subepidermal blistering disease. It is a disease of older adults, with age of onset commonly >60 years and a median age at presentation of 80 years. The incidence of bullous pemphigoid is 4.3 per 100 000 person-years and increases over time, with the average yearly increase reported to be 17%. Clinically, the disease has diverse manifestations. Typically, bullous pemphigoid presents as an extremely pruritic eruption with widespread blister formation. The blisters are typically tense, often filled with clear fluid. The distribution is symmetrical and widespread, although the flexural areas and lower trunk may be favored. Mucous membranes are involved in up to one-third of patients. The blisters often resolve without scarring. Early or atypical lesions may be nonbullous with primarily urticarial lesions.

Bullous pemphigoid is a prototypical organ-specific autoimmune disease with a humoral and cellular immune response targeted against 2 antigens in the hemidesmosome. With the help of autoreactive T cells, pathogenic B cells produce antibodies that target these hemidesmosomal antigens. The antibodies trigger an inflammatory cascade of complement activation, the recruitment of neutrophils and eosinophils, and the elaboration of proteases. Bullous pemphigoid has been associated with medications, including diuretics, analgesics, antibiotics, and ACE inhibitors. Diagnosis is made by clinicopathologic correlation.

Although the disease may last for months to years, it is often self-limited. Treatment should be commensurate to the severity of disease. Limited, localized disease can be treated with potent topical corticosteroids, topical calcineurin inhibitors, and nicotinamide with tetracycline. Systemic corticosteroids are the mainstay of more extensive treatment. Steroid-sparing agents (eg, azathioprine[OL] and cyclophosphamide[OL]) are often used to avoid the adverse events of corticosteroids.

Pruritus

Pruritus, a very common skin complaint, is associated with many cutaneous and systemic conditions. Severe pruritus can compromise quality of life. Pruritus can be idiopathic, related to a primary skin disease, or secondary to a systemic disease. In older adults, xerosis is the most common cause of chronic pruritus. However, evaluation must exclude other underlying pruritic dermatologic conditions, including infestations such as scabies; genetic or childhood diseases such as atopic dermatitis; and autoimmune blistering diseases, including bullous pemphigoid. Pruritus can be caused by medications (eg, dermal hypersensitivity reactions), related to chemical exposures (eg, irritant dermatitis or allergic contact dermatitis), or be a consequence of autosensitization to stasis dermatitis. Pruritus can be secondary to systemic diseases such as renal disease, cholestasis or chronic liver disease, thyroid disease, anemia, and occult malignancies. Finally, generalized pruritus can also be associated with generalized anxiety disorder, depression, and even psychosis, including delusions of parasitosis.

A thorough evaluation of pruritus in an older adult therefore includes a complete history and physical examination to exclude underlying and treatable skin disease. Distribution of the pruritus may help to determine the underlying cause. Involvement of flexural areas suggests atopic dermatitis or bullous pemphigoid, whereas primary involvement of the lower legs suggests an autosensitization to stasis dermatitis. Laboratory evaluation to exclude secondary causes includes a CBC and function tests of the liver, kidneys, and thyroid. It is also important to perform age-appropriate cancer screening, as warranted by the findings of above.

Treatment requires addressing the cause of the pruritus, if known, and relieving symptoms. If there is a primary dermatologic condition or a systemic disease, treatment should be tailored to the underlying disease. For example, prednisone may be warranted for bullous pemphigoid, and topical corticosteroids for atopic dermatitis. In addition, symptomatic relief often requires multiple modalities. Nonpharmacologic measures include open-wet dressings: in brief, a thin, white material such as a bed sheet can be moistened with lukewarm tap water and placed over the skin for 10–15 min; as the water evaporates, it can relieve pruritus. It is important to treat xerosis with frequent applications of emollients. Topical corticosteroids, such as 0.1% triamcinolone ointment, can also relieve xerosis and any underlying inflammation. Topical pramoxine, menthol in calamine preparations, and capsaicin[OL] cream can change the neurologic sensation of pruritus. These topical agents can also be used frequently with minimal adverse events in the short-term. Systemic therapy can include nonsedating oral antihistamines. Most trials investigating their use have used desloratadine in treatment of chronic idiopathic urticaria. It has significantly improved patient-reported pruritus, sleep disruption, and interference with daily activities with a low incidence of adverse events (SOE=A). Cetirizine, fexofenadine, and levocetirizine are also used for this purpose. In severe, refractory cases, including cases secondary to systemic disease, patients can be referred to a dermatologist for UVB phototherapy or oral thalidomide.

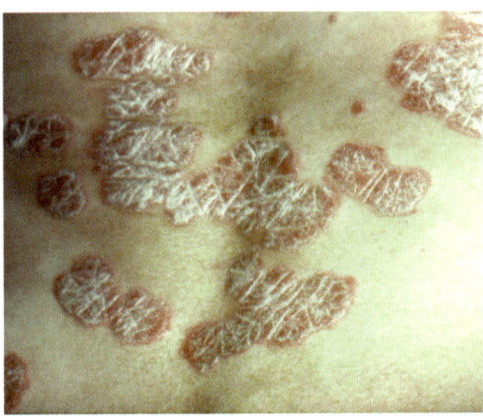

Figure 47.7—Psoriasis. Characteristic well-demarcated beefy red plaques with overlying silvery white scales are evident on the back of this patient.

Psoriasis

Psoriasis (Figure 47.7) is a chronic inflammatory skin disease characterized by well-demarcated plaques with overlying silvery scale. Chronic plaque psoriasis is the most common variant, and it characteristically involves the scalp, the gluteal cleft, and extensor surfaces. Hands and feet can be involved, as well as the nails, which may portend psoriatic arthritis. The other psoriatic subtypes are as follows:

- Inverse pattern, in which lesions develop in skin folds, such as the neck, axillae, and genital area
- Guttate, in which small papules (approximately 1 cm or less) appear over the upper trunk and proximal extremities, usually after an infection
- Pustular, which is acute with generalized eruption of sterile pustules (2–3 mm) and fever
- Palmoplantar pustulosis, in which sterile pustules are confined to the palms and soles
- Erythrodermic psoriasis, in which the patient has generalized erythema

Psoriasis is common, affecting 2% of the population. The incidence is bimodal, first in the mid-20s and then at about 50–60 years of age. The cause is likely multifactorial. There is a strong genetic predisposition, with a multigene mode of inheritance, as well as a role for environmental factors. Triggers that initiate or exacerbate disease include physical trauma (known as Koebner phenomenon), infections (including streptococcal upper respiratory infections), stress, and medications (eg, oral corticosteroids, lithium, β-blockers, ACE inhibitors, NSAIDs). In psoriasis, the risk factors ultimately lead to activation and recruitment of autoreactive Th1 and Th17 T cells to the skin. Cytokines such as tumor necrosis factor-alpha (TNF-α) and IL-23 likely lead to activation of T cells, and IL-22 ultimately leads to increased keratinocyte proliferation.

Psoriatic arthritis, which is characterized by pain, swelling, and stiffness of affected joints, is also seen in 5%–35% of patients. Classically, psoriatic arthritis is an asymmetrical oligoarthritis of the small joints of the hands. Alternative patterns of presentation include inflammation restricted to the distal interphalangeal joints, symmetrical polyarthritis of the hands, and arthritis mutilans with telescoping of the involved digit. Also, some patients suffer from back pain in the form of spondylitis or sacroiliitis.

Because of the wide clinical spectrum of disease, treatment should be tailored to the individual, with special attention paid to the risks and benefits for the older patient. Therapies directed at the skin are appropriate for patients with limited disease. These include topical treatments such as topical corticosteroids, vitamin D derivatives (eg, calcipotriene), topical retinoids (eg, tazarotene), salicylic acid, and tar compounds. Long-term use of topical steroids is limited by the risk of cutaneous atrophy. If topical therapy is unsuccessful or disease is extensive, phototherapy can be of benefit. UV light therapy, including narrow-band UVB therapy and psoralen with UVA light (PUVA), can be used alone or in conjunction with topical therapies. Patients receiving UV light therapy must be able to stand for the duration of the treatment. Risks include increased incidence of skin cancer.

For those with widespread and recalcitrant disease, systemic agents are available. Oral immunosuppressive agents, including cyclosporine and methotrexate, are effective but require careful monitoring for adverse events. Toxicities of cyclosporine include hypertension and renal dysfunction. Toxicities of methotrexate include bone marrow suppression, liver fibrosis, and interstitial lung pneumonitis. Oral retinoids such as acitretin can be used in conjunction with other therapies such as UV light.

Biologics can be effective in patients in whom traditional systemic therapies are either ineffective or contraindicated. Biologics include agents that block the cytokine TNF and T-cell surface molecules, including adhesion molecules and co-stimulatory molecules. The important adverse effects that have been most extensively related to TNF inhibitors include lymphoma, infections (especially tuberculosis reactivation and opportunistic fungal infections), congestive heart failure, demyelinating disease, a lupus-like syndrome, induction of auto-antibodies, and injection site reactions. In general, anti-TNF agents are contraindicated in those with a history of hepatitis C, multiple sclerosis, heart failure, and lymphoma.

Initiation of psoriasis involves both epithelial cells and immune cells; as a result of this interaction, psoriatic skin lesions and/or joint issues may develop, as well as an underlying systemic inflammatory disease with potential cardiovascular implications and risks. Therefore patients with psoriasis should be counseled about diet, exercise, and weight control.

Stasis Dermatitis

Stasis dermatitis can be an early sign of chronic venous insufficiency of the legs. Chronic venous hypertension, caused mostly by incompetency of the venous valves, is the initial trigger for stasis dermatitis. Venous hypertension slows down the flow of blood in the microvasculature, damages the permeability barrier of the small vessels, and allows for the passage of fluid and plasma proteins into the tissue, leading to edema and extravasation of erythrocytes. These processes lead to decreased oxygen diffusion and metabolic exchange and to activation and attraction of inflammatory cells and mediators to the site. Stasis dermatitis typically develops in the medial supramalleolar areas. It is often associated with intense pruritus. Initially, pitting edema to the ankle is noted, which is often worse later in the day. Over time, these events lead to progressive induration and adherence of the skin and subcutaneous tissues. Venous ulcers can develop spontaneously or secondary to trauma, arising most often in the supramalleolar areas.

The goal of therapy is to control the venous hypertension by regularly using compression bandages or stockings, elevating the legs at rest, and exercising the calf muscles to improve venous return. Topical treatment includes the judicious use of corticosteroids and emollients. Sensitization to ingredients in topical medications and emollients, including topical antibiotics, is common and frequently overlooked. Patch testing to exclude contact sensitization to these agents should be considered before use.

INFECTIONS AND INFESTATIONS

Herpes Zoster

Herpes zoster represents reactivation of the varicella zoster virus (VZV), the virus that is responsible for varicella, ie, chickenpox. Classically, it is a disease of older adults, with more than two-thirds of cases in patients >50 years old. The lifetime risk of reactivation of VZV is 20% in healthy adults and 50% in immunocompromised individuals. During primary infection, ie, varicella, VZV establishes a latent infection in sensory ganglia. Partly because of the decline in the cellular immune response associated with age or immunosuppressive conditions, the virus is reactivated and leads to painful ganglionitis. The infection spreads down the sensory nerve and is released around the sensory nerve endings in the skin, producing the characteristic lesions.

Usually, zoster begins with a prodrome of pain. In some people, the prodrome includes sensations of pruritus, tingling, tenderness, or hyperesthesia. The prodrome is followed by a painful eruption of grouped vesicles on an erythematous base, usually in a sensory distribution. In the localized form of zoster, the vesicles rarely cross midline (Figure 47.8). Rarely, prodromal pain is not followed by a cutaneous eruption, a condition called zoster sine herpete.

Herpes zoster infection has been associated with a number of complications, including post-herpetic neuralgia (PHN), scarring ophthalmic zoster, and Ramsay Hunt syndrome. The incidence and severity of PHN increase with increasing age and an immunocompromised state. In 7% of cases of herpes zoster, the ophthalmic branch of the trigeminal nerve is involved. Involvement of the nasociliary branch, which presents as vesicles in the pharynx and on the tip of the nose (known as Hutchinson sign), requires careful ophthalmic examination to monitor for complications, such as neurotrophic keratitis and ulceration, scleritis, uveitis, and ultimately blindness. In the Ramsay Hunt syndrome, the geniculate ganglion is involved. In addition to producing vesicles on the external ear or tympanic membrane, Ramsay Hunt is associated with facial palsy with or without tinnitus, vertigo, and deafness. Zoster is considered disseminated if it involves two noncontiguous dermatomes. In disseminated zoster, meningoencephalitis, hepatitis, and pneumonitis are also complications.

Although the symptoms of herpes zoster can be confused with a variety of conditions causing localized pain (ie, pleurisy, myocardial infarction, renal colic, cholecystitis, and acute glaucoma), the combination of the history and the characteristic physical examination (ie, the dermatomal distribution) facilitate the diagnosis. A Tzanck smear from the base of the vesicle can be performed to confirm the diagnosis. Detection of multinucleated giant cells suggests a herpes simplex or herpes zoster infection. Direct fluorescence antibody testing can be performed to confirm the presence of VZV. Polymerase chain reaction and viral cultures are the most sensitive means to confirm the diagnosis.

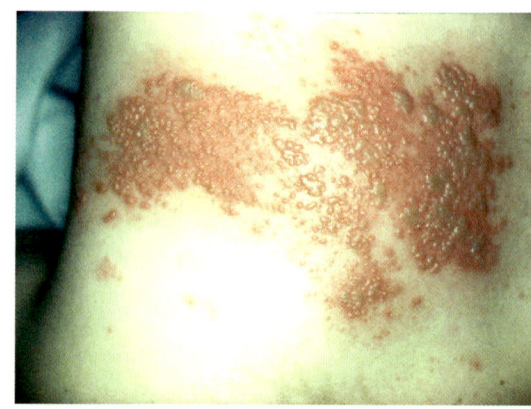

Figure 47.8—Herpes zoster. This patient has clusters of vesicles and pustules on an erythematous base involving a thoracic dermatome.

Early treatment with antiviral therapies, optimally within 72 hours of onset of rash, decreases disease duration and pain (SOE=A). FDA-approved therapies include acyclovir, famcyclovir, and valacyclovir; their use should be monitored in patients who have reduced renal function. A meta-analysis showed no benefit of adding oral corticosteroids to antiviral therapy for improving quality of life or reducing incidence of PHN. Intravenous antiviral therapy is reserved for immunocompromised individuals and for those who demonstrate signs of disseminated disease or complications. Most cases of acute herpes zoster are self-limited, but the probability of developing PHN increases with advanced age. PHN occurs in approximately 20% of zoster patients ≥70 years old and is difficult to treat. Acute herpetic neuralgia refers to pain preceding or accompanying the eruption of rash that persists up to 30 days from its onset. Subacute herpetic neuralgia refers to pain that persists beyond healing of the rash but that resolves within 4 months of onset. PHN refers to pain persisting beyond 4 months from the initial onset of the rash. Prevention of PHN can be attempted by vaccinating to decrease the incidence of acute zoster and PHN, by treating the acute zoster infection itself, or by treating acute zoster very early with preventive pain medications such as tricyclic antidepressants or anticonvulsants. Anticholinergic adverse events of tricyclics are common and may limit their use in older adults. In an animal study, early treatment with gabapentin reduced the incidence of delayed post-herpetic pain, but there are no clinical data in people for evaluating gabapentin in prevention of PHN.

Treatment of PHN can be challenging. Systematic reviews of randomized controlled trials of treatments of PHN with evaluation periods of >24-hour duration found no single best treatment. Tricyclic antidepressants[OL], opioids, topical capsaicin, gabapentin, topical lidocaine, pregabalin, and tramadol can alleviate the pain of PHN, but the long-term benefits of most therapies are not known and adverse events are common. Intrathecal methylprednisolone may relieve pain in patients refractory to the oral and topical measures discussed above.

Candidiasis

Candidiasis has a wide spectrum of presentation. Cutaneous candidiasis is often seen in intertriginous areas; it can be superimposed on intertrigo caused by psoriasis or seborrheic dermatitis. *Candida* pustules can also develop on the backs of bedridden patients and on other areas prone to moisture and occlusion. In these areas, candidiasis is characterized by red patches, sometimes with erosions. Often, there are peripheral satellite pustules. Candidiasis can also affect the scrotum, the nails, the genital area, and corners of the lips, causing perleche. Oral thrush is an example of mucocutaneous candidiasis, seen most commonly in patients on corticosteroid inhalers, antibiotics, or immunosuppressive medications; or with concomitant systemic illnesses, such as diabetes mellitus. A potassium hydroxide preparation of skin scrapings of the involved site can confirm the diagnosis. The presence of spores and pseudohyphae is consistent with candidiasis.

Topical medications are generally effective and should be applied beyond the margins of the lesion. Most commonly used are topical polyenes such as nystatin, and topical azoles such as miconazole, clotrimazole, ketoconazole, and econazole. Other effective topical agents are terbinafine, butenafine, and ciclopirox. Topical therapies can be used twice a day until symptoms resolve and subsequently twice a week for prophylaxis as necessary. Pruritus, pain, and burning generally resolve with use of topical antifungal medications, although a low-dose topical corticosteroid can sometimes be used in conjunction. In patients with widespread candidiasis, oral therapy with an azole has a response rate of 80%–100%. Effective eradication of candidiasis generally also requires treating the underlying intertrigo by keeping the moist areas dry with drying agents and physical barriers to keep the skin folds separated (eg, bed sheets).

Scabies

Human scabies is a pruritic eruption caused by the mite *Sarcoptes scabiei* var *hominis*. The entire 30-day life cycle is confined to the human epidermis. After fertilization, adult female mites lay eggs, which mature over 10 days. For first-time infestations, sensitization can take 2–6 weeks; therefore, symptoms may not be seen until a month after infestation, making it difficult to make a diagnosis before disease spread. Scabies is spread primarily by person-to-person contact and is common in institutionalized older adults.

Scabies is characterized by intense pruritus, worse at night, and a symmetrically distributed cutaneous eruption. The eruption is most often characterized by small erythematous papules, sometimes accompanied by linear excoriations. The pathognomonic sign is a burrow characterized by a wavy, threadlike lesion about 1–10 mm long. The lesions are distributed over the interdigital webs, the flexural wrists, the umbilicus, the wrists, the ankles, and the feet. In men, lesions are also seen on the scrotum and penis. In women, the areolae, nipples, and genital areas are commonly affected. Immunocompromised patients can get crusted scabies, characterized by thousands of mites per gram of epidermis. Other manifestations include vesicles and indurated nodules. The lesions may be nonspecific, and the diagnosis should be considered in anyone with intense pruritus.

Diagnosis can be confirmed by microscopic examination of skin scrapings in mineral oil. This allows direct visualization of the adult mites, nymphs, eggs, or fecal matter (scybala). Occasionally, diagnosis can also be made by skin biopsy. Treatment includes topical creams such as 5% permethrin cream applied head to toe and left on for 8–14 hours, or systemic medications such as ivermectin (200 mcg/kg). Therapies are generally not effective against the eggs; therefore, a second treatment is needed 1–2 weeks later, after the eggs mature. Clothes, linens, and towels should be either washed in hot water and dried in high heat or left in a closed bag for 10 days to prevent reinfestation by fomites. In the absence of human contact, the mite cannot survive. Caregivers should also be treated because they are usually exposed, even though they may not have symptoms.

Louse Infestations

Lice can infest the body (pediculosis corporis), scalp (pediculosis capitis), or pubic hair (pediculosis pubis). With pediculosis corporis or capitis, lice are spread from person to person through physical contact or fomites. Pediculosis pubis is usually spread by sexual contact. In all cases, patients complain of pruritus of the involved areas, and there can be secondary infection. In pediculosis corporis, the lice feed on the body but live on clothing, where they lay eggs, often near the seams. In pediculosis capitis, the lice lay eggs on the proximal part of the hair shaft. The eggs (or nits) are visible as white specks cemented to the hair at an oblique angle. Patients with pediculosis pubis also have nits on the pubic hair and commonly have more organisms.

Treatment involves eradicating the lice and larvae, treating close contacts, and treating the secondary infection. Pyrethrin or its derivatives (permethrin) are ovicidal and can be used as a single 10-minute topical treatment. People who come into contact with the patient, including caregivers and those who share bedding, should be evaluated for lice and treated. Combs, brushes, hats, clothing, bedding, and towels must be washed with hot water.

Bed Bugs

Bed bugs were mostly eradicated in the developed world by the early 1940s. However, since the mid 1950s, their prevalence notably increased likely because of pesticide resistance, governmental bans on effective pesticides, and international travel.

Bed bugs are insects of the cimicid family that feed exclusively on blood. The insects tend to reside inside beds and bedding and are mainly active at night feeding on the unaware sleeping bed occupant(s). Although bed bugs are not known to be disease vectors, multiple bites (red papules with or without vesicles) result in a linear pruritic eruption.

Once bed bugs finish feeding, they return to the mattress or couch. They have been identified in various articles, including (but not limited to) luggage, cars, furniture, and clothes, as well as inside electrical sockets and near computers.

The bites are treated symptomatically with topical steroids and topical or oral anti-itch medications. Treatment of the infestation is more challenging, because there is presently no effective pesticide that is safe for people. Mechanical approaches, such as vacuuming up the insects and heat-treating or wrapping mattresses, have been reported to be effective. Bed bugs cannot usually be starved because they can survive without eating for 100–300 days. Professional pest control services should be called to eradicate bed bugs from a home.

BENIGN GROWTHS

Seborrheic Keratoses

Seborrheic keratoses (Figure 47.9) are benign growths that are extremely common in adults >40 years old. They are tan, gray, or black waxy or warty papules and plaques. They often have a stuck-on appearance with follicular prominence. They can be found anywhere on the body except on mucous membranes, palms, and soles. Occasionally, some lesions are darkly pigmented, and differentiation from a melanoma can be difficult without a biopsy. These growths can be removed for cosmetic purposes with cryosurgery or shave excision if necessary.

Cherry Angiomas

Cherry angiomas are the most common acquired cutaneous vascular proliferations. They usually appear in people in their 20s and increase in number over time. They are round to oval, bright red, dome-shaped or

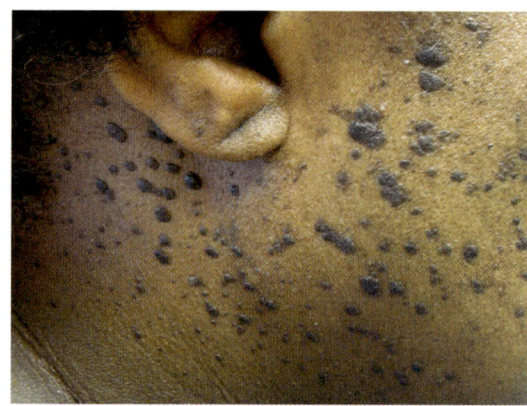

Figure 47.9—Seborrheic keratoses. These lesions present as waxy, warty, stuck-on papules in a variety of colors.

polypoid papules ranging in size from <1 mm to several millimeters. Cherry angiomas are benign, consisting of dilated, congested capillaries and postcapillary venules. However, they can bleed when traumatized. These lesions can be removed with excision, electrodessication, or laser ablation.

Actinic Keratoses

Actinic keratoses (Figure 47.10) are precancerous lesions caused by chronic UV radiation. They are seen in fair-skinned people and characterized by occasionally tender, rough, poorly circumscribed, erythematous papules with white or yellow scaling. They appear most often in areas with prolonged sun exposure, including the face, neck, ears, arms, and the dorsum of the hands. The scalp of alopecic men is commonly affected. Clinical variants include hypertrophic, pigmented, and lichenoid types. Some may have an overlying thick, hard, raised crust known as a *cutaneous horn*. Actinic keratosis or actinic damage of the lips is called *actinic cheilitis*.

Actinic keratoses are considered premalignant growths, precursors of squamous cell carcinoma. It is unclear how many progress to squamous cell carcinoma; reports vary from 0.24% to 20%. Actinic keratoses are treated to prevent progression to squamous cell carcinoma. They may respond to medical and surgical management. They can be easily treated in the office setting with cryotherapy (liquid nitrogen) or photodynamic therapy. Alternatively, they can respond to topical chemotherapeutic agents such as 5-fluorouracil, and immunomodulators such as imiquimod[OL]. When lesions are numerous, topical treatment with 5-fluorouracil or imiquimod is preferred over cryotherapy (SOE=B). These topical therapies are associated with a transient reaction characterized by bright erythema and discomfort.

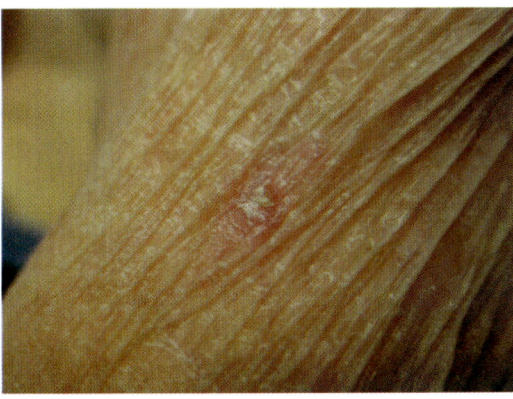

Figure 47.10—Actinic keratosis close up to demonstrate the adherent scale.

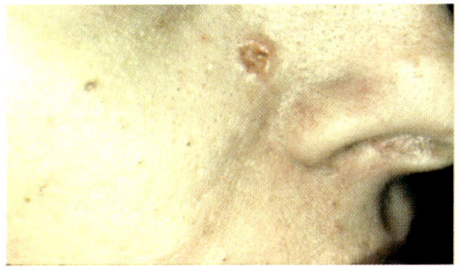

Figure 47.11—Basal cell carcinoma. This pearly, fleshy papule is ulcerated in the center and has a characteristic rolled border.

Skin Cancer

Basal Cell Carcinoma

Basal cell carcinoma (Figure 47.11) is the most common cancer in the United States. Although the tumors may be locally invasive, the risk of metastasis is low. There are many clinical subtypes, including nodular, superficial, and pigmented (which can be confused for melanoma). The three major clinical subtypes are the following:

- Nodular—the most common variant; appears as a waxy, translucent papule with overlying telangiectasias, often with central ulceration

- Morpheaform—has a scar-like appearance and can look atrophic

- Superficial—appears as an erythematous macule or papule with fine scale or superficial erosion often surrounded by telangiectasia

Risk factors for basal cell carcinoma include age, UV exposure, immunosuppression, genetic syndromes, and chemical exposures. Definitive treatment of basal cell carcinoma is surgical excision. Because of its higher cure rate, Mohs micrographic surgery is warranted for basal cell carcinomas that have indistinct borders, are >2 cm in diameter, are recurrent, or have high-risk histologic features (ie, morpheaform). An additional benefit of Mohs micrographic surgery is that it spares tissues and therefore can provide additional cosmetic benefits. Basal cell carcinomas that develop in poor surgical candidates can also be treated with ablative methods such as cryosurgery and radiation. Superficial basal cell carcinomas can be treated with less invasive techniques such as curettage with electrodessication and topical imiquimod therapy.

Squamous Cell Carcinoma

Squamous cell carcinoma is the second most common form of skin cancer. It generally presents as an occasionally tender, erythematous papule, plaque, or nodule with keratotic scale. The lesions can develop scaling and crusting. Squamous cell carcinomas are locally invasive and can cause subsequent tissue destruction. The risk of metastasis is low but higher than that of basal cell carcinomas; the risk increases with size of the tumor, high-risk histologic features (eg, poor differentiation, perineural invasion), depth of invasion, and location. Squamous cell carcinomas on the lip and ear can behave more aggressively. Squamous cell carcinomas also have a propensity to develop in longstanding, nonhealing wounds and in burn and radiation scars; these lesions are known as Marjolin ulcers and are associated with a higher risk of metastasis.

Like other nonmelanoma skin cancers, squamous cell carcinomas are associated with cumulative sun exposure and age. They tend to be found on sites chronically exposed to the sun, such as the face, the dorsum of hands, and arms. Additional risk factors include exposure to arsenic, ionizing radiation, and immunosuppression. Definitive treatment consists of surgical excision. In anatomically sensitive areas or with high-risk tumors, Mohs micrographic surgery is indicated. If surgery is contraindicated, palliative measures with lower cure rates (such as ionizing radiation) can be used.

Melanoma

Melanomas are malignant tumors of melanocytes. They have a higher risk of metastasis than basal cell carcinomas and squamous cell carcinomas. In addition to spreading locally, they are associated with distant metastases to the skin, brain, lung, liver, and small intestine. The tumors present usually as atypical pigmented lesions. There are 4 clinical types:

- Lentigo maligna—an irregularly shaped tan or brown macule that has been enlarging slowly; the type seen most commonly on atrophic, sun-damaged skin of older adults

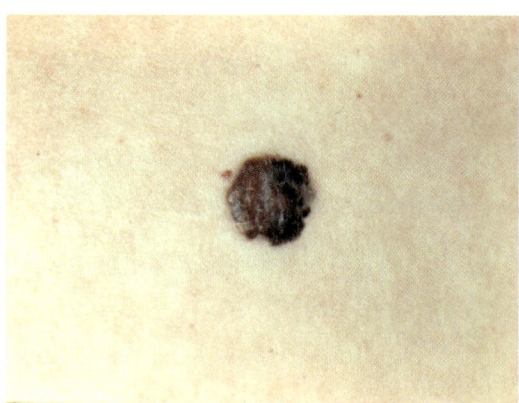

Figure 47.12—Melanoma. This lesion has irregular variegation in pigment (shades of brown and blue-black) as well as irregular borders, suggesting melanoma.

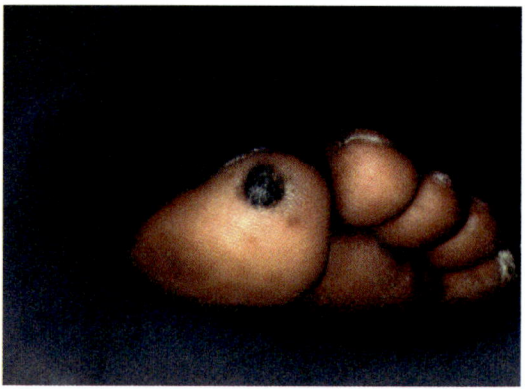

Figure 47.13—Acral lentiginous melanoma. This type of melanoma presents as a dark macular growth with irregular borders on volar surfaces of palms and soles (as in this case) and nails.

- Superficial spreading—an irregularly shaped macule, papule, or plaque with great variation in color (Figure 47.12) and that can occur anywhere but most commonly on the trunk or proximal extremities
- Nodular—a papule or nodule, often brown, black or gray, that has been growing rapidly; can be red or amelanotic
- Acral lentiginous—a dark brown or black patch found on the palms, soles, or nail beds, with a pigmented streak of the cuticle known as Hutchison sign (Figure 47.13) found in all skin types; incidence is highest in adults ≥65 years old

The incidence of melanoma continues to increase. Mortality due to melanoma has also increased but at a lower rate, in part because of earlier detection. Risk factors for melanoma include family history, fair skin type, red hair, history of dysplastic or numerous nevi, and sunlight exposure, particularly intermittent blistering sunburns in childhood.

Melanomas are usually asymptomatic. If detected early, they can be associated with a high rate of cure. Therefore, regular skin examinations and early recognition are important. A new, pigmented skin lesion or a change in the color, size, surface, or borders of a preexisting mole should be biopsied. A useful mnemonic when examining skin for melanoma or atypical moles is ABCD: asymmetry, borders, color, diameter >6 mm.

Risk factors for metastases and mortality due to melanoma are depth of invasion, ulceration, and number of mitoses. Treatment is tailored to the perceived aggressiveness of the tumor. If caught early with a Breslow depth <1 mm, definitive treatment is surgical excision. If Breslow depth is ≥1 mm, standard treatment is wide excision, and sentinel node biopsy may be indicated. Adjuvant therapy such as interferon is sometimes used in cases with lymph node involvement. If there is evidence of distant metastases, treatment options include immunotherapy such as interleukin-2, pegylated interferon alpha-2b, and/or chemotherapy.

Until recently, 95% of patients with stage IV melanoma died within 5 years. In 2010–2011, two breakthroughs in treatment of metastatic melanoma engendered tremendous excitement. The first was FDA approval of ipilimumab, a monoclonal antibody that binds to cytotoxic T lymphocyte–associated antigen 4, which functions as a negative feedback mechanism within the immune system. Ipilimumab blocks this negative feedback and allows the T cells of the immune system to attack the melanoma cells. The second breakthrough was approval of vemurafenib, a drug that can inhibit mutated BRAF protein, which has been identified in >50% of melanomas. Melanoma cells with this mutation depend on activated signaling through the mitogen-activated kinase pathway. Vemurafenib is a potent inhibitor of melanoma cells with the BRAF V600E mutation and thus inhibits the kinase pathway, subsequently blocking proliferation of the melanoma cells. Recently, a new BRAF inhibitor (dabrafenib) in combination with a new MEK kinase inhibitor (trametinib) has shown enhanced clinical responses in patients with metastatic melanoma. Additionally, two drugs (pembrolizumab and nivolombab) that block the programmed cell death 1 (PD-1) receptor have been approved by the FDA for patients with advanced melanoma.

RESOURCES

- Bisgaard E, Tarakji M, Lau F, et al. Neglected skin cancer in the elderly: a case of basosquamous cell carcinoma of the right shoulder. *J Surg Case Rep*. 2016 Aug 17;2016(8).

- Cunningham AL, Lal H, Kovac M. et al. Efficacy of the herpes zoster subunit vaccine in adults 70 years of age or older. *N Engl J Med*. 2016;375(11):1019–1032.

- Kirkland-Kyhn H, Zaratkiewicz S, Teleten O, et al. Caring for aging skin: preventing and managing skin problems in older adults. *Am J Nurs*. 2018;118(2):60–63.

- Murphree RW. Impairments in skin integrity. *Nurs Clin North Am*. 2017;52(3):405–417.

CHAPTER 48—DENTISTRY AND ORAL HEALTH

KEY POINTS

- Disease in the mouth can negatively impact the overall health of an individual. Several studies have found an association between periodontal disease and various systemic diseases, including respiratory disease, diabetes, and cardiovascular disease.

- Teeth may become less sensitive with age, and it is not uncommon to observe profound yet asymptomatic untreated dental decay, including broken teeth, in older adults.

- Periodontitis caused by plaque formation can lead to loss of alveolar bone supporting the tooth, malposition, loosening, and eventual loss of the tooth. Prevention is possible with daily oral hygiene and regular examinations and cleanings.

- Dentures can improve facial esthetics, aid in speech, and improve chewing ability.

- Antibiotic prophylactic coverage before dental procedures that may cause bleeding is indicated only in high-risk individuals to prevent infective bacterial endocarditis.

- Individuals taking antiresorptive agents are at risk of osteonecrosis of the jaw.

- Missing teeth, dental decay, periodontal disease, gingival recession, salivary hypofunction, and dry mouth are not normal age-related changes.

The FDI Dental World Federation defines oral health as follows: "Oral health is multifaceted and includes the ability to speak, smile, smell, taste, touch, chew, swallow, and convey a range of emotions through facial expressions with confidence and without pain, discomfort, and disease of the craniofacial complex."

AGING OF THE TEETH

The anatomy of the tooth and its supporting structures can be seen in Figure 48.1. Most age-related changes in teeth are subtle (Table 48.1) but become significant in the presence of environmental factors or disease. The teeth of older adults are typically less sensitive or wholly insensitive to temperature changes due to a shrinking of the dental pulp. Teeth also tend to darken with age. It is not uncommon to observe profound yet asymptomatic untreated dental disease in older adults.

DENTAL DECAY

Dental *caries*, or decay, is a bacterially caused demineralization and cavitation that can attack teeth throughout life. Older adults are more likely to have decay next to existing restorations or on the root of the tooth. The root may be exposed because of gingival recession from previous periodontal disease or aggressive tooth brushing. The root surface is softer than the enamel-covered crown of the tooth and can be more difficult to clean, so it can decay rapidly. Dental decay in older adults is generally asymptomatic and can become advanced before discovery, often resulting in destruction of much or all of the tooth.

Untreated, advanced caries commonly results in necrosis of the remaining pulp, which usually leads to an acute or chronic dental abscess. These infections may not present with pain, but they should not be ignored because severe infections of dental and oral origin can lead to systemic disease. In particular, α-hemolytic (viridans) streptococci of the oral cavity have long been implicated in nearly one-third of the cases of bacterial endocarditis reported annually in the United States.

The risk factors for dental caries are the same at any age, but many of the risk factors increase in prevalence with age. A primary risk factor is poor oral hygiene, which is common in older adults when visual acuity, manual dexterity, or arm flexibility is impaired, or when salivary flow is diminished. Another risk factor is frequent ingestion of sticky foods with a high sugar content such as cake, candy, and cookies. Other risk factors include lack of dental insurance or financial resources to pay for treatment, lack of transportation, no perceived need for dental care, and limited fluoride exposure.

The prevention of dental caries involves daily oral hygiene (brushing twice a day with a fluoride-containing toothpaste and cleaning between the teeth) and limitation of sugar exposure on the teeth. The treatment of dental caries usually involves removing decay and placing a restoration to fill the defect or rebuild the tooth. Sometimes, topical high-potency fluoride can remineralize early lesions. When dental caries involves the dental pulp, root canal treatment or tooth extraction becomes necessary. Routine professional dental care, including dental prophylaxis and topical fluoride application can also help prevent dental caries. In addition, routine dental examinations can detect decay early and improve the prognosis for maintaining a dentition for a lifetime.

Table 48.1—Clinical Significance of Selected Age-Related Changes in Oral Tissues

Tissue Affected	Nature of Change	Clinical Significance
Tooth dentin	Increased thickness	Diminished pulp space
	Diminished permeability resulting from sclerosis of dentinal tubules	Diminished sensitivity of dentin; diminished susceptibility to effects of bacterial metabolites; increased tooth brittleness
Dental pulp	Diminished volume	Diminished reparative capacity; diminished sensitivity and change in nature of sensitivity
	Shift in proportion of nervous, vascular, and connective tissues	Diminished reparative capacity; diminished sensitivity and change in nature of sensitivity
Salivary glands	Fatty replacement of acini	Possibly less physiologic reserve

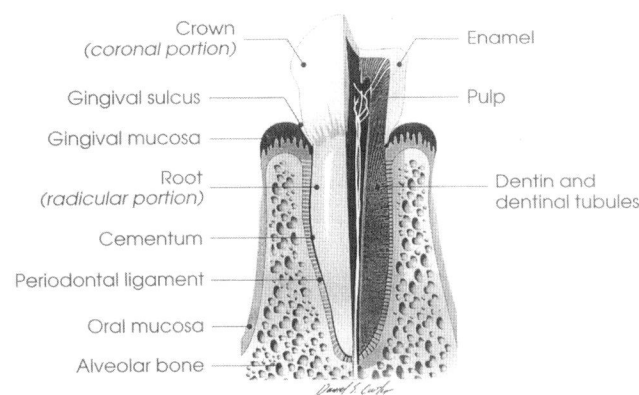

Figure 48.1—Tooth anatomy and surrounding structures

PERIODONTAL DISEASE

The tissues surrounding the teeth, termed the *periodontium*, consist of the gingiva, the alveolar bone, and a collagenous sleeve (termed the *periodontal ligament*) located between the tooth root and the surrounding bone. Periodontal disease occurs when bacterial colonies (*plaque*) form on the teeth near the gingiva and between the gingiva and the root surface within the gingival sulcus. If the plaque is not removed, it can harden and become tarter or calculus, which acts as a further irritant to the gingiva. Gingivitis is a form of gum disease in which the inflammatory reaction to plaque is limited to the gingiva. Gingivitis results in gingival edema and light bleeding on brushing and resolves after plaque removal. If the inflammatory process extends to the periodontal ligament and alveolar bone, the process is termed periodontitis or periodontal disease. In periodontitis, there is destruction of the hard and soft tissues of the periodontium. In advanced cases of periodontal disease, loss of alveolar bone around the tooth leads to the decreased support, malposition, loosening, and eventual loss of the tooth.

Periodontal disease is common in older adults with estimates of 70% of those >65 years old affected. Epidemiologic data and clinical observation support the concept that those who reach advanced age without significant periodontal bone loss will not likely experience a worsening of the disease in senescence. In contrast, other adults who have experienced a more rapid rate of bone loss commonly will have lost teeth in their 40s and 50s. In addition to age, risk factors for periodontitis include smoking and poor oral hygiene. Treating periodontal disease involves removing the plaque and tarter on the teeth and the roots below the gingiva. This is called deep cleaning or scaling and root planing and often requires local anesthetic and sometimes surgical access. Adjunctive therapy with topical antibiotics such as chlorhexidine oral rinse (SOE=B) or systemic antibiotics such as minocycline (SOE=B) or metronidazole (SOE=C) can also be useful in periodontal therapy. Preventing gingivitis and periodontitis involves daily oral hygiene (brushing and interdental cleaning with floss or special brushes) and routine dental examinations and cleanings. Electric toothbrushes can make it easier for older adults and care providers to provide daily oral hygiene.

MISSING TEETH AND DENTURES

Advanced age was once considered synonymous with the need for false teeth, but that stereotype is fading. In the early 1960s, more than 70% of adult Americans ≥75 years old were edentulous. By the 1990s, fewer than 40% of this group were edentulous, and this number has now declined to fewer than 25%. This is most likely because of some level of preventive and restorative dental care in childhood or early adulthood and fluoridated water. But despite the decreased percentages, the number of edentulous older adults is still large because of the increasing population in this cohort. Teeth may need to be extracted because of extensive decay or periodontal disease or the inability or unwillingness to pay for dental treatment necessary to save a tooth. Lack of access to routine dental care may also lead to problems progressing until extraction is the only option.

Some unique problems are associated with being edentulous. Functionally, the teeth aid in mastication and speech. Aesthetically, the teeth support the lips and cheeks and keep the nose and chin a fixed distance apart. When a person has lost all teeth and there are no prosthetic replacements, the facial appearance is dramatically changed because of the lack of tissue support and the diminished vertical height of the lower half of the face. Chewing ability is severely compromised, yet the impact on nutritional intake is difficult to characterize.

Removable dentures can aid in speech and restore diminished facial contours, but they are less predictably successful in restoring the ability to masticate. Edentulous people with dentures can generally eat a wider range of foods than edentulous people without dentures. However, some individuals with complete dentures still have difficulty eating certain foods and may not be able to enjoy the unrestricted diet of individuals with a full complement of natural teeth. Denture wearers also have to chew more times before they swallow food, and they swallow their food in larger particles. Older adults and their clinicians who hope that dentures will restore oral intake in cases of malnutrition or unexplained weight loss are sometimes disappointed, whereas those who hope for a more socially acceptable appearance, clearer speech, and modest improvement in chewing comfort and range of dietary choices are more likely to be satisfied.

Dentures can be a considerable source of discomfort, dysfunction, and embarrassment for older adults. This is because the alveolar bone that originally held the natural teeth continually remodels and decreases in volume once the natural teeth are gone. For most individuals, dentures require professional adjustment and periodic relines or replacement. Alveolar ridge resorption is most severe in the oldest patients who have had the longest time without natural teeth. Denture adhesive may be helpful in holding dentures in place but should not be used to compensate for a poorly fitting denture. Dental implants that integrate with the jaw bone are another option to retain dentures but require surgical placement and significantly increase the cost of treatment. Implants can greatly improve the retention of dentures for appropriate candidates and can also be used to provide fixed (nonremovable) dental replacements for individual or multiple teeth.

Individuals without teeth will not develop dental decay or periodontal disease but can develop other problems related to wearing complete or partial (some natural teeth remain to anchor the denture) dentures. Dentures that do not fit properly can become loose or cause denture sores. Dentures that are not routinely removed from the mouth and cleaned each day can lead to oral fungal infections. Individuals with broken or ill-fitting dentures should see a dental professional. Poorly fitting dentures in a cognitively impaired individual may result in the person not eating or having behavior changes due to constant pain. Resolving the pain by adjusting the denture may eliminate behavior changes and allow the individual to eat again. These same changes can occur in people with teeth, and the mouth should always be considered as a potential source of pain.

Taking care of partial or complete dentures involves removing them from the mouth every day to clean them with a mild dishwashing liquid and a denture brush. Soaking them in a denture cleanser a couple of times a week will also help to remove stains and keep the dentures clean. Dentures should be left out of the mouth for some time every day, with overnight being best. When not in the mouth, dentures should soak in water.

SALIVARY FUNCTION IN AGING

Saliva is critical for protecting the tissues of the oral cavity and maintaining their function in speech, mastication, swallowing, and taste perception. Saliva buffers the intraoral pH, contains a wide spectrum of antimicrobial factors, remineralizes and lubricates the oral cavity, and keeps the taste pores patent. In the absence of disease, the major salivary glands undergo regressive histologic changes with age. Yet data from the Baltimore Longitudinal Study on Aging and the Veterans Affairs Dental Longitudinal Study have demonstrated that with healthy aging, flow from the parotid glands under both resting and stimulated conditions remains essentially unchanged. In both studies, flow from the submandibular glands did not change with age. Data from other centers has shown a measurable but clinically minor decrease. It has been suggested that the major salivary glands demonstrate "organ reserve," in which the capacity of youthful glands exceeds ordinary demands, but that with age-related changes, functional reserves dwindle. By extreme old age, healthy glands function adequately under normal conditions but are more susceptible to factors that impede function, such as dehydration or drug-induced hypofunction.

Complaints of dry mouth are very common among older adults. The leading cause is an adverse reaction to medication. Commonly implicated are medications with anticholinergic effects, including antimuscarinic agents for urinary incontinence, tricyclic antidepressants, opioids, antihistamines, antihypertensives (including diuretics, ACE inhibitors, calcium channel blockers, and both α- and β-blockers), and antiarrhythmic agents. Separate studies have found that 72% of institutionalized older adults received at least one (and some as many as five) potentially xerostomic medications daily and that 55% of >4,000 rural community-dwelling older adults took at least one potentially xerostomic medication daily. Dry mouth can also be due to local disease, such as salivary gland tumors and blocked ducts, or to systemic disease. Sjögren syndrome affects approximately

3 million Americans, predominantly women, ≥50 years old. Cevimeline (30 mg q8h), a cholinergic agent, is approved for dry mouth in patients with Sjögren syndrome. Another agent for Sjögren syndrome is oral pilocarpine 5 mg 4 times daily. Depression has been reported to diminish saliva flow, as have poorly controlled diabetes mellitus and hypothyroidism.

Dry mouth is also an adverse consequence of head and neck radiation. As a result, patients who have undergone radiation of the head and neck can experience rapidly destructive dental caries. These individuals should have a dental evaluation before radiation and be started on an aggressive preventive program, including daily fluoride application. Treatment of older adults with dry mouth is usually palliative. If the cause is an adverse effect of medication and the medication can be changed, then the problem may completely resolve. However, many older adults have several chronic medical conditions requiring numerous medications. Changing or eliminating medications may not be possible and may not matter if the salivary glands are damaged because of disease or previous radiation. Sipping on water throughout the day is a simple and inexpensive approach for dealing with a dry mouth but may not be the best solution for someone with urinary incontinence. Saliva substitutes and oral lubricants, available without prescription and used as needed, can provide transient relief but replenish none of the protective properties of saliva. If hard candy or gum is used for relief, it should be sugar free or sweetened with xylitol, which will not cause decay. Medications such as pilocarpine and cevimeline also have adverse effects and add one more drug to what may already be a long list. Patients should understand the reason for their dry mouth and increased risk of dental decay and be educated on the need to limit dietary sugar exposure and optimize daily oral hygiene practices. These individuals should have a dental evaluation and usually require more frequent dental visits to prevent and treat dental problems.

COMMON ORAL LESIONS

Several oral lesions (Table 48.2) may be seen in older adults. It is important to recognize the appearance of a healthy mouth so abnormalities can be identified. The most common, periodontal disease and dental caries, can both result in abscess formation. This can present as a firm or fluctuant swelling inside the mouth or on the face. An elevated nodule representing a localized collection of pus in gingival soft tissue, or parulis, may be seen on the gingiva near an abscessed tooth and represents a fistula associated with the infection. These are often asymptomatic but need to be treated by root canal therapy or dental extraction. Antibiotics will not resolve these and are not recommended if there are no other symptoms.

Exostoses, called torus (singular) or tori (plural), can form on the palate and on the lingual aspects of the mandible. Tori can grow slowly throughout adulthood and sometimes reach dimensions that can predispose to trauma from food and impede swallowing. They can also create problems for denture wearers.

The parotid ducts enter the mouth under small flaps of tissue termed Stenson's papillae, which are located inside the cheek opposite the maxillary second molars. These can be distinguished from pathologic polypoid structures by applying gentle pressure to the preauricular area—saliva will be excreted only if the structure is Stenson's papilla.

The dorsum of the tongue in some individuals displays irregular patterns of hyperkeratotic and denuded reddened areas lacking lingual papillae. This presentation is variously termed geographic tongue (because the pattern looks map-like) and migratory glossitis (because the patterns change over time) and is no basis for concern. Increased varicosities may be noted on the ventral surface of the tongue and are also not a concern.

Candidiasis presents as diffusely erythematous mucositis, cracking at the corners of the mouth (angular cheilitis), curd-like white patches (thrush), or erythema in denture-bearing areas (denture stomatitis); it can be wholly asymptomatic or result in taste dysfunction, burning, itching, and pain. Older adults are particularly susceptible to candidiasis because of denture use, salivary hypofunction, the prevalence of diabetes mellitus, and the use of antibiotics for pulmonary and urologic diseases. Use of inhaled corticosteroids places oropharyngeal structures in the path of the spray, increasing their risk of localized candidal colonization. Management of candidiasis involves first excluding any immunopathologic cause for the disease, followed by administering topical or systemic antifungal agents and optimizing oral and denture hygiene.

Herpes simplex is a virus that resides preferentially in the trigeminal ganglion and periodically causes intraoral outbreaks. These outbreaks are limited to the palate, the gingiva, and the extraoral aspects of the lips. They begin as clusters of small, circular, red-rimmed yellowish blisters that burst and coalesce into irregular denuded lesions. They are highly contagious until healed.

Aphthous ulcers represent another episodic, painful oral outbreak. They tend to appear as isolated lesions and form only on the movable oral mucosa (ie, inner aspects of the cheeks and lips, floor of the mouth, and lateral border of the tongue). Aphthous ulcerations are not known to be contagious.

Table 48.2—Common Oral Lesions

Lesion	Description	Treatment
Dental caries	Destruction of tooth	Dental restoration
Gingivitis	Gingival inflammation	Remove plaque
Periodontal disease	Gingival inflammation and alveolar bone loss	Remove plaque and tartar
Parulis (gum boil)	Solitary, soft nodule on gingiva associated with nonvital tooth	Root canal therapy or extraction
Torus (tori)	Bony exostosis	No treatment
Angular cheilitis	Red, cracked labial commissures	Nystatin–triamcinolone cream
Candidal infection	White plaques easily wiped away or mucosal erythema, especially on denture-bearing surfaces	Various antifungal agents
Herpes simplex	Small vesicles that rupture to form ulcers located on attached mucosa	Various antiviral agents
Aphthous ulcers (canker sore)	Ulcer with erythematous border on nonattached (movable) mucosa	Topical anesthetic or mild steroid
Traumatic ulcer	Superficial ulcer associated with traumatic injury	Remove offending etiology, topical anesthetic
Squamous cell carcinoma	Indurated ulcer of long duration	Wide excision, chemotherapy, radiation

Traumatic ulcers are commonly seen in older adults and can be associated with broken teeth, ill-fitting dentures, or any other mouth trauma. The cause of the lesion should be identified and, if it does not resolve within a couple of weeks of correcting the problem, additional evaluation including biopsy may be indicated.

An idiopathic disruption of the desquamation of tongue filiform papillae (normally about 1 mm long), which seems to become more prevalent with advancing age, results in elongation of the papillae (to ≥3 mm) and the appearance of a "hairy tongue." This condition is prone to staining from a variety of foods (eg, tea, coffee), from tobacco use, and from medications (eg, bismuth). "Hairy tongue" can also serve as a substrate for bacterial and/or fungal growth. Any of these, all of which are exacerbated by salivary hypofunction, can confer on the tongue notable colorations (eg, "black hairy tongue"), but none is associated with symptoms.

Burning mouth syndrome is a chronic orofacial pain disorder usually without other clinical signs. It typically affects women ≥50 years old, particularly in Asian Americans and Native Americans. The pain most commonly affects the lips, tongue, and palate. Multiple causes have been suggested, including xerostomia, denture use, candidiasis, nutritional deficiencies, and psychiatric disorders. Treatment is symptomatic and empirical.

Oral malignancies can appear clinically as painless red, white, or mixed red and white areas of the oral mucosa that may be ulcerated or indurated. Red and mixed lesions (termed *erythroplakia*) display cellular atypia in as many as 93% of cases and should be biopsied immediately. White lesions (*leukoplakia*) are malignant or premalignant <10% of the time and merit close monitoring; biopsy is indicated if a lesion does not resolve in 14 days or is increasing in size. Less invasive diagnostic tools can be used for determining whether a white or red lesion in the mouth merits biopsy, such as scraping (exfoliative cytology) and in situ staining. Early identification markedly improves outcome.

CHEMOSENSORY PERCEPTION

Olfactory function declines with age. A decreased ability to identify odors and to rank their intensities affects both older men (to the greater extent) and women. Several medications have been implicated in olfactory dysfunction, as has Alzheimer disease, among other disorders common among older adults. Impaired olfaction in older adults has been anecdotally implicated as a risk factor for eating spoiled food or failing to notice gas leaks or domestic fires.

Taste perception changes with aging. The subjective perception of saltiness and sweetness blunts with advancing age. This change potentially has clinical significance, possibly playing a role in the tendency to oversalt foods or crave sweets.

Complaints of taste and smell dysfunction are common among older adults. Often the complaint derives from medication use, but other causes are possible (Table 48.3 and Table 48.4). Some medications may have no primary effect on taste but reduce saliva flow and lead to impaired taste perception. The sense of "taste" can actually be more accurately termed "flavor," ie, the full range of sensations that accompany eating, including temperature, texture, sound, and smell in addition to the perception of sweet, salt, sour, and bitter.

Table 48.3—Medications That Interfere With Gustation (Taste) and Olfaction (Smell)

Gustation[a]		
Allopurinol	Diclofenac	Ofloxacin
Amiloride	Dicyclomine	Nifedipine
Amitriptyline	Diltiazem	Pentamidine
Ampicillin	Doxepin	Phenytoin
Baclofen	Enalapril	Propranolol
Buspirone	Fenoprofen	Ritonavir
Captopril	Hydrochlorothiazide	Saquinavir
Chlorpheniramine	Imipramine	Sulfamethoxazole
Desipramine	Nabumetone	Tetracyclines
Dexamethasone	Nelfinavir	Zidovudine

Olfaction[b]		
Amitriptyline	Dexamethasone	Morphine
Amphetamine	Enalapril	Pentamidine
Beclomethasone dipropionate	Flunisolide	Pirbuterol
Codeine	Flurbiprofen	
	Hydromorphone	

[a] Source lists >250 agents reported to disturb the sense of taste; agents listed are limited to those for which taste disturbance was determined objectively through threshold or intensity scaling or both, using one or more standardized solutions.
[b] Source lists >40 agents reported to disturb the sense of smell; agents listed are limited to those for which olfactory disturbance was determined objectively through experiment or clinical trial.

SOURCE: Data from Schiffman SS, Zervakis J. Taste and smell perception in the elderly: effect of medications and disease. *Adv Food Nutr Res.* 2002;44:247–346.

Table 48.4—Nonpharmacologic Causes of Taste and Smell Dysfunction in Older Adults

Gustatory dysfunction
Oral causes:
  Burning mouth syndrome (chronic orofacial pain disorder without clinical signs)
  Candidiasis
  Laceration
  Malignancy
  Salivary hypofunction
  Therapeutic irradiation of head
  Thermal or chemical burn
Other causes:
  Alzheimer disease, other neurodegenerative disorders
  CNS tumor
  Endocrinopathies (eg, diabetes mellitus, Cushing syndrome, adrenocortical insufficiency, hypothyroidism)
  Head trauma
  Nutritional deficiencies (vitamin B_{12}, zinc)
  Psychiatric disorders
  Stroke

Olfactory dysfunction
Upper aerodigestive and respiratory causes:
  Dental infection
  Periodontal disease
  Poor oral hygiene, including poor denture hygiene
  Sinusitis
  Tobacco smoking or use of nasal snuff
  Tumor of airway or sinus
  Upper respiratory infection (bacterial or viral)
Other causes:
  Alzheimer disease, other neurodegenerative disorders
  CNS tumor
  Exposure to volatile or particulate toxins
  Head trauma
  Nutritional deficiencies (niacin, zinc)
  Psychiatric disorders
  Stroke

Older adults are prone to impaired flavor perception because of changes in olfaction and oral stereognosis, salivary hypofunction, and the presence of dentures, which present physical and thermal barriers. Flavor enhancement strategies have had positive effects on both food preference and caloric intake among frail older adults.

THE RELATIONSHIP BETWEEN ORAL HEALTH, GENERAL HEALTH, AND THE IMPACT OF MEDICATIONS ON THE ORAL CAVITY

Numerous studies have found an association between periodontal disease and systemic diseases such as respiratory disease, diabetes, and cardiovascular disease. Periodontal disease and the pathogens responsible for it have been linked epidemiologically and immunologically with coronary artery disease, peripheral vascular disease, cerebrovascular disease, and pneumonia. In addition, medications prescribed to older adults can have an impact on the oral cavity and providing dental care.

Aspiration pneumonia can result when bacteria in the mouth enter the lungs. Older adults with numerous chronic conditions and a compromised immune system may be unable to deal with the insult. In addition, those individuals may have poor oral hygiene because they are unable to clean their own mouth and do not receive proper oral hygiene from a caregiver. Pneumonia is a significant problem in older adults. Correlation between length of stay in nursing homes, hospitals, and ICUs, and colonization of dental and oral mucosal plaque with known pulmonary pathogens (SOE=B) is compelling justification for ensuring daily oral care is a required nursing task. Direct care staff should receive training, and the daily practice of such care carefully monitored as a component of infection control (SOE=B). Numerous reports in the dental, infectious disease, and critical care literature demonstrate increasing prevalence of pulmonary pathogens from dental and oral plaque with increasing length of stay (SOE=B). Several studies have demonstrated significantly reduced incidence of institution-acquired pneumonia, reduced mortality, and reduced length of hospital stay in patients on ventilators (SOE=B) and those in nursing homes (SOE=C) when a program of daily oral hygiene is instituted. Daily oral hygiene improves oral health and could reduce pneumonia.

Periodontitis has long been reported to be worse in patients with poorly controlled diabetes mellitus. Investigations also support the contention that periodontitis, as a cause of chronic inflammation, impedes effective control of diabetes. Periodontal disease can negatively impact glycemic control because inflammation and infection can increase blood glucose. Individuals with poorly controlled diabetes can have more severe periodontal disease because hyperglycemia can decrease the body's ability to kill bacteria. Also, hyperglycemia can lead to increased glucose in the crevicular fluid around the teeth, which feeds the bacteria.

Two potential mechanisms explain the association between periodontal disease and cardiovascular disease. There can be direct infection from oral bacteria, which causes an inflammatory response and leads to plaque formation in the blood vessel. In addition, some periodontal pathogens can cause platelet aggregation, which can result in clot formation.

The mouth contains $\sim 10^{11}$–10^{13} microorganisms, and the rich vascular supply beneath the relatively delicate mucosal covering predisposes to episodes of orally seeded bacteremia. Approximately one-third of the reported cases of infective endocarditis are caused by organisms normally found only in the mouth. Case reports of prosthetic implants infected by organisms originating in infected oral tissues have for years compelled physicians and dentists to administer antibiotics prophylactically before invasive dental care for patients with such history. However, the 2007 recommendations from the American Heart Association reflect that tooth brushing and eating in the presence of gingival inflammation are recognized to present, over time, as much as or a greater source of bacteremia than dental care and that there is growing concern that widespread, short-term antibiotic treatment promotes the emergence of drug-resistant strains of microorganisms. Prophylactic coverage is now recommended only in specific individuals who are at increased risk of complications if endocarditis develops (Table 48.5). Routine antibiotic prophylaxis before dental treatment is not indicated for individuals with prosthetic joint replacements.

Anticoagulants normally do not need to be discontinued before routine dental care, including most dental extractions. For individuals taking warfarin, an INR should be obtained within 24 hours of the procedure. Generally, if the INR is ≤3.5, the risk of uncontrolled oral hemorrhage is minimal and outweighed by the protective effects of anticoagulation (SOE=B).

Case reports in the medical and dental literature describe apparently spontaneous aseptic osteonecrosis of the mandible in patients who had been treated with bisphosphonates for management of bony metastases.

Table 48.5—Prevention of Bacterial Endocarditis

Indications	■ Individuals with prosthetic heart valves ■ Individuals with history of previous endocarditis ■ Individuals with congenital heart disease (CHD): unrepaired cyanotic CHD, completely repaired CHD defect with prosthetic material for first 6 months, repaired CHD with residual defects at site of or adjacent to site of prosthetic patch ■ Cardiac transplant recipients who develop cardiac valvulopathy
Antibiotic regimen options	■ Amoxicillin 2 g, po, 30–60 minutes before procedure ■ Clindamycin 600 mg, po, 30–60 minutes before procedure ■ Cephalexin 2 g, po, azithromycin 500 mg, po, or clarithromycin 500 mg, po, may also be used 30–60 minutes before procedure if penicillin allergy

SOURCE: Adapted from Wilson W, Taubert KA, Gewitz M, et al. Prevention of infective endocarditis: guidelines from the American Heart Association: a guideline from the American Heart Association Rheumatic Fever, Endocarditis, and Kawasaki Disease Committee, Council on Cardiovascular Disease in the Young, and the Council on Clinical Cardiology, Council on Cardiovascular Surgery and Anesthesia, and the Quality of Care and Outcomes Research Interdisciplinary Working Group. *Circulation.* 2007;116(15):1736–1754.

Because the reports are relatively uncommon, formal epidemiologic determination of risk factors has been challenging. However, it does appear that bisphosphonates administered for osteoporosis rarely lead to osteonecrosis, that women are more likely affected than men, and that the mandible is more likely to be affected than the maxilla (SOE=C). Individuals who begin treatment with an antiresorptive agent should receive a dental evaluation and treatment before starting the drug. If dental surgery is undertaken in a patient with a history of high-dosage bisphosphonate therapy, such as treatment for metastatic cancer, the patient should be advised of the increased risk of osteonecrosis-related complications.

Gingival enlargement may be seen in people taking phenytoin, cyclosporins, and calcium channel blockers. If the medication cannot be changed, this adverse effect can be minimized by good oral hygiene.

Hundreds of medications list dry mouth as a potential adverse effect. The complications and treatments have been discussed (above).

ORAL ASSESSMENT

Asking about dental problems, the last dental visit, and the presence of a dry mouth should be a routine part of a history and physical examination. This should be followed by a thorough oral assessment.

The assessment should begin outside the mouth with a visual inspection and manual palpation of the head and neck region. Intraorally, first impressions may be a good indicator of overall oral health. Dentures, if worn, should be removed so that the oral mucosa and teeth can be better visualized. A tongue blade can be used to retract the cheeks and tongue. The buccal mucosa, gingiva, palate, floor of the mouth, and all surfaces of the tongue should be examined. Inflammation, white or red patches, and ulcerations should be evaluated.

Referral for a complete dental evaluation is indicated when "something does not look right," or when the person has not had routine dental care, has broken or decayed teeth, reports a dry mouth, or has any oral lesion without a definitive benign diagnosis.

ORAL HYGIENE IN LONG-TERM CARE FACILITIES

Adequate oral hygiene for residents in nursing facilities is often a concern. Many reasons have been cited as to why this basic care is not performed, including lack of training, not recognizing its importance, and high turnover of aides. Regardless, oral care is a significant part of general care and should be performed every day. The main goals of providing daily oral care are to disrupt the plaque that accumulates on the teeth and to check for any problems. Brushing and flossing are ideal but may not be practical, because flossing is difficult to accomplish on another individual. Interdental brushes are often easier to use than floss and may be better tolerated by the individual. A power toothbrush with a standard toothbrush head is often a best option for care providers because the brush does the work. It is only necessary to hold the bristles against the teeth and move the brush around the mouth.

If brushing in front of a sink is not possible, using a towel to cover the resident and providing a basin to spit in is a workable arrangement. Standing behind or to the side of the resident gives good access to brush teeth. However, for individuals with dementia, standing in front to perform oral hygiene may be beneficial because it allows them to see what is happening. A toothbrush with a fluoride-containing toothpaste should be used to brush all the tooth surfaces. The resident should be asked to spit out after brushing. Rinsing is not necessary, and leaving more of the fluoride in contact with the teeth may be beneficial. Dentures should be removed before the mouth is cleaned.

Performing oral care for a cognitively impaired or uncooperative individual may be more of a challenge. Sometimes, spending a little more time or choosing the right time during the day is all that is necessary. If today's attempt is unsuccessful, things may be better tomorrow. Oral care should be attempted every day.

Fingers should not be used to hold the mouth open; safer options include a second large handle tooth brush, a stack of tongue blades, or a mouth prop. When the person opens his or her mouth, the second brush can be inserted between the teeth. Disrupting the plaque is the goal and more important than proper technique, so chewing on the toothbrush is also beneficial. Oral care swabs (ie, "foam on a stick") should not be used in place of a toothbrush but are appropriate for cleaning an edentulous mouth. Numerous online videos demonstrate oral care for nursing-home residents and individuals with dementia (https://youtu.be/AVsMmppYXrI; www.youtube.com/watch?v=jnxQsGg3R3w [accessed Feb 2019]).

Nursing directors and administrators should understand that oral care is not just brushing teeth but an important part of infection control that may have a substantial impact on general health and overall quality of life of the resident.

RESOURCES

- Rantzow V, Andersson P, Lindmar U. Occurrence of oral health problems and planned measure sin dependent older people in nursing care. *J Clin Nurs.* 2017;27:4381–4389.

- Sollecito TP, Abt E, Lockhart PB, et al. The use of prophylactic antibiotics prior to dental procedures in patients with prosthetic joints: evidence-based clinical practice guideline for dental practitioners—a report of the American Dental Association Council on Scientific Affairs. *JADA.* 2015;146(1):11–16.

- Tonetti MS, Bottenberg P, Conrads G, et al. Dental caries and periodontal diseases in the ageing population: call to action to protect and enhance oral health and well-being as an essential component of healthy ageing – Consensus report of group 4 of the joint EFP/ORCA workshop on the boundaries between caries and periodontal diseases. *J Clin Periodontol.* 2017;44(Suppl18):S135–S144.

CHAPTER 49—PULMONOLOGY

KEY POINTS

- With age, forced vital capacity (FVC), forced expiratory volume in 1 second (FEV_1), and PaO_2 all decrease, while the alveolar-arterial gradient (A-a gradient) increases.

- Clinically significant dyspnea is often underreported and unrecognized in older adults.

- There is a second peak prevalence of asthma for people ≥65 years old.

- COPD is the third leading cause of death in older adults. Pharmacologic treatment of COPD chiefly consists of inhaled bronchodilators and steroids.

- Use of fixed FEV_1/FVC as a criterion for COPD diagnosis risks overdiagnosis in older adults.

- Smoking cessation will slow the decline in lung function at any age.

- Because most patients with DVT/PE are asymptomatic, clinicians must maintain a high index of suspicion.

AGE-RELATED PULMONARY CHANGES

Studies of age-specific changes in pulmonary function are limited because of potential confounding by common, important comorbidities experienced by older adults, including smoking-related diseases, occupational and industrial exposures, heart failure, sarcopenia, or physical deconditioning. These study limitations notwithstanding, decrements in various aspects of pulmonary function have been demonstrated with aging.

Because of changes in connective tissue with age, the size of the airways is reduced and the alveolar sacs become shallower. Chest wall compliance decreases as a consequence of kyphoscoliosis, calcification of the costal cartilage, and arthritic changes in the costovertebral joints. Sarcopenia leads to intercostal muscle atrophy, and diaphragmatic strength is reduced by 25%. These processes result in a decline of FVC and FEV_1 of 25–30 mL/year in nonsmokers and approximately double that (60–70 mL/year) in smokers ≥65 years old. The normal A-a gradient increases with age and can be approximated by the following formula: (age/4) + 4 (in mmHg). The PaO_2 decreases with age and can be estimated by the equation: $PaO_2 = 110 - (0.4 \times age)$.

COMMON RESPIRATORY SYMPTOMS AND COMPLAINTS

There is a common misperception that older adults tend to overestimate or exaggerate respiratory symptoms; however, the opposite is more often true. Many older adults and their clinicians underestimate the importance of dyspnea, the cause of which may go undiagnosed until disease is advanced. This is partly because dyspnea is blamed on deconditioning and "normal" aging. Older adults often reduce their activity level to compensate for the often insidious decline in lung function and resultant dyspnea. (Unfortunately, with increasing amounts of sedentary time, deconditioning may become a significant contributor to the problem.) Such changes in lifestyle often go unnoticed by family, the clinician, and even the patient. Pulmonary or cardiac disorders, or both, may underlie such modifications in lifestyle, and testing (eg, pulmonary function tests, chest radiography, or cardiac echocardiography) can reveal major abnormalities such as asthma, emphysema, pulmonary fibrosis, or pulmonary arterial hypertension. Another complicating feature of symptom recognition in older adults is that there is often more than one explanation for their conditions. A patient may have overlapping symptoms of dyspnea, cough, and wheezing because of a combination of diseases such as asthma or emphysema, obstructive sleep apnea, heart failure, and gastroesophageal reflux.

Rhinosinusitis

Rhinitis complaints of older adults include a constant need to clear the throat, a sense of nasal obstruction, nasal crusting, facial pressure, and a decreased sense of taste and smell. Some changes in physiology and function of the nose accompany aging. As people age, the nose lengthens and the tip begins to droop secondary to weakening of the supporting cartilage. These physiologic changes can restrict nasal airflow. Narrowing of nasal passages can lead to complaints of nasal obstruction, which has been referred to as geriatric rhinitis.

There are no data to determine if either acute or chronic rhinosinusitis manifests any differently in older adults than in younger adults, so guidelines from the American Academy of Otolaryngology–Head and Neck Surgery do not advise different approaches to diagnosis or treatment based on age. Acute (<4 weeks duration), subacute (4–12 weeks duration), and chronic (>12 weeks duration) rhinosinusitis are further subclassified as uncomplicated, when inflammation is restricted to the nasal cavity and sinuses, or complicated, when inflammation extends beyond these areas (eg, with soft-tissue or neurologic involvement). Bacterial rhinosinusitis is associated with purulent nasal discharge and facial pain or pressure. Treatment may focus on pain relief with simple analgesics, as well as on relief of nasal obstruction by saline irrigation. Antibiotics are generally not prescribed when illness is mild but are advised if symptoms persist for ≥7 days or if the symptoms worsen at any time. Early treatment with antibiotics in those with mild disease has been shown to be harmful (SOE=B). In patients with clear nasal discharge, the cause of the rhinosinusitis is likely viral, and treatment should be symptomatic only. Although topical α-adrenergic decongestants may be effective, their use should be restricted in older adults, particularly those with hypertension or voiding symptoms from prostate disease. Chronic rhinosinusitis may be treated with a variety of topical approaches. A Cochrane review demonstrated that saline irrigation is more effective than placebo and is a safe approach for many older adults. Topical nasal steroids are more effective than saline irrigation but may cause epistaxis and local irritation. Allergic causes of rhinosinusitis are best treated by avoiding the inciting allergens if possible, although topical nasal steroids are often required. Anti-allergy medications may also have a role in treatment of allergic rhinosinusitis in older adults but should be used judiciously, because antihistamine formulations may also have undesired anticholinergic effects.

Dyspnea

Dyspnea becomes prominent in end-stage lung diseases such as COPD and idiopathic pulmonary fibrosis. Importantly, the level of dyspnea is the best predictor of quality of life, yet it does not correlate with either oxygenation or pulmonary function test results. A thorough history and physical examination can help tailor both testing and empirical treatment choices. For example, in an older adult presenting with dyspnea and associated nocturnal cough, common diseases such as asthma, emphysema, allergic rhinitis with postnasal drip, and gastroesophageal reflux disease should be considered first. Minimal testing (eg, pulmonary function tests only) followed by an empiric trial directed toward the most likely cause would be a reasonable approach. In the same patient, the presence of significant weight loss or constitutional symptoms (eg, fever, night sweats) could suggest other disease, such as malignancy or tuberculosis. At times, the specific words the patient chooses to describe the dyspnea can be revealing, such as "heavy" for cardiac dysfunction or deconditioning or "tight" for asthma. Common causes of dyspnea to consider in older adults include COPD, cardiac disease, asthma, interstitial lung disease, anemia, and deconditioning.

Table 49.1—Potential Causes of Chronic Cough in Older Adults

Postnasal drip (common)
Asthma (common)
Gastroesophageal reflux (common)
Medication effects (especially ACE inhibitors)
COPD/chronic bronchitis
Congestive heart failure
Laryngeal dysfunction
Bordetella pertussis infection
Other bacterial infections
Viral upper respiratory infection
Bronchiectasis
Central airway tumors
Interstitial lung disease

Chronic Cough

Fortunately, most patients can be reassured that chronic cough, although annoying, usually has a benign cause in individuals without a history of chronic lung disease or smoking. A careful history and physical examination should help direct the diagnostic evaluation or empiric treatment. By far, the most common causes of chronic cough are postnasal drip, asthma, and gastroesophageal reflux. These three diagnoses account for >90% of the causes identified in most series, so a reasonable approach to treatment of chronic cough is empiric treatment for these conditions (SOE=C). Combinations of these conditions may contribute to an individual's cough, and treatment for multiple causes may be warranted when single therapies are ineffective. In older adults, the possibility of silent aspiration also needs to be considered, especially in patients with frequent pneumonias or neurologic deficits or who live in extended-care facilities. In these cases, videofluoroscopy (modified barium swallow) can evaluate oropharyngeal and esophageal aspiration. Fiberoptic endoscopic evaluation of swallowing can also be used to evaluate swallowing problems in the pharyngeal or laryngeal areas and can be performed at the bedside. For additional, less common yet important differential diagnostic considerations of cough in older adults, see Table 49.1.

Wheezing

Although asthma is a common cause of wheezing in all age groups, it is not the principal cause in older adults, particularly if it is not associated with cough or dyspnea. Wheezing in older adults is more commonly caused by COPD or heart failure. ("Cardiac asthma" refers to wheezing arising from heart failure.) Other common causes of wheezing include postnasal drip and uncontrolled gastroesophageal reflux disease.

Table 49.2—Example of an Asthma Action Plan

Green zone: Doing well	Patient Action
No cough, wheeze, chest tightness, or shortness of breath during day or night Can do usual activities *Peak flow:* ≥80% of my best peak flow	Take these long-term medications as prescribed: Medicine 1: how much, when to take it Medicine 2: how much, when to take it
Yellow zone: Getting worse	**Patient Action**
Cough, wheeze, chest tightness, or shortness of breath, *or* Waking at night due to asthma, *or* Can do some, but not all, usual activities *Peak flow:* 50%–79% of my best peak flow	Keep taking your Green zone medications and add quick-relief medication (a short-acting β_2-agonist). If your symptoms return to Green zone after 1 hour of above treatment, continue monitoring. If your symptoms do *not* return to Green zone after 1 hour of treatment, take another dose of the short-acting β_2-agonist and add oral steroid.
Red zone: Medical alert	**Patient Action**
Very short of breath, *or* Quick-relief medications have not helped, *or* Cannot do usual activities, *or* Symptoms are the same or get worse after 24 hours in the Yellow zone *Peak flow:* <50% of my best peak flow	Take a short-acting β_2-agonist and oral steroid. Then call your doctor *now*. Go to the hospital or call an ambulance if you are still in the Red zone after 15 minutes *and* you have not reached your doctor.

MAJOR PULMONARY DISEASES

Asthma

Following childhood, the prevalence of asthma peaks again after the age of 65 years (late-onset asthma); 5%–10% of older adults meet criteria for airway obstruction and bronchial hyperreactivity, particularly in nonsmokers. Atopy and obesity are common in older adults with long-standing asthma. Asthma deaths in older adults account for >50% of asthma fatalities annually, and older adults with the disease have a 5-fold greater overall mortality than younger adults. This is likely due to reduced awareness of bronchial constriction on the part of the older adults (with attendant delays in seeking medical attention), as well as underrecognition and undertreatment on the part of clinicians. Asthma significantly affects the quality of life of many older adults.

Population studies of asthma in older adults have shown that, unlike younger adults, who may need only symptomatic treatment, most older adults require continual treatment programs to control their disease (SOE=B). Overall, however, the principles of asthma management do not differ between older and younger people. Inhaled corticosteroids (or other controller drugs such as leukotriene-receptor antagonists) are the mainstay of therapy in both older and younger patients. The lowest effective dosage should be prescribed, and a spacer and counseling on rinsing of the oropharynx are important to avoid thrush. Oral corticosteroids are discussed under COPD (see below). The bronchodilator response to inhaled β-agonists decreases with age, but β-agonists are still the mainstay as-needed reliever medication for asthma treatment. The potential for adverse events of β-agonists (eg, hypokalemia or possible QT prolongation in cardiac patients on digoxin or other medications) warrants adequate controller drug use in older asthmatic patients to minimize overreliance on the β-agonist. Use of long-acting β-agonists is helpful for long-term maintenance therapy and nocturnal symptoms. Anticholinergics can be considered in those who cannot tolerate β-agonists. In older adults, use of theophylline is fraught with adverse events and drug interactions; therefore, theophylline should be considered a third-line medication. It should be prescribed for use only once daily in the evening, for severe asthma or COPD, with a target serum level of 5–15 mg/L if tolerated.

In addition to pharmacologic treatment, asthma "action plans" should be developed and addressed in the event of worsening pulmonary symptoms. For an example of an asthma action plan, see Table 49.2. Patients should keep a copy of such a plan in a convenient location for easy reference.

Asthma and Allergic Disease Treatment

Patients with asthma frequently experience allergies that can exacerbate their airway symptoms. Conversely, patients with rhinosinusitis are also at increased risk of developing airway disease such as asthma. These observations have led to the "one airway" hypothesis, which proposes treating asthma and allergic rhinosinusitis as disease entities that coexist on the same spectrum. Thus, treatment of asthma and allergy can be approached in concert. Specifically, identification and avoidance of allergic triggers is paramount in allergic asthma control. Aspirin sensitivity should be considered in patients who are receiving aspirin for primary or secondary prevention of coronary artery disease. For patients who require long-

Table 49.3—GOLD[a] Guidelines for COPD

Key Factors for Considering a Diagnosis of COPD

Dyspnea	Progressive over time Worse with exercise Persistent (present daily) Described as "increased effort to breathe," "heaviness," "air hunger," "gasping"
Chronic cough	May be intermittent and nonproductive
Sputum production	Any pattern of chronic sputum production can indicate COPD
Risk factors	Tobacco smoke Occupational dusts and chemicals Smoke from home cooking and heating fuel Family history, genetic variant (α-1 antitrypsin deficiency)

Spirometric Classification of Airflow Obstruction in COPD (Post-Bronchodilator FEV_1)
$FEV_1/FVC < 70\%$[b] applies to each category

Mild	$FEV_1 \geq 80\%$ predicted
Moderate	$50\% \leq FEV_1 < 80\%$ predicted
Severe	$30\% \leq FEV_1 < 50\%$ predicted
Very severe	$FEV_1 < 30\%$ predicted or $FEV_1 < 50\%$ predicted and chronic respiratory failure[c]

NOTE: FEV_1 = forced expiratory volume in 1 sec; FVC = forced vital capacity
[a] GOLD=Global Initiative for Chronic Obstructive Lung Disease
[b] Using the criteria $FEV_1/FVC < 70\%$ may overdiagnose COPD in older, nonsmoking adults; some experts recommend using as the lower limit of normal the 5th percentile of the normal distribution of the FEV_1/FVC ratio for the reference (older) population. The Global Lung Initiative recommends using this 5th percentile value as the cutoff. Most recent GOLD recommendations for COPD diagnosis and severity assessment are to use a combination of spirometric classification, symptoms, and exacerbation history.
[c] Chronic respiratory failure entails the need for chronic invasive or noninvasive ventilator support.

term aspirin treatment, aspirin desensitization may be necessary. Intranasal as well as inhaled glucocorticoids should be considered to control asthma symptoms. Oral antihistamines and leukotriene inhibitors can also reduce asthma symptoms for patients with concurrent allergic rhinosinusitis. For patients with more severe asthma and IgE levels between 30 and 700 IU/mL, omalizumab has been shown to have efficacy in older adults similar to that in younger adults in improving lung function and asthma symptoms, reducing asthma exacerbations and emergency department visits. However, anti-IgE therapies were discontinued more frequently in older adults than in younger adults.

Chronic Obstructive Pulmonary Disease

COPD is estimated to affect 12.7–14.7 million adults in the United States, based on responses to the National Health Interview Survey and the Behavioral Risk Factor Surveillance System. COPD is the third most common cause of death after heart disease and cancer. The prevalence of COPD in adults ≥75 years old is at least 10%. Both the prevalence of COPD and its mortality are increasing, especially in older adults. Episodes of acute respiratory failure that require mechanical ventilation are associated with mortality rates ranging from 11% to 46%. The National Heart, Lung and Blood Institute estimate that annual direct costs of COPD/asthma exceed $50 billion, with $20 billion required for prescription medications and $13 billion spent on inpatient hospitalizations. COPD is a leading cause of hospitalization in the United States; it accounts for about 20% of the total hospitalizations for patients 65–75 years old and 18% for patients >75 years old. In one study, patients >65 years old who were admitted to an ICU with COPD had a hospital mortality of 30% and a 1-year mortality of 59%.

Airflow limitation is a key feature of COPD, yet no single item or combination of items from the history and clinical examination can exclude it. For criteria often used to make the diagnosis of COPD, see Table 49.3. Because the FEV_1/FVC ratio decreases with age, using a fixed ratio to separate normal from obstructive creates a risk of over-diagnosis of COPD in older adults. Up to one-fifth of current smokers and one-seventh of individuals >50 years old who have never smoked can be misidentified as abnormal when a fixed cut-off is used. Other approaches to staging severity of COPD include using the lower limit of normal based on survey-derived airflow measurements or distribution of Z-scores, similar to the strategies used in measuring bone mineral density or pediatric growth charts. The most recent recommendations for diagnosing COPD from the Global Initiative for Chronic Obstructive Lung Disease (GOLD) are to use the combined "ABCD" assessment approach. The ABCD assessment includes spirometric assessment of airflow obstruction (FEV_1), respiratory symptoms using validated dyspnea scales, and exacerbation history including frequency of hospitalization. Disease severity is then ranked from least (A) to most (D) severe.

Table 49.4—Inhaled Bronchodilators and Corticosteroids for COPD

Class	Medications	Duration (hours)	Dosage
Short-acting			
β₂-Agonists	Albuterol sulfate, levalbuterol, pirbuterol	4–6	2 puffs q6h
Anticholinergic	Ipratropium bromide	4–6	2 puffs q6h
Long-acting			
β₂-Agonists	Formoterol fumarate, salmeterol xinafoate	8–12	1 puff q12h
	Arformoterol	8–12	15 mcg nebulized q12h
	Indacaterol maleate	24	1 puff q24h
	Olodaterol	24	2 puffs q24h
	Vilanterol	24	1 puff q24h
Anticholinergic	Tiotropium bromide	>24	1 puff q24h
	Aclidinium	12	1 puff q12h
	Umeclidinium	24	1 puff q24h
	Glycopyrrolate	12	Inhale contents of 1 capsule q12h
Inhaled corticosteroid	Beclomethasone diproprionate	12	1 or 2 puffs q12h
	Fluticasone[OL]	12	1 or 2 puffs q12h[a]
	Budesonide[OL]	12	Nebulized, or 2 puffs q12h
	Mometasone furoate	24	1 or 2 puffs q24h

[OL] Off-label when used alone (not as a component of a combination product) for treatment of COPD.
[a] Also available in diskus form in 3 strengths, dosed 1 puff q12h.

Current guidelines recommend against screening asymptomatic older adults for COPD. In smokers, chronic cough is the most commonly reported symptom associated with COPD diagnosis. Wheezing noted on physical examination is the most potent predictor of airflow limitation; individuals with obstructive airflow limitation are 36 times more likely to have wheezing than those without this problem. Other findings associated with an increased likelihood of airflow limitation include a barrel-shaped chest, hyperresonance on percussion, and a forced expiratory time of >9 seconds measured during a clinical bedside examination.

Smoking cessation at any age slows the decline in lung function, and aggressive cessation efforts are appropriate even in the oldest patients. The "Five A's" method, from the Agency for Health Care Policy and Research, is a commonly used approach for addressing smoking cessation:

- Ask patients about use of tobacco at every office visit.
- Advise patients to quit.
- Assess readiness to quit.
- Assist patients in the quit attempt with aids such as a local cessation program and pharmacologic agents such as bupropion, nicotine replacement, or varenicline.
- Arrange both a quit date and a follow-up visit or contact to discuss the quit attempt.

The chief components of daily medication therapy in COPD consist of a β-agonist, ipratropium bromide or a long-acting anticholinergic medication (tiotropium, umeclidinium, aclidinium), or both in combination (Table 49.4 and Table 49.5). For more severe disease, the use of the long-acting anticholinergic tiotropium with albuterol-only rescue inhalers or long-acting β-agonists such as salmeterol can achieve long-term control. Symptoms can be controlled in some patients with monotherapy, potentially improving long-term adherence by reducing the number of maintenance inhalers by one. Concern has been raised over risk of cardiovascular events associated with anticholinergic medications, although in a randomized controlled trial of 6,000 patients with COPD, tiotropium use was associated with decreased cardiovascular events compared with treatment with β-agonists, inhaled corticosteroids, and/or theophylline. Use of inhaled corticosteroids has been associated with some improvement in airway reactivity, frequency of exacerbations, and respiratory symptoms, but they have not been shown to impact the rate of decline in lung function (SOE=A). Combination therapy with inhaled corticosteroids and a long-acting β-agonist has been associated with better lung function and symptom control but not survival benefit. A landmark investigation documented that use of systemic corticosteroids (intravenous followed by oral) reduces

Table 49.5—COPD Therapy[a]

Class	Treatment
Mild COPD	
$FEV_1 \geq 80\%$	Short-acting β_2-agonist or combination of short-acting β_2-agonist and anticholinergic, prn Smoking cessation
Moderate COPD	
$50\% \leq FEV_1 < 80\%$	Long-acting β_2-agonist or anticholinergic if needed for added benefit or if ≥2 exacerbations per year Smoking cessation Rehabilitation
Severe COPD	
$30\% \leq FEV_1 < 50\%$	Regular treatment with one or more bronchodilators[b], preferably long-acting β_2-agonist or anticholinergic Inhaled steroids[c] if significant symptomatic and PFT response or if ≥2 exacerbations per year Smoking cessation Rehabilitation
Very severe COPD	
$FEV_1 < 30\%$ or	Regular treatment with one or more bronchodilators[b], preferably long-acting β_2-agonist or anticholinergic (Consider adding a phosphodiesterase-4 inhibitor, eg, roflumilast, if chronic bronchitis or frequent exacerbations.)
$FEV_1 < 50\%$ plus chronic respiratory failure[d]	Inhaled steroids[c] if significant symptomatic and PFT response or if repeated exacerbations Smoking cessation Treatment of complications Long-term oxygen therapy if respiratory failure
COPD exacerbation	
(acute increase in breathlessness, wheezing, cough, and sputum beyond normal day-to-day variation and leads to change in medication)	Increase dosage and/or frequency of β_2-agonists with or without anticholinergics. Use spacers or nebulizers for improved medication delivery. Add steroid (eg, oral prednisolone 30–40 mg/d for 5 days). Add antibiotics if increased sputum volume, increased purulence, and/or increased dyspnea or requiring mechanical ventilation (for specific agents, consider local bacterial resistance patterns and/or patient's prior sputum culture results). Serum procalcitonin–based protocols to guide antibiotic prescription may reduce antibiotic use without affecting outcomes, including mortality, but require further study. Supplemental oxygen (target saturation 88%–92%), monitor arterial blood gas CBC, chest radiograph, ECG *Indications for noninvasive mechanical ventilation:* severe dyspnea (respiratory accessory muscle use, paradoxical motion of abdomen, intercostal space retraction), respiratory rate ≥25 breaths/min, arterial pH ≤7.35, or pCO_2 >45 mmHg *Indications for invasive mechanical ventilation:* unable to tolerate noninvasive (with or without hypoxemia), respiratory or cardiac arrest, loss of consciousness, gasping for air, massive aspiration, inability to clear respiratory secretions, severe hemodynamic instability, life-threatening ventricular arrhythmias

NOTE: PFT = pulmonary function test
[a] $FEV_1/FVC < 70\%$ for all levels of severity
[b] β_2-agonists, ipratropium, slow-release theophylline (caution in older adults with other conditions and taking other medications). Inhaled bronchodilators are preferred over oral because of efficacy and adverse effects. Avoid inhaled anticholinergics (ipratropium, tiotropium) in men with lower urinary tract obstructive symptoms.
[c] Consider osteoporosis prophylaxis.
[d] Chronic respiratory failure entails the need for chronic invasive or noninvasive ventilator support.
SOURCE: Data from *Global Initiative for Chronic Obstructive Lung Disease (GOLD)*; 2017. www.goldcopd.org (accessed Feb 2019).

the duration and recurrence of acute exacerbations of COPD for up to 6 months (SOE=A). Importantly, there is no benefit to a course of systemic steroids for >14 days for acute exacerbation of COPD.

A subset of patients with recalcitrant COPD experience frequent exacerbations or persistent symptoms despite the use of maximal inhaler therapy, and they may benefit from trial of additional treatments. Phosphodiesterase-4 inhibitors, such as roflumilast, have been shown to reduce exacerbations and improve quality of life when used as adjuvant therapy in patients with severe COPD. Prophylactic antibiotics may reduce exacerbation frequency but carry substantial risk of increasing bacterial drug resistance or secondary infections such as *Clostridium difficile* diarrhea. Theophylline may also be considered in patients with refractory COPD but should be used cautiously. Chronic systemic steroids are required for relatively few patients (5%–10%). The risks of peptic ulcer disease, hypertension, cataracts, diabetes mellitus, osteoporosis, psychosis, poor wound healing, infections, and aseptic necrosis of the hip must be carefully considered in these patients. Appropriate preventive measures should be taken in circumstances of prolonged use, such as monitoring for signs of osteopenia or osteoporosis; using the lowest possible dosage of corticosteroids; and using supplemental vitamin D, calcium, and perhaps a bisphosphonate for those at risk of osteoporosis. Patients with frequent exacerbations may benefit from prescription of a "rescue pack" composed of a 5-day supply of systemic corticosteroid with antibiotic, allowing for ready access to treatment at any time.

Long-term oxygen therapy benefits patients who have a resting PaO_2 of ≤55 mmHg on ambient air (SOE=A). Use of oxygen for at least 15 hours per day improves survival, exercise tolerance, sleep, and cognitive function. Other possible beneficial interventions in older adults with COPD include pulmonary rehabilitation via exercise training, and respiratory therapy and education. Home-based, self-administered exercise and strength-building programs may also have a role in pulmonary rehabilitation of older adults with COPD. Both major depressive disorder and anxiety are present in up to 40% of patients with COPD; these diagnoses should be screened for and treated appropriately. In older adults, anxiety is associated with diminished physical functioning and is a major predictor of emergency department visits and hospitalization. Pulmonary rehabilitation can improve respiratory function, as well as relieve depression and anxiety in patients with refractory COPD. By stimulating nasopharyngeal mechanoreceptors, a stream of air from an electric fan can help to relieve dyspnea in patients with refractory symptoms. When dyspnea persists despite these measures and maximal bronchodilator therapy, low-dose oral opiates can be used. Careful monitoring must accompany this treatment with attention to somnolence, neuropsychiatric adverse effects, and constipation.

Paramount to the care of older adults with asthma or COPD is adequate instruction in proper use of peak expiratory flow meters and inhalers. Neurologic, muscular, and arthritic diseases in older adults can lead to suboptimal timing and lack of coordination in proper use of inhaler devices. Only 60% of older adults have been reported to show adequate technique with a metered-dose inhaler; this proportion decreases to 36% when objective criteria are used. Although the use of spacers improves technique, 85% of older adults do not use the spacer when it is prescribed. Breath-activated dry-powder inhalers demand less coordination but require a certain minimal peak inspiratory flow for adequate drug delivery. The clinician should observe the patient actually using the inhaler; pharmacists may provide instruction in inhaler technique as well. Cost is another additional barrier to adherence in over one-quarter of patients with COPD, particularly when out-of-pocket costs exceed $20.

Patients with advanced-stage COPD and recalcitrant dyspnea may benefit from referral to palliative care. Characteristics of patients who may satisfy hospice prognostic criteria are dyspnea, hypoxemia despite supplemental oxygen, weight loss, poor functional status, and disease progression (manifested by repeated emergency department visits or hospitalizations).

Obstructive Sleep Apnea

Sleep-related breathing disorders are very common in older adults, and obstructive sleep apnea (OSA) is the most frequent. OSA is more common in men in both older and younger patients. The estimated prevalence of OSA in older men ranges from 13% to 28% and in women from 4% to 20%. Age-related changes of respiratory anatomy and physiology, such as increased deposition of adipose tissue in the upper airway and pharyngeal bony changes, may predispose older adults to sleep apnea. Body habitus as a risk factor for apnea is less important in older patients than in younger patients. In the Heart Health Study, although the overall prevalence of OSA did not differ by racial group, black women were significantly younger than white women at time of diagnosis. Black patients with OSA are more obese and have higher rates of hypertension than white patients with OSA. Medications, alcohol consumption, and abnormal upper airway configuration are additional risk factors for OSA, with the latter issue particularly relevant in older adults. OSA has been associated with cerebrovascular accidents, myocardial infarctions, and a 3-fold increase in mortality (SOE=B). Untreated OSA is associated with significant cognitive impairment, including executive dysfunction, as well as depression in older patients. Most patients with OSA remain undiagnosed and therefore do not receive treatment for this life-threatening, yet potentially treatable disease. Clinicians should consider the diagnosis in patients who have complaints of daytime somnolence, frequent daytime napping, or drowsiness while driving. A history of snoring or witnessed apneas or hypopneas by a bed partner should also prompt further evaluation. Treatment options include addressing upper-airway obstruction via weight loss, avoiding alcohol and sedatives, sleeping on one's side or upright, correcting metabolic disorders such as hypothyroidism, and using continuous positive-airway pressure (CPAP) via a nasal mask. To increase adherence to the use of CPAP, the treatment can be ordered with "nasal pillows" to increase comfort, and "ramping technique" to give a delayed rise in the applied pressure after the individual has fallen asleep. Electronic monitoring chips can be used to determine appropriate pressure settings and overall compliance with the CPAP machine. Diagnosis and treatment issues are generally the same for both young and old, and the major consideration for the primary clinician is to maintain a high index of suspicion for this disease.

Idiopathic Pulmonary Fibrosis

Among older adults, idiopathic pulmonary fibrosis (IPF) is the most common of the >100 causes of interstitial lung diseases. It has a mean age of onset of 55 years and is increasing in prevalence with the aging population. The disease shows a relentless progression; median survival is 3–5 years. Survival is even worse in patients with both IPF and pulmonary hypertension. Disease presentation is normally one of insidious dyspnea (often unrecognized because of a decrease in the patient's activity level) and nonproductive cough, with dry inspiratory rales on examination. Clubbing is often a prominent finding on physical examination in IPF (40%–70%), as opposed to emphysema, which rarely causes clubbing. (Discovery of clubbing in an emphysematous patient should prompt a search for another disease, such as occult lung cancer.) Older adults often present with advanced disease because of the insidious onset of symptoms. IPF should be considered in older adults with a restrictive ventilatory defect or a reduced diffusing capacity on pulmonary function testing, or both. Chest radiographs often show reticular opacities in the mid and lower lung zones. High-resolution CT scans show characteristic areas of subpleural reticulation and honeycombing. Experienced pulmonologists and radiologists can often make the diagnosis based on clinical and radiographic findings.

In the past, oral corticosteroids (dosed at 0.5 mg/kg/d for 3–6 months) had been commonly used as initial therapy, but only 10%–20% of patients respond to these agents and adverse events are common. High-dose steroids are commonly used for acute exacerbations, although data supporting their use are lacking. Combination therapy with oral corticosteroids, azathioprine, and N-acetylcysteine had been used for several years, but recent trials showed that mortality, hospitalizations, and adverse events were higher in those treated with this combination. However, although there currently is no medical cure for IPF, there have been some promising therapeutic discoveries. Treatment of patients with mild to moderate IPF with pirfenidone or nintedanib significantly reduced disease progression compared with placebo; pirfenidone may reduce mortality. Although older age was not a specific focus in this research, the mean age of patients enrolled in these trials was 66–68 years. GI adverse effects (nausea, diarrhea, increased liver function tests) were the most common adverse drug-related events in trials of these drugs. In patients with IPF and pulmonary hypertension, a therapeutic trial of sildenafil may be reasonable in patients without contraindications. Treatment of GI reflux disease may also slow progression of disease.

Lung transplantation is the only treatment for end-stage IPF. However, risks associated with transplantation need to be carefully considered, especially in patients ≥65 years old whose survival after the surgery is lower than that of younger patients. With the advent of new treatment options for IPF, early referral to a subspecialist experienced in fibrotic lung diseases may be warranted. The primary care provider may initiate the evaluation by obtaining a detailed history and searching for evidence of chemical exposure, smoking, asbestosis, connective tissue syndromes, chronic aspiration, or a family history of lung diseases. Chest CT and pulmonary function tests are helpful in guiding subsequent management decisions. Patients with advanced disease may benefit from a palliative care approach, although these referrals often occur only days before death for most patients with IPF. Earlier involvement of palliative services may benefit these patients.

Ventilatory Disorders

A variety of disorders affecting the bellows function of the respiratory system can affect older adults. Common causes of hypoventilation are neurologic diseases (motor neuron disease, quadriplegia, Guillain-Barré syndrome, myasthenia gravis), bilateral diaphragmatic paralysis, morbid obesity, kyphoscoliosis, and severe abdominal ascites. Certain restrictive lung disorders (in addition to IPF, described above) may impair ventilation as well, such as lymphangitic carcinomatosis, rheumatoid lung disease, silicosis, severe sarcoidosis, or drug- or radiation-induced lung injury.

Patients with ventilatory disorders may experience daytime hypercapnia with somnolence, or, particularly with restrictive lung diseases, dyspnea with exertion. Treatments for ventilatory disorders generally include strategies to reduce the work of breathing (eg, weight loss in obese patients), supplemental oxygen, and assisted ventilation.

Venous Thromboembolic Disease

The incidence of venous thromboembolism (VTE), including deep venous thrombosis (DVT) and pulmonary embolism (PE), increases in older adults because of age-related risk factors, including changes in the hemostatic system that predispose to thrombosis; venous stasis related to illness, injuries (eg, hip fracture), and immobility (especially hospitalization and residence in long-term care); incompetence of the superficial and deep veins, including failure of the venous valves; and the high prevalence of systemic illnesses associated with thrombogenesis (eg, heart failure, cancer, neurologic diseases). Established risk factors for VTE include age

>60 years, indwelling central venous catheters, surgery, trauma, chronic lung disease, dehydration, history of VTE, having a first-degree relative with VTE, increased fibrinogen level, activated protein-C resistance due to factor-V Leiden gene mutation, inflammatory bowel disease, obesity, rheumatoid arthritis, or treatment with various medications (aromatase inhibitors, hormone replacement therapy, megestrol acetate, selective estrogen-receptor modulators, or erythroid-stimulating agents with hemoglobin concentration >12 g/dL). The incidence of PE triples between the ages of 65 and 90 years and has a reported 10% recurrence rate within 1 year. Age >70 years has been independently associated with missed antemortem diagnosis of PE.

Symptoms and signs of VTE are similar in older and younger patients, but it is important to recognize that most patients with DVT or PE, or both, are asymptomatic; therefore, a high index of suspicion for these conditions must be maintained, particularly in hospitalized patients and in residents of transitional-care facilities and nursing homes. Physical examination findings of DVT include limb pain, tenderness, warmth, and edema. The clinical diagnosis of venous thrombosis is generally insufficiently accurate to exclude additional testing, because the signs and symptoms are nonspecific. The utility of most routine tests, including blood tests, arterial blood gases, chest radiographs, ECGs, and echocardiography for diagnosing VTE is quite low, and the presence of "normal" findings on each of these tests does not exclude a diagnosis of DVT or PE. The plasma d-dimer level, when performed using ELISA, has a high sensitivity for VTE but very low specificity in older adults; therefore, a normal d-dimer level in an older patient with low clinical suspicion for VTE essentially excludes the diagnosis. The upper limit of normal for d-dimer increases with age and can be estimated (in ng/mL) by multiplying age (in years) by 10. Increased d-dimer levels are common in older and hospitalized patients, particularly after surgery or in those who have been diagnosed with malignancy or renal insufficiency. Serum brain natriuretic peptide (BNP) and troponin are not sensitive or specific for PE but can inform risk stratification for patients with suspected PE.

Noninvasive tests for DVT include upper and lower extremity venous Doppler examinations, impedance plethysmography, and CT of the legs; rarely, contrast venography may be required to establish the diagnosis. When positive, noninvasive tests provide presumptive evidence for VTE, but negative tests do not exclude DVT or PE, especially in patients for whom the clinical suspicion is high. Similarly, ventilation/perfusion lung scanning and spiral CT of the chest are useful when the findings are unequivocally normal or abnormal. However, indeterminate ventilation/perfusion scans are common in older patients, and 2%–10% of patients with PE have false-negative spiral CT scans, depending on whether multidetector or single-detector scanners are used. Therefore, in patients in whom clinical suspicion of PE is high but noninvasive evaluations (which might include lower extremity ultrasound studies) are negative, pulmonary angiography should be performed as the definitive diagnostic procedure. Although clinicians are often reluctant to recommend pulmonary angiography, data from the PIOPED study indicate that this procedure is generally well tolerated by older adults and that the risks of the procedure are lower than those of either empiric anticoagulation in patients without PE or failing to anticoagulate patients with PE. Magnetic resonance pulmonary angiography is reserved for patients who cannot undergo spiral ventilation/perfusion scans or CT scans for PE evaluation. However, the sensitivity and specificity of these scans are limited, especially for subsegmental emboli; thus, scan results should not be used to exclude PE if clinical suspicion is high.

Anticoagulants are central to VTE therapy, and their use is generally guided by the same principles for patients of any age. Because of reduced cardiopulmonary reserve in older patients, achieving satisfactory anticoagulation quickly may be particularly urgent to avoid major adverse hemodynamic or oxygenation defects. The trend toward increased use of low-molecular-weight heparin preparations for outpatients, while achieving anticoagulation with warfarin, is supported by large, well-designed randomized controlled trials (SOE=A). Weight-adjusted dosage of low-molecular-weight heparin can be safely used in older patients, except for those weighing <45 kg. Full-dose low-molecular-weight heparin adjusted for weight and renal function, subcutaneous fondaparinux adjusted for weight and renal function, and intravenous unfractionated heparin to maintain the activated partial thromboplastin time in the range of 50–70 seconds (1.5–2 times the control value) have been the mainstay of initial therapy (SOE=A for all). Because of risk of hemorrhage and mortality, unfractionated heparin is less favorable than low-molecular-weight heparin and fondaparinux. The oral factor Xa inhibitors apixaban, rivaroxaban, and edoxaban may also be used for initial therapy of VTE.

Long-term therapy for VTE may include warfarin, low-molecular-weight heparin, apixaban, rivaroxaban, edoxaban, or the direct thrombin inhibitor dabigatran. If warfarin is chosen, administration may begin on the same day as the initial (fast-acting) anticoagulant. The initial anticoagulant (eg, low-molecular-weight heparin) should be used for at least 5 days, which should include 1–3 days of overlap with warfarin while the INR is therapeutic. For patients with VTE and malignancy who do not have abnormalities in kidney function or contraindications to anticoagulation, clinical practice guidelines recommend low-molecular-weight heparin as both initial and chronic therapy for at least 6 months. Patients who are not candidates for anticoagulation should be considered for an inferior vena cava filter, recognizing that such devices reduce the risk of PE but may increase the risk of recurrent DVT and post-phlebitic syndrome.

Factor Xa inhibitors and direct thrombin inhibitors do not require routine blood work (ie, INR monitoring) and, unlike warfarin, do not require prolonged bridging therapy before becoming effective. Until recently, these agents did not have specific antidotes to treat significant and life-threatening bleeding events, leaving providers to consider expert opinion for the use of prothrombin complex concentrates for this purpose. However, idarucizumab, an antibody fragment, has been shown to rapidly reverse the anticoagulant effects of dabigatran, with the effect evident within minutes and potentially lasting up to 24 hours. Andexanet is the antidote for apixiban and rivaroxaban. It has a rapid onset.

Long-term anticoagulation (≥6 months) is preferred to shorter term (eg, 3 months) unless there are increased risks of bleeding. Patients with multiple ongoing risk factors for pulmonary thromboembolic disease may be considered for anticoagulation therapy for up to 2 years or longer. Recurrent pulmonary thromboembolism is usually treated with lifelong anticoagulation therapy (SOE=C). In addition to the above measures, regular exercise, such as walking, is recommended to reduce the risk of recurrent DVT.

VTE prophylaxis with subcutaneous unfractionated or low-molecular-weight heparin, fondaparinux, or intermittent pneumatic compression of the calves is indicated in all hospitalized older adults who are not fully ambulatory, as well as in transitional care and long-term care residents at increased risk of VTE.

RESOURCES

- Lavorini F, Mannini C, Chellini E, et al. Optimizing pharmacotherapy for elderly patients with chronic obstructive pulmonary disease: importance of delivery devices. *Drugs Aging*. 2016;33(7):461–473.

- Skloot GS, Busse PJ, Braman SS, et al. An official American Thoracic Society Workshop report: Evaluation and Management of Asthma in the Elderly. *Ann Am Thorac Soc*. 2016;13(11):2064–2077.

CHAPTER 50—CARDIOVASCULAR DISEASE

KEY POINTS

- Increasing age is associated with extensive changes throughout the cardiovascular system that lead to a progressive decline in cardiovascular reserve capacity and to substantive alterations in the clinical presentation, response to therapy, and prognosis of cardiovascular disease in older adults.

- Older adults account for the majority of patients hospitalized with acute coronary syndromes (ACS), and approximately 80% of deaths attributable to ACS occur in patients ≥65 years old. Although the benefits of current treatments for ACS are generally similar in older and younger patients, older patients are at increased risk of major complications from therapeutic interventions.

- Atrial fibrillation (AF), the most common sustained dysrhythmia in clinical practice, increases in prevalence with age, and >50% of all patients with AF are ≥75 years old. Most older adults with AF respond to rate-control medications in conjunction with antithrombotic therapy, but some patients require antiarrhythmic drug therapy or other intervention to maintain sinus rhythm and alleviate symptoms.

- Calcific aortic stenosis (AS) is the most common valve disorder requiring intervention in older adults. Surgical aortic valve replacement (SAVR) is the primary treatment for AS in healthier older adults, while transcatheter aortic valve replacement (TAVR) is an effective alternative to SAVR in older adults at intermediate or high risk of surgery because of comorbidity, frailty, or other factors.

- The prevalence of peripheral arterial disease (PAD) increases progressively with age, and the presence of PAD is often predictive of concomitant coronary artery and cerebrovascular disease. Management of patients with PAD should therefore include appropriate treatment of hypertension, dyslipidemia, diabetes, and tobacco abuse in accordance with existing practice guidelines.

Note: Heart failure, hypertension, and cerebrovascular disease have dedicated chapters elsewhere in the *Geriatrics Review Syllabus*.

EPIDEMIOLOGY

The prevalence of cardiovascular disease (CVD) increases progressively with age, exceeding 80% in both men and women >80 years old (Table 50.1). Because of the high prevalence of CVD in older age, adults ≥65 years old account for 71% of hospitalizations for CVD in the United States, including more than 50% of percutaneous and surgical coronary revascularization procedures, 60% of defibrillator implantations, 71% of arterial endarterectomies, and 82% of permanent pacemaker insertions.

Over the past 50 years, lifestyle changes and medical advances have led to a progressive decline in age-adjusted mortality rates from CVD. Nevertheless, CVD remains the leading cause of death in the United States, accounting for approximately 31% of all deaths in 2013. Notably, cancer is the leading cause of death among adults up to age 75, and it is only after age 75 that CVD becomes the dominant cause of death. Thus, among 800,937 deaths in the United States from CVD in 2013, 81% occurred in adults ≥65 years old and 65% occurred in those ≥75 years old. Mortality rates from CVD are higher in men than in women at all ages, but women account for more than 50% of CVD deaths among adults ≥65 years old. CVD mortality rates are highest in black Americans, followed by non-Hispanic whites, Hispanic Americans, Native Americans, and Asians/Pacific Islanders. With the aging of the population, it may be anticipated that the absolute number of cardiovascular deaths in older adults will increase markedly over the next several decades.

EFFECTS OF AGING ON CARDIOVASCULAR FUNCTION

Normal aging is associated with diverse changes throughout the cardiovascular system (Table 50.2), and these changes are accentuated by common comorbid conditions, particularly hypertension, diabetes, obesity, and atherosclerosis.

Age-related changes in other organ systems have important implications for diagnosis and treatment of cardiovascular disorders in older adults. These changes interact with the cardiovascular system to substantially alter the clinical features, response to therapy, and prognosis of older adults with prevalent cardiovascular diseases.

CARDIOVASCULAR RISK FACTORS

In general, the 4 major modifiable risk factors for cardiovascular disease—hypertension, diabetes mellitus, dyslipidemia, and smoking— exert significant influence on cardiovascular risk, even in older adults. In addition, because the incidence and prevalence of cardiovascular diseases are higher in older than in younger individuals, the absolute number of cases attributable to a given risk factor tends to increase with age. Moreover, because the prevalence of hypertension, diabetes mellitus, and dyslipidemia all increase with age, older adults are more likely to have multiple risk factors that act in concert with age-related cardiovascular changes to promote development and progression of heart and vascular disorders.

Hypertension

Pulse pressure (the difference between systolic and diastolic blood pressure) increases with age, and isolated systolic hypertension is the dominant form of hypertension in older adults. Increased systolic blood pressure has been identified as the strongest risk factor for incident cardiovascular disease in older adults, including those >80 years old (SOE=A). While there is continued debate over optimal blood pressure targets in older adults, the SPRINT trial demonstrated a reduction in the risk of major adverse cardiovascular events and all-cause mortality with more intensive systolic blood pressure lowering in patients at increased cardiovascular risk, including those ≥75 years old. The 2017 American College of Cardiology/American Heart Association (ACC/AHA) High Blood Pressure Guidelines recommended pharmacologic therapy in patients with a blood pressure of ≥130/80 mmHg and estimated 10-year atherosclerotic cardiovascular disease risk of ≥10% (using the ACC/AHA pooled cohort equations). This means essentially all patients ≥ 75 years old with blood pressure ≥130/80 warrant therapy, because age confers strong risk in the pooled cohort equations. Decisions on intensity of pharmacologic therapy need to take into account patient goals of care (as acknowledged by the new guidelines), as well as potential adverse effects (common in older adults).

Diabetes Mellitus

The prevalence of diabetes mellitus increases with age, and approximately half of all patients with diabetes in the United States are ≥65 years old. As in younger individuals, the impact of diabetes confers a significant risk of cardiovascular disease in older patients (approximately doubling the general risk of CVD). Notably, the excess risk associated with diabetes in the Framingham Heart Study was greater in both men and women >65 years old than in younger individuals. Despite the association of diabetes with cardiovascular risk, the AGS has recommended that for older adults with multiple chronic conditions, ADL impairment, or cognitive impairment, more lenient hemoglobin A_{1c} targets (eg, <8%) are reasonable given limited life expectancy and the risk of hypoglycemia with overly aggressive therapies.

Table 50.1—Prevalence (percent of population) of Cardiovascular Disease in Americans by Age and Sex

Age Cohort	Men	Women
20–39 years old	11.9	10.0
40–59 years old	40.5	35.5
60–79 years old	69.1	67.9
≥80 years old	84.7	85.9

SOURCE: Data from NHANES 2009–2012.

Dyslipidemia

Low HDL-cholesterol levels (<40 mg/dL in men, <50 mg/dL in women) and high total cholesterol to HDL-cholesterol ratios (≥5.5 in men, ≥5 in women) are independently associated with coronary events among adults at least up to age 85 years (SOE=A). Clinical trials have demonstrated beneficial effects from LDL-lowering therapy with statins in moderate- and high-risk patients, ie, those with established coronary heart disease, diabetes, or multiple other risk factors up to 85 years of age (SOE=A). More recently, therapy with PCSK-9 inhibitors, in addition to statin therapy, has been shown to reduce the risk of major adverse cardiovascular events in patients with established cardiovascular disease, via lowering of LDL levels to extremely low values. Indeed, the current evidence indicates that in high-risk populations, the risk of cardiovascular events declines with LDL concentration, in accordance with the so-called "LDL hypothesis." To date, however, the benefits of PCSK-9 inhibition have not been tested specifically in older populations. The value of lipid-lowering therapy for primary prevention of cardiovascular disease in older adults, especially those >80–85 years old, remains uncertain.

Smoking

Unlike other risk factors, the prevalence of smoking declines with age, in part because of successful smoking cessation and in part because of premature deaths attributable to smoking. In 2013, the prevalence of smoking was <5% among individuals >85 years old. Nonetheless, smoking remains a strong and independent risk factor for cardiovascular events among older adults, and cessation is associated with substantial reductions in cardiovascular risk.

Other Risk Factors

Obesity is associated with increased cardiovascular risk in young and middle-aged people, in part because of its association with hypertension, diabetes mellitus, and dyslipidemia. The importance of obesity as a cardiovascular risk factor among older adults, especially those >80 years old, is less clear. Indeed, among older

Table 50.2—Principal Effects of Aging on the Cardiovascular System

Age Effect	Clinical Implication
↑ Arterial stiffness	↑ Afterload and systolic blood pressure
↓ Myocardial relaxation and compliance	↑ Risk of diastolic heart failure and atrial fibrillation
↓ Responsiveness to β-adrenergic stimulation	↓ Maximum heart rate and cardiac output; impaired thermoregulation
↓ Sinus node function and conduction velocity in the atrioventricular node and infranodal conduction system	↑ Risk of sick sinus syndrome, atrioventricular block, left anterior fascicular block, and bundle branch block
↓ Endothelium-dependent vasodilation	↑ Demand ischemia and risk of coronary artery disease and peripheral arterial disease
↓ Baroreceptor responsiveness	↑ Risk of orthostatic hypotension, falls, and syncope
↓ Exercise response (↓ maximal heart rate, maximal cardiac output, Vo_2 max, coronary blood flow, peripheral vasodilation)	↓ Exercise capacity and ↑ cardiac complications (ischemia, heart failure, shock, arrhythmias, death) with illness

adults with CAD, heart failure, or renal insufficiency, there is evidence that being overweight or mildly obese (ie, BMI 25–35 kg/m²) exerts a favorable effect on prognosis, while being underweight (BMI <20 kg/m²) confers the highest mortality risk (SOE=B).

Low levels of physical activity are associated with increased risk of cardiovascular and all-cause mortality in people of all ages, and participating in a regular exercise program reduces risk across the age spectrum. Additional benefits of regular exercise include improved functional capacity and quality of life, improved control of other risk factors, and reduced depressive symptoms. Strength and balance training also reduce the risk of falls and fractures in older adults. In the absence of contraindications, older adults with or without CVD should be encouraged to participate in a regular exercise program that includes both aerobic and strengthening activities.

Increased levels of the inflammatory marker C-reactive protein (CRP) are associated with increased risk of incident CAD events and cardiovascular death in older adults, but the clinical utility of CRP in guiding management is undefined, and routine measurement of CRP is not currently recommended.

The utility of assessing coronary artery calcium content by CT scanning is uncertain but appears to be best suited to more precisely risk-stratify patients who are deemed to be at intermediate risk of cardiovascular events by readily available scoring systems, such as the Framingham risk score or the ASCVD score of the ACC. Coronary artery calcium scores increase with age, while the correlation of calcium scores with the severity of clinically significant coronary artery stenoses declines with age. Nonetheless, calcium scores ≥100 (Agatston method) are associated with increased risk of incident coronary events in older adults, and higher scores predict greater risk. Despite this, routine use of CT scans to screen for CAD is not recommended, even in patients with multiple risk factors.

In the Cardiovascular Health Study, several subclinical markers of cardiovascular disease identified individuals at increased risk of subsequent cardiovascular events. These included increased carotid artery intima-media thickness assessed by carotid ultrasonography, increased left ventricular mass by echocardiography, borderline or decreased left ventricular ejection fraction, and decreased ankle-brachial index. As with CT scanning, the clinical use and cost-effectiveness of these measures require further study, but in patients with diabetes or multiple other risk factors, the presence of any of these markers may identify those likely to benefit from more aggressive management (SOE=C).

Pre-frailty and frailty are associated with increased risk of developing CVD, possibly because of the interplay of shared mechanisms, including chronic low-level inflammation and insulin resistance. The presence of frailty is also linked to increased morbidity, functional decline, and mortality in older adults with CVD. In particular, among patients who have suffered a myocardial infarction, there is a significant correlation between frailty and subsequent mortality. Whether interventions aimed at reducing frailty can diminish the risk of CVD and, conversely, whether prevention of CVD can reduce the risk of frailty, remain to be determined.

Coronary Artery Disease

Epidemiology

In the United States, the incidence of nonfatal and fatal CAD has declined markedly over the past 5 decades. Nonetheless, autopsy studies indicate that up to 70% of adults ≥70 years old have significant CAD, defined as ≥50% obstruction of one or more coronary arteries. In men, the prevalence of clinically diagnosed CAD increases from 6.3% in those 40–59 years old, to 19.9% among those 60–79 years old, and 32.2% after age 80; among women, prevalence increases from 5.6% to 9.7% and 18.8% across these age ranges. Notably, the annual incidence of nonfatal myocardial infarction (MI) or fatal coronary heart disease is higher in men than in women up to age 85, but after age 85 the reverse is true. The prevalence of angina pectoris increases with age and exceeds 10% in both men and women >80 years old. The incidence of angina pectoris peaks between the ages of 65 and 84 and decreases modestly thereafter. Of an estimated 700,000–800,000 fatal and nonfatal MIs occurring annually in the United States (excluding silent MIs), approximately two-thirds are in adults ≥65 years old, including more than 40% in those ≥75 years old. The proportion of MIs occurring in women increases progressively with age, exceeding 50% in those ≥75 years old. Mortality after acute MI also increases with age. Up to 80% of MI deaths occur in adults ≥65 years old, and approximately 60% among those ≥75 years old.

ACUTE CORONARY SYNDROMES

The acute coronary syndromes (ACS) comprise unstable angina, non-ST-elevation MI (NSTEMI), and ST-elevation MI (STEMI). Unstable angina and NSTEMI are often considered together, because they are pathophysiologically similar and clinically difficult to distinguish at the time of presentation; the distinction depends on analysis of cardiac biomarker proteins (ie, troponin or creatine kinase).

Presentation

The proportion of patients with ACS who present with chest pain declines with age, especially after age 80, and shortness of breath is the most common initial symptom in patients >80–85 years old. Older ACS patients are more likely than younger patients to present with altered mental status, confusion, dizziness, or syncope. The time from onset of symptoms to initial presentation at a medical facility also tends to be longer in older patients, in part due to the decreased prevalence of chest pain, although other factors likely contribute to delays.

The initial ECG is more likely to be nondiagnostic of ACS in older than in younger patients due to the higher prevalence of prior MI, conduction abnormalities (especially left bundle-branch block), left ventricular hypertrophy, and paced rhythm. In addition, the proportion of ACS associated with ST elevation declines with age, further reducing the diagnostic accuracy of the ECG. Importantly, the combination of presentation delays, altered symptomatology, and nondiagnostic ECGs often results in slowed initiation of treatment, thereby limiting the potential benefits of current therapies and contributing to higher complication rates and worse outcomes.

Therapy

All patients with suspected ACS, regardless of age, should immediately receive aspirin 160–325 mg (SOE=A). Oxygen should be administered to maintain an arterial oxygen saturation of at least 92% (SOE=B), but routine use of oxygen in patients with arterial oxygen saturations >92% is of unproven value and may be harmful (SOE=C). Patients with ongoing chest discomfort should receive intravenous or sublingual nitroglycerin initially, unless there is evidence of potential right ventricular infarction, given the need in that case to assure adequate preload. Intravenous morphine should be used if nitroglycerin is ineffective for controlling chest pain. Patients with ACS can also be started on β-blocker therapy within 24 hours of presentation, although attention should be paid to potential contraindications (ie, bradycardia, hypotension, advanced heart block, moderate or severe heart failure, or active bronchospasm). β-Blocker therapy in the early to intermediate postinfarction period can decrease the risk of malignant ventricular arrhythmias, reduce infarct size, and inhibit myocardial remodeling. However, very early initiation of β-blocker therapy during ACS presentation, particularly in patients who have not yet undergone revascularization, has not been reliably shown to improve outcomes and may increase the risk of development of cardiogenic shock, especially in patients with larger infarct sizes or evidence of heart failure on presentation. Most patients presenting with ACS should also be discharged from the hospital on an ACE inhibitor (or ARB if intolerant to ACE inhibitors), especially those with left ventricular (LV) systolic dysfunction, anterior wall myocardial infarction, heart failure, diabetes mellitus, or hypertension (SOE=A). Aldosterone receptor antagonist therapy has been shown to improve long-term mortality (SOE=A) for patients who are post-MI with left ventricular ejection fraction ≤40% and who have clinical heart failure and/or diabetes. Early administration of high-intensity statin therapy (eg, atorvastatin 80 mg) has been associated with improved outcomes in some but not all studies, and some experts recommend its routine use; data in patients >75–80 years old are, however, very limited (SOE=C).

In addition to aspirin, current Class I recommendations for antithrombotic therapy in patients with ACS include a combination of a P2Y12 inhibitor (clopidogrel 300 mg or 600 mg loading dose followed by 75 mg daily, or ticagrelor 180 mg loading dose followed by 90 mg twice daily) and a parenteral anticoagulant (enoxaparin, unfractionated heparin, bivalirudin, or fondaparinux). The anticoagulant is generally stopped after revascularization. Enoxaparin and bivalirudin require dose reduction in patients with creatinine clearance <30 mL/min. Fondaparinux is not approved in the United States for treatment of ACS, and it is contraindicated in patients with creatinine clearance <30 mL/min and in those weighing <50 kg. Prasugrel and glycoprotein IIb/IIIa inhibitors are not recommended for routine use in ACS but may be appropriate in selected patients. Prasugrel has been associated with increased bleeding risk in patients ≥75 years old and is generally not recommended for routine therapy in this patient population. In patients receiving clopidogrel, ticagrelor, or prasugrel who require coronary bypass surgery, these drugs are usually discontinued for at least 5 days (clopidogrel, ticagrelor) or 7 days (prasugrel) before surgery, if feasible, to reduce the risk of perioperative bleeding.

Reperfusion therapy with percutaneous coronary intervention (PCI) or a fibrinolytic agent is indicated in patients presenting within 12 hours of onset of STEMI (Class I recommendation) or within 24 hours if there are signs or symptoms of ongoing ischemia (Class IIa recommendation). PCI is the preferred reperfusion strategy; it has been associated with superior outcomes relative to fibrinolysis in patients up to 85 years old. Fibrinolytic therapy reduces mortality in STEMI patients <75 years old, as well as in carefully selected patients ≥75 years old. However, risk of intracranial hemorrhage after administration of a fibrinolytic agent increases considerably with age, especially after age 75. For patients who present with STEMI to non-PCI capable hospitals, guidelines generally recommend transfer to a PCI-capable hospital for primary PCI if the time from first medical contact to PCI-mediated reperfusion is expected to be <120 minutes. Furthermore, patients who are being considered for fibrinolytics must be carefully evaluated to ensure they do not have any contraindications to this therapy, such as poorly controlled hypertension, recent ischemic stroke, recent major surgery, prolonged CPR, recent noncompressible arterial puncture, or active bleeding.

In the setting of non-ST-elevation ACS, early PCI has been associated with improved outcomes in high-risk patients, including older adults, especially those with ongoing ischemia, extensive ECG changes, decreased LV systolic function, or hemodynamic instability (SOE=A). For hemodynamically stable older patients without active chest pain or major ECG abnormalities, an initial strategy of either optimal medical therapy or coronary angiography is appropriate. However, invasive management is not recommended for patients with extensive comorbidities in whom the benefits of revascularization are unlikely to outweigh the risks.

Routine use of antiarrhythmic agents, including lidocaine and amiodarone, is not recommended in patients with ACS. Dihydropyridine calcium channel blockers are contraindicated in patients with acute MI (SOE=A), and use of the nondihydropyridine calcium channel blockers, diltiazem and verapamil, should be limited to the treatment of supraventricular tachyarrhythmias (including atrial fibrillation and atrial flutter) in patients with preserved ventricular function who are unresponsive to or intolerant of β-blockers.

Digoxin should be used cautiously in patients with ACS, because it may increase myocardial oxygen demand and thus worsen ischemia, although it may be used to slow a rapid ventricular response in patients with atrial fibrillation (especially if associated with severe LV systolic dysfunction).

After documented ACS, patients should be maintained on aspirin (Class I recommendation), a β-blocker (Class I recommendation), an ACE inhibitor (or ARB (Class I recommendation after anterior STEMI, Class IIa recommendation after other STEMI, Class IIb recommendation after NSTEMI), and a high-intensity statin (Class I recommendation) in the absence of contraindications (SOE=A). Clopidogrel 75 mg/d, ticagrelor 90 mg twice daily, or prasugrel 10 mg/d (for patients <75 years old) is recommended for at least 12 months for all patients with ACS, whether or not PCI is performed. For patients at high risk of bleeding after stent placement for ACS, discontinuation of dual antiplatelet therapy (DAPT) after 6 months may be considered. However, select patients may benefit from extended DAPT for up to 30 months. The DAPT risk score (http://tools.acc.org/DAPTriskapp/#!/content/calculator/) enables calculation of the risks and benefits of prolonged DAPT in a given patient.

Patients with large anterior MIs associated with apical wall motion abnormalities may be considered for anticoagulation with warfarin for 3–6 months to maintain an INR of 2–3 to reduce the risk of mural thrombus formation and embolization (Class IIa recommendation). In addition, counseling on modifiable cardiovascular risk factors, including recommendations about diet and exercise, should be performed before hospital discharge. Whenever feasible, patients should be referred to a structured cardiac rehabilitation program, because such programs have been associated with improved functional, emotional, behavioral, and clinical outcomes, including 25%–30% reduction in mortality, and the beneficial effects are at least as great in older as in younger patients (SOE=A).

CHRONIC CORONARY ARTERY DISEASE

Presentation and Diagnosis

As is the case with ACS, older patients with chronic CAD are more likely than younger patients to present with exertional fatigue or shortness of breath rather than classical angina pectoris. Withdrawal from usual activities and other atypical manifestations of ischemia are also more common in older adults. In addition, older patients tend to present later in the course of disease, in part because more sedentary lifestyles result in delays in symptom onset or reduced symptom severity. Coronary angiographic studies and autopsy series indicate that older patients tend to have more severe and diffuse CAD, including more triple-vessel and left main CAD, as well as higher prevalence of prior MI and associated LV dysfunction.

The diagnosis of CAD is similar in older and younger adults, except that older adults have, on average, a higher pretest probability of having significant coronary obstructions. As a result, false-positive rates on stress tests tend to be lower in older adults, whereas false-negative rates tend to be higher. Diminished exercise capacity can also contribute to higher false-negative rates on exercise stress tests (but not pharmacologic stress tests) in older patients.

In most patients with stable symptoms thought likely to be due to coronary ischemia, a stress test is the initial diagnostic test of choice. When feasible, an exercise test is preferable to a pharmacologic test because it is more physiologic and provides additional prognostic information based on exercise tolerance and the hemodynamic response to exercise not afforded by pharmacologic testing. In patients unable to exercise because of poor physical conditioning or comorbid illness (especially orthopedic or neurologic disorders), pharmacologic stress tests with imaging, such as dobutamine echocardiography or regadenoson nuclear perfusion provide equivalent diagnostic sensitivity and specificity relative to exercise tests.

In patients with accelerating symptoms or a markedly abnormal stress test in whom coronary revascularization may be an appropriate therapeutic option, coronary angiography provides definitive information about the precise location and severity of coronary stenoses. Although the risks of coronary angiography increase slightly with age, in experienced centers the procedure can be performed with very low risk of major complications (<1% combined risk of all major complications, including death), even in patients of very advanced age. The risk of serious bleeding is substantially lower when angiography is performed via the transradial rather than the transfemoral approach. The radial approach also confers the benefit of early ambulation, because postprocedural immobilization for several hours is not required.

Medical Therapy

Control of risk factors is the foundation for reducing CAD progression in patients of all ages. Diabetes, hypertension, and lipid abnormalities should be treated in accordance with published guidelines. Individuals who smoke should be strongly encouraged to discontinue use of all tobacco products, and behavioral or pharmacologic support, or both, should be routinely offered to all patients who express an interest in smoking cessation. A diet low in saturated fat and cholesterol but high in fruits, vegetables, and whole-grain products should be prescribed, and patients should be encouraged to engage in at least 30 minutes of aerobic exercise, such as walking, at least 5 days per week. Modest weight reduction is advisable in patients who are markedly overweight (BMI ≥35 kg/m^2), but as noted above, the value of weight loss in older adults with lesser degrees of obesity has not been established.

All patients with chronic CAD should receive aspirin 75–162 mg/d (SOE=A). Lower dosages are associated with decreased incidence of GI intolerance and bleeding complications but possibly higher risk of aspirin resistance. In the small percentage of patients with true aspirin allergy or intolerance, clopidogrel 75 mg/d is a reasonable alternative. Although the combination of aspirin with either clopidogrel or warfarin is somewhat more effective than aspirin alone in reducing the risk of ACS in patients with CAD, the additional expense and higher risk of major hemorrhage makes combination therapy less desirable in the absence of specific indications (eg, clopidogrel after PCI or warfarin for atrial fibrillation). In patients with an indication for therapeutic anticoagulation after PCI (eg, atrial fibrillation), the combination of a full-dose anticoagulant plus one antiplatelet agent (preferably a P2Y12 inhibitor) leads to less bleeding and equal protection against cardiovascular events relative to so-called "triple therapy" with an anticoagulant plus DAPT.

Statin therapy is indicated for all patients with CAD, because statins have been shown to reduce mortality and major cardiac events regardless of the pretreatment LDL-cholesterol level (SOE=A). For older adults with established CAD, current guidelines recommend therapy with a moderate-intensity (if >75 years old) or high-intensity (if ≤75 years old) statin, including atorvastatin 40–80 mg and rosuvastatin 20–40 mg. Guidelines no longer recommend treating to specific cholesterol targets but instead advise therapeutic decisions based on predicted CVD risk. Statins have been shown to improve clinical outcomes in trials involving CAD patients up to 85 years old. Although altered hepatic metabolism and the use of multiple medications may place older patients at increased risk of statin-related adverse events, studies have not consistently shown an increased incidence of major statin toxicity in older adults. However, there is some evidence that statin-associated myalgias may be more common in older adults, perhaps because of reduced muscle mass.

ACE inhibitors have been shown to reduce mortality and cardiovascular morbidity in patients up to 85 years old with CAD, peripheral arterial disease, or diabetes. Routine use of ACE inhibitors is recommended for patients with established CAD who also have hypertension, diabetes mellitus, LVEF ≤40%, or chronic kidney disease, in the absence of contraindications (SOE=A). ARBs are an acceptable alternative in patients unable to tolerate ACE inhibitors. ACE inhibitors and ARBs should be used cautiously, if at all, in patients with estimated creatinine clearance <30 mL/min (unless receiving dialysis). Renal function and serum potassium levels should be monitored carefully when starting or titrating these medications.

Patients should be treated with a β-blocker for at least 3 years after an MI in the absence of contraindications or limiting adverse effects (SOE=A). In addition, specific β-blockers are indicated for all patients with an LV ejection fraction ≤40%, regardless of cause. β-Blockers that have been shown to improve mortality in patients with reduced LVEF include metoprolol succinate, carvedilol, and bisoprolol. β-blockers are also the most effective anti-ischemic agents and should be considered the medications of first choice for treatment of anginal symptoms. The dosage of β-blocker should be titrated to maintain a resting heart rate of 50 to no more than 70 beats per minute. Up to 20%–30% of patients are unable to tolerate β-blockers because of adverse events, but there is no convincing evidence that older patients experience more adverse events than younger patients.

Calcium channel blockers are effective anti-ischemic agents, either as first-line therapy in patients unable to take β-blockers, or in combination with either β-blockers or long-acting nitrates. Calcium channel blockers are relatively contraindicated in patients with heart failure or an LV ejection fraction <40%. Leg edema due to venodilation is a common adverse effect of dihydropyridine calcium channel blockers, whereas constipation is more common with the nondihydropyridines, especially verapamil; both problems appear to be more common in older patients.

Long-acting nitrate preparations, such as isosorbide mononitrate, are less effective anti-ischemic agents than β-blockers or calcium channel blockers, in part because of the high rate of tolerance that develops during long-term use and the need for a daily nitrate-free interval of at least several hours. These agents are therefore best used as adjunctive therapy in patients with persistent symptoms despite treatment with a β-blocker, calcium channel blocker, or both. Headache is the most common adverse effect associated with nitrates, but most cases resolve with continued use. Occasionally, patients develop hypotension, dizziness, falls, or syncope, most commonly on initiation of nitrate therapy.

Ranolazine, alone or in combination with conventional antianginal medications, reduces angina and improves exercise tolerance in patients with symptomatic CAD. In addition, the benefits of ranolazine are similar in older and younger patients. Ranolazine is generally well tolerated, although adverse events, including constipation and dizziness, tend to be more common in patients >70 years old than in younger patients. Ranolazine increases the QT interval slightly, but a significant proarrhythmic effect has not been reported.

Revascularization

Adults >65 years old currently account for over half of all PCIs and coronary bypass operations performed in the United States, and both of these procedures are now routinely performed in older adults (a paradigm shift from several decades ago). In patients with chronic CAD, the principal indications for coronary revascularization are to ameliorate symptoms that have not responded to maximally tolerated medical therapy, and to reduce mortality in select patients with high-risk coronary disease or ischemic cardiomyopathy with reduced LVEF. In patients <70 years old, clinical trials conducted more than 20 years ago demonstrated that coronary bypass surgery decreased mortality relative to medical therapy in patients with stenosis of the left main coronary artery and in patients with severe multivessel CAD and LV systolic dysfunction. Additionally, a large meta-analysis spanning trials from the years 1980 to 2013 showed a mortality reduction in patients with stable CAD who were treated with coronary bypass surgery or new generation drug–eluting stents as compared with medical therapy alone. However, complication rates, including mortality, increase with age after both PCI and coronary bypass surgery, especially among patients >80 years old. Nevertheless, despite the lack of direct evidence for a reduction in mortality with revascularization procedures in older patients with stable CAD, some trials have demonstrated improved symptoms and quality of life in those who did not respond adequately to aggressive medical therapy (SOE=A). Therefore, it is appropriate to offer revascularization on an individual basis to older patients with persistent symptoms and impaired quality of life attributable to coronary ischemia. Finally, in select older patients with ischemic cardiomyopathy and reduced LVEF, particularly those with good functionality and >10 years of remaining life expectancy, revascularization should be considered for mortality reduction.

Short-term mortality, major complication rates (including cognitive dysfunction), hospital length of stay, and convalescence time are all increased with coronary bypass surgery relative to PCI, but there is evidence that surgery is superior to PCI with regard to long-term mortality, particularly in patients with diabetes or with higher-complexity coronary lesions. In all cases, the benefits and risks of all major therapeutic options—continued medical therapy, PCI, or bypass surgery—should be discussed in detail with the patient and family before deciding the best course of treatment. An important consideration in assessing the risk of bypass surgery is the potential for postoperative cognitive impairment and functional decline. Up to 50% of older patients undergoing bypass surgery using extracorporeal circulation experience measurable cognitive impairment after surgery (SOE=B). Although most patients recover completely within 3–6 months, a small percentage demonstrate persistent cognitive dysfunction. Functional decline is also common after major cardiac surgery, and return to the preoperative functional status often takes several months; some patients experience irreversible functional loss. To minimize functional deficits, rehabilitation should be started in the hospital as soon as possible after surgery, and patients should be referred to a structured cardiac rehabilitation program after hospital discharge whenever possible.

VALVULAR HEART DISEASE

Valvular heart diseases include aortic stenosis (AS), aortic regurgitation (AR), mitral stenosis (MS), and mitral regurgitation (MR).

Epidemiology

The prevalence of AS increases with age, approaching 15% in octogenarians, and AS is the most common valvular abnormality requiring intervention in older adults. AS in patients >70 years old is usually due to fibrosis and calcification of a previously normal trileaflet aortic valve, rather than to a congenitally bicuspid valve or rheumatic disease, which are the most common causes in middle-aged adults.

AR may be acute or chronic, and the incidence of both increases with age. Although up to 30% of older adults have some degree of AR detectable by echocardiography, only rarely is it severe enough to require surgical intervention. The most common causes of acute AR in older adults include infective endocarditis, dissection of the ascending aorta, malfunction of a previously implanted prosthetic valve (eg, dehiscence or thrombosis), and chest trauma. Chronic AR may be due to pathology of the valvular apparatus (eg, calcific or rheumatic valve disease, prior endocarditis, chronic malfunction of a valve prosthesis) or to dilatation of the aortic root resulting in poor coaptation of the valve leaflets (eg, from ascending aortic root aneurysm, sinus of Valsalva aneurysm, chronic ascending aortic dissection).

Rheumatic MS is uncommon in older adults in the United States, but occasionally patients in their 70s or 80s will present with symptoms attributable to previously undiagnosed rheumatic disease. Alternatively, the diagnosis may be established incidentally when a patient undergoes echocardiography for another reason (eg, new-onset atrial fibrillation). More commonly, MS in older adults is due to nonrheumatic calcification of the mitral valve annulus and subvalvular apparatus, leading to a narrowed orifice and decreased excursion of the valve leaflets.

MR of at least mild severity is common in older adults, but only a small proportion require surgical intervention. As with AR, MR may be acute or chronic. Causes of acute MR include papillary muscle dysfunction or rupture due to acute myocardial infarction, rupture of chordae tendinae related to myxomatous degeneration (ie, mitral valve prolapse), destruction of the valvular apparatus due to infective endocarditis, and malcoaptation of the mitral leaflets due to wall motion abnormalities as a result of an acute MI. Chronic MR may be due to myxomatous degeneration, annular dilation associated with ischemic or nonischemic dilated cardiomyopathy, chronic LV wall motion abnormalities, mitral annular calcification, rheumatic mitral valve disease, or prior endocarditis.

Diagnosis, Clinical Features, and Treatment

The echocardiogram is the procedure of choice for diagnosing valvular disorders. For AS, echocardiography is essential for assessing disease severity, evaluating left ventricular function, and determining the presence of associated valvular lesions. Severe AS is indicated by a maximum aortic jet velocity >4 meters/second, a mean transvalvular pressure gradient ≥40 mm Hg, or an aortic valve area <1 cm². Occasionally, technical considerations preclude accurate echocardiographic assessment of AS severity; in these cases, measurements made via right- and left-heart catheterization are definitive. Further, some patients with calculated aortic valve areas ≤1 cm² on resting echocardiography have transvalvular pressure gradients or aortic jet velocities that are less than severe, as a result of LV systolic dysfunction. In such cases, low-dose dobutamine stress echocardiography can be used to transiently increase LV stroke volume and help verify the presence of severe aortic stenosis by hemodynamic parameters.

In patients with acute severe AR, echocardiography demonstrates a short duration AR jet with rapid deceleration, and premature closure of the mitral valve. In patients with severe chronic AR, the AR jet is typically more prominent and of longer duration, often persisting throughout diastole. In chronic severe AR, the left ventricle is usually dilated. Untreated, chronic, severe AR may eventually lead to reduced LV ejection fraction.

Echocardiography is the definitive test for diagnosing MS, quantifying disease severity, and evaluating for the presence of other valvular lesions, especially MR. Severe MS is indicated by a mitral valve area <1.5 cm^2 or a mean transvalvular gradient of ≥10 mmHg.

Echocardiography with Doppler assists in determining the cause and severity of either acute or chronic MR, and helps to differentiate primary (pathology involving the valvular apparatus itself) or secondary MR (eg, malcoaptation of leaflets due to LV dilation or wall motion abnormalities). Echocardiography also provides important information about left ventricular size and function, left atrial size, pulmonary artery pressure, and the presence and severity of other valvular lesions.

For symptoms, clinical findings, and treatment recommendations for aortic and mitral valve diseases, see Table 50.3.

Transcatheter Aortic Valve Replacement (TAVR)

Until recently, surgical aortic valve replacement (SAVR) was the only effective treatment for severe AS, and numerous studies have demonstrated excellent outcomes after SAVR in appropriately selected older adults, including octogenarians. However, many older patients are either not suitable candidates for SAVR or decline to undergo the procedure due to high perioperative risk attributable to comorbidity or frailty. Recently, transcatheter aortic valve replacement (TAVR) with a bioprosthesis has been shown to be associated with improved outcomes relative to medical therapy in older adults who are not candidates for SAVR. TAVR is performed through an arteriotomy or transapically and does not require either a median sternotomy or extracorporeal circulation. As a result, hospital length of stay is shorter and functional recovery faster than with SAVR. In patients who are high-risk for SAVR, TAVR has demonstrated similar or better outcomes up to at least 3–5 years, including risk of stroke, vascular complications, and all-cause mortality.

Infective Endocarditis

Since the early part of the 20th century, infective endocarditis has undergone a transformation from a disease of young adults with rheumatic or congenital valve anomalies to one of older adults with degenerative valve disorders or prosthetic valves. Native-valve endocarditis is most commonly caused by streptococci viridans or *Staphylococcus aureus*. Enterococcal species and gram-negative bacilli, including gastrointestinal and genitourinary organisms, are also common causes of native valve endocarditis in older adults. Less frequently, infections are due to HACEK organisms (a group of gram-negative rods that primarily inhabit the oral cavity and include the genera *Haemophilus*, *Actinobacillus*, *Cardiobacterium*, *Eikenella*, and *Kingella*) or other atypical pathogens. Coagulase-negative staphylococci are a common cause of prosthetic-valve endocarditis, particularly in the first 60 days after valve replacement.

Endocarditis is often difficult to diagnose in older adults. Fever is less common than in younger patients, occurring in 55% versus 80%, respectively, as is leukocytosis, occurring in 25% versus 60%. Rates of positive blood cultures do not vary by age, but the sensitivity of transthoracic echocardiography is reduced to 45% in older patients (versus 75% in younger patients) because of the increased prevalence of calcific valve disease and prosthetic valves. Transesophageal echocardiography (TEE) improves the diagnostic yield for infective endocarditis, but the lack of positive findings on TEE does not exclude the diagnosis.

Antibiotic treatment of infective endocarditis is directed at the identified pathogen or at the most likely causes if blood cultures are negative. Therapy is administered intravenously for 4–6 weeks. Surgical therapy should be considered in the presence of severe valvular dysfunction, evidence of persistent infection despite appropriate antibiotic therapy, recurrent emboli, marked heart failure, myocardial abscess formation, high-degree AV block, vegetations >1 cm in diameter on left-sided valves, or fungal endocarditis. In the absence of major comorbidities, age does not appear to play a major role in mortality risk, with a 2-year survival of 75% for infective endocarditis in all age groups.

Recommendations for preventing endocarditis after dental procedures focus on providing prophylaxis only in the highest-risk patients (ie, those with a prosthetic valve, prior endocarditis, certain congenital heart diseases, or cardiac transplantation with valve disease). Recent guidelines have eliminated recommendations for prophylaxis for those undergoing gastrointestinal or genitourinary procedures.

CARDIAC ARRHYTHMIAS

Epidemiology

Age-related changes in the cardiac conduction system, coupled with the increasing prevalence of cardiovascular diseases at older age, lead to a progressive increase in the incidence and prevalence of conduction abnormalities and heart rhythm disturbances in older adults. Among healthy adults ≥65 years old, occasional supraventricular ectopy, ventricular ectopy, short runs of SVT, and consecutive premature ventricular beats are common. In the absence of structural heart disease, the presence of supraventricular and ventricular arrhythmias generally does not affect mortality or predict cardiac events, except that exercise-induced supraventricular tachycardia has been associated with an increased risk of atrial fibrillation. Conversely, in patients with prevalent cardiovascular disease, increased ventricular (but not supraventricular) ectopy has been associated with an increased risk of cardiovascular mortality. Furthermore, atrial fibrillation, whether paroxysmal or persistent, is an independent predictor of increased mortality in both men and women (SOE=A).

Age-related degenerative changes in and around the sinoatrial and atrioventricular (AV) nodes lead to an increase in bradyarrhythmias with advancing age. Although resting heart rate is unaffected by age in healthy individuals, the incidence and prevalence of sinus node dysfunction ("sick sinus syndrome") and AV-nodal block increase progressively with age. As a result, >75% of permanent pacemakers are implanted in patients ≥65 years old, and approximately half are in patients ≥75 years old. The prevalence of infranodal conduction disorders, including bundle-branch and fascicular block, also increases with age.

Atrial Fibrillation

Atrial fibrillation (AF) is the most common sustained arrhythmia encountered in clinical practice. The incidence and prevalence of AF increase exponentially with age, such that the prevalence of AF in octogenarians is approximately 10%. Among older patients with valvular heart disease or HF, the prevalence of AF is even higher, approaching 30%. Currently, about half of patients with AF are ≥75 years old, and it is projected that by 2050 half will be ≥80 years old. AF confers relative risks of mortality of 1.10–1.15 in men and 1.20–1.25 in women.

The proportion of strokes associated with AF also increases exponentially with age, rising from 1.5% of strokes in patients 50–59 years old to 23.5% of strokes in patients 80–89 years old. Women with AF are at particularly increased risk of stroke, especially after age 75; their relative risk of stroke is 1.8 compared with that in men in this age group.

Clinical Features

Symptoms related to AF are highly variable. Most commonly, patients experience palpitations, shortness of breath, or impaired exercise tolerance. However, some patients are entirely asymptomatic, whereas others present with acute pulmonary edema. Less commonly, stroke, transient ischemic attack, or acute coronary syndrome may be the initial manifestation. Physical examination reveals an irregularly irregular rhythm with heart rates ranging from <60 beats per minute (eg, in patients with AV nodal dysfunction or those taking a β-blocker) to >150 beats per minute. Pulmonary crackles may be present in patients with acute HF, and a heart murmur may be heard in patients with valvular heart disease. Rarely, an enlarged or nodular thyroid may be detected, or signs of deep venous thrombosis may be evident, reflecting the association of hyperthyroidism and venous thromboembolism with this dysrhythmia.

Diagnosis and Evaluation

In patients with ongoing AF, the standard 12-lead ECG is diagnostic. Additional laboratory studies should include evaluation of serum electrolytes (especially potassium and magnesium) and an assessment of thyroid function. A transthoracic echocardiogram is indicated in all patients with new-onset AF to evaluate LV size and function, left atrial size, pulmonary artery pressure, and the cardiac valves. Further evaluation in selected cases might include a chest radiograph, serial cardiac biomarker proteins to exclude acute MI, a brain natriuretic peptide level, a d-dimer level, lower-extremity venous Doppler studies, and an evaluation for pulmonary embolism.

Management

The objectives of therapy for AF include relieving symptoms and minimizing risk of thromboembolic events, particularly stroke. The principal strategies for relieving symptoms are control of heart rate and maintenance of normal sinus rhythm. Several clinical trials comparing "rate control" with "rhythm control" have consistently demonstrated that in patients who are asymptomatic or minimally symptomatic, therapy directed at controlling the heart rate with AV-nodal blocking agents such as a β-blocker, diltiazem, verapamil, or digoxin, alone or in combination, is associated with fewer hospitalizations and favorable trends in stroke and mortality rates relative to therapy directed at maintaining sinus rhythm using antiarrhythmic medications (SOE=A). Based on these findings, rate control in conjunction with systemic anticoagulation is the preferred treatment for AF patients with minimal or no symptoms. In general, β-blockers are the most effective agents for rate control, followed by diltiazem and verapamil. Digoxin is not recommended as first-line therapy but may be a useful adjunct in patients with persistently increased heart rates despite β-blockers or calcium channel blockers, as well as in those with symptomatic LV systolic dysfunction. In the Rate Control Efficacy (RACE-II) trial, lenient heart rate control (resting heart rate <110 beats per minute) was not inferior to strict heart rate control (resting heart rate <80 beats per minute) with respect to major clinical outcomes in patients with chronic AF (mean age 68 years). Based on these

Table 50.3—Cardiac Valvular Conditions

Condition	Signs and Symptoms	Findings	Treatment
Aortic stenosis (AS)	Angina, DOE, heart failure, light-headedness, presyncope/syncope	*Physical examination*: mid/late systolic ejection murmur radiating to carotids, S4 gallop, left ventricular heave *ECG*: LVH	*Medical*: no effective therapy *Percutaneous*: for symptomatic severe AS, transcatheter aortic valve replacement in selected patients at intermediate to high surgical risk[a] *Surgical*: AVR[b] for severe AS with symptoms or LVEF <50%; bioprosthetic valves preferred in older patients[c]
Aortic regurgitation (AR)	Can be acute or chronic; asymptomatic or minimally symptomatic in mild/moderate AR; DOE, heart failure, angina in severe AR	*Physical examination*: ↑ pulse pressure, bounding/collapsing pulses, diastolic decrescendo murmur, systolic ejection murmur *ECG*: LVH (severe chronic AR), tachycardia (acute AR) *Chest radiograph*: cardiomegaly (severe chronic AR), pulmonary congestion (acute AR)	*Medical* (less severe cases): control of hypertension, preferably with a dihydropyridine calcium channel blocker, ACE inhibitor, or angiotensin receptor blocker (SOE=B); β-blocker in patients with symptoms or LV systolic dysfunction (SOE=B) *Surgical*: AVR[b] indicated for acute severe AR, symptomatic severe chronic AR, asymptomatic severe chronic AR with LVEF <50% or left ventricular end-systolic dimension ≥5 cm (all SOE=B)
Mitral stenosis (MS)	Gradually worsening DOE early, orthopnea and leg edema late, progressive decline in exercise capacity, fatigue	*Physical examination*: early diastolic opening snap, low-pitched ("rumbling") diastolic murmur at apex, pulmonary hypertension, right heart failure	*Medical*: diuretics for volume overload and β-blockers for decreased exercise tolerance associated with tachycardia *Indication for intervention*: symptomatic severe MS *Percutaneous*: balloon valvuloplasty preferred if valvular morphology is amenable, but most older adults are not good candidates because of extensive calcification and commissural fusion or concomitant mitral regurgitation *Surgical*: MVR[b] effective but with 5%–15% operative mortality in older patients
Mitral regurgitation (MR)	Can be acute or chronic; marked shortness of breath, orthopnea in acute severe MR; progressive DOE in chronic MR	*Physical examination*: pulmonary rales, tachycardia, narrow pulse pressure, S3, and short harsh systolic murmur in acute severe MR; holosystolic murmur radiating to axilla, S3, pulmonary hypertension, right heart failure in chronic severe MR	*Medical*: medical therapy as for heart failure with systolic dysfunction in patients with symptomatic chronic MR and LVEF ≤60% who are not candidates for intervention (SOE=B) *Percutaneous*: transcatheter mitral valve repair in selected patients (SOE=B) *Surgical*: mitral valve repair preferred over MVR[b] (SOE=B); bioprosthetic valves[c] preferred over mechanical valves in older patients; all effective with 5%–15% operative mortality in older patients. Operative mortality is lower for repair than replacement. Surgical intervention is indicated: ■ Urgently for acute severe MR with heart failure ■ Symptomatic patients with severe, chronic MR as long as LVEF >30% (SOE=B) ■ Asymptomatic patients with severe chronic MR and LVEF 30%–60% and/or left ventricular end-systolic dimension ≥4 cm (SOE=B) ■ When mitral valve repair is deemed likely to be successful in asymptomatic patients with severe chronic MR and an LVEF ≥60% (SOE=B) ■ In patients with severe chronic MR and pulmonary artery systolic pressure >50 mmHg or new-onset atrial fibrillation with high likelihood of successful MV repair (SOE=B)

NOTE: DOE = dyspnea on exertion; LVH = left ventricular hypertrophy; LVEF = left ventricular ejection fraction; AVR = aortic valve replacement; MVR = mitral valve replacement
[a] Based on comorbidities and frailty.
[b] Older adults being considered for AVR and MVR should have coronary angiography first, because significant coronary artery disease is present in >50% of patients.
[c] After AVR with a bioprosthetic valve, antithrombotic therapy with aspirin 75–100 mg/d is recommended in the absence of risk factors for thromboembolism (SOE=B). After MVR with a bioprosthetic valve, anticoagulation to maintain INR of 2–3 is recommended for 3 months (SOE=C), followed by maintenance therapy with aspirin 75–100 mg/d in the absence of risk factors for thromboembolism (SOE=B).

findings, guidelines have been modified to reflect the safety and efficacy of lenient rate control.

Patients who experience significant shortness of breath, fatigue, or exercise intolerance attributable to AF may be best managed with antiarrhythmic drug therapy aimed at maintaining sinus rhythm. Selection of an antiarrhythmic agent in older adults is challenging. Amiodarone is the most effective medication available, but it is associated with multiple adverse events (eg, thyroid dysfunction, neurologic disorders, pulmonary toxicity, ophthalmologic disturbances, liver function abnormalities), some potentially serious, as well as numerous drug interactions. Dronedarone, an amiodarone analogue, is less effective than amiodarone but has fewer adverse events. However, dronedarone is contraindicated in patients with advanced heart failure, and it may be associated with increased mortality, stroke, and hospitalizations for heart failure in older patients with chronic (permanent) AF. Sotalol is less effective than amiodarone and is contraindicated in patients with significant renal insufficiency. Flecainide and propafenone are contraindicated in patients with CAD or heart failure. Quinidine and procainamide have limited efficacy and are accompanied by relatively frequent adverse events, whereas disopyramide is generally contraindicated in older adults because of its anticholinergic effects. Dofetilide is moderately effective, but its use is restricted in the United States, and it may be dispensed only by pharmacies and health care settings that are specially certified. Initiation of the drug requires hospitalization for a minimum of 2–3 days.

Alternatives to antiarrhythmic drug therapy for maintenance of sinus rhythm include catheter ablation of the arrhythmogenic foci, usually through pulmonary vein isolation, and the surgical maze procedure. Pulmonary vein isolation has been associated with "cure" rates of >80% in younger patients with paroxysmal AF, but experience is limited with this procedure in older patients with persistent AF. Nonetheless, catheter ablation may be considered in older patients with refractory symptoms attributable to AF in whom antiarrhythmic drug treatment has not been successful or tolerated. There is emerging evidence that catheter ablation of AF is associated with clinically significant improvements in outcomes among appropriately selected patients; for example, the CASTLE-AF trial demonstrated reduced mortality in patients with severe LV systolic dysfunction (≤35%) and AF who were randomized to catheter AF ablation as compared with conventional medical therapy. The maze procedure results in long-term maintenance of sinus rhythm in >90% of cases but requires open heart surgery; however, it is a reasonable option for older patients with AF undergoing open heart surgery for other indications if a surgeon with expertise in performing the procedure is available.

All older patients with paroxysmal or persistent AF require consideration for stroke prophylaxis, regardless of whether a rate-control or rhythm-control strategy is adopted. Prior to 2010, the two main options for stroke prophylaxis were warfarin, titrated to maintain an INR of 2–3, and aspirin 75–325 mg/d, alone or in combination with clopidogrel. In patients with nonvalvular AF, numerous trials have shown that warfarin reduces the risk of stroke by 65%–70%, whereas aspirin reduces the risk by 20%–25% (SOE=A). Additionally, the ACTIVE-W trial demonstrated the superiority of warfarin to the combination of aspirin and clopidogrel in terms of both risk of ischemic stroke and major bleeding in patients with AF.

In the past several years, 4 direct oral anticoagulants (DOACs) have been approved for use in the United States: dabigatran, rivaroxaban, apixaban, and edoxaban. All except dabigatran (a direct thrombin inhibitor) are factor Xa inhibitors. The DOACs are all at least as effective as warfarin for stroke prevention in patients with nonvalvular AF, and are not inferior to warfarin with respect to overall risk of major bleeding. In addition, all four DOACs have been associated with reduced risk of intracranial hemorrhage (ICH) relative to warfarin. The DOACs are administered in fixed dosages (with adjustment for renal function as described below) and do not require routine monitoring of INR or other coagulation parameters. The DOACs also have fewer interactions with other medications and foods than does warfarin. Idarucizumab, an antibody fragment, has been approved by the FDA as an antidote to dabigatran, and andexanet is approved to reverse the effects of apixiban and rivaroxaban. For the characteristics and dosing of the 4 DOACs available for prevention of cardioembolic events in patients with AF, see Table 50.4.

Selection of a strategy for stroke prophylaxis is often challenging in older adults, who are at higher risk of both stroke and hemorrhagic complications than are younger patients. To aid in the decision-making process, it is helpful to stratify AF patients according to stroke risk. In patients with nonvalvular AF (ie, AF not related to significant mitral stenosis), the CHA_2DS_2-VASc score is widely used. CHA_2DS_2-VASc assigns 1 point for chronic heart failure, hypertension, age ≥65 years (2 points for age ≥75 years), diabetes, 2 points for prior stroke or transient ischemic attack, and 1 point each for cardiovascular disease and female gender. CHA_2DS_2-VASc has been shown to be more accurate than the $CHADS_2$ score in identifying patients at low risk of stroke. In general, patients with a CHA_2DS_2-VASc score of 0 are at very low risk of stroke, and the risks of systemic anticoagulation are generally thought to outweigh the benefits; therefore, either no antithrombotic treatment or aspirin only is appropriate in these patients. Similarly, patients with a CHA_2DS_2-VASc score of 1 are at relatively low risk of stroke, and current guidelines indicate that such patients can be managed with aspirin, warfarin, a DOAC, or no antithrombotic therapy. However, all women ≥65 years old and all men ≥75 years old have a CHA_2DS_2-VASc score of at least 2, and in most of these cases the beneficial effects of systemic anticoagulation outweigh the risks in the absence of clear contraindications. Importantly, among patients ≥75 years old, the value of aspirin, alone or in combination with clopidogrel, for reducing the risk of thromboembolic events is uncertain. In patients with AF in the setting of significant mitral stenosis, anticoagulation with warfarin should be initiated unless there is a significant contraindication, given the increased risk of cardiac thromboembolism in these patients regardless of CHA_2DS_2-VASc score.

One of the most common reasons for not prescribing anticoagulation for older patients with AF is concern about the risk of falls with the potential for serious bleeding complications, particularly ICH. However, in most older patients with a CHA_2DS_2-VASc score ≥2, the risk of thromboembolic stroke is thought to outweigh the risk of fall-related intracranial bleeding. Therefore, in most cases the perception of high fall risk alone is insufficient justification for withholding anticoagulation. The HAS-BLED score may be a useful adjunctive tool to promote informed decision making by estimating a patient's annual risk of major bleed. Also, a useful online calculator for estimating the risk of ischemic stroke and major bleed in patients with AF on various anticoagulant/antiplatelet regimens is available at www.sparctool.com/. Notably, these calculators do not incorporate history of falls and do not predict risk of fall-related major bleeding. Given the limitations of current tools, decisions in practice need to be individualized. For selected cases, consideration should be given to percutaneous left atrial appendage closure (via the Watchman device, which requires a limited duration of postprocedural anticoagulation), which was shown in the PROTECT-AF trial to be noninferior to chronic warfarin therapy for prevention of stroke.

Other Supraventricular Arrhythmias

Atrial flutter most often occurs in older patients with concomitant AF, and both anticoagulation and rate control considerations are similar to those for AF as discussed above. Patients with typical atrial flutter (due to a macro-reentrant circuit around the tricuspid valve within the right atrium) that is either symptomatic or refractory to pharmacologic rate control should be considered for a catheter atrial flutter ablation (Class I recommendation). This procedure is successful in alleviating typical atrial flutter in most cases, although some patients subsequently develop atrial fibrillation.

Atrial tachycardia, AV-nodal reentrant tachycardia, atrioventricular reentrant tachycardia, and multifocal atrial tachycardia are less common than AF and atrial flutter in older patients, especially after age 75. Management is similar for older and younger patients with these arrhythmias and generally involves treatment of the underlying condition and pharmacotherapy aimed at rate control or arrhythmia suppression. In selected patients with recurrent symptomatic episodes, antiarrhythmic medications or catheter ablation may be considered.

Ventricular Arrhythmias

In general, frequent ventricular premature beats, ventricular couplets, and short runs of nonsustained (<30 seconds) ventricular tachycardia require no specific therapy unless highly symptomatic, in which case β-blockade is the treatment of first choice. Patients with longer episodes of ventricular tachycardia associated with dizziness or syncope should be referred to a cardiologist or electrophysiologist for consideration of antiarrhythmic drug therapy, catheter ablation, or implantation of a cardiac defibrillator for secondary prevention.

Bradyarrhythmias

Increasing age is associated with a progressive increase in the prevalence of bradyarrhythmias. Patients with mild bradycardia (resting heart rate 50–60 beats per minute) are often asymptomatic; indeed, bradycardia may protect against the development of angina pectoris in patients with CAD. Patients with more marked bradycardia (resting heart rate 40–50 beats per minute) may experience fatigue, lightheadedness (especially on standing), or reduced exercise tolerance. Presyncope or syncope may occur in patients with profound bradycardia, manifested by a heart rate of <40 beats per minute or asystolic pauses of ≥3 seconds, whether due to sinus node dysfunction or heart block within the AV node or infranodal conduction system.

Diagnostic evaluation of patients with suspected symptomatic bradycardia should start with exclusion of significant electrolyte abnormalities, measurement of thyroid function to exclude hypothyroidism, and a review of the patient's medications (including OTC medications and dietary supplements). The most commonly used medications associated with bradycardia in older adults are β-blockers (including eye drops), diltiazem, verapamil, clonidine, amiodarone and other antiarrhythmic agents, and cholinesterase inhibitors. Patients with otherwise unexplained presyncope or syncope should undergo carotid sinus massage to evaluate for carotid hypersensitivity. An abnormal response to carotid massage is defined as unequivocal

Table 50.4—Direct Oral Anticoagulants for Prevention of Cardioembolic Events in Atrial Fibrillation

	Dabigatran	Rivaroxaban	Apixaban	Edoxaban
Mechanism of action	Direct thrombin (factor IIa) inhibition	Direct factor Xa inhibition	Direct factor Xa inhibition	Direct factor Xa inhibition
Standard dose	150 mg q12h	20 mg/d	5 mg q12h	60 mg/d
Dosing in renal impairment	CrCl 15–30 mL/min: 75 mg q12h CrCl <15 mL/min or HD: contraindicated	CrCl 15–50 mL/min: 15 mg/d CrCl <15 mL/min or HD: contraindicated	2.5 mg q12h if two of the following are present: Cr ≥1.5 mg/dL, ≥80 years old, or weight ≤60 kg HD: 5 mg q12h unless ≥80 years old or weight ≤60 kg	CrCl 15–50 mL/min: 30 mg/d CrCl <15 mL/min or HD: contraindicated CrCl >95 mL/min: contraindicated
Geriatric dosing	If ≥65 years old and CrCl <30 mL/min: contraindicated If ≥75 years old: use with extreme caution or consider another anticoagulant because of increased bleeding risk.	If ≥65 years old and CrCl 30–50 mL/min: reduce dose* If ≥65 years old and CrCl <15 mL/min: contraindicated	As above, if ≥80 years old	If ≥65 years old and CrCl 30–50 mL/min: 30 mg/d
Evidence-based comparison with warfarin				
Ischemic stroke	Lower risk	Similar risk	Similar risk	Similar risk
Hemorrhagic stroke	Lower risk	Lower risk	Lower risk	Lower risk
Systemic embolism	Similar risk	Similar risk	Similar risk	Similar risk
Major bleeding	Similar risk	Similar risk	Lower risk	Lower risk

CrCl = creatinine clearance, HD = hemodialysis
*Specific dose adjustment not provided by manufacturer.

reproduction of the patient's symptoms (eg, syncope), asystole ≥3 seconds, or a decrease in systolic blood pressure ≥50 mmHg in the absence of symptoms or ≥30 mmHg in association with symptoms (eg, dizziness, presyncope).

For patients with intermittent symptoms, it is essential to establish a correlation between symptoms and bradyarrhythmias before considering pacemaker implantation. If symptoms occur daily or almost every day, an ambulatory monitor (for 24–48 hours) may be helpful for confirming or excluding bradycardia (or other heart rhythm disorder) as the proximate cause. In patients whose symptoms occur at least once a month (but not daily), a 30-day event monitor may provide a definitive diagnosis. In patients with rare (ie, less than monthly) but recurrent symptoms of a serious nature (eg, syncope with injury), an implantable loop recorder may be considered. These devices, which may be left in place for a year or longer, have increased diagnostic yield in patients with infrequent syncopal events.

In patients with unexplained syncope and a nondiagnostic noninvasive evaluation, electrophysiologic testing may be helpful, especially in those with structural heart disease and/or an abnormal resting ECG (eg, right or left bundle-branch block). In such cases, electrophysiologic testing may distinguish syncope due to bradycardia (eg, high-grade infranodal AV block) from that due to a tachyarrhythmia (eg, supraventricular tachycardia or ventricular tachycardia), thus facilitating appropriate therapy.

Management of bradycardia includes correction of any treatable causes (eg, hypothyroidism) and elimination of potentially offending medications, if possible. In patients with confirmed symptomatic bradycardia not amenable to conservative management, permanent pacemaker implantation is warranted. For Class I indications for permanent pacing, see Table 50.5. In patients with sinus rhythm and preserved atrioventricular conduction (ie, normal PR interval and narrow QRS complex), atrial pacing is the preferred pacing mode. Patients with sinus rhythm but impaired atrioventricular conduction are often best served by dual-chamber (ie, atrial and ventricular) pacing. Patients with bradycardia in the context of atrial fibrillation or atrial flutter should receive a single-chamber ventricular pacemaker. Dual-chamber pacemakers have been associated with reduced incidence of atrial fibrillation and heart failure relative to single-chamber ventricular pacemakers, but beneficial effects on mortality and stroke have not been demonstrated.

Tachy-Brady Syndrome

The tachy-brady syndrome is a common variant of "sick sinus syndrome," in which patients manifest both tachyarrhythmias (most commonly supraventricular tachycardia or atrial fibrillation) and bradyarrhythmias, either or both of which can result in symptoms. Treatment of the tachyarrhythmias with AV-nodal blocking agents or antiarrhythmic medications often exacerbates symptoms related to bradycardia, for which pacemaker implantation may be required.

PERIPHERAL ARTERIAL DISEASE

Peripheral arterial disease (PAD) encompasses disorders of the abdominal aorta, renal and mesenteric arteries, and the iliofemoral-popliteal arterial tree. The prevalence of PAD increases with age and is higher in men than in women. In one study, the prevalence of PAD increased from 5.6% in adults 38–59 years old, to 15.9% in adults 60–69 years old, and to 33.8% in adults 70–82 years old. In addition to age, risk factors for PAD include hypertension, diabetes, smoking, and, to a lesser extent in older adults, family history.

Abdominal aortic aneurysms (AAA) are usually asymptomatic in the early stages. As an aneurysm enlarges, a patient may notice abdominal pulsations or experience back pain or abdominal discomfort. Symptoms of lower extremity PAD include claudication with exertion and skin changes related to chronically impaired circulation. In advanced cases, rest pain, ulcers, or dry gangrene may develop. Physical findings associated with PAD may include a pulsatile abdominal mass, bruits over the renal or femoral arteries (or both), diminished or absent peripheral pulses, and skin changes ranging from hair loss and pallor to ulcers and gangrene.

Diagnosis

It is estimated that at least 50% of patients with PAD are either asymptomatic or attribute their symptoms to another disorder (eg, arthritis); this proportion is likely even higher in older adults because of a more sedentary lifestyle. Diagnosis of PAD therefore requires a high index of suspicion and a proactive approach. Current guidelines recommend a formal history and physical examination to screen for symptoms and signs of PAD in all adults 50–69 years old with risk factors for atherosclerosis, as well as in all individuals ≥70 years old with or without risk factors (SOE=C). Men ≥60 years old with a family history of AAA and men 65–75 years old who have ever been smokers should undergo an abdominal ultrasound to screen for the presence of AAA (SOE=B).

Individuals with symptoms or physical findings suggestive of PAD should undergo assessment of the ankle-brachial index (ABI), the ratio of the systolic blood pressure obtained at the ankle to the blood pressure obtained over the ipsilateral brachial artery. A normal ABI is 1.0–1.4, and an ABI <0.9 has been reported to be 95% sensitive and 99% specific for leg PAD. An ABI of 0.91–0.99 is considered borderline low, whereas an ABI >1.4 is usually associated with stiff, noncompressible arteries, which are commonly seen in older patients with atherosclerosis or long-standing hypertension. An ABI <0.40 is generally associated with critical PAD and severely impaired perfusion of the distal limb. In most cases, an exercise treadmill test is also recommended, preferably with pre- and postexercise ABIs, to assess for both the degree of functional impairment and for evidence of PAD in patients who have normal or borderline resting ABI but in whom there is clinical concern for PAD.

Patients with moderate or severe symptoms and an abnormal ABI should undergo additional evaluation if percutaneous or surgical revascularization is being contemplated. Imaging procedures that may be useful in selected cases include Doppler flow velocity measurements, ultrasonic duplex scanning, magnetic resonance angiography, and CT angiography. If revascularization is indicated based on symptoms and the results of noninvasive testing, contrast angiography is usually required before a revascularization procedure is performed.

Treatment

PAD is considered a CAD risk-equivalent, indicating that patients with PAD have a ≥20% risk of experiencing a new coronary event within 10 years (SOE=A); in patients with comorbid diabetes or established CAD, the risk is even higher. Indeed, most deaths in patients with PAD are attributable to CAD or its complications (eg, heart failure, arrhythmias) rather than to PAD per se. The importance of PAD as a risk marker for CAD provides the rationale for the proactive approach to diagnosis described above, as well as for the aggressive treatment of prevalent cardiovascular risk factors. Older patients with PAD should be treated with a moderate to high-intensity statin, and blood pressure should be treated in accordance with current guidelines. Smoking cessation should be strongly encouraged, and patients who indicate an interest in quitting should be offered counseling in combination with drug therapy.

In addition to risk factor management, patients with significant lower extremity PAD should engage in a regular exercise program, preferably under supervision (SOE=A). Exercise should include walking for at least 30–45 minutes at least 3 times a week for a minimum of 12 weeks (SOE=A). Data from multiple randomized trials and at least one large meta-analysis indicate that the beneficial effects of exercise on maximal walking capacity exceed those of available pharmacotherapies. The greatest improvements in walking ability occur in individuals who exercise to near maximal pain threshold for a period of at least 6 months.

Pharmacotherapy for PAD includes aspirin 75–325 mg/d to reduce the risk of MI, stroke, or vascular death (SOE=A). Clopidogrel 75 mg/d is a reasonable alternative to aspirin in selected patients (SOE=B). The combination of aspirin and clopidogrel may be considered in patients at high risk of vascular events and acceptably low risk of bleeding (SOE=B). In addition to antiplatelet therapy, routine treatment with an ACE inhibitor or ARB for the prevention of cardiovascular events is reasonable in patients with symptomatic PAD (SOE=B).

Currently, the only pharmacologic agent that has been shown to improve symptoms and walking distance in patients with claudication is the phosphodiesterase inhibitor (type III) cilostazol. At dosages of 100 mg q12h, cilostazol increases maximal walking distance by 40%–60%, and a therapeutic trial of this agent is recommended for patients with lifestyle-limiting claudication (SOE=A). Although cilostazol is generally well tolerated, it is not recommended in patients with heart failure. Pentoxifylline is another agent approved for use in patients with symptomatic PAD, but the clinical effectiveness of this drug appears marginal (SOE=C).

Revascularization is indicated for patients with severe symptoms attributable to PAD that have not responded to a trial of aggressive risk factor modification, exercise, and pharmacotherapy. Revascularization is also indicated for patients with critical-limb ischemia, defined as rest pain, ulceration, or gangrene; in this context, revascularization has been shown not only to improve symptoms but also to reduce the likelihood of subsequent amputation. The choice of revascularization procedure, ie, percutaneous transluminal angioplasty with or without stenting versus surgical revascularization, depends on lesion location and severity, likelihood of success, risk of major complications, and experience and technical expertise of the interventionalist and surgeon. Importantly, these two therapeutic approaches should be viewed as complementary rather than competing strategies, and the choice of procedure should be tailored to individual patient circumstances and preferences.

Indications for AAA repair include development of symptoms, rapid aneurysmal dilatation detected during serial assessments (≥1 cm in 1 year), and aneurysms ≥5.5 cm in diameter. Patients with asymptomatic AAAs 4–5.4 cm in diameter should undergo repeat evaluations at intervals of 6–12 months. The choice of open or endovascular surgical repair of AAAs is based on location of the lesion and patient comorbidities and prognosis. Open repair is favored for suprarenal

Table 50.5—Class I Indications for Permanent Pacemaker Implantation for Bradyarrhythmias

Sinus node dysfunction with documented symptomatic bradycardia, including frequent sinus pauses that produce symptoms (SOE=C)

Symptomatic chronotropic incompetence (inability to increase heart rate commensurate with increased activity level) (SOE=C)

Symptomatic sinus bradycardia or advanced AV block that results from required drug therapy for medical conditions (SOE=C)

Third-degree or advanced second-degree AV block associated with symptomatic bradycardia or ventricular arrhythmias presumed to be due to AV block (SOE=C)

Third-degree or advanced second-degree AV block in awake, symptom-free patients in sinus rhythm with periods of asystole ≥3 seconds or any escape rate <40 beats per minute, or with an escape rhythm that is below the AV node (SOE=C)

Third-degree or advanced second-degree AV block in awake, symptom-free patients in atrial fibrillation with 1 or more periods of asystole ≥5 seconds (SOE=C)

Second-degree AV block with associated symptomatic bradycardia (SOE=B)

Third-degree AV block after catheter ablation of the AV junction (SOE=C)

Second- or third-degree AV block during exercise in the absence of myocardial ischemia (SOE=C)

Asymptomatic persistent third-degree AV block with average awake ventricular rates of 40 beats per minute or faster if cardiomegaly or left ventricular dysfunction is present or if the site of block is below the AV node (SOE=B)

Third-degree or advanced second-degree AV block at any anatomic level that is due to cardiac surgery and is not expected to resolve postoperatively (SOE=C)

AAAs and for patients with fewer comorbidities and a remaining life expectancy of >10 years, because this procedure has reduced rates of long-term leakage and rupture (SOE=B). Endovascular repair is suitable for patients with infrarenal AAAs and for those who have a higher surgical risk or shorter remaining life expectancy, because it is associated with lower perioperative complications and mortality (SOE=B).

SHARED DECISION MAKING IN CARDIOVASCULAR DISEASE

Biomedical advances provide patients and clinicians with a growing range of treatment options for cardiovascular diseases. These treatment options vary widely in invasiveness, as well as in potential benefits, risks, complications, and burdens. Because the choice among treatments can be not just clinically complex but also highly dependent on patients' individual values and preferences, it is critical for patients to play an active role in decision making. Ensuring a process of shared decision making is particularly crucial in

> ### CHOOSING WISELY® RECOMMENDATIONS
>
> *Cardiology/Coronary Artery Disease*
>
> - Do not order coronary artery calcium scoring for screening purposes in low-risk, asymptomatic individuals except those with a family history of premature CAD.
> - Do not use coronary artery calcium scoring for patients with known CAD (including stents and bypass grafts).
> - Do not routinely order coronary CT angiography for screening asymptomatic individuals.
> - Do not perform stress cardiac imaging or advanced noninvasive imaging in the initial evaluation of patients without cardiac symptoms unless high-risk markers are present.
> - Do not obtain screening exercise ECG testing in individuals who are asymptomatic and at low risk of coronary heart disease.
> - Do not perform routine annual stress testing after coronary artery revascularization.
>
> *Cardiology/Valvular Heart Disease*
>
> - Do not perform echocardiography as routine follow-up for mild, asymptomatic native valve disease in adult patients with no change in signs or symptoms.
>
> *Cardiology/Peripheral Arterial Disease*
>
> - Do not perform percutaneous or surgical revascularization of peripheral artery stenosis in patients without claudication or critical limb ischemia.

the care of older patients, who frequently prioritize maintaining physical function and symptom relief over prolonging life. When done well, such shared decision making entails patients expressing their preferences and values, and clinicians providing relevant details of the risks and benefits of possible treatments.

Translating these principles into practice has been gaining prominence in cardiovascular medicine, and a number of tools have been developed to promote shared decision making. Investigators at the University of Colorado, for example, have developed patient decision aids for ICD and LVAD implementation (https://patientdecisionaid.org/). Mayo Clinic researchers have developed a decision aid that allows clinicians and patients to weigh the potential benefits of statin therapy, based on a risk factor profile (https://statindecisionaid.mayoclinic.org).

At least 2 limitations are recognized with current decision aid paradigms. First, the risks and benefits for treatments or devices are typically derived from studies involving relatively young populations, as data on benefits in older adults are often limited. Second, decision aids generally assume that conversations are limited to a patient and a clinician, but with older patients (particularly those with limited decision-making capacity), family members and caregivers commonly play a prominent role. The development of decision aids specifically targeted toward cardiovascular interventions in older patients is an important area for future research.

RESOURCES

- Amsterdam EA, Wenger NK, Brindis RG, et al. 2014 AHA/ACC Guideline for the management of patients with non-ST-elevation acute coronary syndromes. *J Am Coll Cardiol*. 2014;64(24):e139–228.

- Chalmers SW, Champion CR. Pharmacotherapeutics in cardiovascular dysrhythmias. *J Nurs Pract*. 2019;15(1):132–138.e1.

- January CT, Wann LS, Alpert JS, et al. 2014 AHA/ACC/HRS guideline for the management of patients with atrial fibrillation. *J Am Coll Cardiol*. 2014;64(21):e1–76.

- Murphy N, Alderman P, Harvey KV, et al. Women and heart disease: an evidence-based update. *J Nurs Pract*. 2017;13(9):610–616.

- Nishimura RA, Otto CM, Bonow RO, et al. 2014 AHA/ACC guideline for the management of patients with valvular heart disease. *J Am Coll Cardiol*. 2014;63(22):e57–185.

- Oliver-McNeil S. Management of valvular heart disease in adults: implications for nurse practitioner practice. *J Nurs Pract*. 2019;15e(1):65–72.

CHAPTER 51—HEART FAILURE

KEY POINTS

- Heart failure (HF) is the leading cause of hospitalization in older adults and a major source of chronic disability.

- Compared with younger patients, older patients with HF are more likely to be women and more likely to have preserved left ventricular systolic function.

- ACE inhibitors, angiotensin-receptor blockers (ARBs), β-blockers, ARBs/neprilysin inhibitors (ARNIs), aldosterone antagonists, and in selected patients hydralazine/nitrates reduce morbidity and mortality from HF with reduced ejection fraction (HFrEF). No pharmacotherapy for HF with preserved ejection fraction (HFpEF) has been definitively shown to reduce mortality.

- Optimal management of HF in older patients often requires a multidisciplinary approach.

EPIDEMIOLOGY

Heart failure (HF) currently affects approximately 6.5 million Americans, with >950,000 new cases diagnosed each year. Costs related to HF in the United States exceed $30 billion annually, half of which is spent on hospitalizations, which number over 1 million annually. Up to 25% of cases are readmitted within 1 month of a hospitalization for HF. By 2030, the projected prevalence of HF and associated costs are expected to rise to >8 million Americans and almost $70 billion annually, respectively. The incidence and prevalence of HF increase progressively with age, and HF is the leading cause of hospitalization and rehospitalization in older adults. The median age of patients hospitalized with HF is 75 years, and approximately two-thirds of deaths attributable to HF occur in patients ≥75 years old. Approximately 14% of men and 13% of women >80 years old have HF. Among older adults with HF, three-fifths have ≥5 additional chronic conditions, more than half have functional impairment and mobility disability, and more than a quarter have cognitive impairment and frailty. Although the incidence of HF is somewhat higher in men, women comprise 55% of prevalent HF cases.

ETIOLOGY AND PATHOPHYSIOLOGY

The syndrome of HF in older adults is often multifactorial in origin. Hypertension is the most common antecedent cardiovascular condition, closely followed by coronary artery disease (CAD). Other common causes of HF in older adults include valvular heart disease and nonischemic dilated cardiomyopathy. Less commonly, hypertrophic cardiomyopathy, restrictive cardiomyopathy (eg, from amyloidosis), or pericardial disease induce HF. The rising prevalence of HF with increasing age reflects both age-related changes in cardiovascular structure and function that diminish cardiovascular reserve, and greater prevalence of those cardiovascular diseases (especially hypertension and CAD) that predispose to HF.

Distinguishing between HF patients with a left ventricular ejection fraction <40% (heart failure with reduced ejection fraction [HFrEF]) and those with a left ventricular ejection fracture >40%–50% (heart failure with preserved ejection fraction [HFpEF]) is clinically important. The terms HFrEF and HFpEF have supplanted the previous labels of "systolic" and "diastolic" heart failure. (One reason HFrEF is a more descriptive term than "systolic HF" is that patients with this condition generally have impaired diastolic as well as systolic function.) HFpEF comprises approximately 50% of total HF prevalence and is associated with female sex, obesity, CAD, diabetes, dyslipidemia, atrial arrhythmias, and, most importantly, hypertension. Although nearly 90% of HF patients <65 years old have HFrEF, approximately 40% of men and two-thirds of women >65 years old with HF have HFpEF. The rising prevalence of HFpEF in older patients is due to age-related changes in left ventricular diastolic function and increased prevalence of hypertension, particularly in women.

CLINICAL FEATURES

As in younger patients, exertional shortness of breath, fatigue, orthopnea, and leg edema are the most common symptoms of HF in older adults. Exertional symptoms, however, may be less prominent in older patients because of a more sedentary lifestyle. Conversely, the prevalence of atypical symptoms increases with age, and older HF patients may present with decreased mental acuity, confusion, lethargy, irritability, anorexia, abdominal discomfort, or altered bowel function, including both constipation and diarrhea.

Classical physical findings of HF in younger patients include tachycardia, narrowed pulse pressure, increased jugular venous pressure, hepatojugular reflux, an S3 gallop, moist pulmonary crackles, diminished breath sounds at the lung bases (due to pleural effusions), and pitting edema of the legs. Many or even all of these findings may be absent in older HF patients. In addition, pulmonary crackles in older patients may be due to comorbid chronic lung disease or atelectasis, and peripheral edema may arise from hepatic or renal disease, venous insufficiency, hypoalbuminemia, or medications (especially calcium channel blockers).

Because the symptoms and signs of HF in older adults are often atypical and nonspecific, it is important for clinicians to maintain a high index of suspicion when an older patient presents with complaints that are vague, or the origins of which appear unrelated to the circulatory system.

DIAGNOSIS

The diagnosis of HF may be established on clinical grounds in patients presenting with a constellation of classical symptoms and signs. However, the diagnosis is often uncertain, and additional testing is required.

The standard chest radiograph remains a useful initial test for determining the presence of HF, with the appearance of cardiomegaly, pulmonary congestion, or pleural effusion suggesting the diagnosis. Competing diagnoses such as pneumonia can also be excluded. However, the chest radiograph may be difficult to interpret in older adults with chronic lung disease, kyphoscoliosis, or poor inspiratory effort. Importantly, the absence of pulmonary congestion on a chest radiograph does not exclude a diagnosis of HF.

The ECG may show evidence of left ventricular hypertrophy, acute ischemia or prior myocardial infarction, left atrial enlargement, or atrial fibrillation—all of which predispose to development of HF—but the ECG is not usually helpful in establishing a diagnosis of either acute or chronic HF. Similarly, although it is appropriate to obtain a CBC, routine chemistry panel, thyroid studies, and in selected cases, biomarkers of cardiac ischemia (ie, troponin) in patients with suspected HF, in most cases these tests are insufficient to confirm or exclude the diagnosis.

B-type natriuretic peptide (BNP) and its precursor N-terminal pro-BNP (NT-proBNP) are generated by cardiac myocytes in response to myocardial stretch and are thus valuable laboratory tools for establishing the diagnosis of volume overload due to HF (either HFrEF or HFpEF), as well as for distinguishing shortness of breath due to HF from that attributable to noncardiac causes. BNP and NT-proBNP levels increase with age (especially in women) and with decreasing renal function. As a result, the specificity of increased levels of these peptides for diagnosing HF decreases with age, and the clinical significance of an isolated increase of BNP or NT-proBNP in an older adult may be difficult to interpret. Despite these caveats, a BNP level <100 pg/mL in an older adult with suspected acute HF makes the diagnosis very unlikely (negative likelihood ratio approximately 0.1), whereas a BNP level ≥500 pg/mL is consistent with active HF (positive likelihood ratio approximately 6). Finally, BNP and NT-pro-BNP levels are lower in obesity and therefore may be less helpful in excluding the diagnosis of HF.

Once a diagnosis of HF has been established, it is important to determine the cause and to assess left ventricular function because these factors affect management. Echocardiography with Doppler is the preferred method for evaluating left ventricular function because it provides detailed assessment of left and right ventricular size and wall thickness, systolic and diastolic function, atrial size, valvular function, intracardiac pressures, and the pericardium. MRI may be used, when not contraindicated by the presence of implanted ferromagnetic devices or advanced kidney disease, in patients with inadequate echo images or to assess for infiltration or scarring of the myocardium. Radionuclide ventriculography is another alternative for quantification of left ventricular ejection fraction (LVEF) in patients with inadequate echo images. In patients with suspected CAD who are suitable candidates for revascularization (including willingness to undergo further testing and interventions if clinically indicated), a stress test (echo or nuclear medicine) should be performed, followed by coronary angiography should the stress test suggest severe—especially multivessel—CAD.

MANAGEMENT

The goals of HF management are to decrease symptoms, improve quality of life, reduce acute exacerbations requiring hospitalization, and prolong survival. Hypertension, hyperlipidemia, and diabetes should be treated in accordance with current guidelines. Smoking cessation should be strongly encouraged and supported, and alcohol intake should be limited to no more than 2 drinks/day in men and 1 drink/day in women. NSAIDs should be avoided because they promote water and sodium retention, and they antagonize the effects of diuretics and renin-angiotensin system inhibitors. CAD should be treated with anti-ischemic medications and, if indicated, percutaneous or surgical revascularization. Similarly, valvular lesions should be managed in accordance with established practice guidelines. In patients with atrial fibrillation, the heart rate should be controlled, preferably with β-blockers. In selected cases, restoration and maintenance of sinus rhythm may be considered using either a pharmacologic or catheter-based approach, recognizing that rhythm control is not superior to rate control in patients with HF (SOE=B). Finally, patients should be tested for anemia and thyroid dysfunction, and appropriate therapy started if indicated.

Nonpharmacologic Therapy

HF patients have long been counseled to restrict dietary sodium intake to no more than 2 grams/day (SOE=C), but

Table 51.1—Characteristics of Heart Failure Disease Management Programs

Program Components	Description
Delivery personnel	Varies from single providers (usually nurses) to large interprofessional teams comprising nurses, physicians, pharmacists, social workers, dietitians, physical therapists, case managers, and care coordinators
Assessments	Ability to perform self-care (health literacy, cognitive function, depression, etc), motivation to perform self-care, social supports, caregiver burden, root causes of hospitalization (if applicable)
Intervention content	Development of individualized care plans, patient/caregiver education, medication management, care coordination, discharge support, caregiver support, remote monitoring (weight, vital signs, symptoms)
Methods of communication	In person, telephonic, mixed
Duration and intensity of follow-up	Highly variable from days to months; program ideally tailored to HF severity and individual patient needs
Clinical outcomes	Hospitalizations, rehospitalizations, symptoms, quality of life, knowledge/skills attainment, self-efficacy

low-sodium diets have been linked to worse outcomes in several clinical trials and little data exist on optimal sodium intake. Sodium allowances should likely be individualized, taking into account volume status, serum sodium level, and severity of HF, particularly in older patients predisposed to hyponatremia. Fluid restriction is not usually necessary except in patients with advanced HF or hyponatremia, but patients should be advised to avoid excess fluid intake (ie, the oft-quoted dictum to drink 8–10 glasses of water every day does not apply to individuals with HF, renal insufficiency, or other fluid-retaining states). Exercise training or regular physical activity (eg, walking, stationary cycling, swimming, or water aerobics) has favorable effects on functional status in HF patients and is recommended by current HF guidelines (SOE=B). Exercise duration and intensity should be adjusted to the individual patient's level of conditioning, severity of HF, and comorbidities, but should be gradually increased over time, if possible, to achieve 30–60 minutes of aerobic exercise most days of the week. These activities should be complemented by stretching and strengthening exercises, as well as by gait and balance exercises if indicated. Cardiac rehabilitation for patients with stable symptoms and an LVEF ≤35% has been approved by CMS and most private insurance companies as an effective therapy for older HF patients. Payers generally do not provide coverage for cardiac rehabilitation for patients with HFpEF.

Patients should be instructed to keep an ongoing record of their daily weight. Weights should be measured in the morning without clothes after going to the bathroom but before eating. A "dry weight" should be established (based on the home scale, not the office scale), and patients should be instructed to contact their clinicians if the weight varies by more than 2–3 pounds above or below the dry weight. Selected patients may be provided with detailed instructions for self-adjustment of diuretic dosages based on daily weights.

Older patients with moderate or advanced HF, multiple comorbidities, or a recent HF exacerbation requiring hospitalization may benefit from participation in a structured HF disease management program. While significant variation exists across programs, they often involve enhanced education and care coordination, usually by an HF nurse specialist or interprofessional team, in some cases supplemented by telemonitoring devices. Common program characteristics are described in Table 51.1. Multicomponent interventions delivered in person with high intensity have been shown to reduce hospitalizations and inpatient costs, as well as to improve quality of life in older HF patients (SOE=A) (see Recurrent Hospitalization section below for further discussion).

Pharmacotherapy of HFrEF

ACE inhibitors, ARBs, aldosterone antagonists, and β-blockers have been shown to improve outcomes and reduce mortality in multiple large prospective trials involving a broad range of HF patients with decreased left ventricular systolic function (SOE=A), and these agents are now considered the cornerstone of therapy for HFrEF. In addition, combination therapy involving the ARB valsartan with sacubitril, a neprilysin inhibitor, reduced mortality and HF hospitalization in a single large prospective trial (SOE=B). This ARNI combination is now considered an alternative to ACE inhibitors and ARBs for appropriately selected patients. Although older patients, especially those with multiple comorbid conditions, have been markedly under-represented in these studies, the available evidence indicates that the beneficial effects of these agents likely extend to them.

For a list of ACE inhibitors approved for the treatment of HF, along with recommended initial and maintenance dosages, see Table 51.2. In general, treatment of older HF patients should be started at the lowest dosage and gradually titrated to the maintenance

Table 51.2—Recommended Dosages of ACE Inhibitors, Angiotensin II Receptor Blockers, β-Blockers, and Neprilysin Inhibitor Plus Angiotensin II Receptor Blocker in Patients with Heart Failure with Reduced Ejection Fraction (HFrEF)

Agent	Starting Dosage	Target Dosage
ACE Inhibitors		
Benazepril[OL]	2.5 mg/d	40 mg/d
Captopril	6.25 mg q8h	50 mg q8h
Enalapril	2.5 mg/d	10–20 mg q12h
Fosinopril	5–10 mg/d	40 mg/d
Lisinopril	2.5–5 mg/d	20–40 mg/d
Moexipril[OL]	3.75 mg/d	15 mg/d
Perindopril[OL]	2 mg/d	8–16 mg/d
Quinapril	5 mg q12h	10–20 mg q12h
Ramipril	1.25–2.5 mg/d	10 mg/d
Trandolapril	1 mg/d	4 mg/d
Angiotensin II Receptor Blockers		
Candesartan	4 mg/d	32 mg/d
Eprosartan[OL]	400 mg/d	400 mg q12h
Irbesartan[OL]	75 mg/d	150–300 mg/d
Losartan[OL]	25 mg/d	50–100 mg/d
Olmesartan[OL]	20 mg/d	40 mg/d
Telmisartan[OL]	20 mg/d	80 mg/d
Valsartan	20–40 mg q12h	160 mg q12h
β-Blockers		
Bisoprolol[OL]	1.25 mg/d	10 mg/d
Carvedilol	3.125 mg q12h	25–50 mg q12h
Carvedilol ER	10 mg/d	80 mg/d
Metoprolol XL	12.5–25 mg/d	200 mg/d
Neprilysin Inhibitor + Angiotensin II Receptor Blocker		
Sacubitril + Valsartan	24/26 mg q12h	97/103 mg q12h

dosage as tolerated. Contraindications to ACE inhibitors include known intolerance to these agents, hyperkalemia (serum potassium ≥5.5 mEq/L), hypotension (systolic blood pressure <80 mmHg), and severe renal insufficiency (estimated creatinine clearance <30 mL/min) in patients not currently undergoing dialysis. Common adverse events include cough in 5%–10% of patients during long-term treatment, mild worsening of renal function (often transient), hyperkalemia, hypotension, GI distress, and rarely angioedema. Renal function and potassium concentrations should be monitored at least weekly during initiation and titration of ACE inhibitor therapy.

ARBs are indicated as an alternative to ACE inhibitors in HF patients unable to tolerate the latter class of medications because of cough, allergic reactions, or GI disturbances (Table 51.2). Contraindications and adverse events associated with these agents are otherwise similar to those of ACE inhibitors. In particular, the incidence of renal insufficiency, hyperkalemia, and hypotension is comparable with equivalent dosages of ACE inhibitors and ARBs. Combination therapy with an ACE inhibitor and an ARB increases the probability of adverse events without providing clear clinical benefit.

β-Blockers counteract the deleterious effects of chronic activation of the sympathetic nervous system in HF patients and have been shown to improve ventricular function and symptoms while reducing the risk of both sudden and non-sudden cardiac death (SOE=A). Unlike the case with ACE inhibitors and ARBs, the reduction in mortality of β-blockers is not thought to be a class effect and has been demonstrated only for carvedilol, metoprolol succinate, and bisoprolol. The treatment strategy of β-blockers is like that for ACE inhibitors and ARBs: the patient should be started at the lowest available dosage, which should be gradually titrated to the maintenance dosage over several weeks (Table 51.2). The benefit of β-blockers is proportional to the degree of heart-rate reduction achieved, but there is no established "optimal" heart rate, and the potential benefit of dose escalation should be weighed against the risk of adverse effects. Contraindications to β-blocker therapy include severe decompensated HF, active bronchospastic lung disease, marked bradycardia (heart rate <45–50 beats per minute), relative hypotension (systolic blood pressure <90–100 mmHg), significant atrioventricular nodal block (PR interval ≥240 msec or higher degrees of block), and known intolerance to β-blockers. Occasionally, HF symptoms will worsen on initiation or titration of a β-blocker (and patients should be warned about this possibility), but in most cases this is a transient phenomenon, and >80% of HF patients are able to tolerate long-term β-blocker therapy when judiciously initiated and titrated, even those whose treatment is started before discharge (during hospitalization for HF).

Valsartan plus sacubitril, an ARNI, is the first medication in its class. Sacubitril acts to raise the levels of several endogenous vasoactive peptides, including natriuretic peptides, bradykinin, and adrenomedullin. A clinical trial comparing valsartan plus sacubitril with the ACE inhibitor enalapril in symptomatic patients with HFrEF found that the ARNI significantly lowered rates of mortality and hospitalization (SOE=B). Valsartan plus sacubitril can be used as an alternative to ACE inhibitors or ARBs in patients with HFrEF and New York Heart Association (NYHA) Class II–III symptoms (Table 51.3) who have previously tolerated treatment with ACE inhibitors or ARBs. As with ACE inhibitors and ARBs, the use of ARNIs may be associated with mild worsening of renal function, hyperkalemia, and hypotension.

Hypotension, in particular, may limit the use of ARNIs in patients with low blood pressure before treatment. ARNIs may also rarely cause angioedema and are contraindicated in patients with a history of this complication. ARNIs should not be administered concomitantly with ACE inhibitors or additional ARBs. To minimize the risk of angioedema, an ARNI should not be started within 36 hours of the last dose of an ACE inhibitor.

Diuretics are usually a necessary component of HF therapy, and they remain the most effective agents for relief of congestion and edema. Except for aldosterone antagonists (see below), diuretics have not been shown to reduce mortality. In general, the diuretic dosage should be adjusted to maintain euvolemia, manifested by the absence of pulmonary rales, an S3 gallop, increased jugular venous pressure, hepatojugular reflux, and peripheral edema. In patients with equivocal findings, serial measurement of BNP may be useful for tracking volume status. Some patients with mild HF respond satisfactorily to a thiazide diuretic, but most require maintenance therapy with a loop diuretic, such as furosemide, bumetanide, or torsemide. Patients with advanced HF, concomitant renal insufficiency, or both, may be resistant to conventional dosages of loop diuretics; in these patients, the addition of metolazone at 2.5–10 mg/d is often effective, but careful monitoring of electrolytes is required. The principal adverse events associated with diuretic therapy are electrolyte disturbances, including hypokalemia, hyponatremia, and hypomagnesemia; close monitoring of these electrolytes, as well as renal function, is therefore warranted. Thiamine deficiency may occur during long-term treatment with loop diuretics and can contribute to apparent diuretic resistance. Although routine monitoring of thiamine levels is not recommended, supplemental thiamine in the form of a multivitamin is reasonable in older patients who require long-term therapy with a loop diuretic (SOE=D). Older patients as a group are also at increased risk of dehydration during diuretic treatment because of attenuation of the thirst response and diminished oral fluid intake, especially during periods of illness or increased ambient temperatures. Therefore, clinicians should remain vigilant for possible signs of dehydration, including excess weight loss during daily weight monitoring.

The aldosterone antagonist spironolactone has been shown to reduce mortality and hospitalizations in patients with NYHA class III–IV HF (Table 51.3) and an LVEF <30% (SOE=A), with similar benefits observed in older and younger patients. Similarly, the selective aldosterone antagonist eplerenone has been associated with improved outcomes in patients with recent myocardial infarction complicated by HF or an LVEF <40%, as well as in patients with NYHA class II HF and an LVEF ≤35% (SOE=A). Based on these

Table 51.3—New York Heart Association Functional Class

Class	Symptoms
I	No symptoms and no limitation in ordinary physical activity, but structural heart disease present. Walking, climbing stairs, or doing household chores does not cause undue shortness of breath, palpitations, chest discomfort, or fatigue.
II	Slight limitation of physical activity. Ordinary physical activity causes shortness of breath, palpitations, chest discomfort, or fatigue; able to walk more than 2 blocks and climb 2 flights of stairs.
III	Marked limitation of physical activity. Less than ordinary physical activity (eg, walking less than 2 blocks) causes shortness of breath, palpitations, chest discomfort, or fatigue; no symptoms at rest.
IV	Severe activity limitation. Unable to carry out any physical activity (eg, walking in the house, dressing, bathing, toileting) without shortness of breath, palpitations, chest discomfort, or fatigue; symptoms may be present at rest.

studies, spironolactone 12.5–25 mg/d or eplerenone 25–50 mg/d is recommended for patients with NYHA class II–IV HF and an LVEF ≤35%. Spironolactone and eplerenone are contraindicated in patients with serum creatinine ≥2.5 mg/dL or serum potassium ≥5 mEq/L. Older adults are at increased risk of worsening renal function and hyperkalemia during aldosterone antagonist therapy. Potassium levels and renal function should be checked within 2–3 days and again at 7 days after initiating treatment. Subsequent monitoring should generally occur at least monthly during the first 3 months and every 3 months thereafter. Potassium supplementation can usually be discontinued in patients receiving an aldosterone antagonist, especially in combination with an ACE inhibitor or ARB. Up to 10% of patients develop painful gynecomastia during long-term treatment with spironolactone compared with <1% with eplerenone.

Before the advent of ACE inhibitors and β-blockers, the combination of hydralazine and isosorbide dinitrate was shown to reduce mortality relative to placebo in patients with HFrEF. Although a subsequent study showed reduced mortality in patients treated with the ACE inhibitor enalapril compared with those treated with hydralazine and nitrates, retrospective analysis revealed that this difference was not evident in black participants. This observation led to a prospective trial conducted exclusively in self-described blacks that demonstrated additional survival benefit when hydralazine and nitrates were added to background therapy that included ACE inhibitors/ARBs and β-blockers. Based on these studies, the combination of hydralazine and nitrates is recommended for HF patients with contraindications to ACE inhibitors and ARBs (eg, severe renal insufficiency), and in blacks with advanced HF as an adjunct to ACE inhibitor and β-blocker therapy (SOE=A). The benefit of adding hydralazine and nitrates to ACE inhibitors and β-blockers in non-black patients has not been established. The starting dosage of hydralazine is 25–50 mg q8h, titrating to a maximal dosage of 100 mg q8h. The starting dosage of isosorbide dinitrate is 10 mg q8h, titrating to a maximal dosage of 30–40 mg q8h. Common adverse events associated with hydralazine include palpitations, nausea, and dizziness; rarely, a drug-induced lupus syndrome may occur during prolonged therapy at high dosage (≥300 mg/d). The most common adverse event from isosorbide dinitrate is headache, which usually resolves with continued use.

Digoxin improves symptoms and reduces HF hospitalizations in patients with HFrEF but does not decrease mortality. It is a reasonable therapeutic option in patients with persistent limiting symptoms or recurrent hospitalizations in whom the measures discussed above have not resulted in a satisfactory response. Retrospective analyses based on a large randomized trial suggest that the optimal digoxin serum concentration for improving clinical outcomes is 0.5–0.9 ng/mL, which is substantially lower than the "therapeutic range" previously reported by most clinical laboratories. Concentrations above this level may be associated with increased mortality. Therefore, digoxin should be dosed to maintain a serum concentration <1 ng/mL, and a dosage of 0.125 mg/d is likely to be sufficient for most older patients with relatively preserved renal function. A lower dosage (0.125 mg every other day) might be required in patients with renal insufficiency or low lean body mass. Adverse effects of digoxin include nausea, visual disturbances, and cardiac arrhythmias (bradyarrhythmias as well as supraventricular and ventricular tachyarrhythmias). However, with appropriate monitoring of the serum digoxin concentration, serious digoxin toxicity is infrequent, and there is no convincing evidence that older patients are at increased risk of life-threatening digitalis intoxication. Amiodarone, quinidine, and verapamil, as well as several other medications, are associated with up to a 2-fold increase in serum digoxin concentrations, and the dosage of digoxin should be reduced by 50% in patients receiving these drugs.

Previous guidelines suggested consideration of antiplatelet or anticoagulant therapy for HF patients in normal sinus rhythm, even in the absence of compelling indications for treatment. However, although HFrEF patients are at increased risk of thromboembolic events, the only placebo-controlled trial of antithrombotic therapy in these patients showed no difference in a composite outcome that included stroke. Randomized trials comparing different antithrombotic strategies (aspirin, clopidogrel, warfarin) have also shown no benefit of one strategy over another. Moreover, among HF patients >60 years old, warfarin has been associated with increased bleeding without a corresponding reduction in thromboembolic events. Current guidelines therefore recommend against routine anticoagulation in HF patients in the absence of atrial fibrillation. For HF patients with comorbid atrial fibrillation, which includes nearly 30% of the geriatric HF population, long-term anticoagulation with warfarin or one of the newer oral anticoagulants is indicated in most cases.

From the preceding, it is apparent that optimal treatment of HFrEF usually requires a minimum of 3 medications and, in some cases, up to 7. Because HF in older patients almost never occurs as an isolated disease process, almost all patients are taking one or more additional medications for other coexisting illnesses. Thus, pharmacotherapy of the older HF patient is problematic from the perspective of adherence, potential for drug interactions and adverse events, and cost. It is therefore essential that therapy be individualized, taking into consideration the multiple and often competing factors that influence quality of life and other clinical outcomes in older adults with multiple chronic illnesses and limited life expectancy.

Pharmacotherapy of HFpEF

In contrast to HFrEF, no trials looking at HFpEF have demonstrated a clear reduction in mortality with any pharmacologic intervention. Several antagonists of the renin-angiotensin system have shown a trend toward reduced hospitalizations, including the ARB candesartan (SOE=A) and the ACE inhibitor perindopril (SOE=B). In contrast, a large trial of the ARB irbesartan showed no effect on mortality, hospitalizations, or other cardiac outcomes in older adults with HFpEF (SOE=A). The TOPCAT trial showed that the aldosterone antagonist spironolactone did not reduce a composite outcome of cardiovascular death or hospitalization, but a small reduction in HF hospitalizations was noted (SOE=A). Conversely, a large retrospective registry study failed to demonstrate improved clinical outcomes, including hospitalizations, with the use of aldosterone antagonists among HFpEF patients ≥65 years old (SOE=B). Digoxin may reduce hospitalizations due to HF in patients with HFpEF, but this appears to be at the expense of increased hospitalizations for unstable angina (SOE=B). In a study of HF patients ≥70 years old, the β-blocker nebivolol was associated with an overall reduction in a composite outcome of all-cause death or hospitalization, but this difference was not statistically significant in a subgroup analysis of patients with LVEF ≥35% (SOE=B). The phosphodiesterase-5 inhibitor sildenafil had no effect on functional or clinical outcomes in the RELAX trial (SOE=B), whereas the endothelin A-type receptor antagonist sitaxsentan had a modest but significant effect on exercise performance in the ESS-DHF trial (SOE=C). Isosorbide mononitrate resulted in worsening functional capacity in the NEAT-HFpEF trial and should not be used (SOE=B). Based on the available evidence, optimal therapy for HFpEF remains undefined. Current recommendations include aggressive treatment of hypertension and other risk factors, appropriate management of comorbid CAD, and maintenance of sinus rhythm or effective rate control in patients with atrial fibrillation (SOE=D). Diuretics should be used judiciously to maintain euvolemia while avoiding over-diuresis, because patients with HFpEF are often "volume-sensitive." The addition of an ACE inhibitor or ARB, and possibly a β-blocker (especially in patients with CAD), is appropriate to reduce the risk of hospitalization, recognizing that the impact of these agents on other clinically relevant outcomes is unproved.

Device Therapy, Mechanical Circulatory Support, and Heart Transplantation

The implantable cardioverter-defibrillator (ICD) has been shown to reduce mortality from sudden cardiac death in patients with HF (whether ischemic or nonischemic) and an LVEF of ≤35% (SOE=A). However, few older patients were enrolled in the ICD randomized trials, and a meta-analysis suggested that the benefit of ICDs in reducing mortality is lower in older than in younger patients, probably because of the higher risks of death from both non-arrhythmic causes and "non-shockable" rhythms like asystole and pulseless electrical activity (SOE=A). In addition, major complications related to ICD implantation are 2-fold greater in patients ≥80 years old than in younger patients (SOE=B). Nonetheless 40%–45% of ICDs in the United States are implanted in patients ≥70 years old. Importantly, ICDs have not been shown to improve survival in patients with NYHA class I or IV HF, and there is no survival benefit within the first 12–18 months after implantation. Also, quality of life is impaired in patients who receive one or more ICD shocks, and up to 10% of shocks are inappropriate, ie, occurring in the absence of a life-threatening tachyarrhythmia. Rates of inappropriate shock may, however, be lower with newer devices and programming algorithms.

Based on available evidence, prophylactic ICD placement is recommended in patients with NYHA class II or III HF, an LVEF ≤35%, and a remaining life expectancy with good functional status of at least 1 year. ICD implantation should be deferred for at least 40 days after acute myocardial infarction and for at least 90 days after a new diagnosis of dilated cardiomyopathy (in the latter case because left ventricular function often improves after initiation of β-blocker and ACE inhibitor therapy).

Given that HF patients >75–80 years old have limited remaining life expectancy, especially if they have multiple comorbid illnesses or frailty, and that ICDs may not reduce mortality in this age group, the selection of older patients for ICD therapy must be individualized, and a shared decision-making approach is recommended. Patients should be advised about the potential benefits and risks of ICD implantation, including the possibility of an adverse effect on quality of life. Although many older patients elect to forego ICD implantation after an informed discussion, those who desire an ICD should not be denied one solely on the basis of age, assuming that appropriate indications for the device are present. In these patients, it is appropriate to discuss circumstances under which the patient would want to have the device disabled, especially at end of life due to progressive HF or other terminal illness.

Cardiac resynchronization therapy (CRT) has been shown to improve symptoms, exercise tolerance, quality of life, and survival in selected patients with advanced HFrEF and persistent severe symptoms (NYHA class III or IV) despite conventional medical therapy (SOE=A). CRT involves placement of a biventricular pacemaker with one lead in the right ventricle and a second lead inserted retrograde into the coronary sinus to stimulate the left ventricle. CRT is indicated in patients with dyssynchronous left ventricular contraction, most commonly related to left bundle-branch block, which is present in up to 30% of patients with HFrEF. The basis for CRT, as the name implies, is to "resynchronize" left ventricular contraction, thereby increasing myocardial efficiency, stroke work, ejection fraction, and cardiac output. Although few older patients have been enrolled in the CRT trials, observational studies indicate that the benefits of CRT are age-independent (SOE=B). Therefore, because the main objective of CRT is to improve symptoms and quality of life, and because the risk of CRT is modest, it seems reasonable to offer such treatment to older patients with severe left ventricular dysfunction, advanced HF symptoms, and evidence of left ventricular dyssynchrony (ie, left bundle-branch block with QRS duration ≥150 msec).

An advance in the management of HF patients who remain highly symptomatic despite optimal medical and device therapy is the development of implantable mechanical left ventricular assist devices (LVADs). LVADs reduce symptoms, increase exercise tolerance, and improve quality of life and survival in selected patients with HF and severe systolic dysfunction, including adults in their 70s and 80s. Although originally reserved for use as a "bridge" to heart transplantation, LVADs are now often implanted (ie, used as "destination therapy") to alleviate symptoms and improve quality of life in patients who are not transplant candidates. As a result, an increasing number of older adults are receiving LVADs, and this trend is likely to accelerate as the safety and efficacy of these devices continue to improve. Older patients are at increased risk of LVAD-related complications, particularly GI bleeding, and patients with advanced comorbidities or frailty may not be suitable candidates. Nonetheless, small studies of LVADs in highly selected septuagenarians and octogenarians have reported favorable effects on quality of life and survival, so age alone should not be considered an absolute contraindication to LVAD implantation.

RECURRENT HOSPITALIZATION

Recurrent hospitalization is common among patients admitted with HF. Approximately 20%–25% of such patients are readmitted within 30 days of discharge, and up to 50% are readmitted within 6 months. Prediction and prevention of early readmission has proved challenging, in part because only one-third of patients readmitted within 30 days have HF as the primary reason for rehospitalization. Common alternative reasons for readmission include pneumonia, COPD, sepsis, and other cardiovascular conditions, including acute myocardial infarction. Efforts to predict and prevent readmission have intensified following the October 2012 implementation of the Hospital Readmissions Reduction Program under the Affordable Care Act, which requires CMS to reduce payments to hospitals with excess readmissions.

Contributors to readmission may include biological factors (severity of heart failure, number and severity of comorbidities), patient behavioral factors (adherence to pharmacotherapy, adherence to diet and lifestyle), and health-care system factors (quality of inpatient care, discharge practices, care transitions, outpatient care resources). Providers should consider the impact of therapeutic choices on comorbid conditions, with particular attention to renal function, anticoagulation, lung disease, and drug interactions. Patients who experience recurrent HF hospitalization should be questioned carefully and educated appropriately about adherence to the medication regimen, use of over-the-counter medications (especially NSAIDs and "dietary supplements"), dietary choices, and daily fluid intake. Patients should also be asked if they have been monitoring their weight and if there have been any recent changes. In patients who acknowledge nonadherence to the medication regimen or to sodium restriction, reasons for nonadherence should be explored. Reasons for medication nonadherence often include concerns about adverse events, cost, efficacy, and excessive number of pills. Nonadherence to sodium restriction may be rooted in lack of knowledge about the salt content of foods, inability to acquire low-sodium foods, frequent eating out, and altered sense of taste. If possible, strategies should be developed to overcome these barriers, and the importance of future adherence as a means to prevent subsequent admissions emphasized. An interprofessional team approach, including the physician, HF nurse specialist (if available), dietitian, social worker, pharmacist (preferably with expertise in geriatric drug prescribing), home-health representative, and case manager, is most likely to result in significant changes in health behavior, thereby fostering improved adherence, self-efficacy, and decreased risk of early readmission (SOE=A). When feasible, the patient's partner and family should be actively engaged in the evaluation and teaching process.

Health services research in the care of patients with HF is helping to clarify factors that reduce readmission risk. Practitioner-level factors associated with reduced readmissions include discharging patients on evidence-based therapies for chronic HF, such as ACE inhibitors and β-blockers (SOE=B). Hospital-level practices associated with fewer readmissions include partnering with community doctors and other hospitals to develop consistent strategies for reducing readmission, nursing supervision to coordinate medications, scheduling follow-up appointments before patient discharge, sending discharge information to the patient's primary care provider, and contacting patients about test results received after discharge (SOE=B). HF disease management programs, as described above and in Table 51.1, may have a positive impact on near-term outcomes. However structured telephone support and telemonitoring programs, when used in isolation, do not clearly reduce mortality or rehospitalizations (SOE=B). Implantable hemodynamic monitoring is a new technology that may play a role in following advanced HF patients and reducing readmissions (SOE=C), although to date only one device has received FDA approval.

PROGNOSIS

The prognosis of older patients with HF is poor, with median survival rates of 2–3 years. These outcomes are worse than for most cancers. However, prognosis is also heterogeneous, with 25%–30% of patients dying within 1 year after initial diagnosis, 50% surviving 1–5 years, and 20%–25% surviving >5 years. Increasing age plays a critical role in prognosis; eg, in a study of Medicare beneficiaries hospitalized with HF in 2008, 1-year mortality rates in patients 65–74, 75–84, and ≥85 years old were 22.0%, 30.3%, and 42.7%, respectively. Older adults discharged to a skilled-nursing facility have especially high mortality rates of 14.4% and 53.5% within 30 days and 1 year of discharge, respectively. Women have somewhat better survival rates than men, as do patients with

HFpEF versus those with HFrEF, but other outcomes, including hospitalization rates, functional status, and quality of life, do not differ significantly among these subgroups. Other factors that adversely affect prognosis include symptom severity (eg, higher NYHA functional class), lower systolic blood pressure, presence of CAD (an important factor contributing to worse outcomes in men), diabetes (especially in women), peripheral arterial or cerebrovascular disease, cognitive impairment or dementia, renal insufficiency, anemia, and hyponatremia. Patients with higher BNP also have a worse prognosis, especially if the BNP remains substantially increased despite aggressive therapy.

END-OF-LIFE CARE

In light of the poor prognosis of older HF patients, it is appropriate to initiate discussions about end-of-life care early in the course of treatment and to readdress these issues as clinical circumstances evolve. Hospitalization for HF, in particular, can be viewed as a sentinel event. Clinicians should be aware of the poor prognosis associated with HF and learn how to compassionately share this information with their patients. These communications can motivate the preparation of advance directives, which may include the appointment of a surrogate decision maker and the delineation of interventions desired or to be avoided in the event of clinical worsening and approaching death. Patients with ICDs should be asked to indicate under what conditions they would want the ICD turned off to avoid repetitive painful shocks at the end of life. For patients with particularly poor prognosis and remaining life expectancy of <6 months (eg, NYHA class IV symptoms despite appropriate medical therapy), clinicians should offer the option of a transition to palliative care and hospice as part of a candid discussion of prognosis and goals of care.

> **CHOOSING WISELY® RECOMMENDATIONS**
>
> *Heart Failure/Device Therapy, Mechanical Circulatory Support, and Heart Transplantation*
>
> - Do not implant an ICD for the primary prevention of sudden cardiac death in patients unlikely to survive at least 1 year because of non-cardiac comorbidity.
>
> - Do not leave an ICD activated when it is inconsistent with the patient/family goals of care.
>
> - Avoid NSAIDs in individuals with hypertension, HF, or chronic kidney disease of all causes, including diabetes.

RESOURCES

- Arnett DK, Goodman RA, Halperin JL, et al. AHA/ACC/HHS strategies to enhance application of clinical practice guidelines in patients with cardiovascular disease and comorbid conditions: from the American Heart Association, American College of Cardiology, and US Department of Health and Human Services. *Circulation*. 2014;130(18):1662–1667.

- Bowers MT. Chronic heart failure: impact of the current guidelines. *J Nurs Pract*. 2019; 15(1):125–131.e2.

- Duncan K, Pozehl B, Hertzog M, et al. Psychological responses and adherence to exercise in heart failure. *Rehabil Nurs*. 2014;39:130–139.

- Yancy CW, Jessup M, Bozkurt B, et al. 2017 ACC/AHA/HFSA. Focused Update of the 2013 ACCF/AHA Guideline for the Management of Heart Failure: A Report of the American College of Cardiology/American Heart Association Task Force on Clinical Practice Guidelines and the Heart Failure Society of America. *J Card Fail*. 2017;23(8):628–651.

CHAPTER 52—HYPERTENSION

KEY POINTS

- Age-related changes in blood pressure regulation lead to greater variability in blood pressure and postural changes. Multiple blood pressure readings, including home and postural measurements, may be needed to accurately diagnose and safely manage hypertension.

- Treating hypertension is beneficial, independent of age, and reduces stroke, heart failure, and cardiovascular and overall mortality.

- Initial antihypertensive drug therapy should be selected according to the individual patient's comorbidities.

- Caution is needed in treating frail older adults with antihypertensives. "Start low and go slow." Monitoring for falls, decrease in orthostatic blood pressure, and other adverse drug events is essential.

EPIDEMIOLOGY AND PHYSIOLOGY

Systolic blood pressure (SBP) progressively increases with age, whereas diastolic blood pressure (DBP) plateaus in the fifth to sixth decade. According to the National Health and Nutrition Examination Survey (NHANES) 2011–2012, 65% of noninstitutionalized adults ≥60 years old had hypertension. Over the last few decades, awareness and control rates of hypertension have improved significantly. The number of adults ≥60 years old who were aware of their hypertension was 86%, and the number of those receiving treatment was 82% in the same period. Close to 50% of older adults have their hypertension controlled.

The association between hypertension and cardiovascular, cerebrovascular, and renal diseases is well documented in older adults (SOE=A). Increased SBP, especially in midlife, may also increase the risk of both age-related cognitive decline and cognitive disorders (SOE=B). Many observational studies have documented that the risk associated with hypertension does not decrease with age, although the association between hypertension and mortality is weaker in the very old. The 2014 Report from the Panel Members Appointed to JNC-8 did not address the definition of hypertension but recommended an age-based approach for managing hypertension (discussed below). Many factors contribute to poor rates of blood pressure control, including lack of awareness of having hypertension and misinformation on desired normal blood pressure goals; these issues appear to be particular barriers among older black and Hispanic women. Factors related to health care providers' practices and concepts about hypertension in older adults also contribute to the age-related disparities in control rates.

Vascular structural changes and neurohumoral alterations contribute to the progressive increase in blood pressure with aging. Large vessels become less distensible with age. This is related to structural changes in the media (elastin fracture, collagen deposition, and calcification), atherosclerosis, and endothelial dysfunction. These changes lead to increased peripheral vascular resistance and decreased vascular compliance, the physiologic hallmark of hypertension in older adults. Decreased sensitivity of the baroreflex, perhaps related to decreased arterial distensibility, contributes to an increase in blood pressure variability and sympathetic nervous system activity. The dynamic regulation of vascular tone is affected by impairments in vasodilator systems (eg, production of nitric oxide by vascular endothelial cells and vasodilation mediated by β-adrenergic receptors) and by heightened vasoconstriction mediated by α-adrenergic receptors. Changes in kidney function as well as in systems involved in sodium balance, such as the renin-angiotensin system, lead to an increase in salt sensitivity and the blood pressure response to dietary sodium. Approximately two-thirds of hypertensive older adults have salt-sensitive hypertension.

In addition to the increase in blood pressure level, blood pressure dysregulation in aging renders older adults at increased risk of orthostatic and postprandial hypotension. Maintaining normal blood pressure and cerebrovascular and coronary perfusion in the face of hypotensive stimuli related to postural challenge, meals, or medications requires the integrated coordination of multiple compensatory mechanisms both centrally and peripherally. The age-associated decline in baroreflex sensitivity and changes in sympathetic nervous system function impair the dynamic regulation of blood pressure. Because of the blunted sensitivity of the baroreflex, a greater decrease in blood pressure occurs before heart rate increases and other compensatory mechanisms are activated. Other pathophysiologic changes that impair blood pressure regulation include arterial and cardiac stiffness and a decrease in early diastolic filling. Finally, changes in the circadian control of blood pressure predisposes older adults to higher relative night-time blood pressure and greater early morning blood pressure rise, both leading to increased risk of stroke and myocardial infarction.

CLINICAL EVALUATION

Accurate measurement of blood pressure is the most critical aspect of diagnosis of hypertension in older adults. Because variability in blood pressure increases with age, the diagnosis of hypertension requires at least 3 blood pressure readings taken on 2 separate visits. Ambulatory (home) 24-hour blood pressure monitoring is recommended for patients with extreme blood pressure variability or possible "white-coat" hypertension. Ambulatory blood pressure monitoring is also recommended for evaluation of resistant hypertension and when there is concern regarding hypotensive episodes, including postural hypotension. Additional clinically useful information derived from ambulatory blood pressure monitoring is the mean blood pressure over a 24-hour period and the diurnal blood pressure rhythm. A diminished nocturnal fall in blood pressure (<10% of waking values)—the non-dipping pattern—has been associated with higher cardiovascular risk. If 24-hour ambulatory blood pressure monitoring is not possible or not available, home-based blood pressure measurements using a calibrated blood pressure monitor may provide important information about the patient's blood pressure in the nonclinical setting. Further, the use of home blood pressure monitoring facilitates partnerships between patients and their providers and family members. This provides an important aspect of the patient-centered medical home, in which both providers and patients are intimately involved in chronic disease management.

Indirect or cuff blood pressure measurements correlate very well with direct, intra-arterial measures in most older adults. In rare individuals, extreme rigidity of the peripheral arteries may prevent complete compression of the brachial artery when the cuff is inflated, resulting in a falsely high blood pressure measurement. This is referred to as pseudohypertension and should be considered in cases of what appears to be resistant hypertension or when there are marked adverse events—especially hypotension-related symptoms—when antihypertensive therapy is started. Clinicians should also be aware of an auscultatory gap, which can lead to underestimation of the true SBP and can indicate arterial stiffness. This can be avoided by inflating the blood pressure cuff 40 mmHg higher than the pressure required to occlude the brachial pulse.

Once hypertension has been diagnosed, the remainder of the clinical evaluation focuses on excluding secondary forms of hypertension and risk stratification by identifying target-organ damage, other cardiovascular risk factors, and the presence of comorbid conditions. Although most hypertensive older patients have essential hypertension, secondary forms of hypertension should be suspected in the presence of malignant hypertension, a sudden increase in DBP, new worsening level of blood pressure control, or resistant hypertension (poorly controlled blood pressure on a regimen of 3 antihypertensive medications, including a diuretic). Renovascular disease is the most common secondary form of hypertension among older adults. Hyperaldosteronism, obstructive sleep apnea, and use of NSAIDs are other causes of secondary hypertension that can be reversed. Treatment decisions are based on both risk stratification and overall evaluation of the patient's remaining life expectancy and functional status. Higher risk strata are those with target-organ damage (eg, left ventricular hypertrophy) or comorbid illnesses such as diabetes mellitus and hyperlipidemia, renal disease, or congestive heart failure. In older adults, risk stratification should also include an overall evaluation of functional abilities, life expectancy, and personal health care wishes. Those who have a short remaining life expectancy or are extremely frail should be counseled and monitored closely for adverse events to medications. Final decisions regarding treatment or target blood pressure should be based on goals of care and patient/family preferences.

Hypertensive older adults should always be counseled about lifestyle modification because doing so may decrease the need for antihypertensive medications. Smoking history, dietary intake of sodium and fat, alcohol intake, and level of usual physical activity are essential factors to be addressed. Contrary to common belief, older adults are able and willing to change their lifestyle but require specific education and monitoring.

TREATMENT

Evidence for Treatment

Treatment of hypertension in healthy and robust older adults is safe and effective. Meta-analyses of more than 40 randomized clinical trials of antihypertensive therapy have provided compelling evidence that treatment is effective in reducing cardiovascular (eg, chronic heart failure) and cerebrovascular (eg, stroke) morbidity and mortality (SOE=A). In a meta-analysis of outcome trials in systolic hypertension among older adults, treatment was associated with significant reductions in overall mortality by 13%, cardiovascular events by 26%, and stroke by 30% (SOE=A). The treatment effect was greatest in men, in those ≥70 years old, and in those who had higher pulse pressures.

In those ≥80 years old, the evidence is not as consistent. The Hypertension in the Very Elderly Trial (HYVET) study was one of the first randomized controlled trials specifically conducted in those ≥80 years old (N=3,845). The study was stopped early when a significant 21% reduction in total mortality (10.1% versus 12.2%, ARR 2.2%, NNT 45 over a median of 1.8 years) was identified in the treatment group (extended-release indapamide plus perindopril if needed to achieve a goal SBP of 150 mmHg) relative to the placebo control group (RR 0.76; CI 95%, 0.62–0.93; $P=.007$). The treatment group also demonstrated improvements in fatal and nonfatal stroke (RR 0.59; CI 95%, 0.40–0.88; $P=.009$) and heart failure and had fewer adverse events. More recently, in a pre-specific subgroup analysis of patients >75 years old (mean age 79.9) in the Systolic Blood Pressure Intervention Trial (SPRINT), which included >9,000 patients with an SBP of ≥130 mmHg, the intensive treatment target of SBP <120 mmHg was associated with a 33% relative risk reduction in the composite outcomes of fatal and nonfatal cardiovascular events (ARR 1.26% per year, NNT 27 over 3.14 years) compared with the standard treatment goal of SBP <140 mmHg. These findings were also statistically significant in the subgroup with the greatest level of frailty or those with impaired gait speed. Unlike the results of the main trial, overall the rate of serious adverse events in those ≥75 years old were comparable between the two treatment groups, including the most frail participants, although the rate of acute kidney injury tended to be higher in the intensive treatment group (5.5% vs 4.0%; hazard ratio 1.41; 95% CI, 0.98–2.04). Those with advanced frailty, cognitive decline, loss of autonomy, or living in a nursing home were excluded from the trial. The generalizability of the SPRINT results to very frail elderly individuals is limited. The study participants were more likely to tolerate blood pressure lowering if they has already been receiving treatment for 3 years with at least three antihypertensive drugs. Additionally, blood pressure measurement in SPRINT was performed 3 times using automated measurement in the office (ie, unobserved). Blood pressure measured by this method is likely to be 5–10 mmHg lower than when measured in community practice.

Participants in most hypertension clinical trials are generally healthier on average than patients in clinical settings. Those with dementia, living in nursing homes, or who have an inability to walk were excluded from most trials, including SPRINT. The JNC-8 recommends treating adults ≥60 years old to achieve a blood pressure below 150/90 mmHg (SOE=A). The below 150 mmHg target has been a source of controversy, and many other guidelines have recommended a target below 140 mmHg in those ≥60 years old. In JNC-8, the Committee considered targeting lower SBP (<140/90 mmHg) acceptable if treatment is not associated with adverse effects on health or quality of life (SOE=D). The Committee also recommended a target below 140/90 mmHg for those with diabetes mellitus using expert opinion evidence (SOE=D). An individual status-based approach to managing hypertension in older adults is recommended in which both age and health status (rather than age alone) are considered when initiating or continuing antihypertensive therapy and in defining the blood pressure target of therapy.

Treatment should focus on SBP because among older hypertensive adults, it is a stronger predictor of adverse outcomes than DBP. Some studies have shown increased mortality with blood pressure reduction below a certain threshold—especially DBP (<60 mmHg)—creating a J-shaped curve in relation to mortality (SOE=B). The significance of these concerns remains controversial. The relationship between lower DBP and increased cardiovascular morbidity when DBP is below 60–70 mmHg was observed in the Systolic Hypertension in the Elderly Trial and in the INVEST trial. The latter included only hypertensive patients with coronary artery disease. In a meta-analysis of individual's data from hypertension trials, a J curve was noted in both treated and untreated patients. It is possible, as concluded by the authors of this meta-analysis, that this J-curve is explained by poor health. Yet it seems reasonable to attempt to avoid excessive reductions in DBP (eg, <60–65 mmHg), especially in individuals with coronary heart disease. Based on JNC-8, it is also reasonable to consider 140/90 mmHg as a target, especially in robust nonfrail older patients or those <80 years old. Also notable is that the Medicare Healthcare Effectiveness Data and Information Set (HEDIS) blood pressure target is <140/90 mmHg for adults 60–85 years old with diabetes.

Further complicating the issue of blood pressure targets for treatment are the preliminary results of SPRINT. In this trial, 9,361 participants >50 years old, 2,636 of whom were ≥75 years old, were randomized to treatment SBP target groups of <140 mmHg and <120 mmHg. In September 2015, SPRINT was stopped early because of an observed 25% relative risk reduction (0.54% per year absolute risk reduction) of cardiovascular events and death in the latter group. The incidence of hypotension, syncope, electrolyte abnormalities, and acute kidney failure was significantly higher in the intensive treatment group, while there was no difference observed in the rate of injurious falls. These findings were consistent across age strata. Patients with diabetes or prior stroke were not enrolled in the trial, and residents of assisted-living facilities and nursing homes were also excluded.

Concerns about falls and use of antihypertensive therapy have been generated from observational studies (SOE=C). Yet, as found in SPRINT, clinical trials have not demonstrated an increased risk of falls. The differences between populations studied may explain this discrepancy, with clinical trial enrollees being healthier than those included in analyses of Medicare or other datasets. Hence, caution should be exercised when treating older adults with antihypertensive medication who report falling or who are at increased risk of falls.

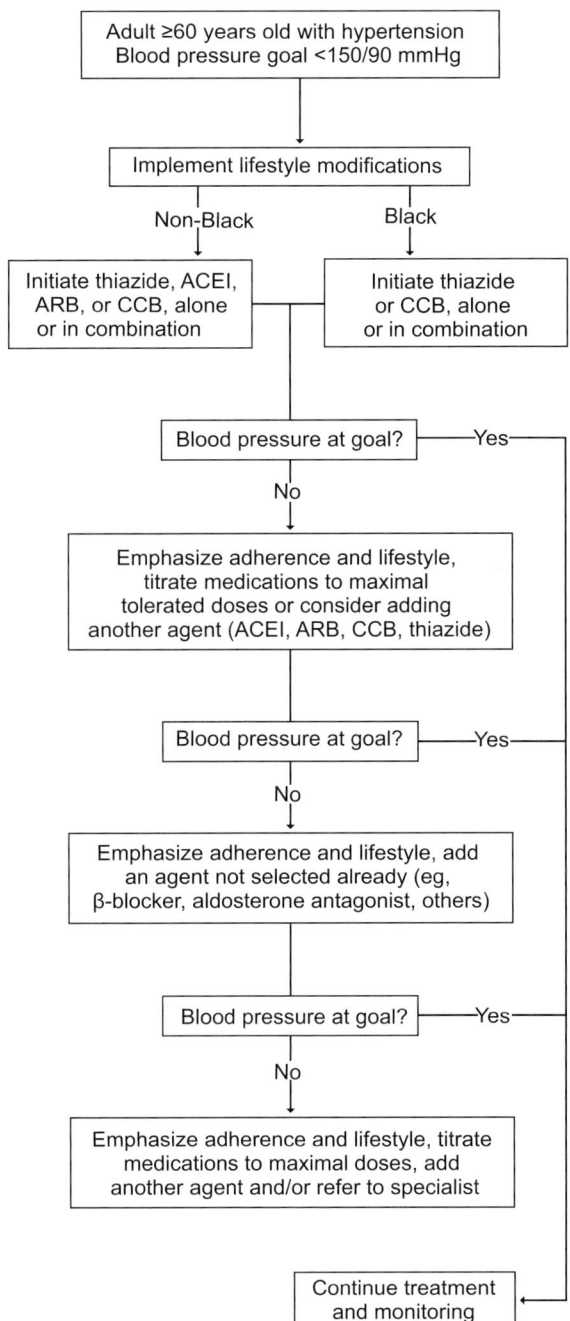

Figure 52.1—JNC-8 Hypertension Guideline Algorithm for Adults ≥60 Years Old

Lifestyle Modification

Nonpharmacologic therapy is an important adjunct to drug treatment in all patients because of synergistic effects with antihypertensive drugs and the benefits realized through reduction in other cardiovascular risk factors. Lifestyle modifications that target the typical characteristics of the older hypertensive adult—overweight, sedentary, and salt-sensitive—are likely to be effective. The randomized Trial of Nonpharmacologic Interventions in Elderly study, which evaluated the effects of dietary sodium restriction and weight loss in older adults, demonstrated that relatively modest reductions in dietary sodium intake (1.8 g/d) and in body weight (4 kg) are accompanied by a 30% decrease in the need to reinitiate pharmacologic treatment. A meta-analysis of randomized trials assessing the effects of dietary sodium restriction demonstrated a significant reduction in SBP (a mean decrease of 3.7 mmHg for each decrease of 2.4 g/d of sodium) but not in DBP (SOE=A). This differential reduction in systolic pressure is particularly well suited for the older hypertensive patient. Stress-reduction techniques and increasing potassium intake in the form of fruits and vegetables also lower blood pressure. Increasing physical activity is particularly critical, because the benefit of exercise may not only lower blood pressure but also improve other domains such as balance and cognitive function (SOE=C).

Table 52.1—Comorbid Conditions Influencing Medication Selection in Hypertension

Indication	Preferred Medication
Heart failure	ACEI/ARB, β-blocker, diuretic, spironolactone
Clinical coronary artery disease or after myocardial infarction	ACEI/ARB and β-blocker
Coronary artery disease	ACEI, β-blocker, diuretic, CCB
Diabetes	ACEI/ARB, CCB, diuretic
Chronic kidney disease	ACEI/ARB
Recurrent stroke prevention	ACEI, diuretic

Pharmacologic Treatment

The general approach to pharmacologic management of older hypertensive adults is similar to that presented in the JNC-8 (Figure 52.1). Initial drug choice is influenced by the presence or absence of comorbid conditions (eg, diabetes mellitus, coronary artery disease or history of myocardial infarction, heart failure, prostatism), cost, and compliance (Table 52.1). A once-a-day regimen with long-acting medications is more likely to be successful. Medications should be started at the lowest dosage and cautiously increased during follow-up visits (every 4–6 weeks). If the response is inadequate or there is evidence of adverse events, a drug from a different class can be substituted. However, before adding new drugs, polypharmacy, nonadherence, and drug interactions should be considered.

Thiazide-type diuretics, calcium channel blockers, angiotensin-receptor blockers (ARBs), and ACE inhibitors are all effective as initial treatment in non-black older adults (SOE=A). In black older adults, thiazide-type diuretics or calcium channel blockers may be preferred (SOE=B).

Centrally acting agents (eg, clonidine, methyldopa) and α-blockers are not recommended as first choice (SOE=A). β-Blockers in noncardiac patients are also not recommended as first-choice agents. Many older patients will not reach their SBP goal on a single medication, and additional medications may be necessary.

Diuretics

Therapy with low-dose thiazide-type diuretics (eg, chlorthalidone ≤25 mg/d, or equivalent) has demonstrated significant benefits in mortality, stroke, and coronary events in randomized clinical trials in older hypertensive adults (SOE=A). The adverse-event profile includes hypokalemia, hyperuricemia, hypomagnesemia, hyponatremia, and possible glucose intolerance. Adverse events are more likely to occur with higher dosages, so lower dosages are recommended. Adequate potassium replacement during diuretic-based treatment decreases the risk of arrhythmias and glucose intolerance. Thiazide diuretics are also well suited for use in combination therapies because of synergistic effects with other classes of antihypertensive medications; however, they increase the risk of gout flare. Loop diuretics may be used for hypertension but are usually reserved for those with heart failure or chronic kidney disease. Their adverse-event profile includes increasing glucose concentration, headaches, ototoxicity, and electrolyte disturbances. Aldosterone antagonists (spironolactone, eplerenone) are also useful in hypertension and may be used in those prone to hypokalemia.

ACE Inhibitors

ACE inhibitors block the production of angiotensin II and are effective in lowering blood pressure in hypertensive older adults. They lower peripheral vascular resistance through their humoral and structural effects on the vasculature without causing reflex tachycardia as seen with direct vasodilators. They are also effective in slowing the progression of hypertension nephrosclerosis and are particularly advantageous in those with concomitant diabetes or heart failure (SOE=A). Their use in African Americans has been questioned, but data from the African American Study of Kidney Disease and Hypertension (AASK) trial showed a significant beneficial effect (SOE=A). Their adverse-event profile includes cough, hyperkalemia, angioedema, renal insufficiency (especially in those with renal artery stenosis), and in rare instances neutropenia and agranulocytosis. Black Americans are at greater risk of cough and angioedema than white Americans.

Angiotensin-Receptor Blockers

ARBs block the effect of angiotensin II on the type 1 angiotensin receptor. ARB therapy may be considered as first line or as an alternative to an ACE inhibitor, especially in those with diabetes, heart failure, or microalbuminuria. ARBs are excellent choices for those who cannot tolerate ACE inhibitors (SOE=A).

Renin Inhibitors

Renin inhibitors (eg, aliskiren) are approved for hypertension treatment. They are as effective as ACE inhibitors or ARBs in their blood pressure lowering effects, with the advantage of no dose-related increases in adverse events in older adults (SOE=B). However, no long-term outcome data are available for older adults, and renin inhibitors are significantly more expensive than other antihypertensives. They are associated with diarrhea, and there are no data on safety in those with a glomerular filtration rate <30 mL/min/1.73 m^2.

Calcium-Channel Antagonists

Therapy with long-acting dihydropyridine calcium-channel antagonists (CCAs) (nifedipine-like) is effective in reducing stroke risk in hypertensive older patients (SOE=A). CCAs in combination with ACE inhibitors have been shown to be superior to the diuretic–ACE inhibitor combination in patients with multiple vascular risk factors. Because of age-related changes in the pharmacokinetics of CCAs, lower dosages should be used. Adverse events are related to vasodilator mechanisms and include ankle edema, headaches, and postural hypotension. CCAs are also associated with constipation. Non-dihydropyridine CCAs can suppress left ventricular function and may precipitate heart block in older adults with conduction defects. Unless there is a strong indication for their use (eg, symptomatic supraventricular tachycardia, rate-controlled atrial fibrillation), they should be avoided as first choice for hypertension management. Short-acting CCAs should not be used to treat hypertension.

β-Receptor Antagonists

Several meta-analyses have questioned the efficacy of β-blockers in treating uncomplicated hypertension. Compared with placebo, β-blockers, especially atenolol, provide no reduction in all-cause mortality and myocardial infarction in older adults, and only modest reduction in stroke, which is smaller than the risk reduction seen with other antihypertensives (SOE=A). Based on available evidence, β-blockers are not preferred as first-line agents, unless there is a strong indication, such as heart failure, prior myocardial infarction, acute coronary syndrome, stable angina, prevention of perioperative cardiac complications, or hypertrophic obstructive cardiomyopathy. Because of their effectiveness in management of symptomatic coronary artery disease, in secondary prevention after myocardial infarction, and in management of heart failure, β-receptor antagonists should be considered for older adults whose hypertension is complicated by these comorbid conditions (SOE=A).

Other Classes

α-Receptor antagonists are not appropriate for first-line therapy of hypertension. The treatment arm that included participants randomized to therapy with the α-receptor antagonist doxazosin in the ALLHAT study was stopped early because of a higher rate of cardiovascular complications, including a 2-fold greater likelihood of being hospitalized for heart failure. α-Receptor antagonist therapy might be considered as part of a multidrug regimen, especially in those with prostatism, because these drugs have been shown to be efficacious in improving obstructive urinary symptoms.

Direct vasodilators (hydralazine and minoxidil) are considered last-line therapy because of their toxic adverse-event profile, which includes tachycardia, arrhythmia, and fluid retention. Centrally acting agents (eg, clonidine) are also poorly tolerated in older adults and can be associated with sedation, bradycardia, and reflex hypertension, as well as tachycardia if abruptly stopped. Alpha-beta blockers have an antihypertensive effect, but their tolerability is an issue in older adults. Labetalol is useful in hypertensive urgencies and carvedilol in heart failure with reduced ejection fraction. Both may be associated with weakness and significant orthostatic hypotension.

Follow-Up Visits

Attempts to reduce blood pressure to target levels too rapidly are unnecessary and likely deleterious. For most patients, an interval of 4–6 weeks between visits is appropriate to determine the need for dosage adjustment. However, it may take up to 10–12 weeks for full pharmacodynamic effect after starting a medication or increasing a dosage. At all follow-up visits, it is imperative to determine both supine and standing blood pressure measurements. It is good practice to adjust antihypertensive drug dosages to achieve the target (seated) blood pressure only after determining whether postural hypotension is present.

Blood pressure monitoring outside the clinic setting may be essential, especially in those who cannot tolerate even small doses of antihypertensives. Home blood pressure monitoring may also aid in promoting adherence to therapy (SOE=B). If available, an interprofessional geriatric team is well suited to provide a well-rounded approach to hypertension management (eg, nurses to provide feedback on degree of blood pressure control, dietitians to review dietary information and adherence, pharmacists to promote adherence to the medical regimen, and social workers to review the financial burden associated with medical therapy).

When a patient's blood pressure has not been successfully reduced to the target level, cautiously increasing the dosage, adding another medication (particularly a thiazide diuretic if the patient is not already taking one), or switching to another class of medication should be considered. Patients should also be counseled to continue their lifestyle modifications. Achieving the target blood pressure goal may take many months. When this goal is not attained despite adherence to a 3-drug regimen, an evaluation for refractory or resistant hypertension (especially renovascular disease, hyperaldosteronism, and sleep apnea) should be considered. After more than a year of appropriate stable blood pressure control, step-down treatment may be considered; dosages may be decreased cautiously, with close blood pressure monitoring. Patients who have successfully modified their lifestyle (eg, weight loss) are most likely to be able to reduce their dosage or eliminate antihypertensive medications.

SPECIAL CONSIDERATIONS

Hypertensive Emergencies and Urgencies

Increased blood pressure per se in the absence of signs or symptoms of target-organ damage does not constitute a hypertensive emergency. Rapidly and too aggressively decreasing blood pressure in a patient with incidentally discovered increased blood pressure is potentially harmful and can cause complications, such as coronary or cerebral hypoperfusion syndromes (SOE=B).

Examples of true hypertensive emergencies in older adults include hypertensive encephalopathy, acute heart failure with pulmonary edema, dissecting aortic aneurysm, and unstable angina. These patients present with symptoms and signs of vascular compromise of affected organs. Management of these emergencies requires an acute hospital setting, with parenteral administration of a short-acting antihypertensive agent and continual blood pressure monitoring to immediately reduce blood pressure, although not initially to a normal target level. Blood pressure should not be lowered emergently more than 25% within the first 2 hours, with a goal of achieving 160/100 mmHg gradually over the first 6 hours of therapy (SOE=D).

Hypertension in the Long-Term Care Setting and Frail Older Adults

Approximately one-third to two-thirds of residents in long-term care facilities have hypertension. Special considerations are warranted in the care of residents with respect to making the correct diagnosis and defining the goals of therapy and its effects on quality of life. Blood pressure measurements in long-term care settings may not be accurate because of measurement errors and the temporal variability in blood pressure, particularly in relation to meals. Blood pressure appears to be highest in the morning before breakfast. Postprandial hypotension is common among long-term care residents, affecting about one-third of this population. It has been associated with otherwise unexplained syncope and found to be a significant independent risk factor for falls, syncope, stroke, and overall mortality.

Several factors should be considered in management of hypertension in this setting. First, the advanced average age and comorbidity of residents in long-term care facilities raises controversy surrounding the question of whether the benefits of antihypertensive therapy extend to this population. If the beneficial effects of treatment are less evident, the potential adverse events and risks of therapy should be weighed more heavily in defining the goals of therapy. Even an intervention as seemingly innocuous as a sodium-restricted diet needs to be evaluated in the context of the high prevalence of protein-energy malnutrition among nursing-home residents. Second, the average resident in long-term care takes 9 or 10 medications, and most have 3 or more comorbid conditions. The addition of an antihypertensive medication increases the possibility of an adverse event in this frail, at-risk group. Hence, avoiding aggressive blood pressure control (eg, avoiding SBP <130 mmHg) is likely to be the safer approach in this population. Third, several studies have identified the use of antihypertensive medications, particularly vasodilators, as a risk factor for falls in this high-risk population, experiencing an average of 2 falls each year (SOE=B). It is therefore important to assess both postural and postprandial blood pressure in this population. Further, the evidence for a mortality or morbidity benefit in frail older adults is lacking. In observational studies, older adults who could not walk more than 6 meters (20 feet) in <8 seconds demonstrated no association between blood pressure and mortality. In particular, in those with severe physical frailty, higher blood pressure may be linked with lower mortality (SOE=B). Therefore, it is critical to assess functional levels and expected survival in frail patients before starting or continuing antihypertensive therapy.

Renal Artery Stenosis

Atherosclerotic renal artery stenosis (defined as ≥50% narrowing) is present in 7% of older adults and in 25% of those with a serum creatinine >2 mg/dL. In older adults, renal artery stenosis is a common contributor to resistant hypertension and may lead to cardiac destabilization syndromes such as heart failure exacerbation, cardiac ischemia, and "flash" pulmonary edema. Detection can be performed by Doppler ultrasonography and CT or MR angiography. Medical therapy includes lifestyle change and blood pressure medications. Percutaneous renal artery revascularization and stenting is an additional treatment option, but the clinical benefit for stenting is limited. Both the Cardiovascular Outcomes in Renal Atherosclerotic Lesions (CORAL; mean age=69.1 years) and Angioplasty and Stenting for Renal Artery Lesions (ASTRAL; mean age=70 years) studies did not demonstrate a benefit for stenting on either cardiovascular or renal outcomes (SOE=B). Better patient selection using dynamic or physiologic effects of the renal artery stenosis (eg, flow reserve or a translational pressure gradient >20 mmHg) may improve clinical response (SOE=C). Clinically, selecting those with resistant hypertension (use of 3 medications including a diuretic), ischemic renal disease with bilateral stenosis, or cardiac destabilization syndromes (flash pulmonary edema or ischemic cardiac events) should be evaluated for potential stenting (SOE=C). Stenting is limited by the development of intrastent restenosis; hence, the risk of secondary interventions should be weighed against the modest clinical benefit observed in clinical trials.

CHOOSING WISELY® RECOMMENDATIONS

Hypertension

- Do not screen for renal artery stenosis in patients without resistant hypertension and with normal renal function, even if known atherosclerosis is present.

RESOURCES

- Aronow WS, Fleg JL, Pepine CJ, et al. ACCF/AHA 2011 Expert Consensus Document on Hypertension in the elderly: a report of the American College of Cardiology Foundation Task Force on Clinical Expert Consensus documents developed in collaboration with the American Academy of Neurology, American Geriatrics Society, American Society for Preventive Cardiology, American Society of Hypertension, American Society of Nephrology, Association of Black Cardiologists, and European Society of Hypertension. *J Am Coll Cardiol.* 2011;57(20):2037–2114.

- Davis LL. Hypertension: how low to go when treating older adults. *J Nurs Pract.* 2018;15(1):1–6.

- Ritchie LD, Campbell NC, Murchie P. New NICE guidelines for hypertension. *BMJ.* 2011;343:d5644.

- Schwinn S, McKay R, Dinkel S, et al. Hypertension management in the oldest old: Findings from a large long-term care facility. *J Am Assoc Nurs Pract.* 2017;29(3):123–129.

CHAPTER 53—GASTROENTEROLOGY

KEY POINTS

- Although physiological changes of aging can affect GI function, most GI symptoms and signs are due to pathologic conditions and should be evaluated accordingly.

- Medications used to treat many illnesses that affect older adults can cause GI symptoms and disorders.

- Geriatric patients often present with atypical symptoms of GI disorders and with more severe disease, creating diagnostic challenges and urgency.

- Older patients can tolerate many treatments for GI diseases as well as younger patients but may be more susceptible to medication adverse events.

The structure and function of the GI tract are affected both by physiological changes of aging and by the effects of accumulating disorders involving many organ systems. In association with advancing age, changes in connective tissue can limit the elasticity of the gut and changes in the nerves and muscles can impair motility. Disturbances of epithelial, muscle, or neural function may all result from age-related enteric neurodegeneration and loss of excitatory enteric neurons. Accumulating chronic conditions are often associated with increased use of medications by older adults, many of which have direct effects on intestinal mucosa and motility. Some disease states, such as atherosclerosis and diabetes mellitus, can adversely influence GI function and lead to symptoms and complications. GI problems can quickly compromise the older adult's ability to maintain adequate nutrition, leading to weight loss and fatigue.

DISORDERS OF THE ESOPHAGUS

Dysphagia

Dysphagia refers to the subjective sensation of difficulty swallowing and may be due to any disruption in the swallowing process. The prevalence of dysphagia in patients ≥65 years old has been reported to be 15%–40% in the outpatient setting and up to 60% in older adults living in nursing homes. Physiological or anatomical abnormalities along any portion of the esophagus, including the upper and lower sphincters, may lead to the sensation of difficulty swallowing. Dysphagia is typically classified as oropharyngeal or esophageal. Although there are physiological changes associated with aging that may lead to dysphagia, this is considered an alarm symptom that must prompt evaluation and should never be attributed to normal aging without an appropriate evaluation.

Oropharyngeal dysphagia (often referred to as transfer dysphagia) is characterized by the inability to initiate a swallow or transfer food from the mouth to the esophagus. In addition to the sensation of dysphagia, typical symptoms include coughing, choking, nasopharyngeal regurgitation, aspiration (with or without subsequent pneumonia), and retained food in the mouth after an attempted swallow. In patients with advanced dementia, oropharyngeal dysphagia may result from apraxia and be misinterpreted as a refusal to swallow. Multiple changes in the physiology of the aging gut as well as specific disorders may lead to oropharyngeal dysphagia. Physiological studies have shown reduced tongue strength, reduced pharyngeal wall contraction, decreased salivary flow, and impaired gag reflexes in healthy older adults, all of which likely contribute to dysphagia. Poor dentition may lead to inadequate mastication of food bolus and contribute as well. Neurologic disorders (such as stroke, Parkinson disease, Alzheimer dementia, myasthenia gravis) and malignancies of the oropharynx are common causes of oropharyngeal dysphagia. Structural abnormalities such as a Zenker diverticulum or prominent cervical osteophytes are also common in this age group.

In contrast, esophageal dysphagia typically presents as the sensation of food getting stuck in the esophagus (or chest) several seconds after initiating a swallow. Age-related physiologic changes such as decreased salivary flow and loss of neurons in the myenteric and submucosal plexus lead to altered motility and contribute to the high rates of dysphagia among older adults, especially those >80 years old. Further, medications can exacerbate these changes, often through anticholinergic effects. The etiology of esophageal dysphagia is usually subclassified into motility disorders, structural disorders, and infectious diseases. Dysphagia for both solids and liquids from the onset usually implies a motility disorder of the esophagus. Common primary motility disorders include achalasia, hypoperistaltic disorders (ineffective esophageal motility) often associated with gastroesophageal reflux disease (GERD), and hypertensive or spastic disorders (jackhammer esophagus, distal esophageal spasm). The most well-described motility disorder, achalasia, does not appear to be seen in greater frequency in older adults; however, it may present later in its course with greater esophageal dilation due to delay in presentation in older adults. Less is known about the epidemiology of the nonspecific motility disorders, which may be the presenting problem in systemic disorders such as scleroderma. In contrast to motility disorders, dysphagia for solids that progresses later to involve liquids suggests mechanical obstruction. In the older age group, multiple causes of mechanical obstruction are seen. Malignancy must be excluded in all patients. The most common cancers tend to be adenocarcinomas occurring in the distal esophagus often in the background of Barrett changes. Benign strictures may be due acid to reflux, prior radiation, or pill-induced esophageal injury. Extrinsic compression may be due to variant vasculature, a large aortic aneurysm, an enlarged left atrium, or extra-esophageal malignancies such as lymphoma. Dysphagia accompanied by odynophagia (painful swallowing) is suspicious for an infectious etiology, such as a viral or fungal infection. Candidal infections are the most common and often seen in the setting of systemic immunosuppression or with use of steroids administered via inhaler. Common viruses are the herpes simplex virus, which can be seen in immunocompetent older adults, and cytomegalovirus, which is typically found only in immunosuppressed patients.

Treatment of dysphagia depends on the underlying cause. A medication review should be done, particularly focusing on anticholinergic drugs that may worsen dysphagia. Treatment of oropharyngeal dysphagia may require swallowing rehabilitation or dietary modifications such as thickening liquids, or careful hand feeding with a spoon, cup, or straw. In cases in which dementia is the cause of dysphagia, the placement of a percutaneous gastrostomy with tube feeding has not demonstrated improvement in survival, function, or symptoms, and tube feeding is recognized as a risk factor for aspiration (SOE=B). Multiple treatment options exist for achalasia. Injection of the lower esophageal sphincter with botulinum toxin may provide months of symptomatic relief in patients who are not surgical candidates or have a very limited remaining life expectancy. In most patients, however, definitive treatment with surgical or endoscopic myotomy is indicated (SOE=A). Calcium channel blockers or phosphodiesterase inhibitors (such as sildenafil[OL]) may provide relief in various spastic motility disorders (SOE=B). Treatment of malignancy is primarily surgical, often with adjunct chemotherapy and/or radiation. However, in nonadvanced cancers or in patients who are not surgical candidates, endoscopic treatments may be available for curative or palliative intent. Strictures are treated with endoscopic dilation, with a very high success rate, although they often require ongoing medical treatment of the underlying cause as well (eg, reflux). Infectious causes require targeted antiviral or antifungal therapy.

Gastroesophageal Reflux Disease

GERD is defined as symptoms or complications resulting from the reflux of gastric contents into the esophagus or beyond to the oropharynx, nasopharynx, larynx, or lung. GERD is the most commonly seen upper GI condition in primary care. Among adults ≥65 years old, symptoms of heartburn or acid regurgitation occur at least weekly in 20% of the population and at least monthly in 59%. Prolonged pH studies show that esophageal acid exposure frequency and duration increases with age, and endoscopic data suggest that esophagitis is more severe in older adults. However, likely because of decreased pain perception in this age group, the severity of symptoms often does not correlate with the severity of disease.

Multiple potential factors aggravate GERD in older adults, including frequent inappropriate transient lower esophageal sphincter relaxations, medications known to decrease lower esophageal sphincter tone, higher prevalence of hiatal hernia, impaired esophageal peristalsis, and decreased salivary volume and bicarbonate concentration.

Heartburn is the characteristic symptom of GERD, described as a "burning" sensation in the chest, often rising from the epigastrium. Symptoms often occur or are worse after a meal, and patients may note certain food triggers (eg, spicy foods, citrus or acidic foods, fats, caffeine, or alcohol) that reliably bring on the symptoms. Older patients may present with atypical or extraesophageal manifestations of GERD, sometimes without accompanying heartburn. These so called atypical or extraesophageal symptoms include dyspepsia, epigastric pain, nausea, bloating, belching, asthma, chronic cough, and laryngitis or voice changes. Many older adults with longstanding disease marked by atypical symptoms delay in seeking care and first present with alarm symptoms such as dysphagia, odynophagia, or vomiting.

Diagnosis of GERD, especially in the older population, may be difficult. Guidelines allow for a presumptive diagnosis of GERD in the setting of typical symptoms and recommend initial treatment with an empiric trial of acid-suppression therapy. In the general population, empiric treatment with a proton-pump inhibitor (PPI), as a test for GERD, has a sensitivity of 68%–83% (SOE=A). Current guidelines do not differentiate diagnosis in older adults from any other age group. However, adults >60 years old may benefit from earlier endoscopic evaluation, because they may have vague or mild symptoms despite the presence of severe esophagitis and are at higher risk of Barrett esophagus and esophageal adenocarcinoma. Patients with alarm signs or symptoms, or those with longstanding reflux, should undergo endoscopy to exclude severe esophagitis, strictures, Barrett esophagus, dysplasia, and malignancy. Patients who do not respond to a trial of PPI and/or do not have endoscopic findings to explain their symptoms warrant further testing. Evaluation with 24-hour pH-impedance testing can confirm or exclude acid and nonacid reflux. Prolonged pH monitoring for 48–96 hours using a wireless pH capsule can identify acid reflux in patients who do not have daily symptoms. Esophageal manometry is used to document the presence of effective esophageal peristalsis in patients in whom antireflux surgery is being considered and to exclude an underlying esophageal motility disorder, such as achalasia, as the cause of the symptoms.

The primary goals of treatment are to reduce symptoms and prevent complications. Although evidence for the effectiveness of lifestyle and dietary modifications is limited, these nonpharmacologic interventions are still considered first-line therapy. Obesity has been associated with increased risk of GERD, and weight loss has been shown to decrease reflux symptoms; thus, for obese patients with GERD, weight loss is recommended. Elevating the head of the bed and avoiding meals within 2–3 hours before bedtime should be recommended for patients with nocturnal symptoms. Medications that reduce lower esophageal sphincter tone or acidify gastric contents should be avoided when possible. These include anticholinergics, benzodiazepines, opiates, nitrates, and calcium channel antagonists. Elimination of food triggers such as chocolate, caffeine, spicy foods, citrus foods, or carbonated beverages is recommended only in patients who can identify an exacerbation in symptoms with specific foods. Antacids, alginic acid, or OTC histamine$_2$-receptor antagonists (H$_2$RAs) may be helpful in relieving mild, transient reflux symptoms (SOE=B). The duration of action of each of these is limited, as is their ability to achieve healing of erosive esophagitis.

Antisecretory therapy in the form of PPIs remain the treatment of choice for patients with moderate to severe GERD or GERD with any complication (SOE=A). PPIs achieve healing of erosive esophagitis in >80% of patients, compared with 50%–60% with H$_2$RAs, regardless of age. Available PPIs include omeprazole, esomeprazole, lansoprazole, dexlansoprazole, pantoprazole, and rabeprazole. Omeprazole, esomeprazole, and lansoprazole are currently available as OTC formulations. There are no clinically important differences in symptom relief with any of the above PPIs given once daily. As recommended in current guidelines, an 8-week course of once-daily PPI should be administered in most patients. PPIs should be taken 30–60 minutes before a meal for maximal pH control. If acute medical therapy alleviates symptoms, a trial off medication can be considered after symptoms have resolved. Maintenance PPI therapy should be administered for GERD patients who continue to have symptoms after PPI is discontinued, and in patients with complications including erosive esophagitis and Barrett esophagus. Recurrence of symptoms is common after therapy is stopped, and lifelong therapy may be needed. Intermittent therapy with an H$_2$RA or PPI may be successful in some patients with mild to moderate symptoms, while maintenance daily PPI therapy is needed in those with severe symptoms. A dosage increase or change in PPI can be attempted in patients who only partially respond to a PPI. Patients who do not respond to PPIs should be referred for evaluation with endoscopy, pH monitoring, and/or manometry.

Antisecretory therapy, specifically with PPIs, is associated with a number of risks. Case reports have shown association between long-term PPI use and lowered vitamin B$_{12}$ levels in older adults. A relationship between antisecretory therapy and infections, specifically enteric infections (particularly *Clostridium difficile*), has been raised because of the loss of the gastric acid barrier; however, the data are mixed. Concerns have also been raised regarding blunted calcium absorption in the setting of acid suppression and long-term effects of PPIs on bone mineral density. However, the data regarding this association have been conflicting and favor no increased risk. Current guidelines state that even patients with known osteoporosis can stay on PPIs and that concern for hip fractures and osteoporosis should not affect the decision to use PPIs in the average patient. Regardless, it is reasonable to adjust the regimen in patients with known osteoporosis risk factors such as smoking. For PPI users who require calcium supplementation, a soluble form such as calcium citrate is preferred. Concerns have been raised about the interaction between PPIs (which inhibit the hepatic cytochromic P450 system) and the antiplatelet medication clopidogrel. This concern was borne out of pharmacokinetic platelet aggregation studies as well as observational data that suggested an increased risk of cardiovascular events in patients taking PPIs. However, a large number of subsequent studies, including several randomized controlled trials and meta-analyses, showed no increased risk of cardiovascular or cerebrovascular events or mortality and revealed a lower rate of GI bleeding in PPI users. Thus, it is not recommended to routinely stop or avoid PPI use in patients on clopidogrel or dual antiplatelet therapy. Concerns have been raised regarding PPIs and risk of dementia, chronic kidney disease, cardiac disease, stroke, and even "early" death. All of these associations require further study to determine if they are clinically important or due to confounding of some sort. It is difficult to determine if aging itself is an independent risk factor. Because these adverse associations have not been adjudicated, most agree it is prudent to use the lowest effective dose possible in patients needing long-term PPI therapy.

Drug-Induced Esophageal Injury

Several medications are known to cause direct injury to the esophageal mucosa. Older adults are at increased risk of pill-induced injury because of several factors, including polypharmacy, impaired esophageal peristalsis, and decreased salivary flow. Increased age alone has been shown to be a risk factor for pill retention. Injury is commonly at the level of the aortic arch, an enlarged left atrium, or the esophagogastric junction, areas with a potentially decreased lumen circumference.

Tetracyclines, particularly doxycycline, are the most common antibiotics that induce esophagitis. All NSAIDs, including aspirin, potassium chloride, ferrous sulfate, quinidine, and bisphosphonates are most common. Bisphosphonates appear to be of particular concern, because they have been reported to induce severe esophagitis, often with an affected surface area much larger than that of the offending tablet. Gelatin capsules are of particular concern.

The diagnosis of pill esophagitis is often clinical. The typical presenting symptom is odynophagia. Patients often recall having ingested a medication known to cause injury, often with little or no water or immediately preceding bedtime. Endoscopy is needed if the diagnosis is not clear from the clinical history or in cases of severe symptoms, and may reveal a discrete ulcer of variable size with normal surrounding mucosa.

Symptoms tend to resolve quickly if the offending medication is avoided; specific treatment is not typically required. Acid suppression (with PPIs or H_2RAs), topical anesthetics (such as lidocaine), and sucralfate suspension or slurries (to provide a protective coating) are often given, but their use is off-label and little evidence exists to show efficacy. In severe disease, patients may be unable to tolerate any oral intake and should be admitted for parenteral hydration. Underlying dysmotility should be evaluated and treated if suspected to prevent recurrence as should strictures, which may be the cause of or result of pill-induced injury.

Patients should be instructed to drink plenty of water (at least 8 ounces) with each pill and to sit or stand upright for at least 30 minutes after pill ingestion. For patients with known esophageal disorders, alternative medications or liquid forms should be considered.

DISORDERS OF THE STOMACH

Dyspepsia

Dyspepsia implies chronic or recurrent pain or discomfort in the upper abdomen, more specifically bothersome postprandial fullness, epigastric pain, or epigastric burning. These symptoms are common (with up to 40% of the general population affected during their lifetime), and the differential diagnosis for these symptoms is broad, which often makes diagnosis difficult. The most common diseases associated with dyspepsia are peptic ulcer disease, gastroesophageal reflux, biliary colic, or medication-induced discomfort. Some would consider gastritis due to *Helicobacter pylori* as a potential cause of symptoms, but this is debated. Esophageal, gastric, or duodenal malignancies have all been seen in patients presenting with dyspepsia. Patients in whom structural disease is excluded meet the criteria for functional dyspepsia.

Although an empiric trial with antisecretory therapies is often used, prompt endoscopy should be considered in older adults because of the increased rate of organic disease (including malignancy) in this age group. Endoscopy for evaluation of dyspepsia in older adults has been shown to obtain diagnostic information in >90% of patients and is associated with a significant reduction in PPI use and an improvement in quality-of-life measures (SOE=B). Endoscopy has been shown to be safe in older adults who are otherwise healthy. The risk of endoscopy in older patients with cardiac, pulmonary, or other systemic disease depends on disease severity. The decision to perform endoscopy should be made on a case-by-case basis.

H pylori testing should be performed in all patients with dyspepsia, with a 13C-urea breath test or fecal antigen test along with biopsies at the time of endoscopy. Treatment for *H pylori* in patients with ulcers will result in healing and elimination of symptoms in a large majority of patients. Large or nonhealing ulcers should be biopsied to exclude malignancy. Data are conflicting on whether treating *H pylori* in patients with nonulcer or functional dyspepsia reduces symptoms. Many in practice treat these patients in hope that eradication will reduce or eliminate symptoms. Those who are negative for *H pylori* should be given a 2-month empirical trial of a PPI (SOE=B).

Patients with a normal upper endoscopy should be considered for further testing (including abdominal imaging and a gastric emptying study). Imaging should include an abdominal sonogram to exclude hepatobiliary disease, which can mimic dyspepsia. Ultimately, patients with no identified organic disease are classified as having functional dyspepsia. These patients can also be given a trial of PPI, although the rate of symptom improvement is low.

NSAID-Induced Gastric Complications

All NSAIDs, including aspirin, can cause considerable injury to the gastric and duodenal mucosa. Age is an independent risk factor for NSAID-induced complications, and older adults experience considerable morbidity and mortality due to this class of medications.

The common gastroduodenal adverse effects of NSAIDs are dyspepsia (associated with gastritis and duodenitis) and peptic ulcer disease (PUD), with associated pain, bleeding, and perforation. The pathogenesis of NSAID-induced injury appears to be due to the systemic effect of the medications, although local effects do play a role. Many NSAIDs are carboxylic acids and exert local injury on contact with gastric and duodenal mucosa. However, most NSAID toxicity appears to occur through the cyclooxygenase pathway. Cyclooxygenase-1 (COX-1) is used by healthy gastric and duodenal mucosa in production of mucosal-protective prostaglandins. Prostaglandins protect the upper GI mucosa by various mechanisms, and NSAIDs induce injury by inhibiting COX-1 and disrupting these protective actions.

Risk factors for NSAID-induced disease include age ≥65 years, high-dose NSAID use, a prior history of PUD, and concurrent use of two NSAIDs (typically, low-dose aspirin in addition to another NSAID). Patients also taking anticoagulants, glucocorticoids, antiplatelet medications (such as clopidogrel), or SSRIs (which have weak antiplatelet activity) appear to have an increased risk of bleeding with NSAIDs. The presence of *H pylori* infection appears to have a synergistic effect on the risk of ulcer disease and bleeding in the setting of NSAID use. Several preventive strategies are available to minimize risk of GI complications in patients who must use NSAIDs. Enteric-coated NSAID formulations appear to reduce endoscopic evidence of injury but do not protect against GI bleeding, and their use is not enough to provide adequate protection in patients at risk. Switching to NSAIDs that selectively inhibit COX-2 (such as celecoxib) is associated with a 40% reduction in bleeding risk but at a potentially higher risk of cardiovascular events. Concurrent use of PPIs while on NSAIDs has been shown to be a safe and effective strategy in reducing complications, with some case series showing no gastric ulcers in patients using PPIs while on NSAIDs. Similarly, the prostaglandin E analogue misoprostol has been shown to reduce serious GI complications by >50% (SOE=A). The AGS Beers Criteria® recommend the use of PPIs or misoprostol in older adults requiring chronic NSAID therapy.

Peptic Ulcer Disease

Peptic ulcers are GI mucosal defects created in part by acid injury. Although ulcers can be seen throughout the GI tract, the term peptic ulcer usually refers to ulcers in the stomach and duodenum. Ulcers in the esophagus may be acid related but are not typically called peptic. Rates of PUD have been falling over the past several decades. Nonetheless, PUD is still a common disorder, and the incidence and complications of PUD both increase with age. In the United States, *H pylori* infection is responsible for about 80% of duodenal ulcers and 60% of gastric ulcers. The vast majority of ulcers in *H pylori*–negative patients are due to NSAIDs. Ulcers may be asymptomatic and found on upper endoscopy performed for other indications. In symptomatic PUD, common presentations are dyspepsia, bleeding, anemia, and acute abdominal pain.

Peptic ulcers are diagnosed via endoscopy, which has a sensitivity of >90% and also allows for treatment of bleeding lesions (and lesions at high risk of bleeding). Equally important, endoscopy allows for biopsies to differentiate benign ulcers from gastric cancers as well as to exclude an underlying *H pylori* infection. Clinicians should have a low threshold for repeat endoscopy in older patients with gastric ulcers to confirm ulcer healing and to exclude malignancy, because initial biopsies for gastric cancer can have a sensitivity as low as 70%.

Once a diagnosis of PUD is made, PPI therapy should be instituted. All PPIs are effective in inducing ulcer healing with rates of 80%–100% at 8 weeks (SOE=A). All patients with peptic ulcers who are infected with *H pylori* should undergo therapy to eradicate the infection. In such patients, PPI therapy can be stopped after *H pylori* treatment if ulcers were small and the patient is otherwise at low risk of bleeding. *H pylori* eradication should be confirmed with a post-treatment urea breath test or fecal antigen test. Patients with NSAID-induced PUD should remain on antisecretory therapy indefinitely if they are to remain on NSAIDs. PPI treatment once a day is sufficient in these patients.

Biliary Disease

Gall stones primarily form in the gallbladder and are often asymptomatic. However, when they obstruct the cystic duct, common bile duct, or ampulla, symptoms and complications can occur.

Gall stone disease encompasses a variety of disorders, including biliary colic, cholecystitis, cholangitis, and gall stone pancreatitis. Biliary colic is typically due to a stone transiently obstructing the cystic duct (during a gallbladder contraction) and results in severe, epigastric or right upper quadrant pain that lasts for ~30–60 minutes. Cholecystitis and cholangitis are due to stones obstructing the cystic duct and common bile duct, respectively, and are associated with inflammation and/or infection of the biliary tree. In addition to pain, these may cause a full spectrum of infectious symptoms, including fever, delirium, and shock. Older adults may present atypically, without pain or fever, and with only advanced symptoms such as delirium or hypotension.

The evaluation of biliary disease includes appropriate blood tests (including liver function tests, amylase, and lipase) as well as imaging. The initial imaging of choice in all patients is an abdominal ultrasound, which can have a sensitivity of >80% and a specificity of nearly 100% for gall stone disease. Abdominal CT can better visualize the pancreas and can identify common bile duct stones often missed by ultrasound. Magnetic resonance cholangiography is a highly sensitive imaging modality for the biliary system and may be used when suspicion of ductal stones is high, but the above imaging studies are nondiagnostic. Advanced imaging, with endoscopic ultrasound or endoscopic retrograde cholangiopancreatography, is limited to cases with a very high suspicion of gall stone disease and negative imaging or for those patients requiring endoscopic therapy.

Gallstones can be found in 35% of women and 20% of men by 70 years of age because of an age-related increase in the lithogenicity of bile. Although many older adults with cholelithiasis are asymptomatic, biliary disease is the predominant indication for urgent abdominal operations in this population; in adults >80 years old, hepatobiliary disease accounts for 20% of all abdominal surgeries. In general, asymptomatic patients with gallstones can be observed. Patients with symptomatic cholelithiasis should undergo laparoscopic cholecystectomy if they are surgical candidates because of the high rate of complications such as cholecystitis, cholangitis, and pancreatitis. In the rare older patient who is unable to undergo surgery, treatment with ursodeoxycholic acid or lithotripsy, or both, may be attempted, although efficacy rates are low. In patients with common bile duct obstruction due to gallstones, endoscopic sphincterotomy and bile ductal drainage is adequate in preventing recurrent cholangitis, and the gallbladder may be left in situ. Older patients with multiple comorbidities (and a high risk of complications from anesthesia) may undergo a percutaneous cholecystostomy. In older adults presenting with biliary pain who have had a cholecystectomy, a retained common bile duct stone should be suspected and evaluated by endoscopic retrograde cholangiopancreatography, magnetic resonance cholangiography, or endoscopic ultrasonography.

The possibility of cancer should be considered in any older adult with biliary symptoms. For patients with malignant jaundice, treatments are mostly palliative, with either surgery or percutaneous or endoscopic stenting. Such drainage improves quality of life, decreases pruritus, and improves nutritional state but does not improve survival.

Pancreatitis

Acute pancreatitis is any acute inflammatory process affecting the pancreas. It is a common cause of presentation to the emergency department for abdominal pain and can range in severity from mild to life threatening. The epidemiology of pancreatitis is complex due to the multiple underlying etiologies. However, the incidence does appear to increase with age.

The 3 most common causes of pancreatitis are alcohol use disorder, gallstones, and medications. Alcohol, the most common cause of pancreatitis in the young, appears to cause only a minority of acute pancreatitis in patients >65 years old. Gallstones are a common cause of pancreatitis in all age groups but become increasingly prevalent with age. Finally, a significant portion of older patients are classified as having an "idiopathic" cause, although the vast majority of these are likely to be medication induced. Medications associated with pancreatitis include loop diuretics statins, certain antibiotics, and many cardiac medications.

Patients with pancreatitis typically present with epigastric abdominal pain radiating to the back and worsening with food intake. As in many diseases, geriatric patients may present with delirium. The diagnosis requires any 2 of the 3 following criteria: classic pain, increase in the serum amylase or lipase to ≥3 times than the upper limit of normal, or classic findings of acute pancreatitis on imaging (CT, MRI or ultrasound). Once the diagnosis is made, the evaluation of acute pancreatitis is typically straightforward. Routine history-taking is needed to assess the patient's alcohol exposure and medication use. Hepatic enzymes levels should be obtained, with an increase in the transaminases or bilirubin suggesting gallstones as the cause of the pancreatitis. A sonogram of the gallbladder should be obtained to identify gallstones.

The bedrock of treatment for acute pancreatitis is volume resuscitation with intravenous fluids. Fluid replacement should be aggressive, because patients are often severely volume depleted. Fluid status should be checked regularly, with blood tests and lung examinations to ensure adequate replacement without inducing fluid overload. Pain control with opiates is important, because uncontrolled pain can trigger further hemodynamic instability. Nutrition has been an area of debate. Although bowel rest is critical in the initial stages of pancreatitis, recent data have shown that early refeeding (24–48 hours in most cases) is beneficial. Management of severe pancreatitis, such as necrotizing pancreatitis, pancreatitis with evidence of other end-organ compromise, or pancreatitis that does not appear to be improving in the first 24 hours or with any other concerning features, should be managed by a specialist. In these cases, consultation with the gastroenterologist soon after admission is critical.

DISORDERS OF THE COLON

Constipation

Chronic constipation affects about 30% of adults ≥65 years old, more commonly women. The rate can be even higher in hospitalized or nursing-home patients (with up to 50% of patients affected). Constipation has been defined as a fecal frequency of <3 times per week. However, some individuals may complain of lumpy or hard feces, straining at defecation, or a sense of incomplete defecation despite a daily bowel movement.

Common primary causes of constipation include functional constipation (in which no specific etiology is identified), slow-transit constipation (or colonic inertia), and pelvic floor dyssynergia. Metabolic causes include hypothyroidism, hypercalcemia, and diabetes. Structural lesions, such as strictures, malignancy, and rectal prolapse are relatively uncommon but important to exclude. Many medications have been implicated in constipation. Calcium supplements (and antacids containing calcium or aluminum), iron supplements, anticholinergics, opiates, and smooth muscle relaxants (such as calcium channel blockers) are commonly used medications with known constipating effects. In many older adults, lack of mobility, poor diet with limited fiber intake, and inadequate fluid intake play a major role in constipation.

Evaluation of constipation relies foremost on the history and physical examination. Patients should be asked about fecal frequency and consistency, straining, and if they use any maneuvers to assist with defecation. Alarm signs or symptoms, such as bleeding, weight loss, or a recent change in fecal caliber, should be elicited. A complete review of medications, including nonprescription medications, should be performed. Further evaluation can be pursued, if needed, based on this initial basic assessment. For many older adults, adjusting medications and/or a trial of fiber or laxatives may be sufficient to treat the constipation. If this empiric trial is not successful, more invasive testing is required. A basic metabolic evaluation, including measurements of thyroid-stimulating hormone and calcium should be considered. Patients with alarm signs or symptoms, patients with abrupt onset of symptoms, or those who have never had colorectal cancer screening should be counseled about undergoing colonoscopy. In patients who do not respond to dietary changes, fiber supplementation or a trial of laxatives as outlined below, anorectal manometry and a rectal balloon expulsion test to exclude dyssynergia or pelvic floor dysfunction, and a colonic transit study (Sitz marker study) to assess colonic motility could be considered. The reported prevalence of pelvic floor dysfunction is as high as 50% in older patients with constipation. There are conflicting data on the prevalence of slow colonic motility in this age group, although it is considered a common problem.

Management of constipation depends on the results of the above evaluation and is often multimodal. In all patients, medications should be reviewed and adjusted as needed to eliminate those that may induce constipation. An increase in fluid intake, dietary fiber intake, and physical activity should be recommended, often with a fiber supplement as well (typically psyllium husk). Patients who respond poorly or who do not tolerate fiber may require laxatives. Osmotic laxatives, such as polyethylene glycol, are safe and effective used on a daily basis. Use of stimulant laxatives such as bisacodyl and senna 2 or 3 times a week is generally safe, although they can be associated with cramping and have been associated with electrolyte abnormalities with long-term use. Fecal softeners, such as docusate sodium, have minimal to no effect and should generally be avoided (SOE=B). Saline laxatives (such as magnesium hydroxide) have not been well studied in the geriatric population, are associated with a risk of hypermagnesemia, and should be avoided if possible.

Patients with slow-transit constipation should be treated similarly. If first-line laxatives fail, newer pharmacologic agents, typically colonic secretagogues such as lubiprostone or linaclotide, should be considered (SOE=A). Although they appear to be safe and effective in the general population, these agents have not yet been studied extensively in older adults and should be used with caution. Patients with slow-transit constipation with severe, longstanding symptoms who do not respond to these therapies may ultimately require surgery (typically a subtotal colectomy). However, this is considered a treatment of last resort.

Patients with defecatory disorders identified by anorectal manometry and a balloon expulsion test should be referred for pelvic floor retraining and biofeedback. This can be done in addition to the therapies used in normal-transit and slow-transit constipation.

Depending on the response to each step, the underlying colonic motility, or any identified anorectal disorders, these treatments can be combined or attempted in concert with one another.

Fecal impaction is common in older adults with constipation of any etiology. This should be treated first by manual disimpaction to fragment large fecal boluses and then followed by several warm-water enemas to help evacuate the rectum. Soap suds enemas have been associated with a chemical colitis (sometimes severe, with hemorrhage) and should be avoided. After local disimpaction, a polyethylene glycol preparation should be used to cleanse the entire colon. Long-term management involves treating the underlying cause of constipation and typically adding a daily polyethylene glycol laxative to the patient's medication regimen. Weekly cleansing enemas can be considered in those with recurrent fecal impaction.

Fecal Incontinence

Fecal incontinence is a disturbing disability, affecting quality of life and often leading to social isolation. Multiple definitions of fecal incontinence exist, but in general it is defined as the involuntary passage or the inability to control passage of fecal material through the anus. This problem can be subcategorized as major incontinence (involuntary excretion of feces) or minor incontinence (seepage of liquid feces, staining of undergarments, or inadvertent escape of flatus). Fecal incontinence affects 2%–7% of adults, mostly older adults in poor general health, and is a common cause of nursing-home placement. Women are disproportionately affected. Patients are reluctant to discuss this disorder with clinicians because of embarrassment and social stigma, resulting in substantial delays in treatment.

Fecal continence depends on many factors, such as physical and mental function, fecal consistency, colonic transit, rectal compliance, internal and external anal sphincter function, and anorectal sensation and reflexes. Normal defecation is a complex sequential process that starts with the entry of feces into the rectum, leading to reflex relaxation of the internal anal sphincter. If defecation is desired, the anorectal angle is voluntarily straightened, and abdominal pressure is increased by straining. This results in descent of the pelvic floor, contraction of the rectum, and inhibition of the external anal sphincter, which causes evacuation of the rectal contents. Fecal incontinence may thus occur with a disruption of any of the above processes and it is often a multifactorial issue.

The history and physical examination often provide clues to the cause of fecal incontinence. A description of the incontinence should be obtained. The history should determine if the incontinence is of a large volume of feces, small volume, or simple staining of the underwear and if it occurs chronically or only with increased intra-abdominal pressure (such as with laughing or coughing). Additional important historical details to obtain include coexisting diarrhea, an obstetric history, and concomitant conditions such as diabetes, neurologic disorders, and spinal cord injury. The examination should note sphincter tone, appropriate perineal descent, any rectal prolapse, and perineal sensation. A flexible sigmoidoscopy may be considered to exclude inflammation or tumor. The next step is anorectal manometry, which measures resting anal sphincter tone, squeeze pressure, the rectoanal inhibitory reflex, rectal sensation, and rectal compliance. This test requires complete cooperation by the patient and will not be appropriate for many patients, particularly those with moderate or advanced dementia. The results often identify pelvic floor disorders that may be treated with physical therapy aimed at the specific abnormalities identified. Pelvic floor physical therapy also requires intensive cooperation and involvement by the patient and would not be recommended for patients who would have difficulty with the exercises. Abnormalities of the anal sphincters, the rectal wall, and the puborectalis muscle identified on anorectal manometry can be further evaluated by use of endorectal ultrasound. Typically, a defect in the internal anal sphincter is associated with low resting sphincter pressure, whereas defects in the external sphincter are associated with lower anal squeeze pressure.

Medical therapy is aimed at treating the underlying cause when possible, improving fecal consistency, and reducing fecal frequency. Fecal bulking agents (eg, methylcellulose) and antidiarrheal medications (including loperamide and diphenoxylate/atropine) can be effective first-line agents. Diphenoxylate/atropine should be used with caution in older adults because of its anticholinergic effects. Biofeedback therapy, which includes anal sphincter strengthening and rectal sensory conditioning, is painless, safe, and often effective in patients who have no structural defect. Patients in whom conservative measures are ineffective, or who have anal sphincter defects, may benefit from injectable sphincter bulking agents or surgery. Bulking agents are injected submucosally at the site of sphincter weakness and may be best reserved for those with mild incontinence (SOE=B).

Chronic Diarrhea

Chronic diarrhea is defined as a decrease in fecal consistency lasting for >4 weeks. Diarrhea is associated with decreased quality of life and significant morbidity and sometimes mortality in older adults. There are many potential causes of chronic diarrhea, and evaluation can be challenging. The presenting history is essential in narrowing the differential diagnosis and helping to target the evaluation.

Common causes of chronic diarrhea are irritable bowel syndrome, lactose or other food intolerance, inflammatory bowel disease (typically Crohn disease), malabsorption syndromes (such as celiac disease, small-intestinal bacterial overgrowth, and chronic pancreatitis), and chronic infections (such as recurrent *C difficile*, amebiasis, giardiasis, *Cryptosporidium*, Whipple disease, and *Cyclospora*). Microscopic colitis (lymphocytic and collagenous colitis) is common in this age group and should be strongly considered in those with endoscopically normal colons. Many medications, including OTC medications, herbs, and supplements are associated with development of diarrhea. Common medications include SSRIs, PPIs, and certain oral hypoglycemic and chemotherapeutic agents. OTC medications or supplements include vitamin C or magnesium-containing antacids. Clinicians should be aware that diet drinks, foods, or even chewable medications containing sorbitol or other artificial sweeteners can cause chronic diarrhea.

A thorough medical history is essential to define fecal consistency, volume, and frequency, and the presence of urgency or fecal soiling. Fecal incontinence is frequently confused with diarrhea in older adults. Malodorous feces and weight loss may suggest fat malabsorption, whereas visible blood suggests inflammatory bowel disease. If the diarrhea occurs during fasting or at night, a secretory etiology (eg, neuroendocrine tumor) needs to be considered. Large-volume watery diarrhea is more likely to be due to a small-intestinal disorder or microscopic colitis, whereas small-volume frequent diarrhea with tenesmus reflects distal colonic inflammation. All medications must be reviewed and patients asked specifically about nonprescription medications and "sugar-free" or diet food products.

Depending on the initial history and physical examination, the diagnostic approach to chronic diarrhea is complex and multifaceted, involving fecal analyses, exclusion of infectious causes, structural evaluation by colonoscopy with appropriate biopsies, small-bowel capsule endoscopy and/or radiography, and abdominal CT imaging. Treatment of chronic diarrhea depends on the underlying diagnosis and may require referral to a specialist.

Diverticular Disease

The prevalence of diverticular disease is age dependent, seen in 30% by age 60 and increasing to 65% by age 85. Although most patients remain asymptomatic, 20% develop diverticulitis, and 10% may develop diverticular bleeding. Therefore, the mere presence of diverticulosis does not require specific therapy. A diet high in fiber appears to be associated with a reduced risk of developing diverticular disease and may reduce the risk of subsequent complications.

Uncomplicated diverticulosis is often an incidental finding on screening sigmoidoscopy, colonoscopy, or cross-sectional imaging, such as a CT scan. Some patients may complain of nonspecific abdominal cramping, bloating, flatulence, and irregular bowel habits. Diverticular bleeding is usually painless and self-limited, and it rarely coexists with acute diverticulitis. Diverticulitis usually presents with left lower quadrant pain, although nausea, vomiting, constipation, diarrhea, and dysuria or frequency may occur, particularly in women. The physical examination usually reveals left lower quadrant tenderness, a tender mass, and abdominal distention. Generalized tenderness suggests perforation and peritonitis. Low-grade fever and leukocytosis are common, but their absence in older adults does not exclude the diagnosis. Urinalysis may reveal sterile pyuria induced by adjacent colonic inflammation; the presence of mixed colonic flora on urine culture suggests a colovesical fistula. Other potential complications include perforation, obstruction, and abscess formation.

CT scanning is the optimal imaging choice in suspected acute diverticulitis. CT can also identify peritonitis, obstruction, and fistula to the bladder, vagina, and abdominal wall. However, in approximately 10% of patients, diverticulitis cannot be distinguished from colon cancer, because both may show focal thickening of the bowel wall. In such cases, on resolution of the acute inflammation, a colonoscopy is indicated.

Most (85%) patients with simple diverticulitis respond to medical therapy. Patients with complicated diverticulitis usually require surgery.

Mild diverticulitis with left lower quadrant pain, low-grade fever, and minimal physical findings is often treated on an outpatient basis, with clear liquids and oral antibiotics, such as ciprofloxacin 500 mg q12h or metronidazole 500 mg q8h, or both. Hospitalization is needed only if no improvement is seen. Once the episode resolves, solid food is reintroduced and the colon evaluated, preferably by colonoscopy. For patients with moderate to severe symptoms, treatment with bowel rest, fluids, and intravenous antibiotics is initiated, with the aim to avoid urgent surgery. Antibiotics should be active against gram-negative rods and anaerobes. If there is no improvement, either the diagnosis is incorrect, or an abscess, peritonitis, fistula, or obstruction is present. Older immunosuppressed patients with multiple underlying medical conditions may present with minimal symptoms or signs, even in cases of frank peritonitis, and the diagnosis is commonly delayed. In such cases, early surgical intervention should be considered. Diffuse peritonitis requires fluid resuscitation, broad-spectrum antibiotics, and emergency laparotomy. Colonic resection removes the septic focus, corrects the obstruction or fistula formation, and restores bowel continuity.

Irritable Bowel Syndrome

Irritable bowel syndrome (IBS) is a functional GI disorder with remissions and exacerbations, characterized by abdominal pain, bloating, and either constipation or diarrhea, or both. Although the pathogenesis is incompletely understood, IBS appears to result at least partly from altered bowel motility, visceral hypersensitivity, and enhanced perception by the brain of many visceral stimuli. A common mediator for all these abnormalities is serotonin, and serotonin-receptor agonists and antagonists are used in management of IBS. Although psychosocial factors are commonly involved in IBS, they are not known to have a causative role. The prevalence of IBS in geriatric patients has been reported to be as high as 20%. Thus, this diagnosis should be considered in older patients with chronic symptoms consistent with IBS.

Because the clinical symptoms characteristic of IBS are not specific, it is important to be mindful of features that are not consistent with IBS. These include weight loss, first onset of symptoms after age 50, nocturnal diarrhea, family history of cancer or inflammatory bowel disease, rectal bleeding or obstruction, and laboratory abnormalities (eg, anemia, leukocytosis, abnormal chemistries, positive fecal cultures, or the presence of parasites in the feces). In older patients, the diagnosis should be made only after other conditions (ie, ischemia, diverticulosis, colon cancer, or inflammatory bowel disease) have been carefully excluded. An appropriate evaluation of an older adult with symptoms consistent with IBS should include a colonoscopy and often an upper endoscopy. A CT scan of the abdomen should be considered. Small-bowel imaging, either with CT enterography, MRI enterography, or video capsule endoscopy should be performed in patients with symptoms, signs, or laboratory values suggestive of possible small-bowel disease. These include patients with weight loss, iron-deficiency anemia, or diarrhea that is unexplained by endoscopy and colonoscopy.

If the history, physical examination, and laboratory or imaging studies are negative, the diagnosis of IBS can then be made and subcategorized as IBS with constipation (IBS-C), IBS with diarrhea (IBS-D), or IBS with alternating constipation and diarrhea (IBS-M or IBS mixed).

Treatment depends on IBS subtype. Reassurance is necessary in all subtypes to clarify that, although it may impact quality of life, IBS is not life threatening and repetitive testing is unnecessary and may be harmful. Dietary changes may be useful in all subtypes of IBS, with many patients responding well to increased fiber intake. In patients with diarrhea, a 3- to 6-week trial of a lactose-free diet may identify patients with concomitant lactose intolerance (calcium supplementation should be considered in patients on a long-term lactose-free diet). Some specific diets have been studied for IBS. A gluten-free diet has been shown to be helpful in some randomized trials, although no specific data are available in older adults. A diet low in fermentable oligo-, di- and monosaccharides and polyols (FODMAP diet) has been shown to be effective in reducing IBS symptoms in a few high-quality trials, but again no data exist specifically in the geriatric population. These diets should be instituted with the aid of a nutritionist, because they can be very restrictive and difficult to maintain and pose a risk of nutritional deficiencies. Probiotics (specifically, bifidobacterium-containing formulations) have been used in treatment of all subtypes of IBS with anecdotal efficacy, but available data do not support routine use. Antibiotics have been used, with randomized trials showing significant improvement in global symptoms of IBS with a short course of the nonabsorbable antibiotic rifaximin (SOE=A). However, the long-term efficacy of rifaximin is unknown. Antispasmodic agents, typically short-acting intestinal smooth-muscle relaxants, should be used with caution to treat the pain of IBS, because they act via anticholinergic properties and may have systemic adverse effects. Tricyclic antidepressants have been shown to be efficacious in treatment of global symptoms of IBS in younger populations, but these drugs should be used with caution in older adults. Less consistent data are available for nontricyclic antidepressants such as SSRIs.

IBS-C can be treated similarly to chronic constipation. Of the constipation medications, specific consideration should be given to linaclotide, because in the general population it appears to have an analgesic effect independent of its effect on constipation (SOE=A). However, its use in older adults has not been systematically evaluated. IBS-D may respond to fiber-bulking agents such psyllium, because they help normalize fecal consistency. Loperamide, an antidiarrheal opiate agonist, has been shown to be effective in randomized controlled trials. Bile acid sequestrants, such as cholestyramine or colestipol, can be effective as well. They should not be taken with other medications, because they can bind and block absorption of those drugs. Finally, a serotonin antagonist, alosetron, available on a compassionate use basis from the FDA, is highly effective but should be used with extreme caution, because it may precipitate intestinal ischemia.

Occult Gastrointestinal Bleeding

Older adults commonly have a positive fecal occult blood test (FOBT) or are diagnosed with unexplained iron-deficiency anemia, or both. Although colorectal cancer is a leading concern, other causes (of which there are many) include esophagitis, peptic ulcers, esophageal and gastric malignancies, intestinal or colonic angiodysplasia, benign colon polyps, inflammatory bowel disease, or hemorrhoids. A positive FOBT should not be attributed to esophageal varices or colonic diverticula, because it is rare for such lesions to bleed in an occult fashion. The presence of a positive

FOBT warrants evaluation and should not be attributed to aspirin or other antiplatelet or anticoagulant use.

Detection of fecal occult blood using a standard guaiac-based test has a low sensitivity and a high rate of false-positive results, leading to more invasive and expensive tests. Newer fecal immunochemical tests are more specific (they respond only to human globin and not to animal source of heme), but they miss upper GI sources of blood loss (as the globin is digested in transit) and can be expensive. Despite these limitations, an annual FOBT is currently recommended as one method of screening for colon cancer and has been associated with up to a 33% reduction in mortality from colon cancer. Because of the high prevalence of colorectal cancer and/or adenomatous polyps in older adults with a positive FOBT, a colonoscopy should be performed and, if negative, consideration given to an upper endoscopy. If symptoms of upper GI disease are present, there is a high likelihood for a positive endoscopy. However, in older adults at risk of colon cancer, the presence of an upper GI lesion should not preclude evaluation of the colon. Patients with normal upper and lower endoscopy should be considered for evaluation for a small-bowel source using video capsule endoscopy, followed if necessary by balloon enteroscopy. The most common cause of bleeding from the small bowel is angiodysplasia, followed by tumors or ulcers that are commonly caused by NSAIDs. Unrecognized gluten-sensitive enteropathy can result in iron-deficiency anemia, because iron is absorbed in the proximal small bowel, and multiple biopsies should always be taken from the duodenum to confirm this diagnosis histologically.

In one prospective study in which patients with iron-deficiency anemia were evaluated with colonoscopy and endoscopy, followed by radiographic examination of the small intestine if these tests were negative, a source of bleeding was identified in 62% of cases. A lesion was seen on colonoscopy in 25%, on upper endoscopy in 36%, and on both in 1% of patients. Peptic ulcer disease was the primary abnormality in the upper GI tract, but cancer was detected on colonoscopy in 11% of patients.

Colonic Angiodysplasia

The terms *angiodysplasia*, *arteriovenous malformation*, and *vascular ectasia* are often used interchangeably. These aberrant vessels are dilated, thin-walled vascular structures in the mucosa and submucosa that are lined by endothelium or by smooth muscle. Although they are mostly tortuous veins, arteriovenous communications or enlarged arteries may be present, leading to brisk bleeding. The pathogenesis of angiodysplasias is not well understood. They are commonly seen in association with certain systemic disorders, including end-stage renal disease and aortic stenosis, and appear to increase with age. When angiodysplasias occur in the setting of a known syndrome, such as Osler-Weber-Rendu syndrome or scleroderma CREST variant, they are typically referred to as telangiectasias.

Angiodysplasias are seen most often in the cecum and ascending colon, where they may cause bleeding, particularly in patients ≥60 years old. However, angiodysplasias are seen throughout the GI tract and may be multiple or coexist in several different regions of the GI tract. They may be asymptomatic or cause occult or clinically overt GI bleeding.

Angiodysplasias are usually diagnosed during endoscopy or colonoscopy but can also be diagnosed by angiography. If they are serendipitously detected during routine endoscopy or colonoscopy, angiodysplasias do not require treatment. However, an actively bleeding angiodysplasia should be treated. Whether angiodysplasias were the cause of bleeding in patients who have stopped bleeding and, in particular, in patients who are found to have both angiodysplasias and diverticula is a more difficult problem. In such cases, bleeding from angiodysplasias is almost always from the cecum or ascending colon.

Iron supplementation should be given to all patients with chronic bleeding from angiodysplasias and may be the only treatment needed in patients with limited, occult bleeding (SOE=B).

Colonic Ischemia

Ischemic colitis is the most common form of intestinal ischemia and typically affects patients >65 years old. Colonic ischemia usually occurs in the setting of an acute but temporary reduction in blood flow to the colon. In the vast majority of cases, the effect is transient, and symptoms resolve without long-term sequela. However, up to 15% of patients can present with life-threatening ischemia or colonic gangrene, which is associated with high mortality.

Any low-flow state can cause ischemic colitis, including dehydration, infection, or medication-induced hypotension. Risk factors for colonic ischemia include known cardiovascular disease, prior vascular surgery, hemodialysis, and thrombophilia. Ischemia usually affects "water-shed" segments of the colon, such as the splenic flexure and the rectosigmoid junction, where collateral blood flow is limited.

The presentation of ischemic colitis depends on the severity of hypoperfusion. In the typical, nonocclusive presentation, patients will complain of acute, crampy abdominal pain followed by hematochezia. Diagnosis is often made radiographically, with CT showing segmental thickening of the affected watershed region in the appropriate clinical setting. Colonoscopy, if performed, reveals segmental edema, hemorrhages, gray-black pseudomembrane formation, and focal ulcers, mostly in the region of the splenic flexure and typically sparing the rectum.

Treatment is mostly supportive with intravenous fluids and treatment of the underlying cause of the low-flow state. In the minority of cases when life-threatening ischemia occurs (suggested by peritoneal signs, fever, marked leukocytosis, increased lactate, and/or a lack of response to fluid resuscitation), emergent surgery and broad-spectrum antibiotics are required. However, in these cases, morbidity and mortality can be as high as 75%, even with rapid surgical intervention.

Acute Colonic Pseudo-Obstruction

Acute colonic pseudo-obstruction (Ogilvie syndrome) is manifested by massive dilation of the colon without evidence of mechanical obstruction. In older adults, it is often related to neurologic disease such as Parkinson or cerebrovascular disease, trauma, recent orthopedic surgery, or use of opioids. Infections, particularly *C difficile*, and colonic ischemia can cause colonic dilation and need to be excluded. Ogilvie syndrome presents clinically with abdominal distention, often with accompanying pain. Patients may have a lack of fecal output or a paradoxical "postobstructive" diarrhea. The diagnosis is made with an abdominal radiograph and confirmed with a CT scan to exclude an underlying obstruction. Treatment is initially supportive and aimed at addressing underlying precipitating factors such as poor mobility, opioid use, or metabolic disturbances that may exacerbate gut dysmotility (such as hypokalemia or hypomagnesemia). Patients who do not respond to conservative measures in the first 24 hours, who have abdominal pain, or who have significant (>10 cm) dilation of the colon should receive further care. Treatment with neostigmine, an acetylcholinesterase inhibitor, can produce rapid and sustained colonic decompression but must be performed in a monitored setting because of the risk of bradycardia and hypotension. In extreme cases (or when neostigmine is contraindicated), colonoscopy can provide temporary decompression. Placement of a colonic tube at the time of colonoscopy can provide longer-term decompression. Surgical decompression is rarely used and reserved for only severe cases unresponsive to all other measures.

CHOOSING WISELY® RECOMMENDATIONS

Gastroenterology

- For pharmacologic management of GERD, use lowest dosage needed to achieve symptom control.

- For diagnosis of IBS, exclude ischemia, diverticulosis, colon cancer, and inflammatory bowel disease by physical examination and testing (colonoscopy, CT scan, or small-bowel series). Do not repeat CT unless major changes in clinical findings.

RESOURCES

- Baker NR, Blakely KK. Gastrointestinal disturbances in the elderly. *Nurs Clin North Am*. 2018;52(3):419–431.

- Crogan NL. Nutritional problems affecting older adults. *Nurs Clin North Am*. 2017;52(3):433–445.

- Loozen CS, van Ramshorst B, van Santvoort HC, et al. Acute cholecystitis in elderly patients: a case for early cholecystectomy? *J Visc Surg*. 2018;155(2):99–103.

- Schnoll-Sussman F, Katz PO. Managing esophageal dysphagia in the elderly. *Curr Treat Options Gastroenterol*. 2016;14(3):315–326.

CHAPTER 54—NEPHROLOGY

KEY POINTS

- With aging, kidneys become less able to maintain homeostasis in response to physiologic stress.

- Serum creatinine is a poor marker of kidney function. Kidney function is better approximated by the estimated glomerular filtration rate (eGFR).

- Causes of acute kidney injury are divided into prerenal azotemia, urinary tract obstruction, and intrinsic kidney disease, which may be glomerular, tubulointerstitial, or vascular in origin.

- Chronic kidney disease (CKD) is very common in older adults and is classified into stages based on eGFR. Preventing progression of CKD is important at any age.

- Patients with CKD are at increased risk of cardiovascular disease and should be carefully evaluated for modifiable risk factors.

- For those with CKD, referral to a nephrologist is recommended when eGFR decreases to <30 mL/min (Stage 4 CKD) for help in management of CKD-related complications and discussions regarding dialysis and transplantation. Referral is also recommended earlier for many high-risk groups, including those with substantial proteinuria, unexplained hematuria or rapidly declining renal function.

KIDNEY ASSESSMENT

Measures of Kidney Function

Direct measurement of glomerular filtration rate (GFR) is not practical in the clinical setting. Serum creatinine, which is freely filtered at the glomerulus but not reabsorbed or metabolized and only minimally secreted by the tubule, has traditionally been used to approximate GFR. However, creatinine level alone can be misleading. Muscle mass, the source of serum creatinine, declines with age, especially in frail older adults. Therefore, kidney function can be profoundly impaired despite having a serum creatinine that remains near or even within the normal range in a person with low muscle mass.

Formulas for estimating GFR have been developed to account for some of the key variables known to be related to muscle mass and thus serum creatinine (age, sex, race). The Cockcroft-Gault formula is mathematically straightforward but generally overestimates creatinine clearance; thus, other formulas are preferred. The Modified Diet in Renal Disease (MDRD) equation was developed from a mostly white cohort with an average eGFR of 40 mL/min/1.73 m^2. It is less accurate when GFR is >60 mL/min/1.73 m^2 and may also be less accurate among non-whites. The more recent CKD-Epi equation is a variation of the MDRD that is more accurate across the spectrum of GFR values and race/ethnicities.

All creatinine-based eGFR estimating equations have important limitations. First, not all the variability in muscle mass from patient to patient can be accounted for by measurement of age, sex, and race. For example, muscle mass may also be related to body habitus, exercise habits, and chronic illness. Another way to estimate GFR is by measuring creatinine clearance based on a 24-hour urine collection. However, under most circumstances, a 24-hour urine collection is not recommended because of frequent errors in collection that can cause substantially misleading results.

Thus, there is an ongoing search for novel endogenous molecules that might prove useful in better assessing kidney function. The best studied of these is cystatin C, a small protein that derives from all nucleated cells. Similar to creatinine, it is cleared by the kidneys such that the serum level increases as kidney function decreases. In contrast to creatinine, because it comes from all nucleated cells rather than just muscle, it is less affected by the changes in muscle mass with aging. There are 2 variations of the CKD-Epi formula that use cystatin C. Although cystatin C–based eGFR estimates certainly have some potential advantages (eg, improved accuracy in estimating GFR in the setting of abnormal muscle mass), they also have some substantial limitations, such as the lack of standardization between laboratories. Currently, cystatin C–based eGFR estimates are often used in clinical practice as a confirmatory test in patients with suspected moderate CKD. These estimates may also be useful in those with substantially abnormal muscle mass or sarcopenia. Of note, all eGFR-estimating equations rely on the assumption of a stable serum level of creatinine or cystatin C and, thus, can be misleading in the setting of acute kidney injury (AKI).

The National Kidney Foundation (NKF) recommends that laboratories report eGFRs calculated with the CKD-EPI Equation. The NKF has an online calculator that provides an estimate of GFR using several equations including CKD-Epi (www.kidney.org/professionals/KDOQI/gfr_calculator). A close approximation of a patient's GFR is essential for medication dosing, as well as for avoiding nephrotoxins that pose increased risk to patients with already tenuous renal function.

Table 54.1–Changes in Kidney Function with Aging

Function	Clinical Significance
↓ GFR	↑ Risk of chronic kidney disease ↑ Risk of acute kidney injury
↓ Diluting capacity (generally mild)	↑ Risk of hyponatremia
↓ Concentrating ability	↑ Risk of hypernatremia Poor compensation for volume depletion Nocturia
↓ Sodium conservation when sodium intake is low	↑ Risk of volume depletion
↓ Sodium excretion when sodium intake is high	↑ Risk of salt-sensitive hypertension Edema
↓ Potassium excretion	↑ Risk of hyperkalemia
↓ Capacity to excrete acid	↑ Risk of metabolic acidosis

Measures of Urinary Protein Excretion

Proteinuria is an important sign of kidney damage, as well as a risk factor for vascular events and progression of CKD. There are several methods of measuring urinary protein excretion. The standard urine dipstick is a simple screening test but is insensitive for low levels of proteinuria. The urine albumin/creatinine ratio (ACR) has been recommended as the best screening test for low levels of proteinuria in high-risk individuals. Moderately increased albuminuria is defined as 30–300 mg/g creatinine, and severely increased albuminuria as >300 mg/g creatinine. This range of albuminuria was previously called microalbuminuria, but this term has fallen out of favor because it may be misleading. The ACR provides an estimate of 24-hour albumin excretion but may miss nonalbumin proteinuria (eg, monoclonal gammopathy–related proteinuria). A 24-hour urine collection for albumin and/or protein is the gold standard method of measuring proteinuria but is infrequently done because errors in technique are common and render misleading results.

METABOLIC AND VOLUME DISORDERS

Older adults are vulnerable to metabolic and volume derangements for a number of reasons. Age-related anatomic, hemodynamic, and hormonal changes affect crucial functions that maintain homeostasis of fluids, electrolytes, volume, and acid-base balance. Under normal conditions, the aging kidney is usually able to maintain homeostasis; however, under stress, the adaptive response to maintain homeostasis is impaired. See Table 54.1 for examples of kidney-related physiologic changes with aging.

Disorders of Water Balance: Hyponatremia and Hypernatremia

Dysnatremias are common among older adults. Water balance is regulated through the effects of ADH, or vasopressin, which is released from the posterior pituitary in response to increased blood tonicity. ADH binds receptors in the kidneys, leading to reabsorption of water through water channels, thus diluting the blood and concentrating the urine. ADH should be high in hypernatremia, leading to retention of water and excretion of concentrated urine. ADH should be suppressed in hypoosmolar hyponatremia, leading to a dilute urine and excretion of excess water. Severe volume depletion, through the action of baroreceptors in the aortic arch and carotid bodies, is a nonosmotic stimulus for ADH release and causes retention of water to avoid exacerbating volume depletion at the expense of maintaining a normal serum sodium concentration. In older adults, alterations in the ADH system have clinical implications, as discussed below.

Hyponatremia

Hyponatremia has been reported in approximately 8% of all older adults and up to 11% of hospitalized geriatric patients. Older adults are generally thought to have adequate ADH secretion in response to changes in serum osmolality. However, they frequently exhibit a decreased ability to maximally dilute urine in response to hyponatremia, likely due to a lower GFR and consequent lower maximal free water clearance. Older adults are also at increased risk of being both volume depleted and on medications that cause or exacerbate hyponatremia.

Early recognition and treatment of hyponatremia are critical to avert serious complications and neurologic sequelae, so it is essential to be aware of its varied symptoms and signs. Hypoosmolar hyponatremia causes an osmotic shift of water from the extracellular to the intracellular space, which can lead to brain edema and symptoms of apathy, disorientation, lethargy, muscle cramps, anorexia, nausea, agitation, headache, seizures, and coma. Even when mild and apparently asymptomatic, hyponatremia is associated with deficits in gait and attention, falls, and increased fracture risk in older adults (SOE=A). Overt symptoms are more likely to develop when the sodium concentration acutely falls below 125 mEq/L. The only manifestations of chronic hyponatremia may be lethargy, confusion, and malaise.

The first step in determining an underlying cause is obtaining the serum osmolality. Hyperosmolar, isoosmolar, and hypoosmolar hyponatremia are distinctly different with regard to differential diagnosis and treatment. The most common type of hyponatremia by far is hypoosmolar hyponatremia. After excluding isoosmolar and hyperosmolar hyponatremia, the next step in diagnosis is determining the patient's volume status.

Hyponatremia with Volume Depletion
Older adults are prone to volume depletion because of a number of factors, including comorbid conditions, medications (particularly thiazide diuretics), and hormonal changes. As mentioned above, significant volume depletion leads to release of ADH in response to signals from baroreceptors in the aortic arch and carotid bodies. Often, patients appear volume depleted with clinical signs such as orthostatic hypotension, dry mucus membranes, and dry axillae, but occasionally hypovolemia is less apparent by clinical examination. Once intravascular volume is repleted, ADH is suppressed and the kidneys excrete the excess water, correcting the hyponatremia.

Hyponatremia with Volume Overload
Common conditions include heart failure, cirrhosis, and the nephrotic syndrome. In these conditions, a decrease in effective arterial volume stimulates both ADH release and the renin-angiotensin-aldosterone system (RAAS), thus promoting salt retention and edema. The urine quantity is generally small in these cases, and urine sodium concentration is also low as the kidneys are maximally reabsorbing both water (mediated by ADH) and sodium (mediated by aldosterone).

Treatment includes fluid restriction and loop diuretics. Under the care of a nephrologist or cardiologist, a direct ADH (V2) receptor antagonist may also be considered in extreme cases. V2-receptor antagonists are contraindicated in cirrhosis and should be started in the hospital because of the risk of overcorrection and need for close monitoring.

Hyponatremia with Normal Extracellular Fluid Volume
There are many causes of euvolemic hyponatremia, including kidney disease, hypothyroidism, adrenal insufficiency, the syndrome of inappropriate antidiuretic hormone (SIADH), low-solute diet, primary polydipsia, and a reset osmostat. A few etiologies of particular significance for older adults are discussed below.

SIADH is a common cause of hyponatremia in older adults. Most cases are mild and relatively asymptomatic but, as stated above, may increase the risk of falls, gait impairment, and difficulty sustaining attention. In this condition, ADH is released despite euvolemia and hyponatremia. Because the patient is euvolemic, there is no stimulus for sodium retention, and urine sodium excretion reflects sodium intake. Pulmonary and brain pathology, including infections and malignancy, may cause SIADH. Medication-related causes include SSRIs, sulfonylureas, carbamazepine, oxcarbazepine, and tricyclic antidepressants. SIADH is managed by discontinuing offending medications, treating underlying pathology (eg, pneumonia), and restricting fluid. Salt tablets and loop diuretics are sometimes added depending on severity. Treatments such as 3% hypertonic saline and/or ADH receptor antagonists can also be used but should be done in the hospital in collaboration with a nephrologist.

Low-solute diet is a prominent etiology of hyponatremia in older adults. It occurs when a patient eats a diet low in protein and salt (eg, beer potomania, or tea and toast) but maintains a normal or high fluid intake. This causes hyponatremia, more frequently in older patients because of their impaired diluting capacity that necessitates a larger minimum solute intake to excrete the same amount of water as a person with normal diluting capacity.

Reset osmostat is a syndrome in which ADH secretion remains high at a normal serum osmolality (approximately 280 mOsmol/kg, which corresponds to a sodium of about 140 mEq/L) but becomes suppressed when the serum osmolality reaches a slightly lower level. In this situation, serum sodium is stably maintained but at a lower than normal value. This is in contrast to SIADH, in which ADH continues to be released regardless of serum osmolality.

Treatment of Severe or Symptomatic Hyponatremia
Urgent or emergent treatment is indicated when hyponatremia is severe or symptomatic and warrants admission to the hospital for management. Because hyponatremia is usually caused by an inability of the kidneys to excrete a water load, free water restriction is a consideration in managing all forms of hyponatremia. In patients with hypovolemia, solute intake or isotonic saline is generally sufficient to correct the hyponatremia, because euvolemia restores osmotic regulation of ADH. In patients with severe SIADH, administration of isotonic saline can worsen hyponatremia as the salt is excreted and water is retained. Such patients may warrant treatment with intravenous hypertonic saline. In patients treated with either isotonic or hypertonic saline urine output, volume status, and sodium levels should be reassessed frequently. Overly rapid correction of chronic hyponatremia can result in osmotic demyelination and a devastating locked-in syndrome called central pontine myelinolysis. The goal is to increase serum sodium concentration by approximately 6 mEq/24 hours, although in severe symptomatic hyponatremia, a nephrologist may recommend a small bolus of 3% saline given over minutes to acutely raise the sodium a few mEq/L. This is generally safe and can alleviate symptoms. The 24-hour goal remains the same in these cases.

Hypernatremia

Serum sodium concentration can increase from either a net loss of water or a gain of sodium from ingestion. Despite normal to increased ADH secretion, older adults have diminished sensitivity to ADH, which impairs ability to concentrate the urine. Furthermore, older adults sometimes have an impaired thirst mechanism that can result in inadequate fluid intake despite dehydration. Patients with a diminished level of consciousness or immobility with decreased ability to obtain access to free water are at greatest risk of dehydration and hypernatremia. Comorbidities such as infections, fever, dementia, and neurologic disorders increase risk of hypernatremia. In addition, medications that can cloud the sensorium, osmotic diuretic agents, tube feedings containing high protein and glucose, and bowel cathartics increase risk of hypernatremia in older adults and should be used carefully.

Hypernatremia can lead to severe neurologic sequelae, including obtundation, stupor, coma, and death. Free water deficits should be corrected by encouraging oral fluid intake, or if the patient is unable to take adequate fluid by mouth, administration of intravenous or enteral free water. Chronic hypernatremia should be corrected slowly to prevent cerebral edema.

Disorders of Sodium Balance: Hypovolemia and Hypervolemia

Hypovolemia differs from dehydration in that it implies a sodium deficit rather than a water deficit. Older adults are at increased risk of volume depletion precipitated by many causes, but medications and acute illness are two common etiologies. Symptoms include dizziness and fatigue. Signs include low blood pressure, tachycardia, orthostatic hypotension, and decreased skin turgor, although mild volume depletion can be clinically subtle. Laboratory clues may include metabolic alkalosis and increased BUN/creatinine ratio, but these are both nonspecific. Treatment is aimed at replacing sodium, generally with an isotonic fluid such as normal saline, an isotonic crystalloid solution, or lactated Ringer's solution.

Hypervolemia is a common problem and may be related to underlying conditions such as congestive heart failure and other conditions that cause a low effective arterial volume leading to RAAS activation and sodium retention. Excessive sodium intake exacerbates hypervolemia as do a number of medications that can lead to sodium retention, especially NSAIDs, thiazolidinediones, and vasodilators such as calcium channel blockers, hydralazine, and minoxidil. Treatment generally consists of treating underlying conditions, restricting sodium, discontinuing offending medications if possible, and judicious using diuretics.

Loop diuretics are usually effective, whereas thiazide diuretics alone are often insufficient, particularly in the setting of diminished GFR. In diuretic-resistant cases, combinations of diuretics may be necessary, but combined use of loop and thiazide diuretics can lead to profound hypokalemia and hypomagnesemia.

Disorders of Potassium Balance

Most potassium in the body is intracellular. Derangements in serum potassium concentrations may be caused by shifts of potassium in or out of cells, as well as by inappropriate potassium intake or losses. Kidneys regulate potassium concentrations in the collecting tubule where aldosterone stimulates sodium reabsorption, thereby creating an electrochemical gradient drawing potassium and protons into the urine.

Hyperkalemia may be spurious due to hemolysis of the specimen, so measurements should be repeated if values are abnormal. Pseudohyperkalemia refers to hyperkalemia that develops in the serum separator tube in the setting of markedly increased WBC or platelet counts as seen in some hematologic malignancies. In this situation, the potassium level should be checked in a sample from a heparinized tube to avoid spurious hyperkalemia.

Several factors contribute to the increased risk of hyperkalemia in older adults. Medications, including ACE inhibitors, angiotensin receptor blockers, NSAIDs, and potassium-sparing diuretics all increase serum potassium levels (Table 54.2). Older adults are thought to have lower Na^+-K^+-ATPase activity, which may lead to slightly higher extracellular potassium levels. They have also been observed to have slightly lower average levels of renin, which may contribute to hyperkalemia and may also exacerbate hyporeninemic hypoaldosteronism secondary to other causes (frequently diabetes but can also be seen in chronic interstitial nephritis or other causes of CKD).

The urgency of treatment of hyperkalemia in older adults varies with the cause, duration, and presence of signs indicating cardiac toxicity (peaked T waves, widened QRS interval, arrhythmias). In cases of severe hyperkalemia, hospital admission is warranted. Calcium is given intravenously to stabilize the myocardium while medications, including intravenous insulin and glucose are given to shift potassium into cells. Medications that remove potassium include diuretics and sodium polystyrene sulfonate. For patients who are volume depleted, volume repletion with normal saline alone may result in substantial potassium wasting, because increasing sodium delivery to the collecting duct will allow aldosterone-mediated potassium wasting. Dialysis may be necessary in severe cases, especially when kidney function is poor.

Table 54.2—Common Medications that Cause Hyperkalemia

Medication	Mechanism
ACE inhibitors, angiotensin II receptor blockers	Decreased sodium reabsorption and potassium excretion in the aldosterone-sensitive distal nephron secondary to decreased angiotensin-mediated aldosterone production
Amiloride, triamterene	Decreased sodium reabsorption and potassium excretion in the aldosterone-sensitive distal nephron secondary to blockage of the epithelial sodium channel (ENaC) that is linked to potassium excretion
β-blockers	Decreased β receptor–mediated shift of potassium into cells
Cyclosporine, tacrolimus	Multiple mechanisms
Digitalis	Na^+-K^+-ATPase inhibition leads to more extracellular potassium
Heparin	Interferes with aldosterone production
NSAIDs	Multiple mechanisms
Spironolactone, eplerenone	Decreased sodium reabsorption and potassium excretion in the aldosterone-sensitive distal nephron secondary to blockade of aldosterone's receptor (mineralocorticoid receptor)
Trimethoprim, pentamidine	Triamterene-like effect (see above)

In less severe and chronic cases, offending medications should be decreased or stopped. Additional treatment includes a low potassium diet, and possibly diuretics to increase renal potassium excretion. Sodium polystyrene sulfonate should not be used on a chronic basis because of the risk of bowel toxicity. However, patiromer also binds potassium in the colon and may be appropriate for longer term therapy although data are limited. In the OPAL-HK trial, patients with CKD and mild to moderate hyperkalemia while on RAAS inhibition therapy were maintained on patiromer for up to 12 weeks. Patients randomized to patiromer had a lower incidence of recurrent hyperkalemia thanthe placebo group (15% versus 60%) and very few of them required RAAS inhibitor discontinuation (6% versus 56%). The most common adverse effect was constipation; hypokalemia and hypomagnesemia were also reported in a minority of participants. The mean age in the OPAL-HK trial was just over 64 years old, but those >80 years old were excluded.

Secondary Hypertension and Renal Artery Disease

The prevalence of hypertension increases with advancing age, affecting about two-thirds of patients >60 years old. Proposed mechanisms for age-related hypertension include increased arterial stiffness and impaired sodium handling leading to salt sensitivity. Most hypertension is idiopathic, or essential, but occasionally secondary causes are discovered, such as renal artery disease, obstructive sleep apnea, mineralocorticoid hypertension (Conn syndrome), hypercortisolism (Cushing syndrome), or pheochromocytoma. CKD is a more common cause of secondary hypertension. Secondary causes should be suspected in patients with new onset, very severe, or accelerated hypertension.

There has been a great deal of controversy over blood pressure targets for hypertensive patients. The most recent guideline issued by the Eighth Joint National Committee, published 2014, significantly relaxed blood pressure targets to ≤150/≤90 mmHg for nondiabetic patients ≥60 years old without CKD. For diabetic patients and those <60 years old, as well as all patients with CKD, the recommended target is ≤140/≤90 mmHg. Since that time, a landmark trial published in 2015 (Systolic Blood Pressure Intervention Trial [SPRINT]) suggested potential benefit to lower blood pressure thresholds, and a planned subgroup analysis of patients with CKD showed a lower death rate among those participants randomized to the lower blood pressure goal. The 2017 ACC/AHA guidelines recommend those with CKD maintain a blood pressure of <130/80 mmHg. The same target is recommended for all ages of ambulatory community-dwelling patients, although a specific recommendation is made to use clinical judgment in managing hypertension in older adults who have substantial comorbidities. Blood pressure targets in CKD is an active area of research and debate.

Renal Artery Disease

Atherosclerotic renovascular disease is primarily an illness of older adults, while fibromuscular dysplasia renovascular disease is much less common and generally presents earlier in life. Similar to the risk factors for other atherosclerotic diseases, those for atherosclerotic renal artery stenosis (RAS) include smoking and hyperlipidemia. RAS is a common cause of secondary hypertension. Diagnostic test options include duplex Doppler ultrasonography, CT or MR angiography, or renal angiography, the gold standard. The decision to image rests on whether a diagnosis would change management.

In the past, patients with hypertension thought to be secondary to atherosclerotic RAS frequently underwent angioplasty with stenting. However, the CORAL trial, a 2014 landmark study, showed no benefit for renal artery stenting in addition to medical management (ie, antihypertensives) in terms of major cardiovascular or renal outcomes. In the CORAL trial, the first-line antihypertensive was candesartan unless a contraindication existed; additional agents were added as needed. Thus, the general treatment of patients with hypertension secondary to atherosclerotic RAS is medical management to correct the hypertension. Angiography with stenting may still have a role in treatment of atherosclerotic RAS in several instances, including those with new-onset hypertension, those who cannot tolerate or are refractory to medications, and those with either flash pulmonary edema or progressive renal failure thought secondary to RAS. Thus, before pursuing diagnostic imaging of a hypertensive patient with suspected RAS, providers should consider whether the patient would be a candidate for angiography and stenting or not. If not, it would be reasonable to forgo imaging and focus on blood pressure management, including, unless not tolerated, an ARB or ACE inhibitor.

HEMATURIA

Hematuria may be microscopic, seen only by urinalysis, or gross, visible to the naked eye as pink, red, or brown urine. Urinary blood can come from anywhere along the urogenital tract, from the kidneys, to the collecting system, to the external genitalia. Hematuria from glomerular disease is often associated with proteinuria and is sometimes distinguishable on urinalysis by dysmorphic red cells (acanthocytes) and red cell casts. Blood from elsewhere in the urinary tract may be due to infection, nephrolithiasis, arteriovenous malformations, or neoplasms. The likelihood of an associated malignancy increases with age.

The evaluation for hematuria includes a urine culture and microscopic evaluation of the urine. Imaging depends on the clinical setting. A plain abdominal radiograph (kidney, ureter, bladder) may be sufficient to detect kidney stones, particularly those both large and radiopaque. Ultrasound is another option for evaluating nephrolithiasis, which has the advantage of avoiding radiation completely. Both radiographs and ultrasound are less sensitive for detection of nephrolithiasis than a CT scan without contrast. A CT scan with contrast is helpful to exclude an enhancing kidney or other mass. Urology consultation and cystoscopy is often recommended to further exclude a bladder or other collecting system malignancy, particularly in the absence of evidence suggesting a glomerular etiology of hematuria (eg, proteinuria or decreasing GFR).

ACUTE KIDNEY INJURY

Acute kidney injury (AKI) is defined as an acute increase in creatinine or decrease in urine output to <5 mL/kg/hr for at least 6 hours. AKI occurs with increased frequency in the geriatric population, and even minor acute increases in creatinine have been associated with increased risk of prolonged hospitalization and death. In the setting of severe AKI, dialysis is sometimes indicated to support patients while underlying conditions are treated, awaiting recovery of renal function. Recovery of renal function after dialysis-requiring AKI is variable and depends on baseline renal function and the specific cause of the injury. The decision whether to undertake dialysis should be individualized and is discussed in detail below.

The differential diagnosis of AKI is typically categorized into prerenal, intrinsic renal, and postrenal causes. Intrinsic renal disease is divided into tubulointerstitial, glomerular, and vascular disease.

Prerenal Azotemia

Prerenal azotemia is a common cause of AKI in older adults. It is a reversible functional decrease in GFR related to hypoperfusion. Hypoperfusion is often secondary to intravascular volume depletion or a low effective arterial blood volume (eg, in decompensated heart failure). Selective renal hypoperfusion secondary to excessive intrarenal vasoconstriction and/or bilateral RAS can also cause prerenal AKI. Medications that may reduce GFR, such as ACE inhibitors, ARBs, and NSAIDs, sometimes precipitate prerenal azotemia, particularly in patients with an additional cause of renal hypoperfusion.

Older adults are at increased risk of prerenal azotemia for a number of reasons. Physiologic changes described earlier (Table 54.1) can contribute to volume depletion, as can diuretic use. Acute illness leading to poor oral intake, GI fluid loss, and comorbidities such as heart failure and renal artery disease are additional risk factors. ACE inhibitors, ARBs, and NSAIDs decrease glomerular filtration pressure by impairing renal autoregulation that aims to maintain GFR when renal blood flow is decreased. Finally, older adults may have reduced access to nutrition because of cognitive, physical, and/or environmental factors.

The diagnosis is suspected based on history and physical examination. Laboratory results such as a bland urine sediment and fractional excretion of sodium (FE_{Na}) <1% suggest the diagnosis. It should be noted that a low FE_{Na} can be seen in other conditions, such as acute glomerulonephritis, contrast nephropathy, interstitial nephritis, and urinary tract obstruction. Therefore, a low FE_{Na} is not necessarily diagnostic of prerenal azotemia.

Treatment involves discontinuing or reducing offending medications and restoring intravascular effective circulating volume. If the AKI is purely prerenal, kidney function should improve rapidly with correction of the renal hypoperfusion.

Obstructive Uropathy

Urinary tract obstruction is a common and often reversible cause of AKI in older adults. Obstruction can occur either at the level of the bladder outlet or the ureters. Because one kidney is usually sufficient to maintain GFR, unilateral ureteral obstruction does not tend to cause severe AKI unless a patient has a solitary functioning kidney.

Bladder outlet obstruction is more frequent in men but can occur in both genders. In men, bladder outlet obstruction from benign prostatic hyperplasia is the most common cause of obstructive uropathy. Symptoms may include urinary hesitancy, a sensation of incomplete emptying of the bladder, and nocturia. Even partial obstruction can lead to back pressure through the collecting system and decreased kidney function. Other causes of bladder outlet obstruction with a higher prevalence in older adults include bladder carcinoma and urethral stricture. Functional bladder outlet obstruction can occur in both genders and is often secondary to medications, particularly those with anticholinergic effects, or spinal cord injury. Ureteral obstruction is often caused by stones, strictures, or retroperitoneal malignancies. Urinary obstruction is usually diagnosed by ultrasound. Treatment of obstructive uropathy depends on both the cause and level of the obstruction.

Intrinsic Renal Disease

Tubulointerstitial Disease

Acute Tubular Necrosis

Acute tubular necrosis (ATN) can be caused by ischemia, sepsis, and nephrotoxins. ATN is the most common cause of AKI among hospitalized patients. Prerenal azotemia and ischemic ATN occur on a continuum depending on the severity and duration of hypoperfusion. Medications and toxins have been associated with ATN, including aminoglycoside antibiotics, cisplatin, heme pigment (eg, in rhabdomyolysis), and iodinated radiocontrast agents.

ATN is associated with urine sediment findings that include renal tubular epithelial cells and granular "muddy brown" casts. In the setting of oliguria, calculating FE_{Na} can help distinguish prerenal azotemia from ATN. In prerenal azotemia, the kidneys are sodium avid, and FE_{Na} is <1%. In ATN, the kidneys are not able to retain sodium, and FE_{Na} is >2%. Diuretics impair sodium retention by the kidneys, so a high FE_{Na} in a patient on diuretics is not helpful in distinguishing between prerenal azotemia and ATN. However, a low FE_{Na} despite diuretics points to sodium avidity and argues against ATN.

Treatment of patients with ATN is generally supportive. Interventions should include optimization of hemodynamics to ensure renal perfusion and avoidance of nephrotoxins. Medication dosing should be adjusted to the level of renal function to prevent toxicity and further renal injury. Diuretics can be used to manage volume status in hypervolemic patients, but their use is not thought to alter renal prognosis. Aggressive diuresis leading to volume depletion should be avoided. In patients with normal baseline renal function, ATN is often reversible over days to weeks. Dialysis may be required to support patients with severe ATN.

Acute Interstitial Nephritis

Acute interstitial nephritis (AIN) is common in older adults. It is most commonly due to an allergic response to medication, although there are other causes such as infections, heavy metal exposure, and rheumatologic conditions. A diagnostic clue is sterile pyuria, with or without WBC casts on urinalysis. The CBC with differential may show eosinophilia. Although patients with allergic AIN often have an eosinophilic infiltrate on renal biopsy specimens, checking for urine eosinophils is generally not diagnostically useful.

Although any medication can cause interstitial nephritis, antibiotics and NSAIDS are the most common culprits. Proton-pump inhibitors also cause AIN and are worthy of mention because of their widespread use. For drug-induced interstitial nephritis, therapy consists of discontinuing the offending agent. Recent retrospective data suggest that a course of corticosteroids may speed recovery and lead to a more complete resolution of kidney injury. A kidney biopsy is usually indicated to confirm the diagnosis before initiating high-dose steroids because of their toxicity.

Dysproteinemias: Multiple Myeloma and Other Plasma Cell Dyscrasias

Multiple myeloma is a plasma cell dyscrasia with increasing prevalence in advancing age. It is associated with a number of renal manifestations, including AKI. AKI in the setting of dysproteinemia is caused by pathologic plasma cell–produced proteins. Clinical clues to dysproteinemia may include acute or chronic kidney disease, a low serum anion gap, hypercalcemia (in myeloma), and a high globulin gap. Laboratory testing includes serum and urine electrophoresis, immunofixation studies, serum free light chains, β-2 microglobulin, and serum immunoglobulins. In the case of myeloma, a skeletal survey may show characteristic lytic bone lesions. Bone marrow biopsy is generally undertaken.

Dysproteinemia can cause kidney injury in a number of ways. The most common tubulointerstitial cause of AKI in the setting of dysproteinemia is cast nephropathy. In this disorder, the pathologic plasma cells generate protein that obstructs renal tubules. Of note, because the proteinuria in cast nephropathy is caused by a nonalbumin protein, there is often a very large discrepancy between the albumin (minimal) and total protein (high) levels. In myeloma specifically, severe hypercalcemia resulting from lytic bone lesions can cause renal vasoconstriction and subsequent AKI. Abnormal proteins can also deposit in the renal parenchyma, termed light-chain or heavy-chain deposition disease, or form fibrils that deposit as AL amyloid. Extensive deposits in the glomeruli will cause substantial proteinuria. Dysproteinemias with glomerular deposition are further discussed under the nephrotic syndrome (below).

Treatment of the AKI associated with dysproteinemia generally involves treatment of the underlying disorder as well as supportive renal care.

Vascular Disease

Atheroembolic disease occurs when cholesterol emboli lodge in the small arteries of the kidneys and cause progressive damage. Risk factors for atheroembolic AKI include older age, smoking, hypertension, and high cholesterol. The embolization is frequently caused by an inciting event, most often an angiographic procedure such as cardiac catheterization. Occasionally, atheroembolic disease is thought to be spontaneous or is associated with something other than angiography such as anticoagulation or hemodynamic compromise. Patients may exhibit skin manifestations of atheroembolism, or livedo reticularis. Eosinophilia may be present, and serum complements can be transiently decreased.

Occasionally, occlusion of arteries can occur that are unrelated to atherosclerosis. This can be due to a thromboembolus, for example in the setting of atrial fibrillation, or to renal arterial injury or a hypercoagulable state. Occasionally, the etiology is idiopathic. Flank pain is a common symptom, sometimes accompanied by hematuria and/or loss of GFR. If the infarction is unilateral and the other kidney is still functioning well, the decrease in GFR is often not dramatic, and kidney function tends to improve as the functioning kidney hyperfilters to compensate for lost renal parenchyma. Increased lactate dehydrogenase is a diagnostic clue. It is generally diagnosed by a noncontrast CT scan showing a wedge-shaped defect.

Thrombotic microangiopathy causes AKI because platelet microthrombi occlude small renal arterioles. The diagnosis is suspected in the setting of hemolytic anemia and progressive thrombocytopenia. Classic examples include thrombotic thrombocytopenic purpura (TTP) and hemolytic uremic syndrome (HUS), but a similar presentation can occur in a number of other disease processes that cause thrombotic microangiopathy, including drug-induced TTP and atypical HUS (a disease of complement dysregulation). Other systemic disorders that present with macroangiopathic hemolytic anemia, for example malignant hypertension, catastrophic antiphospholipid antibody syndrome, and scleroderma renal crisis should be excluded, because they can present similarly but have different treatments.

Glomerular Disease

Glomerulonephritis can cause both AKI and CKD. Glomerulonephritis (GN) is divided into nephritic syndromes and nephrotic syndromes. Glomerular diseases generally, although not always, require a renal biopsy to diagnose. Older age alone is not a contraindication to renal biopsy.

Nephrotic-Range Proteinuria and Nephrotic Syndromes

Nephrotic-range proteinuria is defined as urinary excretion of >3.5 g of protein per day. Nephrotic syndrome consists of nephrotic-range proteinuria associated with hypoalbuminemia and edema. Patients with nephrotic syndrome often have hyperlipidemia and lipiduria as well. Hematuria is occasionally present but is not part of the classic presentation. Nephrotic syndrome is associated with a hypercoaguable state and increased risk of deep-vein and renal-vein thrombosis as well as pulmonary embolism. Progressive declines in GFR can also be seen. In most cases of nephrotic syndrome, a renal biopsy is indicated for early diagnosis and appropriate therapy. Patients with nephrotic proteinuria generally have pathologic findings in the glomeruli on renal biopsy. In a case series of patients >80 years old who underwent renal biopsy, nephrotic syndrome was the reason for biopsy in approximately 23%. Supportive therapy for nephrotic syndrome includes blood pressure control, use of RAAS blockers, sodium restriction, and statins for hyperlipidemia. Anticoagulation is sometimes undertaken when plasma albumin is <2–3 g/dL depending on the cause of the patient's nephrotic syndrome, the individualized risks and benefits of anticoagulation, and the degree of hypoalbuminemia Nephrotic syndrome can result from primary glomerular disease or be secondary to systemic diseases. The most common cause of nephrotic-range proteinuria is **diabetic nephropathy**, although diabetic nephropathy is less frequently associated with the nephrotic syndrome. Diabetic nephropathy generally progresses slowly over many years and is often associated with other small vessel disease such as diabetic retinopathy. Renal biopsy is sometimes deferred in patients with a classic presentation for diabetic nephropathy and without evidence of other possible causes of renal disease.

Other systemic diseases that commonly present with nephrotic syndrome include **systemic lupus erythematosus** and **dysproteinemias**, including both multiple myeloma and AL amyloidosis, as well as other types of **amyloidosis**. Multiple myeloma can cause nephrotic-range proteinuria in the setting of cast nephropathy or as deposition of paraproteins in glomeruli. Amyloid deposition can occur in many settings other than dysproteinemia. For example, patients with longstanding inflammation can get AA amyloidosis, which causes deposition of amyloid fibrils.

Membranous nephropathy is the most common primary nephrotic disease found in the geriatric population. Although most patients have idiopathic disease, the 2 most common causes of secondary membranous nephropathy are NSAID use and malignancy. Primary membranous nephropathy has been associated with an antibody to the phospholipase A2 receptor-1. Anti-PLA2R antibodies can be measured and are generally negative in the setting of other renal diseases, including secondary membranous nephropathy. Serum testing is not yet widely available. Approximately 7%–20% of patients with membranous nephropathy have had solid organ tumors, particularly of the lung, colon, rectum, breast, and kidney, which are sometimes discovered after nephrotic syndrome develops. Therefore, malignancy should be considered in older adults with membranous nephropathy.

Other primary nephrotic syndromes include **minimal change disease**. Minimal change, more commonly a cause of nephrotic syndrome in children, can also be seen in adults. It can be idiopathic or associated with hypersensitivity reactions, hematologic malignancies, or drugs, particularly NSAIDs.

Focal segmental glomerulosclerosis (FSGS) in older adults is more often secondary than primary, although both are seen. Primary FSGS is idiopathic, whereas secondary causes include infections such as HIV and medications, including interferon and bisphosphonates. Secondary FSGS can also occur in morbid obesity and many forms of advanced CKD as remaining nephrons are injured as they hyperfilter to maintain GFR. FSGS is particularly common among black patients.

CHRONIC KIDNEY DISEASE

Kidney function as measured by GFR declines on average 8 mL/min per decade after age 40; however, some people do not experience any decline at all. Renal glomerular and tubulointerstitial fibrosis increases with age, leading to nephron dropout and CKD. CKD has many causes in older adults, including diabetes, hypertension, glomerulonephritis, obstructive uropathy, and chronic interstitial nephritis often due to medications such as NSAIDs. CKD in older adults frequently manifests with a decompensation of preexisting medical illness such as heart failure, diabetes mellitus, hypertension, or dementia.

Data from the National Health and Nutrition Examination Survey (NHANES) 2007–2012 suggest that 33% of patients >60 years old have CKD and 23% have an eGFR <60 mL/min. The incidence varies among ethnic and racial groups. Diabetes and hypertension, both important causes of CKD, are more common in black, Hispanic, and some Native American populations.

The U.S. Preventive Services Task Force, noting a paucity of data to weigh risks and benefits, does not make a recommendation about screening asymptomatic adults for CKD. However, this recommendation does not apply to those with hypertension or diabetes. The NKF recommends screening all patients with CKD risk factors for CKD. CKD screening generally involves checking a serum creatinine, spot urine albumin, and spot urine creatinine. From these, an eGFR and ACR can be calculated (see also Measures of Kidney Function above).

Classification

In 2002, the NKF, through the Kidney Disease Quality Initiative (KDOQI), established a classification system for CKD and issued related clinical practice guidelines (Figure 54.1). CKD is defined as either kidney damage or decreased kidney function, with an eGFR <60 mL/min for ≥3 months. The NKF KDOQI staging system is based on estimated GFR. Most older adults have a GFR <60 mL/min, and there is ongoing debate whether this represents disease or is related to normal aging. Revisions to the KDOQI classification used in the Kidney Disease: Improving Global Outcomes (KDIGO) CKD Work Group 2012 Guidelines divided Stage 3 CKD into 3A and 3B, again based on GFR, and added a term for the degree of proteinuria. Of note, older patients with Stage 3A CKD (eGFR 45–59 mL/min) and no albuminuria are unlikely to suffer complications of CKD or to progress to ESRD.

Management

In older adults, treatment approaches should be based on preserving remaining renal function and limiting complications. Basic treatment principles include correcting reversible causes, controlling blood pressure, using RAAS blockers to decrease proteinuria, controlling diabetes, and moderately restricting dietary protein. Detailed clinical guidelines are available on the NKF website at www.kidney.org/professionals/guidelines/guidelines_commentaries/chronic-kidney-disease-classification (accessed Feb 2019).

Declines in GFR are accompanied by a broad range of complications, including hypertension, anemia,

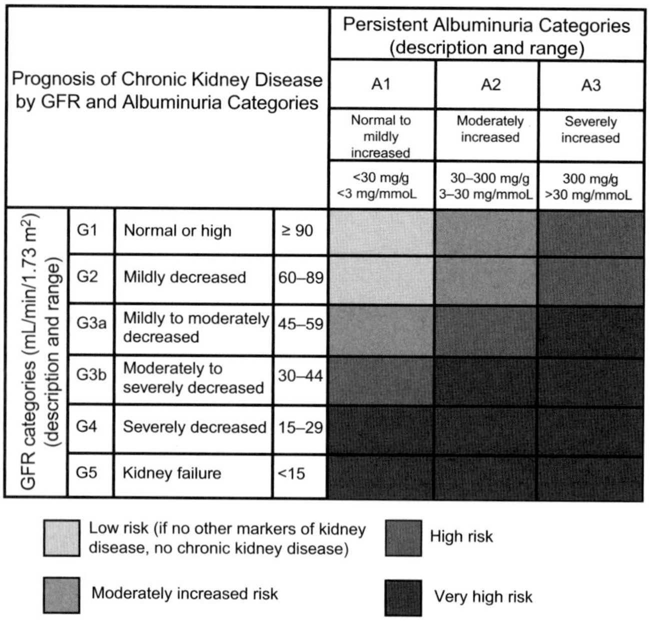

Prognosis of Chronic Kidney Disease by GFR and Albuminuria Categories			Persistent Albuminuria Categories (description and range)		
			A1 Normal to mildly increased <30 mg/g <3 mg/mmoL	A2 Moderately increased 30–300 mg/g 3–30 mg/mmoL	A3 Severely increased 300 mg/g >30 mg/mmoL
GFR categories (mL/min/1.73 m²) (description and range)	G1	Normal or high	≥ 90		
	G2	Mildly decreased	60–89		
	G3a	Mildly to moderately decreased	45–59		
	G3b	Moderately to severely decreased	30–44		
	G4	Severely decreased	15–29		
	G5	Kidney failure	<15		

■ Low risk (if no other markers of kidney disease, no chronic kidney disease)
■ Moderately increased risk
■ High risk
■ Very high risk

Figure 54.1—Stages of Chronic Kidney Disease
SOURCE: KDIGO Guidelines, 2012. Reprinted with permission.

malnutrition, metabolic bone disease, neuropathy, depression, impaired functional status, and increased cardiovascular morbidity and mortality. Early recognition of impaired kidney function allows for screening and management of these complications, improving outcomes. NKF guidelines recommend referral to a nephrologist when a patient reaches Stage 4 CKD for management of complications such as acidosis, phosphorus retention, and anemia. A nephrologist can also guide discussions regarding dialysis preparation and options for transplantation.

Risk of Cardiovascular Events
Patients with CKD of all stages are at increased risk of cardiovascular events, including myocardial infarction, stroke, and death. Older adults with CKD are generally more likely to die of cardiovascular disease than to require dialysis. Reduction of morbidity and mortality in CKD therefore requires aggressive management of cardiovascular disease risk factors. This includes blood pressure control, lipid-lowering therapy, smoking cessation, and attention to diet and exercise.

Medication Use in Chronic Kidney Disease
Prescribing medications for older patients with CKD is complicated by diminished renal clearance compounded by age-associated changes in pharmacokinetics and pharmacodynamics. Many medications or their metabolites are renally excreted, and extreme care must be taken to dose these medications appropriately to avoid renal and systemic toxicity. Dose adjustments may vary based on GFR, and some may be contraindicated at low GFRs. A good practice is to verify appropriate dosing in renal disease of any new medication being prescribed.

Additionally, certain medications, particularly NSAIDs, are potentially nephrotoxic and should be avoided or used with extreme care in patients with CKD. NSAIDs can predispose to prerenal azotemia and ATN, cause acute and chronic interstitial nephritis, and exacerbate hypertension and fluid overload. Other examples of nephrotoxic agents include iodinated contrast agents, lithium, aminoglycosides, and sodium phosphate–containing bowel preparations. Gadolinium is not nephrotoxic, but its use in advanced CKD has been linked to nephrogenic systemic fibrosis, a debilitating and generally irreversible fibrotic disorder.

Anemia
Anemia screening should start no later than when patients reach Stage 3A CKD. Anemia of CKD is typically normocytic and normochromic. When anemia is identified, patients should be evaluated for other common causes of anemia before starting erythropoiesis-stimulating agents, because anemia of CKD is a diagnosis of exclusion. KDIGO guidelines recommend the following as initial investigation of anemia in a patient with CKD and no other specific risk factors for anemia: CBC with differential, reticulocyte count, transferrin saturation, , and levels of ferritin, B_{12}, and folate.

Erythropoiesis-stimulating agents (ESAs), such as recombinant erythropoietin, are often used to treat CKD-associated anemia. The main goal of this therapy is to prevent the need for blood transfusions, which carry the risk of allosensitization of potential kidney transplant recipients, transfusion-related infections, and iron overload. Several large trials have been conducted to evaluate ESA use among CKD patients. The 2009 TREAT trial is the largest and demonstrated that attempts to normalize hemoglobin with erythropoietin increased vascular events, particularly stroke. Current guidelines recommend individualized consideration of ESA initiation in CKD nondialysis-dependent patients when the hemoglobin concentration is <10 g/dL. The guidelines also recommend against maintaining hemoglobin levels >11.5 g/dL through ESA use. Of note, the FDA labels advise against ESA use to achieve and maintain hemoglobin levels >11 g/dL. ESAs are generally avoided in patients with active malignancy.

For ESAs to be effective, patients must have adequate iron stores to support accelerated erythropoiesis. Among those with iron deficiency, iron should be replaced before starting ESA therapy. Patients with frank iron deficiency without recent GI evaluation may also warrant endoscopy. Patients may receive iron orally or intravenously in CKD. In very advanced kidney disease, intestinal iron absorption is impaired. Newer iron preparations (eg, sucrose) have lower rates of anaphylaxis than iron dextran when administered intravenously.

Calcium, Phosphorus, and Renal Bone Disease

Abnormalities of calcium, phosphorus, and parathyroid hormone (PTH) are common in patients with a GFR <60 mL/min/1.73 m² and begin early in CKD. Screening for metabolic derangements should begin in Stage 3 CKD. These abnormalities have been associated with increased risk of vascular calcification and cardiovascular morbidity and mortality in patients with CKD. Patients with CKD are at risk of several bone diseases, including osteitis fibrosis cystica (a high turnover bone disease) and adynamic bone disease (low turnover). CKD alone is a risk factor for fracture, but patients with these bone diseases are at a further increased risk. Older adults with CKD may also have concomitant osteoporosis. Osteoporosis in advanced CKD can be difficult to diagnose, given concomitant mineral bone disease, and also harder to treat because bisphosphonates are generally discouraged if the eGFR is <30mL/min/1.73 m².

Depression

Depression is common in any population suffering from chronic disease but has been underrecognized in the CKD population, especially those on dialysis. Estimates of depression prevalence in CKD have varied widely, but a recent meta-analysis suggested a prevalence of approximately 20%. Depression can be difficult to diagnose in the dialysis population, because the vegetative symptoms can be similar to those of uremia or insufficient dialysis. Functional and cognitive decline are particularly common presenting symptoms in older adults with kidney disease. As with all medications, the dosage of antidepressants should be adjusted based on renal function.

Nutrition

Dietary requirements for patients with CKD are complex. Intake of protein, phosphorus, and potassium all need to be controlled while maintaining adequate energy intake. Once a patient reaches Stage 4 CKD, an experienced renal dietitian should be involved in nutritional management.

END-STAGE RENAL DISEASE (ESRD)

Patients ≥75 years old have the highest incidence of ESRD in the United States. Recently, the incidence of ESRD appears to have fallen among all age groups, although those who choose conservative care are generally excluded from these estimates.

When a patient is nearing ESRD, renal replacement therapy options versus conservative care should be discussed. The decision to pursue dialysis or renal transplant is highly individualized and should always include a cogent discussion regarding the patient's goals of care, potential benefits and harms, and the prognosis with and without therapy. Depending on the situation, including family members, and primary care and/or palliative care providers in the discussion, along with the patient and nephrologist, may be helpful.

Renal Replacement Therapy (Dialysis)

Historically, patients were often started on dialysis in early Stage 5 CKD, but this has not shown a benefit in morbidity or mortality. Dialysis is generally now initiated when clear indications arise, usually with an eGFR <10 mL/min.

Dialysis ameliorates many symptoms and complications of ESRD, including metabolic abnormalities, difficulty with blood pressure and fluid management, and eventually symptomatic uremia with anorexia, nausea, sleep disturbance, myoclonic jerks, serositis, and altered mental status. It also can prolong life in patients with ESRD and has the potential to improve both quality of life and functional status. However, the benefit of dialysis may be diminished in older adults, especially those with poor functional status. In one study that described a cohort of 3,702 nursing-home residents as they initiated dialysis, the 1-year mortality rate was 58%, and only 1 in 8 patients had a stable or improved functional status after 12 months of dialysis versus after 3 months of dialysis.

Both hemodialysis and peritoneal dialysis also have disadvantages to consider. Hemodialysis-related difficulties include a substantial time commitment, the need to travel to a dialysis facility, discomfort related to muscle cramps, fatigue after treatment, and dangerous variations in blood pressure that may lead to subacute cognitive decline and cardiac damage. Peritoneal dialysis–related difficulties include the need to store supplies at home, daily dialysis often requiring assistance from caregivers, increased protein loss, and risk of infection.

Kidney Transplantation

More than 90,000 patients are currently on the kidney transplant wait list in the United States, and the list grows every year. Patients >65 years old are increasingly considered for transplantation. As in younger patients, mortality rates in older patients with transplants are considerably lower than in those on dialysis, although of course, older patients who are healthy enough to receive transplants are different than those who remain on dialysis. Potentially suitable older patients and their families should be encouraged to explore the option of transplantation before the need for dialysis arises. Living donation is encouraged and does not require wait time. Those who elect to be listed on the deceased donor list can be listed when their eGFR is ≤20 mL/min.

Conservative Care

Some patients with ESRD choose conservative therapy as the primary treatment, while others make the decision to pursue conservative care after a time on dialysis. Conservative care includes management of symptoms and communication regarding prognosis and end-of-life preferences. Management of symptoms frequently involves diuretics to control fluid overload and hyperkalemia. Antiemetics for nausea and iron and erythropoietin for symptomatic anemia are also frequently used. Patients considering conservative care may benefit from early palliative care consultation.

When a chronic dialysis patient stops dialysis, death usually occurs within 10 days; however, time to death can be substantially longer, particularly among those with substantial residual renal function. Dialysis withdrawal is relatively common—approximately 20% of the dialysis cohort withdraws from dialysis in any given year. Clinicians with expertise in the care of older adults have an important opportunity to guide nephrologists, as well as patients and their families, when conservative care and/or hospice may be the best option.

> **CHOOSING WISELY® RECOMMENDATIONS**
>
> *Nephrology*
>
> - Do not initiate chronic dialysis without ensuring a shared decision-making process between patient and their families and physicians.
> - Do not place peripherally inserted central catheters in Stage 3–5 CKD patients without consulting nephrology.
> - Avoid NSAIDs in individuals with hypertension or heart failure or CKD of all causes, including diabetes mellitus.
> - Do not initiate erythropoiesis-stimulating agents in patients with CKD with Hgb ≥10 g/dL without signs or symptoms of anemia.
> - Do not perform routine cancer screening for dialysis patients with limited life expectancies without signs or symptoms.

RESOURCES

- Cheung AK, Rahman M, Reboussin DM, et al. for the SPRINT Research Group. Effects of intensive BP control in CKD. *J Am Soc Nephrol.* 2017;28(9):2812–2823.

- Thorsteinsdottir B, Swetz KM, Albright RC. The ethics of chronic dialysis for the older patient: time to reevaluate the norms. *Clin J Am Soc Nephrol.* 2015;10(11):2094–2099.

CHAPTER 55—GYNECOLOGY

KEY POINTS

- Gynecologic issues in older women have a significant impact on quality of life and are often treatable, but often underdiagnosed.

- Genitourinary syndrome of menopause is common in postmenopausal women and is readily reversed with administration of vaginally applied estrogen.

- Nonsurgical management of pelvic organ prolapse can improve comfort and bladder function in some older women with pelvic organ prolapse.

- Any abnormal genital bleeding in a postmenopausal woman should be evaluated.

Many older women do not receive regular gynecologic care partly because of their reticence to discuss personal gynecologic problems as well as the hesitation of primary care providers to question women about gynecologic or sexual symptoms. Consequently, important and treatable disorders often go undiagnosed until they become severely disabling. For example, although pelvic floor disorders affect at least 25% of women in the United States and is more common among postmenopausal women, women often delay evaluation for several years. Full gynecologic examination should be a routine part of a complete history and physical examination for all older women who are amenable to screening.

HISTORY AND PHYSICAL EXAMINATION

The American College of Obstetrics and Gynecology recommendations for primary care of women ≥65 years old include inquiring about not only routine gynecologic issues but also menopausal symptoms, involuntary loss of urine or feces, pelvic organ prolapse, and issues related to sexual dysfunction. The history should also include inquiry about abdominal distention, early satiety, new onset pelvic pain, and abnormal vaginal discharge or bleeding (signs of gynecologic malignancies).

Nongynecologic medical problems that can have significant gynecologic effects should also be noted in the history. Notable examples include effects of breast cancer treatment such as urogenital atrophy, increased risk of endometrial hyperplasia among obese women due to peripheral conversion of androgens to estrogen, the impact of pregnancy on the development of pelvic floor disorders, and vulvovaginal presentations of dermatologic conditions.

If a woman is on systemic hormone replacement therapy (HRT), the regimen should be reviewed annually to ensure adherence and benefit, need for continued therapy, and absence of adverse events. If the uterus is present, estrogen must be combined with a progestin to prevent development of endometrial hyperplasia. The route of administration of estrogen therapy may be reassessed because of observed differences of oral and non-oral therapy on the vascular and other systems, particularly the use of vaginal preparations for treatment of vulvovaginal atrophy.

A review of sexual function and possible barriers to enjoyable sexual activity is an important aspect of the gynecologic history. Over half of women continue to engage in sexual activity after the age of 60 years, and 85% of adults want to discuss sexual function with their clinician. Yet, less than half of providers routinely ask patients if they are sexually active, let alone inquire about satisfaction or problems. The gynecologic interview provides an opportunity to address this important aspect of many women's lives, and specific issues related to sexual activity such as atrophy-related dyspareunia, postcoital bleeding, and sexually transmitted diseases should be addressed.

Performing a complete pelvic examination is necessary unless limiting comorbidities, or a patient's own desire, would prevent intervention on any subsequent diagnoses. Most ambulatory older women can assume the lithotomy position preferred for completion of a systematic pelvic evaluation. However, the position does require flexion and external rotation of the hips while in a supine position. Patients with skeletal lordosis and other spine disorders may require varying degrees of head elevation, and some women with osteoarthritis will find the lithotomy position uncomfortable or impossible to assume. For these women, an alternative position should be used. A common technique involves the patients assuming a left lateral decubitus position with knees flexed. The upper hip (right) is flexed to a greater degree and the right leg is elevated, exposing the perineum. An adequate speculum and bimanual examination can usually be done in this position. A bedbound patient can be examined by positioning an inverted bedpan under the sacrum to elevate the pelvis. Some very immobile women can be examined in the supine position by carefully inserting a speculum upside down. Because the vaginal introitus can be small and stenotic, smaller speculums may be needed. Loss of vaginal depth may not allow full insertion of the speculum, and digital palpation before inserting the speculum is a useful maneuver. Water-based lubricants facilitate the examination and can be used even if a Pap smear will be performed.

Pelvic examination of older women should include the following:

- Examination of the vulva for excoriations, changes in surface texture, abnormal pigmentation, erythema, or lesions
- Examination for signs of urogenital atrophy including pale or dry vaginal mucosa, loss of vaginal rugae, reduced vaginal caliber and depth, or the presence of a urethral caruncle
- Evaluation for transurethral loss of urine or pelvic organ prolapse with the Valsalva maneuver
- Careful palpation for pelvic masses or ovarian enlargement on bimanual examination
- A Pap smear if indicated
- A rectal examination to identify masses, detect occult bleeding, and evaluate the anal sphincter

Ovaries become smaller in the postmenopausal period, and any palpable adnexal tissue should prompt consideration of malignancy. Although uterine fibroids are common, any increase in uterus size should be investigated. An ovarian or uterine mass should be evaluated by transabdominal or, anatomy permitting, transvaginal pelvic ultrasound to elucidate details such as size and location, sonolucency, and vascular flow. Additional investigation with the use of MRI as well as serum tumor markers can be useful. In some cases, a benign nature cannot be established with confidence, and further surgical evaluation ultimately depends on clinical judgment as well as the patient's goals and preferences.

MENOPAUSAL SYMPTOMS

Menopause is the permanent cessation of menstruation, the onset of which is established as 1 year after the last menstrual period. In the United States, the median age at menopause is 51 years. With a life expectancy of approximately 80 years, the average American woman is postmenopausal for at least one-third of her life. Along with mood changes and sleep disorders, vasomotor symptoms, or hot flushes, are the most common symptoms of the period of menopausal transition, also known as the climacteric. Occurring in up to 80% of perimenopausal women, vasomotor symptoms persist on average 5–10 years, and most (87%) of those affected experience daily symptoms. In a small minority of women, symptoms may be lifelong. The pathophysiology of the vasomotor response remains incompletely understood, but symptoms appear to be associated with black race, obesity, and smoking.

The most effective treatment for vasomotor symptoms is systemic hormone therapy with estrogen alone or in combination with progesterone for women with an intact uterus given concern for endometrial hyperplasia due to unopposed estrogen effects on the endometrium (SOE=A). Vasomotor symptoms are usually relieved within the first few weeks of HRT.

Concerns stemming from the Women's Health Initiative (WHI) trial regarding the risks associated with systemic HRT (SOE=A) have led to hesitation on the part of many patients and providers to initiate therapy. The initial study, published in 2002, presented data supporting slightly increased risks of thromboembolic events, breast cancer, coronary heart disease, and stoke among women taking combined HRT. For women on estrogen only, the risk was limited to thromboembolic events. However, clinicians should be aware of more recently published reassuring data, including WHI stratification studies. Specifically, the initial study was conducted among women 5077 years old. A reanalysis of the results among women <60 years old and within 10 years of menopause demonstrated a possible cardioprotective effect of HRT. Furthermore, 18-year cumulative follow-up data found that all-cause mortality was similar between the HRT and placebo arms.

Subsequent studies have noted that the 2- to 5-fold increased risk of thromboembolic events is mitigated by the administration of transdermal estrogen and that the absolute risk of venous thromboembolism is age dependent. Risk factors for thromboembolic events include coronary artery disease, obesity, fracture, renal disease, prothrombotic mutations, and acquired thrombophilic conditions. Caution should be used when considering HRT for women with these underlying conditions.

In summary, when considering hormonal treatment of systemic menopausal symptoms, individualization of therapy is essential. HRT should not be used for primary disease prevention but may be considered for treatment of menopausal vasomotor symptoms. Treatment should be with the lowest effective dose for the shortest duration required to adequately address symptoms and well-being (SOE=A). The American College of Obstetricians and Gynecologists states that "the decision to continue HT should be individualized and be based on a woman's symptoms and the risk-benefit ratio, regardless of age" (SOE=C).

When estrogen is contraindicated or not acceptable, effective alternatives for the treatment of menopausal vasomotor symptoms include SSRIs, SNRIs, clonidine, and gabapentin (SOE=A). Paroxetine is the only FDA approved nonhormonal therapy for treatment of vasomotor symptoms. Phytoestrogens, methyldopa, vitamin E, herbal remedies such as yams and black cohosh, and lifestyle modifications have also been tried with inconsistent evidence of efficacy (SOE=B). Currently, there are no data to support the use of progestin-only treatments, testosterone, or compounded bioidentical hormones in treatment of menopausal symptoms (SOE=B). The FDA has warned the compounding pharmaceutical industry against making claims that "bio-identical compounded" hormone preparations are more effective and/or safer than traditional FDA-approved hormone products because of lack of head-to-head comparison trials.

GENITOURINARY SYNDROME OF MENOPAUSE

The lower genital tract is exquisitely sensitive to estrogen. Proliferation and maturation of the vaginal epithelium depends on adequate estrogen stimulation, the absence os which leads to tissue atrophy. With reduced estrogen production, genital blood flow decreases, leading to further decline in delivery of estrogen to those tissues. This reduction in microvascularity leads to vaginal dryness, mucosal pallor, decreased rugation, mucosal thinning, inflammation with discharge, and ultimately decreased vaginal caliber and depth. With progressive atrophy, there is a histologic decrease in mucosal superficial cells and an increase in intermediate and basal cells, commonly measured as the vaginal maturation index. Vaginal pH can be measured using pH paper; a reading >5.0–5.5 usually denotes significant atrophy.

An estimated 10%–40% of women will experience symptoms related to vaginal atrophy. Many women experience burning, discharge, bleeding, or irritation. Subsequent dyspareunia can be severe and debilitating, affecting sexual function, self-esteem, and quality of life. An increase in the vaginal pH (>5.0–5.5) may alter the vaginal flora, decreasing the proportion of lactobacillus genera and leading to urogenital infections. Further urethral mucosal atrophy may lead to urinary urgency and frequency and increase the risk of recurrent UTIs. In addition, symptoms of vaginal atrophy may be misinterpreted as a UTI and can result in antibiotic misuse; therefore, atrophy should be considered in patients with these symptoms.

These changes are readily reversed by administration of topical estrogen (SOE=A). The intravaginal use of low-dose estrogen cream or tablets, as infrequently as 2 nights per week, allows topical estrogen therapy with minimal absorption into the circulation, endometrial proliferation, or other systemic effects. The use of vaginal estrogen is not associated with an increased risk of cancer recurrence among women currently undergoing treatment for, or with a personal history of, breast cancer. The available prescription estrogen creams appear to be therapeutically equivalent. The estrogen ring can be used for 3 months per ring. Estrogen cream is also an excellent lubricant for use during pessary insertion. In women concerned about systemic absorption of locally administered estrogen, serum estradiol levels can be monitored at baseline and 6–8 weeks after initiation of therapy; dosage can be reduced if any significant increase in levels is noted. Alternatives to vaginal estrogen include ospemifine, a selective estrogen receptor modulator that is FDA approved for treatment of dyspareunia related to atrophic changes, and the prasterone vaginal insert, a steroid hormone that is converted to estradiol and testosterone and is used to treat moderate to severe dyspareunia due to menopause. Fractional carbon dioxide (CO_2) laser therapy has recently gained recognition as a viable treatment modality for vulvovaginal atrophy. Although FDA approved for a variety of dermatologic conditions, it is not specifically cleared for gynecologic use, and data used to support this particular administration are derived from preliminary observational studies only.

VULVOVAGINAL INFECTION AND INFLAMMATION

Alterations to vaginal mucosa and pH and subsequent changes to the vaginal microbiome in the postmenopausal period lead to an increased risk of vulvovaginal fungal infections. candidal infection, common in diabetic and obese patients who are plagued with moisture and irritation, can be treated with oral, intravaginal, and topical antifungal agents. Increasing resistance of *Candida* spp to commonly used azole therapy, including miconazole, terconazole, and oral fluconazole, has been reported. This is especially problematic in non-*albicans* species, including *C glabrata*, *C tropicalis*, *C parapsilosis*, and several even rarer species. When prescribing vaginal therapy, women should be questioned about their ability to insert a vaginal applicator before beginning therapy. For women with severe stenosis, a syringe (10 mL) can be filled with antifungal cream and attached to a urethral catheter (14 Fr.) for intravaginal administration. Topical corticosteroids can be used to hasten relief of symptoms of vulvar irritation but should be avoided as sole agents in vulvovaginal infections.

Other vaginal infections such as *Trichomonas* and *Gardnerella* vaginosis that are common in women of reproductive age are less common in older women, likely because of the higher vaginal pH. Bacterial vaginosis is rarely seen in postmenopausal women. A wet preparation revealing sheets of inflammatory cells without bacterial forms can represent advanced atrophy rather than an infectious cause. In women with inflammatory atrophy, the vagina will look inflamed with the presence of petechiae and serous exudate, rather than thin, pale, and dry as is typical in advanced atrophy. Local estrogen cream may thus need to be considered as well. Clinicians should not be hesitant to inquire about sexual practices when a woman presents with recurrent vaginal infections, vesicular lesions, or other changes suggestive of a sexually transmitted infection, and testing for sexually transmitted infections should not be avoided when indicated.

DISORDERS OF THE VULVA

With aging, the skin of the vulva loses elasticity, and the underlying fat and connective tissues undergo degeneration, with loss of collagen and thinning of the epithelial layer. Consequently, postmenopausal women are predisposed to a variety of dermatologic disorders. The assessment of vulvar complaints must include direct examination. Any pigmented lesion should be carefully evaluated by a gynecologist or dermatologist knowledgeable in gynecologic skin lesions. Most will prove to be benign lentigo or postinflammatory hyperpigmentation. The vulva, however, representing only 1% of the total skin surface, will contain 2% of all melanomas. Biopsy should always be considered in uncertain cases.

Vulvar skin irritation can result from a variety of agents and causes burning, itching, and edema. Hygienic products used for urinary and fecal incontinence can lead to chemical irritant dermatitis. Treatment of incontinence and protection of the delicate mucosa and skin with fastidious hygiene and topical emollients is important. Vulvar burning or pain is rarely due to estrogen deficiency, and this complaint should be investigated rather than treated with ever-increasing dosages of estrogen.

Vulvodynia, a chronic vulvar pain syndrome, is seen in both pre- and postmenopausal women. The International Society for the Study of Vulvovaginal Diseases (ISSVD) categorizes vulvodynia as either generalized or localized. The condition is further divided into provoked (sexual, nonsexual), unprovoked, or mixed. Treatment of vulvodynia can be challenging and should be approached in a comprehensive manner that may include tricyclic antidepressants, GABA-analogues, certain muscle relaxants, SSRI and SNRI agents, local anesthetic agents (all off-label), and others. Other treatment modalities may include pelvic floor rehabilitation therapy, administered by a therapist specifically trained in pelvic disorders. Additionally, sexual counselors, mental health care providers, and pain management specialists should be incorporated into the patients' treatment plan. A thorough evaluation should be performed to exclude disorders presenting with a similar clinical picture such as pudendal neuralgia, contact irritant mucositis, vulvar vestibulitis, and other neuropathic disorders.

Vulvar excoriation can result from scratching of an inflamed vulva, often with lichen simplex chronicus. Local corticosteroids such as hydrocortisone 1% ointment applied daily, and sitz baths, combined with fastidious genital hygiene, can help alleviate vulvar irritation. Any chronically irritated area should be biopsied to exclude a malignancy.

Non-neoplastic Vulvar Lesions

Lichen sclerosus causes over one-third of all vulvar dermatoses and can extend beyond the vulva to the perirectal areas. Squamous cell carcinoma of the vulva can arise in 4%–5% of patients with untreated lichen sclerosus. There is epithelial thinning with edema and fibrosis of the dermis. It can progress to shrinkage and resorption of the labia and severe clitoral phimosis with reduction in introital caliber. Lesions are typically shiny, white or pink, and parchment-like; they can be asymptomatic but typically cause itching, vaginal soreness, and/or dyspareunia. Diagnosis is confirmed on biopsy of the involved vulvar areas. Recommended treatment involves application of an ultra-potent topical corticosteroid such as clobetasol propionate 0.05%. Patients should be counseled on the proper use of these ointments, ie, initially twice a day and gradually less frequently. Once improvements are noted, reducing the strength of the steroid or the frequency of application should be advised. Periodic visits to assess compliance, exclude new lesions, and monitor for skin thinning are important. Further measures include wearing cotton underwear and avoiding irritant soaps. Topical emollient agents can also be helpful.

Lichen simplex chronicus, known for very intense pruritus, including nocturnal itching, has been previously described by many other terms, including neurodermatitis and squamous hyperplasia. Lichen simplex chronicus is a localized type of atopic dermatitis that can arise from either extrinsic or intrinsic insults. This condition can present as hyperplastic, corrugated, and elevated areas found only on keratinized skin. Biopsy may precede treatment, although many specialists recognize and treat the disorder without tissue sample. Topical mid-potency corticosteroids such as triamcinolone 0.1% twice daily for a few weeks (or longer with thick lesions) typically resolve the lesions; intermittent therapy may be necessary to sustain the therapeutic effect. It is essential not only to remove all irritants or allergens but also to control itching with the cautious use of antihistamines to allow for healing of the involved skin. Cloth gloves are still often recommended to reduce skin trauma from inadvertent scratching during sleep.

Other problematic vulvar lesions include lichen planus, which presents as bright red, moist lesions of the vulva or vagina that can also be erosive, and often result in significant discomfort and scarring. Ultra-potency corticosteroids applied topically and hydrocortisone

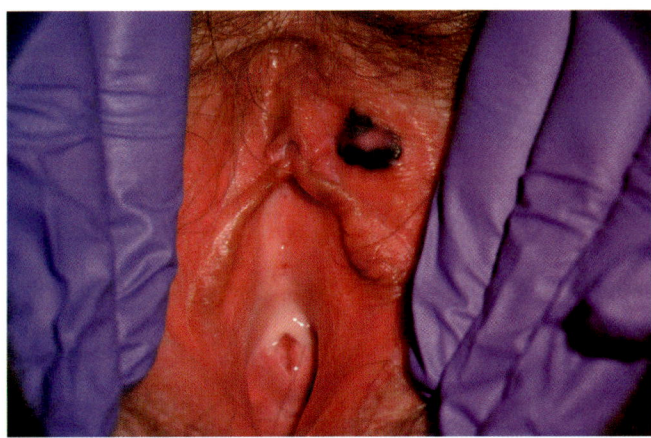

Figure 55.1—Vulvar melanoma, typical appearance of this unusual pigmented lesion

applied intravaginally are recommended. Bacterial infection is quite common with vaginal lichen planus and should be cultured and treated appropriately. Compromised coital ability due to infection a well as severe stenosis of the vagina is often addressed through surgery or vaginal dilation. Although lichen planus and certain cases of lichen sclerosus may sometimes be difficult to distinguish clinically, the hallmark distinction is that lichen sclerosus does not involve the vagina and extragenital lesions are rare, whereas lichen planus frequently involves the vagina and extragenital sites such as the oral cavity.

Vulvar Neoplasia

The classification system used by the ISSVD revised the nomenclature of vulvar intraepithelial neoplasia (VIN) in 2015. Older terms included VIN usual type (commonly associated with human papilloma virus) and differentiated VIN or d-VIN (often seen within a background of lichen sclerosus). In order to unify the nomenclature of human papilloma virus–associated lesions of the genital tract, VIN usual type was reclassified as high-grade squamous intraepithelial lesion of the vulva.

Because benign, premalignant, or malignant vulvar lesions may have similar clinical appearances, all suspicious, unusual, or symptomatic vulvar lesions should be biopsied. Referral to a gynecologic oncologist should be considered if malignancy is suspected. The gold standard for treatment of high-grade squamous intraepithelial lesion (HSIL) is wide local excision because of concern for occult invasion even when biopsy is negative for carcinoma. If carcinoma is excluded, treatment can include excision, laser ablation, or topical application of imiquimod (off-label use). Surveillance for recurrence is recommended, because recurrence rates vary from 9% to 50%. Vulvar HSIL is associated with a slow rate of progression; thus, surveillance is recommended 6 and 12 months after initial therapy and then annually. The prognosis of d-VIN is less predictable, but it does tend to be more aggressive in progression to invasive squamous cell carcinoma.

Invasive cancer of the vulva is an age-related malignancy; half of all cases occur after age 70. The vast majority are squamous cell carcinomas. Malignant melanoma, sarcoma, basal cell carcinoma, and adenocarcinoma account for <20% of cases. See Figure 55.1 for a typical appearance of vulvar melanoma. Treatment typically involves surgery (radical vulvectomy), occasionally accompanied by radiation.

PELVIC FLOOR DISORDERS

Pelvic Organ Prolapse

The prevalence of pelvic organ prolapse identified on examination ranges from 41% to 50% in the United States. Genetic predisposition, age, parity, vaginal delivery, obesity, menopausal status, chronic constipation, chronic heavy lifting, and connective tissue disorders are risk factors for development of prolapse. Prior hysterectomy, commonly thought to increase the risk of developing subsequent prolapse, does not appear to impact its development. While commonly noted on examination, the prevalence of symptomatic prolapse is much lower (3%–6%) and may include bothersome bulge and pressure symptoms, sexual dysfunction, lower urinary tract dysfunction, or defecatory dysfunction. Thus, treatment strategies should be focused on goals for treatment, symptomatic relief, and return of function instead of objective measurements of support on provider examination (SOE=B).

Vaginal or uterovaginal prolapse is often referred to as a pelvic organ hernia and is typically the result of pelvic floor support dysfunction. Traditional classification of vaginal prolapse includes differentiated protrusion of the posterior vaginal wall (enterocele or rectocele), the anterior vaginal wall (cystocele), or the vaginal apex or cervix. These conditions are demonstrated by having the patient bear down or cough while in the dorsal lithotomy position and may be more easily delineated using one half of a bivalve speculum to evaluate each wall separately. The full extent of prolapse may be better appreciated with a standing Valsalva maneuver.

The International Continence Society and the American Urogynecologic Association adopted a rather complex prolapse classification system (Pelvic Organ Prolapse Quantification [POPQ]) that is based on measurement of the distance between vaginal anatomic sites and the hymenal ring, as well as on vaginal length and perineal dimensions. The purpose of this classification, which is used by specialty societies, is to more objectively and reproducibly describe the degree of prolapse. For illustrations of complete uterine and vaginal vault prolapse, see Figure 55.2a and Figure 55.2b.

Anterior vaginal wall prolapse (often referred to as a "cystocele") does not always lead to bladder dysfunction and should not be assumed to be the cause of urinary incontinence. However, advanced prolapse can lead to urinary retention or incomplete bladder emptying, which can lead to the need to "splint" or push on the bulge during voids. Severe retention may eventually lead to kidney damage. Reduction of the prolapse can improve bladder function and prevent further renal implications. Conversely, correcting advanced prolapse can cause or exacerbate urinary incontinence by "unkinking" the urethra or bladder neck. Similarly, posterior vaginal wall prolapse may contribute to defecatory dysfunction and the need to vaginally "splint" during bowel movements. However, in cases of preexisting constipation, restoring the vaginal anatomy may not improve symptoms.

Nonsurgical Management

Nonsurgical management of pelvic organ prolapse should be offered to all patients and may be the most appropriate option for women who wish to avoid surgery or for whom surgery is deemed high risk. In some cases, behavioral or lifestyle changes may be effective at alleviating symptoms associated with pelvic organ prolapse. For example, among women with posterior vaginal wall prolapse and difficult defecation, fiber supplementation or laxative administration may improve symptoms. Urinary incontinence may be decreased with timed voids or more accessible toilet facilities such as bedside commodes. Pelvic floor muscle strengthening, often performed under the guidance of a physical therapist, may improve bulge symptoms and slow the rate of progression (SOE=C).

Vaginal pessaries should be offered to all women considering treatment for pelvic organ prolapse (SOE=B) and can successfully provide comfort and restore function. They may be used in an effort to delay or avoid surgery, or as long-term therapy, depending on the patient's preferences and surgical risk profile. Most commonly used pessaries are made of silicone and are available in a variety of shapes (donuts, rings, cubes, inflatable balls, and foldable models) and sizes designed for a variety of uses. The types of pessaries are divided into "support pessaries" (rings, foldable models) and "space-occupying pessaries" (gellhorns, cubes, donuts, inflatable balls).

The choice of pessary is influenced by the degree of prolapse, presence of incontinence, type of accompanying tissue relaxation, and ease of care. If

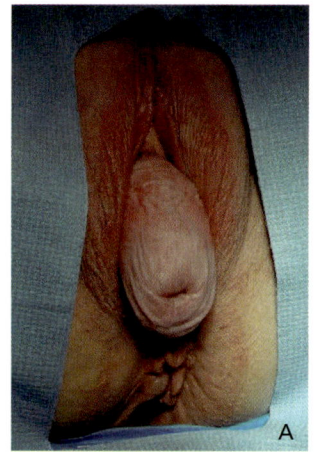 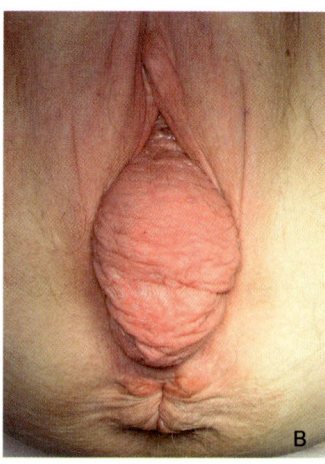

Figures 55.2a and 55.2b—Complete uterine and vaginal vault prolapse representing complete eversion of vaginal canal

possible, using a pessary that the patient can remove and replace independently is ideal. This is most often accomplished with a "support" pessary such as a ring with support. Patients with stress incontinence may benefit from a pessary with a knob that sits under the urethra to provide support during Valsalva maneuvers or a foldable lever-type, which restores bladder neck support. For those with advanced degrees of apical or anterior wall prolapse, a more rigid pessary (ie, gelhorn) may be needed. Although more difficult to insert and remove, making self-care more challenging, this pessary type is popular because of its high degree of efficacy. Cube pessaries should be used with caution because they can adhere to the vaginal walls with suction and are associated with an increased risk of vaginal ulcerations or erosions. These pessaries should be removed and replaced on a daily basis.

While up to 92% of women can be successfully fitted, pessary selection is a learned art. Even in experienced hands, it often proceeds by trial and error and may require multiple office visits. The optimal pessary fits snugly but comfortably and allows voiding and defecating without difficulty (Figure 55.3). Typically, there is one fingerbreadth of space between the circumference of the pessary and the surrounding vaginal wall. Having patients walk around the room, bend and sit, and use the commode before leaving the clinic may help the clinician determine if a pessary is appropriate and may save a return visit. After pessary selection and insertion, clinical follow-up within a few weeks is essential to ascertain satisfactory usage. After initial fitting and recheck, pessaries should be removed, cleaned, and the vaginal walls inspected.

Pessary care requirements often influence the selection of a device and the amount of follow-up required. If a patient's mobility or manual dexterity permits, she should remove the pessary at least one night

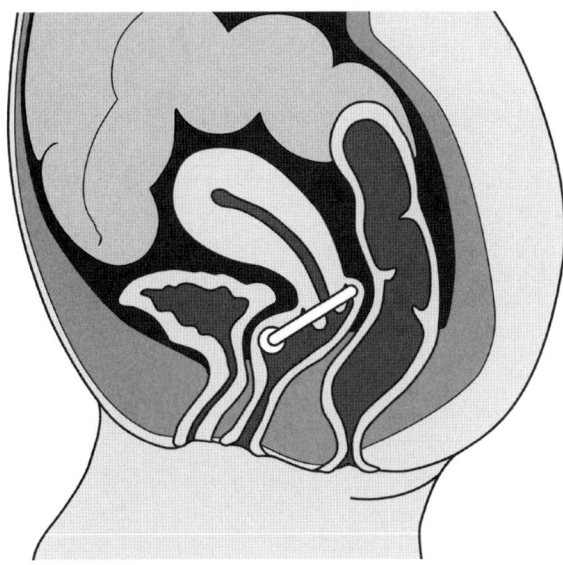

Figure 55.3—Incontinence ring with support pessary in place

per week, wash it with soap and water, and reinsert it with a water-soluble lubricant after arising in the morning. Women who cannot perform this level of self-care should be assisted at periodic office visits (ie, every 3–4 months) or by a visiting nurse. All women with pessaries should be instructed to report any unusual odor, discharge, bleeding, or discomfort, and any changes in bladder or bowel function, and all should have a pelvic examination once or twice a year. If discomfort is present or the device becomes uncomfortable, a different size or type should be tried. For patients with dementia, a caregiver should be cognizant and supportive of the need for routine management. For women using a pessary for long-term management, vaginal estrogen may be prescribed. Although not consistently demonstrated to decrease vaginal erosions or irritation, vaginal estrogen may improve rates of continued pessary use. A nonhormonal, pH-lowering vaginal jelly may be used and can decrease the amount of bothersome vaginal discharge experienced by some patients. If a pessary is left in place for long periods without monitoring, fistulas (while rare) can develop, or fibrous tissue can form around the pessary, requiring removal under anesthesia. If a pessary is found incidentally in patients with dementia in whom it has been in place for an unknown period of time, clinicians may elect to monitor rather than remove, depending on a patient's goals of care and overall prognosis.

Surgery for Prolapse

Surgical treatment of vaginal prolapse can be classified as either reconstructive or obliterative. Reconstructive procedures are designed to restore normal anatomy and may be performed through a vaginal or abdominal route. The use of mesh in transvaginal prolapse repair became popular in the 1990s with the development of prolapse repair "kits." However, because of mesh-related complications, including exposure through the vaginal walls and painful contraction, its use has markedly decreased and become controversial. There is no evidence that mesh augmentation of posterior vaginal wall prolapse repair improves outcomes, and it is associated with increased morbidity when used in the anterior wall (SOE=A). Transabdominal surgery, if possible, should be completed via a minimally invasive approach (eg, laparoscopy or robotic-assisted laparoscopy).

Obliterative procedures result in the narrowing, shortening, or complete closure of the vaginal canal. They are associated with high success rates, low morbidity, and patient satisfaction but are reserved for women who no longer wish to engage in penetrative vaginal intercourse. A colpocleisis does not prevent a woman from being sexually active or intimate with a partner. In a LeFort colpocleisis, performed without a concomitant hysterectomy, the anterior and posterior vaginal walls are sutured together, obliterating the vaginal canal. Two slender "canals" are left along the vaginal sidewalls to allow for recognition of infection or uterine bleeding.

Depending on the vaginal segment prolapsed and its degree of prolapse, success rates after surgical repair can vary from 60% to 90% (SOE=A). Urinary and fecal incontinence procedures can also be performed at the time of the prolapse surgery.

Age, in itself, is not a contraindication to surgery for genital prolapse. When a proven protocol for perioperative care, including preoperative medical clearance, regional anesthesia, infection prophylaxis, and deep-vein thrombosis prophylaxis, is followed, vaginal surgery offers a safe alternative to pessary use for older women with symptomatic genital prolapse who wish to pursue surgery as an option.

POSTMENOPAUSAL VAGINAL BLEEDING

Endometrial cancer, specifically type 1 or endometrioid endometrial carcinoma, is the most common type of gynecologic cancer in the United States. It commonly presents with postmenopausal vaginal bleeding. Risk factors include an excess of unopposed endogenous or exogenous estrogen, obesity, HRT with estrogen only, tamoxifen therapy, nulliparity, diabetes mellitus, and hypertension. However, most symptomatic women who experience vaginal bleeding do not have a malignant etiology. In the evaluation of a patient with postmenopausal bleeding (or bleeding after 1 year of amenorrhea), the challenge is not only to exclude gynecologic malignancies but also to alleviate the symptoms and eliminate the cause of benign conditions. Causes of bleeding can be grouped according to

Table 55.1—Causes of Postmenopausal Vaginal Bleeding

Cervical	Carcinoma
	Cervicitis
	Polyp
Endocrine	Exogenous hormones
	Perimenopausal ovarian function
Ovarian	Functioning ovarian tumor
Uterine	Endometrial atrophy
	Hyperplasia
	Neoplasia
	Polyp
	Submucosal leiomyoma
Vaginal	Atrophy
	Inflammation
	Tumor
	Ulceration
Vulvar	Carcinoma
	Laceration or ulceration
	Urethral caruncle
Other	Coagulation disorder
	Rectal lesion
	Urinary tract infection

anatomic areas and endocrine dysfunction (Table 55.1). Not all complaints of postmenopausal bleeding are related to the reproductive organs. Rectal or urinary tract bleeding may be misinterpreted by the patient or her caregiver as genital bleeding and require assessment as potential etiologies. For confirmed postmenopausal genital bleeding, proper evaluation involves a complete pelvic examination (looking for any vulvar, vaginal, cervical, or uterine source) and directed diagnostic studies. The endometrium should be evaluated initially by measuring endometrial thickness on transvaginal ultrasound if possible. An endometrial thickness of <4 mm has a high negative predictive value for endometrial cancer (99%–100%) and can be used to effectively exclude this diagnosis. While not indicative of cancer, an endometrial thickness of >4 mm should typically be evaluated with histologic sampling via an endometrial biopsy, dilation and curettage, or a sonohysterography. Both endometrial biopsy and dilation and curettage have sampling limitations, with approximately 60% of specimens sampling less than half of the endometrial cavity and resulting in similar rates of cancer detection. Diffuse thickening is usually more amenable to office endometrial biopsy, whereas focal lesions are better evaluated and biopsied hysteroscopically.

If endometrial cancer or precancerous lesions (endometrial intraepithelial neoplasia) are diagnosed or suspected, the patient should be referred to a gynecologic oncologist for management. Decisions regarding surgical or medical management depend on overall patient goals; functional status; a risk-benefit calculation; and assessment based on tissue histology, degree and depth of invasion, and tumor grade. Surgery typically involves a total hysterectomy with bilateral salpingo-oopherectomy and pelvic lymph node sampling performed abdominally often via minimally invasive laparoscopic or robotic-assisted laparoscopic approaches. Minimally invasive approaches are associated with decreased postoperative morbidity, including reduced blood loss, lower rate of ileus, and shorter hospital stay. Nonsurgical management of endometrial hyperplasia, endometrial intraepithelial neoplasia, or low-grade adenocarcinoma involves the use of progesterone to stabilize and limit the mitogenic effects of unopposed estrogen. The route of administration may be oral, intramuscular, or vaginal, or via an intrauterine device. Although there is no consensus regarding the optimal route, dosage, or length of therapy, hyperplasia regression rates associated with progesterone treatment ranges from 67% to 90%.

Noncancerous structural lesions of the uterus or cervix such as polyps or fibroids can be addressed surgically, or observed if not causing persistent bleeding that is poorly tolerated or is resulting in anemia. The most common cause of postmenopausal uterine bleeding is an atrophic endometrium. As suggested above, cervical lesions, including infections, polyps, and malignancies, must be excluded. Of major importance, abrasions and lacerations that may be due to sexual assault or abuse must be carefully excluded, irrespective of the history provided by patient or caregivers. If abuse is suspected, reporting to local authorities is mandatory.

Exogenous hormone replacement is also a common cause of benign postmenopausal bleeding. Women using combined estrogen-progesterone replacement therapy (assuming adequate dosing of progesterone) actually have a lower risk of uterine cancer than women not using HRT. However, any unscheduled or otherwise suspicious bleeding should be evaluated. Women on cyclic hormone therapy who bleed at predicted and anticipated progestin-withdrawal times generally do not require evaluation, unless the characteristics of the withdrawal bleeding substantially change. Some specialists recommend biopsy if any bleeding, even in the presence of a normal ultrasound, persists longer than 6 months.

RESOURCES

- Buchsbaum GM, Lee TG. Vaginal obliterative procedures for pelvic organ prolapse: a systematic review. *Obstet Gynecol Surv.* 2017;72(3):175–183.

- Committee on Practice Bulletins: American College of Obstetricians and Gynecologists. American Urogynecologic Society. Practice Bulletin #185. Pelvic organ prolapse. *Obstet Gynecol.* 2017;130(5):1170–1172.

CHAPTER 56—PROSTATE DISEASE AND CANCER

KEY POINTS

- A number of treatment options exist for benign prostatic hyperplasia (BPH), including watchful waiting, medications, minimally invasive procedures, and more extensive operations. The choice is influenced by the extent of symptoms, the presence of complications from outflow obstruction, and patient preferences.

- The use of 5α-reductase inhibitors for BPH is indicated especially when the prostate gland is large.

- Men should be well informed about the risks and benefits of prostate-specific antigen (PSA) screening before making a decision whether or not to be screened for prostate cancer.

- Several treatment options exist for men with localized prostate cancer, including watchful waiting, resection of the gland and seminal vesicles, and radiation therapy. How the patient balances the potential benefits and burdens of the various options will influence the choice of therapy.

- For patients with chronic prostatitis, efforts should be made to identify the causative organism, and even with a prolonged course of appropriate antibiotics, a cure can be expected in fewer than half the patients.

With advancing age, the prevalence of prostate diseases increases dramatically. The three most common conditions are BPH, prostate cancer, and prostatitis. Self-reported prostate disease affects about 3 million American men. BPH develops in over half of men ≥65 years old and affects the overwhelming majority of men >85 years old. Prostate cancer is the second leading cause of cancer death in men, and many men have asymptomatic or low-grade tumors that cause few or no health problems. The prevalence of prostatitis is similar to that of ischemic heart disease or diabetes mellitus.

BENIGN PROSTATIC HYPERPLASIA

Epidemiology

BPH is a noncancerous enlargement of the epithelial and fibromuscular components of the prostate gland. The epithelial component normally makes up 20%–30% of prostate volume and contributes to the seminal fluid. The fibromuscular component comprises 70%–80% of the prostate and is responsible for expressing prostatic fluid during ejaculation. Age and long-term androgen stimulation induce development of BPH. Microscopic appearance of BPH can be seen as early as age 30, is present in 50% of men by age 60, and is present in 90% of men by age 85. In half of these cases, microscopic BPH develops into palpable macroscopic BPH. Of those with macroscopic BPH, only half develop clinically significant disease that is brought to medical attention. BPH is one of the most common conditions in aging men; in the United States annually it accounts for more than 1.7 million office visits and 250,000 surgical procedures.

Prostatism, or Lower Urinary Tract Symptoms

The symptoms of BPH are nonspecific; other diseases can result in identical symptoms. The pathophysiology of BPH symptoms is not completely understood, but presumably it involves the periurethral zone of the prostate gland, which results in obstructed urine flow and compensatory responses of the bladder, such as hypertrophy and decreased capacity. The urethral obstruction has both mechanical (obstructing mass) and dynamic (smooth muscle contractions) components. The resulting lower urinary tract symptoms are divided into irritative (eg, frequency, urgency, nocturia) and obstructive (eg, hesitancy, intermittency, weak stream, incomplete emptying) manifestations. These 7 lower urinary tract symptoms compose a quantitative symptom index for assessing severity and monitoring treatment response, which was developed by the American Urological Association (AUA) and adopted by the World Health Organization, known as the International Prostate Symptom Score. Although tracking symptom severity is useful in the longitudinal management of patients, symptom severity has not been found to correlate with prostate size, urine flow rates, or postvoid residual volume. BPH primarily affects quality of life, although complications such as recurrent urinary tract infection, bladder stones, urinary retention, chronic renal insufficiency, and hematuria can develop.

Diagnosis

Differential diagnosis of lower urinary tract symptoms includes endocrine disorders (especially diabetes mellitus), neurologic disorders, urinary tract infections, sexually transmitted diseases, kidney or bladder stones, overactive bladder, and medications (especially medications with antimuscarinic and diuretic effects). Overactive bladder and BPH are both very common and may coexist. If the lower urinary tract symptoms are primarily storage issues (frequency, urgency, nocturia), then overactive bladder may be considered the primary diagnosis. When voiding symptoms, such as poor flow or

Table 56.1—Management Options for Benign Prostatic Hyperplasia

Category	Interventions	Rationale	Comments
Lifestyle modification	Reduce nighttime fluids to manage nocturia; eliminate bladder irritants (eg, caffeine, alcohol, nicotine)	Factors outside the urinary tract contribute to urinary symptoms	Often sufficient management for mild symptoms; complements management for moderate to severe symptoms
Pharmacologic management	α-Adrenergic antagonists Selective $α_1$: prazosin^{OL} Long-acting selective $α_1$: terazosin, doxazosin Slow-release, long-acting selective $α_1$: tamsulosin, silodosin, alfuzosin	Relaxation of smooth muscle in hyperplastic prostate tissue, prostate capsule, and bladder neck decreases resistance to urinary flow	Adverse events: dizziness, mild asthenia, headaches, postural hypotension (reduced with careful dosage titration, not present with slow release selective $α_1$ agents), abnormal ejaculation, rhinitis
	5α-Reductase inhibitors: finasteride, dutasteride	Reduced tissue levels of dihydrotestosterone result in prostate gland size reduction	Most effective for men with larger prostates (>40 g); results may not be evident for up to 6 months
	Phosphodiesterase-5 inhibitor: tadalafil	PDE-5 activity in bladder neck, prostatic urethra, and prostate musculature contributes to urinary symptoms	Effective for men with or without erectile dysfunction; only drug that can treat both conditions
Surgery	Transurethral resection of the prostate; transurethral incision of the prostate; open prostatectomy; transurethral vaporization of the prostate; stent placement	Removal or expansion of periurethral prostate tissue reduces obstruction to urinary flow	Indicated for recurrent urinary tract infection induced by benign prostatic hypertrophy, recurrent or persistent gross hematuria, bladder stones, renal insufficiency

hesitancy are present, then the focus is placed on BPH. Digital rectal examination (DRE) can be unremarkable or reveal an enlarged, smooth, rubbery, symmetrical gland. Urinalysis is routinely performed to evaluate for urinary tract infection, hematuria, and glycosuria. This minimal testing is usually sufficient for a provisional diagnosis and empiric therapy. Additional subsequent tests include postvoid residual urine volume (often done by office or bedside bladder scan), urine flow rates, and pressure flow studies. These tests can be considered when the diagnosis is uncertain or an invasive treatment is being planned.

Treatment Approaches

BPH therapy depends on the patient and is driven by the impact of symptoms on the patient's quality of life (Table 56.1). All patients should be educated regarding lifestyle modification by adjusting fluid intake (eg, avoiding caffeine) and avoiding medications (especially antimuscarinics) that aggravate symptoms. Men with mild to moderate symptoms may be satisfied with lifestyle modification only. Both medical and surgical treatments are also available, with medication the usual first approach. Indications for surgical treatment include patient preference, dissatisfaction with medication, and refractory urinary retention, as well as renal dysfunction, bladder stones, recurrent urinary tract infections, or hematuria if these are clearly due to prostatic enlargement.

Medical Treatment

The two main pharmacologic approaches are α-adrenergic antagonist and 5α-reductase inhibitor therapy (SOE=A).

α-Adrenergic antagonists, or α-blockers, are directed at the dynamic component of urethral obstruction. Smooth muscle of the prostate and bladder neck has a resting tone mediated by α-adrenergic innervation. α-Blockers relax the smooth muscle in the hyperplastic prostate tissue, prostate capsule, and bladder neck, thus decreasing resistance to urinary flow. Of the two major α-adrenergic receptors, α1 receptors predominate in the prostate. α-Blockade development for BPH therapy has progressed from selective α1 agents (eg, prazosin) to long-acting selective α1 agents (terazosin, doxazosin) and then to slow-release, long-acting selective α1 agents (tamsulosin, alfuzosin, silodosin). The most common adverse events of α1 agents are dizziness, mild asthenia (fatigue or weakness), and headaches. Postural hypotension occurs infrequently and can be minimized by careful dosage titration of terazosin and doxazosin; slow-release agents do not require dose titration. Ejaculatory dysfunction is common with these agents, but alfuzosin does not have this effect. For patients undergoing cataract surgery, intraoperative floppy iris syndrome (IFIS), characterized by sudden intraoperative iris prolapse and pupil constriction, is a potential risk of all α-blockers, with the greatest frequency and severity of IFIS among those using tamsulosin (SOE=B).

The enzyme 5α-reductase is required to convert testosterone to the more active dihydrotestosterone. Finasteride and dutasteride are inhibitors of 5α-reductase and reduce tissue levels of dihydrotestosterone, thus reducing prostate gland size. Improvements in symptom scores and urine flow rates may not be evident for up to 6 months. The 5α-reductase inhibitors are most effective in men with larger prostates (>40 g, about the size of a plum) (SOE=A). Because 5α-reductase inhibitors reduce serum PSA levels by an average of 50%, after 6 months of therapy men receiving prostate cancer surveillance will need a new baseline serum PSA determination.

When used together over years, the α-adrenergic antagonists combined with 5α-reductase inhibitors have been shown to be safe and to reduce clinical progression of BPH better than either agent alone (SOE=A). In particular, a lower risk of urinary retention, urinary incontinence, renal insufficiency, and recurrent bladder infections is associated with combination therapy. Trials of BPH therapy with the herbal preparation *Serenoa repens*, or saw palmetto, show conflicting results. Limited data from smaller studies suggested that it improves urinary symptoms and flow measures in men with BPH. However, a Cochrane review found that compared with placebo, *S repens* monotherapy does not improve urinary symptoms or maximal urinary flow rate even at double and triple the usual dosage.

Antimuscarinic agents have a role in managing lower urinary tract storage symptoms in men with BPH. Used alone, or in combination with α-blockers, antimuscarinic medications do not seem to significantly increase postvoid residual urine volumes or provoke acute urinary retention (SOE=A).

Many men experience both BPH and erectile dysfunction, and BPH medications can negatively impact erectile function. Shared pathogenetic mechanisms have been proposed for BPH/lower urinary tract symptoms and erectile dysfunction. Tadalafil is now FDA approved for both BPH and erectile dysfunction. Research continues to explore the role of phosphodiesterase-5 (PDE-5) inhibitors alone, or in combination with conventional BPH treatments, in relieving lower urinary tract symptoms in men with BPH, with or without erectile dysfunction. Caution is advised when using PDE-5 inhibitors and α-blockers because of possible additive effects of hypotension.

Surgical Treatment

Surgical management includes transurethral resection of the prostate (TURP), transurethral incision of the prostate (TUIP), open prostatectomy, transurethral vaporization of the prostate, and device insertion such as stent placement. Surgical approaches offer the best chance for symptom improvement but also have the highest rates of complications. The benefits of various surgical treatments are generally considered equivalent, but complication rates differ. TURP is the standard of care to which other BPH treatments are compared, and it has an 80% likelihood of successful outcome in properly selected patients (SOE=A). Usually performed under spinal anesthesia, TURP involves passage of an endoscope through the urethra to surgically remove the inner portion of the prostate. Long-term complications can include retrograde ejaculation, urethral stricture, bladder neck contracture, incontinence, and impotence. TUIP is an endoscopic procedure via the urethra to make one or two cuts in the prostate and prostate capsule, relieving urethral constriction. Limited to use in small prostate glands (<30 g), TUIP offers lower rates of retrograde ejaculation, bleeding, and contractures. Open prostatectomy involves removal of the inner portion of the prostate through a retropubic or suprapubic incision. It is best used for patients with larger prostates or with complicating conditions such as bladder stones or urethral strictures. Open prostatectomy is associated with incisional morbidity, longer hospitalization, and greater risk of impotence. Transurethral vaporization of the prostate uses a high-energy electrode inserted via the urethra to vaporize the prostate. This approach has little bleeding but creates more prolonged irritative voiding. Prostatic stents are used to maintain expansion of the prostatic urethra and have both temporary and permanent uses.

Management of Acute Urinary Retention

Acute urinary retention (AUR), considered a urologic emergency, is characterized by a sudden and painful inability to pass urine. Up to a third of men undergoing TURP present with AUR. AUR may be the result of natural progression of BPH, or it may be precipitated by surgical procedures, infection, or medications. Immediate management of AUR consists of bladder decompression, usually with a urethral catheter. Subsequently, conservative management is common with a trial of catheter removal after 1–3 days. Starting therapy with $α_1$-blockers before catheter removal improves the chances of success (SOE=B). The catheter should be removed as soon as possible, because this is the most effective means of reducing the incidence of catheter-associated urinary tract infections.

PROSTATE CANCER

Incidence and Epidemiology

Prostate cancer is the most common noncutaneous cancer and the second leading cause of cancer deaths among men in the United States. Since 2010, it has been estimated that 150,000–200,000 men would be diagnosed with and 25,000–30,000 men would die annually from prostate cancer. In recent years, the incidence of prostate cancer and related deaths are declining likely because of the large screening efforts that were undertaken. Incidence increases with age; prostate cancer is rare in men <40 years old. A prevalence study, reported in 2008, of 340 healthy men scheduled for organ donation found the prevalence of prostate cancer was 0.5% in men <50 years old, 23.4% in men 50–59 years old, 35% in men 60–69 years old, and 45.5% in men >70 years old. Earlier autopsy studies that included debilitated men had found prevalence rates as high as 80% in men >80 years old. The incidence of disease varies according to race, with black Americans having the highest risk in the world. Among black men, prostate cancer occurs at an earlier age, has a higher mortality rate, and tends to be at a more advanced stage at diagnosis. Family history is a contributing factor. Men with one first-degree relative affected have more than a 2-fold increased risk (SOE=B). Androgens are necessary for prostate cancer pathogenesis; the disease does not occur in men castrated before puberty. History of sexually transmitted infection can be associated with an increased risk of prostate cancer (SOE=B). The association between prostate cancer and omega-3 fatty acid intake, alcohol intake, or vasectomy is inconclusive.

Symptoms

Cancer usually arises in the peripheral zone of the prostate. Most men, especially those with early-stage, potentially curable disease, are asymptomatic. Prostate cancer spreads by 3 routes: direct extension, the lymphatics, and the bloodstream. Direct invasion of the urethra and bladder can lead to irritative voiding symptoms, urinary incontinence, and hematuria. Extension of disease to adjacent nerves can cause impotence and pelvic pain. Nodal metastasis can cause extrinsic ureteral obstruction. Leg edema can develop from lymphatic obstruction. Hematogenous metastasis to bone can cause severe local pain, normochromic normocytic anemia, pathologic fractures, and spinal cord compression. Less commonly, hematogenous metastasis involves viscera, namely the lung, liver, and adrenal glands.

Screening Controversy

The benefit of early detection and the best approach to treatment of prostate cancer are controversial. There is a large reservoir of prostate cancer that does not need to be diagnosed because most men with prostate cancer die with the disease, not from it. However, the well-recognized burden of progressive prostate cancer is a potential impetus for early detection and management.

Results of two prospective, randomized controlled trials of prostate cancer screening report somewhat conflicting findings. The Prostate, Lung, Colorectal, and Ovarian Cancer (PLCO) Screening Trial found no significant difference in prostate cancer mortality between screened and unscreened groups after 7–10 years of follow-up. However, about 50% of men in the PLCO control group had PSA testing before enrollment and close to 90% had PSA testing during the trial. Thus, PLCO researchers described this as a comparison of "opportunistic versus systematic screening". The European Randomized Study of Screening for Prostate Cancer, which was actually a collection of smaller trials in 8 different European countries, found an 11% absolute risk reduction in prostate cancer mortality at 13 years of follow-up. Number needed calculations showed that 781 men would need to be screened and 27 additional cases of prostate cancer treated for every prostate cancer death prevented. Approximately 6% of men in the control arm and about 10% of men in the screening arm were diagnosed with prostate cancer, with most of the excess cancers identified by screening as being low-grade Gleason 6 tumors. The authors concluded that overdiagnosis of indolent cases and concerns about overtreatment and related harms prevent support of organized prostate cancer screening as a public health measure. Both trials documented significantly increased prostate cancer incidence associated with screening. Men who were >74 years old at baseline were not enrolled in either trial. The two trials had significant methodologic differences, particularly for inclusion criteria, enrollment size, frequency and mode of screening, definition of a positive PSA level, and follow-up.

Screening for prostate cancer remains a somewhat controversial topic with different recommendations and guidelines from various task forces and specialty societies. In 2012, the U.S. Preventive Services Task Force issued updated recommendations giving routine screening for prostate cancer a "D" rating, meaning that "there is moderate or high certainty that the service has no benefit or that the harms outweigh the benefits." The U.S. Preventive Services Task Force (USPSTF) noted that "The reduction in prostate cancer mortality 10 to 14 years after PSA-based screening is, at most, very small, even for men in the optimal age range of 55 to 69 years." In May 2018, the USPSTF issued an updated recommendation stating, "For men aged 55–69 years; the decision to undergo periodic prostate-specific antigen (PSA)-based screening for prostate cancer should be an individual one. Before deciding whether to be screened, men should have an opportunity to discuss the potential benefits and harms of screening with their clinician and to incorporate their values and preferences in the decision." This 2018 statement has a "C" rating, meaning that there is moderate certainty that the net benefit for some men aged 55–69 is small. The USPSTF notes "How each man weighs specific benefits and harms will determine whether the overall net benefit is small." Major guidelines from oncology, urology, and primary care recommend some level of shared decision making for PSA screening for prostate cancer. The American Cancer Society guideline recommends that men discuss screening with their clinicians to make an informed decision, starting at age 50, or younger if risk factors are present. The AUA guideline recommends shared decision making for screening in men aged 55–69 years old, with the screening decision based on patient values and preferences. The American College of Physicians guideline recommends that clinicians inform men 50–69 years old about limited potential benefits and substantial harms of screening for prostate cancer, and recommends against PSA screening in men who do not express a clear preference for screening.

Screening and Diagnostic Tests

DRE allows palpation of the posterior surfaces of the lateral lobes of the prostate, where cancer most often begins. Cancer characteristically is hard, nodular, and irregular. Although DRE is less sensitive than PSA in detecting prostate cancer, it can sometimes detect cancers in men who have a normal PSA level. However, its use as a single screening test is greatly limited, because parts of the prostate gland cannot be palpated. About half of the cancers thought to be limited to the prostate on the basis of DRE are found during surgery to have already spread. DRE has many false-positive results; only about one-third of men with positive DRE tests have prostate cancer on biopsy. Local extension of prostate cancer into the seminal vesicles can often be detected by DRE, which may be valuable in staging of disease. Thus, despite its limitations, DRE has a role in prostate cancer staging and in screening asymptomatic patients who choose to be screened.

The serum PSA test is not specific for prostate cancer. PSA increases in benign conditions of the prostate, namely, hypertrophy and prostatitis, and in transient response to conditions such as ejaculation and prostatic massage. The sensitivity of the PSA test is also imperfect. Decreased PSA values have been associated with acute hospitalization and use of medications such as 5α-reductase inhibitors and saw palmetto. PSA levels are normal in 30%–40% of men with cancer confined to the prostate (ie, false-negative tests). The reported positive predictive value of PSA in screening studies is 28%–35%; about one-third of men with increased PSA levels have prostate cancer demonstrated by fine-needle biopsy.

Several approaches to improve the accuracy of PSA testing have been developed. PSA density is derived from the PSA concentration divided by the volume of the prostate gland (measured by ultrasound). Prostate cancer results in higher PSA levels per unit volume than BPH and should therefore yield a higher PSA density. The PSA rate of change or velocity is more specific for prostate cancer than a single PSA measurement. Using a PSA velocity value of ≥0.75 ng/mL/year achieves 90% specificity, whereas using a single PSA level >4 ng/mL achieves 60% specificity. This high specificity for PSA velocity is realized even in serum PSA levels in the normal range (<4 ng/mL). Another approach involves age-adjusted PSA reference ranges, because PSA values increase with age. Finally, the ratio of free to complexed PSA can be measured, recognizing that PSA bound to α1-antichymotrypsin accounts for a larger proportion of total PSA with prostate cancer than with BPH.

Advances in DNA sequencing have led to commercial development of several genomic assays that may be used to predict prostate cancer outcomes and therapeutic responses. These tests are expensive and lack long-term data on comparative effectiveness. Understanding how and when to use these tests is still evolving.

Abnormal DRE or PSA tests lead to transrectal ultrasound (TRUS)-guided biopsy of the prostate for pathologic diagnosis. To avoid excessive testing and overdiagnosis, the AUA advocates prostate biopsy be considered only after PSA increase is confirmed (SOE=C). Many PSA values revert to normal when repeated several months later. In the past, core needle biopsies were routinely taken from the base, middle, and apex of each lobe (6 samples total, termed sextant biopsy). Sextant biopsy has been enhanced by extended biopsy schemes that sample more gland areas, particularly the lateral aspects with variable core numbers. Prostate biopsy schemes that consist of 10 to 12 cores with apical and laterally directed sampling of the peripheral zone increase cancer detection rates, reduce the need for repeat biopsies, and predict pathologic features on prostatectomy (SOE=B).

Multiparametric MRI (mpMRI) is a combination of standard anatomical T1 and T2 weighted imaging supplemented by any functional form of imaging such as dynamic contrast-enhanced MRI or diffusion-weighted imaging. Compared with ultrasound, mpMRI has superior imaging ability; mpMRI-guided prostate biopsy may improve detection of significant prostate cancer with reduced diagnosis of insignificant cancer (SOE=B).

MRI ultrasound fusion-guided biopsy involves the creation of a detailed 360 degree prostate map that merges previously captured MRI images with live TRUS images from the inserted ultrasound wand to guide more precise sampling of tissue. Fusion imaging requires specialized knowledge, equipment, and software that is not yet widely available.

Grading

The Gleason grading system is based on the histologic appearance of prostate cancer. The Gleason grade ranges from 1, or well differentiated, to 5, or poorly differentiated. The Gleason score is the sum of the two most common Gleason grades observed. The Gleason score ranges from 2 to 10. Gleason scores were sometimes grouped as 2–4, well differentiated; 5–7, moderately differentiated; and 8–10, poorly differentiated. Well-differentiated tumors have a favorable prognosis; poorly differentiated tumors,

Table 56.2—Localized Prostate Cancer Risk Stratification and Treatment Recommendations

Risk Category	Criteria	Recommended Treatment
Very low risk	PSA <10 ng/mL *and* Grade Group 1 *and* clinical stage T_1-T_{2a} *and* <34% of biopsy cores positive *and* no core with >50% involved *and* PSA density <0.15 ng/mL/cc	Active surveillance (SOE=A)
Low risk	PSA <10 ng/mL *and* Grade Group 1 *and* clinical stage T_1-T_{2a}	Active surveillance (SOE=B) Definitive treatment for select patients (SOE=B)
Intermediate risk	PSA 10 to <20 ng/mL *or* Grade Group 2–3 *or* clinical stage T_{2b-c} Favorable: Grade Group 1 (with PSA 10 to <20) *or* Grade Group 2 (with PSA <10) Unfavorable: Grade Group 2 (with either PSA 10 to <20 *or* clinical stage T_{2b-c}) *or* Grade Group 3 (with PSA <20)	Radical prostatectomy *or* radiation therapy with ADT (SOE=A) Favorable: active surveillance possible (SOE=C), comes with higher risk of metastases
High risk	PSA >20 ng/mL *or* Grade Group 4–5	Radical prostatectomy *or* radiation therapy with ADT (SOE=A)

Definitive treatment = radical prostatectomy or radiation therapy
ADT = androgen deprivation therapy
SOURCE: For further details, see Clinically Localized Prostate Cancer: AUA/ASTRO/SUO Guideline: American Urological Association; 2017; www.auanet.org/guidelines/clinically-localized-prostate-cancer-new-(aua/astro/suo-guideline-2017).

an unfavorable prognosis (SOE=A). Most clinically detected tumors are moderately differentiated. The World Health Organization now recommends a new grading system with 5 distinct Grade Groups as follows: Grade Group 1 = Gleason score ≤6, Grade Group 2 = Gleason score 3+4=7, Grade Group 3 = Gleason score 4+3=7, Grade Group 4 = Gleason score 8, Grade Group 5 = Gleason scores 9 and 10.

Staging

Clinical staging of prostate cancer is necessary for planning disease management. The tumor, regional node, metastasis (TNM) system is widely used. Usually detected by transurethral resection of the prostate, incidentally discovered cancers are stage T_1. Stage T_{1c} reflects the growing number of tumors detected because of an increased PSA level. Tumors detectable by DRE and confined to the prostate are stage T_2. Staging is also based on the degree of extension and invasion of surrounding structures in tumors that extend beyond the prostatic capsule (T_3 to T_4) and on presence of lymph node involvement (N) and distant metastasis (M).

For localized cancer (clinical stage T_1–T_2, N0 or NX, M0 or MX; X=cannot be assessed), the AUA advocates risk stratification of prostate cancer aggressiveness based on PSA, DRE, Grade Group, amount of cancer on biopsy (ie, number of cores involved, maximum involvement of any single core), PSA density, and imaging. These criteria allow segregation into a limited number of risk groups to form the basis of clinical decision making (Table 56.2).

In the past, CT scans, MRI scans, pedal lymphangiography, and pelvic lymph node dissection were routinely used in various combinations to evaluate the extent of prostate cancer. In the initial staging evaluation of patients with prostate cancer, these tests should be eliminated, because they have been associated with unacceptably high false-negative and false-positive results.

Management of Localized Disease

Localized cancer lends itself to cure, but the prevalence of men dying with prostate cancer (often asymptomatic) but not from the disease questions the necessity of treatment. There remains a lack of evidence that treatment prolongs life when treatment is compared with watchful waiting. Thus, 3 approaches to localized prostate cancer are routinely advocated: watchful waiting, radical prostatectomy, and radiation therapy (Table 56.3).

Watchful waiting (also called *expectant* or *conservative management; surveillance*) is the approach offered most commonly to men with <10 years of remaining life expectancy, who have significant medical comorbidities, or whose tumor is small and well to moderately differentiated. Conservative management studies have shown that 10-year disease-specific survival is 89%–96% for men with Gleason score 2–5 tumors, 70%–82% for men with Gleason score 6 tumors, 30%–58% for men with Gleason score 7 tumors, and 13%–40% for men with Gleason score 8–10 tumors. Because most men with prostate cancer are asymptomatic, watchful waiting attempts to spare men the burden of unnecessary treatment. However, waiting for symptoms in men with prostate cancer before starting treatment means sacrificing the opportunity for cure. Patients are offered palliation if and when symptoms develop. Active surveillance combines the concept of expectant management with the option for deferred curative intent treatment. The optimal selection criteria and surveillance strategy for active surveillance have not been defined. Active surveillance selection criteria include cases detected by PSA screening with Gleason scores <7 and

Table 56.3—Management Approaches for Prostate Cancer

Management	Description	Comments	Selected Potential Adverse Effects
Localized			
Watchful waiting	Prostate cancer is not treated until symptoms develop.	Offered to men with <10 years of remaining life expectancy; significant medical comorbidities; small, well-differentiated tumors; or unwillingness to bear treatment burdens. Awaiting symptoms sacrifices opportunity for cure.	Anxiety
Active surveillance	Prostate cancer treatment is delayed until evidence of disease progression.	Offered to men with cancer detected by PSA screening, Gleason score <7, small volume involvement	Anxiety, discomfort of serial PSA, DRE, and prostate biopsies
Radical prostatectomy	Surgical removal of entire prostate gland and seminal vesicles	Offered to men who have no surgical contraindications. Adverse effects realized immediately.	Erectile dysfunction, urinary incontinence
External beam radiation therapy	Standard regimen delivers 6,000–7,000 rads of pelvic radiation over 5- to 8-week period.	Radiation reaches tissues outside the prostate, including pelvic lymph nodes. Adverse effects occur initially from radiation-induced inflammation, then develop over time as scar tissue develops.	*Acute:* proctitis, urethritis *Chronic:* erectile dysfunction, urinary incontinence, bowel dysfunction
Brachytherapy	Radioactive seeds (eg, iridium, palladium) are implanted into the prostate gland using CT scan guidance.	Improvements in prostate imaging allow uniform distribution of seed, overcoming past limitations. Adverse effects occur initially from radiation-induced inflammation, then develop over time as scar tissue develops.	*Acute:* prostatitis, urinary retention, hematuria *Chronic:* erectile dysfunction, urinary incontinence, bowel dysfunction
Locally Advanced			
Radiation therapy	See external beam radiation (above).	Offered to men with prostate cancer extending beyond capsule or into seminal vesicles. Asymptomatic cancer period may be prolonged.	See external beam radiation (above).
Androgen deprivation	Hormone therapy can be combined with radiation therapy.	Neoadjuvant androgen deprivation provides additional benefit toward increased survival and freedom from metastases; because of adverse effects, controversy exists regarding early versus delayed use of androgen deprivation.	Erectile dysfunction, loss of libido, loss of stamina, increased fatigue, hot flashes, diminished muscle mass, premature osteoporosis
Advanced/Metastatic			
Complete androgen ablation	Combined approach of reducing androgens to castration levels and inhibiting binding of androgen to its receptor	Includes orchiectomy or LHRH agonists with antiandrogens	Erectile dysfunction, loss of libido, loss of stamina, increased fatigue, hot flashes, diminished muscle mass, premature osteoporosis
Orchiectomy	Surgical castration	Oldest, safest, least expensive approach; rejected by half of American men	Erectile dysfunction, loss of libido, loss of stamina, increased fatigue, hot flashes, diminished muscle mass, premature osteoporosis
LHRH agonists	Chemical castration	Alternative to surgical castration, equally effective; causes initial increase in serum testosterone levels	Erectile dysfunction, loss of libido, hot flashes, gynecomastia, insomnia, GI upset, dizziness
Antiandrogens	Inhibit binding of androgen to its receptor	Used at initiation of LHRH-agonist therapy to block effect of increased testosterone levels; used after castration to block effect of residual small amount of androgen being produced by adrenal glands	Erectile dysfunction, loss of libido, gynecomastia, insomnia, GI upset, dizziness
Chemotherapy with docetaxel	Antimitotic agent, inhibits cell division	Used at initiation of androgen deprivation or for cancer progression despite androgen deprivation	Nausea, vomiting, diarrhea, alopecia, anemia, asthenia
Other	Symptom-specific approaches used as indicated	For example, focal radiation therapy can be provided to the site of a bony metastasis to reduce both pain and risk of fracture.	Intervention specific

NOTE: LHRH = luteinizing hormone-releasing hormone

small volume involvement (<3 of 6 biopsy cores, <50% malignant involvement within each core). The National Comprehensive Cancer Network guidelines for active surveillance suggest serum PSA measurement at least every 6 months, DRE at least annually, and repeat prostate biopsy considered annually (SOE=C).

Radical prostatectomy involves surgical removal of the entire prostate gland and the seminal vesicles. It can be performed through a perineal (incision near the rectum) or retropubic (lower abdominal incision) approach. The perineal approach allows an easier vesicourethral anastomosis and less bleeding, whereas the retropubic approach allows access to the pelvic lymph nodes and spares the neurovascular supply to the corpora cavernosa (with improved potency). The major complications of radical prostatectomy are urinary incontinence and erectile dysfunction. Surgery is thought to have the highest incidence of sexual dysfunction after treatment. In a population-based study of 1,291 men undergoing radical prostatectomy for clinically localized prostate cancer, 59.9% reported erections not firm enough for sexual intercourse and 8.4% were incontinent 18 months later (SOE=C). After radical prostatectomy, men are more likely to experience stress incontinence, with symptoms ranging from occasional leakage to no urinary control. Bladder neck contractures also occur, resulting in obstructive voiding symptoms and urinary retention. The relationship between these symptoms and sense of bother is not direct; for example, those with the most leakage may have little bother, whereas those with minimal leakage may report substantial bother.

Radiation therapy is provided through external beam radiation or through implantation of radioactive sources (known as *brachytherapy*). The standard regimen of external beam radiation delivers a total of about 6,000–7,000 rads over 5–8 weeks. Hypofractionated schemes use higher doses per fraction that achieve biologically similar doses over 4–5 weeks. Pelvic lymph nodes can be radiated as well. Proctitis and urethritis are common acute adverse events. Chronic complications include erectile dysfunction, urinary incontinence, and chronic proctitis. The incidence of urinary stress incontinence after radiation therapy is significantly less than with surgery but that of irritative voiding dysfunction is greater. Bowel dysfunction, uncommon after surgery, affects more than half of patients after radiation. Bowel symptoms include diarrhea, rectal urgency, and fecal soiling. Most patients classify these bowel symptoms as minor with little to no effect on quality of life. Conformal radiation therapy is a mode of high-precision external-beam radiation that uses high-resolution CT scan data and advanced computer technology to conform the radiation dose to the 3-dimensional configuration of the tumor. This newer technology shows promise in reducing complications and adverse events. Local control and cancer survival rates appear to be comparable to those of radical prostatectomy, at least for the first 5–8 years (SOE=C). Comparisons between treatments are difficult, because men undergoing radiation treatment tend to be older, less medically fit, and usually have not been pathologically staged.

Brachytherapy involves retropubic or perineal implantation of radioactive seeds, usually iridium or palladium. Improvements in 3-dimensional imaging of the prostate through CT scan or ultrasound guidance have allowed more uniform distribution of seeds throughout the prostate and overcome many of the past limitations of brachytherapy. Potency is better preserved with seed implants. Urinary symptoms include frequency, dysuria, and urge incontinence. Bowel symptoms include rectal urgency and rectal bleeding. The morbidity of seed implants appears to improve over time after the initial seed placement and associated prostate inflammation and swelling. In retrospective series, it appears that brachytherapy is comparable to radical prostatectomy and external beam radiation for low-risk disease. However, brachytherapy outcomes appear less favorable for men with tumors that have a higher Gleason score or with higher pretreatment PSA levels (SOE=C).

In the Prostate Testing for Cancer and Treatment (ProtecT) trial, 1643 men 50–69 years old with PSA-detected localized prostate cancer were randomized to active monitoring, radical prostatectomy, or external beam radiation therapy. With a 10-year median follow-up, no significant difference in prostate cancer–specific or overall mortality was detected among the 3 groups. The rates of prostate cancer death were low and likely relate to the study population's favorable disease characteristics (median PSA 4.6 ng/mL, and >75% with clinical stage T1c and Gleason score 6 disease). Disease progression and development of metastases was higher in the active monitoring group. Patient-reported outcomes differed among the 3 groups. Prostatectomy had the greatest and most persistent negative impact on urinary continence and sexual function. At 6 months, radiotherapy had the worst impact on urinary voiding, nocturia, and bowel and sexual function with subsequent improvement. At 2 years follow-up, compared with active monitoring, treating 4 men with prostatectomy or 8 men with radiation therapy would cause one additional case of erectile dysfunction; treating 5 men with prostatectomy or 143 men with radiation therapy would cause one additional case of urinary incontinence (SOE=B).

Management of Locally Advanced Prostate Cancer

Locally advanced prostate cancer extends beyond the capsule or invades the seminal vesicle, without evidence of distant or nodal metastasis. Radiation therapy is the recommended treatment, and neoadjuvant androgen deprivation provides additional benefit toward increased survival and freedom from metastases (SOE=B). However, controversy exists as to when androgen deprivation should be started. Patients may have a prolonged asymptomatic cancer period, but significant negative quality-of-life changes from long-term androgen deprivation occur, including loss of stamina, increased fatigue, hot flashes, diminished muscle mass, and premature osteoporosis. Although radiation therapy with neoadjuvant androgen deprivation is a standard approach for locally advanced disease, some advocate that patients should be given the choice of early versus delayed androgen deprivation.

Management of Advanced Disease

Advanced disease is treated with androgen ablation and symptom-specific approaches, such as focal radiation therapy to painful bone metastasis. Androgen ablation aims to eliminate prostate cancer growth stimulation and includes orchiectomy or luteinizing hormone-releasing hormone (LHRH) agonists with antiandrogens. Orchiectomy and LHRH agonists are equally effective at reducing androgens to castration levels. Orchiectomy is the oldest, safest, least expensive approach but is rejected by nearly half of American men. LHRH agonists such as leuprolide and goserelin result in castration levels about 1 month after an initial increase in serum testosterone levels. Antiandrogens (eg, flutamide) are often given before starting LHRH agonists to blunt the effects of the initial testosterone increase. Antiandrogens inhibit the binding of androgen to its receptor. After castration, a small amount of adrenal androgen exists and may allow continued stimulation of prostate cancer growth. Antiandrogens can be combined with chemical or surgical castration, a practice called *complete androgen ablation*. Survival rates for antiandrogens alone are inferior to those for chemical or surgical castration alone; complete androgen ablation offers slight improvement in survival over that offered by castration only (SOE=B).

Chemotherapy with docetaxel helps delay disease progression and enhances overall survival in metastatic, hormone-sensitive prostate cancer (SOE=A). Giving 6 cycles of docetaxel at the start of androgen deprivation is becoming a first-line treatment of metastatic, hormone-naive prostate cancer. Docetaxel may also be used in metastatic prostate cancer patients who progress while on androgen-deprivation therapy.

Radiation therapy is useful for relieving the pain of isolated bone metastasis and reducing the risk of fracture of bones with significant destruction. Diffuse bone metastases require alternative approaches. Bone-seeking radiopharmaceuticals such as strontium or radium can be beneficial for pain control (SOE=B). Androgen deprivation decreases bone pain in two-thirds of symptomatic patients (SOE=B). Bisphosphonates also decrease bone pain (SOE=B).

PROSTATITIS

Etiology

Prostatitis is an inflammatory condition of the prostate that can result from acute bacterial, chronic bacterial, or nonbacterial causes. The most common sources of acute or chronic infection are ascending urethral infection or reflux of infected urine into the prostatic ducts, or both. Direct seeding can occur at the time of transrectal prostate biopsy. Direct extension or lymphatic spread from the rectum or hematogenous spread also occurs. Acute prostatitis is an infectious process that is more common in younger men than in older men. Uropathogens are the most common cause, predominantly *E coli*. In sexually active men, *Neisseria gonorrhea* and *Chlamydia trachomatis* should be considered. In older men, acute prostatitis is associated with indwelling urethral catheter use, and coliforms are the suspected bacterial cause. In >80% of patients with prostatitis, no infectious agent is identified.

Diagnosis

Acute bacterial prostatitis is characterized by fever, chills, dysuria, and a tense or boggy, extremely tender prostate. Because bacteremia can result from manipulation of the inflamed gland, minimal rectal examination is indicated. Gram stain and culture of the urine can identify the causative agent.

Chronic bacterial prostatitis presents classically as recurrent bacteriuria caused by the same organism, although most patients do not have this presentation. Patients have varying degrees of obstructive or irritative voiding symptoms and perineal pain. The prostate often feels normal. First-void or midstream urine is compared with expressed prostatic secretion or urine collected after prostatic massage. The expressed sample should reveal leukocytosis and the causative agent. Sterile expressant with leukocytosis suggests nonbacterial prostatitis.

Treatment

Acute bacterial prostatitis is treated with antibiotics and can require hospitalization. The severe inflammation allows antibiotics to penetrate the prostate, and prompt response to empiric therapy is expected. CT or MRI should be considered to evaluate for an abscess if recovery is delayed. Antibiotic selection should be based initially on results of a urine Gram stain, with subsequent consideration of sensitivity profiles. Fluoroquinolones are highly effective in most cases.

Antibiotics are less effective for chronic bacterial prostatitis because of their poor penetration of the prostate. Prolonged therapy (6–16 weeks) offers a cure rate of 30%–40%. Continuous low-dose antibiotic suppression therapy can be offered to those with frequent symptomatic relapse. Total prostatectomy offers cure but at a high risk-to-benefit ratio. Transurethral resection of the prostate is safer but cures only one-third of patients.

Nonbacterial prostatitis is treated symptomatically. A small percentage of cases can involve occult infections, and empiric antibiotic therapy is often used. Efforts to reduce pain and discomfort include anti-inflammatory agents, sitz baths, fluid adjustments (avoid caffeine), antimuscarinic agents, and α-adrenergic antagonists.

Choosing Wisely® Recommendations

Prostate Disease

- Do not perform PET, CT, and radionuclide bone scan in the staging of early prostate cancer at low risk of metastasis.
- A routine bone scan is unnecessary in men with low-risk prostate cancer.
- Do not order creatinine or upper-tract imaging for patients with benign prostatic hyperplasia.
- Do not treat an increased PSA with antibiotics for patients not experiencing other symptoms.

RESOURCES

- Cadet M. An overview of prostate cancer screening recommendations and shared decision-making process model to guide nursing practice. *Med Surg Nurs*. 2018;27(5):301–304.

- Hamdy FC, Donovan JL, Lane JA, et al. 10-Year outcomes after monitoring, surgery, or radiotherapy for localized prostate cancer. *N Engl J Med*. 2016;375(15):1415–1424.

- US Preventive Services Task Force. Screening for Prostate Cancer: US Preventive Services Task Force Recommendation Statement. *JAMA*. 2018;319(18):1901–1913.

CHAPTER 57—SEXUALITY

KEY POINTS

- Normal age-associated changes lead to decreased sexual interest and ability; however, complete sexual dysfunction is not a part of healthy aging.

- Physiologic changes in sexual response occur in both men and women. It is important to distinguish between normal age-associated changes and pathologic conditions that can be related to medications or medical disorders.

- Sexual activity in older adults typically must be planned. Success requires privacy, longer foreplay, help with vaginal lubrication, and understanding of the impact of aging and disease on sexual function.

- Many older women have sexual dysfunction but do not report it to their primary care providers unless asked.

- Multiple effective options are available to treat male and female sexual dysfunction.

- Prevention of sexually transmitted infection is still important despite older age.

- Sexuality is an important part of quality of life for many older adults; treatment of sexual dysfunction can improve well-being.

- Long-term care facilities need to be sensitive to the sexual needs of their residents and should have a sexual activity policy.

SEXUALITY AND AGING

Although older men and women are still interested in sex, sexual activity declines with age. In a large study of community-living older adults, the National Social Life, Health, and Aging Project (NSHAP), people 57–85 years old were surveyed. In the younger group (age 57–65 years), overall 62% of women and 85% of men reported they were sexually active the prior year, while among those with a partner 81% of women and 91% of men reported sexual activity. At age 75–85, only 17% of women and 39% of men reported sexual activity, while almost half of those with a partner were still sexually active.

Several factors may cause some older couples to stop sexual activity, including poor health, psychosocial issues (eg, aging sexual stigma that causes ambivalence toward sexuality, lack of privacy when living in adult child's home or long-term care setting), depression, decreased libido, and changes in sexuality with aging. In women, changes in sexual response include requiring longer clitoral stimulation, decreased genital engorgement, reduced vaginal lubrication, and, occasionally, painful uterine contractions during orgasm. Despite these changes, many older women can still achieve multiple orgasms. In men, sexual response changes include delay in achieving an erection, prolonged plateau stage, diminished duration and intensity of orgasm, prompt detumescence, and prolonged refractory period.

MALE SEXUALITY

Erectile Physiology and Dysfunction

Penile rigidity results from a complex interaction between the brain, spinal cord, testosterone, neurotransmitters, arterial inflow, and venous outflow. In brief, testosterone, mental health, and an attractive partner typically stimulate sexual interest (libido). Fantasy, visual, tactile, or other erotic stimuli (eg, scents or sounds) trigger neural impulses from the brain or spinal cord to the penis. Neural impulses cause release or synthesis of various neurotransmitters (eg, nitric oxide, cGMP), which induce arterial vasodilation and increased penile arterial inflow. Increasing arterial inflow results in penile tumescence, which impedes venous outflow. As the intrapenile (intracavernosal) pressure equilibrates to mean arterial pressure, the penis becomes rigid. Thus, there are many steps along the path that can be broken and result in erectile dysfunction (ED).

ED, the inability to achieve or maintain an erection adequate for intercourse, is the most common sexual problem of older men. By age 70, the prevalence of ED increases to 67%. This high prevalence is important; in a study comparing affected and unaffected men, men with sexual dysfunction reported impaired quality of life. For a summary of the causes of sexual dysfunction in men, see Table 57.1.

The most common cause (30%–50%) of ED in older men is vascular disease (SOE=A). Risk of vascular ED increases with traditional vascular risk factors, eg, diabetes mellitus, hypertension, hyperlipidemia, and smoking. In fact, ED is a predictor of future major atherosclerotic vascular events (ie, myocardial infarction and stroke).

Obstruction from atherosclerotic arterial occlusive disease likely impedes the intracavernosal blood flow and pressure needed to achieve a rigid erection. In addition, atherosclerotic disease can cause ischemia of trabecular smooth muscle and result in fibrotic changes leading to failure of venous closure mechanisms,

Table 57.1—Causes of Sexual Dysfunction in Older Men

Causes (in order of prevalence)	Characteristics
Vascular disease	■ Gradual onset Vascular risk factors: diabetes mellitus, hypertension, hyperlipidemia, tobacco use
Neurologic disease, eg, radiation therapy, spinal cord injury, autonomic dysfunction, surgical procedures	■ Gradual onset for progressive conditions; sudden onset for injury or surgery Neurologic risk factors: diabetes mellitus; history of pelvic injury, surgery, or irradiation; spinal injury or surgery; Parkinson disease; multiple sclerosis; alcoholism Loss of bulbocavernosus reflex
Medications, eg, anticholinergics, antihypertensives, cimetidine, antidepressants	■ Sudden onset Lack of sleep-associated erections or lack of erections with masturbation Temporal association with a new medication
Psychogenic, eg, relationship conflicts, performance anxiety, childhood sexual abuse, fear of sexually transmitted diseases, "widower's syndrome"	■ Sudden onset Sleep-associated erections or erections with masturbation are preserved
Hypogonadism	■ Gradual onset Decreased libido more than erectile dysfunction Small testes, gynecomastia Low serum testosterone concentration
Endocrine, eg, hypothyroidism, hyperthyroidism, hyperprolactinemia	■ Rare, <5% of cases of erectile dysfunction

ie, inability to impede venous outflow necessary for equilibration to mean arterial pressure causing penile rigidity. Venous leakage leading to vascular ED can also result from Peyronie disease, arteriovenous fistula, or trauma-induced communication between the glans and the corpora. In anxious men who have excessive adrenergic-constrictor tone and in men with injured parasympathetic dilator nerves, ED can result from insufficient relaxation of trabecular smooth muscle.

The second most common cause of ED in older men is neurologic disease (17%–37%). Disorders that affect the parasympathetic sacral spinal cord or the peripheral efferent autonomic fibers to the penis impair penile smooth muscle relaxation and prevent the vasodilation necessary for erection. In patients with prostate cancer, treatment frequently causes neurogenic erectile failure (brachytherapy or external radiation, 50%; radical prostatectomy with nerve sparing, 45%–80%) and pain on orgasm (SOE=B). Common health problems such as diabetes mellitus, stroke, and Parkinson disease can cause autonomic dysfunction that results in erectile failure. Finally, surgical procedures such as cystectomy and proctocolectomy commonly disrupt the autonomic nerve supply to the penis, resulting in postoperative ED.

Numerous commonly used medications have been associated with ED for which the mechanism, for the most part, is unknown. In approximately 5% of men with ED, the ED is drug-induced. Medications with anticholinergic effects, such as antidepressants, antipsychotics, and antihistamines, can cause ED by blocking parasympathetic-mediated penile artery vasodilatation and trabecular smooth muscle relaxation. Almost all antihypertensive agents have been associated with ED; of these, clonidine and thiazide diuretics have higher incidence rates, whereas ACE inhibitors and angiotensin-receptor blockers have lower incidence rates (SOE=B). One mechanism by which antihypertensives can cause ED is lowering blood pressure below the threshold needed to maintain sufficient blood flow for penile erection, especially in those men who already have penile arterial disease. OTC medications such as cimetidine and ranitidine can also cause ED. Cimetidine, an H_2-receptor antagonist, acts as an antiandrogen and increases prolactin secretion; thus, it has been associated with loss of libido and erectile failure. Ranitidine can also increase prolactin secretion, although less commonly than does cimetidine.

The prevalence of psychogenic ED correlates inversely with age. In approximately 9% of men ≥65 years old with ED, the ED is psychogenic. Psychogenic ED can develop via increased sympathetic stimuli to the sacral cord, inhibiting the parasympathetic dilator nerves and thus inhibiting erection. Common causes of psychogenic ED include relationship conflicts, performance anxiety, childhood sexual abuse, and fear of sexually transmitted diseases. Older men may have "widower's syndrome," in which the man involved in a new relationship feels guilt as a defense against subconscious unfaithfulness to his deceased spouse (may also occur in women ["widow's syndrome"]).

Hyperthyroidism, hypothyroidism, and hyperprolactinemia have been associated with ED. However, <5% of ED is caused by endocrine abnormalities. Thus, endocrine evaluation of men with ED but intact libido is of limited value (SOE=B).

The role of androgens in erection is becoming clearer. Hypogonadism is moderately common in older men. Hypogonadal men show smaller and slower developing erections in response to fantasy, which is improved with androgen replacement. However, even men with castrate levels of testosterone can attain erections in response to direct penile stimulation. It may be that erection from direct penile stimulation is less androgen dependent, whereas erection from fantasy is more androgen dependent. Nevertheless, testosterone is necessary for intracavernosal nitric oxide synthesis. Thus, testosterone plays a large role in libido and a smaller role in erectile function. For example, hypogonadal men do respond better to phosphodiesterase inhibitors after testosterone replacement therapy. However, men with ED and normal testosterone serum concentrations do not benefit from testosterone therapy. Rather, giving eugonadal men testosterone therapy may increase libido and vascular risk without improving erectile function.

Evaluation of Erectile Dysfunction

The initial step is to obtain a sexual, medical, and psychosocial history. Requesting permission to ask about sexuality is recommended for both sexually active older men and women. Without making assumptions about behavior, clinicians can then ask questions, in a straightforward and non-judgmental fashion, about number of partners, sexual orientation (eg, "Do you have sex with men, women, or both?"), sexual identity (eg, "Do you consider yourself trans [transgender, transsexual, or a person with a history of transitioning sex]?")", and sexual practices. In men, sexual history should clarify whether the problem consists of inadequate erections, decreased libido, or orgasmic failure. The onset and duration of ED, the presence or absence of sleep-associated erections, and the associated decline in libido are clues to the likely cause.

Sudden onset (in the absence of pelvic surgery) suggests psychogenic or drug-induced ED. A psychogenic cause is likely if there is a sudden onset but retention of sleep-associated erections or if erections with masturbation or a different partner are intact (SOE=A). If sudden-onset erectile failure is accompanied by lack of sleep-associated erections and lack of erection with masturbation, temporal association with new medication should be investigated. A gradual onset of ED associated with loss of libido suggests hypogonadism. Gradual onset associated with intact libido (most common presentation) suggests vascular, neurogenic, or other organic causes.

Medical history is directed at discerning those factors likely to be contributing to ED. Vascular risk factors include diabetes mellitus, hypertension, coronary artery disease, peripheral arterial disease, hyperlipidemia, and smoking. Neurogenic risk factors include diabetes mellitus; history of pelvic injury, surgery, or radiation; spinal injury or surgery; Parkinson disease; multiple sclerosis; or alcoholism. A thorough medication review, including OTC medications, is essential. Finally, the psychosocial history should assess the patient's relationship with the sexual partner, the partner's health and attitude toward sex, economic or social stresses, living situation, alcohol use, and affective disorders.

On physical examination, attention should be paid to signs of vascular or neurologic diseases. Peripheral pulses should be palpated. Signs of autonomic neuropathy (eg, orthostatic hypotension and absent heart rate response to standing) and loss of the bulbocavernosus reflex suggest neurologic dysfunction. The genital examination includes palpating the penis for Peyronie plaques and assessing for testicular atrophy. A femoral bruit and diminished (or absent) pedal pulses suggests arterial insufficiency. An absent bulbocavernosus reflex suggests penile neuropathy. A loss of secondary sexual characteristics, small testes, and gynecomastia suggest hypogonadism or hyperprolactinemia.

Appropriate laboratory evaluations are those that target relevant comorbid conditions such as diabetes mellitus and vascular disease or that evaluate neurologic disorders if suggested by the physical examination. The measurement of serum testosterone should be considered in the setting of other symptoms of androgen deficiency. As in older women, older men at risk of sexually transmitted infections (STIs) should be offered counselling and testing for HIV and other STIs. In 2009, the American College of Physicians recommended universal HIV screening up to age 75; in 2015, the CDC recommended universal HIV screening up to age 64 and screening adults ≥65 years old only if at increased risk of infection. Sexually active men who have sex with men should be screened for HIV and other STIs at least annually.

An at-home therapeutic trial of a phosphodiesterase inhibitor (sildenafil or vardenafil) is considered first-line evaluation and treatment. The initial dose should be low (sildenafil 25–50 mg or vardenafil 5–10 mg) in men suspected of having neurogenic ED. A poor response suggests vasculogenic ED. Further therapeutic trial with sildenafil at 100 mg or vardenafil at 20 mg may prove to be effective. An at-home therapeutic trial using tadalafil (5–10 mg) can be considered, but its long half-life complicates matters if an adverse event occurs with the first dose.

More extensive diagnostic tools are available but not commonly used. Nocturnal penile tumescence testing is of little value, except to confirm a psychogenic cause. The penile-brachial pressure index can be helpful in assessing arteriogenic ED. This index measures

Table 57.2—Treatment Options for Erectile Dysfunction

Treatment	Route/ Administration	Onset	Duration of Action	Dosage	Selected Adverse Events
Sildenafil	Oral	60 min	4 h	25–100 mg	Headache, flushing, rhinitis, dyspepsia, transient color blindness; contraindicated with nitrate use and α-blockers
Vardenafil	Oral	45 min	4 h	5–20 mg	Headache, flushing, rhinitis, dyspepsia; contraindicated with nitrate use and α-blockers
Tadalafil	Oral	45–60 min	24–36 h	5–20 mg	Headache, dyspepsia, flushing, rhinitis; contraindicated with nitrate use and α-blockers
Avanafil	Oral	30 min		100 mg	Headache, flushing, prolonged erection; contraindicated with nitrate use and α-blockers
Vacuum device	External	<5 min	30 min	—	Petechiae, bruising, painful ejaculation
Papaverine^{OL}	Intracavernosal	10 min	30–60 min	15–60 mg	Prolonged erection, fibrosis, ecchymosis
Alprostadil	Intracavernosal	10 min	40–60 min	5–20 mcg	Prolonged erection, pain, fibrosis
Phentolamine^{OL}	Intracavernosal	10 min	30–60 min	0.5–1 mg	Prolonged erection, fibrosis, headache, facial flushing
Medicated urethral system for erection (MUSE)	Intraurethral	10–15 min	60–80 min	250–1,000 mcg	Penile pain or burning, hypotension
Penile prosthesis	Surgical		replacement in 5–10 years	—	Infection, erosion, mechanical failure
Sex therapy	Counseling	weeks	years	weekly	Anxiety

NOTE: Above treatments, excluding sex therapy, are effective for neurogenic causes and may be helpful for arteriogenic and venogenic etiologies. Vacuum device and sex therapy are effective for psychogenic causes.

the loss of systolic pressure between the arm and the penis. When measured before and after exercise, it can be used to assess for a pelvic steal syndrome, which is the loss of erection associated with initiation of active pelvic thrusting, presumably due to the transfer of blood flow from the penis to the pelvic musculature. More invasive and expensive tests such as Doppler ultrasound to assess penile arterial function, dynamic infusion cavernosometry to assess venous leakage syndrome, and penile arteriography are generally reserved for research or penile vascular surgery candidates.

Treatment of Erectile Dysfunction

Multiple effective therapeutic options are available for the treatment of ED. Treatment should be individualized and based on cause, personal preference, partner issues, cost, and practicality (Table 57.2).

Oral therapy for ED with sildenafil, vardenafil, tadalafil, or avanafil has revolutionized treatment of male sexual dysfunction. Sildenafil is a type-5 phosphodiesterase inhibitor that potentiates the penile response to sexual stimulation. It improves the rigidity and duration of erection. It is taken 1 hour before sexual activity and has no effect until sexual stimulation occurs. Because absorption is attenuated when sildenafil is ingested with a fatty meal, patients need to be educated about this issue. Vardenafil is a more potent and specific phosphodiesterase inhibitor. A lower effective dose and better adverse-event profile (no effect on color vision) make vardenafil a reasonable option. Tadalafil is a longer-acting phosphodiesterase inhibitor with an adverse-event profile similar to that of vardenafil but with the added potential problem of muscle pain. Avanafil is a more recently approved phosphodiesterase inhibitor; it is taken 30 minutes before sexual activity. All four of these agents are contraindicated for concomitant use with nitrate medications, because the combination can produce profound and fatal hypotension. In addition, combined use of α-blockers with phosphodiesterase inhibitors should be done with caution, starting with the lowest dose of either. Choosing among these phosphodiesterase inhibitors should likely be based on price and patient preference. All phosphodiesterase inhibitors result in sufficient penile rigidity for an approximately 50% success rate at intercourse. Because of the longer duration of action of tadalafil, men tend to select it when given the choice (SOE=B).

Vacuum-assisted erection devices are another option. The apparatus consists of a plastic cylinder with an open end into which the penis is inserted. A vacuum device attached to the cylinder creates negative pressure within the cylinder, and blood flows into the penis to produce penile rigidity. A constriction ring placed at the base of the penis then traps the blood in the corpora cavernosa to maintain an erection for about 30 minutes. The vacuum device is effective for psychogenic, neurogenic, and venogenic ED, but it requires manual dexterity. Local pain, swelling, bruising, coolness of penile tip, and painful ejaculation are potential adverse events. It is important to remove the constriction ring after 30 minutes. This device is not recommended for men on anticoagulant therapy or with a history of bleeding disorders.

Intracavernosal injection of vasoactive drugs such as papaverine, phentolamine, and alprostadil are effective in producing erections adequate for sexual activity (SOE=A) but are used much less frequently since oral therapy has become available. Alprostadil, which is the only agent approved by the FDA for intracavernosal injection, produces erections that last 40–60 minutes. Phentolamine[OL] is mainly used in combination therapy with papaverine[OL] or alprostadil, or both. Potential adverse events are bruising, ecchymoses or hematoma, local pain, fibrosis from repeated injections, and priapism. Alprostadil appears to cause less scarring and priapism than papaverine. If an erection lasts >4 hours, detumescence is necessary by aspiration of blood from the corpora cavernosa or injection of phenylephrine because of the potential for intracavernosal hypoxia and fibrosis of trabecular smooth muscle, which can prevent future erections. In general, intracavernosal therapy should probably be reserved for patients in whom oral therapy with a phosphodiesterase inhibitor is not effective. Alprostadil can also be administered intraurethrally using a medicated urethral system for erection (MUSE). This system contains a small pellet of alprostadil that is placed within the urethra and is absorbed through the urethral mucosa to produce an erection within 10–15 minutes. Possible adverse events are penile pain, urethral burning, and a throbbing sensation in the perineum. The sexual partner may also experience burning or irritation if the intraurethral alprostadil is expelled during sexual activity.

Testosterone therapy (TT) increases libido and can improve ED in men with true hypogonadism (SOE=B). However, as mentioned above, it has little value in eugonadal men with ED. Testosterone is available as an intramuscular injection (short-acting: testosterone enanthate or cypionate; long-acting: undecanoate), buccal patch, intranasal, transdermal patch, and gel. Possible adverse events associated with TT include polycythemia, prostate enlargement, gynecomastia, and fluid retention. It is important to perform a digital rectal examination to assess the prostate and obtain a baseline prostate-specific antigen (PSA) level and hematocrit before beginning TT. If PSA or hematocrit increases with TT, it usually does so within 6 months. Therefore, these levels should be checked every 3 months during the first year of therapy, then every 12 months thereafter. It is important to discontinue TT until further assessment if hematocrit is >54% (markedly increased hematocrit may require phlebotomy) or PSA is increased. Of note, several retrospective studies have suggested that TT increases the risk of cardiovascular disease. Also, in a randomized, placebo-controlled trial in older men with symptomatic hypogonadism, TT was associated with a significantly greater increase in coronary artery plaque volume than placebo. However, there are meta-analyses that found no increase in the risk of cardiovascular disease in hypogonadal men treated with testosterone compared with placebo. Similarly, while TT is commonly believed to increase the risk of prostate cancer or worsen lower urinary tract symptoms, recent studies in hypogonadal men do not support this. Patients should be informed of the potential risks and benefits before starting TT.

Surgical implantation of a penile prosthesis is another therapeutic option. Mechanical failure, infection, device erosion, and fibrosis are possible complications. However, since the availability of alprostadil and, more recently, phosphodiesterase inhibitors, surgical implantation of a penile prosthesis is rarely done (ie, used in men with severe arterial occlusive disease). Nevertheless, long-term patient satisfaction with penile prosthesis is actually higher than with oral therapy (SOE=B). Penile revascularization surgery has limited success.

Men with psychogenic ED should be referred to a mental health or other professional specializing in treatment of sexual disorders for further evaluation and treatment.

FEMALE SEXUALITY

Female Sexual Dysfunction

For the most part, menopause is accompanied by decreased sexual function, with decreased sexual interest, responsiveness, and coital frequency. In addition, there is an increase in urogenital symptoms, often not discussed with the clinician. For example, in the NSHAP, among women 75–85 years old who were sexually active, the most common sexual problem was lack of interest (49.3%), followed by difficulty with lubrication (43.6%), inability to climax (38.2%), lack of pleasure during sex (24.9%), and dyspareunia (11.8%).

Dyspareunia, defined as pain with intercourse, can be due to organic or psychologic factors, or a combination. For example, a woman can experience an episode of dyspareunia because of postmenopausal vaginal atrophy. With each subsequent sexual encounter, she anticipates pain, causing inadequate arousal with decreased lubrication. Because of this cycle, she continues to experience dyspareunia, even after the vaginal atrophy has been treated. The most common organic cause of dyspareunia is vaginal atrophy (also referred to as vulvovaginal atrophy or atrophic vaginitis) due to estrogen deficiency. The term *genitourinary syndrome of menopause* encompasses both vulvovaginal and bladder-urethral symptoms due to estrogen deficiency. It affects up to 45% of postmenopausal women. Because of lack of estrogen, the vaginal epithelium becomes thinner and pH rises from a premenopausal value of 3.5–4.5 to a postmenopausal range of 5.0–7.5, which increases the risk of bacterial colonization and urinary tract infections. Other causes of dyspareunia include inadequate lubrication, localized vaginal infections, cystitis, Bartholin cyst, retroverted uterus, marked uterine prolapse, endometriosis, pelvic tumors, excessive penile thrusting, or vaginismus (involuntary muscle spasms).

Local estrogen therapy can improve symptoms of vaginal atrophy, but it has little effect on libido or sexual satisfaction (SOE=B). Androgens have more of a role in libido in women. The ovaries and adrenals are the main sources of androgens in women. The effects of female androgen deficiency were originally identified in women treated for advanced breast cancer with oophorectomy and adrenalectomy. When deprived of androgens, these women reported loss of libido. Hypoactive sexual desire disorder (HSDD) is defined as decreased libido that causes personal distress and is not due to a psychiatric or medical illness or a substance (such as medication). HSDD is thought to be due to low testosterone. Because there are no normative data on plasma total and free testosterone in women and no well-defined clinical syndrome of androgen deficiency, the Endocrine Society has not recommended making a diagnosis of androgen deficiency in women.

Older women commonly have multiple medical conditions, some of which affect sexuality. However, scientific studies on the effect of chronic diseases and medications on the sexuality of older women are limited. Women with diabetes mellitus are less likely to be sexually active, and report decreased libido and lubrication and longer time to reach orgasm. Rheumatic diseases affect sexuality via functional disability. After mastectomy for breast cancer, 20%–40% of women experience sexual dysfunction, possibly because of disruption of body image, marital and family problems, spousal reaction, adjuvant therapy, or the psychologic impact of a breast cancer diagnosis. Several drugs can adversely affect sexual function, including antidepressants (with higher rates for SSRIs and lower rates for bupropion), antihypertensives, antipsychotics, antiestrogens, antiandrogens, anticholinergic drugs, narcotics, alcohol, and illicit/recreational drugs.

Evaluation and Treatment

In sexually active older women, as in men, taking a sexual health history is the most important step of the evaluation. The history should include questions about number of sexual partners, sexual orientation, identity, and practices. Careful and sensitive questioning can detect problems that a woman might not otherwise volunteer. In a survey of postmenopausal women, 43% experienced menopause-related vaginal discomfort; of these, 40% reported it affected their sex life but 66% did not discuss the condition with their clinician because of embarrassment and 33% expressed preference for the clinician to initiate the discussion. About half of the women did not know that topical treatments are available for vaginal discomfort. Clinicians should ask about dyspareunia, lack of vaginal lubrication, quality of the relationship and sexual communication with the partner, and previous negative experiences, such as rape, child abuse, or domestic violence. Medications should be carefully reviewed. A woman with dyspareunia should undergo a pelvic examination to exclude organic causes.

Older women who are sexually active should be counselled about risk factors for sexually transmitted infections (STs) and about testing for HIV and other STIs if they are at risk. It is important to note that older adults have increased potential to acquire STIs. Longer, more active living combined with increased rates of divorce increases the number of new sexual partners and a new sexual partner within the last 3 months is an indication for screening for STIs. Postmenopausal atrophic changes in the vaginal mucosa may lead to microabrasions during intercourse and therefore increase risk of STIs. Older adults may find negotiating safer sex unfamiliar and challenging, lack knowledge about HIV/AIDS risk factors, and be less likely to use condoms. Women who have sex with women should be educated that STIs can spread between female sex partners through exchange of cervicovaginal secretions or by direct mucosal contact. Sex toys can transmit STIs; in fact, the human papilloma virus has been detected on vibrators even after standard cleaning. Preventive measures to limit exchange of bodily fluids include washing hands, not sharing sex toys, and/or using protective barriers such as gloves for digital-vaginal sex, condoms for vaginally inserted toys, and dental dams for oral-vaginal or oral-anal sex.

Decreased lubrication, vaginal discomfort, itching, and dyspareunia due to vaginal atrophy respond well to topical estrogen therapy (SOE=A). In the United States, there are three topical estrogen formulations that are considered "low-dose," because they cause minimal systemic absorption without significant proliferation of the endometrial lining. A low-dose conjugated estrogen cream regimen is 0.5 g once daily 21 days on/7 days off (cyclic regimen) or 0.5 g twice weekly (continuous regimen). The plastic applicator is calibrated in 0.5-g increments with a minimum of 0.5 g and a maximum of 2 g. It can be difficult for an older woman to self-administer the 0.5-g dose accurately, but doses >0.5 g are not considered "low-dose" and may have systemic effects. The low-dose vaginal estradiol ring releases estradiol at 7.5 mcg/d; the ring is replaced by the patient or provider every 90 days. Although the ring is left in the upper third of the vagina for 3 months, it does not interfere with intercourse. The estradiol vaginal tablet (10 mcg) is placed in the vagina daily for 2 weeks, then 1 tablet twice a week. The estradiol ring and tablet are better tolerated than topical estrogen creams because of ease of use and comfort. In the 2013 Position Statement on the management of vulvovaginal atrophy, the North American Menopause Society recommends discussing with the patient's oncologist before starting a woman with breast cancer on topical estrogen because of lack of safety data beyond 1 year. The AGS Beers Criteria® notes that vaginal estrogens for the treatment of vaginal dryness are safe and effective; women with a history of breast cancer who do not respond to nonhormonal therapies are advised to discuss the risk and benefits of low-dose vaginal estrogen (dosages of estradiol <25 mcg twice weekly) with their health care provider.

In 2016, the FDA approved topical prasterone, a synthetic dehydroepiandrosterone (DHEA), for dyspareunia due to vulvovaginal atrophy. Prasterone as 6.5 mg (0.5%) daily vaginal tablet improved symptoms of dyspareunia in a 12-week randomized trial (SOE=B). It caused a slight increase in DHEA, testosterone, and estrone plasma levels but all within the normal postmenopausal values. As with low-dose topical estrogens, prasterone should be used with caution in women with estrogen-sensitive malignancies.

For mild symptoms of vaginal atrophy or if the patient is not a candidate for topical hormones, vaginal moisturizers with the addition of lubricants during intercourse can provide some relief but are not effective in reversing the atrophic changes. An alternative for women with atrophic vaginitis who do not like to use topical agents is the oral selective estrogen-receptor modulator ospemifene. It is approved by the FDA for moderate to severe dyspareunia due to vaginal atrophy. In a 12-week randomized trial, ospemifene administered orally at 60 mg/d improved symptoms of dyspareunia and improved vaginal epithelium and pH. It caused a slight increase in endometrial thickness from baseline, but biopsies did not show endometrial hyperplasia or carcinoma. Although ospemifene is effective, long-term safety data are lacking. Systemic adverse effects include hot flashes and increased risk of thromboembolism.

Importantly, local stimulation through regular intercourse helps maintain a healthy vaginal mucosa. Longer foreplay allows more time for vaginal lubrication in older women, just as older men often need longer and more direct stimulation to achieve an adequate erection.

Decreased libido without identifiable cause may respond to testosterone, but no androgen preparation is approved by the FDA for hypoactive sexual desire disorder in women. In several placebo-controlled, randomized trials, low-dose testosterone patch[OL] delivering 300 mcg/d dosed twice weekly or daily improved sexual desire in women with natural or surgical menopause and on systemic estrogens. Androgenic adverse events such as acne and hirsutism were mild, and concentrations of high-density lipoprotein cholesterol did not decrease as in studies with oral methyltestosterone. The testosterone patch was also effective in women with natural or surgically induced menopause who had decreased libido and were not taking estrogens. Although the testosterone patch seems effective (SOE=B), there are only limited data on its long-term safety in women. As mention above the topical androgen DHEA is FDA approved only for dyspareunia, not for decreased libido.

Finally, older women should receive education about male sexual aging in addition to female sexual aging. Otherwise, an older woman might mistakenly attribute her partner's diminished erection and need for more genital stimulation to her own inability to arouse her partner. Other psychologic issues, including depression, history of sexual abuse, and relationship problems, should be addressed and treated with antidepressants, psychotherapy, and marital therapy, as necessary (SOE=C). A sex therapist can be identified on the website of the American Association of Sex Educators, Counselors, and Therapists (www.aasect.org). For a summary of treatments for female sexual dysfunction, see Table 57.3.

SEXUALITY IN LONG-TERM CARE

Despite evidence of the contrary, the myth of older adults as asexual beings still persists, especially in the nursing-home setting, where sexual needs of residents are frequently ignored. Sexual expressions are often considered behavioral problems that need to be suppressed. The need for love, touch, companionship, and intimacy continues in older age. In a survey of nursing-home residents, most reported sexual thoughts and feelings but lacked the opportunity for sexual activity. Nursing-home residents are faced with multiple barriers to express their sexuality: lack of privacy, lack of a partner, staff and family members' attitudes, mental

Table 57.3—Treatment Options for Sexual Dysfunction in Older Women

Symptom	Possible Cause	Therapy
Decreased desire	Low testosterone from natural or surgical menopause Chronic illness Depression Relationship problems Medications	Testosterone[OL] is not recommended by the Endocrine Society Treatment of underlying illness Antidepressant medication Marital therapy Review of drug regimen
Decreased lubrication	Vaginal dryness or atrophy from postmenopausal status	Longer foreplay, regular intercourse, moisturizers/lubricants, low-dose topical estrogens
	Antiestrogens and anticholinergic medications	Review of medications, including OTC drugs
Delayed or absent orgasm	Neurologic disorders, diabetes Psychologic problems	Treatment of underlying illness Cognitive-behavioral therapy, masturbation, Kegel exercises
Pain with intercourse	Organic cause Vaginal dryness, atrophy	Treatment of underlying physical condition Longer foreplay, regular intercourse, moisturizers/lubricants, low-dose topical estrogens or topical DHEA, oral estrogen-receptor modulator (ospemifene)
	Vaginismus (involuntary vaginal contractions)	Psychotherapy, cognitive-behavioral therapy

and physical illness, adverse effects of medications, feeling of being unattractive, and an insufficient understanding of sexuality. The most common sexual behaviors observed in nursing homes are hand holding, kissing, caressing, and masturbation.

Sexuality in the nursing home poses difficult legal and ethical dilemmas. A goal of the nursing home is to promote quality of life and autonomy. Because adults have the right to consensual sexual activity, the nursing home should provide appropriate accommodation for consensual and private sexual relationships. However, the nursing home also has a duty to protect residents from harm, including evaluating the risk of sexually transmitted diseases and protecting against sexual abuse if the resident is not capable of consenting to sexual activity. Furthermore, nursing homes are designed to facilitate observation of the residents with the priority of providing medical care, nutrition, hygiene, and a safe environment; this makes it difficult to provide privacy for sexual activity. In addition, both nursing home staff and family members come from varied cultural, moral, and religious backgrounds and may have negative views of sexuality in the residents.

A 2016 national survey of 366 nursing directors of U.S. nursing homes found that the majority (71%) had experienced issues of residents' sexuality; 58% reported sexual activity between residents, 22% reported sexual activity between residents and visitors, and 60% reported resident masturbation. In addition, 57% required next-of-kin approval of sexual activity of a cognitively impaired resident, and 12% required next-of-kin approval even if the resident was cognitively intact. Despite the high prevalence of sexual activity, only 37% of the nursing homes had a policy about sexual activity.

The medical director should ensure that the nursing home has a written sexual activity policy to help the interdisciplinary team create an individualized care plan that addresses sexuality. The first step is to determine whether the resident has capacity to consent to sexual activity. According to the 2016 American Medical Director Association (AMDA) white paper "Capacity for Sexual Consent in Dementia in Long-Term Care" (http://bit.ly/2y97LbS), a diagnosis of dementia does not necessarily imply lack of capacity for sexual consent, which should be viewed along a continuum of sexual activities, from touching to penetrative intercourse. A higher degree of intimacy and risk requires a higher degree of capacity to consent, with a lower threshold for consent for engaging in hand holding or kissing. The most commonly used criteria to assess consent include knowledge of the facts, including risks and benefits; understanding or reasoning consistent with the individual's values (which may change over time); and voluntariness of the consent, free from coercion. While there is no validated instrument to assess sexual consent capacity, Lichtenberg suggests these 3 elements: 1) resident awareness of relationship (Is the resident aware of who is initiating the relationship or have a delusional belief that the other person is his or her spouse?), 2) resident ability to avoid exploitation (Is this relationship consistent with former beliefs/values, and is the resident capable of rejecting unwanted sexual contact? The ability to refuse sexual advances is an important consideration in assessment of capacity to consent.), and 3) resident awareness of potential risk (Does the resident realize the relationship may be temporary and can describe how he or she will react when it will end?).

The issues of family involvement in the decision regarding sexual activity in residents with cognitive impairment is challenging, The nursing home must balance the family's desire to be informed, with the resident's desire for privacy if it is determined that he or she has capacity to consent to sexual activity. Education and counseling of both family and staff on the sexual activity policy is essential. Several studies have shown that sexual sensitivity training of nursing staff improves attitudes. Capacity may decline with time and therefore will need to be reassessed periodically. When the resident has lost capacity to consent, the next-of-kin or proxy decision maker must be informed of any sexual interaction and decide whether it should continue. Additional resources for the most challenging cases include ombudsmen, ethics committees, and psychiatric consultation.

The concept of what is inappropriate sexual behavior (ISB) depends on religious and societal views and has been defined as "disruptive behavior characterized by a verbal or physical act of an explicit or perceived sexual nature, which is unacceptable within the social context in which it is carried out." Residents with dementia may manifest sexual behaviors that can be considerate appropriate (such as masturbating in private or sitting next to another resident and kissing or stroking on the face, hands, or arms when both are capable of consent) or inappropriate (such as public masturbation, exposing, touching staff's or other resident's breasts or genitalia, and explicit sex talk). The staff should be educated to interpret ISB as inappropriate choices regarding sexuality, which is a basic need in human life, rather than as an offensive behavior. Some behaviors such as public shedding of clothing or touching of one's own genitals might be due to restlessness/agitation from discomfort, feeling hot, under stimulation, an unfamiliar environment, or stereotyped movements associated with dementia rather than due to sexual urges. ISB could also be due to the lack of the usual partner, misidentification of someone as the usual partner, or misinterpretation of nonsexual acts such as routine nursing care. Instruments, such as the St. Andrew's Sexual Behaviour Assessment, can help standardize documentation of severity of the ISB. If the inappropriate behavior is new, the resident should be evaluated for possible delirium. Medications that can contribute to the inappropriate behavior include dopamine agonists, androgen supplements, and benzodiazepines. Once medical conditions are excluded, behavioral management should be attempted with environmental and behavioral strategies. Some examples include removing precipitating factors, using clothing that opens in the back, redirecting, distracting with activities that keep the hands busy, providing dolls, ensuring opportunities for affection from family and pets and private conjugal visits if possible to satisfy the resident's need for love and intimacy (SOE=C).

There are little data on pharmacologic management of inappropriate sexual behaviors in residents with dementia, consisting mainly of case reports and cases series. Serotoninergic drugs (especially SSRIs) are considered first choice, followed by other antidepressants. Use of hormonal agents is considered controversial, because their use is viewed as a chemical castration. These agents include antiandrogens (cyproterone acetate, medroxyprogesterone), LHRH agonists, and estrogens. Finasteride blocks conversion of testosterone to dihydrotestosterone and decreases libido. Other drugs include anticonvulsants, antipsychotics, cholinesterase inhibitors, and β-blockers (SOE=C). Use of these medications for inappropriate sexual behavior is considered off-label, and risks and benefits should be discussed in detail with family members.

LESBIAN, GAY, BISEXUAL, AND TRANSGENDER OLDER ADULTS IN LONG-TERM CARE

Although data are limited on lesbian, gay, bisexual, and transgender (LGBT) people, it is estimated that they range from 5% to 10% of the general population. As LGBT older adults become frail, they have the same needs for public programs and assistance as heterosexual older adults. Since the 2015 Supreme Court decision, Obergefell v. Hodges made same-sex marriage legal in every state, and same-sex married couples receive the same Medicare and Medicaid coverage as heterosexual couples, including the spousal impoverishment protection that allows one spouse to keep the residence when the other needs to "spend down" to become Medicaid eligible to pay for nursing-home care.

LGBT older adults often face prejudice and ignorance when they enter a nursing home. Lack of sensitivity for sexual activities is even stronger than it is for homosexual expressions. The first form of discrimination LGBT older adults may encounter is heterosexism, or the assumption that every resident is or should be heterosexual; therefore, data on sexual orientation and gender identity/transgender status are not collected on admission. Even if a sexual history is taken, LGBT older adults might choose not to disclose their sexual orientation or identity even if they were living "out of the closet" before entering the nursing home.

In a survey, LGBT individuals suspected that staff and residents of long-term care facilities discriminate against LGBT older adults and felt they would have to hide their sexual orientation if admitted to a nursing home. They also felt that LGBT sensitivity training and possibly LGBT-specific retirement facilities would be beneficial for LGBT older adults. Being "in the closet" has negative psychological and health effects for LGBT individuals. LGBT individuals become more isolated and depressed when they cannot talk about their lives and if they have to hide pictures or other signs of their identity in fear of discrimination. Even when providers feel compassionate toward LGBT older adults, they might not have the training necessary to know how to provide care in a culturally competent way or how to handle difficult situations, such as when a heterosexual resident or other staff member make homophobic comments regarding an LGBT resident.

Directors of long-term care communities have several resources available to provide LGBT cultural competence training to their staff, for example the National Resource Center on LGBT Aging provides a free online learning tool: "Building Respect for LGBT Older Adults" (www.lgbtagingcenter.org). Services and Advocacy for LGBT Elders (SAGE) in New York City offers LGBT competency for businesses that want to train their staff and receive a "SAGECare Credential" that indicates employees have completed training on LGBT aging by SAGECare (http://sageusa.care).

RESOURCES

- Link D. Let's talk about sex. *J Nurs Pract*. 2018;14(3):213–214.

- National Institute on Aging. Intimacy and Sexuality: Resources for Dementia Caregivers. www.nia.nih.gov/health/intimacy-and-sexuality-resources-dementia-caregivers#pro (accessed Feb 2019).

CHAPTER 58—MUSCULOSKELETAL PAIN

KEY POINTS

- The most common cause of pain in older adults is related to musculoskeletal issues.

- Back problems are the third most common reason for clinician visits by older adults.

- Lumbar spinal stenosis pain is characterized by back pain radiating into the buttocks or legs that is worse on standing and walking, particularly downhill, and is relieved with sitting.

- About 25% of women will experience a vertebral compression fracture in their lifetime.

- Laboratory tests and diagnostic imaging procedures should not be performed until potential diagnoses have been narrowed from the history and physical examination.

GENERAL PRINCIPLES FOR DIAGNOSIS

Pain is a major issue for many older adults, and the most common cause is a musculoskeletal problem. Systemic analgesics have significant adverse effects in older adults and are often ineffective in position-associated musculoskeletal pain. The best way to manage pain is to find its source. The search for this cause can be both challenging and rewarding. Laboratory tests and diagnostic imaging studies may identify abnormalities, but they do not indicate whether these findings are the cause of the patient's pain. In the words of a sage clinician "you can't read pain on an x-ray." The search for the source of pain requires knowledge of the referral patterns of pain for musculoskeletal conditions as well as the ability to take a careful and well-focused history and perform an appropriate joint and manual muscle examination. The history should thoroughly review the characteristics, chronology, intensity, and precipitants of the patient's pain. What symptoms accompany the pain? What brings on the pain? Is the pain exacerbated when going from lying to sitting, ascending or descending stairs, standing, or walking? Is the pain worse in the morning, midday, or nighttime? Does the pain radiate? Does the pain cause the patient to cease the activity associated with the pain?

The pattern of the pain is also important. Pain that is gradual at onset and progressively worsens raises concern for a systemic condition such as a tumor or infection. Pain that is relatively abrupt at onset and related to position is more typical of mechanical pain. Some mechanical pain, such as rotator cuff tendonitis, is worse at night, interrupting sleep. Many musculoskeletal conditions produce pain at sites quite distant from the structure involved. The referral patterns of musculoskeletal conditions have been mapped out by numerous investigators. Neck conditions produce pain throughout the trapezius and retroscapular region. Shoulder and neck disease can cause pain throughout the arm. Lumbar spine disease can produce discomfort in the back and legs, whereas pain in the buttock, thigh, groin, and knee may originate from the hip.

Once the clinician has used this history to target likely causes of pain, the patient must be observed and examined to complete the assessment.

When an older adult presents with pain in more than one joint, a systemic process should be considered; however, older adults often have multiple mechanical problems in different sites of the body. For example, many older adults may have osteoarthritis of the knees and hips along with tendonitis of the rotator cuff structures. Others might have inflammatory arthritis with involvement of the knees and shoulders. An examination of the joints is the best method of distinguishing a systemic process from multiple mechanical problems.

A thorough physical examination should focus on an assessment of joints and muscle groups. A manual muscle examination can identify patterns of weakness associated with musculoskeletal problems. The joint examination should focus on malalignment and swelling of joints, whether the swelling is soft tissue or bony enlargement, decreased range of motion, and patterns of joint involvement consistent with specific conditions. For example, generalized osteoarthritis affects the distal interphalangeal joints, proximal interphalangeal joints, the first carpal-metacarpal joint, hips, knees, and tarsal-metatarsal joints of the foot. This condition does not involve the metacarpal-phalangeal joints, wrists, shoulders, or ankles.

Careful observation of the patient's mobility is an essential part of the examination in the search for the cause of the pain. Does the patient have a limp, spending less time on one leg than the other when walking? Does he or she have difficulty picking up a leg when going from a sitting to a supine position? Is the pain reproduced by ascending or descending stairs?

Laboratory tests or diagnostic imaging procedures should not be performed until the list of potential diagnoses has been narrowed from the history and physical examination. The incidence of abnormalities of diagnostic imaging tests on asymptomatic older patients is very high. Obtaining these studies early in the evaluation process can mislead the clinician, often directing the process down the wrong path. If the clinician feels that mechanical internal derangement of the knee is the most likely cause of the patient's complaint, then meniscal abnormalities on an MRI can be helpful. If the patient is more likely to have a systemic inflammatory process, these same abnormalities are incidental and should not direct therapy.

EVALUATION AND MANAGEMENT OF REGIONAL MUSCULOSKELETAL COMPLAINTS

Neck Pain

When a patient complains of "shoulder pain," it is important to know exactly where the individual feels pain and what activities exacerbate the symptoms. Both the cervical spine and shoulder structures can cause pain in this area. If the pain is felt predominantly in the trapezius and retroscapular region and brought on by rotating the neck with such activities as backing an automobile out of a driveway, the neck is the likely source of the pain. Shoulder conditions are more apt to produce pain when the upper arm is moved in such maneuvers as putting on a jacket or a coat or reaching above the head.

A number of systemic conditions, such as polymyalgia rheumatic, rheumatoid arthritis, and other inflammatory conditions, can cause neck pain. Pain with these conditions is usually worse in the morning, associated with joint complaints elsewhere in the body, and with systemic symptoms and signs. Examination of the neck may not diagnose these conditions; however, inflammation in the small joints of the hands and wrists can lead the clinician to the correct diagnosis.

The extent of pain at onset and the presence of radicular symptoms are the most important predictors of outcome in patients with mechanical neck disease. The severity of radiographic abnormalities does not predict this outcome.

The myelopathy produced by cervical stenosis does not usually cause neck pain. Rather, it is often characterized by a spastic gait disturbance and weakness in the lower extremities with upper motor neuron signs, including hyperreflexia, increased muscle tone, and positive Babinski signs. This condition can also produce lower motor neuron findings in the upper extremities. Thus, physical examination findings of lower motor neuron disease in the upper extremities and upper motor neuron disease in the lower extremities suggest cervical stenosis. The same neurologic pattern can be seen in amyotrophic lateral sclerosis. Bladder symptoms of cervical stenosis include urgency, frequency, or retention. This condition should be identified as early as possible, because it is a potentially reversible cause of leg weakness and spasticity.

Cervical radiculopathy is characterized by pain in the neck and arm, sensory loss, loss of motor function, and reflex changes in the affected nerve-root distribution. It is usually due to encroachment of the neuroforamina of the cervical spine. The C7 nerve root is most frequently affected. Pain that is reproduced by rotating the head or bending it toward the symptomatic side suggests this diagnosis. Most patients improve with symptomatic treatment, and only a relatively small number require surgery.

Most older adults with neck pain have nonspecific mechanical disease of the cervical spine. Cervical disc displacement appears to be a frequent cause of these complaints. Cervical disc disease can be referred into several regions. C2-C3 disease is felt in the occiput; C3-C4 and C4-C5 problems are referred into the posterior and lateral aspects of the neck; C5-C6 lesions are referred into the trapezius and upper cervical regions; C6-C7 disease is felt in the retroscapular region, often as far down as the mid to lower thoracic region. Cervical spine disease produces not only pain in those regions but also local muscle spasm and tenderness. This referred tenderness is often mistaken for the "trigger points" of fibromyalgia. Physical examination often shows asymmetric loss of range of motion of the cervical spine and weakness of the muscles innervated by cervical nerve roots, such as elbow extension and finger abduction in patients with C7, C8, and T1 disease.

There are little hard data on the effectiveness of one therapy versus another in the management of nonspecific neck pain. The Bone and Joint Decade 2000–2010 Task Force on Neck Pain suggested that manual therapy and exercise are more effective than alternative strategies. Although several studies have shown that spinal manipulation and exercise programs are helpful, virtually all these studies were done on patients ≤65 years old. Surgery is rarely if ever indicated for pain and should be considered only if there are significant, persistent, and worsening neurologic signs.

Shoulder Pain

Most shoulder pain is due to lesions affecting the periarticular components of this structure. The shoulder girdle is composed of 3 bones (the clavicle, scapula, and proximal humerus) and 3 joints (the glenohumeral, sternoclavicular, and acromioclavicular). Periarticular structures that often cause shoulder pain include the 3 rotator cuff tendons that insert on the greater tuberosity of the humerus (the supraspinatus, infraspinatus, and teres minor tendons), the subacromial bursa, and the biceps tendon. Joint problems can affect the acromioclavicular joint and the glenohumeral joint.

The first step in examination of the shoulder is to assess the passive range of motion of the glenohumeral joint. The examiner places one hand on the superior spine of the scapula and passively abducts the arm. The point at which the scapula starts to rise is the point of glenohumeral abduction. This is normally approximately 90 degrees. External or lateral rotation is checked by rotating the arm in that direction until tightness is felt. External rotation is usually approximately 90 degrees, and internal rotation, approximately 80 degrees.

At the same time that the examiner is abducting the arm, he or she should check for the presence of a "painful arc." This sign is present if the patient has discomfort when the arm is passively abducted from 45 degrees to 120 degrees. This finding indicates disease of 3 of the rotator cuff tendons (supraspinatus, infraspinatus, teres minor) or the subacromial bursa.

Although most patients with shoulder pain have painful arcs because of rotator cuff disease or subacromial bursitis, shoulder pain can also be due to biceps tendonopathy, tendon rupture, glenohumeral disease, adhesive capsulitis, and acromioclavicular disease.

Rotator Cuff Tendonopathies and Tears

These conditions are characterized by shoulder pain that is aggravated by pulling, lifting, or holding the arm above the shoulder level, as well as by lying on the affected side. Tendonitis is suggested if the pain can be reproduced by resisting the active range of motion of the affected tendon (abduction for supraspinatus, and external rotation for infraspinatus and teres minor). The pain from both conditions is usually felt in the deltoid area and often down as far as the elbow. The supraspinatus is the most common tendon involved, and it can be evaluated with the "empty can" sign. The patient places a straight arm in 90 degrees of abduction and 30 degrees of forward flexion and then internally rotates the arm until the thumb is pointing down. The patient resists the clinician's attempts to push down the arm. Pain without weakness is consistent with tendonopathy, whereas weakness is consistent with a tendon tear.

Rotator cuff tendonitis is typically treated with NSAIDs, physical therapy, and/or local subacromial corticosteroid injections. Corticosteroid injections for painful shoulders are more effective than placebo and a bit more effective than NSAIDs. Because of the complications of NSAIDs in older adults, corticosteroid injections may be a more practical treatment for this condition. Although such injections may be helpful in reducing pain early on, mobilizing exercises alone are a reasonable approach.

Patients with persistent rotator cuff tendon symptoms may have tears of the tendon. Rotator cuff tears are common in older adults and may be insidious in onset. They cause recurring shoulder pain as well as loss of function. Rotator cuff tears are diagnosed if active range of motion is less than passive range of motion of the glenohumeral joint, there is a positive "drop arm" sign (patient is unable to hold the arm in the abducted position against gravity), or the patient has significant weakness when performing the "empty can" sign. MRI is a definitive method of diagnosing these tears. Surgery should be considered if patients have substantial functional loss from a tendon tear or persistent pain that has not responded to conservative therapy.

Biceps Tendonopathy and Tendon Rupture

Tendonitis of the biceps muscle results in pain over the anterior aspect of the shoulder that is aggravated by lifting and pulling. This condition is diagnosed if pain is reproduced by resisting elbow flexion, shoulder flexion (bringing the arm forward with the elbow straight), or wrist supination with the patient's elbow by his or her side. The biceps muscle has a long and short head, and the long head often ruptures. This rupture produces an indention of the proximal biceps and a palpable mass of the distal biceps (positive "Popeye" sign). The strength loss with this rupture is relatively insignificant and does not require surgical repair.

Osteoarthritis of the Glenohumeral Joint

Although generalized osteoarthritis does not affect the shoulder, many patients do develop osteoarthritis of the glenohumeral joint. This condition is characterized by global shoulder pain, loss of active shoulder movement, and significant loss of the passive range of motion of the glenohumeral joint. The diagnosis is made by plain radiograph. The therapy is symptomatic; severe disease may require a shoulder replacement.

Adhesive Capsulitis (Frozen Shoulder)

Adhesive capsulitis is characterized by loss of passive range of motion of the glenohumeral joint without intrinsic disease of the bone or cartilage of this joint. Patients with shoulder injuries, tendonitis, or other conditions often lose mobility in this structure. Radiographs are normal. The natural history of this condition is good, although it may take up to a year to restore the range of motion of the shoulder.

Acromioclavicular Disease

The acromioclavicular joint is often affected by trauma as well as osteoarthritis. Patients complain of anterior shoulder pain. Pain is often produced when the extended arm is adducted across the chest.

Elbow Pain

Elbow pain can be referred from the neck or shoulder. Intrinsic conditions of the elbow include arthritis of this joint, olecranon bursitis, and epicondylar pain on the medial or lateral aspect of the elbow.

Involvement of the elbow joint itself is the only condition that limits flexion and extension of the elbow. If this movement is limited, the clinician must evaluate the synovial structure of the elbow. To do so, the examiner should follow the lateral aspect of the humerus down the forearm with his or her thumb until finding the lateral epicondyle. There should be an indentation below that epicondyle and then a second bony structure below that indentation. If that structure rotates when the patient's wrist is rotated, it is the radial head. The examiner should run his or her thumb between the radial head and the olecranon. This space is where the synovial outpouching of the true elbow joint is felt. Swelling or induration of this region indicates an elbow joint process.

Olecranon bursitis causes swelling over the tip of the olecranon. This condition can be caused by trauma, gout, calcium pyrophosphate deposition disease (CPPD), or infection. Asymptomatic swelling of that bursa can also occur. Infection of the bursa usually results from contiguous spread of infection from the skin, whereas infection of the elbow joint itself usually comes from a systemic source. The best method of determining the cause of either bursitis or arthritis is to aspirate the bursa or joint and to examine the fluid for white cells, infection, or crystals.

"Tennis elbow," or lateral epicondylitis, is due to irritation of the wrist extensor tendons close to their insertion on the lateral epicondyle of the humerus. Tenderness may be found over the lateral aspect of the elbow. This diagnosis is made if the patient's elbow pain is reproduced by resisting extension of the patient's wrist.

"Golfer's elbow" occurs over the medial epicondyle. This condition is diagnosed if the patient's elbow pain is reproduced by resisting flexion of the wrist and is often accompanied by tenderness over the medial epicondyle. Infection of the olecranon bursa can be treated with oral antibiotics and drainage of the bursa (outpatient). Although steroid injections may relieve pain in the short term, they are inferior to other therapies in the intermediate and long term. Physical therapy and counter-force braces placed 6–10 cm distal to the elbow joint are often suggested for this condition (SOE=B). Arthritis of the elbow joint should be treated in a manner appropriate for the underlying condition. Local corticosteroid injections are often helpful for patients with gout or CPPD of this joint.

Hand and Wrist Pain

A variety of rheumatic and neurologic conditions can cause hand and wrist pain. The pattern of joint involvement helps to distinguish generalized osteoarthritis from inflammatory arthritis or from mechanical conditions of the hand and wrist.

Generalized osteoarthritis involves the distal and proximal interphalangeal joints as well as the first carpal-metacarpal joints at the base of the thumb. This condition does not affect the metacarpal phalangeal joints or wrists. Rheumatoid arthritis characteristically involves the proximal interphalangeal joints, metacarpal phalangeal joints, and wrists. It usually does not involve the distal interphalangeal joints. Osteoarthritis in the hand is characterized by medial or lateral deviation of the involved joint along with bony enlargement. Inflammatory arthritis produces synovial thickening of the affected joints. Symmetric decreased range of motion of the wrists also suggests inflammatory joint disease.

Monoarticular arthritis of the wrist is frequently caused by gout or CPPD. In older adults, gout frequently affects the distal and proximal interphalangeal joints that are already involved in generalized osteoarthritis. Crystal-induced arthritis of the wrist (gout or CPPD) can be effectively treated with a local steroid injection into the wrist.

De Quervain tenosynovitis produces pain along the radial aspect of the wrist, increased when grasping objects. This condition is caused by stenosing inflammation of the tendon sheath located over the radial styloid, which contains the abductor pollicis longus and extensor pollicis brevis tendons. Pain is produced when a clinched fist is deviated quickly in an ulnar direction. De Quervain tenosynovitis responds well to a corticosteroid injection into the tendon sheath.

Carpal tunnel syndrome is a common cause of hand pain. Patients complain of numbness and pain over the palm of the hands. Classically, the thumb, index and middle fingers, and the radial half of the ring finger are involved, but most patients cannot make this distinction. The pain is often increased in the morning; patients often drop objects because of this pain, which may radiate up the arm. The Tinel test for carpal tunnel syndrome involves tapping the medial aspect of the wrist with a reflex hammer. The test is positive if the hand has pain or paresthesias in the fingers innervated by the median nerve. In the Phalen maneuver, the patient hyperflexes his or her wrist by placing the backs of the hands against each other with the elbows in a flexed position. Pain or paresthesias in the fingers with 1 minute of wrist flexion is a positive test. The usual approach to treatment of carpal tunnel syndrome is splinting of the wrist. If splinting is ineffective, a corticosteroid injection into the carpal tunnel space can be tried. If this therapy is ineffective, surgery is the next option.

Ulnar neuropathies are common and can also be caused by trauma at the elbow area. Patients develop numbness and tingling on the lateral aspect of the hand. The diagnosis is confirmed if the patient has weakness of finger abduction but not elbow extension.

A "trigger finger" causes difficulty opening up a flexed finger. The syndrome is due to a combination of a flexor tendon nodule and thickening or fibrosis of the sheath in which this tendon travels. This combination results in a "mouse trapping" effect, in which the tendon is caught in a flexed position.

Dupuytren contraction of the palm of the hand produces painless deformities. These contractions cause thickening and fibrosis of the palmar fascia sheath, often with "puckering" of the skin over the flexor tendon. Flexion contractures of the fingers may result.

Thigh Pain

Thigh pain can be caused by such conditions as hip or back disease, trochanteric bursitis, a hernia, referred pain from abdominal viscera, femoral neuropathy, bone conditions, and vascular insufficiency.

Hip disease is a common cause of thigh pain as well as pain in the groin, buttock, and knee. The pain often comes on with walking and is relieved with sitting and lying. Patients may complain of significant pain on the first few steps after getting up from a sitting position. If the pain is significant, the patient usually limps, spending less time bearing weight on the affected side. If the disease is severe, it produces a short stride, because the hip is the "hinge" joint that controls the length of the stride. If the patient develops a flexion contracture of the hip, he or she will bend forward while walking.

The physical examination is the best method to diagnose hip disease. If the range of motion of the hip is normal, it is unlikely that the hip joint is the cause of the pain. The patient should be placed in a supine position. The examiner places one hand on the pelvis and gently abducts the hip. Abduction of the hip is reached when the pelvis starts to tilt. This is normally approximately 40 degrees. The examiner should also be able to flex the hip beyond 110 degrees. With the hip flexed, the foot should be moved toward the midline (external rotation). Normal external rotation should be 50–60 degrees. Internal rotation is when the heel is moved away from the midline and is normally 15–20 degrees.

The most common cause of hip disease in older adults is osteoarthritis. Plain radiographs of the hip may not display characteristic joint space narrowing and osteophytosis in patients with early osteoarthritis, because cartilage can be seen only on an MRI. If the patient has significant signs and symptoms of hip arthritis with an unimpressive radiograph, then an MRI may be indicated.

Medical therapies for osteoarthritis of the hip are limited. In one study, physical therapy did not result in better improvement in pain or function than sham treatment. Although NSAIDs are effective in the treatment of osteoarthritis, adverse effects limit their use in older adults. Corticosteroid injections, given under fluoroscopic guidance, can be an effective treatment of pain in hip osteoarthritis, with benefits lasting up to 3 months. Although medical therapies have a limited role in this condition, surgical approaches can be very effective. The success rate of a hip arthroplasty for osteoarthritis of the hip is high.

Lumbar spine disease commonly causes thigh pain, which often occurs with standing and walking. Pain can be felt on the lateral aspect of the hip and into the thigh region. The physical examination is key to this diagnosis, because many patients with lumbar spine disease will have subtle weakness of the great toe extensor, hip abductor, and hip extensor, because the L4-L5 and L5-S1 regions are the most common ones involved in lumbar spine disease.

Trochanteric bursitis pain is felt in the lateral thigh and may radiate down the lateral aspect to the knee. It is usually worse when rolling over on that side at night or after prolonged sitting, and it may be reproduced by resisting abduction of the hip. The most characteristic physical feature is local tenderness. This tenderness is usually felt approximately 1.5 inches below the superior portion of the trochanter.

Diseases of the femoral nerve can produce pain in the thigh area, particularly in patients with diabetes, retroperitoneal hemorrhages, or metastatic cancer. Patients have pain over the anterior aspect of the thigh, not affected by movement. These patients may have altered sensation over the anterior aspect of the thigh and a decreased quadriceps reflex. This condition causes focal weakness of the hip flexor and knee extensor muscles, because both of these muscle groups are innervated by the femoral nerve.

Pain in the groin and upper thigh area may be due to an inguinal or femoral hernia. Discomfort is increased when intra-abdominal pressure is increased, which can occur with straining, prolonged standing, or heavy lifting. Although incarceration and strangulation of these hernias are rare, this complication requires urgent attention and surgery. The diagnosis of an inguinal or femoral hernia is best made on physical examination with the finding of a groin bulge or a discrete groin impulse that increases with cough or a Valsalva maneuver.

A number of visceral problems in the abdomen can produce leg pain. A psoas abscess can produce hip and leg pain. This pain is increased when the psoas muscle is stretched or extended, which occurs with extension of the hip. Psoas abscess pain is typically diminished with hip flexion.

Although peripheral arterial disease typically causes calf pain, it can cause thigh and buttock pain. Two studies have demonstrated that approximately 40% of patients with claudication have pain in the proximal aspect of the leg. Claudication produces pain and discomfort in the legs when walking but not when standing or sitting. The pain worsens if the patient walks up a hill quickly and should disappear within 10 minutes after standing still.

Patients with bone disease of the pelvis or femur can also develop pain in the thigh. A number of cancers, such as breast, prostate, lung and kidney, can produce metastatic lesions in these bones.

Knee Pain

Knee pain greatly limits the function of many older adults and can also be referred from the hip and back. The most common cause of this pain is osteoarthritis. In some cases, however, patients may have radiographic findings of osteoarthritis of the knees, but their pain may be caused by other conditions such as gout, CPPD, or anserine bursitis.

Several structures around the knee can cause knee pain. The prepatellar bursa is located directly on top of the patella. The infrapatellar bursa is just inferior to the patella. The patient can often localize the site of the pain over the anterior, medial, or posterior aspect of the knee. Anterior pain can be due to prepatellar or infrapatellar bursitis or to irritation of the patellofemoral compartment of the knee. Patellofemoral pain can be reproduced by placing fingers firmly on the superior aspect of the patella and then asking the patient, lying supine, to press his or her knee into the bed. This maneuver contracts the quadriceps muscle, and the patella is a sesamoid bone within this muscle. When the quadriceps muscle contracts, the patella moves in a superior fashion. Pressure on the patella will reproduce pain from the patellofemoral component of the knee. Patellofemoral pain often radiates down to the anterior aspect of the lower leg and is usually worse on prolonged knee flexion (eg, sitting in a theater or airplane) or when the patient is descending stairs.

Pain on the medial aspect of the knee can be caused by conditions such as osteoarthritis of the medial compartment of the knee, medial meniscal disease, irritation at the attachment of the medial meniscus to the medial collateral ligament, or from irritation of the anserine bursa. Patients with a varus or "bow-legged" appearance have significant medial joint space narrowing due to osteoarthritis. Meniscal disease can be diagnosed by reproducing the patient's pain with a combination of extension and rotation of the knee. Patients with irritation at the attachment of the medial meniscus to the medial collateral ligament often have night pain in the medial aspect of the knee. There is usually tenderness along the medial joint line, and patients frequently put a pillow between their knees at night.

The first step in management of osteoarthritis of the knee should be quadriceps-strengthening exercises and weight reduction. NSAIDs can be effective, but their use is limited by their adverse effects in older adults. Interarticular injections of corticosteroids are effective but on average last only 4 weeks, although response is more prolonged in some patients. Although the use of hyaluronic acid injections is somewhat controversial, their adverse effects are limited and they may offer a more prolonged response than corticosteroid injections. They can be considered in patients for whom surgical intervention is not an option. These injections have fewer adverse effects than daily use of NSAIDs.

The evidence of meniscal disease in a patient with osteoarthritis may not call for a surgical intervention. Recent studies have demonstrated that arthroscopic partial meniscectomies were no more effective than physical therapy for meniscal tears in patients with osteoarthritis of the knee.

Anatomists, noting that the combined insertion of the medial hamstring muscles (gracilis, semitendinosis, and semimembranosus) on the tibia resembled a "goose's foot," named this region "pes anserine." The anserine bursa is located directly over that combined insertion, approximately 2 finger breadths below the medial joint line on the medial aspect of the tibia. Marked local tenderness at the region can indicate a bursitis. This condition often responds to a local injection of a corticosteroid and lidocaine.

Pain is often felt in the popliteal region if there is significant swelling or inflammation of synovial tissue. Sometimes this swelling can produce an outpouching in the popliteal area known as a popliteal or Baker cyst. This diagnosis is made by palpating a cystic mass in the popliteal space. These cysts sometimes rupture, causing swelling and pain in the calf, producing a "pseudothrombophlebitis" syndrome.

It is important to determine if the patient has a knee effusion, signifying that the problem is likely intra-articular. If there is pain and a joint effusion, the most important step is to aspirate the joint fluid and have it analyzed, looking for WBCs, crystals, and infection. The WBC count in the synovial fluid is very important. Patients with a mechanical disease such as osteoarthritis and meniscal irritation will have a bland fluid with a WBC count of <2,000 cells/mL. Any condition that produces inflammation of the joint, such as rheumatoid arthritis, gout, CPPD, or infection, will produce a synovial fluid WBC count of ≥2,000 cells/mL.

Back Pain

Back problems are the third most common reason for clinician visits by older adults. The evaluation of back pain in older adults requires a careful history, because

Table 58.1—Conditions Causing Back Pain in Older Adults

Condition	History	Examination	Laboratory Tests, Imaging
Tumor	Persistent, progressive pain at rest; systemic symptoms	No focal abnormalities	Anemia, increased ESR, abnormal bone scan or MRI
Infection	Persistent pain, fever; at-risk patient (eg, indwelling catheter)	Tender spine	Increased ESR, WBC count; positive bone scan or MRI
Lumbar spinal stenosis	Pain on standing and walking relieved by sitting and lying	Immobile spine; L4, L5, S1 weakness	MRI or CT scan showing stenosis
Sciatica	Pain in posterior aspect of leg; may be incomplete	Often positive straight leg raise; L4, L5, S1 weakness	Variable diagnostic imaging findings
Vertebral compression fracture	Sudden onset of severe pain; may resolve in 2–3 months, but many patients have persistent pain	Pain on any movement of spine; no neurologic deficits	Vertebral end-plate collapse; compression fracture seen on plain film
Osteoporotic sacral fracture	Sudden lower back, buttock, or hip pain	Sacral tenderness	Best identified on CT scan, bone scan, or MRI

NOTE: ESR = erythrocyte sedimentation rate

systemic conditions have a history quite distinct from that of mechanical pain (see Table 58.1). Several of the specific mechanical causes of back pain have characteristic historical features. Although systemic causes of pain are uncommon, they are more prevalent in older adults than in younger ones. There are also a number of specific causes for pain in older adults, including lumbar spinal stenosis, osteoporotic vertebral compression fractures, and osteoporotic sacral factures, that are rarely seen in younger individuals. The acuity and positional relationship of the pain provide useful diagnostic historical clues (see Table 58.2).

Low back pain is rarely associated with inflammatory arthritis. Although ankylosing spondylitis, psoriatic arthritis, and Reiter syndrome can produce back pain, this involvement is not seen with rheumatoid arthritis, systemic lupus, polymyalgia rheumatica, or other inflammatory conditions. Systemic conditions such as tumors and infections of the spine generally have an insidious onset of pain that becomes more and more persistent and severe over time. This pain is usually nonpositional, can occur at night, and may be associated with systemic symptoms or signs. The likelihood of cancer as a cause of back pain increases in adults >50 years old, those with a previous history of cancer, and those with pain that persists for longer than 1 month.

Fever, discrete local vertebral tenderness, pain in the upper lumbar or thoracic area, and nonpositional pain may indicate vertebral infection. Approximately 10% of older adults with endocarditis have back pain. Infection should be evaluated as a source of back pain in patients at risk of endovascular infections, such as those on hemodialysis, with chronic indwelling intravenous access catheters, or with a history of intravenous drug abuse.

A number of visceral problems, such as abdominal aortic aneurysm, bladder distention secondary to urinary

Table 58.2—Assessment of Lower Back Pain in Older Adults

Symptoms	Conditions
Acute pain	Vertebral compression fracture Disc displacement Osteoporotic sacral fracture Visceral origin (eg, aortic aneurysm)

Positional pain
  Increased with standing and walking and relieved with sitting
  Brought on by bending, lifting, or unguarded movements
	Lumbar spinal stenosis
	Mechanical back disease

Persistent pain (gradually increasing, nonpositional)	Tumor Infection

retention, uterine fibroids, pancreatic cancer, or other intra-abdominal infections or tumors, can present with back pain. Referred pain from these conditions should be suggested by the historical pattern of the pain, the absence of positional changes, and a normal examination of the lumbosacral spine. Patients with a known cancer with likelihood of spread to the bones should be urgently evaluated if they develop back pain.

On physical examination of older adults with back pain, the back, hips, legs, and gait should be evaluated. Examination of the hips, described above, is important, because many patients with back, buttock, and leg pain have hip disease. Gait evaluation should note if the patient bends forward as he or she walks, has a short stride, or spends less time on one leg than the other (limp).

The patient should next be examined in the upright position. The back should be moved through all 4 planes

Table 58.3—Physical Examination of Older Adults with Lower Back Pain

Sign	Condition
Paravertebral muscle spasm	Mechanical disc disease*
Asymmetric range of motion of the lumbar spine	Mechanical disc disease
Spinal tenderness	Vertebral compression fracture Infection
Weakness of L4-L5 and L5-S1 muscles	Mechanical disc disease Lumbar spinal stenosis
Normal examination of lumbar spine	Osteoporotic sacral fracture Hip disease Tumor Referred visceral pain

*Not caused by tumor, infection, spinal stenosis, or fracture

Table 58.4—Innervation of Lower Extremities

Function	Muscle	Nerve Root
Great toe dorsiflexion	Extensor hallucis longus	L5
Ankle dorsiflexion	Tibialis anterior	L4, L5
Ankle eversion	Peroneus longus, brevis	L5, S1
Ankle plantar flexion	Gastrocnemius, soleus	S1, S2
Knee extension	Quadriceps	L3, L4
Hip flexion	Iliopsoas	L2, L3
Hip adduction	Adductor magnus, brevis, longus	L3, L4
Hip abduction	Gluteus medius	L4, L5
Hip extension	Gluteus maximus	L5, S1

of movement of the lumbar spine: side flexion to the right, side flexion to the left, forward flexion, and extension. The pain of lumbar spinal stenosis is often produced by spinal extension. Asymmetric limitation of the range of motion of the lumbar spine, or reproduction of the pain with these maneuvers, may indicate mechanical disease of the lumbar spine (see Table 58.3).

The most helpful physical finding in patients with possible back disease is subtle weakness of the L4-L5 and L5-S1 muscles. L4-L5 weakness is demonstrated by weakness of the great toe extensor and hip abductor. The ankle dorsiflexor is also innervated by L4-L5, but this muscle is quite strong and subtle weakness may be difficult to elicit. L5-S1 weakness is demonstrated by involvement of the hip extensors. This is easily tested by attempting to pull up the leg at the ankle when the patient is trying to hold the leg on the bed. Normally, the patient can successfully resist this maneuver. The level of neurologic injury can often be discerned by physical examination (see Table 58.4).

In the setting of acute back pain, the *Choosing Wisely* recommendation to wait 6 weeks before performing diagnostic imaging tests is appropriate to limit the use of CT scans, MRIs, and plain radiographs in younger patients, but older adults commonly have red flags that warrant imaging without delay. A plain radiograph of the lumbar spine can detect a vertebral compression fracture and should be obtained in older women, and in older men with risk factors for osteoporosis, if the discovery of a compression fracture will change management. Other red flags that would prompt early imaging include acute neurologic deficit, bowel or bladder dysfunction, fever, and history of cancer.

Specific Conditions Causing Back Pain in Older Adults

Lumbar Spinal Stenosis

Lumbar spinal stenosis is a common cause of back pain in older adults and the most frequent indication for spinal surgery in people >65 years old. It is important, however, for the clinician to ensure that the patient truly has the clinical symptoms of lumbar spinal stenosis, because it is frequently seen on spine imaging in asymptomatic patients.

The stenosis results from a narrowing of either the central or lateral aspect of the lumbar spinal canal. Osteophytes of the facet joints often impinge on nerve roots of the lower lumbar region when they travel in the lateral recess of the canal. This space can also be compromised by lumbar disc displacement into the canal.

These patients report pain in the lower back, buttock, thighs, and legs. The pain is positional, because it occurs with standing and extending the spine, is worsened by walking, and relieved by sitting or forward flexion of the spine. Patients report that their symptoms often improve when they are walking with a shopping cart. The anatomy of the lumbar spine explains the symptoms: flexion of the lumbar spine results in an increase in spinal canal volume and a decrease in nerve root bulk, whereas extension of the lumbar spine results in a decrease in spinal canal volume and an increase in nerve root bulk. Therefore, positions that flex the spine, such as sitting, bending forward, walking uphill, or lying in a flexed position, all relieve symptoms. Positions that extend the spine, such as prolonged standing, walking, and walking downhill, exacerbate the symptoms.

Patients with lumbar spinal stenosis may develop sciatic pain with standing and walking. Pain in the calf when walking can mimic the claudication of arterial insufficiency and is referred to as pseudoclaudication. It can be difficult to distinguish neurogenic claudication from vascular claudication. The combination of pain with standing, relief with sitting, symptoms located above the knees, and a positive "shopping cart sign" have been associated with neurogenic claudication. Patients who had symptoms in the calf that were relieved by standing still were more likely to have vascular claudication. Patients with lumbar spinal stenosis often have subtle weakness of the muscles innervated by the L4, L5, and S1 nerve roots.

The variable natural history of this condition makes it difficult to evaluate therapeutic options. Most patients have stable symptoms for up to 8 years of follow-up, while others deteriorate and some improve. Although physical therapy, exercise regimens, and medications are used in the treatment of this condition, there is no clear evidence that they alter the natural history of the condition. A study of epidural steroid injections for spinal stenosis demonstrated minimal or no short-term benefit. Most studies have shown that surgical treatment was more effective than conservative therapy. Some studies have shown that, although interspinous spacers may provide some benefit, they are associated with a much higher incidence of reoperation then decompression laminectomies. For patients who do not respond to conservative therapy and are not candidates for spinal surgery, the use of a rolling walker with an attached seat can be quite helpful in improving mobility and quality of life.

Sciatica

Although sciatica is most common in the fourth to fifth decades of life, it also frequently occurs in older individuals. Unfortunately, there are no published data about this syndrome in older patients. This pain differs from the leg pain seen in spinal stenosis in that it occurs spontaneously and usually does not require the patient to be standing. Sciatica usually resolves without treatment in one-third of patients within 2 weeks and in three-quarters of patients within 3 months of onset. Diagnostic imaging is not helpful in prognosis. No consistent evidence favors one therapeutic option over another.

Osteoporotic Vertebral Compression Fractures

About 25% of women will experience a vertebral compression fracture in their lifetime. Although symptoms are seen in only one-third of patients with these fractures, these symptoms can be quite severe. The onset of pain is typically abrupt, with pain felt deep in the site of the fracture. The pain is usually worse on standing and walking and relieved with lying down. Although the pain may radiate to the flank or legs, neurologic sequelae are unusual. The diagnosis is usually made on a plain radiograph of the lumbar or thoracic spine.

Studies of the natural history of this syndrome vary. Many studies show a significant decrease in pain by 6 weeks. A Japanese study, however, found that patients still had a good deal of pain and disability 6 and 12 months after the fracture. It is unclear whether these fractures are markers of frailty or contribute to disability; patients with fractures are more likely to have further fractures, become more disabled, and have a higher mortality rate than those without fractures.

Therapy of these fractures remains controversial. A Cochrane review in 2015 "does not support a role for vertebroplasty for treating osteoporotic vertebral fractures in routine practice." Other reviews maintain that patients do better with vertebroplasty than with conservative therapy. Currently, there is still no convincing evidence that these procedures should be a standard of care for vertebral compression fractures. However, a number of studies have shown that calcitonin significantly reduces the severity of acute pain in patients with acute vertebral fractures. Probably the most important intervention is to treat the underlying osteoporosis to help prevent such conditions as hip fractures.

Sacral Insufficiency Fractures

Sacral insufficiency fractures occur without trauma. They can be a cause of significant back pain, usually felt in the buttock and low back region. There is often significant tenderness on sacral compression. Most patients have a history of significant osteoporosis. These fractures can also be seen after radiation to this area. Plain radiographs are often negative. CT identifies approximately 70% of these fractures, while bone scans and MRIs almost always demonstrate these fractures. Patients have difficulty with weight bearing and often have severe pain when sitting. Full recovery can take 6–12 months. If patients do not respond to conservative therapy, then many clinicians do a sacroplasty, which involves the injection of bone cement into the fracture site of the sacrum. Although observational studies seem to indicate good results with this technique, there are no controlled trials of this procedure.

Nonspecific Low Back Pain

Many older adults have nonspecific low back pain that is mechanical in origin. Although much has been learned about specific conditions that affect the back in older adults, such as lumbar spinal stenosis and vertebral compression fractures, little is known about nonspecific mechanical low back pain, other

Chapter 58: Musculoskeletal Pain **483**

than that it is quite common and relatively short in duration. In the Framingham study, 22% of patients ≥68 years old had back pain on most days. A 10-year study of 550 community-dwelling adults ≥70 years old documented 1,528 episodes of low back pain severe enough to restrict activity. Of these episodes, 80% lasted <1 month and only 6.4% lasted >3 months.

As in younger individuals, the best way to determine the probable cause of the pain in older adults is the history and physical examination. Diagnostic images demonstrate many abnormalities in asymptomatic patients. It is thus difficult to ascribe the pain to one of these abnormalities.

Mechanical pain usually has a relatively sudden onset and is exacerbated by positions that stress the lumbar spine such as going from supine to sitting, getting in and out of bed, bending, lifting, or putting on socks and shoes. If there is weakness of the L4-5 and L5-S1 innervated muscles, the pain is likely due to a displacement of disc material. Herniation of the nucleus pulposus is unlikely in older adults, because the water content of this structure decreases dramatically with age. It is no longer gel-like and, therefore, much less apt to herniate.

Given that the natural history of mechanical back pain in older individuals is good, the most important action for the clinician is to explain this prognosis and avoid aggressive interventions.

> **CHOOSING WISELY® RECOMMENDATIONS**
>
> *Musculoskeletal Pain*
>
> - Avoid NSAIDs in individuals with hypertension, heart failure, or chronic kidney disease of all causes, including diabetes mellitus.
>
> - Do not perform imaging for lower back pain within the first 6 weeks unless red flags are present (severe or progressive neurologic deficits or when serious underlying conditions are present).

RESOURCES

- Cohen SP. Epidemiology, diagnosis, and treatment of neck pain. *Mayo Clin Proc*. 2015;90(2):284–299.

- Lurie J, Tomkins-Lane C. Management of lumbar spinal stenosis. *BMJ*. 2016 Jan 4;352:h6234.

- Metzger RL. Evidence-based practice guidelines for the diagnosis and treatment of lumbar spinal conditions. *Nurse Pract*. 2016;41(12):30–37.

- Saccomano SJ. Osteoarthritis treatment: decreasing pain, improving mobility. *Nurse Pract*. 2018;43(9):49–55.

CHAPTER 59—RHEUMATOLOGY

KEY POINTS

- Osteoarthritis is the most common cause of chronic pain among older adults and leads to considerable morbidity and disability.

- History and physical examination remain the most important tools in diagnosing and distinguishing among the rheumatologic diseases, although laboratory tests and imaging studies can be helpful to confirm clinical suspicion.

- When developing treatment plans for older adults with rheumatologic disease, it is important to keep in mind each patient's comorbid medical conditions, functional status, and the potential for drug-drug and drug-disease interactions.

- Interventions ideally use a multimodal approach, including pharmacologic and nonpharmacologic treatments as well as rehabilitation modalities.

OSTEOARTHRITIS

Osteoarthritis (OA) is the most common source of joint pain, and chronic pain, among older adults. Recent estimates suggest OA affects >30 million people in the United States alone. Depending on the source of data and which joint is involved, OA is present in 50%–90% of older adults. OA is the principal cause of knee, hip, and back pain in older adults, and it is expected to increase in both incidence and prevalence as the population ages. Yet, caution needs to be exercised to avoid the reflexive conclusion that all joint pain in the geriatric age group is necessarily the result of underlying OA. Differential diagnosis of OA includes inflammatory and crystal arthritides, as well as septic arthritis and bone pain due to malignancy.

Cartilage degeneration is the hallmark of OA, with fibrillation and ulceration that begins superficially and eventually extends into deeper layers. However, evidence indicates that OA is not a purely degenerative disease restricted to the cartilage; subchondral bone abnormalities and focal synovial inflammation have also been seen in pathologic specimens. These pathologic characteristics are thought to arise as a result of repetitive cycles of degradation and repair responses that eventually become inadequate to maintain joint health. Inflammatory cytokines, matrix-degrading metalloproteinase enzymes, and chondrocyte apoptosis are likely contributors to this process.

OA commonly affects the hands, knees, hips, and cervical and lumbar spine, but it can develop in any joint that has suffered injury or other disease. On examination, bony enlargement and crepitus suggest OA. In the fingers, bony enlargement occurs in the distal interphalangeal joints (Heberden nodes) and in the proximal interphalangeal joints (Bouchard nodes). Osteophytes are the radiographic counterpart of this enlargement, and asymmetric joint space narrowing is common (Figure 59.1). Joint tenderness and warmth may appear, but true synovitis suggests an alternative or concomitant diagnosis.

Imaging is not required to make a diagnosis of OA in patients with typical symptoms (usage-related pain, short duration of morning stiffness, age >40, symptoms affecting one or a few joints) (SOE=C). When imaging is obtained, weight-bearing plain radiographs are most useful. Advanced imaging studies are generally not indicated in patients with OA, and should not be used as an initial diagnostic tool in the evaluation of chronic joint pain. Rather, advanced imaging is typically reserved for patients who are experiencing atypical symptoms such as rapidly progressive pain, symptoms of inflammation, or night or rest pain, or for those who are considering surgical intervention.

The objectives of OA management are to alleviate painful symptoms, prevent disease progression, maximize function, and minimize disease-related complications. Patient education and shared decision making are important when developing the treatment plan. Self-management programs have been shown to improve pain and function (SOE=A). Obesity is a modifiable risk factor for OA, and weight reduction can help reduce pain and improve function in patients with OA of the knee, hip, or spine. Use of thermal agents is recommended for relief of pain and stiffness related to hand, knee, and hip OA, although patients should be cautioned regarding the risk of burning the skin if heating agents are used.

Assessment of older adults with OA should include evaluation of the ability to perform daily activities. Many assistive devices can be recommended, including jar or bottle openers, walking aids, braces, and insoles, depending on the activity that is most difficult for the patient. In knee OA, braces can alleviate patellofemoral symptoms by improving patellar tracking and can provide a greater sense of joint stability by improving joint proprioception (SOE=A). Specific orthoses designed to reduce medial knee pain by "unloading" the medial compartment of the knee include a valgus unloader brace and a lateral wedge insole. A well-designed running shoe can also lessen pain and damage by decreasing the impact transmitted during ambulation. Finally, a properly fitted and used cane can provide

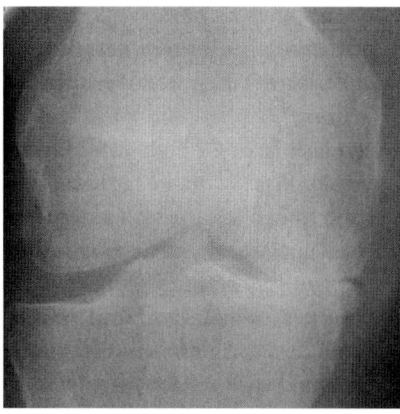 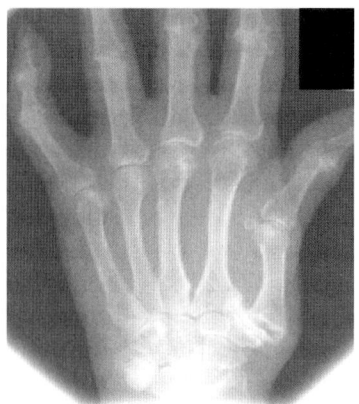

Figure 59.1—*Left:* Radiographic osteoarthritis of the knee with medial compartment osteophytes, joint space narrowing, and sclerosis. *Right:* Radiographic osteoarthritis of the hand with osteophytes, asymmetric joint space narrowing, and sclerosis of varying degrees of the thumb base (carpometacarpal joint) and proximal interphalangeal joints

stability as well as "unloading" the symptomatic knee or hip.

Physical activity is a critical component in the treatment of OA-related pain. Regular physical activity is associated with decreased pain and improvement in functional status (SOE=A). For example, one study found walking >6,000 steps per day to be protective against developing functional limitation related to OA. Additionally, regular physical activity has the benefit of promoting weight loss, which can further improve pain control. Chair yoga has been shown to improve pain, fatigue, and gait speed, specifically in older adults (SOE=B). The CDC and Arthritis Foundation recommend a minimum of 150 minutes (2.5 hours) of moderate intensity aerobic exercise along with 2 days of muscle strengthening exercise per week to improve pain and functioning in patients with OA, although these guidelines do not apply specifically to older adults. For patients with significant pain and disability, achieving this level of activity may initially be difficult. A multimodal interdisciplinary approach, including referral to physical and occupational therapy, is key in managing chronic pain related to OA. Physical and occupational therapists can help older adults maintain and often improve their functional status by implementing individualized therapy programs, assessing ability to perform activities of daily living, providing recommendations about assistive devices to improve functioning, and training patients and caregivers in fall prevention.

The American Geriatrics Society 2009 guidelines on management of persistent pain is an appropriate resource to consult when managing OA-related pain. Traditionally, first-line therapy has been "around the clock" dosing of acetaminophen, with a maximum daily dose of 4 g in 24 hours; however, more recent evidence suggests that this therapy is not as effective as previously thought and when compared with placebo may have an increased risk of mortality as well as cardiovascular, GI, and renal adverse events. Topical therapies (eg, analgesic balms, capsaicin, topical NSAIDs) can be helpful in hand or knee OA, with the strongest evidence for topical diclofenac (SOE=A). Oral NSAIDs should be used with caution in older adults because of known GI, renal, and cardiovascular adverse effects. NSAIDs can be used for an acute flare of OA, but use should be limited to the lowest dose and shortest duration possible. Age >65 years is a risk factor for NSAID-related peptic ulcer disease, and the use of a proton-pump inhibitor should be considered in conjunction with NSAID therapy, especially if patients have additional risk factors for peptic ulcer disease. Tramadol can be tried for pain refractory to optimal acetaminophen or NSAID dosing. Low-dose narcotic medications may be considered in those who do not respond to acetaminophen, NSAIDs, or tramadol. Use of opioid medications for OA should be limited to those whose quality of life is significantly impacted by pain, and risks and benefits of use must always be considered. Duloxetine may also be tried as an adjunct for chronic pain associated with OA (SOE=A). Studies evaluating glucosamine and chondroitin sulfate for pain have conflicting results. A recent meta-analysis found that glucosamine was not superior to placebo for hip or knee OA (SOE=A). Glucocorticoid injections have been considered a reasonable treatment option for knee OA, but a recent randomized controlled trial found limited long-term pain relief from intra-articular triamcinolone compared with placebo and potentially more cartilage loss with triamcinolone injected every 3 months. Hyaluronic acid and hyaluronan polymers given in a series of weekly injections in the knee are approved for intra-articular viscosupplementation therapy, although evidence for efficacy is mixed (SOE=B). For hip OA, glucocorticoid injections have been shown to provide only temporary relief as compared with placebo. Prior studies have suggested that use of intra-articular steroids for hip OA could increase risk of postoperative infection after hip arthroplasty; however, evidence of this association is limited. Imaging can be useful for injections of joints that are difficult to access (such as the hip), or in obese patients.

Rheumatoid Arthritis

Although less prevalent than OA, rheumatoid arthritis (RA) is an important disease in older adults. Up to 40% of patients with RA are >60 years old; some of these individuals have aged with the disease, whereas 20%–55% develop RA later in life. As with OA, the incidence and prevalence of RA in older adults is expected to increase as the population ages. Compared with the general population, patients with RA have an increased incidence of cardiovascular disease and an increased risk of premature death, and their cardiovascular risk should be formally evaluated at least once every 5 years. In models that do not incorporate rheumatoid arthritis as a risk factor, risk can be adjusted for patients with RA by a 1.5 multiplication factor (SOE=B).

Most older adults with late-onset RA present similarly to young adults, with acute seropositive inflammatory polyarthritis that involves the small joints of the hands and feet. Those who develop RA in later life have marked early morning stiffness and prominent upper extremity pain, especially involving the shoulders, wrists, metacarpophalangeal and proximal interphalangeal joints. Two additional seronegative presentations are unique to older adults. The "RS3PE" syndrome consists of remitting seronegative symmetrical synovitis with pitting edema, and accounts for approximately 10% of late-onset inflammatory arthritis cases. Additionally, there is an acute onset, seronegative, inflammatory arthritis of the shoulder and hips similar to polymyalgia rheumatica (PMR), which accounts for approximately 25% of late-onset RA cases and can be difficult to distinguish from PMR. In fact, descriptive studies suggest that late-onset RA should be considered in the differential diagnosis of PMR and vice versa. Other diseases that mimic RA include calcium pyrophosphate dihydrate deposition disease (CPPD) and polyarthritis related to malignancy.

As with young adults, the diagnosis of RA relies on history, physical examination, radiologic, and laboratory criteria. Older adults present more frequently than younger adults with constitutional symptoms such as malaise, fever, fatigue, and weight loss, in addition to the characteristic synovitis of RA. Older adults with RA are also more likely to have a higher initial erythrocyte sedimentation rate (ESR). Evaluation of possible RA in older adults should include checking autoantibodies, including rheumatoid factor (RF), and anti-cyclic citrullinated peptide/protein antibodies (anti-CCP or ACPA). However, prevalence of autoantibodies increases with age, so caution should be exercised in interpreting individual laboratory abnormalities, particularly a positive RF. A positive anti-CCP antibody is more specific than a positive RF alone. Radiographic evaluation can be helpful to demonstrate erosions or deformities that appear in more aggressive and long-standing disease.

Assessment of disease activity in RA includes symptoms (including reports of impairment or disability), physical examination, laboratory data, and imaging. This should be done on the initial visit and routinely thereafter to assess response to treatment. Symptoms to assess include pain intensity and location, duration of morning stiffness, severity of fatigue, and functional status. Physical examination includes a systematic examination of the number of tender and swollen joints, as well as evaluation for extra-articular manifestations, including rheumatoid nodules and other cutaneous manifestations, interstitial lung disease, pleuropericardial disease, vasculitis, ocular disease, and neuropathy. Routine laboratory monitoring includes acute phase reactants, such as ESR and C-reactive protein (CRP), which can serve as markers of disease activity, as well as CBCs, metabolic panels, and liver function tests to evaluate for potential toxicity if the patient is on disease-modifying antirheumatic drugs (DMARDs). Radiographs may be obtained periodically to assess for disease progression.

Patients with RA should be treated by a rheumatologist, and patient education is an important component of treatment (SOE=A). Descriptive studies suggest that patients with seropositive RA, even if of late onset, should be managed aggressively, including use of DMARDs and biologics (SOE=B). Similar to that in younger adults, management of RA in older adults should be started as soon as the diagnosis is made, with the goal of achieving remission or the lowest level of disease activity possible, "a treat to target" strategy (SOE=A). Treating to target requires frequent follow-up (every 1–3 months) in patients with active disease, with adjustments in therapy if the target is not reached within 3–6 months (SOE=B). An oral DMARD is recommended as the initial treatment in all DMARD-naive patients, regardless of severity or duration of disease activity. If disease activity remains moderate or high on DMARD monotherapy, additional DMARDs or biologics should be added. Glucocorticoids at the lowest possible dose for the shortest possible duration may be used for disease flares and should be considered as a bridge therapy when starting or changing oral DMARDs (SOE=A). Therapies should be continued in patients when low disease activity is achieved, but tapering may be considered when remission is achieved. However, it is recommended that some therapy be continued even in remission.

In younger adults, the first-line oral DMARD is methotrexate, followed by leflunomide or sulfasalazine in patients in whom methotrexate is contraindicated (SOE=A). Methotrexate is well tolerated, but older adults may require a lower dose; it should be given with daily folic acid supplementation. Cases of lymphoproliferative disease have been reported with long-term methotrexate treatment. Hydroxychloroquine is well tolerated, but patients must be monitored for retinal toxicity, which is problematic if macular degeneration is present at baseline. Safety and efficacy of sulfasalazine in older adults appears to be similar to that in younger adults, although dosing should be adjusted for renal function. Leflunomide has been demonstrated to prevent radiographic progression in younger adults, but experience is minimal in older adults (SOE=B). It has a relatively fast onset of action (about 4 weeks) compared with other DMARDs; however, its half-life is longer. Older agents, such as penicillamine, gold, and cyclophosphamide, are less well tolerated by older adults and are rarely used.

Many biologic agents for RA are now available, but experience with these agents in older adults is limited, so their use is generally reserved for those in whom conventional triple therapy with oral DMARDs has not been effective. These agents work by inhibiting tumor necrosis factor α (etanercept, infliximab, adalimumab, golimumab, and certolizumab), antagonizing the interleukin-1 receptor (anakinra), antagonizing the interleukin-6 receptor (tocilizumab), serving as a fusion protein co-stimulation modulator via inhibition of CD28 (abatacept), inhibiting janus kinase (tofacitinib), or binding the CD20 antigen on B-lymphocytes (rituximab). Of these medications, only tofacitinib is administered orally; the rest require either intravenous or subcutaneous administration. Infliximab, adalimumab, and rituximab all increase the risk of granulomatous infections with organisms such as *Mycobacterium tuberculosis*, atypical mycobacteria, yeast, *Listeria*, and *Nocardia*. Infliximab can also cause postinfusion fever, chills, headache, chest pain, and dyspnea. All of the biologic agents have been associated with bacterial respiratory tract infections. B lymphocyte–depleting therapies, such as rituximab, have been associated with reactivation of hepatitis B, especially when used in combination with prednisone. Patients taking these medications should be screened before initiating therapy, as there are now excellent medications for suppressing reactivation (eg, entecavir or lamivudine). Also, it is recommended that patients receive the zoster vaccine before treatment with a biologic agent is started (SOE=C).

Low-dose prednisone (10–20 mg/d) may be used as the primary treatment for seronegative PMR-like disease and the "RS3PE" syndrome. However, in contrast to classic PMR, late-onset RA may not respond promptly to low-dose prednisone. Further, prednisone alone is often not sufficient in managing seropositive RA but may be useful as an adjunctive agent. In general, chronic use of prednisone should be avoided, because its use is associated with increased risk of infectious complications (notably herpes zoster reactivation), fluid retention, and osteoporosis.

GOUT

Gout is a crystal-induced arthropathy that is more common in older adults than in younger adults. The global burden of gout is increasing, particularly in high-income countries; this has been attributed both to the aging of the population as well as rising rates of obesity. Hyperuricemia and gout are associated with cardiovascular disease and metabolic syndrome. Women generally do not develop gout until menopause, at which time the rate in women approaches that in men. Polypharmacy, including diuretic use, and higher incidence of renal and hepatic impairment also predispose older adults to accumulation of uric acid and development of gout.

Gout can cause both severe pain and disability. The clinical characteristics of gout can differ appreciably in older adults. Gout can present as a subacute smoldering oligoarthritis affecting larger joints (eg, knee, wrist, shoulder, ankle) rather than as an acute, monoarticular, and incapacitating attack, as in classic podagra affecting the first metatarsophalangeal joint. Tophaceous deposits in the distal and proximal interphalangeal joints can be mistaken for, or coexist with, osteoarthritis. Similarly, tophi at the extensor surfaces can be confused with rheumatoid nodules. Acute attacks can be precipitated by trauma, acute nonarticular illness requiring hospitalization, and abrupt changes in uric acid concentration (as can be seen with dehydration and particularly after surgery or admission for congestive heart failure with aggressive diuresis). An acute gout flare is characterized by abrupt onset of intense inflammation and pain, typically reaching maximum intensity within 12–24 hours, with resolution of symptoms within 7–10 days, even without treatment.

In 2015, the ACR and EULAR jointly published classification criteria that are 92% sensitive and 89% specific for gout diagnosis. The diagnosis may be made with at least one episode of swelling, pain, or tenderness in a peripheral joint or bursa with demonstration of monosodium urate crystals from the joint or bursa or a tophus. Monosodium urate crystals are needle-shaped and strongly negatively birefringent and can be demonstrated in synovial fluid obtained during an acute flare or in the intercritical phase. If monosodium urate crystals are not demonstrated, the diagnosis of gout may still be made by applying the additional classification criteria, which take into account symptom characteristics, time course of symptoms, presence of tophus, serum uric acid levels, and imaging findings on radiographs, ultrasound, or dual-energy CT. Online calculators are available at http://goutclassificationcalculator.auckland.ac.nz and also on the ACR and EULAR websites. Radiographs may show juxta-articular erosions of the involved joints. An overhanging edge (Martel sign) can be seen and is helpful in distinguishing gout from RA erosions. With rare exception, asymptomatic hyperuricemia precedes the development of gouty arthritis. Increased serum uric acid, along with a clinical history of episodic mono- or oligoarthritis, is highly suggestive of gouty arthritis. However, hyperuricemia is not uniformly present at the time of an acute gout attack, and the presence of hyperuricemia alone neither confirms a diagnosis of gout nor necessitates starting urate-lowering medication.

Patients with gout should be counseled regarding lifestyle modifications that can help prevent recurrent episodes of gout. These interventions include weight loss; avoidance of purine-rich foods such as shellfish, mollusks, organ meats, and full-fat dairy products; and avoidance of alcohol, particularly beer, which is especially purine rich (SOE=B). The importance of these lifestyle modifications should be reinforced at each follow-up visit, because these changes can be difficult to implement and sustain but can be invaluable in prevention of future attacks. Topical therapy with ice is an important and effective adjunctive therapy for an acute gout attack (SOE=B). In patients with recurrent attacks, discontinuation of medications that increase uric acid accumulation should be considered (SOE=C); however, this is not always feasible in older adults with multiple comorbidities. Diuretics, niacin, and low-dose aspirin are among the medications that may predispose a patient to developing a gout attack.

Treatment of gout in older adults must be individualized, taking into account the potential for drug-drug and drug-disease interactions. An acute gout attack may be managed with a short-acting NSAID (SOE=A) in those who can tolerate it, keeping in mind the potential for serious cardiovascular, GI, and renal adverse effects in older adults. Of note, indomethacin is listed as a drug to avoid in the AGS Beers Criteria® for potentially inappropriate medication use in older adults because it has the most adverse effects of all the NSAIDs. Cyclooxygenase-2 inhibitors have been shown to be as effective as nonselective NSAIDs for managing acute gout attacks with fewer adverse events (SOE=A). Intra-articular glucocorticoids (assuming septic joint has been excluded) are preferred for attacks involving one joint such as the knee, ankle, or wrist (SOE=B). Alternatively, short-term oral glucocorticoids tapered over 5–10 days are preferred in managing a polyarticular gouty flare (SOE=A). Glucocorticoids may be preferable to NSAIDs in the treatment of gout in older adults with multiple comorbidities, because the typical complications of steroid use are generally not seen with short courses. Colchicine can also be used to treat an acute gouty attack, although its use is often limited by the presence of renal impairment (SOE=A). Previously, colchicine was dosed every 1–2 hours until resolution of symptoms or onset of adverse effects; however, this aggressive regimen has proved to be both excessive and poorly tolerated in older adults. Current evidence suggests that doses as low as 0.6 mg every 8–24 hours can be effective in treating an acute attack.

Medications such as allopurinol, febuxostat, or probenecid are uric acid–lowering therapies used for longer term management. Chronic use of uric acid–lowering agents should be considered in patients with >2 attacks in a year, evidence of tophi, erosive disease (SOE=A), or chronic kidney disease stage 2 or higher (SOE=C). Historically, these medications are not initiated during an acute gout attack; however, there is limited evidence showing that doing so would worsen the acute attack (so long as abortive therapy is also prescribed). Allopurinol and febuxostat lower serum uric acid via inhibition of xanthine oxidase and are considered first-line therapies in management of chronic gout (SOE=A). Allopurinol dosage should be adjusted in patients with renal impairment. Probenecid works as a uricosuric agent and may be used as an alternative first-line therapy if at least one of the xanthine oxidase inhibitors is not tolerated or contraindicated, but probenecid is not recommended if creatinine clearance is <50 mL/min (SOE=B). Because uric acid–lowering therapy is initiated with the goal of lowering serum uric acid levels to 5–6 mg/dL (SOE=A), it is important to educate the patient that this drop in serum uric acid may precipitate a flare. Therefore, it is reasonable to use a prophylactic agent such as colchicine at dosages as low as 0.6 mg/d, renal function permitting, or low-dose prednisone for several months as the uric acid–lowering therapy is titrated up (SOE=A). If the patient develops an acute gout attack while on a uric acid–lowering agent, it is important to continue taking the medication daily while adding an abortive treatment (SOE=C). While patients are on uric acid–lowering therapies, serum uric acid as well as renal and liver function should be monitored. During dosage titration, these values should be checked every 1–2 months, but frequency of testing may be reduced once on a consistent dose if uric acid is at goal and other values remain stable. If the goal uric acid level is not achieved with up-titration of the xanthine oxidase inhibitor to the maximum dose, a uricosuric agent such as probenecid, fenofibrate, or losartan may be added (SOE=B). Pegloticase may be tried in patients with severe gout refractory to appropriate urate-lowering therapy (SOE=A).

Calcium Pyrophosphate Dihydrate Deposition Disease

Calcium pyrophosphate dihydrate deposition disease (CPPD), like gout, is a crystal-induced arthropathy that is more common in older adults. CPPD, also known as "pseudogout," causes synovitis that can mimic RA, inflammatory osteoarthritis, gout, or septic arthritis. CPPD is associated with disorders of calcium metabolism (eg, hypomagnesemia, hypophosphatemia, and hyperparathyroidism), hypothyroidism, and hemochromatosis. CPPD of the wrist can mimic RA but can be distinguished by prominent synovitis and chondrocalcinosis of the wrist and/or metacarpophalangeal joints with a negative RF and anti-CCP antibody. CPPD can also mimic inflammatory osteoarthritis but with rapid joint destruction of the wrist, patellofemoral knee compartment, and hip joint.

CPPD can result in an acute, intermittent inflammatory arthritis of the knee, hip, wrist, and metacarpophalangeal joints, with elbow, shoulder, and ankle involvement less common. CPPD can mimic an acute gout attack with sudden onset of pain and swelling that coincide with or immediately follow an acute illness or traumatic event such as surgery. When fever is present, distinguishing CPPD from septic arthritis is imperative, and diagnostic arthrocentesis is indicated.

Arthrocentesis with crystal analysis is diagnostic and useful to distinguish CPPD from gout and infection. CPPD crystals are weakly positively birefringent rhomboids or squares. CPPD is commonly suspected by the radiographic finding of chondrocalcinosis on plain films (Figure 59.2), which appears as a stippled or linear calcification of the articular cartilage of the knee, wrist, hip, shoulder, and symphysis pubis. However, radiographic chondrocalcinosis is not diagnostic of CPPD in the absence of clinical arthritis.

Intra-articular steroid injection can result in significant relief of painful symptoms with CPPD and may be the preferred management option if one joint is involved. Short-acting NSAIDs and oral steroidal agents are also useful in management of CPPD in patients who can tolerate them (SOE=C). Evidence for the use of colchicine in CPPD is limited, and its use is largely based on anecdotal evidence and extrapolation from gout treatment. Oral colchicine may be used to treat acute flares of CPPD and is typically dosed 0.6 mg every 8–24 hours, similar to acute gout treatment. Colchicine can also be useful to prevent future acute episodes of CPPD, typically at doses of 0.6 mg every 12–24 hours (SOE=C). Unfortunately, there are currently no disease modifying treatments for CPPD.

Polymyalgia Rheumatica

Polymyalgia rheumatica (PMR) is an inflammatory rheumatic disease unique to older adults. PMR occurs almost exclusively in patients ≥50 years old, with 90% of affected patients >60 years old. It is twice as common in women as in men, and whites are the most commonly affected ethnic group. PMR is a relatively common condition, second in incidence only to RA among all of the inflammatory autoimmune rheumatic disorders. Approximately 50 new cases develop per 100,000 persons per year, with an estimated prevalence of 600 cases per 100,000 and higher prevalence with increasing age. Approximately 15%–20% of patients with PMR also have giant cell arteritis (GCA), whereas up to 40%–60% of patients with GCA will have symptoms of PMR. As such, diagnosis of one condition should prompt evaluation for the other.

PMR is characterized by persistent pain or stiffness of the neck, bilateral upper arms, shoulders, hips, or thighs that is accompanied by significant morning stiffness and constitutional symptoms of fatigue, low-grade fever, anorexia, and weight loss. In 2012, ACR and EULAR released guidelines for the classification of PMR. Although these criteria were developed as a research tool rather than as specific diagnostic criteria, this classification system can be helpful in assessing patients with suspected PMR. The differential diagnosis of PMR is broad, including RA (particularly the RS3PE and polymyalgia rheumatic variations), dermatomyositis, polymyositis, fibromyalgia, drug-induced myalgia or myositis, multiple myeloma, osteoarthritis, depression, vasculitis, hypothyroidism, and endocarditis. Initial evaluation in older adults with suspected PMR should focus on history, physical examination, and laboratory findings to exclude alternative diagnoses. The physical examination in PMR is nonspecific and may be normal. There may be mild muscular tenderness to palpation, and range of motion may be limited by pain, but there should be no true muscular weakness. Normal muscle bulk and strength distinguishes PMR from the inflammatory myopathies. One-third of patients will have a mild, symmetric, nonerosive polyarthritis of the hands, wrists, and knees. Over half of patients will have synovitis of the glenohumeral joint and biceps tenosynovitis. Laboratory evaluation in PMR is typically characterized by increased ESR and/or CRP, along with negative RF, anti-CCP, ANA, and normal CPK. However, it is important to keep in mind the increasing prevalence of positive RF and ANA with age, independent of the presence of autoimmune disorders. Plain radiographs of involved joints should not reveal abnormalities, and the arthritis of PMR is not characterized by erosions. As noted in the ACR/EULAR

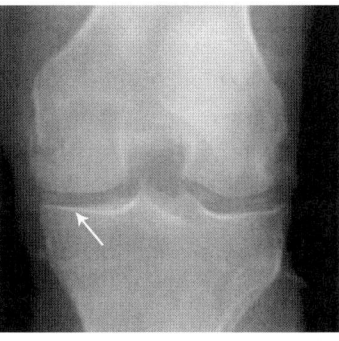 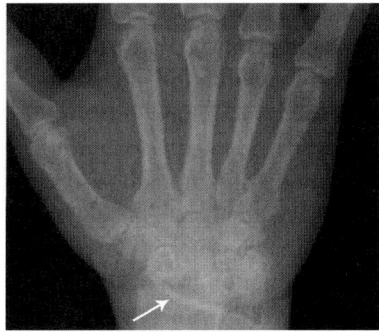

Figure 59.2—*Left:* Chondrocalcinosis of the meniscus. *Right:* Chondrocalcinosis of the triangular fibrocartilage of the wrist distal to the ulna

criteria, ultrasound can be helpful in differentiating PMR from other noninflammatory conditions.

Corticosteroids are the cornerstone of treatment of PMR. Doses required for treatment of PMR are much lower than those used in treatment of GCA. ACR and EULAR published joint recommendations for the management of PMR in 2015. The recommended initial dose is 12.5–25 mg of prednisone equivalent daily, with doses at the higher end of this range recommended for patients at higher risk of relapse and low risk of adverse effects from steroids, and doses at the lower end of the range for patients at increased risk of adverse effects from steroids, such as those with diabetes, osteoporosis, or glaucoma. Intramuscular methylprednisolone may be considered as an alternative to oral prednisone. The minimum effective dose should be used (SOE=B). Symptoms should improve within 2 weeks with near complete resolution after 4 weeks. Concomitant GCA or an alternative diagnosis should be considered in patients whose response to therapy is incomplete or not sustained. The ACR/EULAR guidelines strongly recommend individualizing the steroid taper, based on regular monitoring of symptoms, inflammatory markers, and adverse effects of steroids. The steroid taper should begin once remission is achieved, reducing the dose gradually to 10 mg daily within 4–8 weeks. Then, the dose should be further tapered by 1 mg every 4 weeks. If relapse occurs, the dose should be increased to the pre-relapse dose and then decreased again gradually over 4–8 weeks to the dose at which relapse occurred. Treatment may take 12–18 months or longer to complete, following these guidelines. Osteoporosis prevention is critical in these patients, especially if anticipated doses of prednisone exceed 7.5 mg/d for >3 months. *Pneumocystis* pneumonia prophylaxis may be considered in patients receiving daily prednisone doses of ≥20 mg for longer than 1 month. Oral methotrexate at dosages of 7.5–10 mg/week should be considered as an adjunctive, steroid-sparing agent in patients at high risk of relapse or adverse effects of glucocorticoids (SOE=B). Tumor necrosis factor α–blocking agents have not been shown to be effective in PMR (SOE=B).

GIANT CELL ARTERITIS

Giant cell arteritis (GCA) is a granulomatous vasculitis that involves large and medium-sized arteries. Like PMR, GCA is a disease unique to older adults, occurring almost exclusively in patients ≥50 years old and increasing in incidence with age. The incidence in the United States is estimated at 18 per 100,000, and it is twice as common in women than in men. As noted previously, the overlap between GCA and PMR is considerable; therefore, patients with PMR with any symptoms above the neck should have a temporal artery biopsy to evaluate for GCA.

The most well-known presentation of GCA is that of cranial arteritis that may result in visual loss; however, GCA may also present initially with extracranial arteritis, systemic inflammatory symptoms, PMR, or any combination of these manifestations. PMR is the presenting symptom of GCA in 25% of patients. Head and neck manifestations of GCA include headache, scalp tenderness, jaw or tongue claudication, diplopia, and prominent tender, erythematous, or nodular temporal arteries, which are typically pulseless. Constitutional symptoms, including fatigue, malaise, weight loss, and fever, are common and may be the only manifestations of GCA. Optic nerve pallor or swelling portends ischemia with impending blindness that warrants immediate glucocorticoid therapy. GCA can also present as sudden blindness with no prior systemic illness. GCA may present with claudication in the arms, respiratory symptoms, transient ischemic attack, stroke, peripheral neuropathy, syncope, ischemic necrosis of tongue or scalp, or rarely myocardial infarction. Aortic aneurysm, predominantly thoracic, is a late manifestation of GCA even when previously appropriately treated. The incidence of aneurysm in GCA has been reported to be up to 8%, although the time period of maximal risk for aneurysm development is unclear.

Laboratory evaluation of patients with suspected GCA is characterized by increased ESR and/or CRP. Patients may have other laboratory manifestations of systemic inflammatory disease, including anemia of chronic inflammation, thrombocytosis, leukocytosis, hypoalbuminemia, and increased alkaline phosphatase. Serologic tests are generally not helpful in establishing the diagnosis of GCA, although a proportion of patients are anti-phospholipid or anti-ferritin antibody positive.

Radiographic findings in GCA include hypermetabolic activity in vascular walls seen on PET-CT with ^{18}F-FDG, evidence of inflammation on MRI, and hypoechoic changes representing edema of the temporal artery walls, called a "halo sign," on Doppler ultrasound. Magnetic resonance angiography or CT angiography may be used to evaluate aortic dissection or occlusion. However, imaging findings alone are not sufficient to make the diagnosis.

Although presumptive diagnosis of GCA is made based on history, physical examination, and laboratory findings, temporal artery biopsy is the gold standard for diagnosis. In fact, biopsy is the only test able to definitively diagnose GCA. Histologic examination shows vasculitis at the intima-media junction with mononuclear cell infiltrates and usually with giant cells. Care should be taken to differentiate the histologic findings of GCA from the normal changes in vascular histology that occur with aging.

The most recent ACR classification criteria for GCA are from 1990. A diagnosis of GCA can be made with 94% sensitivity and 91% specificity if at least 3 of 5 criteria are present: age at onset ≥50 years, new headache, temporal artery tenderness or decreased pulsation, increased ESR, and artery biopsy consistent with GCA.

Preferably with a positive biopsy confirming GCA, but often with a convincing history and symptoms (and negative biopsy), patients suspected of having GCA should start treatment with prednisone to reduce the risk of sudden blindness. If necessary, prednisone may be started before biopsy; fortunately for diagnostic purposes, pathologic evidence of GCA persists for up to 2 weeks after prednisone therapy has been started. Prednisone is given at a dosage of 40–60 mg/d and should be maintained for 4–8 weeks or until symptomatic relief and normalization of the ESR and/or CRP before considering dosage reduction. Initial treatment with intravenous glucocorticoids may be considered in patients presenting with transient or permanent vision loss, diplopia, transient ischemic attack, or stroke. Treatment typically continues for approximately 1–3 years. Relapses during steroid taper often present with PMR symptoms, and steroid dose should be temporarily increased to treat the symptoms before resuming the taper. ESR should be monitored along with symptoms to assess disease activity. A persistently increased ESR without symptoms should prompt evaluation for silent aortitis. Long-term glucocorticoid therapy warrants prophylaxis for osteoporosis and possibly for *Pneumocystis* pneumonia if daily prednisone doses exceed 20 mg for >1 month. Published studies of methotrexate as a steroid-sparing agent have not consistently demonstrated a benefit, but the highest quality studies suggest that it is helpful and should be considered for patients at high risk of glucocorticoid-related adverse effects (SOE=B). Other immunomodulatory agents such as etanercept (SOE=B) may be useful as adjunctive steroid-sparing agents. Interleukin-6 is thought to play a role in pathogenesis, which is supported by recent research demonstrating the efficacy of tocilizumab in the treatment of GCA. A phase 2, randomized, placebo-controlled trial has demonstrated the efficacy of tocilizumab in addition to glucocorticoids for inducing and maintaining remission of GCA and for decreasing the cumulative glucocorticoid dose (SOE=B). In addition, concomitant administration of low-dose aspirin has been shown to decrease the risk of vision loss and cranial ischemic complications. Even after immunosuppression is discontinued, the clinician should remain vigilant for development of aortic aneurysm.

SYSTEMIC LUPUS ERYTHEMATOSUS

Systemic lupus erythematosus (SLE) is an autoimmune multisystemic disease that most commonly affects women of child-bearing age, yet up to 20% of cases are seen in older adults. When onset is after 50 years of age, the condition is referred to as "late-onset lupus." Late-onset lupus shows less of a female predominance than traditional SLE. Of note, data from the UK suggests that the peak incidence of lupus occurs in women 50–54 years old and men 70–74 years old. There is no corresponding data from the United States.

In contrast to SLE in younger patients, late-onset lupus is characterized by a more insidious onset, less major organ involvement, and lower disease activity, making definitive diagnosis challenging. Late-onset lupus may present initially with vague symptoms, including fatigue, fever, weight loss, arthralgia, and myalgia, invoking a broad differential diagnosis. Late-onset lupus should be considered in the differential diagnosis of rash (need not be malar in distribution), nonerosive arthritis, serositis (pleuritis, pericarditis), cytopenias (leukopenia, hemolytic anemia, or thrombocytopenia), neuropsychiatric symptoms (cognitive, seizures), sicca symptoms (in the absence of medication-induced dry mouth), and Raynaud phenomenon. Renal involvement (eg, urinary casts, proteinuria) is less common in older lupus patients than in younger ones. Additional physical findings can include periungual or palmar erythema, asymptomatic oral or nasal ulcers, and livedo reticularis; when present, these may raise suspicion of antiphospholipid antibody syndrome (venous or arterial thromboembolic phenomena).

The more characteristic features of SLE, such as malar rash, photosensitivity, arthritis, and nephritis, are less common at presentation of late-onset lupus, and older patients typically fulfill fewer ACR criteria for the classification of SLE than younger patients. In contrast, pulmonary involvement and serositis seem to be more common in late-onset lupus. These differences in the presentation of late-onset lupus can contribute to a significant delay in diagnosis.

Diagnosis of SLE, particularly in older adults, requires a detailed history, thorough physical examination, and laboratory investigation. In late-onset lupus, patients are less likely to have positive anti-ribonucleoprotein or anti-Smith antibodies, but they are more frequently positive for rheumatoid factor (RF), ANA, anti-Ro/Sjögren syndrome (SS) A, and anti-La/SSB. Anti-double-stranded DNA and hypocomplementemia, both useful in monitoring disease activity in younger patients, are less frequently found in older patients.

Given the frequency of polypharmacy in older adults, it is especially important to distinguish late-onset lupus from drug-induced lupus erythematosus, although this is often clinically difficult. Both have a positive ANA test, although drug-induced lupus erythematosus is associated with a speckled pattern with antihistone antibodies.

In 2014, a multispecialty international task force published recommendations for a "treat to target" approach in SLE, which is the concept that the remission of symptoms or the lowest possible disease activity should be achieved using the lowest possible dose of medication to minimize drug toxicities while optimizing quality of life. This concept is particularly important when caring for older adults. Exercise (both aerobic and strength training) has been shown to be an effective method of reducing fatigue in SLE patients (SOE=A). The treatment recommendations below are based entirely on extrapolation from younger adults; no studies of these therapies have been conducted specifically in older adults with lupus (SOE=D). If not contraindicated, short-acting NSAIDs can be used to treat arthritis and serositis in older adults who can tolerate them. It is important to use a gastroprotective proton-pump inhibitor if NSAID use is prolonged. Hydroxychloroquine is effective in managing skin and joint manifestations (200–400 mg/d). To minimize risk of hydroxychloroquine-associated retinal toxicity, the maximal recommended daily dose is 5 mg/kg of actual body weight. Before starting hydroxychloroquine, patients should undergo a baseline ophthalmologic examination. In the absence of major risk factors for retinal toxicity (daily dose >5 mg/kg, renal disease, tamoxifen use, or underlying retinal or macular disease), annual ophthalmologic screening should begin after 5 years of hydroxychloroquine use (SOE=A). Low-dose corticosteroid use may be considered in patients with symptoms refractory to hydroxychloroquine, although long-term use of steroids in older adults is associated with significant adverse effects that may outweigh potential benefits. Depending on the organ system involved and disease manifestation, methotrexate^{OL}, azathioprine^{OL}, mycophenolate mofetil^{OL}, or cyclosporine^{OL} can be of benefit as corticosteroid-sparing agents, although safety of these drugs has not been studied specifically in older adults.

SJÖGREN SYNDROME

Sjögren syndrome is a systemic, multiorgan chronic disease characterized by lymphocytic infiltration of exocrine glands. The estimated incidence is 7 per 100,000 persons per year with an estimated prevalence of 70 per 100,000 people. It is approximately 10 times more common in women than in men with an average age of 56 years at time of diagnosis (SOE=A). Sjögren syndrome may develop alone or in conjunction with other rheumatologic diseases, including RA, SLE, scleroderma, or inflammatory myopathy, in which case it is classified as secondary Sjögren syndrome. The presence of palpable purpura and C4 hypocomplementemia are recognized as potential predictors for development of lymphoma.

The most well-known manifestations of Sjögren syndrome are signs of keratoconjunctivitis sicca, including ocular and oral dryness (xerophthalmia and xerostomia, respectively), which result from destruction of lacrimal and salivary glands. These signs are relatively common in older adults, and initial evaluation should focus on excluding drug-induced sicca symptoms, particularly due to anticholinergic adverse effects, as well as age-related exocrine gland fibrosis or fatty infiltration, or other underlying connective tissue syndromes. It is important to remember that Sjögren syndrome is not limited to the lacrimal and salivary glands; it may present with dysphagia, weight loss, vaginal dryness, or sexual dysfunction. Sjögren syndrome may also cause extraglandular disease, including pulmonary, renal, bladder, liver, biliary, thyroid, nervous system, articular, and skin manifestations. As such, Sjögren syndrome should be considered in patients with interstitial lung disease; malabsorption; CNS disease that mimics multiple sclerosis; unexplained renal, liver, or thyroid disease; or rash.

Patients should be counseled on the importance of maintaining good dental health to prevent caries (they are at higher risk with xerostomia), gum disease, and dental erosions. Pilocarpine and cevimeline can be used to treat xerostomia; however, their use in older adults is limited by cholinergic adverse effects. Symptomatic treatment of xerophthalmia consists of lubricating ointments and artificial tears. Ophthalmic cyclosporine or lifitegrast can be added to artificial tears if symptom relief is inadequate (SOE=A). Under the direction of an ophthalmologist, a short course of topical steroids can be given for severe refractory symptoms (SOE=B). Punctal plugs can be tried to retain tears (SOE=B). Treatment of an underlying inflammatory disease (eg, RA, SLE, myositis, or scleroderma) will usually improve symptoms as well.

POLYMYOSITIS AND DERMATOMYOSITIS

Inflammatory muscle diseases, including polymyositis and dermatomyositis, form a heterogeneous and uncommon group of skeletal muscle diseases. Incidence of these diseases peaks in adults in their 50s, but they can occur at any age, and studies suggest that up to 20% of cases occur in adults ≥65 years old. Inclusion body myositis is another type of idiopathic inflammatory myopathy that can be seen in older adults. In contrast to polymyositis and dermatomyositis, inclusion body myositis may be more insidious in onset, affects men more frequently than women, and causes both proximal and distal muscle weakness. Response to steroids or other immunosuppressive therapy is generally poor in inclusion body myositis, with disease progression despite treatment.

Muscle weakness is the central feature of polymyositis and dermatomyositis, and it is most prominent in the proximal muscle groups. Patients report difficulty with tasks such as standing from a chair, ascending stairs, or lifting a light package above the head. Muscle tenderness is usually not a manifestation and should increase suspicion of other conditions. Arthritis, when present, is inflammatory and occasionally erosive, suggesting overlap with RA. Esophageal dysmotility can cause dysphagia, hoarseness, and aspiration. Arrhythmia, symptoms of congestive heart disease, dyspnea on exertion, or persistent cough can also be present and suggest cardiac muscle involvement or coexistent interstitial lung disease. Pulmonary involvement, including interstitial lung disease and diaphragmatic insufficiency, is a poor prognostic sign associated with increased morbidity and mortality. Raynaud phenomenon or Sjögren syndrome can also be present.

Dermatomyositis is characterized by several skin findings that can help distinguish it from polymyositis: a heliotrope rash that is erythematous to violaceous and involves the eyelids; Gottron papules, which are areas of skin thickening over the metacarpophalangeal and interphalangeal joints; and a photo-distributed rash over the neck, upper chest, and upper back. "Mechanic's hands" or thickened and fissured skin on the fingers may be seen in either dermatomyositis or polymyositis. Amyopathic dermatomyositis is dermatomyositis limited to the skin, in which patients have the classic cutaneous manifestations of dermatomyositis but do not have muscle weakness. The antisynthetase syndrome can be seen in patients with dermatomyositis or polymyositis; classic features include antibodies to aminoacyl-transfer ribonucleic acid (tRNA) synthetase enzymes, constitutional symptoms, interstitial lung disease, myositis, nonerosive arthritis, Mechanic's hands, and Raynaud phenomenon, all typically with acute disease onset.

Differential diagnosis of myositis includes endocrine, metabolic, musculoskeletal, and medication-related disorders, including thyroid disorders, diabetes, vitamin D deficiency, electrolyte abnormalities, polymyalgia rheumatica, and medication adverse effects from steroids or statins. Statins are perhaps the most widely used medication with risk of toxic myopathy, with increased risk in older adults, especially with longer duration and higher doses. Statins have been associated with myalgias in 5%–10% of patients, myositis in 1%, and rhabdomyolysis in 0.1%, and up to 25% may develop exercise-related muscle cramping or pain. In patients with suspected myositis, initial evaluation should focus on excluding other more common causes of muscle weakness before pursuing invasive testing with muscle biopsy. Serum levels of muscle enzymes (creatine kinase, aldolase, and sometime transaminases) are usually increased in myositis; normal levels suggest an alternative diagnosis. ANA is often positive, as well as various myositis specific autoantibodies which can be predictive of the patient's phenotype and symptoms. Electromyographic testing is used to exclude neuropathy and to identify the presence of an irritable myopathy. MRI using fat-suppression sequences helps to confirm myositis and can help to select which muscle to biopsy. Muscle biopsy remains the gold standard to confirm the diagnosis and also to distinguish among the subtypes of myositis. A diagnosis of polymyositis warrants an evaluation for cardiac and pulmonary disease. Dermatomyositis and polymyositis have been associated with increased incidence of underlying colon, lung, breast, prostate, ovarian, and uterine cancers. However, extensive evaluation for occult malignancy is costly and is not without risks. It is recommended that patients with dermatomyositis and polymyositis simply undergo age-appropriate cancer screening, although clinicians should keep in mind this increased incidence of malignancy when evaluating any new or abnormal signs or symptoms.

Concurrent with pharmacologic management, a supervised exercise program over 6-week and 6-month study periods has proved beneficial in polymyositis

(SOE=B), improving function without aggravating underlying disease. Response to therapy in older adults with polymyositis and dermatomyositis is lower than that in younger adults. Glucocorticoids are the initial therapy for polymyositis and dermatomyositis. Oral prednisone at 1 mg/kg/d is a typical starting dosage; for severe disease, an initial dose of methylprednisolone 1,000 mg IV is often used over 3 consecutive days. Prednisone can be tapered after an initial phase of improved muscle strength and normalized muscle enzyme concentrations. However, prolonged glucocorticoid use at high dosages can result in a myopathy with resultant proximal muscle weakness. Therefore, tapering the total dose by 10%–20% per month should be attempted. High dose or prolonged glucocorticoid use necessitates osteoporosis prevention and possibly *Pneumocystis* pneumonia prophylaxis (discussed in detail in PMR and GCA sections of this chapter.) Methotrexate[OL] (SOE=B) or azathioprine[OL] (SOE=B) may be used in combination with prednisone as steroid-sparing agents. Because of hepatic and pulmonary toxicity of methotrexate, azathioprine[OL] may be preferred in patients with interstitial lung disease or underlying liver disease. In patients without an adequate response to glucocorticoids in combination with either methotrexate or azathioprine, rituximab[OL] (SOE=B) and intravenous immunoglobulin (IVIG)[OL] (SOE=B) may be considered as alternative therapies. However, older adults are at increased risk of renal failure and thrombotic events with IVIG.

FIBROMYALGIA

Fibromyalgia is a pain syndrome that incorporates both physical and psychological components. Because of its heterogeneous presentation, fibromyalgia can be challenging to diagnose and manage, particularly in older adults. Generalized body pain is the hallmark of fibromyalgia, which can be associated with various other complaints, including mood disturbance, fatigue, cognitive disorders, and a variety of somatic symptoms, including but not limited to irritable bowel syndrome, fatigue, muscle pain, headache, and sleep disturbance.

Fibromyalgia is a clinical diagnosis, which was redefined by the 2010 ACR criteria. Diagnosis is made on the basis of Widespread Pain Index and Symptom Severity scores, with symptoms present for at least 3 months and no other explanation for symptoms. Diagnosis of fibromyalgia no longer includes tender point examination, which was previously included in 1990 diagnostic criteria. Thorough history and physical examination are central to the diagnosis of fibromyalgia. Aside from generalized soft-tissue sensitivity, physical examination in patients with fibromyalgia should be normal for age. Importantly, patients with fibromyalgia will not have evidence of inflammation or synovitis on physical examination. Likewise, laboratory abnormalities such as an increased ESR or CRP should prompt investigation for an alternative diagnosis.

It is especially important in older adults to ensure that the diagnosis of fibromyalgia is accurate and that symptoms cannot be attributed to another condition. Diagnosis of fibromyalgia is complex in older adults, because widespread pain is more common in this population, and older adults may have multiple comorbid conditions with overlapping symptoms. Chronic pain from a variety of sources, including osteoarthritis, neuropathy, and degenerative spinal disease, may coincide with fibromyalgia, making differentiation of the source of chronic pain challenging. Differential diagnosis in fibromyalgia includes musculoskeletal, endocrine, psychiatric, and medication-related disorders, including RA, PMR, myositis, osteoarthritis, hypothyroidism, vitamin D deficiency, depression, and medication adverse effects (eg, from statins, bisphosphonates, and proton-pump inhibitors).

Pathophysiology of fibromyalgia remains unclear, but current theories suggest central pain sensitization as a result of dysregulation of pain processing. Although up to one-third of patients may have a clear inciting event, most patients with fibromyalgia have no identifiable cause.

Treatment of fibromyalgia, particularly in older adults, should be focused on nonpharmacologic therapies. Studies have shown that physical activity (SOE=A), patient education (SOE=A), cognitive-behavioral therapy (SOE=A), meditation, acupuncture, and hydrotherapy can improve symptoms. When encouraging physical activity in patients with chronic pain syndromes, it can be helpful to distinguish between "hurt" and "harm." Although increasing activity may temporarily cause increased physical pain, it can be reassuring to emphasize that pain is not necessarily harmful, and that in the long-term, physical activity is an essential component of managing this condition. Increasing physical activity slowly and in small increments that are easily sustainable in daily life is critical. It is important to use a multimodal approach to treat fibromyalgia; chronic pain, sleep disturbances, and depression and anxiety must each be addressed individually to optimize efficacy of treatment.

Few pharmacologic treatments have proved effective in treatment of fibromyalgia. There are 3 FDA-approved medications for fibromyalgia: pregabalin, duloxetine, and milnacipran (SOE=A). Other medications, including acetaminophen, anticonvulsants, antidepressants, muscle relaxants, and weak opioids such as tramadol, have been used in treatment of fibromyalgia, although studies have not specifically evaluated their use in older adults. Most medications used in treatment of fibromyalgia provide only modest benefits despite carrying considerable risk of adverse effects, including sedation, cognitive deficits, insomnia, balance impairment, and falls. Pharmacologic therapy should be individualized based on specific symptoms, and medication regimens should be frequently reassessed to evaluate for effectiveness and adverse effects. Perhaps the most crucial aspect of treatment of fibromyalgia is formation of a therapeutic alliance between clinician and patient. By setting realistic expectations, expressing commitment to finding solutions, and, most importantly, being available to provide support and reassurance, clinicians can ultimately help improve treatment outcomes for their patients with chronic pain syndromes.

Choosing Wisely® Recommendations

Rheumatology

- Do not test ANA sub-serologies without a positive ANA and clinical suspicion of immune-mediated disease.

- Do not perform MRI of the peripheral joints to routinely monitor inflammatory arthritis.

- Do not prescribe biologics for rheumatoid arthritis before a trial of methotrexate (or other conventional nonbiologic DMARDs).

- Do not routinely repeat DXA scans more often than once every 2 years.

RESOURCES

- Buttgereit F, Dejaco C, Matteson EL, et al. Polymyalgia rheumatica and giant cell arteritis: a systematic review. *JAMA*. 2016;315(22):2442–2458.

- Huges L, Adair J, Feng F, et al. Nurse practitioners' education, awareness, and therapeutic approaches for the management of fibromyalgia. *Orthop Nurs*. 2016;35(5):317–322.

- Minnock P, McKee G, Kelly A, et al. Nursing sensitive outcomes in patients with rheumatoid arthritis: a systematic literature review. *Int J Nurs Stud*. 2018;77:55–129.

- Rosenthal AK, Ryan LM. Calcium pyrophosphate deposition disease. *N Engl J Med*. 2016;374(26):2575–2584.

CHAPTER 60—DISORDERS OF THE FOOT

KEY POINTS

- Foot and ankle problems are common in older adults. Early diagnosis and effective treatment are critical to maintaining function and quality of life.

- Long-term effects of common structural foot deformities, including collapsing pes plano valgus, cavus foot, and equinus deformity of the ankle and forefoot, cause significant disability in older adults.

- Skin disorders of the foot are common in older adults. Complete assessment of the skin of the foot is necessary to identify skin conditions and potential malignancies.

- Systemic diseases can have long-term effects on the foot and ankle.

- Structural changes not improved with shoe changes and/or OTC inserts may require referral for prescription footwear, orthoses, or ankle/foot orthoses.

- Surgical intervention for treatment of foot deformities can alleviate pain and improve function in older adults who are appropriate surgical candidates. Many surgical interventions in older adults can be performed under local anesthesia or with moderate sedation.

Foot problems can have a significant effect on the functional capacity of older adults and negatively impact their quality of life. Left untreated, these problems can lead to inactivity, morbidity, and even death.

Foot problems vary in severity from dry xerotic skin on the plantar surface of the foot to an infected, limb-threatening diabetic foot ulcer in a patient with peripheral neuropathy and arterial disease. In general, most foot problems are musculoskeletal and/or dermatologic in nature, although vascular, neurologic, and systemic diseases can also affect the foot. Complicating the situation is the fact that many older adults are not in the habit of inspecting their feet or may lack the flexibility and mobility to do so effectively. Unless older adults are experiencing pain or discomfort, they may not notice or may ignore pathologic changes that are developing.

Therefore, clinicians treating older adults should be conscious of the potential for foot problems and make an effort to determine whether any of these conditions or predisposing factors exist. The prevalence of diabetes in middle-aged and older populations intensifies the need for this inspection. Once identified, specific problems should be treated or the patient referred to the appropriate specialist, depending on the preliminary presentation or diagnosis.

Not all older adults are similarly affected by foot problems. The prevalence of foot problems in older adults varies by level of disability and site of care. Studies of a variety of health care settings (including nursing homes, inpatient facilities, and outpatient settings) and examination of age- and morbidity-specific populations show that the prevalence of foot pathology increases with age. Approximately one-third of the geriatric population has some foot pathology, and incidence is higher in those residing in a medical facility such as a nursing home or hospital.

The most common problems identified are nail disorders, corns/calluses, hammertoes, plantar fasciitis, hallux valgus, and flat feet. Studies of the geriatric population demonstrate that foot complaints can inhibit daily activities such as getting out of a chair, walking, and climbing stairs. The resulting decrease in mobility can exacerbate other age-related conditions and lead to loss of muscle, a decrease in cardiovascular function, and weight gain. Foot pathologies are also associated with increased risk of falling in the aging population.

THE ROLE OF THE PRIMARY CARE CLINICIAN IN FOOT CARE

Because older adults may not always be vigilant when it comes to the health of their lower extremities, primary care clinicians should regularly assess their geriatric patients' feet. Practitioners should pay close attention to foot conditions and the complications of systemic diseases (such as arthritic changes, neurologic disorders, diabetes mellitus, peripheral arterial disease, and mental health issues) that can manifest as foot symptoms and signs. Primary care clinicians should recognize common foot problems and refer patients for podiatric care and management in a timely and appropriate manner. The health, quality of life, and functional capacity of older adults can be significantly improved by early detection and comprehensive management of foot problems (SOE=D).

COMMON DEFORMITIES OF THE FOOT

Most foot deformities derive from the longstanding effects of a pathologic foot. A pathologic foot is one in which pressure distribution and force is abnormally concentrated or directed because of acquired or congenital morphology/physiology. Over an extended period, this physical stress on the foot may result in arthritis, tissue atrophy, and subluxation of the joints of the foot and ankle.

Disability is, broadly, created by two pathologic foot types: collapsing pes plano valgus (low arch morphology) and the rarer cavus foot (high arch morphology). A higher than normal arch (cavus deformity) can lead to pes cavus, which is commonly associated with neurologic change. In older adults, excessive pressure is usually placed on the metatarsal heads. With atrophy of the plantar fat pad and displacement, pressure is increased, which can predispose to pain and ulceration. Equinus, the effect of a tight Achilles tendon (or gastrocnemius-soleus muscle complex), or bone obstruction, is a deforming force that can be identified in both pes planus and pes cavus foot types. Collapsing pes plano valgus is a foot type with an unstable medial longitudinal arch, which leads to a "flat foot." A flat arch (pes planus) can lead to collapsing pes plano valgus, ie, a flattening of the medial longitudinal arch (flat feet) along with pronation, demonstrated by a lateral deviation of the Achilles tendon and an outward and rotational deformity of the foot. The instability can occur in the talonavicular joint, the navicular cuneiform joint, and/or the first metatarsal cuneiform joint. This instability causes the hindfoot and leg to internally rotate on a plantigrade foot, leading to the appearance of an abducted or externally rotated forefoot. Rearfoot eversion or valgus positioning relative to the ankle joint and leg is then observable. When the patient bears weight, the longitudinal arch collapses, resulting in compression and/or subluxation of joints and soft-tissue strain, arthrosis, and finally arthritis.

While moderate planus deformity is considered the norm in childhood (ages 1–10), if the tendency is retained into adolescence and adulthood, it may be associated with symptoms. When the foot is flexible, symptoms are generally manageable with prescription or OTC shoe inserts/orthoses. However, with age, rigidity, or spastic deformity, the foot becomes less tolerant of excessive stress, and conservative modalities may prove ineffective. Patients with this type of foot often have other associated deformities, including posterior tibial tendon dysfunction (tendonitis or tendinosis), hallux valgus (bunion deformity), lesser metatarsal phalangeal joint (MTPJ) dislocations (chronic dislocation of the toe joints), hammertoes, and neuromas.

The cavus foot type is generally more rigid and is a very poor shock absorber. It also can be, rarely, congenital. If acquired later in life, it usually has a neurologic origin. The cavus foot often has a component of metatarsus adductus (inward orientation of the metatarsal bones). Older adults with this foot type generally experience loss of the fat pad in both the heel and the submetatarsal head region or ball of the foot due to accumulated stress. Associated deformities include hallux hammertoe,

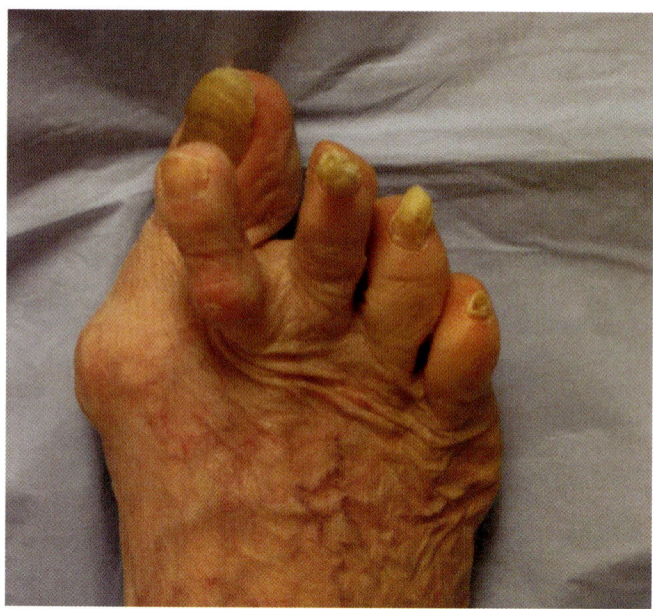

Figure 60.1—Hallux abducto valgus with crossover toe deformity

sagittal/dorsal dislocation of the MTPJs, mid-foot dorsal exostoses (bone spurs), and rigid hammertoe deformities.

An equinus deformity is commonly seen in a pes planus or cavus foot, but it can also be seen in a foot with a normal appearance. Ankle equinus causes decreased plantar pressure at the heel during gait, and increased pressure and loading velocity of the forefoot. Functional equinus may evolve from tightness of either the gastrosoleal complex or the gastrocnemius muscle complex or may be related to bone obstruction at the anterior tibio-talar joint. Equinus is associated with Achilles tendinitis, plantar fasciitis, metatarsalgia, and hammertoe deformities. It is also considered to be a risk factor for development of acquired flatfoot deformity in adults.

Common Associated Deformities

Specific associated deformities can develop due to the pathomechanics of the general deformities. See Table 60.1.

Chronic Dislocated Metatarsal Phalangeal Joint

The end-stage of a hammertoe deformity is a chronic, fixed, dislocated joint, a condition that is not uncommon in older adults and is caused by long-term flexor versus extensor imbalance across the lesser MTPJs. This is also seen sometimes at an earlier age in patients who have rheumatoid arthritis. The proximal phalanx dislocates dorsally onto the metatarsal head, which in turn causes a retrograde pressure on the metatarsal head, increasing local plantar pressure. When this occurs on the second toe, it is frequently associated with a hallux valgus deformity and can result in a cross-over deformity, as

Table 60.1–Common Disorders of the Foot

Location/Disorder	Definition or Description
Forefoot	
Bunion	Prominent dorsal and/or medial eminence of the first metatarsal; associated with hallux valgus, ie, deviation of the great toe, or main axis of the toe, toward the fibular or lateral side of the foot
Digiti quinti varus	Valgus displacement or splaying of the fifth metatarsal, with a resulting varus or inward deviation of the fifth toe
Dislocation of lesser metatarsal phalangeal joint	A progressive loss of capsular and ligamentous constraint at lesser MTPJs, allowing dorsal and medial or lateral subluxation and dislocation of the digit. Associated with hallux valgus, rheumatoid arthritis and diabetes.
Hallux abducto valgus	An alternative term for hallux valgus, or bunion. There is adductus of the first metatarsal relative to the second metatarsal with valgus rotation and abductus deformity of the phalanges of the great toe. The condition is more common in women than men and affects up to 35% of individuals >65 years old.
Hallux limitus and rigidus	A degenerative joint change involving the first MTPJ, resulting from dorsal spurs, with a marked limitation or absence of range of motion. The difference between hallux limitus and rigidus is based on radiographic interpretation and measurement of joint motion.
Hammertoe	Muscle tendon imbalance causing contraction of the proximal or distal interphalangeal joint, or both
Tailor's bunion	Prominence of the dorsal lateral aspect of the fifth metatarsal head caused by exostosis formation or splaying of the metatarsals
Valgus position	Frontal plane position in which the center of pressure is directed toward the midline/line of progression
Varus position	Frontal plane position in which the center of pressure is directed away from the midline/line of progression
Midfoot	
Metatarsalgia	A nonspecific term describing pain in the forefoot near the heads of the metatarsals
Morton foot	A congenital shortening of the first metatarsal shaft, which creates an abnormal metatarsal arc. Excessive weight is placed on the second metatarsal head during gait and stance. The dynamics and mechanics of the foot are modified and can lead to hallux valgus, abducto valgus, or rotational deformity of the hallux and dislocation of the second digit at the MTPJ.
Tibialis posterior dysfunction	A general term describing degenerative change of supporting soft tissue structures of the medial hindfoot associated with developing or chronic pes planus. This is most commonly seen among middle-aged and older individuals, frequently women, who are obese and meet the definition of metabolic syndrome (up to 10% of all cases fit this description).
Rear foot	
Calcaneal spur/heel spur	A calcification of the attachment of the plantar fascia, usually at the medial plantar tuberosity of the calcaneus. The spur projects anteriorly and is the consequence of chronic repetitive trauma or stress. The presence of the exostosis is common (as high as 45% of participants in one study), especially in adults >40 years old, and does not consistently correlate to symptoms. Traction of the plantar fascia at the attachment (ie, enthesis) of the medial tubercle is the cause of most plantar heel pain, although other diagnoses should be considered in older adults.
Equinus	A functional or structural loss or restriction of ankle joint dorsiflexion
Haglund deformity	A hyperostosis of the posterior and superior portion of the calcaneus, enlarging the calcaneus, which is often accompanied by calcific change within the distal Achilles tendon. The presence of the deformity can produce a pressure area for the heel counter of the shoe. It is easily demonstrated on a lateral radiograph of the foot and can be associated with tendinitis or bursitis anterior to the tendon.
Plantar fasciitis	Inflammation and pain involving repetitive microtrauma to the plantar fascia, particularly at its inferior calcaneal attachment, associated with pathomechanical function of the foot. It may be associated with plantar calcaneal exostosis, partial tear of the fascia, and fat pad atrophy.
Plantar fasciosis	A degenerative condition, causing heel pain, that describes the noninflammatory phase of heel pain caused by degeneration of the plantar fascia, usually as a result of repetitive stress.
Tarsal tunnel syndrome	An entrapment neuropathy of the posterior tibial nerve. This may be related to valgus positioning of the hindfoot or to compression of the nerve bundle by lipoma, ganglion, or other mass inferior to the nerve.
Other	
Rheumatic and other degenerative disorders	Mono-articular, symmetrical, or regional joint pathology may exist as a consequence of trauma, chronic postural stress, or inflammatory arthritis. Radiographs and other studies will reveal changes consistent with these disorders such as erosion, joint space narrowing, and/or dislocation/deviation.
Entrapment syndrome	Occurs when a nerve is compressed by ligamentous or other soft-tissue inflammation, resulting in pain and possibly numbness and neuropathic symptoms; most common sites are the posterior tibial nerve and the intermetatarsal nerve, plantarly.
Capsulitis/tenosynovitis	Inflammation of the synovial sheath of a tendon complex or joint, due to microtrauma, chronic postural stress, or inflammatory disease.

well as symptomatic rupture of the plantar MTPJ capsule (plantar plate) (Figure 60.1).

MTPJ dislocations can be a source of chronic pain and contribute to development of plantar ulcerations at the metatarsal heads, especially in those who suffer from neuropathy, peripheral arterial disease, and/or diabetes. Patients developing MTPJ dislocations usually require shoes with increased toe box height to reduce dorsal pressure. Surgical reconstruction of the joint(s) offers predictably positive results, which may restore function and decrease disability, and is indicated when conservative modalities fail.

Hallux Limitus

Hallux limitus is an arthritic condition involving the first MTPJ. Normal motion of the first MTPJ generally ranges from 35 to 75 degrees. Hallux limitus occurs when osseous or soft-tissue compression has decreased the functional range of motion at the joint. There may be early clinical or radiographic findings of arthritis, including crepitus and pain. Hallux rigidus is an end-stage degenerative change that describes very little or absent motion and pronounced arthritic deformity.

The cause of hallux limitus is thought to be sagittal plane instability in the first metatarsal (the first metatarsal has increased dorsiflexion on weightbearing), resulting in hypermobility at the metatarsal-cuneiform joint. This elevation makes necessary dorsiflexion of the hallux on the first metatarsal head more difficult, resulting in compression at the opposing dorsal joint surfaces. Traditional treatment consists of orthoses that limit motion at the first MTPJ and thereby relieve pain. In a study of >700 patients, more than half were successfully treated with conservative orthotic therapy, indicating that this is a viable approach as an initial treatment (SOE=B).

Surgical treatment of hallux limitus/rigidus can range from removal of bone spurs (cheilectomy) to hemi or total joint implants to osteotomies and arthrodesis of the joint. Surgery can successfully reduce symptoms and increase function (SOE=B).

Hallux Valgus

One-third of people >65 years old have a hallux valgus deformity, or bunion. The hallux valgus deformity is a subluxation of the first MTPJ, resulting from the adduction of the first metatarsal and the abduction of the hallux. This deformity progresses throughout a person's lifetime, often associated with hypermobility of the first metatarsal cuneiform joint. The medial prominence and subluxation can be painful, especially when wearing shoes, because of the pressure applied by the shoes to the bunion deformity and because of the abduction and valgus stress applied to the first MTPJ.

Chronic hallux valgus deformities are frequently arthritic. The great majority of cases, even in young patients, include radiographically evident lateral/abducted cartilage adaptation of the first metatarsal head. These deformities are treated conservatively by adapting the shoe to the deformity, ie, instructing the patient to wear wider shoes with a wider toe box and to use various padding techniques. Surgery may be considered if the deformity is symptomatic and unresponsive to conservative management. The types of procedures undertaken depend on the severity of the deformity and on the patient's health and activity level.

Surgical correction of hallux valgus is undertaken with consideration of the cause of the deformity as well as the fundamental nature of the patient's symptoms. Surgical reconstruction in early adult life is not considered to be a life-long correction; recurrence is not uncommon. For older patients in whom deformity may be more advanced, surgical recommendations might also be adapted to simplify procedures, which may be considered acceptable to alleviate symptoms and reduce the demands of surgery and recovery.

As with younger patients, surgical procedures around the first MTPJ focus on the medial eminence of the first metatarsal head, where revision is required to eliminate a symptomatic prominence. However, joint adaptation as noted above, can only be modified by procedures that realign the articular cartilage away from its fibular deviation. This requires an osteotomy of the distal metatarsal head and, therefore, complicates/prolongs recovery and requires bone density that many older adults no longer have. Severely arthritic joints are addressed in essentially two ways: joint arthroplasty (usually without implantation) or MTPJ arthrodesis, which is both durable and effective but again requires a more complex operative and postoperative course.

Studies evaluating orthopedic quality-of-life indicators and Short Form-36 after repair of hallux valgus showed that patients experienced reduced symptoms and were once again able to wear shoes comfortably. In most instances, this positive outcome was seen regardless of the surgical approach. These findings were consistent across all age ranges (SOE=B).

Hammertoe Deformities

Hammertoes are caused by a muscle-tendon imbalance that occurs around the MTPJ. Hammertoes involve a buckling or contraction at the proximal interphalangeal joint (PIPJ) or the distal interphalangeal joint (DIPJ) of the lesser toes. In a "classic" hammertoe, there is a flexor contracture at the PIPJ. A mallet toe is a hammertoe that contracts at the DIPJ. A claw toe is a hammertoe that contracts at both the PIPJ and the DIPJ.

Hammertoes can be flexible and easily reducible, or they can be rigid and nonreducible. Rigid hammertoes are generally more painful and create problems when the patient is wearing shoes. When hammertoes press against the shoe, a callus or corn is created at the dorsal joint margin, causing pain and occasionally ulceration. Treatment of hammertoes may include padding of the affected area, a wide toe box in shoes or custom shoes, palliative debridement, or surgical correction of the deformity. Surgical correction is achieved by joint arthroplasty (one or more joints), frequently in conjunction with arthrodesis or implantation. Concurrent procedures on the metatarsal or adjacent soft tissues are often required to fully remediate the deformity and assure longevity. When hallux valgus is present, surgical repair of that deformity may also be required to allow successful repositioning of lesser digits.

Extra depth or soft, adaptable shoes with more toe box height may also help alleviate symptoms. When irritation occurs at the distal end of the tuft or toe, a crest pad can help elevate the front of the digit and reduce pressure (SOE=C). Deep accommodative insoles may also assist in off-loading painful distal digital deformities.

Neuromas

A neuroma is a benign growth of a peripheral nerve, caused by chronic entrapment. Neuromas are often seen in the foot between the third and fourth metatarsal heads, where they are referred to as Morton neuromas. It is theorized that the metatarsal nerve is entrapped by the deep intermetatarsal ligament as it courses underneath the ligament and forms the digital nerve branches. Tight shoe gear is also commonly implicated in the development of these lesions.

Conservative treatment of neuromas may involve metatarsal pads, orthoses, corticosteroid injections, cryotherapy, or sclerosing alcohol injections. Alternatively, the patient may require surgical release of the intermetatarsal ligament or primary excision of the neuroma. A comparative review of surgical intervention consistently demonstrates favorable results, with 80% of patients reporting a high level of satisfaction after surgery (SOE=B).

Posterior Tibial Tendon Dysfunction

Posterior tibial tendon dysfunction, also known as adult acquired flatfoot deformity, is a condition defined as the gradual tearing and/or rupturing of the tibialis posterior tendon. The tibialis posterior muscle arises from the posterior aspect of the leg, and its tendon runs posteromedially across the ankle joint and inserts primarily into the medial and plantar aspects of the navicular bone, with small connections to lesser tarsal bones. In a healthy foot, this muscle serves as a powerful inverter and plantar flexor (off-weightbearing) and a primary decelerator of internal tibial rotation and hindfoot eversion in weight-bearing gait. Loss of its function creates significant pain and disability, especially in obese patients, and is sometimes accompanied by disruption of the deltoid ligament, which is a strong supportive structure at the medial ankle. This condition causes collapse of the medial longitudinal arch, which in turn leads to subluxation of the rearfoot tarsal joints and eventually the ankle joint.

The dysfunction is classified in 4 stages. Stage I is a tendinitis of the tibialis posterior tendon without observable foot deformity. Stage II is tearing or rupturing of the tibialis posterior tendon, which creates a flexible, reducible deformity. Stage III involves a deformity that has become rigid and arthritic. Stage IV occurs when the pronatory forces weaken the deltoid ligament, resulting in a valgus ankle deformity. These deformities result in a progressively debilitating gait.

Conservative treatment, including NSAIDs, physical therapy, eccentric muscle rehabilitation, or judicious and limited use of injected corticosteroid, may be effective in reducing pain in stage I deformity. In-shoe orthoses that place the foot in a less pronated position (stage I or II only), or bracing with an ankle-foot orthosis (stages III and IV) that may be hinged or rigid at the ankle, may also be effective, although usage compliance with ankle-foot orthoses is not high. Surgical treatment varies, depending on the stage of deformity. Stage I deformity is treated with synovectomy and repair/augmentation of the tendon. Stage II frequently requires a calcaneal osteotomy that medializes the calcaneus relative to the leg. Stage III deformity may require arthrodesis of the sub-talar joint, or the sub-talar joint and the calcaneal navicular and calcaneal cuboid joints. Stage IV disorders require a pan-talar arthrodesis or malleolar osteotomy to fully reduce the deformity. Stage I and II repairs can improve function and reduce symptoms; stage III and IV repairs are complex and require significant rehabilitation and investment of time and are considered salvage procedures (SOE=B).

Plantar Fasciitis and Heel Pain

Heel pain is common in older adults, with as many as 7% of the population >65 years old reported to complain of plantar heel pain. Patients generally have two different symptoms: a painful heel on first weight-bearing of the morning or after rest, or a painful plantar heel while walking.

The first condition is commonly referred to or diagnosed as plantar fasciitis, and is related to traction of the plantar fascia at the medial tuberosity of the calcaneus. The plantar fascia is a dense, inelastic structure that originates at the calcaneus and inserts distally in slips in proximity to the MTPJs. It provides mechanical support to the arch of the foot. When the patient walks, tension increases in the fascia through heel lift and dorsiflexion of the MTPJs. If the foot pronates or everts excessively, traction force will be increased as the foot tends to elongate and deviate medially. The medial arch collapses at the expense of the fascia, which is overly stressed longitudinally. Reactive bone formation occurs at the calcaneal tubercle, resulting in the classic heel spur, which is visible on lateral radiographs.

A tight Achilles tendon causes functional equinus and predisposes patients to this process. Initial treatments include reducing inflammation through use of oral NSAIDs, steroid injections, and/or physical therapy. Second-tier and more preventive therapies include reducing traction forces with inserts (custom or OTC), night splints, and stretching exercises such as rolling the arch of the foot over a frozen water bottle.

Heel pain is often associated with fat pad atrophy, which is common in older adults and in patients with diabetes. As the plantar cushion thins, direct bone-to-skin contact occurs because of the lack of the intermediary cushion, causing pain. Direct palpation demonstrates lack of the fat pad, and keratotic lesions may be present at pressure points. Symptoms increase during barefoot ambulation and decrease with the use of cushioned shoes or inserts. Treatment for fat pad atrophy is accommodative shoes and inserts, which act as external shock absorbers.

Third-tier management strategies for heel pain include the use of extracorporeal shock wave therapy or injected platelet-rich plasma. Surgical remediation by partial or total (rarely done) fascia sectioning (done endoscopically) may bring relief for recalcitrant heel pain symptoms *not* associated with plantar fat pad atrophy.

General Treatment Strategies

Orthoses

Orthoses are external devices placed either on the foot/ankle or into the shoe to accommodate a foot deformity or to alter the function of the foot to relieve physical stress on a certain portion of the foot. Orthoses placed on the foot include temporary felt padding or silicone/putty spacers to accommodate structural deformities (eg, hallux valgus, hammertoes, tailor's bunion).

Orthoses placed in the shoe can be either OTC or custom made. OTC devices are generally made of lightweight polyethylene foam, soft plastics, or silicone. A custom-made device is constructed from an impression of a person's foot. Impressions may be made using negative plaster casting of the foot in a subtalar joint neutral position or with other media, including fiberglass and, increasingly, 3D laser or optical scanning. The devices are then made from the impression, with prescriptive recommendations made by the prescribing clinician. These devices are generally made from a variety of flexible and rigid plastics (eg, polypropylene, carbon fiber) and can be quite durable. Less rigid prescriptions rely on foam, cork, or ethyl vinyl acetate composites and may be better tolerated by older adults, although their bulk may require significant modification in shoe design or size.

Shoes

Because of physical changes that develop in the foot with age, shoes usually do not fit well in older adults and can be a cause of foot pain. Studies have indicated that approximately 75% of adults ≥65 years old wear shoes that are too small. It is common for feet to flatten and widen with age, and feet should be measured routinely. Older adults should be advised to purchase a well-fitting shoe that has a sturdy heel counter, a firm beveled heel, and good traction. With expansion of the wider shoe size market, shoes that fit well and are structurally sound are available OTC. Athletic and walking sneakers also offer older adults accommodative designs with structural support.

Narrow high heels should be avoided. A wide heel that is <6 cm high can be appropriate for women who have tight heel cords and have been wearing high-heeled shoes all their lives. This shoe type will also suit some individuals who have plantar fasciitis. Older adults wearing heels that are >6 cm high are at a greater risk of falls. Proper shoes and inserts that reduce pressure can decrease pain, protect the foot from injury, and improve function (SOE=B) (Table 60.2).

Most patients can be fitted with OTC shoes, except when significant structural changes occur or systemic diseases change the foot. Extra-depth shoes can help accommodate foot changes that prevent regular use of shoe wear. In diabetes, intrinsic muscle weakness causes hammering of the digits and bunion formation. Extra-depth shoes have one-and-a-half times the toe box height and soft leather or synthetic material, which prevents irritation to the dorsal contracted digits. When structural changes are severe, as seen in patients with end-stage rheumatoid arthritis, a custom molded shoe may be required. These shoes are manufactured from plaster molds of the patient's feet to allow for the severe changes and to prevent skin breakdown.

Surgical Considerations of Foot Deformities

Foot surgery in older adults has increased substantially in the past 30 years, mainly because of the growth of this population segment. Poor surgical outcomes usually reflect the overall health of an individual rather than his or her chronological age. When relief of pain and restoration of function are the goals, surgery may be a better alternative for foot problems that are not alleviated by conservative methods. Most podiatric surgical procedures for older adults can be performed under local anesthesia with monitored sedation, thereby minimizing surgical risk.

Complications of foot surgery include delayed healing, increased risk of non-union when osteotomies

Table 60.2—Shoe Terms

Term	Definition or Description
Custom-made molded shoes	Made from an impression of the foot either by a plaster cast, laser scan, or foam imprint
Extra depth shoe	Provides additional vertical space in the shoe; useful when adding prescribed insoles to the shoe
Heel counter	The (more) rigid portion of the shoe posteriorly; the heel fits against this material; shoes with a stiffer and higher heel counter are considered more stable.
Rocker bottom sole	Modification of the sole to facilitate sagittal plane motion
Shock-absorbing heel	Hard but absorbent material that provides shock absorption; good for patients with a cavus foot and for obese patients
Thomas heel modification	A distal medial extension of the heel that provides stability of the arch
Toe box	The forward portion of the shoe that envelops the forefoot; important when considering conservative management of digital/forefoot deformity

are performed, infection, and secondary morbidities such as deep venous thrombosis caused by necessary postoperative weight-bearing restrictions. Increasing complexity of the surgical procedure and osseous fixation increase healing times and the potential for failure, either through non-union or infection. Still, patients who present with intractable pathology and who are medically stable, with adequate peripheral circulation and appropriate home-based support, may be considered good surgical candidates.

SKIN AND NAIL DISORDERS

Skin Lesions

Skin lesions on the foot are common in older adults but are rarely malignant; several common benign lesions are described below. Suspicious lesions require biopsy.

Keratotic lesions are calluses or corns often seen over sites of pressure. Common types are heloma durum (hard corn), heloma molle (soft corn), and tyloma (widespread callus). Treatment options include surgical debridement by a podiatrist or medical professional with experience. In older adults, OTC treatments are limited because of the acid base of these products. Self-care can include using a pumice stone or foot file after bathing to help reduce the thickness of these lesions. The use of nonmedicated OTC padding may be useful, but only when the risk of skin tear secondary to adhesive material is low.

Plantar verruca is the most common skin disorder of the foot, although incidence decreases dramatically with age. This viral infection of the plantar aspect is caused by a strain of the human papilloma virus. Lesions are circular, punctated, flat, and commonly contain thrombosed vessels. It is important to differentiate these lesions from keratotic lesions. Clinically, verrucae demonstrate interrupted skin lines, pinpoint bleeding with debridement, and increased lateral compression pain when compared with keratosis. A cluster of the lesions is referred to as a mosaic wart. Treatments include application of topical salicylic acid, bleomycin injections, cryotherapy, CO_2 laser treatment, and surgical excision, which must be used with caution in older adults who have reduced circulation and impaired healing. Treatment of verrucoid lesions in older adults may require mixing approaches and treating associated complications, eg, treating hyperkeratosis with keratolytic agents such as urea (SOE=B).

Epidermal inclusion cysts are created by a portion of the epidermis proliferating in the dermis.

Dermatofibromas are flat-topped, raised, and firm lesions that generally are not treated unless located across a joint or irritated by shoe wear. Recurrence rate after excision is high.

Hemangiomas are common vascular tumors that manifest as flat-topped, red lesions that contain abundant capillaries. They are typically seen on the plantar aspect of the foot.

Malignant lesions are uncommon in the foot but can easily go undiagnosed and generally have a poor outcome. Pigmented lesions of the foot should be fully evaluated, and any suspicious lesions biopsied. Characteristics of a potentially malignant lesion include a new lesion in a patient ≥60 years old, or a lesion that changes in shape, color, or diameter. Lesions not responding to conservative therapy and slow or nonhealing ulcerations of the foot should be biopsied to exclude a potential underlying neoplasm. Morbidity associated with these lesions increases at age 60 and beyond. Malignant lesions identified in the foot include basal cell carcinoma, Bowen disease, squamous cell carcinoma, and malignant acral lentiginous melanoma. The incidence of melanoma (plantar and interdigital in particular) in dark-skinned individuals is higher than in less pigmented individuals and is not characteristically related to sun exposure. Such individuals should be carefully evaluated during routine assessments.

Xerosis

Excessive dryness, or xerosis, is associated with a lack of hydration and lubrication. The number of sebaceous and sweat glands decrease in older adults and plantar skin lacks sebaceous glands, so it is common for fissures to develop on the heel, resulting in dryness and increased stress in that area.

The goal in managing xerosis is to prevent infection and other complications. Urea cream or solution (10%, 20%, or 40%) or ammonium lactate (12%) may be helpful as a mild and safe keratolytic. A heel sleeve or pad made with mineral oil or a heel cup can help minimize trauma to the heel, thereby reducing the potential for complications. Urea and/or lactic acid–based emollients have been shown to be effective but must be used daily and applied after bathing (SOE=C).

Eczema

Eczema is inflamed skin that is not infected. The most common types in older adults are xerotic eczema, venous stasis eczema, and drug-induced eczema. Treatment is generally a combination of emollients and steroid creams, with or without occlusive dressings.

Nail Disorders

Nail disorders are the most common disorders of the foot.

Ingrown Nails and Paronychia

Onychocryptosis, the incurvation of the edge of the nail plate into the nail groove, is generally seen in the distal portion of the nail groove. This condition can result from long-term improper nail cutting (too short), narrow shoes, and/or genetically incurvated nail matrixes. A chronically ingrown nail is best treated either with a partial nail avulsion or a permanent matricectomy, which is done either by applying a caustic (usually phenol but possibly sodium hydroxide) to the proximal nail matrix or by surgically excising the matrix and/or adjacent hypertrophic skin. The need for partial (margins) or total nail removal is determined by the clinical presentation and history of discomfort and infection. Assessment of the underlying pathology may be necessary when the morphology of the nail plate or distal aspect of the digit suggests the presence of a subungual exostosis.

Paronychia, a localized infection caused by the nail embedding into the nail groove, requires incision and drainage of the abscess with removal of the nail spicule. All infected granulation tissue is resected. Depending on the presence of cellulitis or comorbidities, antibiotic treatment may be needed. If paronychia is long-standing, the toes should be radiographed to exclude underlying osteomyelitis, especially in patients with diabetes or peripheral arterial disease.

Onychomycosis

Approximately one-third of the older population has onychomycosis, a fungal infection of the nail plate. An increased incidence is seen in older adults with obesity, immunodeficiency, diabetes, peripheral arterial disease, chronic tinea pedis, and/or psoriasis. By the age of 65, approximately 20% of men and 10% of women are affected; these values are doubled in those with diabetes. Dermatophytes account for 80% of infections, with the remainder caused by saprophytes or yeast.

Onychomycosis results in thickening of the nail plate and can cause pain. In patients with neuropathy, onychomycosis can be a source of nail bed ulcerations. Treatment includes topical and oral antifungal medications, as well as permanent excision of the nail. A decision to treat is usually made because of one of the following: the cosmetic concern of a yellow friable nail, other comorbidities (particularly diabetes mellitus, in which the break in the epidermal barrier due to the fungal infection can serve as a route for bacterial infections), and occasionally pain.

Topical antifungal treatments with amorolfine[OL], ciclopirox, and tioconazole have shown efficacy in improving and curing onychomycosis (SOE=C) but require 24–48 weeks of treatment, often at considerable out-of-pocket expense, for cure rates that are <25%. Oral antifungals such as terbinafine, fluconazole, and itraconazole are effective for onychomycosis, but their duration of treatment, adverse-event profile, and high rate of relapse after discontinuation warrant careful consideration for use in older adults. These agents are primarily metabolized by the liver and, except for terbinafine, can interact with many medications commonly taken by older adults. Treatment can take 3–4 months, and the rate of relapse is high. Onychomycosis should not be considered a benign event in vulnerable populations (ie, those with diabetes or peripheral arterial disease), and nail deformity as a cause of pain should not be underestimated. Treatment, at least with periodic debridement and, when possible, definitive pharmacologic modalities is recommended.

FALL RISK AND PODIATRIC INTERVENTION

The repercussion of falls is well known, with the CDC reporting that the unintentional fall death rates among adults ≥65 years old increased from 41 per 100,000 to nearly 58 per 100,000 between 2004 and 2013. Risk factors for falls include obesity, diabetes (neuropathic change), adverse pharmacologic reactions, arthritis, vision change, shoe gear/walking surface challenges (high friction interfaces are to be avoided), pain, and fear of falling. For CDC guidelines for assessment and management of fall risk see (www.cdc.gov/steadi.index.html). All medical practitioners should incorporate these practices into their evaluation of at-risk patients, and individuals with foot-related risk factors should be referred for management. In one study, simple intervention consisting of molded foot orthosis, palliative management of painful plantar or digital keratotic lesions, and patient education reduced falls by 36% compared with no intervention.

SYSTEMIC DISEASES AFFECTING THE FOOT AND ANKLE

Diabetes Mellitus

Diabetes is the number one disease affecting foot health in older adults. Complications of diabetes can cause loss of limb and significant disability. Currently 1 in 10 diabetic patients who develop ulceration eventually undergo some form of amputation, which is a strong predictor of early fatality. It has been estimated that 50%–75% of all amputations in patients with diabetes could be prevented by foot health education, periodic clinician assessment, and early intervention. The ocular complications of diabetes can decrease the ability of patients to see ingrown toenails, corns, and ulcers. Other complications of diabetes that contribute to poor foot health include neuropathy, vascular insufficiency, dermopathy, atrophy of the muscles and soft tissues, and deformity. Neuropathy, especially sensory impairment, is considered the dominant precursor to incurring wounds. Paresthesias, decreased vibratory sense, and loss of sensation and proprioception are among the most important neuropathic changes that contribute to ulcer formation in older diabetic patients.

Arterial insufficiency is represented by pallor, a loss or decrease in the posterior tibial and dorsalis pedis pulses, cool skin temperature, dependent rubor, and decreased capillary filling time in the toes. Severe vascular disease can result in nocturnal rest pain Loss of the plantar metatarsal fat pad is associated with vascular insufficiency and predisposes to ulcerations at the plantar forefoot.

Foot ulcers are a common result of the multiple pathologies found in patients with diabetes. Prevention and early recognition are the most important strategies in managing foot ulcers. Older diabetic patients should have their feet examined at least annually. Diabetic patients are often instructed to remove their shoes at all visits so that the clinician can visually inspect the feet and the areas between the toes to ensure there has been no skin breakdown. Patients and caregivers should be instructed in the importance of daily foot inspections. Preventive strategies include optimizing glycemic control and monitoring and treating peripheral neuropathy, arterial disease, limited joint mobility, bony deformities, hyperkeratosis, and onychodystrophy (SOE=C).

Prevention of foot ulcers in diabetic patients is both cost-effective and limb saving in this high-risk population (SOE=A). Assessing vibratory sensation using the Semmes-Weinstein monofilament and monitoring reflex changes help the clinician determine a patient's risk of development of ulcers. If a diabetic patient's risk is high, appropriate steps should be taken to prevent ulcers, including reducing excessive pressure, shock, and shear by accommodating, stabilizing, and supporting deformities through weight diffusion and dispersion (SOE=C). Early intervention with proper shoes and foot care reduces complications in high-risk feet, as demonstrated by the Lower Extremity Amputation Prevention (LEAP) program and the Medicare Loss of Protective Sensation (LOPS) program.

Initial assessment of an ulcer should focus on duration, inciting event or trauma, history of prior ulceration, previous attempts at wound care, and the use of pressure off-loading procedures. The examination should include an assessment of the location and depth of the ulcer, the presence of infection, ischemic or neuropathic changes, edema, and the vulnerability of the patient to Charcot neuroarthropathy. Imaging should be performed to exclude osteomyelitis (SOE=B) and may include plain radiography, CT, technetium bone scans, indium or gallium scans, and MRI. Noninvasive vascular studies include Doppler and transcutaneous oxygen tension are useful. The ankle-brachial pulse index (ABI) strongly correlates to outcomes of wound healing and risk of amputation. Consultation with a vascular specialist may be needed when ABI is low and healing is seen to be delayed. Open surgical or endovascular intervention may significantly modify the potential for wound healing and reduce overall risk.

The general management principles the high-risk foot include debridement, off-loading, appropriate wound dressings, treatment of infection with antibiotics, negative-pressure therapy, management of ischemia, medical management of comorbidities, and hospitalization and surgical management when necessary. Weight bearing can be modified by the use of crutches and wheelchairs as well as total contact casts, walkers, braces, surgical boots, and surgical shoes. Wounds that are not complicated by a dysvascular status or infection should reduce by 50% within a 4-week period. If a wound is reducing as planned, then regular follow-up care and prevention are required. Nonreducing wounds require reassessment of the patient's medical condition, and well as his or her vascular, infectious, and nutritional statuses. Adjunctive therapies such as bioengineered graft or skin substitutes may be indicated if there is no infection and the patient's vascular status is adequate. Hyperbaric oxygen chambers can also aid in closure of difficult-to-heal wounds in diabetic patients (SOE=B).

Empiric antibiotic therapy should be started early when infection is suspected, followed by more specific therapy based on results of culture and sensitivity. Hospitalization is usually indicated in cases involving osteomyelitis or limb-threatening infection. The choice of antibiotic is based on the clinical symptoms; culture and sensitivity; presence of deep infection, bone exposure, or sepsis; and whether soft tissue or bone is infected (SOE=B).

Peripheral Arterial Disease

Older adults with peripheral arterial disease demonstrate many of the same signs and symptoms as those with diabetes mellitus. In contrast to neuropathic ulcers, vascular ulcers are extremely painful.

Arthritis

Osteoarthritis is common in older adults. It causes pain, swelling, stiffness, limitation of movement, and deformity in weight-bearing joints. It may be worsened by chronic trauma, strain, or obesity. Gouty arthritis is often monoarticular and is most common in the first MTPJ. In its early stages, it results in intense pain and erythema, followed later by joint damage. It may be associated, in older adults, with concurrent use of diuretic medications, which makes a medication review vital for controlling acute episodes.

Rheumatoid arthritis affects the hands and feet equally and is usually symmetric in its presentation. It can result in muscle wasting and marked deformity. The MTPJs become dislocated or subluxed; there is increased protrusion of the metatarsal heads, and walking becomes painful. If conservative treatment with orthotics and special shoes does not relieve the pain, surgical excision by arthroplasty of affected joints may help to allow less painful ambulation.

RESOURCES

- Bakker K, Apelqvist J, Lipsky BA, et al; International Working Group on the Diabetic Foot. The 2015 IWGDF guidance documents on prevention and management of foot problems in diabetes: development of an evidence-based global consensus. *Diabetes Metab Res Rev*. 2016;32 Suppl 1:2–6.

- Bubra PS, Keighley G, Rateesh S, et al. Posterior tibial tendon dysfunction: an overlooked cause of foot deformity. *J Family Med Prim Care*. 2015;4(1):26–29.

CHAPTER 61—NEUROLOGY

KEY POINTS

- A new-onset seizure in late life is frequently a symptom of an underlying brain disease or injury, but may not need to be treated with medications, if no cause is found. Recurrent seizures can be prevented with medications. Newer antiepileptic drugs are better tolerated.

- Parkinson disease and other common movement disorders seen in older patients are diagnosed clinically and can be effectively managed medically.

- Peripheral neuropathy is common in older adults, and diabetes is the most common cause in the United States. Several medications are approved by the FDA for the treatment of painful diabetic neuropathy.

- New onset of headaches in older adults should prompt a search for a secondary cause, including brain tumor, systemic illness, temporal arteritis, or medication-induced causes.

Note: Stroke has a dedicated chapter elsewhere in the *Geriatric Nursing Review Syllabus*.

Neurologic diseases and disorders are increasingly common with advancing age. The most prevalent neurologic disorders include Alzheimer disease (AD) and related dementias, gait disorders, cerebrovascular disease, epilepsy, Parkinson disease (PD), and peripheral neuropathy. In the United States, almost half (40%–50%) of the population >85 years old suffer from dementia, and a similar percentage of hospitalized patients of this age have a gait disorder caused by a neurologic condition. Other U.S. population data include the following: 7.5% of adults 60–79 years old and 15% of those ≥80 years old have had a stroke, 1% of adults >60 years old and 3% of those >80 years old have been diagnosed with PD, 3% of adults by age 75 and close to 10% of the nursing-home population have epilepsy, and up to 10% of adults >65 years old have some signs of a peripheral polyneuropathy. This chapter will cover epilepsy in older adults, PD and other movement disorders, and other common neurologic conditions, including neuromuscular disorders, myelopathy, and headaches.

Individual neurologic disorders in older adults can be challenging to differentiate, given that it is common for a patient to have more than one such disorder or sequela when examined. Pharmacologic treatment of neurologic disorders must account for the unique metabolism of older adults and the potential for drug-drug interactions. Furthermore, because neurologic disorders add substantially to the burden of functional dependency, acknowledging the psychosocial aspects of these conditions is vital in constructing treatment plans to improve functional abilities and quality of life.

EPILEPSY

A seizure is caused by excessive and synchronous discharges of cortical neurons producing a transient disruption of normal brain function. Recurrent seizures are the defining feature of epilepsy. Seizures are broadly classified as partial or generalized, depending on whether the seizure discharges involve only a portion of the cortex or the entire cortex. Partial seizures are subdivided on the basis of whether the seizure is associated with impaired consciousness. Simple partial seizures do not impair consciousness, but complex partial seizures do. Most commonly, simple partial seizures involve focal rhythmic motor twitching. Complex partial seizures are often preceded by an aura, followed by loss of awareness and responsiveness typically manifested as staring off into space. Automatisms and other minor motor manifestations can occur with complex partial seizures. After the event, patients display postictal confusion and amnesia for the seizure. Generalized seizures involve the entire cortex and typically cause tonic-clonic convulsions (ie, generalized tonic-clonic, or "grand mal," seizures). A seizure may start as a complex partial seizure and secondarily progress into a generalized seizure. In critical care settings, a generalized seizure may manifest as a nonconvulsive continuous seizure (ie, nonconvulsive status epilepticus) in which a patient shows persistent alteration in mental status without convulsive movements.

The incidence of epilepsy follows a bimodal pattern with respect to age, with an initial peak within the first year of life and a second peak after the age of 60. The annual incidence of epilepsy peaks at 135 per 100,000 in those >80 years old. Secondary causes of seizures, ie, those with an underlying discernible cause, are more common among older adults. In this demographic group, about 70% of new-onset seizures are secondary. Common causes include cerebrovascular disease, space-occupying lesions, brain trauma, neurodegenerative diseases, and alcohol withdrawal. It is estimated that cerebrovascular disease causes 50% of known causes of late-onset seizures, with tumors, trauma, and degenerative dementias each causing 10%–20% of cases. Cortical or hemorrhagic strokes are more likely to cause seizures than other types of stroke. AD increases the risk of seizures, although seizures in AD are relatively uncommon, occurring in 2%–5% of patients.

Seizures in AD are seen more often in advanced stages of dementia and in young-onset AD. The incidence of partial epilepsy (which frequently has an underlying cause) increases in older adults, whereas the incidence of primary generalized epilepsy (generally idiopathic or genetic) is more common in pediatric populations.

It is important that older adults with new-onset seizures undergo diagnostic evaluation to exclude an underlying treatable condition. The neurologic history and examination should aim to clinically characterize the seizure and localize its source, as well as to elicit other signs of a focal lesion or a metabolic disturbance (eg, uremia, hepatic failure). Blood studies (comprehensive metabolic panel, magnesium, calcium), brain imaging (MRI is preferable to CT), and electroencephalography play important roles. Brain imaging should be obtained with and without contrast to identify and characterize structural brain lesions.

Once the appropriate evaluation has been done, the decision to begin an antiepileptic drug should be made carefully to maximize benefit and minimize risk. On average, 30% of patients with a single unprovoked seizure have another seizure, but 70% do not. The presence of a focal brain abnormality on brain imaging or epileptic changes on an electroencephalogram (EEG) raises the likelihood of recurrence and should prompt consideration of pharmacologic therapy. If a patient has a second unprovoked seizure, then the probability of further seizures increases to 70%, and pharmacologic therapy should generally be initiated.

There have been only 3 randomized, double-blind, comparative clinical trials in older adults with newly diagnosed epilepsy. In a Department of Veterans Affairs (VA) study that compared lamotrigine, gabapentin, and carbamazepine, seizure control was similar among these 3 drugs, but carbamazepine was significantly less well tolerated than the other 2. Discontinuation rates due to adverse events were 12% with lamotrigine, 22% with gabapentin, and 31% with carbamazepine in this 52-week study. Two other trials compared lamotrigine to carbamazepine. As in the VA trial, both drugs effectively prevented recurrent seizures, but lamotrigine was significantly better tolerated. This difference in tolerability was not found in a third study in which a controlled-release form of carbamazepine and flexible dosing design were used. Several of the other newer antiepileptic drugs have been examined in open-label trials in older populations, including studies with oxcarbazepine, levetiracetam, and low-dose topiramate. These agents have demonstrated good seizure control and tolerability. Thus, there is growing evidence that use of one of the newer antiepileptic drugs described above is preferred to the use of older antiepileptic drugs in the older population because of improved tolerability and compliance (SOE=A).

The incidence of adverse effects and drug-drug interactions increases with age. This is particularly true with the older antiepileptic drugs, such as phenobarbital, carbamazepine, phenytoin, and valproate. For example, phenobarbital can cause cognitive adverse effects, phenytoin can cause ataxia, carbamazepine can cause hyponatremia, and valproate can cause weight gain, tremors, and parkinsonism. Many of the older antiepileptic drugs, including phenobarbital, phenytoin, and carbamazepine, are potent inducers of the cytochrome P450 system, which increases the risk of drug-drug interactions. Also, each of these 3 agents has been associated with increased bone loss with age. Finally, changes in hepatic function or binding protein levels in older adults can alter the metabolism of older antiepileptic drugs, active drug levels, and risk of adverse effects. Clinical pharmacists can help to resolve complex issues of drug interactions, dosages, and adverse events, especially when using older antiepileptic drugs.

Antiepileptic drug doses are best started at low levels and increased very slowly in older adults to avoid problematic adverse effects. Older adults may have difficulty with adherence to antiepileptic drug schedules for a variety of reasons. It is particularly important when treating older adults to involve caregivers so that the goals of treatment, adverse events, and monitoring of response are understood. Final medication dose is determined by consideration of both seizure control and adverse events. Ideally, drug doses are increased to a level that eliminates seizures but does not result in adverse effects. Some antiepileptic drugs do not require laboratory monitoring. Common causes of breakthrough seizures in individuals known to be epileptic are systemic infections, metabolic disturbances, sleep deprivation, and medication noncompliance. Providers should consider discontinuing antiepileptic drugs if a patient has not had a seizure for ≥2 years, particularly if the original seizure was a single or poorly characterized event and if a recent EEG does not show epileptic activity.

MOVEMENT DISORDERS

A simple definition of movement disorder is the presence of abnormal involuntary movements. These movements result not from weakness or sensory deficits but from dysfunction of the extrapyramidal motor systems. Movement disorders can be classified as hypokinetic (paucity of movement) or hyperkinetic (excessive movement). The hypokinetic movement disorders include PD and the related Parkinson-plus syndromes (eg, multiple system atrophy, progressive supranuclear palsy). Hyperkinetic movement disorders include conditions that produce chorea (eg, Huntington disease), dyskinesias (eg, tardive dyskinesias), dystonia, and tremor (eg, essential tremor). Movement disorders are especially common among older adults.

Parkinson Disease (PD)

PD is a progressive neurodegenerative disease that results in neuronal dysfunction and neuronal loss in pathways of the brainstem, basal ganglia, and cerebral cortex. The pathologic hallmark of the disease is the Lewy body, an intracellular inclusion body originally found in dopaminergic neurons of the substantia nigra. These neurodegenerative changes cause a constellation of clinical signs, including tremor at rest, bradykinesia, rigidity, and postural instability. As the disease progresses, neurodegeneration and Lewy body pathology extends into the cortex (limbic region and neocortex), causing neuropsychiatric and cognitive symptoms (ie, PD with dementia).

The incidence and prevalence of PD increase with age. Prevalence rates in the United States rise from 1% of the population at age 60 to 3% at age 80. Aging, environmental factors, and genetics are thought to be involved in the pathogenesis of PD. Risk factors associated with increased risk of PD include exposure to pesticides, welding as a profession, exposure to manganese, age, and family history. Smoking and caffeine consumption have been associated with decreased risk. A small proportion of PD cases (5%–10%) are the result of a causative genetic mutation, while a larger proportion of patients may have inherited a susceptibility gene that increases risk. Approximately 10 genes have been associated with PD, either as causative mutations or susceptibility genes. Idiopathic PD (ie, parkinsonism not attributable to strokes, medications, or other primary causes) most commonly appears clinically between the ages of 50 and 79 years. Dementia in PD occurs in 30%–40% of PD patients and is more common with longer duration of disease, more severe motor symptoms, an akinetic-rigid presentation, and older age of onset of motor symptoms.

Diagnosis of PD

Recent clinical diagnostic criteria continue to highlight the central role of the motor signs of PD and the importance of the physical examination in making a clinical diagnosis. To make a diagnosis of PD, there should be evidence of parkinsonism, defined as the presence of bradykinesia in combination with either resting tremor, rigidity, or both. The term *bradykinesia* describes either a slowness in initiating movement (ie, a paucity of spontaneous movements) or slow movements themselves. This can be manifested clinically as reduced frequency and amplitude of fine finger movements, decreased facial expression or blinking, and micrographia (small handwriting). The tremor of idiopathic PD is generally asymmetric, involving one hand more than the other, and has a slow frequency (usually 4–6 Hz). It is present at rest and typically resolves or decreases with active, purposeful movement. Muscular rigidity is usually readily evident on passive movement of a limb when the patient is relaxed. Passive movement may demonstrate a smooth resistance ("lead pipe" rigidity) or superimposed ratchet-like jerks (ie, "cogwheel" phenomenon, which is caused by tremor superimposed on the rigidity). The fourth cardinal motor feature of PD is impaired postural reflexes, which can be elicited with a pull test (pulling a standing patient backward and assessing his or her ability to maintain balance). Impaired postural balance is a feature present later in the course of idiopathic PD; the presence of early postural imbalance and frequent falls often signals a Parkinson-plus syndrome.

Additional clinical features that are supportive of a diagnosis of idiopathic PD include a clear improvement in motor symptoms with dopaminergic medications and a loss of the sense of smell. Standardized tests are available to quantify a patient's olfactory function (eg, University of Pennsylvania Smell Identification Test [UPSIT]). However, loss of sense of smell is not specific to PD and can be seen in other neurodegenerative disorders (including AD), or in those with paranasal sinus disease or a history of head trauma. Recent studies using the UPSIT demonstrated sensitivities of 78%–84% and specificities of 68%–83% in differentiating patients with PD from healthy controls, depending on age and gender. Of note, similar sensitivities and specificities have been seen in patients with Alzheimer disease as compared with healthy controls, using the UPSIT. It is appropriate to refer patients to a neurologist with movement disorder expertise if atypical features are present or the diagnosis is unclear.

Treatment of PD

Patients who are functionally disabled by tremors, bradykinesia, or rigidity should be offered pharmacologic treatment. Drug therapy is effective in reducing these symptoms but does not improve postural instability or nonmotor symptoms of PD. Patients who respond well to initial pharmacologic treatment are generally well managed by primary care providers, but those with advanced disease or suboptimal response to drug therapy may benefit from referral to neurologists with movement disorder expertise and who are familiar with the increasing variety of available treatments. Nonpharmacologic therapy should include a regular exercise program. Many older adults benefit from a course of physical therapy aimed at restoring their confidence in walking and maintaining balance, often with instruction in PD-focused physical therapy programs (eg, the "Training BIG" program) or symptom-focused therapy (eg, for coping with disabling freezing episodes). Physical therapists can also help, when needed, with selection of appropriate canes or walkers. A home visit by an occupational therapist can help to evaluate safety and equipment needs in the home, such as appropriate placement of wall rails, grab bars, and other such assistive devices that reduce the risk of falling.

Levodopa therapy for PD motor symptoms: The most effective pharmacologic treatment of patients with PD is levodopa combined with carbidopa (SOE=A). Levodopa is converted to dopamine in both the CNS and the periphery via dopa decarboxylase. Peripheral conversion is reduced by combining levodopa with carbidopa (a dopa decarboxylase inhibitor), which does not cross the blood-brain barrier. This formulation decreases adverse events associated with peripheral conversion. Treatment usually begins with a half tablet of the immediate-release 25/100 combination (ie, 25 mg carbidopa to 100 mg levodopa) administered every 8–12 hours. Every 1–2 weeks, the dose can be increased by one-half tablet, to reach a dosage of one full tablet three times a day (commonly 30 minutes before meals). The duration of action of this formulation is typically 4 hours. If disabling bradykinesia, rigidity, or resting tremor is still present, the dosage can be gradually increased further, with cautious observation for adverse events. Older adults, particularly those who are cognitively impaired, rarely tolerate total levodopa doses >1,000 mg/d. Additional formulations include a "controlled-release" form (available as 25/100 and 50/200) that generally requires a slightly higher total daily dose than immediate-release, and an "extended-release" form, which is dosed at 1.5–2 times higher than immediate-release. To convert from immediate-release to extended-release, the prescriber should use the conversion table in the manufacturer's labeling. Common adverse events of levodopa-carbidopa include nausea, abdominal cramping, orthostatic hypotension, and visual hallucinations.

Managing PD symptoms with medications becomes more challenging as the disease progresses, because the therapeutic window narrows, making it difficult to control motor symptoms without undesirable adverse effects. After 5 years of treatment for PD, up to 50% of patients develop motor fluctuations or dyskinesias (involuntary choreiform movements). PD patients are commonly described as "on" (symptoms well controlled), "on with dyskinesias" (symptoms controlled but complicated by dyskinesias), or "off" (parkinsonism not well controlled). End-of-dose "off" symptoms are common and can be treated by increasing the dosing frequency of levodopa to every 3–4 hours or by adding an enzyme inhibitor such as rasagiline or entacapone (described below) to increase the duration of action of levodopa. Peak dose "on" dyskinesias are common and are treated by increasing the interval between levodopa doses or lowering the total daily dose of dopaminergic medications. The incidence and severity of dyskinesias can be reduced by introducing a dopamine agonist (described below) early in the treatment of PD, either as monotherapy or in combination with levodopa when daily dosages exceed 400 mg/d. This is an important consideration in patients <75 years old who are expected to have a long duration of disease and treatment. An intestinal gel form of carbidopa-levodopa is available for continuous administration via a pump through a percutaneous endoscopic gastrostomy (PEG)-jejunum tube for treatment of motor fluctuations in advanced PD.

Other medications for PD motor symptoms: Medications other than levodopa that can be used to treat PD motor symptoms include enzyme inhibitors, amantadine and anticholinergic medications, and dopamine agonists. Enzyme inhibitors include the catechol-O-methyl-transferase (COMT) inhibitor entacapone. COMT inhibitors block breakdown of levodopa, thereby increasing its bioavailability at the synapse. Entacapone increases the duration of action of levodopa, resulting in greater "on" time for a given dose of levodopa, but it can also exacerbate dyskinesias (SOE=A). Adverse events of COMT inhibitors are similar to those of levodopa. A second class of enzyme inhibitors are the monoamine oxidase B (MAO-B) inhibitors, which also block one of the enzymes responsible for dopamine breakdown. Rasagiline is a newer selective MAO-B inhibitor that has been approved by the FDA as early monotherapy or as adjunct therapy (SOE=A). Selegiline, an older MAO-B inhibitor, was shown in controlled trials to delay the need for additional antiparkinsonian agents (SOE=A). A neuroprotective role of MAO-B inhibitors in PD has been investigated but not established. Although chemically related to nonselective monoamine oxidase inhibitors, the selective MAO-B inhibitors, rasagiline and selegiline, do not require dietary restrictions. MAO-B inhibitors are generally well tolerated, although some patients can experience adverse events, including nausea, insomnia, confusion, or anxiety. Other medications used to treat motor symptoms of PD include amantadine and anticholinergic medications such as trihexyphenidyl. Amantadine, which has multiple pharmacologic properties, can provide mild improvement in PD motor symptoms and decreased dyskinesias (SOE=B). Older adults, especially with impaired renal clearance, can develop confusion and hallucinations with amantadine. Anticholinergic medications can modestly improve some PD symptoms, but adverse events such as dry mouth, urinary retention, and confusion outweigh benefits in most older adults.

Dopamine agonists may be used initially as monotherapy to treat motor symptoms of PD, or may be added to levodopa when its dosage exceeds 400 mg/d. The agents may be particularly useful for younger PD patients with milder disease and no signs of dementia (SOE=A). Slow upward titration of dopamine agonists is required to reduce the occurrence of common adverse effects such as nausea, sleepiness, orthostatic hypotension, and hallucinations. When compared with levodopa, dopamine agonists are less effective in controlling motor symptoms and are associated with more adverse events. However, early use of dopamine agonists can delay the emergence of levodopa-induced dyskinesias (SOE=A). Commonly used dopamine agonists include ropinirole, pramipexole, and rotigotine transdermal patch. All dopamine agonists, and to a lesser extent levodopa, have been associated with sudden sleep attacks in which patients may doze off abruptly while driving. Additionally, dopamine agonists have been associated with compulsive behaviors such as pathologic gambling. Patients should be warned of these rare but potentially serious adverse events, and clinicians should ask about these behaviors during routine follow-up visits.

Nonmotor Symptoms of PD

Nonmotor symptoms are common in PD and can be a target of treatment. These include urinary incontinence, constipation, drooling, seborrhea, anxiety, depression, visual hallucinations, sleep disorders, and cognitive impairment. PD patients are also at higher risk of melanoma and may benefit from screening for the condition and counseling about sun exposure. For PD patients who develop visual hallucinations or delusions, dopaminergic regimens should be reviewed and doses reduced. If symptoms are severe, the addition of low-dose clozapine may be considered, because this atypical antipsychotic agent is least likely to exacerbate PD motor symptoms. However, clozapine requires frequent laboratory monitoring to look for neutropenia. Pimavanserin, a new medication with a different mechanism of action, has been FDA approved for treatment of psychosis (hallucinations and delusions) in patients with PD. Pimavanserin improved psychosis without worsening motor function in patients with PD and does not require laboratory monitoring. PD patients who develop dementia symptoms can be treated with a cholinesterase inhibitor. Rivastigmine has been FDA approved for treatment of the dementia associated with PD (SOE=A).

"Parkinson-plus" Syndromes

"Parkinson-plus" or parkinsonian syndromes are a group of disorders with some motor features of PD (eg, bradykinesia, rigidity, postural imbalance) but that also have additional distinct and distinguishing features atypical for idiopathic PD. As a group, these disorders are much less responsive to pharmacologic treatment with dopaminergic medications than idiopathic PD. The parkinsonian syndromes described in some detail below include multiple system atrophy (MSA) and progressive supranuclear palsy (PSP). Other Parkinson-plus syndromes include dementia with Lewy bodies; corticobasal degeneration; vascular parkinsonism, in which small-vessel ischemic strokes in the basal ganglia produce parkinsonism; and medication-induced parkinsonism, in which dopamine-receptor blocking medications (typically antipsychotic or antiemetic drugs) produce parkinsonism.

Multiple System Atrophy

A histopathologic understanding of 3 parkinsonian syndromes, olivopontocerebellar atrophy, Shy-Drager syndrome, and striatonigral degeneration, has permitted these overlapping syndromes to be included within the rubric of one disease called multiple system atrophy (MSA). MSA produces degeneration in 3 distinct neuronal systems, the basal ganglia, cerebellum, and autonomic nervous system. MSA is characterized by parkinsonism, autonomic failure (eg, severe orthostatic hypotension, constipation, incontinence, erectile dysfunction, impaired sweating or temperature control), and cerebellar dysfunction (eg, ataxia, dysmetria). Other features that can accompany MSA are upper motor neuron signs, severe dysarthria, stridor, dystonia, and restless legs syndrome. The diagnosis is clinical, and MSA can initially be indistinguishable from idiopathic PD, but the degree of autonomic dysfunction, disappointing response to levodopa, and cerebellar signs all support a diagnosis of MSA. The mean age of onset for MSA is 55 years; it is slightly more common in men, and it progresses to death in approximately 7 years on average. MSA accounts for approximately 3% of cases of parkinsonism. Orthostatic hypotension is often the most disabling symptom of MSA. Nonpharmacologic management of autonomic dysfunction includes eating small meals, arising to standing position slowly, using compressive elastic stockings, and increasing salt and fluid intake. Medications may be needed to treat severe orthostatic hypotension and include midodrine, fludrocortisone, and droxidopa (SOE=A). Use of these medications may result in supine hypertension, which requires close blood pressure monitoring and medication adjustments. Levodopa may initially help with some symptoms of rigidity and bradykinesia, but the improvement is not as significant as in idiopathic PD, and dopamine replacement may worsen orthostatic hypotension.

Progressive Supranuclear Palsy

Progressive supranuclear palsy (PSP) accounts for approximately 4% of cases of parkinsonism. PSP is marked by an akinetic-rigid form of parkinsonism with early loss of postural balance causing frequent falls (afflicted persons typically fall backward). As the disease progresses, supranuclear gaze palsy (described below) becomes apparent, and patients eventually develop spasticity, dystonia, dysarthria, dysphagia, and a subcortical-frontal dementia. Usual age of onset is the late 50s or early 60s. The disease typically progresses rapidly, with marked incapacity occurring within 3–5 years and death within 6–8 years, generally as a result of aspiration, infection, or complications of immobility. Progressive supranuclear palsy derives its name from progressive impairments of voluntary, vertical gaze. Most patients develop eye movement restrictions approximately 3–4 years into the disease course. Patients are unable to voluntarily look up or down, with down gaze impairment more specific for PSP. Resting tremor is typically absent, and the rigidity is more pronounced in the neck and trunk (axial rigidity). Patients with PSP often have a fixed facial expression due to facial dystonia that causes them to keep their eyebrows elevated in a look of surprise or furrowed in a persistent scowl. The dysarthria of PSP is distinct from that of PD, with mixed spastic (strangled) and hypophonic features. Gait is disturbed early in the course, and falls are frequent in most patients. Cognition, particularly involving executive function or judgment, is often affected, and personality changes may arise as well. Treatment with levodopa may partially reduce the rigidity, but the dramatic response to levodopa seen in patients with early PD is lacking.

Hyperkinetic Movement Disorders

Chorea

Chorea is a flowing, continuous, random movement that migrates from one part of the body to another. A variety of conditions are associated with chorea in older adults. The pathologic basis for chorea is dysfunction of the striatum. Huntington disease (HD) is the most common cause of chorea in adults. In HD, a patient's family history will suggest an autosomal dominant mode of inheritance, and other family members may have a genetically confirmed diagnosis. Sometimes, however, suggestive family history is lacking, or the patient may be the first family member to display a late onset of the disease with mild features. The age of onset of HD is normally distributed around a mean age of 40 years, but there are reported cases of symptom onset as late as 75–80 years. The diagnosis of HD can be made by genetic testing of the huntingtin gene. Other causes of choreiform movements include drug-induced chorea (eg, from levodopa, antiepileptics, estrogen), which is common and optimally treated by reducing or removing the offending agent. Chorea may arise from ischemic injury to the basal ganglia (ie, vascular chorea). Idiopathic choreiform movements may occur as an isolated symptom in adults ≥60 years old, a condition termed senile chorea if other causes of chorea have been excluded. Chorea can be treated with dopamine receptor–blocking medications (eg, risperidone[OL], haloperidol[OL]), but possible benefit must be weighed against adverse effects, including risk of development of tardive dyskinesia (SOE=B). Two medications, tetrabenazine and deutetrabenazine, are currently approved by the FDA for treatment of chorea in HD (SOE=A) and have been used to treat other causes of chorea. These drugs block the storage and release of dopamine presynaptically. They are not associated with an increased risk of tardive dyskinesia. Patients taking tetrabenazine or deutetrabenazine need to be monitored closely for signs of depression and medication-induced parkinsonism.

Dystonia

Dystonia is a hyperkinetic movement disorder that results in sustained muscle contractions causing twisting movements or abnormal postures. Dystonia may occur as an isolated disorder, on a genetic basis, or as part of another movement disorder (eg, PD, corticobasal degeneration). Common focal dystonias seen in older adults include cervical dystonia (spasmodic torticollis), blepharospasm, spasmodic dysphonia, or focal hand dystonia (writer's cramp). Medications such as anticholinergics (eg, trihexyphenidyl) or muscle relaxants (eg, baclofen) may be tried, but improvement in symptoms is typically limited and adverse effects are common (SOE=B). Botulinum toxin injections into contracted muscle can provide effective, but temporary, relief of dystonia (SOE=A).

Drug-Induced Movement Disorders

Several different types of involuntary movements can arise as a result of the use of medications. It is important to distinguish among medication effects that are acute, chronic but reversible, and chronic and irreversible. One acute effect that may occur with antipsychotic medications is an acute reaction resulting in dystonia of the mouth, tongue, or neck. If the dystonia is severe enough, treatment with intravenous diphenhydramine or lorazepam may be required, although this approach in older adults should be exercised with caution because of the risk of adverse effects. Chronic reversible drug effects include action tremor (eg, lithium, theophylline, valproic acid), parkinsonism (eg, antipsychotic or antiemetic medications), chorea (eg, antiepileptic medications, estrogen, levodopa), or dystonia (dopamine replacement therapy in PD). Chronic irreversible drug effects or tardive phenomena often begin after the medication (usually an antipsychotic medication) has been used for weeks to months; movements can include orobuccal dyskinesias, dystonia, akathisia (sensation of needing to move), myoclonus, and tics. Advanced age and duration of treatment with antipsychotic medications are the only well-established risk factors for developing tardive movement disorders. Once the diagnosis of a tardive phenomenon is established, the dosage of medication should be reduced or the medication should be discontinued. Treatment for tardive dyskinesia or tardive dystonia includes anticholinergic agents (eg, trihexyphenidyl[OL]), valbenazine, baclofen[OL], and tetrabenazine[OL], all of which must be used with caution in older adults. In cases of severe tardive dystonia, intramuscular injections of botulinum toxin can reduce the frequency and severity of abnormal movements.

Essential Tremor

Essential tremor (ET) is the most common form of tremor. The tremor of ET is an action tremor and postural tremor, which is present when the limbs are in active use (eg, while writing or holding a cup). The tremor most commonly involves the arms, although the head and voice may be affected also. Other less affected areas of the body include the chin, tongue, and legs. Typically, the tremor in ET is symmetric, but it may be slightly worse in one arm than the other. The severity of the action tremor may vary significantly depending on the type of movement. The tremor disappears when the arms are relaxed, such as when the person is sitting with hands at rest in the lap, or standing with arms held at the sides. Functionally, the tremor may interfere with many daily activities, such as eating, writing, or fastening buttons. Stress or anxiety often exacerbates the tremor. The frequency of the tremor is in the range of 4–12 Hz, which is faster than the rest tremor of PD. The prevalence of ET increases with advancing age, with as many as 5% of adults >60 years old affected. The age of onset seems to have a bimodal distribution, with peaks in the teens through 20s and in the 50s through 70s. Prevalence rates among men and women are similar. Affected individuals commonly report they have an affected relative, suggesting a familial or genetic cause. Familial forms of the tremor have been linked to regions on chromosomes 2p and 3q. Familial and sporadic forms of ET have no apparent clinical differences. Alcohol may decrease the severity of ET.

The main indication for treatment of ET is functional disability due to the tremor (eg, difficulty writing, using a cup or spoon, trouble holding objects). It is important to educate the patient about exacerbating factors such as caffeine, stress, and fatigue. The first-line options for pharmacologic treatment of ET are nonselective β-blockers (propranolol, nadolol[OL]) or primidone[OL] (SOE=A). Propranolol is the only drug approved by the FDA for treatment of ET. Each of these drugs improves the severity of tremor in most patients by approximately 30%–50%. Other medications, including baclofen[OL], gabapentin[OL], mirtazapine[OL], pregabalin[OL], and topiramate[OL], have been described as effective in some patients, but results have not been consistent (SOE=B/C). Occupational therapy and specialized equipment may provide complementary benefit for patients whose tremor threatens function (eg, use of weighted utensils or electronic "tremor-cancelling" utensils). Some patients with severe, medically refractory tremor may undergo DBS. DBS stimulation in the ventral intermediate nucleus of the thalamus provides significant improvement in tremor control in most patients (SOE=A). Potential adverse events are similar to those of DBS in PD (described above). Unilateral thalamic ablations (eg, MRI-guided focused ultrasound) has been FDA approved as a treatment option for ET.

Restless Legs Syndrome

Restless legs syndrome (RLS) is a condition in which a patient feels an uncontrollable urge to move the legs at night, usually accompanied by an uncomfortable and unpleasant sensation of the legs that worsens with inactivity and improves with movement. The symptoms occur while the person is awake, and symptoms may also involve the arms. The diagnosis is based on the patient's description of the symptoms; polysomnography is not required. There may be a family history of the condition, particularly in patients with an earlier age of onset of RLS. Some patients have an associated, underlying medical disorder (eg, anemia, or renal or neurologic disease). Because iron deficiency can trigger RLS, this should be excluded with a check of serum ferritin level. RLS is 1.5 times more common in women than men, and evidence suggests that RLS prevalence increases with age. Periodic limb movements of sleep (PLMS), which entail involuntary limb movements while asleep, occurs in most (80%–90%) patients with RLS. RLS may also be seen in demented patients who may not be able to adequately describe the symptoms. Such patients may demonstrate behaviors such as rubbing or massaging of legs, increased motor activity (eg, pacing, wandering), particularly in the evening and/or with inactivity; improvement is evident with movement of the legs. Many medications may aggravate or induce RLS symptoms, such as antiemetics, antipsychotics, SSRIs, tricyclic antidepressants, and diphenhydramine. Clinicians should carefully review the medication regimens of patients with new or worsening RLS.

Several effective medications are available if pharmacologic treatment for RLS or PLMS is indicated (because of severity of symptoms or significant effects on quality of life). For example, a dopamine agonist (eg, pramipexole, ropinirole, or rotigotine, all FDA approved for treatment of RLS) about 1–2 hours before bedtime is effective in the treatment of RLS and PLMS (SOE=A). A nighttime dose of carbidopa-levodopa[OL] may also be effective (SOE=A) and can be used for patients who need medication infrequently (ie, for as-needed use). However, some patients describe a shift of their symptoms to daytime hours with successful treatment of symptoms at night; this problem (termed augmentation) appears more frequently when carbidopa-levodopa is used on a regular basis but can also be seen with dopamine agonists. An extended-release form of gabapentin (gabapentin enacarbil) and pregabalin[OL] have been shown to be effective in improving RLS symptoms (SOE=A). In a blinded, head-to-head comparison, pregabalin was as effective as the dopamine agonist pramipexole in controlling RLS symptoms but less likely to produce augmentation. RLS symptoms may improve with iron replacement in patients with iron deficiency (SOE=B). Benzodiazepines[OL] and opioids[OL] have also been used for RLS but likely have more adverse events in older adults than the FDA-approved agents. Dopamine agonists may cause "hangover" fatigue or sleepiness, orthostatic hypotension, confusion, or dyskinesias.

NEUROMUSCULAR DISORDERS, PERIPHERAL NEUROPATHY, AND MYELOPATHY

The prevalence of peripheral neuropathy in older adults has been estimated to be as high as 10%. Peripheral neuropathy can be particularly devastating in older adults, because it may cause gait impairment from sensory and motor deficits with a resulting propensity to fall. In developed countries, diabetic neuropathy is the most common form of the condition; up to 30%–60% of diabetic patients >60 years old have peripheral neuropathy. Several types of neuropathy are associated with diabetes mellitus, including a distal symmetric neuropathy; asymmetric neuropathies that may involve cranial nerves, roots, or plexi; and mononeuropathy multiplex.

The history and physical examination are the most important tools in diagnosis of a peripheral neuropathy. Questions from the history should be geared toward identifying possible causes and risk factors. If the patient is not known to be diabetic, risk factors for diabetes or insulin resistance should be assessed. The past history and review of systems may give clues to a systemic disease that could contribute to a peripheral nerve disorder. A history of gastric bypass, eating disorder, or hemodialysis could indicate a possible nutritional deficiency. A thorough medication history should be taken to look for possible causes. The social history may uncover evidence of a possible exposure, such as alcohol or an occupational toxin. The family history should include inquiries for possible genetic forms of peripheral neuropathy. The neurologic examination focuses on establishing evidence of a length-dependent loss of sensory and/or motor function that is maximal distally in the limbs, associated with decreased reflexes and atrophy in affected regions.

Electrodiagnostic studies (ie, electromyography and nerve conduction studies) are considered an extension of the neurologic examination. They may yield valuable information in classifying the neuropathy, which may help to narrow a complicated differential diagnosis. First, these studies can differentiate between lesions affecting a single nerve, a nerve root, or a peripheral polyneuropathy. Next, they can help classify a polyneuropathy as axonal, demyelinating, or mixed. This distinction is important because certain neuropathies affect nerves in characteristic ways. For instance, a diabetic neuropathy is predominantly axonal, as are many of the toxic neuropathies such as alcohol and heavy metal exposure. In contrast, the hereditary and immune-mediated neuropathies more commonly cause peripheral demyelination. Acute, atypical, rapidly progressive, or severe forms of neuropathy should be referred to a neurologist with neuromuscular medicine expertise, who may perform tests of small fiber function, tests of autonomic function, peripheral nerve biopsy, and epidermal skin biopsy.

Treatment of the neuropathy depends on the underlying cause and ranges from withdrawal of the causative agent (eg, alcohol, medications) to nutritional supplementation (in the case of nutrient deficiency), to treatment of a primary cancer (in the setting of paraneoplastic neuropathy). There is evidence that optimizing glucose control can lessen the severity of diabetic neuropathy. Topical agents such as capsaicin cream and local anesthetic medications (eg, lidocaine patch) may provide relief for some patients with peripheral neuropathy (SOE=B). Systemic treatment of neuropathic pain may include the use of tricyclic antidepressants[OL] or antiepileptic medications such as gabapentin and pregabalin. Gabapentin and pregabalin are approved for use in treatment of post-herpetic neuralgia, and pregabalin is also approved for use in diabetic neuropathy and fibromyalgia (SOE=A). Two other FDA-approved medication options for use in patients with diabetic neuropathic pain are duloxetine, which is a serotonin-norepinephrine reuptake inhibitor antidepressant, and tapentadol, which also blocks reuptake of serotonin and norepinephrine and has additional agonist effects at mu-opioid receptors (SOE=A). In addition, tramadol[OL], which has properties similar to those of tapentadol, and opioids[OL] may be used to treat neuropathic pain (SOE=B). Combination therapy with effective medications that have different mechanisms of action are often needed to control symptoms adequately.

Radiculopathy

Radiculopathy results from compression of a spinal root as it exits the spinal canal. Among older adults, this can be the result of herniated discs or osteophyte formation. Symptomatic nerve root compression may result in complaints of pain radiating down the neck, back, arm, or leg, and on neurologic examination, this can be accompanied by motor and sensory deficits as well as by diminution of reflexes in the distribution of a particular spinal root or roots. MRI imaging of the involved nerve root may determine a structural cause of radiculopathy. Progressive involvement of lumbosacral nerve roots may be seen in meningeal carcinomatosis. MRI imaging with contrast and lumbar puncture with cytology may help to make this diagnosis. An acute, immune-mediated form of polyradiculopathy is acute inflammatory demyelinating polyradiculoneuropathy (AIDP), also termed Guillain Barré syndrome. AIDP is treated with immunotherapy acutely, using either plasma exchange or intravenous immunoglobulin therapy (IVIG). Chronic inflammatory demyelinating polyneuropathy is a chronic counterpart of AIDP and requires long-term immunotherapy. Patients with diabetes may present with diabetic amyotrophy, which is a lumbosacral polyradiculitis and plexopathy that starts with subacute onset of severe neuropathic pain in the thighs, which is often asymmetric, followed by proximal muscle weakness in the legs and eventual atrophy. Referral to a neuromuscular specialist is recommended for atypical and severe cases of radiculopathy.

Myopathy

Myopathies are characterized by proximal limb weakness, muscle wasting, and diminished or absent reflexes. Typically, they are accompanied by an increase in serum concentrations of muscle enzymes (eg, creatine kinase), a myopathic pattern on electromyogram, and abnormalities on muscle biopsy. Older adults may attribute mild to moderate muscle weakness to aging and therefore may not immediately consult a clinician. Proximal muscle weakness, which may result in difficulty rising from a chair, climbing stairs, or washing one's hair, is particularly likely to be falsely attributed to aging or arthritis.

The most common myopathies in older adults are polymyositis, endocrine myopathies, and toxic myopathies. Polymyositis, a disorder of skeletal muscle with diverse causes, is characterized by lymphocytic infiltration of the muscles. Muscle biopsy usually shows signs of both myocyte degeneration and regeneration. Immunotherapy with prednisone is considered the treatment of choice for polymyositis, but it should be used with caution in older adults because of adverse effects of chronic steroid use. In thyrotoxic myopathy, weakness and wasting are greatest in the pelvic girdle muscles and, to some extent, in the muscles of the shoulder region. Reflexes can be normal, and diagnosis is based on the distribution of muscle weakness in an individual with thyrotoxicosis. The myopathy improves with successful treatment of the underlying endocrine disorder. Hypothyroidism may cause a myopathy that improves with thyroid replacement therapy. Creatine kinase levels are significantly increased in the myopathy associated with hypothyroidism. Finally, several medications are known to cause myopathy, including corticosteroids, lipid-lowering agents, colchicine, and procainamide. The treatment of choice for drug-induced myopathy is cessation of the offending medication.

Motor Neuron Disease

Motor neuron disease, also called amyotrophic lateral sclerosis (ALS), is a neurodegenerative condition involving the cell bodies of both upper and lower motor neurons. It is characterized clinically by progressive weakness and wasting of skeletal muscles, often in combination with dysarthria, dysphagia, and respiratory failure. The incidence increases with age but reaches a plateau in the seventh decade of life. To date, age remains the single most clearly identifiable risk factor for this progressive and fatal disorder. Genetic causes of ALS are thought to occur in 5%–10% of patients. Four genes have been identified that can cause ALS. The gene C9ORF72 is the most common cause of familial ALS, accounting for 25%–40% of such cases. Mutations in this gene can also cause frontotemporal dementia, or a combination of ALS and frontotemporal dementia.

Patients with ALS commonly present with gait disturbance, falls, foot drop, weakness in grip, dysphagia, or dysarthria. On neurologic examination, patients may have a combination of upper motor neuron signs (eg, hyperreflexia, clonus, extensor plantar responses) and lower motor neuron signs (eg, weakness, atrophy, fasciculations). Weakness of the face, tongue, and palate are common, but extraocular muscles are usually spared. The electromyogram demonstrates findings consistent with diffuse denervation and poor recruitment of motor units. The differential diagnosis includes lesions at the level of the foramen magnum, a combination of cervical myelopathy associated with cervical and lumbar polyradiculopathies, or a motor predominant peripheral polyneuropathy in a patient with CNS lesions. The prognosis is poor with survival time averaging 2–3 years. The presence of bulbar weakness carries a poorer prognosis. Although most new cases of ALS occur in older adults, it is less common than several other neurologic disorders in this population. Therefore, gait disturbance and focal motor weakness may frequently be incorrectly attributed to the more common conditions. Older adults are also more likely to have coexisting neurologic disorders that might explain symptoms of weakness, adding to the challenge of and delay in diagnosing ALS. In one study, afflicted individuals >65 years old were diagnosed after 19 months, while those <65 years old were diagnosed after 3 months.

Treatment of ALS is primarily supportive. Riluzole, which has demonstrated modest effects on survival or time to tracheostomy (SOE=A), is in widespread use. Riluzole is thought to protect against glutamate toxicity, which may be implicated in the pathogenesis of ALS. Follow-up in a dedicated multidisciplinary ALS or muscular dystrophy clinic has also been shown to improve quality of life of ALS patients and may improve survival (SOE=B). In these settings patients may receive multidisciplinary care from a team, including a neuromuscular subspecialist; respiratory, physical, occupational, and speech therapists; and a social worker. Noninvasive support of ventilation, such as bilevel intermittent positive-airway pressure (BiPAP), has been shown to improve survival in ALS patients with respiratory compromise (SOE=A). Edaravone is a new medication approved by the FDA for treatment of ALS. It is given as an intravenous infusion for 10–14 days in a row, followed by 2 weeks off, and then this cycle is repeated. Edaravone is thought to reduce oxidative stress and was shown to slow progression of disability on an ALS scale (ALSFRS-R) in a subset of patients with milder symptoms of ALS by 33% (SOE=B). The impact of edavarone on long-term outcomes, such as quality of life and survival, is not known.

Myelopathy

Myelopathy or spinal cord dysfunction can be the result of extrinsic compression of the spinal cord or intrinsic spinal cord lesions. The cervical region is affected most commonly. Intrinsic spinal cord lesions may include spinal cord tumors, vascular events (eg, infarcts or hemorrhages), or trauma (eg, central cord syndrome). Extrinsic compressive lesions are more prevalent; common causes among older adults are cervical spondylosis (with resultant osteophyte formation and degenerative disc disease), disc prolapse or herniation, rheumatoid arthritis with vertebral body subluxation, meningioma, or spinal metastases. Nearly 80% of adults ≥70 years old have radiographic evidence of osteophyte formation with some narrowing of the spinal canal, but most are asymptomatic. Cervical spinal stenosis most often arises from spondylosis but may be worsened by disc protrusion or a congenitally narrow canal. Narrowing of the cervical canal can lead to neck stiffness and pain; radicular pain, sensory loss, or weakness in the arms; and weakness with upper motor neuron signs (eg, hyperreflexia, spasticity, Babinski sign) in the legs. Narrowing of the lumbar canal may lead to lower back pain, radicular pain, sensory loss, or weakness and other lower motor neuron signs in the legs. Lumbar spinal stenosis causes neurogenic claudication, manifested by increasing pain with weakness and numbness while walking, relieved by flexion at the waist or sitting.

MRI can be helpful for diagnosis of myelopathy, but results must be viewed with caution because abnormal MRI findings are common in asymptomatic older adults. If the patient cannot tolerate MRI because of the presence of an implanted metallic object (such as a pacemaker) or severe claustrophobia, then spinal CT with intrathecal contrast may be performed. Conservative management includes activity modification, neck immobilization with a cervical collar, massage, heat treatment, physical therapy, and analgesics.

HEADACHES

The prevalence of headaches appears to diminish with age. One study demonstrated that although 74% of men and 92% of women 21–34 years old have headaches, these proportions drop to 22% and 55% after the age of 75 years. Headache is one of the most common medical complaints in young persons, and yet one study suggests that it is only the tenth most common symptom in older women and the fourteenth most common symptom in older men. The incidence of migraine, the most common cause of headaches in younger adults, also declines with age, with only 2% of people developing their first migraine after age 50.

New-onset or persistent headaches in older adults are more likely to represent systemic illness or intracranial lesions (ie, secondary causes). In one study, 10% of headaches among younger patients represented systemic illness or intracranial lesions; in older adults, this proportion was 34%. These secondary causes include intracranial masses (eg, primary or secondary tumors, subdural hematomas), cervical spondylosis, COPD, obstructive sleep apnea, carbon monoxide poisoning, and giant cell arteritis. Brain imaging with contrast (ie, head CT or brain MRI) is indicated in older patients with new-onset or progressive headaches to exclude structural causes.

An important secondary cause of headache specific to older adults is giant cell (temporal) arteritis. This condition does not appear to develop in those <50 years old and peaks in incidence between the ages of 70 and 80. Women are affected twice as often as men. Pain may be centered at the temporal or occipital arteries. Palpation of the scalp arteries may reveal focal tenderness and nodularity. Complaints of visual changes, low-grade fever, polymyalgia, and constitutional symptoms further suggest the diagnosis. Typically, the serum sedimentation rate is significantly increased, and the diagnosis is made with a temporal artery biopsy. If the diagnosis is suspected and biopsy is planned within a few days, then corticosteroids may be started to prevent vascular complications (eg, loss of vision or stroke). In addition to structural and systemic causes of headaches, many commonly used medications may cause headaches that are dull, diffuse, and nondescript, including vasodilators (eg, nitrates), antihypertensives, antidepressant medications, and stimulants.

The common primary headache disorders can be classified into migraine (with or without aura), tension-type headaches, cluster headache, and chronic daily headaches. Migraines are headaches of moderate to severe intensity associated with nausea, vomiting, or photophobia. Half of the time they are unilateral and throbbing, but commonly the pain is bilateral. Auras, when they occur, usually precede the headache and are manifested by transient neurologic symptoms that can be localized to the cerebral cortex or brainstem. Visual phenomena are among the most common types of auras. Migraine headaches in older adults typically present as they do in younger people, but atypical presentations have been described. These include migraine auras without headache (acephalic migraine). The occurrence of an isolated visual or sensory aura in the absence of a headache can be diagnostically challenging, because it can mimic signs of a transient ischemic attack. In contrast to migraines, tension-type headaches typically are more diffuse in distribution, less severe in intensity, have a pressing or a tight quality, and are much less often associated with nausea or vomiting. Cluster headaches are much more common in men, may be associated with tearing and rhinorrhea, and are of shorter duration (15 minutes commonly but may last up to 3 hours) than migraines. They are severe in intensity and tend to recur in clusters during an interval of time (eg, within a day or within a few weeks). Chronic daily headaches are persistent, often bilateral, and have features that overlap with those of both migraine and tension-type headaches.

The treatment of migraine headaches can be categorized as either abortive (treating an attack that has already begun) or preventive. Other than various OTC preparations that contain NSAIDs, migraine-specific abortive therapies include ergotamines or triptans (eg, sumatriptan), which act by central serotonergic mechanisms. These medications are mild vasoconstrictors and thus contraindicated in patients with uncontrolled hypertension, stroke, or coronary artery disease. Generally, safety data in geriatric populations are lacking. Preventive therapies for migraine include nonselective β-blockers (eg, propranolol[OL]), valproic acid, topiramate, tricyclic antidepressants[OL], and calcium channel blockers (eg, verapamil[OL]). Preventive therapies decrease the frequency and severity of migraine over time and should be considered for patients who have disabling migraine headaches ≥2 times per month. The choice of agent should be guided by an effort to avoid adverse events and drug interactions. Treatment of muscle tension headaches includes NSAIDs[OL] as abortive agents and low doses of tricyclic antidepressants[OL] as preventive medication in chronic muscle tension headaches. Muscle relaxants, such as tizanidine[OL], have shown some effectiveness in treating chronic muscle tension headaches in open-label studies but may cause sedation or confusion. Each of the medications above may be contraindicated by comorbidities or existing medication regimens. A referral to a headache specialist should be considered for patients with either cluster headaches or chronic daily headaches.

RESOURCES

- Choi H, Pack A, Elkind MSV, et al. Predictors of incident epilepsy in older adults: The Cardiovascular Health Study. *Neurology*. 2017;88:870–877.

- Dieplinger A, Kundt FS, Lorenzl S. Palliative care nursing for patients with neurological diseases: What makes the difference? *Br J Nurs*. 2017;26(6):356–259.

- Harris M. Cognitive issues: Decline, delirium, depression, dementia. *Nurs Clin North Am*. 2017;52(3):363–374.

- Postuma RB, Berg D, Stern M, et al. MDS clinical diagnostic criteria for Parkinson's disease. *Mov Disord*. 2015;30(12):1591–1599.

CHAPTER 62—STROKE AND CEREBROVASCULAR DISEASE

KEY POINTS

- Cerebrovascular disease is a leading cause of disability and death among older adults.

- Acute stroke treatments can improve outcomes in patients, especially when care is provided soon after stroke symptoms begin and in a multidisciplinary stroke center.

- Primary and secondary stroke prevention can significantly decrease the burden of cerebrovascular disease in older populations.

IMPACT OF CEREBROVASCULAR DISEASE

Stroke is a leading cause of disability and death among older adults. The incidence of stroke increases with advancing age, approximately doubling with each decade. At younger ages, incidence of stroke for women is 25%–30% lower than that for men in comparable age groups, but it surpasses that of men ≥85 years old. Approximately 795,000 new strokes occur each year in the United States, and there are an estimated 6.8 million adults who are stroke survivors. Long-term disability is very common in stroke survivors. Six months after a stroke in those ≥65 years old, 26% are dependent in their ADLs and 46% have measurable cognitive deficits. Although older age is associated with worse functional recovery (measured by independence in performing ADLs), stroke patients at any age can nevertheless benefit from formal rehabilitation.

Besides being the most common acute, serious neurologic disease, stroke is also a leading cause of death. The fatality rate within 1 month of an acute stroke is 20%–30% across all age groups. Survival in part depends on the anatomic location and severity of the stroke. Neurologic causes of death include the brain injury itself or resultant brain edema. Common medical causes of death associated with stroke are myocardial infarction, arrhythmia, heart failure, aspiration pneumonia, and pulmonary embolism.

ISCHEMIC STROKE

Ischemic strokes are caused by occlusion of a cerebral blood vessel causing interruption of blood flow and infarction of the brain. Approximately 80%–85% of strokes are ischemic. Epidemiologic studies suggest that approximately 27% of ischemic strokes are due to cardiac emboli, 19% are due to large vessel disease, 17% are due to small vessel disease, and 35% cannot be classified. These proportions vary by 5%–10% among different study populations because of differences in risk factors, diagnostic studies performed, and race. Knowing the cause of the ischemic stroke helps to guide treatment decisions and to estimate risk and prognosis.

Small Vessel Disease

Small vessel disease causes occlusion of small penetrating vessels due to lipohyalinosis (lipid deposition and hyalinization) or local arteriolosclerosis. Small vessels supply deep white and gray matter structures such as the internal capsule, basal ganglia, thalamus, and pons. Occlusion of these small vessels can result in several well-defined clinical syndromes, including pure motor hemiplegia, pure hemisensory stroke, ataxic hemiparesis, and dysarthria–clumsy hand syndrome. Small vessel disease causes ischemic strokes that are typically <1 cm in size and are termed lacunar infarcts. Risk factors include hypertension, diabetes mellitus, and smoking. Lacunar strokes can occur independently or concurrently with large vessel cerebrovascular disease or other mechanisms of ischemic stroke.

Large Vessel Disease

Large vessel disease is most commonly the result of atherosclerosis and can cause progressive occlusion of cerebral vessels in the anterior and posterior circulation. Ischemic stroke in the setting of large vessel disease is often caused by emboli generated by the atherosclerotic lesion. Complete occlusion of large cerebral vessels can lead to severe and often life-threatening strokes. Strokes caused by large vessel disease can cause recognizable clinical syndromes that are consistent with anatomical distribution of major cerebral vessels (eg, hemiparesis or hemisensory loss associated with aphasia, apraxia, neglect, or visual field deficits). In addition, a lesion at the origin of the internal carotid artery can lead to transient monocular blindness (amaurosis fugax) or a cerebral hemispheric deficit, because both the retina and cerebral hemispheres derive their blood supply from the internal carotid artery. Syndromes associated with vascular lesions in the posterior circulation (vertebral and basilar arteries) can result in dysfunction of the cranial nerves, descending motor or ascending sensory tracts within the brain stem, cerebellar and vestibular pathways, and visual cortex. Signs and symptoms can

Table 62.1—Components of the National Institutes of Health Stroke Scale[a]

Stroke Scale Item	Item Score[b]
Level of consciousness	0–7
Best gaze	0–2
Visual fields	0–3
Facial palsy	0–3
Motor: arms	0–8
Motor: legs	0–8
Limb ataxia	0–2
Sensory	0–2
Best language	0–3
Dysarthria	0–2
Extinction and inattention	0–2
Total	0–42

[a] For full details of criteria for scoring each item, see www.ninds.nih.gov/sites/default/files/NIH_Stroke_Scale.pdf (accessed Feb 2019).
[b] Greater score reflects increased impairment.

include crossed cranial nerve and long-tract findings (eg, complete facial palsy ipsilateral to the lesion and hemiparesis involving the contralateral arm and leg), vertigo, double vision, ataxia, dysarthria, hemianopia or cortical blindness, Horner syndrome (ipsilateral miosis, anhidrosis, and mild ptosis), stupor, or coma. Large vessel disease can be identified by noninvasive imaging of the carotid arteries (Doppler ultrasonography, CT angiography, or magnetic resonance angiography) or conventional angiography. Risk factors for large vessel disease include hypertension, hyperlipidemia, diabetes, and smoking.

Cardioembolic and Cryptogenic Stroke

Cardioembolic strokes are an important, potentially preventable cause of ischemic stroke. Atrial fibrillation is the most common cause of cardioembolic stroke, associated with a 4-to 5-fold increased risk because of thrombus formation in the left atrial appendage and cardioembolism to cerebral vessels. Cardioembolic stroke due to atrial fibrillation accounts for 25%–30% of all ischemic strokes. The estimated stroke risk is similar for persistent and paroxysmal atrial fibrillation. Emboli from the heart tend to occlude medium-sized cerebral vessels (eg, branches of the middle cerebral artery) and often cause multiple cerebral infarcts that involve more than one vascular territory. Cardioembolic strokes often occur without preceding transient ischemic attack (TIA).

A substantial proportion of ischemic strokes do not have a clearly identifiable cause and are classified as cryptogenic. Brain and vascular imaging should, however, provide an indication of the size of the vessel(s) involved. Atypical causes (eg, vasculitis, coagulopathy, mitochondrial disorders) should be considered in the setting of cryptogenic stroke, and prolonged cardiac monitoring is sometimes needed to capture intermittent atrial fibrillation as a potential cause of cryptogenic stroke.

Treatment of Acute Ischemic Stroke

In the setting of acute stroke symptoms, it is important to quickly determine whether the patient is suffering from an ischemic or hemorrhagic event with head CT imaging, and then to assess the severity and pattern of neurologic deficits. The NIH Stroke Scale (NIHSS) is a standardized rating scale used for this assessment (Table 62.1). The severity of deficits on this scale can help to make therapeutic decisions acutely and to determine long-term prognosis during the recovery phase. In general, a NIHSS score of <5 is associated with a very good prognosis. Individuals with a score >20 have a very poor prognosis and a high likelihood of major complications. In the immediate evaluation, non-stroke causes of acute neurologic dysfunction, such as migraine, seizure, and drug intoxication, need to be identified. Recent meta-analyses suggest that patients who are evaluated and treated in a multidisciplinary stroke center have better survival and functional outcomes than those who are not (SOE=B).

The current protocol for acute care of the older stroke patient includes optimizing hydration status; controlling blood pressure while avoiding hypotension; preventing deep-vein thrombosis; detecting and treating coronary ischemia, heart failure, and cardiac arrhythmias; and starting long-term treatment with antiplatelet agents or oral anticoagulation (depending on the presumed cause) to prevent recurrent stroke. Body temperature and blood glucose should be normalized in the acute setting. Dehydration on presentation is common, but rehydration should occur gradually to reduce the risk of cerebral edema. To prevent aspiration pneumonia, all ischemic stroke patients should receive a formal dysphagia evaluation before oral intake is allowed.

Immediately after an ischemic cerebral infarction, treatment of hypertension should be delayed until the situation stabilizes. The eventual goal is to reduce blood pressure gradually (eg, a goal of 15% reduction over the first 24 hours) while avoiding hypotension. The target systolic blood pressure should be 10–20 mmHg higher than the baseline pressure; if the baseline is unknown, systolic pressure should not be lowered below 160 mmHg. Patients treated with thrombolytic agents (see below) require careful blood pressure monitoring, especially during the first 24 hours of treatment. Blood pressure should be lowered and maintained below 185 mmHg systolic and 110 mmHg diastolic in patients who receive thrombolytic agents. Patients with a history of ischemic heart disease or arrhythmia, and patients with embolic strokes should be monitored with telemetry for at least 48 hours. For large, ischemic strokes (eg, involving most of the middle cerebral artery territory, or that of both middle and anterior cerebral arteries) in the setting of atrial fibrillation, anticoagulation therapy is not initiated for 7–14 days after onset because of a high risk of hemorrhagic transformation. Earlier anticoagulation does not improve outcome in these patients.

Recombinant tissue-plasminogen activator (rt-PA, alteplase) is approved for treatment of acute, ischemic stroke by the FDA. Infusion of this medication within 3 hours of stroke onset approximately doubles the chances of a favorable outcome at 3 months (SOE=A, but very limited data in older adults). However, the benefits of rt-PA must be weighed against the increased risk of intracranial hemorrhage, which can be fatal or result in worsened neurologic status. Overall, the literature suggests that approximately one-third of patients treated with thrombolytic therapy have a better outcome, as measured by >1-point improvement in the modified Rankin scale (ie, a clinically meaningful improvement), when compared with placebo. Intracerebral hemorrhage occurs in 6% of patients and is fatal in approximately half of these individuals. Most hemorrhagic events occur among patients with severe strokes (eg, NIHSS score >20).

Use of rt-PA requires careful assessment by a clinician experienced in treatment of stroke. rt-PA should be considered in all patients who present within 3 hours of onset of neurologic deficit and in whom CT confirms the absence of intracranial hemorrhage. Major contraindications include major surgery within the previous 2 weeks, previous intracranial hemorrhage, sustained systolic blood pressure >185 mmHg or diastolic >110 mmHg despite treatment, symptoms of subarachnoid hemorrhage, recent uncontrollable source of bleeding, coagulopathy, thrombocytopenia (platelet count <100,000/mm^3), or INR >1.7. The American Heart Association (AHA) has recommended a prolongation of the window for use of rt-PA in acute stroke to 3–4.5 hours after symptom onset in patients ≤80 years old who have an NIHSS score of ≤25 and no prior history of stroke or diabetes. This AHA recommendation was based on results from the European Cooperative Acute Stroke Study 3, which identified continued benefit in this time window (SOE=B).

Four recent randomized clinical trials have shown that endovascular thrombectomy in patients with proximal, large vessel occlusions of the anterior cerebral circulation provides significant benefit when treatment begins within 6 hours of stroke onset. In these studies, most patients received rt-PA (given IV) before endovascular thrombectomy. This combination therapy is best delivered in a coordinated, comprehensive stroke center. The benefits of this therapy were seen at 24 hours, with a 50% reduction in stroke severity as measured by the NIHSS, and again at 90 days with improvements in functional outcomes as measured by the modified Rankin Scale (mRS). The number needed to treat for a mRS of 0–2 (functional independence) at 90 days ranged between 2 and 4 in these trials (SOE=A).

Transient Ischemic Attack (TIA)

Special consideration should be given to those suffering a TIA, which is defined as a brief episode of neurologic dysfunction caused by focal ischemia to the brain or spinal cord that does not result in acute infarction. The traditional definition suggested that these deficits could last up to 24 hours, but with newer imaging it is clear that a TIA typically lasts <1–2 hours, and longer episodes are commonly associated with acute infarction. TIA is a major risk factor for subsequent stroke. A patient with TIA symptoms should be evaluated emergently. Brain imaging, ideally with MRI, is important to determine whether there has been an acute stroke and, if one is found, its location and type. Noninvasive imaging of the carotid arteries (Doppler ultrasonography or magnetic resonance angiography), electrocardiogram, and an echocardiogram are important tests to obtain to better determine the most likely cause of ischemia. Fasting glucose and lipid levels should be measured, blood pressure monitored, and patients asked about tobacco use to look for modifiable risk factors. Treatment for patients with TIA is focused on completion of diagnostic tests and initiation of treatments for secondary stroke prevention based on the results of the evaluation.

Primary and Secondary Ischemic Stroke Prevention

Throughout the latter half of the 20th century, the incidence of stroke declined in the United States, Canada, and Western Europe. In the past four decades, stroke incidence rates have fallen by 42% in high-income countries but have remained the same or increased in low and middle-income countries. The drop in incidence in high-income countries is attributable in part to better control of modifiable risk factors, including hypertension, heart disease, diabetes mellitus, cigarette smoking, and increased blood lipids. Hypertension is the most prevalent risk factor for stroke, and its treatment substantially reduces that risk. Treatment of isolated systolic hypertension in older adults reduces the risk of stroke by nearly 40% (SOE=A). Initiation of blood pressure (BP) therapy to maintain the systolic BP <140 mmHg and diastolic BP <90 mmHg is recommended for secondary stroke prevention (SOE=A) and for primary prevention in those with other risk factors such as diabetes. Dyslipidemia is another independent risk factor for stroke. Treatment with an HMG coenzyme-A reductase inhibitor ("statin") is recommended for the primary prevention of ischemic stroke in patients estimated to have a high 10-year risk of cardiovascular events based on AHA guidelines (SOE=A). In patients who have had a TIA or stroke believed to be of atherosclerotic origin, high-intensity statin therapy is recommended, regardless of the LDL-C level, to prevent future TIA or stroke (SOE=B). Several studies have confirmed a 2- to 4-fold increased risk of stroke in individuals with diabetes mellitus (SOE=A). Some research suggests that tight control of blood glucose levels in healthier adults might reduce the risk of stroke in individuals with diabetes mellitus, although the evidence for reduction of other diabetic complications (eg, retinopathy, nephropathy) is more compelling. Additionally, aggressive treatment of hypertension and hyperlipidemia in the diabetic population is a crucial component in lowering the risk of stroke. Cigarette smoking independently increases the risk of stroke as much as 3-fold (SOE=A). The incidence of stroke declines significantly even after just 2 years of smoking cessation; after 5 years, the level of risk returns to that of nonsmokers. Thus, counseling and assisting patients to stop smoking is important.

For patients with valvular and nonvalvular atrial fibrillation (AF) at high risk of stroke and low risk of hemorrhagic complications, long-term oral anticoagulation therapy is recommended (SOE=A). Risk stratification scales developed for patients with nonvalvular AF, such as the $CHADS_2$ or CHA_2DS_2-VASc risk scores, can help determine risk. Scores ³2 points imply high risk. A meta-analysis of stroke prevention trials in the setting of nonvalvular atrial fibrillation has shown an average relative risk reduction of 64% for warfarin and 19% for aspirin when compared with placebo. Warfarin dosed to a target INR of 2.0–3.0 is recommended for valvular AF (SOE=A). For nonvalvular AF, first-line anticoagulant options are warfarin with INR 2.0–3.0 (SOE=A) or the novel oral anticoagulants apixaban, edoxaban, rivaroxaban, and dabigatran as alternatives (SOE=A). For patients with nonvalvular AF and low risk of stroke, aspirin can be considered (SOE=C). If possible, oral anticoagulation should be initiated within 14 days of the TIA or stroke in those with AF.

Aspirin is the mainstay of antiplatelet therapy for secondary stroke prevention in patients with noncardioembolic ischemic stroke (SOE=A; relative risk reduction 15%–20%; NNT approximately 60 for prevention of one stroke over 1 year of therapy). Studies on the use of aspirin in stroke prevention suggest that dosages >325 mg/d do not add therapeutic benefit, but the minimal necessary dosage has not been definitively determined. Many clinicians routinely prescribe 81–325 mg/d, although even the lower dosage can cause GI irritation and blood loss. Other antiplatelet medications are available but have not shown consistent superiority to aspirin. These agents include sustained-release dipyridamole combined with aspirin (SOE=A) and clopidogrel (SOE=B). Clopidogrel 75 mg/d is an alternative for patients who cannot tolerate aspirin. Combining clopidogrel and aspirin does not provide additional benefit in the secondary prevention of stroke when initiated days to years after a stroke or TIA (SOE=B). Antiplatelet agents have not been shown to provide significant reduction in stroke risk in primary prevention, but patients with significant cerebrovascular disease on brain imaging who do not have history of TIA or stroke (ie, "silent" cerebrovascular disease) may benefit from antiplatelet therapy, as described above for secondary stroke prevention. In two large trials, no benefit was found for use of warfarin over aspirin for secondary stroke prevention (SOE=A) in the setting of large vessel disease, including intracranial atherosclerotic disease.

For all patients with cerebral atherosclerotic disease, medical management should target modifiable risk factors and should include daily use of an antiplatelet agent and a statin (SOE=B). Whether to recommend surgical management of extracranial carotid atherosclerotic disease depends on the degree of carotid stenosis and whether the patient has had a TIA or stroke in the vascular territory of the stenotic carotid. For patients with ≥70% symptomatic carotid stenosis, carotid endarterectomy (CEA) significantly reduces subsequent stroke risk, provided that endarterectomy is performed at an institution and by a surgeon with extensive experience with the procedure and perioperative risk of morbidity and mortality <6% (SOE=A). For patients with recent TIA or ischemic stroke and ipsilateral moderate (50%–69%) carotid stenosis, CEA can be considered if the patient is a good surgical candidate and the perioperative morbidity and mortality risk is <6%. In this setting, the number needed to treat [NNT] is 15 to prevent one ipsilateral stroke over 5 years of follow-up (SOE=B). Endovascular treatment with carotid artery angioplasty and stenting (CAS) using an embolic-protection device is an alternative to CEA. The relative advantages and disadvantages of CEA versus CAS have not been conclusively determined, but recent meta-analyses suggest that CAS may have a slightly higher risk of periprocedural stroke and 30-day stroke risk (1% difference) but lower risk of cranial nerve injury (3% difference). There was no significant difference in risk of myocardial infarction at 30 days in a recent meta-analysis (SOE=B). CAS can be considered in patients with significant comorbidities (especially those who are high-risk candidates for general anesthesia or who have had prior neck radiation exposure, prior carotid endarterectomy, or contralateral carotid occlusion). It is reasonable to consider performing CEA or CAS in *asymptomatic* patients who have >70% stenosis of the internal carotid artery if the perioperative risk of stroke, myocardial infarction, and death is very low (<3% [SOE=B]). However, the long-term effectiveness of CEA or CAS for asymptomatic stenosis >70% when compared with best "modern" medical management has not been established. Neither CEA nor CAS is recommended for asymptomatic carotid stenosis <70%.

Treatment of cryptogenic stroke includes evaluating and treating modifiable stroke risk factors and initiating antiplatelet therapy. Atypical causes of stroke should be considered, including coagulopathies, vasculitis, metabolic, or genetic causes, and a referral to a vascular neurologist may be helpful in diagnosis and management. If a cardioembolic cause is suspected, then prolonged (eg, 30 days) cardiac rhythm monitoring for AF is reasonable (SOE=B), and oral anticoagulant therapy should be initiated if intermittent AF is found. There are insufficient data to establish whether anticoagulation is equivalent or superior to aspirin for secondary stroke prevention in patients with a patent foramen ovale (PFO) but without AF (SOE=B). However, in the setting of PFO and venous source of embolism, oral anticoagulation is recommended (SOE=A). If anticoagulation is contraindicated in such a patient, then an inferior vena cava filter (SOE=C) can be considered.

The literature supporting management of patients with cryptogenic stroke and PFO is evolving. Three recent clinical trials suggest that transcatheter closure of a PFO may be superior to antiplatelet therapy in such patients (SOE=A). Across the trials, the relative risk reduction was approximately 50%, and the absolute risk reduction of recurrent stroke was approximately 4% over 35 years of follow-up. However, there was 4%–6% increased risk of developing AF in the PFO closure group in 2 of the trials. Prediction scales are being developed to help select patients for possible PFO closure that may include age, presence of cortical stroke, absence of risk factors for atherosclerosis, and characteristics of the PFO (eg, shunt, presence of atrial septal aneurysm).

HEMORRHAGIC STROKE

Hemorrhagic strokes (intracranial hemorrhages) account for 15%–20% of all strokes. There are 4 main subtypes: intracerebral hemorrhage, subarachnoid hemorrhage, subdural hematoma, and epidural hematoma. Intracerebral hemorrhages outnumber subarachnoid hemorrhage by approximately 2 to 1. Subdural hematomas and epidural hematomas are less common than subarachnoid hemorrhages and most commonly arise from trauma. Intracranial hemorrhages present with abrupt onset of focal neurologic symptoms and often are associated with severe headache, vomiting, very high blood pressure, and coma or decreased level of consciousness. However, none of these features is specific enough to distinguish the syndrome from ischemic stroke based on clinical features alone. For this reason, emergent brain imaging (eg, head CT) is needed to determine whether a stroke is hemorrhagic or ischemic. Hemorrhagic strokes carry a higher risk of mortality than ischemic strokes and are best treated in comprehensive stroke centers with neurosurgical expertise and neurointensive care units.

Intracerebral Hemorrhage

The most common risk factor for spontaneous intracerebral hemorrhage (ICH) is uncontrolled hypertension, which is present in 75%–80% of cases. Excessive use of alcohol also increases the risk. The incidence of ICH increases with age, from 36 per 100,000 person-years in those 55–64 years old to 196 per 100,000 person-years in those >84 years old. Common locations for "hypertensive bleeds" are the putamen, thalamus, cerebellar hemisphere, pons, and cerebrum. These are structures supplied by small penetrating vessels that are prone to rupture in the setting of uncontrolled hypertension. Another important cause of spontaneous ICH in older adults is lobar hemorrhage caused by cerebral amyloid angiopathy, which can be visualized as microbleeds on brain MRI scans and can be associated with Alzheimer disease. Intracranial bleeds tend to be recurrent in patients with cerebral amyloid angiopathy. The risk of spontaneous ICH can also be increased by oral anticoagulants, especially warfarin, when the INR exceeds 3.

For patients presenting with acute ICH who have a systolic BP between 150 and 220 mmHg, acute lowering of the systolic BP to 140 mmHg is safe and recommended (SOE=A). Patients on warfarin should receive intravenous vitamin K and therapy to replace vitamin K–dependent clotting factors to normalize the INR (SOE=B). Patients with severe coagulation factor deficiency or severe thrombocytopenia should receive appropriate factor replacement therapy or platelets as needed (SOE=B). All anticoagulant and antiplatelet therapies should be stopped in the acute period. Initial management of ICH patients should occur in an ICU or dedicated stroke unit with neurologic acute care expertise (SOE=B). All patients with ICH should have intermittent pneumatic compression stockings placed on admission to prevent deep-vein thrombosis (SOE=A) and receive formal screening for dysphagia before oral feeding to reduce the risk of aspiration pneumonia (SOE=B). Patients with cerebellar hemorrhage who are deteriorating neurologically, who have brainstem compression, or ventricular obstruction should undergo surgical removal of the hemorrhage as soon as possible (SOE=B). In addition, some large hemorrhages with intraventricular extension may also require neurosurgical intervention.

The most important intervention to prevent recurrent ICH is long-term blood pressure control with a goal of <130 mmHg systolic and <80 mmHg diastolic (SOE=B). The decision to restart anticoagulation or antiplatelet medications after ICH can be difficult. The choice depends on many factors and should take into account the reason the medications were started, the cause of the hemorrhage, the risk of future ischemic events, and the neurologic state of the patient. In those at high risk of future ischemic cerebrovascular events, such as those with mechanical heart valves and prior ischemic stroke, restarting anticoagulation may be needed within 2 weeks of the hemorrhage, but in all others it is not recommended to restart oral anticoagulation for at least 4 weeks to prevent recurrent hemorrhage (SOE=B).

Subarachnoid Hemorrhage

Subarachnoid hemorrhage (SAH) is caused by a rupture of an intracranial aneurysm (80%–85% of the time) or another abnormality of a cerebral vessel (eg, arteriovenous malformation). Some persons are at higher risk of developing intracranial aneurysms, including those with autosomal dominant polycystic kidney disease (3- to 10-fold increase in risk), connective tissue diseases (eg, Marfan syndrome, Ehlers-Danlos syndrome), and certain genetic disorders (Klinefelter syndrome, neurofibromatosis type 1, α_1-antitrypsin deficiency). The incidence of intracranial saccular aneurysms increases with age from 21 per 100,000 person-years at age 60 to 41 per 100,000 person-years at age 80. These aneurysms are more common in women in each age range after age 45. High-risk groups (eg, polycystic kidney disease, strong family history of aneurysm or SAH) should be offered noninvasive screening for saccular aneurysms with CT or MR angiography (SOE=B).

Unruptured cerebral aneurysms are relatively common, with prevalence estimates of 2000–4000 per 100,000, but the incidence of SAH is 10 per 100,000 person-years. Thus, determining what factors increase the risk of rupture is important to effectively manage these unruptured cerebral aneurysms. Meta-analyses have shown that a greater risk of rupture is associated with larger size of the aneurysm, enlargement of the aneurysm over time, older age, female gender, posterior circulation location, and prior SAH. The importance of aneurysm size was shown by a large prospective longitudinal study which documented that the annual risk of rupture was ≤0.5% for aneurysms <7 mm, 1.69% for those 7–9 mm, 4.37% for those 10–24 mm, and 33.4% for those >25 mm. Patients with aneurysms at higher risk of rupture should be referred to a neurosurgeon with expertise in management of cerebral aneurysms. Treatment options for unruptured cerebral aneurysm in high-risk patients include surgical clipping or endovascular coil embolization of the lesion. Location and size of the aneurysm and patient characteristics are considered when deciding on the best approach.

The acute management of SAH is similar to that of ICH but includes both medical and surgical interventions to prevent additional bleeding, and focuses on detection and treatment of arterial vasospasm that commonly complicates SAH. As in ICH, treatment in a multidisciplinary stroke center with neurosurgical expertise and an ICU with neuroscience expertise is needed for best outcomes.

Subdural Hematoma

A subdural hematoma is a collection of blood between the dura and the arachnoid. It is usually due to head trauma, although the trauma may be mild, particularly in older adults. In approximately 15% of cases, the hematomas are bilateral. Some older adults suffer from chronic subdural hematoma that may be symptomatic. The incidence of chronic subdural hematoma increases with age, from 0.13 per 100,000 person-years for those in their 20s to 7.4 per 100,000 person-years for those in their 70s. In 50% of chronic subdural hematomas, there is no history of head injury, and other risk factors include clotting disorders, shunting procedures, and seizures. Symptoms of chronic subdural hematoma are headache, slight to moderate cognitive impairment, and focal neurologic signs (eg, hemiparesis, hemisensory loss). Neuroimaging studies reveal an extra-axial collection of blood or fluid (eg, subdural hygroma). Treatment varies depending on whether the hematoma is symptomatic or an incidental finding on a neuroimaging study. If the patient is symptomatic and clinically worsening, removal of the clot may be attempted. If the patient is asymptomatic or improving, then clinical monitoring is appropriate, because the hematoma may resolve without surgery. Some individuals may develop seizures with or after a subdural hematoma. A history of subdural hematoma may increase the risk of normal pressure hydrocephalus.

> **CHOOSING WISELY® RECOMMENDATION**
>
> *Stroke and Cerebrovascular Disease*
>
> - Do not recommend carotid endarterectomy for asymptomatic carotid stenosis unless the complication rate is low (<3%).

RESOURCES

- Hemphill JC III, Greenberg SM, Anderson CS, et al. Guidelines for the management of spontaneous intracerebral hemorrhage: a guideline for healthcare professionals from the American Heart Association/American Stroke Association. *Stroke*. 2015;46(7):2032–2060.

- Kernan WN, Ovbiagele B, Black HR, et al. Guidelines for prevention of stroke in patients with stroke and transient ischemic attack: a guideline for healthcare professionals from the American Heart Association/American Stroke Association. *Stroke*. 2015;45(7):2160–2236.

- Oertel LB, Fogerty AB. Use of direct oral anticoagulants for stroke prevention in elderly patients with nonvalvular atrial fibrillation. *J Am Assoc Nurs Pract*. 2017;29(9):551–556.

- Wilson SE, Ashcraft S. Ischemic stroke: management by the nurse practitioner. *J Nurs Pract*. 2019;15(1):47–53.e2

CHAPTER 63—INFECTIOUS DISEASES

KEY POINTS

- Immune function wanes with age, and resistance is compromised in older adults not only as a consequence of age-related declines in immunity (ie, immunosenescence), but more importantly because of comorbid disease and increased exposure to nosocomial pathogens.

- Accepted thresholds for "fever" generally do not apply to older adults because of their altered febrile response to infection. Fever can be redefined in frail older adults (temperature >2°F over baseline, single oral temperature >100°F, or repeated oral temperatures >99°F).

- Applying definite criteria for starting antibiotic therapy in residents of long-term care facilities is likely to reduce inappropriate antibiotic use without jeopardizing patient safety.

- Overtreatment of asymptomatic bacteriuria with antibiotics leads to development of multidrug resistant organisms. Providers should be cognizant of susceptibility patterns for urinary isolates, especially when treating urinary tract infections in long-term care residents.

- Vaccinations play an important role in prevention of life-threatening illnesses in older adults, especially influenza and invasive pneumococcal disease.

Infection is a major cause of mortality in adults ≥65 years old, comprising >40% of deaths in this population. Infection is also a significant cause of morbidity in older adults, often exacerbating underlying illness or leading to hospitalization. Pneumonia and other respiratory tract infections, urinary tract infection, and sepsis are all in the top 20 diagnosis-related groups paid by Medicare. Furthermore, older adults are often a "sentinel" population in which new infections (eg, West Nile virus), more virulent strains (*Clostridium difficile* colitis), or the return of annual epidemics (eg, influenza) are first noted. Associations of infection and inflammation with age-related chronic diseases suggest that infectious diseases may play an even larger role in the morbidity and mortality of the older adult population than was previously realized. This chapter explores the biological, cultural, and societal factors that influence susceptibility to infection, addresses the presentation of infectious disease, and offers management suggestions for several common infectious disease syndromes in older adults.

PREDISPOSITION TO INFECTION

The immune system undergoes an age-related decline (Table 63.1), often termed immunosenescence, putting older adults at higher risk of development of infectious diseases, which are also more severe than in younger people. Vaccine efficacy is also lower in older adults because of this phenomenon. Changes in adaptive immunity because of thymic involution involve depressed T-cell function. B cells in older adults can produce antibodies with lower affinity, contributing to the weakened immunogenicity of vaccines. Deficits of innate immunity include decreased macrophage activity, causing infections to have a longer course. The less active macrophages also regulate the adaptive immune response, adding to its impairment in older adults.

Nonspecific host-resistance factors that change with age also increase the risk of infection in older adults. For example, poor skin integrity predisposes to skin and soft-tissue infection, impaired cough or gag reflexes increase the risk of pneumonia, and increased gastric pH and decreased GI motility predispose to diarrheal illnesses. However, all of these changes associated with aging have far less influence on risk of infection than do comorbid diseases. Diabetes mellitus, chronic kidney disease, heart failure, chronic edema due to venous insufficiency, COPD, and stroke are but a few examples of age-related comorbid illnesses that increase risk of infection. Comorbidity further influences the outcomes of and management strategies for infection in older adults. For example, community-acquired pneumonia (CAP) in otherwise healthy adults <50 years old is typically treated on an outpatient basis and rarely causes mortality; however, in older adults with CAP and multiple comorbid conditions, the increased risk of morbidity and mortality often necessitates hospitalization. Several tools, including CURB-65 and the pneumonia severity index, are available to assess severity of CAP and to determine the most appropriate site of care (ie, hospitalization versus outpatient treatment). The CURB-65 score takes into account several factors, including **C**onfusion, **U**rea (blood urea nitrogen >7 mmol/L or 20 mg/dL), **R**espiratory rate ≥30 breaths/minute, **B**lood pressure (systolic <90 mmHg or diastolic ≤60 mmHg); and **A**ge (≥**65** years old). Each criterion is assigned 1 point. The higher the score, the more likely an older adult will need hospitalization. A score of 4 or 5 often necessitates ICU admission. The pneumonia severity index uses variables based on medical history, physical examination, and selected laboratory and radiographic findings at time of presentation.

Table 63.1—Changes in Immune Function Associated with Aging

Type of Immunity	Change With Age	Comment
Innate immunity		
Skin, mucous membranes	↓↓↓	Skin thins and dries with aging
Polymorphonuclear neutrophils		
Adherence, chemotaxis	—	
Ingestion	—	
Intracellular killing	↓	Most changes are due to comorbidity
Adaptive immunity		
Thymic hormones	↓↓↓	
Lymphocyte subsets		
T cells	↓↓↓	Shift from naive to memory subtypes
Natural killer cells	↓↓	Number increases but function declines
Lymphocyte functions		
Proliferative responses	↓↓	
Senescent phenotype	↑↑↑	Refers to oligoclonal expansion of CD8 cells that have replicative senescence, are CD28 negative, and secrete high quantities of proinflammatory cytokines
Cytokine production, secretion		
IL-2, IL-2 receptor	↓↓↓	After stimulation
Interferon-γ	↑	Primarily basal secretion
Prostaglandin E_2	↑↑	Basal and stimulated
Delayed-type hypersensitivity	↓↓	
Autoimmunity	↑↑	Autoantibodies common but of unclear significance

NOTE: — = no age-related changes; ↑ = mild increase; ↑↑ = moderate increase; ↑↑↑ = marked increase; ↓ = mild decrease; ↓↓ = moderate decrease; ↓↓↓ = marked decrease; IL = interleukin

Residing in long-term care or nursing facilities also places older adults at increased risk of epidemic diseases such as influenza. Widespread antibiotic use in these settings increases the likelihood of acquiring diseases caused by multidrug resistant organisms (MDROs); methicillin-resistant *Staphylococcus aureus* (MRSA), vancomycin-resistant enterococci (VRE), and extended spectrum β-lactamase–producing gram-negative rods (ESBLs) are more common causes of infection in institutionalized than in community-dwelling older adults. Resistance issues are augmented in long-term care facilities by debilitated hosts, close proximity of residents, poor staff compliance with prevention strategies (eg, influenza immunization), overutilization of antibiotics, and difficulties in implementing infection-control measures.

DIAGNOSIS AND MANAGEMENT OF INFECTIONS

Fever in Older Adults

Older adults often present without typical signs and symptoms of infection. Fever, generally defined as a single temperature ≥101°F (38.3°C), may be absent in 30%–50% of frail older adults with serious infections, even bacteremia, pneumonia, or endocarditis. The cause of impaired febrile responses in older adults is incompletely understood, but diverse mechanisms of thermoregulation are involved, including a reduced basal body temperature in many older adults and blunted thermogenesis by brown adipose tissue.

To improve the sensitivity of fever to detect infection in older adults, the Infectious Disease Society of America redefined fever in older long-term care residents as a temperature >2°F (1.1°C) over baseline (if a baseline is available), an oral temperature >99°F (37.2°C) or a rectal temperature >99.5°F (37.5°C) on repeated measures, or a single oral temperature >100°F (37.8° C) (SOE=B). This definition of fever has a sensitivity of 82.5% in long-term care residents, and the specificity remains high at 89.9% (Table 63.2). These data were generated in a cohort of frail, older, male veterans in a nursing home. It would seem reasonable to apply the same definitions to frail, older adults of either sex in the community, although the performance characteristics of this definition of fever in otherwise healthy older

Table 63.2—Defining Fever in Frail, Older Residents of Long-Term Care Facilities

Definition	Sensitivity	Specificity	(+) Likelihood Ratio	(−) Likelihood Ratio
T >101°F (38.3°C)	40.0%	99.7%	133	0.6
T >100°F (37.7°C)	70.0%	98.3%	41	0.3
T >99°F (37.2°C)	82.5%	89.9%	8	0.2

NOTE: (+) Likelihood ratio = sensitivity / (1− specificity); (−) Likelihood ratio = (1− sensitivity) / specificity; T = temperature

SOURCE: Data from Castle SC, Yeh M, Toledo S, et al. Lowering the temperature criterion improves detection of infections in nursing home residents. *Aging Immunol Infect Dis*. 1993;4(2):67–76.

adults have not been validated. A more recent study conducted in nursing-home residents concluded that an oral temperature >99.2°F (37.3°C) or a temperature of 1.5°F over an individual's baseline temperature (average of 3 non-illness temperatures) was strongly suggestive of infection in this population.

Atypical Presentation of Infectious Diseases in Older Adults

The absence of fever is only one way that infectious diseases can present atypically in older adults. For example, pneumonia can be signaled by a nonspecific decline in baseline functional status, such as confusion or falling, without cough, sputum production, or shortness of breath. Symptoms of a urinary tract infection may include atypical symptoms such as change in character of the urine and change in mental status. Anorexia and decreased oral intake may be the primary manifestation of infection, or exacerbation of an underlying illness (eg, atrial fibrillation) may become the predominant feature. Cognitive impairment, when present, further contributes to the often confusing presentation of infections in older adults. Many cognitively impaired older adults are unable to communicate symptoms accurately, and clinicians must be ready to pursue objective assessments such as laboratory and radiologic evaluations at a lower threshold, unless advance directives indicate otherwise. Because of the challenges involved with diagnoses of infections in long-term care residents, surveillance definitions have been developed to assist with clinical decision making (Table 63.3).

Antimicrobial Management

Drug distribution, metabolism, excretion, and interactions can be altered with age. Aging in the absence of any comorbid disease is associated with decreased renal function, and antibiotic dosages may need to be reduced in older adults. Furthermore, antibiotics interact with many other medications commonly prescribed for older adults. Digoxin, warfarin, oral hypoglycemic agents, theophylline, antacids, lipid-lowering agents, antihypertensive medications, and H_2-receptor antagonists all have significant interactions with commonly prescribed antimicrobials. Drug concentrations can increase (eg, enhanced digoxin toxicity associated with use of macrolides, tetracyclines, and trimethoprim) or decrease (eg, reduced absorption of some fluoroquinolones with antacids) with concomitant medication administration. Atrophic gastritis, a common problem in older adults, and H_2-blockers or proton-pump inhibitors can reduce the absorption of some antimicrobials, such as ketoconazole or itraconazole. Furthermore, chronic use of proton-pump inhibitors, often prescribed in older adults, has been associated with an increased risk of CAP (SOE=C). Finally, adherence to prescribed regimens may be limited as a consequence of poor cognitive function, impaired hearing or vision, co-prescription of multiple medications, and financial constraints.

The choice and timing of antibiotics is important to minimize morbidity and mortality associated with infection in older adults. In sepsis, pneumonia, and other severe infections, an increasing body of evidence suggests that broad coverage is warranted initially because outcomes (ie, mortality, length of stay in intensive care) are improved when the offending organism is covered by the initial antibiotic regimen. In older adults with pneumonia, data suggest that delaying the start of therapy for ≥4 hours after admission to the hospital is associated with an increased risk of mortality (SOE=B). "De-escalation," a narrowing of antibiotic choice to specific therapy if the offending organism is identified by culture or other diagnostic studies, is essential for antibiotic stewardship and should be done whenever possible. Unfortunately, diagnostic studies (eg, obtaining sputum) are often difficult in older adults or are unavailable in long-term care settings. These factors and the atypical presentation of infection noted above often lead to early initiation of antimicrobials in older adults, particularly in long-term care. However, this practice results in inappropriate use of antibiotics in up to 75% of cases in this setting. The use of strict, minimal criteria (as in Table 63.3) for initiation of antimicrobials in long-term care is likely to reduce inappropriate antibiotic use without jeopardizing patient safety (SOE=C). However, although prompt initiation of antibiotics is important, discontinuing antibiotics when no longer indicated is an equally important practice for health care providers.

Table 63.3—Surveillance Definitions of Infections in Long-Term Care Facilities

Condition	Minimal Criteria
Urinary tract infection, without catheter	Positive urine culture plus at least 1 of the following: ■ Acute dysuria or acute pain, swelling, or tenderness of the testes, epididymis, or prostate ■ Fever or leukocytosis plus 1 of the following: acute costovertebral angle pain or tenderness, suprapubic pain, gross hematuria, new or marked increase in incontinence, frequency, or urgency ■ In the absence of fever or leukocytosis, then 2 of the following symptoms: acute costovertebral angle pain or tenderness, suprapubic pain, gross hematuria, new or marked increase in incontinence, frequency, or urgency
Urinary tract infection, with catheter	Positive urine culture plus at least 1 of the following: ■ Fever, rigors, or hypotension ■ Change in mental status or functional decline ■ New-onset suprapubic pain or costovertebral angle pain or tenderness ■ Purulent discharge from catheter site or acute pain swelling or tenderness of testes, epididymis, or prostate
Skin and soft-tissue infection	At least 1 of the following must be present: ■ Pus present at a wound, skin, or soft-tissue site ■ New or increasing presence of at least 4 of the following: heat, redness, swelling, tenderness or pain, serous drainage or 1 constitutional criteria such as fever, leukocytosis, acute change in mental or functional status from baseline
Pneumonia	All 3 criteria must be present: ■ Interpretation of a chest radiograph showing new infiltrate ■ At least 1 of the following: new or increased cough, sputum production, O_2 saturation <94% on room air or reduction in O_2 saturation of >3% from baseline, new or changed lung examination, pleuritic chest pain, respiratory rate ≥25 breaths/min ■ At least 1 of the following: fever, leukocytosis, acute change in mental status or function status from baseline

SOURCE: Data from Stone ND, Muhammad S, Ashraf, et al. Surveillance definitions of infections in long-term care facilities: revisiting the McGeer Criteria. *Infect Control Hosp Epidemiol.* 2012;33(10):965–977.

IMMUNIZATIONS

Immunizations are particularly important for prevention of infection in adults ≥65 years old, because this population is at increased risk of severe complications from vaccine-preventable illnesses, particularly influenza and pneumococcal disease. Immunization rates for both influenza and pneumococcus in adults ≥65 years old have improved over the past several years, largely due to increased vaccine awareness and national campaigns aimed to improve vaccination rates, such as Healthy People 2020. In 2014, 72% of older adults reported being vaccinated for influenza and 61% of older adults for pneumococcus. Estimated rates of vaccination for herpes zoster (shingles) in older adults ≥60 year old are still low at 27.9%, 2.1 percentage points below the Healthy People 2020 target of 30%.

Influenza Vaccine

In 2009, the FDA approved a high-dose seasonal influenza vaccine for use in adults ≥65 years old, based on data suggesting improved immune response (ie, antibody production) with the high-dose vaccination, which contains 4 times the dose of the same antigens used in the standard-dose vaccine. In a study evaluating the efficacy of the high-dose influenza vaccine for prevention of laboratory-confirmed influenza, the high-dose vaccine provided enhanced protection compared with the standard-dose. In this randomized, controlled trial, adults without moderate or severe illness, ≥65 years old, were assigned to receive either high-dose or standard-dose influenza vaccine. The percentage of adults with laboratory-confirmed influenza who received the high-dose vaccine was 1.4% compared with 1.9% in the standard-dose group (relative efficacy, 24.2%; 95% CI, 9.7–36.5) (SOE=A). The Advisory Committee on Immunization Practices (ACIP) for the CDC has not expressed a preference for which flu vaccine is preferred for people ≥65 years old. However, it is reasonable to offer high-dose influenza vaccine over standard-dose influenza vaccine when available, particularly in the long-term care setting. For current immunization recommendations for older adults, see Table 63.4.

Pneumococcal Vaccine

The incidence of invasive pneumococcal disease and pneumococcal pneumonia continues to be higher in older adults than in younger ones, especially in those

Table 63.4—Immunization Schedule for Adults ≥65 Years Old[a]

Vaccine	Dose Recommendation
Influenza	1 dose annually of standard or high-dose inactivated influenza vaccine
Tetanus, diphtheria, pertussis (Td/Tdap)	Administer Tdap then boost with Td every 10 years
Varicella	2 doses unless immune or previous receipt of 2-vaccine series
Zoster	2 doses 2–6 months apart) of the inactivated subunit vaccine in immunocompetent adults ≥50 years old is preferred over the attenuated zoster vaccine [b] *Alternative:* 1 dose of the attenuated vaccine in adults ≥60 years old.[c]
Pneumococcal (conjugate) (PCV13)	1 dose in adults ≥ 65years old before receiving PPSV23[d] or in those ≥19 years old with certain comorbid conditions[e]
Pneumococcal (polysaccharide) (PPSV23)	1 dose in adults ≥65 years old or 5 years after previous dose if given before age 65
Meningococcal	1 or more doses based on risk factors[f]
Hepatitis A	2 doses based on risk factors[g]
Hepatitis B	3 doses based on risk factors[h]
Haemophilus influenzae type b	1 or 3 doses based on risk factors[i]

[a] Based on recommendations from the CDC Advisory Committee on Immunization Practices 2018. For CDC immunization recommendations, see www.cdc.gov/vaccines/schedules/hcp/imz/adult.html.
[b] Adults who have already received the attenuated herpes zoster vaccine should also receive the inactivated subunit herpes zoster vaccine at least 2 months after receiving the attenuated vaccine. Excludes patients with severe acquired or primary immunodeficiency.
[c] Excludes patients with severe acquired or primary immunodeficiency.
[d] PCV13 should be given before PPSV23 in vaccine-naive adults ≥65 years old, or at least 1 year after adults ≥ 65 years old who have previously received PPSV23.
[e] Only in older adults with chronic renal failure, asplenia, CSF leaks, or cochlear implants.
[f] Risk factors include functional asplenia, persistent complement component deficiencies, travelers to endemic countries.
[g] Risk factors include men who have sex with men, persons who use illicit drugs, persons with chronic liver disease or who receive clotting factor concentrates, travelers.
[h] Risk factors include sexually active persons not in a monogamous relationship, injection drug users, men who have sex with men, those being evaluated for a sexually transmitted infection, diabetic patients, those potentially exposed to blood or body fluids (eg, health care workers), persons with end-stage renal disease (including those on hemodialysis), HIV infection, persons with chronic liver disease, household contacts and sex partners of hepatitis B–positive persons, travelers, all adults in institutions and nonresidential daycare facilities, or persons with developmental disabilities.
[i] One dose should be administered to older adults who have functional or anatomic asplenia, sickle cell disease, or are undergoing elective splenectomy and have not previously received *Haemophilus influenzae* type b vaccination. Vaccination should occur 14 days before splenectomy. Patients receiving hematopoietic stem cell transplant should be vaccinated with 3 doses 6–12 months after transplant in 4-week intervals.

with chronic medical comorbidities. Currently, ACIP continues to recommend vaccination with 23-valent pneumococcal polysaccharide vaccine (PPSV23) in all adults ≥65 years old. Adults who received PPSV23 before age 65 should receive another dose of the vaccine at age 65 or older if at least 5 years have passed since their previous dose (Table 63.4).

Although most professional societies continue to endorse vaccination of older adults with PPSV23 per ACIP guidelines, studies evaluating efficacy of the vaccine, especially in preventing pneumococcal pneumonia in older adults, have demonstrated conflicting results. A meta-analysis published in 2013 sought to evaluate the efficacy of PPSV23 in prevention of invasive pneumococcal disease and pneumococcal pneumonia. The authors found that PPSV23 did reduce the risk of invasive pneumococcal disease (OR 0.26, 95% CI, 0.14–0.45) in the general population, including the subgroup of healthy individuals in high-income countries, which included many older adults (OR 0.20, 95% CI, 0.10–0.39). They did not, however, find a reduction in all-cause pneumonia or all-cause mortality in this subgroup.

Given the lack of known efficacy for PPSV23 in preventing pneumococcal pneumonia, the pneumococcal conjugate vaccine (PCV13), previously indicated only in younger children, was approved by the FDA in 2011 for use in adults ≥50 years old, after a few studies demonstrated increased antibody production after vaccination. In addition, a randomized placebo-controlled trial of approximately 85,000 adults ≥65 years old demonstrated efficacy of the PCV13 vaccine against vaccine-type pneumococcal pneumonia, vaccine-type non-bacteremic pneumonia, and vaccine-type invasive pneumococcal disease in this population. These results, along with immunogenicity studies demonstrating immune responses as good as or better than those seen with PPSV23, prompted ACIP to recommend vaccination with PCV13 for all adults ≥65 years old. Adults ≥65 years old who have not previously received pneumococcal vaccine should receive PCV13 followed by a dose of PPSV23 approximately 12 months later. Adults previously vaccinated with PPSV23 should receive a dose of PCV13 at least 1 year after immunization with PPSV23 (Table 63.4). Immunization of children with PCV13 has reduced the incidence of pneumococcal pneumonia, with serotypes present in this vaccine, even in older adults. Therefore, by adhering to vaccination guidelines for children in close contact with older adults, there may be herd immunity from which older adults can benefit as well.

Varicella-Zoster Virus Vaccine

Two varicella-zoster vaccines are approved for use in older adults, the inactived subunit zoster vaccine and the attenuated zoster vaccine. The inactivated subunit vaccine is now preferred by the CDC over the attenuated vaccine because of higher efficacy (90% effective versus 50%) and longer-lasting immunity.

Inactivated Subunit Zoster Vaccine

The inactivated subunit zoster vaccine, which contains recombinant varicella-zoster virus glycoprotein E in combination with an adjuvant (ASO1B), significantly reduced the risks of herpes zoster and post-herpetic neuralgia in adults ≥70 years old who were followed for a mean of 3.7 years. In this study, 23 participants who received the new vaccine developed herpes zoster compared with 223 of those receiving placebo, resulting in a vaccine efficacy of 89.9% (95% CI, 84.2–93.7). The vaccine efficacy for prevention of post-herpetic neuralgia was 88.8% (CI, 68.7–97.1) (SOE=A). Older adults with a prior history of herpes zoster were excluded in this trial. The CDC now recommends the inactivated subunit zoster vaccine for the prevention of herpes zoster and related complications for the following groups:

- Immunocompetent adults ≥50 years old
- Immunocompetent adults who previously received the attenuated zoster vaccine
- Adults who are taking low-dose immunosuppressive therapy, anticipating immunosuppression, or who have recovered from an immunocompromising illness

There are no recommendations for use of the inactivated subunit zoster vaccine in immunocompromised (eg, autoimmune or transplant recipients) older adults. The inactivated subunit zoster vaccine requires 2 intramuscular injections 2 months apart, potentially impacting adherence. The most common adverse effect reported after administration is injection-site pain (78%), with 9.4% reporting a Grade 3 injection-site reaction (pain, redness, and swelling). Other common adverse effects included myalgia (45%) and fatigue (45%). Systemic symptoms that prevented normal daily activities (Grade 3) were reported in 10.8% of those who received the vaccine and in 2.4% of those who received placebo.

Attenuated Varicella-Zoster Vaccine

The attenuated varicella-zoster vaccine, approved for adults ≥60 years old, reduced the incidence of herpes zoster by 51.3% (95% CI, 47.5–79.2) in a large, placebo-controlled clinical trial of almost 40,000 adults ≥60 years old. In addition, the vaccine decreased the duration of pain and discomfort in patients who developed zoster and decreased the incidence of post-herpetic neuralgia (SOE=A). Older adults with cognitive impairment, significant functional impairment, and <5 years of remaining life expectancy were excluded from the study. In 2012, a follow-up study conducted to assess ongoing efficacy of the vaccine in older adults found that the incidence of herpes zoster continued to decrease by 39.6% (95% CI, 18.2–55.5) through year 5 after vaccination. In a systematic review and meta-analysis published in 2016, the vaccine was effective in preventing cases of herpes zoster, although protection beyond 3 years was uncertain.

The attenuated herpes zoster vaccine has been shown to be safe and well tolerated in adults with a prior history of herpes zoster. Contraindications for vaccination include a history of severe allergic reaction to gelatin or the antibiotic neomycin, severe primary or acquired immunodeficiencies, solid organ transplantation, a CD4 cell count <200 cells/µL in HIV-infected patients, and current chemotherapy or high-dose corticosteroid therapy (defined as ≥2 weeks of daily prednisone [or equivalent] at 20 mg or 2 mg/kg). Patients receiving low-dose immunosuppression (defined as methotrexate ≤0.4 mg/kg/week, azathioprine ≤3 mg/kg/day, 6-mercaptopurine ≤1.5 mg/kg/day, or prednisone <2 mg/kg [maximum ≤20 mg/day] or other steroid equivalent) or HIV-infected older adults with a CD4 count >200 cells/µL with virologic suppression on antiretroviral therapy may still be eligible for vaccination. Primary Care Guidelines for Management of Persons Infected with HIV, published in 2013 by the Infectious Diseases Society of America (IDSA), recommend clinicians consider zoster vaccination in HIV-infected adults >60 years old with CD4 counts ≥200 cells/µL (SOE=C). Studies evaluating safety and efficacy of the vaccine in HIV-infected older adults are still ongoing.

Although recommended by the CDC and multiple professional societies, vaccination rates for herpes zoster remain particularly low compared with rates for other vaccinations (eg, influenza). Few studies have examined barriers to herpes zoster vaccination, with the most frequent barrier reported to be financial. In one study, only 45% of general internists and family medicine physicians who responded to the survey were aware that herpes zoster vaccine was covered through Medicare Part D. Additionally, primary care providers reported that they often face challenges with billing and reimbursement for the vaccine and that patients often have out-of-pocket costs. Efforts to decrease costs associated with administering the herpes zoster vaccine could increase adherence to the recommendation. The herpes zoster vaccine is now free to patients under the Affordable Care Act if given during a preventive care visit.

Tetanus, Diphtheria, Acellular Pertussis Vaccine

ACIP recommends the use of tetanus, diphtheria, acellular pertussis (Tdap) vaccine in older adults to protect children from pertussis infection (Table 63.4).

INFECTIOUS SYNDROMES

Bacteremia and Sepsis

Bacteremia is a common cause of hospitalization in older adults. Older adults with bacteremia are less likely than their younger counterparts to have chills or sweats, and fever is often absent. Gastrointestinal and genitourinary sources of bacteremia are more common; thus, the causative bacteria are more likely to be gram-negative rods or enterococci in older adults than in younger ones.

Bacteremia carries a particularly poor prognosis in older adults. For example, nosocomial gram-negative bacteremia carries a mortality rate of 5%–35% in young adults, but 37%–50% in older adults. Major contributing factors include coexisting diseases that reduce physiologic reserve and the more common use of invasive devices (eg, intravenous or urinary catheters) that make eradication of organisms difficult.

The management of bacteremia and sepsis in older and younger patients is similar. Rapid administration of appropriate antibiotics aimed at the most likely sources is essential, and early "goal-directed" therapy for volume resuscitation has proven benefit in populations of all ages with sepsis (SOE=B).

Pneumonia

Patients aged ≥65 years old account for >50% of all pneumonia cases, and annual hospitalization rates for pneumonia range from 12 per 1,000 among community-dwelling adults ≥75 years old to 32 per 1,000 among long-term care residents. In fact, the cumulative 2-year risk of pneumonia for long-term care residents is approximately 30%. Mortality caused by pneumonia in older adults is 3–5 times that in young adults, but the rate is profoundly influenced by comorbidity. Comorbidity, defined in one study as cancer, collagen vascular disease, or advanced liver disease, was the strongest independent predictor of mortality in CAP in older adults, with a relative risk (RR) of 4.1. Other independent risk factors for pneumonia-related mortality include age ≥85 years old; debility (decreased physical function); serum creatinine >1.5 mg/dL; and the presence of hypothermia (<36.1°F), hypotension (<90 mmHg systolic), or tachycardia (>110 beats per minute) on admission (SOE=A). Long-term follow-up data also suggest that CAP in older adults portends a higher risk of subsequent all-cause mortality over the next 12 years, as a consequence of both recurrent pneumonia (RR 2.1; 95% CI, 1.3–3.4]) and cardiovascular disease (RR 1.4; 96% CI, 1.0–1.9]) (SOE=A).

The causes of pneumonia in younger and older adults tend to differ. In older patients, *Streptococcus pneumoniae* is still the predominant organism, but gram-negative bacilli (eg, *Haemophilus influenzae*, *Moraxella catarrhalis*, *Klebsiella* spp) are much more common than in younger adults, particularly in patients with COPD or who reside in long-term care facilities. *S aureus* and respiratory viruses are also common causes of pneumonia in long-term care residents. Obtaining a microbiologic diagnosis is often difficult in older adults who rarely produce sputum. Blood cultures should be obtained before antimicrobial therapy but are positive in only 10%–15% of patients. Urinary antigen testing for *S pneumoniae* (sensitivity 70%–80%; specificity 77%–97%) or *Legionella pneumophila* (sensitivity 70%–80%; specificity 77%–97%) can be useful diagnostic tests to perform in older adults who are unable to produce sputum. Importantly, the sensitivity of these tests is not affected for up to 24 hours after initiation of antimicrobial therapy. The test for legionellosis detects only serogroup 1, which causes 80% of all *Legionella* infection. The measurement of biomarkers such as procalcitonin has been used to help distinguish between bacterial and viral pneumonia. In patients suspected of having pneumonia, a procalcitonin level <0.1 mcg/L is less suggestive of bacterial etiology, whereas a value of >0.25 mcg/L is more suggestive. However, there are several other reasons for an increased procalcitonin level (malignancy, surgery, trauma), so procalcitonin measurement should only be used as an adjunct test to clinical examination.

Guidelines for pneumonia therapy have evolved to account for emergence of resistant bacteria, particularly drug-resistant *S pneumoniae*, and for the recognition of comorbidities, health care setting versus community-acquired illness, and specific pathogens of interest in certain contexts (eg, *S aureus* after viral influenza infection). Because of their ease of administration and broad activity versus respiratory pathogens, respiratory fluoroquinolones are used often in older adults, and they are one of the first-line therapies suggested by various guidelines. Guidelines of the Infectious Diseases Society of America for treatment of CAP suggest the following as first-line therapy in adults ≥60 years old with or without comorbidity: a β-lactam/β-lactamase combination or advanced-generation cephalosporin (eg, ceftriaxone or cefotaxime) with or without a macrolide. Alternatively, one of the fluoroquinolones with enhanced activity against *S pneumoniae* (eg, levofloxacin, moxifloxacin) may be used. However, several notes of caution are needed regarding fluoroquinolone use in older adults: first, fluoroquinolones kill bacteria better at higher concentrations, and outcomes are better in older adults when high drug concentrations are present (SOE=B). Thus, full-dosage therapy, taking into account renal function, should be provided (ie, the adage of "start low, go slow" often invoked for drug therapy in older adults is *not* appropriate for this class of drugs). Second, if tuberculosis is a realistic possibility, fluoroquinolones should be avoided. Use of fluoroquinolones to treat CAP can lead to delayed diagnosis of tuberculosis (by an average of >40 days) and to fluoroquinolone resistance in the organism. Finally, significant adverse events, including dizziness, cardiac conduction abnormalities (QT prolongation), and risk of Achilles tendon rupture may limit the use of fluoroquinolones in certain older adults. However, fluoroquinolone use in older adults without underlying conduction abnormalities or specific contraindications is quite safe (SOE=B).

In the long-term care setting, polymicrobial infection, often due to aspiration and *S aureus*, is more common than in the community setting. Additionally, risk factors associated with pneumonia caused by an MDRO include: 1) previous antibiotic therapy; 2) recent hospitalization; 3) immunosuppression; 4) pulmonary comorbidity; 5) chronic aspiration; and 5) multiple medical comorbidities. These risk factors are more common in long term care residents. Risk factors for MDRO should guide treatment for pneumonia in this population.

Hospital-acquired pneumonia is defined as pneumonia that occurs ≥48 hours after acute hospital admission without evidence of infection on admission. Pneumonia acquired in a hospital in older adults requires broader initial coverage than does CAP because of the broader spectrum of organisms causing infection. Gram-negative bacilli predominate, but *S aureus* is more common as well and is more likely to affect specific antibiotic choices because of resistance. Outcomes data suggest that response to therapy is greater when the initial antibiotic regimen covers the offending agent. Thus, initial regimens should be broadly inclusive, followed by step-down therapy to more narrow coverage if the causative agent is identified. Importantly, if patients are known to be colonized with MRSA, initial regimens should include vancomycin or linezolid until MRSA is excluded as the causative agent. Daptomycin should not be used to treat MRSA pneumonia due to high failure rates, because the drug binds to surfactant and thus is not an effective treatment. Further, data suggest that patients with clinically improving hospital-acquired pneumonia not caused by nonfermenting gram-negative bacilli (eg, *Pseudomonas*, *Stenotrophomonas*) can be treated with shorter courses of antibiotics (7 or 8 days, rather than the 2 weeks commonly used in the past). Shorter courses (8 days versus 15 days) of antibiotics are associated with equivalent efficacy and less antibiotic resistance (SOE=A). See the 2016 IDSA Guidelines for Management of Adults with Hospital-Acquired and Ventilator-Associated Pneumonia (https://bit.ly/2gbAHJH).

Prevention of pneumonia in older adults is a complex issue, and a multipronged approach is most likely to be effective. Immunization of at-risk individuals is by far the most well-studied measure. Annual influenza vaccine and pneumococcal vaccine should be administered to all older adults. In addition to vaccines, smoking cessation and aggressive treatment of comorbidities (eg, minimizing aspiration risk in patients after stroke, limiting use of sedative hypnotics) can reduce the risk of infection. Although few studies have found that interventions targeting risk factors for aspiration prevented pneumonia in older adults, a large clinical trial in nursing-home residents did not find that an intervention using manual tooth/gum brushing, chlorhexidine oral rinse, and upright positioning during feeding reduced the incidence of first radiographically confirmed pneumonia or lower respiratory tract infection compared with usual care (SOE=A). System changes with attention to infection control (isolation, cohorting patients with the same infection, skin testing for tuberculosis with purified-protein derivative or interferon-gamma release assays, and immunization policies for staff and visitors) can be particularly effective in long-term care facilities.

Influenza

Influenza results in approximately 40,000 deaths annually in the United States, nearly all of which are in the older adult population. The clinical syndrome of influenza is easily recognized by most clinicians, particularly in the setting of local disease activity or outbreaks in long-term care facilities. Although some controversy exists with regard to the effectiveness of influenza vaccine in frail older adults, most data suggest the vaccine is 60%–80% efficacious in older adults for preventing severe disease, hospitalization, and death. Therefore, annual immunization is recommended for all adults (SOE=A).

Several medications are available for treatment and prophylaxis of influenza. M2 inhibitors (amantadine and rimantadine) block the M2 ion channel of influenza and are effective only against influenza A; their use is limited by widespread resistance (>90% of the most virulent strains). Further, amantadine is particularly difficult to use in older adults because of the extensive dosage adjustments required for small changes in kidney function, and frequent adverse events, particularly CNS symptoms. In contrast, neuraminidase inhibitors (zanamivir and oseltamivir) are effective against both influenza A and B; they inhibit the virus by interfering with an essential enzyme, neuraminidase, that cleaves sialic acid to expose host cell receptors for the virus. Oseltamivir, a capsule, is preferred over zanamivir in older adults because zanamivir must be inhaled, and it is difficult for many older adults to properly use the product. Treatment of influenza is effective if started in the first 48 hours, but it is most effective if started within 24 hours of symptom onset (SOE=A). Oseltamivir and zanamivir can also be used for prevention in outbreak situations (eg, in long-term care) when combined with appropriate vaccination strategies (SOE=A). Oseltamivir can cause GI symptoms (eg, nausea, vomiting, and diarrhea) in up to 10%–20% of patients. Adverse effects generally resolve after a few days, and taking the drug with food may help improve tolerance.

Patients with underlying heart disease who contract influenza are at increased risk of developing cardiac complications. One study found that of adults aged ≥ 75 admitted to the hospital with influenza, >60% were found to have a history of underlying cardiac problems. Another study found that underlying cardiac disease was associated with a 2.7-fold increased risk of influenza-related hospitalization. One proposed explanation for this finding is that influenza infection generates an increased release of inflammatory cytokines, leading to destabilization of atherosclerotic plaques, causing occlusion of coronary arteries, resulting in myocardial infarction. A few studies have suggested that influenza vaccination effectively reduces the incidence of cardiovascular-related deaths, although others studies have produced conflicting results. Nevertheless, the potential benefit of vaccination in older adults with established cardiovascular disease is another reason clinicians should strongly recommend the influenza vaccine to their older adult patients.

Urinary Tract Infection

Urinary tract infection (UTI) is among the most common of clinical illnesses in older adults, with an incidence of 10.9 per 100-person years in men and 14 per 100 person-years in women ≥65 years old. Gram-negative bacilli (eg, *Escherichia coli*, *Enterobacter* spp, *Klebsiella* spp, *Proteus* spp) are most common, but there is an increase in more resistant isolates, such as *Pseudomonas aeruginosa*, and in gram-positive organisms, including enterococci, coagulase-negative staphylococci (ie, *Staphylococcus saprophyticus*), and *Streptococcus agalactiae* (group B strep). In patients with indwelling catheters, the microbes listed still predominate, but it is also common to encounter additional organisms, including enterococci, *S aureus*, and fungi, particularly *Candida* spp. The organisms colonizing urinary catheters commonly develop biofilms, and infections are difficult to resolve with the same urinary catheter in place.

Asymptomatic Bacteriuria

Asymptomatic bacteriuria (ASB) in women is defined as the presence of two consecutive urine specimens positive for the same bacterial strain in quantities of ≥105 colony-forming units/milliliter (CFU/mL), in the absence of genitourinary symptoms. Up to 20% of women in the community and 50% of women in nursing homes have ASB. In men, ASB is defined as one voided urine specimen with ≥10^5 CFU/mL in the absence of symptoms. The incidence in men is approximately half that in women. Rates of ASB are even higher with the use of condom catheters (87%) or Foley catheters (nearly 100%). Numerous studies have suggested that there is no clinical benefit from the treatment of ASB, and that treatment is associated with significant adverse events, expense, and potential for selection of resistant organisms. Thus, routine screening and treatment of ASB are not recommended in older adults (SOE=A). Urine studies (eg, urinalysis and/or urine culture) should not routinely be obtained in patients with vague symptoms (eg, fatigue, lethargy) who do not have urinary tract specific symptoms (eg, dysuria) because of the high prevalence of ASB in this population. A positive culture in this clinical scenario is unreliable and often leads to inappropriate antibiotic prescriptions.

Urinary Tract Infection in Community-Dwelling Older Women

In contrast to ASB, symptomatic UTI requires therapy. Diagnosis of UTI in cognitively intact older adults is similar to that in younger adults and is made based on a combination of genitourinary symptoms (eg, new or worsening urgency, frequency, suprapubic pain, gross hematuria) along with evidence of a urine culture growing no more than 2 urinary pathogen in quantities ≥10^5 CFU/mL.

Therapy is based on the location of infection (upper versus lower tract disease) and the likely causative agent. Lower-tract UTI (ie, cystitis) is often treated in young women for 1–3 days, and 3–7 days of therapy is probably sufficient for uncomplicated cystitis in older women (SOE=B). If clinical suspicion for cystitis is high, empiric antibiotic therapy can be started after obtaining a urine culture. However, if the diagnosis is uncertain and the patient is clinically stable, waiting for urine study results to confirm the presence of genitourinary inflammation (eg, pyuria) and the presence of a uropathogen can help minimize unnecessary and/or ineffective antibiotic use. Upper UTI (ie, pyelonephritis), characterized by fever, chills, nausea, and flank pain, is commonly accompanied by lower-tract symptoms and requires a longer period of therapy (7–21 days). According to the International Clinical Practice Guidelines by the Infectious Diseases Society of America and the European Society for Microbiology, first-line therapy for treatment of uncomplicated UTI includes nitrofurantoin 100 mg twice daily for 5 days, or trimethoprim-sulfamethoxazole (TMP-SMX) 160/800 mg twice daily for 3 days, if local resistance rates do not exceed 20%. Nitrofurantoin is contraindicated by the FDA for use in patients with chronic kidney disease (creatinine clearance <60 mL/min), but it has been shown to be safe to administer in patients with creatinine clearance ≥30 mL/min and can be considered for treatment of cystitis in older adults. TMP-SMX is the preferred empiric treatment for UTI in older adults, but caution is warranted in those concurrently receiving warfarin because SMX delays warfarin metabolism or in those with renal disease because of hyperkalemia. Fluoroquinolones, although highly effective for sensitive organisms, are not recommended empirically because of high resistance rates (SOE=C).

Intravenous administration of antibiotics remains the standard of care for patients with suspected urosepsis, those with upper-tract disease due to relatively resistant bacteria such as enterococci, or those unable to tolerate oral medications. Culture and sensitivity data are more useful in guiding antimicrobial therapy in upper-tract UTIs than in lower-tract disease and should be obtained in most cases (SOE=A).

Urinary Tract Infection in Community-Dwelling Older Men

Prostatic disease (primarily hyperplasia) or functional disorders, such as autonomic neuropathy from diabetes mellitus with incomplete bladder emptying, account for most lower and upper UTIs in older men. Therapy should last at least 7–14 days, and if prostatic involvement is suspected (ie, acute or chronic prostatitis), at least 6 weeks (SOE=B). The causative organisms and treatment choices are similar to those outlined above for older women. Fluoroquinolones and TMP-SMX are most widely used when prostatic involvement is suspected and culture data confirm the organism's susceptibility because of the available agents, these two penetrate the prostate best. Because treatment for all UTIs in men is generally longer than in women and the prostate is a common reservoir of organisms responsible for recurrent UTIs, culture and sensitivity data should guide therapy for virtually all UTIs in men (SOE=C).

Urinary Tract Infection in Long-Term Care Residents

Distinguishing symptomatic UTI from ASB in long-term care residents is challenging, because many long-term care residents suffer from cognitive impairment, which limits their ability to effectively communicate genitourinary symptoms. Antibiotics are often inappropriately prescribed for treatment of UTI when residents develop nonspecific symptoms such as changes in functional status. Overuse of antibiotics in this situation has led to the development of multidrug resistant organisms. Several professional societies have developed guidelines to assist clinicians with the diagnosis and treatment of UTI in this population. In 2012, the Society for Healthcare Epidemiology of America updated the current guidelines for diagnosis of UTI to include a combination of genitourinary signs and symptoms, fever or leukocytosis, and a positive urinary culture, although these were primarily developed for surveillance purposes (SOE=C) (Table 63.3). In patients who are cognitively impaired, it is important to carefully assess for new or worsening symptoms such as urinary incontinence and for physical signs such as suprapubic tenderness, as well as to consider other diagnoses that may be responsible for nonspecific symptoms (eg, medications, dehydration, constipation). However, if nonspecific symptoms (eg, mental status changes) persist despite other interventions (hydration, treatment of constipation), obtaining urine studies to evaluate for UTI is reasonable.

Catheter-Associated Urinary Tract Infection

Catheter-associated urinary tract infection (CA-UTI) is the most common health care–associated infection and one of the most common reasons for antimicrobial prescriptions. Adults with indwelling urinary catheters are at high risk of nosocomial infections and are often colonized with MDROs. Several recent studies have highlighted methods aimed to prevent CA-UTI and unnecessary antibiotic use commonly associated with catheter-associated ASB. In a large study in nursing homes, researchers were able to show that a combination of technical interventions (eg, professional development in urinary catheter utilization, catheter care and maintenance, and antimicrobial stewardship) and socioadaptive interventions (eg, empowering facility teams; addressing implementation changes; offering solutions to overcome barriers; and prompting resident and family engagement, resident safety culture, and team building) successfully reduced CA-UTI in settings where utilization was low, but catheter use was prolonged. Another study using a behavioral intervention, "Kicking CAUTI: The No Knee-Jerk Antibiotics Campaign," aimed to reduce urine culture ordering and antimicrobial prescriptions for catheter-associated ASB. This intervention successfully reduced the overall rate of urine culture ordering by 71% and overtreatment of ASB by more than 75% during the study period. The behavioral intervention was designed to impact clinicians' adherence to guidelines by addressing provider knowledge and attitudes.

Prophylaxis for UTI

Prophylactic antibiotics intended to prevent recurrent UTIs in older women are not preferred because of the risk of development of highly resistant organisms; however, if other preventive strategies are ineffective, this treatment modality can be effective. Few small studies have shown benefit of intravaginal estrogen replacement to reduce the recurrence of UTI in postmenopausal women. In 1994, cranberry juice (10 oz) was shown to be efficacious in older adults living in assisted-living facilities and nursing homes and has been used for prevention of bacteriuria and pyuria for several decades, but it is not always well tolerated. Hence, cranberry capsules have been investigated as an alternative intervention strategy. Pilot data on use of cranberry capsules, which contain at least 36 mg of proanthocyanidin, the active ingredient thought to prevent adherence of *E coli* to uroepithelial cells, showed reduction of bacteriuria and pyuria in nursing-home residents. However, in 2016, authors of a randomized clinical trial of older women living in nursing homes did not find evidence that cranberry capsules containing 72 mg of proanthocyanidin compared with placebo significantly reduced the presence of bacteriuria plus pyuria in this population (SOE=A). Hence, cranberry capsules are not recommended for UTI prevention in older adults in nursing homes.

Tuberculosis

Worldwide, approximately 1.7 billion people are infected with *Mycobacterium tuberculosis*; 16 million are in the United States. Adults ≥65 years old account for one-fourth of all active tuberculosis (TB) cases in the United States, most in community-dwelling older adults. However, the rate of infection with TB in long-term care residents is much higher than in community-dwelling adults. Tuberculin skin-test (TST) studies show prevalence rates of skin-test reactivity in the range of 30%–50%. This high prevalence reflects exposure to *M tuberculosis* in the early 1900s, when it was estimated that 80% of all individuals were infected by age 30. Most active cases of TB in older adults are, therefore, due to reactivated disease, but primary infection may account for 10%–20% of cases and is of particular concern in outbreaks in long-term care facilities.

A decline in T-cell mediated immune response in older adults increases the risk that latent TB will become active. Other factors that contribute to the reactivation of TB include chronic comorbid illness (eg, COPD, chronic renal failure, malnutrition) and increased exposure to the health care system, particularly chronic institutionalization.

As with most other infections, TB may not present in the classical fashion (ie, cough, sputum, hemoptysis, fever, night sweats) in older adults. Often, fatigue, anorexia, decreased functional status (eg, changes in activities of daily living, cognitive decline), or low-grade fever are presenting manifestations. Thus, the TB is often mistaken for other more common age-related conditions such as malignancy or failure to thrive. Most tuberculous disease in older adults occurs with lung involvement (75%). Disease that occurs in a subacute manner should particularly raise a high index of suspicion for *M tuberculosis* infection. Older adults are more likely than younger ones to have extrapulmonary disease. Other sites include miliary (disseminated) disease, tuberculous meningitis or osteomyelitis, and urogenital disease, but virtually any body structure or organ system can be involved and can account for the major presenting symptom.

A diagnosis of active disease usually requires isolation of the organism from sputum, urine, or other clinical specimen. Current techniques have improved the speed of diagnosis, particularly for identifying the species of *Mycobacterium* after isolation. This is now typically accomplished within 24 hours of obtaining a positive culture by use of DNA probes. Direct polymerase chain reaction of clinical specimens or other rapid diagnostic techniques are not available or reliable in most local laboratories, but such tests can be available in research settings. They are most likely to be helpful for establishing a diagnosis from cerebrospinal or pleural fluid, which yields positive cultures in only 10%–15% of cases.

A potentially confusing area of TB diagnostics is interpretation of the results of the tuberculin skin test (TST) using 0.1 mL of purified-protein derivative (PPD). For interpretation of TST results, see Table 63.5. Anergy panel testing in conjunction with PPD testing is of little value and is not recommended (SOE=C).

More recently, the use of interferon gamma release assays (IGRAs) have been developed to detect latent TB in most populations. The benefit of using IGRAs instead of TSTs is the ability to have results within 24 hours, without the need for a follow-up visit 2 days later. Thus, IGRAs may be an attractive alternative for older outpatient adults, who often have functional limitations and/or difficulty with transportation. Currently, the CDC recommends use of either the TST or IGRA in most clinical situations. If TST/IGRA is positive, a chest radiograph and clinical evaluation should be performed as soon as possible to evaluate for active TB.

Table 63.5—Interpretation of Results from the Tuberculin Skin Test (TST)

Induration Measurement 48–72 hours After Placement	Population
≥15 mm	Positive result in all populations
≥10 mm	Positive result in ■ Long-term care residents* ■ Employees working in high-risk settings (eg, nursing homes, prisons) ■ Recent converters (eg, previous PPD <5mm) ■ Immigrants from countries with high TB rates ■ Underserved U.S. populations (eg, homeless, IVDU) ■ People with high risk comorbidities (chronic kidney disease, diabetes mellitus, >10% below ideal body weight, malignancy)
≥5 mm	Positive result in ■ HIV-infected persons ■ Recent contact with a person with TB ■ Evidence of fibrotic changes on chest radiograph consistent with prior TB ■ Organ transplant recipients ■ Persons who are immunosuppressed (eg, taking prednisone or TNF-α antagonists)

Source: Centers for Disease Control and Prevention. (www.cdc.gov/tb/publications/factsheets/testing/skintesting.htm)
*Only a single TST is needed in long-term care residents who have had a negative TST done within the previous 12 months. If there is no report of a prior TST, a two-step procedure for PPD testing should be performed during the initial evaluation of residents. Two-step testing requires retesting of patients with <10 mm induration within 2 weeks. If the second skin test results in ≥10 mm of induration or the increase in the size of the induration from the first to the second skin test is ≥6 mm, the patient is considered PPD positive.

The treatment of active TB in older adults is similar to that in younger adults and should always be primarily managed by an infectious disease and/or pulmonary specialist. Active TB is a reportable disease and clinicians should contact their local health department for specific reporting requirements. Four-drug therapy (usually isoniazid [INH], rifampin, pyrazinamide, and ethambutol or streptomycin) is recommended as initial therapy for approxiamately 8 weeks, with tapering to one of several two- or three-drug regimens once susceptibility testing is available for the remainder of treatment. The most common regimen is INH, rifampin, and pyrazinamide for 2 months, followed by INH and rifampin for an additional 4 months. However, adjustments in routine drug treatment protocols are often needed because of comorbidities and drug tolerance in older patients.

Prophylaxis with 9 months of INH for asymptomatic individuals with a positive PPD or IGRA should be provided regardless of age in adults who are recent converters (defined in adults >35 years old as those having a PPD that has gone from <10 mm to ≥15 mm within 2 years), or regardless of duration of PPD positivity if an individual has any of the specific risk factors highlighted above. Patients with a positive PPD or IGRA of unknown duration should receive INH prophylaxis, even those >35 years old (as opposed to recommendations in the 1990s). Older adults should be monitored closely for symptoms and signs of peripheral neuropathy (due to INH and preventable by coadministration of pyridoxine) and hepatitis (due to treatment with INH, rifampin, or pyrazinamide). Shorter-course therapy with 2 months of rifampin and pyrazinamide is effective but has a much higher incidence of hepatotoxicity than INH treatment and thus should be used only in very specific circumstances (SOE=B).

Infective Endocarditis

Since the early part of the 20th century, infective endocarditis has undergone a transformation from a disease of young adults primarily due to rheumatic or congenital valve anomalies to one of older adults associated with degenerative valvular disorders and prosthetic valves. Viridans streptococci and *S aureus* typically cause native-valve endocarditis, and occasional infections are due to HACEK organisms (a group of typically nonfermenting gram-negative rods that primarily inhabit the oral cavity and include the genera *Haemophilus*, *Actinobacillus*, *Cardiobacterium*, *Eikenella*, and *Kingella*). Gastrointestinal and genitourinary organisms, such as enterococci and gram-negative rods, are more common in native-valve infective endocarditis in older adults, and coagulase-negative staphylococci are a common cause of prosthetic-valve endocarditis, particularly in the first 60 days after placement of the valve.

The diagnosis of endocarditis is often difficult in older adults. Fever is less common in older adults than in younger ones, occurring in 55% versus 80%, respectively, as is leukocytosis, occurring in 25% versus 60%. Rates of positive blood cultures do not vary by age; however, degenerative, calcific valvular lesions and

Table 63.6—High-Risk Patients Requiring Antimicrobial Prophylaxis for Endocarditis

- Prosthetic cardiac valves (eg, mechanical, bioprosthetic, homograft valves)
- Prosthetic material used for cardiac valve repair
- Prior history of infective endocarditis
- Unrepaired cyanotic congenital heart disease, including palliative shunts and conduits
- Repaired congenital heart defects with prosthetic material or device, whether placed by surgery or by catheter intervention, during the first 6 months after the procedure
- Repaired congenital heart disease with residual shunts or valvular regurgitation at the site of the prosthetic patch or prosthetic device
- Cardiac transplant recipients with cardiac valvulopathy

SOURCE: Wilson W, Taubert KA, Gewitz M, et al. Prevention of infective endocarditis: guidelines from the American Heart Association: a guideline from the American Heart Association Rheumatic Fever, Endocarditis, and Kawasaki Disease Committee, Council on Cardiovascular Disease in the Young, and the Council on Clinical Cardiology, Council on Cardiovascular Surgery and Anesthesia, and the Quality of Care and Outcomes Research Interdisciplinary Working Group. *Circulation.* 2007;116(15):1736–1754.

prosthetic valves lower the sensitivity of transthoracic echocardiography to 45% in older patients (from 75% in younger patients). Transesophageal echocardiography (TEE) improves the diagnostic yield for infective endocarditis, but the lack of positive findings on TEE never excludes it. TEE is of particular value in investigating *S aureus* bacteremia. Positive findings on TEE support prolonged antibiotic administration (4–6 weeks) versus short-course (2 weeks) therapy. However, TEE is invasive and expensive. Interestingly, age does not appear to play a major role in mortality risk, with a 2-year survival of 75% for infective endocarditis in all age groups unless major comorbidities are also present.

Antibiotic treatment of infective endocarditis is directed at the identified pathogen or at the most likely causes if blood cultures are negative. Therapy is administered intravenously for 2–6 weeks. Surgical therapy should be considered in cases of severe valvular dysfunction, recurrent emboli, marked heart failure, myocardial abscess formation, fungal endocarditis, or when appropriate antibiotic treatment does not yield negative blood cultures.

Recommendations for endocarditis prophylaxis for dental procedures were revised in 2007, focusing on providing prophylaxis only in the highest-risk patients (Table 63.6) and eliminating recommendations for prophylaxis for those undergoing gastrointestinal or genitourinary procedures.

Prosthetic Device Infections

Permanent implantable prosthetic devices are common in older adults. Prosthetic joints, cardiac pacemakers, artificial heart valves, intraocular lens implants, vascular grafts, penile prostheses, and a variety of other devices are placed more often in older than in younger adults. A discussion of all prosthetic device infections (PDIs) is beyond the scope of this chapter, but several general concepts can be summarized.

PDIs are usually separated into early versus late infections, because the causative agents differ significantly. Early PDIs, most commonly defined as occurring <60 days after device implantation, are primarily due to contamination at the time of implantation or to events associated with the acute hospitalization (eg, occult bacteremia caused by intravenous catheters). Thus, coagulase-negative staphylococci predominate, and *S aureus* and diphtheroids are common as well; gram-negative bacilli and fungi are relatively rare causes of early PDI. Late PDIs are usually caused by organisms that commonly cause transient bacteremia (in older adults this is most often skin, respiratory, gastrointestinal, or genitourinary organisms). Staphylococci, including coagulase-negative staphylococci, play a major role in both early and late PDIs, although their relative importance is greater in early PDIs. Thus, empiric staphylococcal therapy should be provided in either early or late PDIs if a specific causative agent is not identified.

In general, hardware removal is required to clear PDIs. However, early antibiotic treatment, in some instances combined with aggressive surgical drainage, can be successful. Small studies in prosthetic joint infection suggest that initial debridement and culture and a brief course (2 weeks) of intravenous antibiotics followed by combination oral two-drug therapy that includes rifampin may obviate the need for device removal. Until more definitive data are available, it is prudent to restrict this approach to patients with a short duration of symptoms (<3 weeks), those who are likely to have difficulty tolerating another surgical procedure, or those in whom return to full functional status is not a realistic goal because of comorbidities. In those older adults in whom full function is the goal, the best chance for cure is a two-stage procedure in which the device is removed and antibiotics are given for an extended period (6–8 weeks), followed by delayed reimplantation. Of course, for life-saving devices, such as mechanical valves or implantable defibrillators, this is not an option. Infected prosthetic devices are usually surrounded by microbial biofilms, such as microbe-derived glycocalyx. Biofilms reduce antibiotic penetration and thus greatly increase the concentrations of antibiotic needed for bactericidal activity. Furthermore, many conditions associated with infected prostheses are also accompanied by poor blood flow to the area. Therefore, it is preferable to use bactericidal antibiotics, often in combination with a second agent that penetrates biofilms and poorly perfused areas (eg, rifampin for staphylococci).

Bone and Joint Infections

Native bone and joint infections in the absence of prostheses occur commonly in older adults. Septic arthritis is more likely to occur in joints with underlying pathology (eg, rheumatoid changes, gout, osteoarthritis), and early arthrocentesis is indicated in any mono- or oligo-articular syndrome to exclude infection. S aureus is the most likely pathogen; gram-negative bacilli and streptococci only rarely cause these infections. Aggressive antibiotic therapy combined with serial arthrocentesis may be as effective as open surgical drainage in uncomplicated septic arthritis, while also preserving better joint function. Surgical drainage is required if this more conservative strategy is not successful.

Osteomyelitis in older adults can be due to hematogenous seeding from bacteremia or contiguous spread from an adjacent focus. S aureus is the predominant organism, but gastrointestinal and genitourinary flora are again more common sources in older adults, emphasizing the advantage of a specific microbiologic diagnosis to guide therapy. Pressure injury infections and diabetic foot infections are very common, particularly in institutionalized older adults, and such infections often require surgical consultation combined with aggressive antimicrobial therapy aimed at mixed aerobic and anaerobic bacteria. Osteomyelitis requires definitive treatment with aggressive debridement/amputation of the infected bone with up to 8 weeks of appropriate (and often intravenous) antimicrobial therapy in consultation with an infectious diseases specialist.

HIV Infection and AIDS

HIV infection in older adults was initially limited to those who had received blood transfusions for surgical procedures. However, increasing numbers of older Americans with HIV have acquired their infection via sexual activity. In addition, improvements in treatment have resulted in a large population of adults aging with HIV infection. Older adults constitute approximately 10% of all new diagnoses of AIDS in the United States, but this group and their clinicians often lack HIV awareness. Nonspecific symptoms such as forgetfulness, anorexia, weight loss, and recurrent pneumonia are often dismissed as age related, delaying HIV testing.

Frailty, a clinical syndrome associated with decreased physiologic function and poor outcomes, is prevalent in HIV-infected older adults and affects patients with HIV earlier than those not infected with the virus. Chronic HIV infection appears to intensify age-associated changes in physiologic reserve, thereby increasing frailty risk. A systematic review found the prevalence of frailty in individuals with HIV to range from 5% to 28.6%. HIV infection was found to be an independent risk factor for frailty. Other factors associated with frailty in HIV-infected individuals include older age, comorbidities, and low nadir and current CD4 count.

Untreated HIV infection in older adults tends to pursue a more rapid downhill course, perhaps because of impaired T-cell replacement mechanisms with advanced age and the impact of additional comorbidities. However, if older adults are treated with aggressive highly active antiretroviral therapy (HAART), the antiviral response is similar to that seen in young adults. In fact, older adults often are more adherent to complicated HAART regimens than young adults. Despite this response, however, increasing data suggest immune reconstitution is less robust in older adults with HIV infection. Recommendations are becoming more aggressive with regard to threshold for initiation of HAART, but these recommendations remain in a state of flux. It is suggested that all patients with HIV be under the care of an infectious diseases specialist to decide when to begin therapy and what agents are most appropriate.

HAART regimens and prophylaxis of opportunistic infections in older adults are similar to those used in younger patients. Indications that HIV therapies can accelerate atherosclerosis and glucose intolerance suggest that an aggressive approach to prevention of cardiovascular disease in older HIV-infected adults is warranted and may lead to specific recommendations in older adults if associations of metabolic changes with specific HIV therapies become clearer. Other age-related comorbidities are also more common in HIV-infected individuals, even those with well-controlled viral replication (ie, a peripheral blood viral load <50 copies/mL). Many types of cancer, osteoporosis, and cirrhosis are all more prevalent in this population and appear to develop about a decade earlier in HIV-infected individuals than in matched, uninfected controls. Older adults also appear to be more susceptible to specific complications associated with HIV infection, such as encephalopathy. Finally, older HIV-infected adults are more likely than uninfected, age-matched adults to have multiple comorbidities, which increases the complexity of their care and the potential for medication interactions.

HIV-associated neurocognitive disorder is a spectrum of neurologic disease ranging from asymptomatic neurocognitive impairment to HIV-associated dementia (eg, AIDS dementia complex). HIV-associated dementia is most often seen in patients with advanced disease without virologic suppression and is characterized by cognitive deficits, behavioral and mood changes, and impaired motor function. The main theuraptic approach to HIV-associated neurocognitive disorders is antiretroviral therapy. As HIV-infected individuals are living longer with advancements in antiretroviral therapy, other dementia syndromes such as Alzheimer disease and vascular dementia must be considered in those presenting with subacute cognitive impairment.

HIV prevention is rarely discussed in the geriatric community but is important if the trend of increasing sexual acquisition of HIV in older adults is to be reversed. Most older women do not believe they are at risk of HIV infection, yet heterosexual activity is the primary mode of infection in this group. The concept of behavior that places one at risk of HIV is not well known among older adults, because HIV was not a problem during their adolescence or young adulthood. Older adults must be included in educational programs aimed at ensuring safe sexual practices and increasing awareness of the benefits of testing and effective HIV therapy.

Miscellaneous Infectious Syndromes

Hepatitis C

Hepatitis C is one of the leading causes of end-stage liver disease in the United States and the most common indication for liver transplantation. Most adults who harbor the hepatitis C virus are asymptomatic and unaware of their infection status. Over the past several years, more effective, better tolerated treatments for hepatitis C have become available and have led to improvement in virologic cure (ie, sustained virologic response). Data from population-based studies have shown that three-fourths of adults who are infected with hepatitis C were born between 1945 and 1965, many of whom remain asymptomatic. Based on this data, the U.S. Preventive Services Task Force (USPSTF) recently updated their recommendations in 2013 to include 1-time screening for hepatitis C virus infection to adults born between those years. Adults in this age group are at potential risk because of possible exposure before universal blood screening (B recommendation). The USPSTF concluded that early detection and intervention for hepatitis C virus infection in this group with antiviral regimens resulted in sustained virologic response and improved clinical outcomes, although there was no direct evidence for reducing overall morbidity and mortality.

Infections of the Central Nervous System

Bacterial meningitis is most common at the age extremes of life, and most meningitis-associated fatalities occur in older adults. *Streptococcus pneumoniae* remains the most common cause in older adults, but gram-negative bacilli (20%–25%), *Listeria* spp (up to 10%), and tuberculosis are more common than in young adults. Because many *S pneumoniae* are resistant to β-lactam antibiotics (up to 30% penicillin resistance and 10% ceftriaxone resistance nationwide), either ceftriaxone or cefotaxime *plus* vancomycin are recommended as empiric therapy for bacterial meningitis in older adults until a specific isolate can be tested for antimicrobial susceptibility. Ampicillin is the drug of choice for *Listeria* spp and is appropriate to add to the empiric antibiotic regimen in older adults, and more resistant gram-negative rods (eg, *Pseudomonas* spp) require ceftazidime or an extended-spectrum penicillin with or without intrathecal aminoglycoside therapy.

Neurosyphilis remains one of the most perplexing diagnoses in medicine. It is often raised as a possible underlying process in stroke or dementia in older adults. Syphilis should also be considered in cases of unilateral deafness, gait disturbances, uveitis, and optic neuritis. In reality, there is no gold-standard test to exclude neurosyphilis. Neurosyphilis can only be "ruled in" by a reactive cerebral spinal fluid (CSF) Venereal Disease Research Laboratory test (VDRL), usually in combination with CSF pleocytosis, elevated protein, and decreased glucose. Suspicion is often first raised when a serum rapid plasma reagent or VDRL is positive. A reasonable diagnostic evaluation after discovery of such a positive test includes confirmation of nonspecific tests (rapid plasma reagent and VDRL) with a specific test (microhemagglutination-*Treponema pallidum*, or fluorescent treponemal antibody absorption); if tests are confirmed, lumbar puncture should be performed for cell counts, glucose, protein, and cerebrospinal fluid (CSF) VDRL. A positive VDRL on CSF is diagnostic of neurosyphilis, but the sensitivity of this test is approximately 75% in most series. Other diagnostic tests are controversial. The ratio of intrathecal to serum-specific treponemal antibody (standardized to the total IgG in CSF and serum) may also be helpful, with ratios ≥3 indicating likely infection. In the absence of these tests, it must be the judgment of the clinician as to whether minor abnormalities in CSF (eg, low-level pleocytosis) and the clinical picture support the diagnosis and warrant therapy for neurosyphilis. Optimal treatment of neurosyphilis remains penicillin G, but a study in HIV-infected patients suggests that ceftriaxone may be an acceptable alternative.

Facial nerve palsy (Bell's palsy) is common in older adults and associated with at least three infectious causes: herpes simplex virus, varicella zoster virus, and *Borrelia burgdorferi* (which causes Lyme disease). There are no strong data at present to suggest benefit of antiviral therapy for facial nerve palsies due to herpes simplex virus, but trials are underway. If facial nerve palsy is seen as part of an episode of varicella zoster virus, treatment is indicated. If Lyme disease is suspected clinically, the patient should receive oral amoxicillin 500 mg q6h for 14 days, oral doxycycline 100 mg q12h for 14 days, or intravenous ceftriaxone 2 g/d for 14 days.

Gastrointestinal Infections

Gastrointestinal infections are common among older adults. Diverticulitis, appendicitis, cholecystitis, intra-abdominal abscess, and ischemic bowel can present diagnostic challenges in the absence of fever or increased WBC counts. A high index of suspicion is necessary in older adults. CT of the abdomen and pelvis is most likely to be of value in establishing the diagnosis of intra-abdominal infection, and ultrasonography is an easy, readily available tool to assist in diagnosing cholecystitis, appendicitis, or abscess. Ischemic bowel often requires angiography for diagnosis.

Infectious diarrhea is also common in older adults. Older patients with achlorhydria (eg, proton-pump inhibitor use, atrophic gastritis) are at particular risk, because a lower bacterial inoculum is necessary to cause disease. Decreased intestinal motility associated with specific medications and advanced age may further increase susceptibility to infection. Epidemics occurring in the long-term care setting are commonly due to *E coli*, viruses, *Salmonella* spp, or *Shigella* spp. Frequent use of antimicrobials in older adults also increases the risk of *Clostridium difficile* colitis, and the risk of severe disease is greatest in this age group.

Clostridium difficile *Infection and Pseudomembranous Colitis*

Clostridium difficile infection (CDI) is becoming increasingly recognized among older hospitalized patients and is the source of epidemics in hospitals and long-term care facilities for older adults. The reasons for this trend are uncertain but likely relate to spread of more virulent strains, widespread use of fluoroquinolone antibiotics, and use of proton-pump inhibitors (SOE=B).

A hypervirulent strain, NAP1/BI/027, has been implicated as the responsible pathogen in selected CDI outbreaks and is capable of enhanced production of toxins A and B. The infection is often precipitated by use of antibiotics, particularly clindamycin, third-generation cephalosporins, and fluoroquinolones.

Older adults often present with watery diarrhea and abdominal cramps, with or without fever. Constipation or ileus can sometimes be the presenting symptom, especially in postoperative patients. Other signs include significant leukocytosis (often >20,000 WBCs/μL), hypoalbuminemia, fecal WBCs, and a distinctive fecal odor.

In many clinical settings, diagnosis is made using polymerase chain reaction for B toxin gene. Alternatively, a combination approach, using antigen detection (enzyme immunoassay method) for the *C difficile* antigen followed by A/B toxin assay, may be used. A negative test excludes the presence of *C difficile*, but a positive test must be interpreted in the context of clinical assessment, because up to 50% of hospitalized patients can be colonized. Testing for *C difficile* should be performed only on unformed stool and should not be repeated during the same episode of diarrhea.

Treatment of CDI, most importantly, begins with discontinuing offending antimicrobial agents as soon as possible. Antibiotics for treatment of CDI include oral vancomycin or oral fidaxomicin. Metronidazole is an alternative if oral vancomycin and oral fidaxomicin are not available.

Metronidazole should not be used beyond the first recurrence of CDI because of the risk of neurotoxicity. Fidaxomicin 200 mg q12h for 10 days has been shown to reduce the rate of relapse compared with oral vancomycin in patients with recurrent CDI; however, it is expensive and often not covered by insurance plans. Multiple relapses of CDI are more common in older adults and can occur in >25% of patients. Fecal microbiota transplantation (FMT) has recently been used for treatment of recurrent CDI in those with severe recurrent infection not responsive to antibiotic therapy. In a 2013 study, 91% of patients who received FMT reported either complete resolution or improvement in diarrhea, with no definite adverse effects. Thus, restoration of normal flora with FMT may be a safe, effective method for resolving CDI in patients with severe, recurrent CDI (SOE=C). Probiotics have increasingly been used as a method to prevent *C difficile*–associated diarrhea through several mechanisms, including restoring intestinal flora disrupted by antibiotic use, preventing the binding of *C difficile* to intestinal epithelial cells, and through antimicrobial activity. Although there have been few smaller studies suggesting a benefit to using probiotics for prevention of CDI, a large randomized clinical trial did not demonstrate efficacy in preventing CDI in adults ≥65 years old with recent antibiotic exposure.

Prevention of transmission of CDI, particularly in hospitals and long-term care facilities is of utmost importance, because this population is at greatest risk of complications from CDI. The mainstay of CDI prevention is compliance with hand washing with soap and water after contacting patients with CDI (SOE=A). Other strategies include contact precautions with gloves and gowns on entry into a patient room and the use of private rooms for patients infected with *C difficile*.

FEVER OF UNKNOWN ORIGIN

Fever of unknown origin (FUO) is defined as temperature >101°F (38.3°C) that lasts for at least 3 weeks and is undiagnosed after 1 week of medical evaluation. Several studies have examined this syndrome in older patients and demonstrated differences between older and younger adults. The presence of fever is more likely to be related to a serious infection or illness in older adults than in younger adults or children.

The cause of FUO can be determined in 70%–90% of cases in older adults, and one-third have treatable

Table 63.7—Evaluation of Fever of Unknown Origin in Older Adults

Sequential Step	Details
1. Confirm fever	Temperature >38°C for ≥3 weeks
2. Comprehensive history	Specifically include travel history, other possible exposures to *Mycobacterium tuberculosis*, place of residence (eg, long-term care facility), and current/past sexual history (often not obtained in older adults). Review all medications, including OTC medications and recently discontinued medications (eg, antibiotics).
	Detailed review of systems should focus on new-onset or recent changes in symptoms, including constitutional symptoms, and symptoms of giant cell arteritis (ie, scalp pain and tenderness, vision loss, jaw pain).
	Consider obtaining history from family members or caregivers, especially if patient has cognitive impairment.
3. Comprehensive physical examination	Include detailed dental examination, temporal arteries and shoulders if symptoms are suggestive of polymyalgia rheumatica, abdomen (tenderness may subtle), skin (including back and sacrum to evaluate for pressure injury), digital rectal exam (to exclude perirectal abscess), and lymph nodes.
4. Initial laboratory evaluation	CBC with differential, liver enzymes, erythrocyte sedimentation rate, blood cultures × 3, procalcitonin, chemistry panel, chest radiograph, urinalysis, antinuclear antibody, C reactive protein, HIV-antibody, PPD skin testing, or IGRA.
If no obvious source based on history and all nonessential or concerning medications have been discontinued:	
5. Initial imaging evaluation	Chest or abdomen CT; can consider FDG-PET/CT scan or indium-111 labeled WBC scan
6. Further testing	■ If CT or WBC scan is positive, consider biopsy of identified pathology. If no pathology identified, consider empiric diagnostic tests listed below: ■ Temporal artery biopsy should be obtained if any symptoms or signs are consistent with giant cell arteritis or polymyalgia rheumatica (eg, increased erythrocyte sedimentation rate or tenderness on palpation of temporal arteries). ■ Consider liver biopsy if liver function tests are abnormal. Bone marrow biopsy if abnormal CBC (include Gram stain and cultures [acid-fast bacilli, fungal, and bacterial]).

infections, such as intra-abdominal abscess, bacterial endocarditis, tuberculosis, perinephric abscess, dental abscess, or occult osteomyelitis, with an incidence of infection similar to that in younger patients. In contrast, collagen vascular diseases are more common causes of FUO in older than in younger patients. These are primarily due to giant cell arteritis, polymyalgia rheumatica, and polyarteritis nodosa, and rarely to granulomatosis with polyangitis (formerly known as Wegner granulomatosis). In several published series, 28% of all FUOs in older adults were due to collagen vascular diseases. Neoplastic disease accounts for another 20%, but with rare exceptions, fever due to cancer is primarily caused by hematologic malignancies (eg, lymphoma and leukemia) and not solid tumors. Medications are another cause of FUO in older adults. Rare causes in this age group include deep-vein thrombosis with or without recurrent pulmonary emboli, and hyperthyroidism.

For a diagnostic approach to FUO in older adults, see Table 63.7.

CHOOSING WISELY® RECOMMENDATIONS

Infectious Diseases

■ Do not use antimicrobials to treat bacteriuria in older adults unless specific urinary tract symptoms are present.

RESOURCES

■ Cunningham AL, Lal H, Kovac M, et al. Efficacy of the Herpes Zoster Subunit Vaccine in adults 70 years of age or older. *N Engl J Med.* 2016;375(11):1019–1032.

■ Mody L, Greene MT, Meddings J, et al. A National Implementation Project to Prevent Catheter-Associated Urinary Tract Infection in Nursing Home Residents. *JAMA Intern Med.* 2017;177(8):1154–1162.

CHAPTER 64—ENDOCRINOLOGY

KEY POINTS

- Thyroid-stimulating hormone (TSH), or thyrotropin, levels may normalize within 1–2 years in up to half of older adults with a single mildly increased TSH level; therefore, hypothyroidism should be confirmed by the combination of a persistently increased TSH concentration and a decreased free T_4 level.

- In older adults with mild subclinical hypothyroidism, levothyroxine supplementation has not been shown to be beneficial for relief of symptoms, or to reduce the risk of cognitive dysfunction or cardiovascular events. Individuals with more marked symptoms and TSH levels of at least 10 mIU/L are more likely to experience symptomatic improvement with levothyroxine.

- Chronic adrenal insufficiency presents with nonspecific symptoms such as anorexia, nausea, weight loss, abdominal pain, weakness, hypotension, and impaired function. It should be considered as a cause of unexplained cachexia, loss of mobility, and hypotension, even in the absence of hyponatremia and hyperkalemia.

- Vitamin D deficiency is common and not only contributes to bone loss due to osteoporosis and osteomalacia but also has been associated with muscle weakness and falls. In meta-analyses of randomized, controlled trials (RCTs), reduced hip fracture and mortality risk with vitamin D supplementation in older adults living in institutions has been reported, but reduced risk of falls or fractures in community-dwelling older adults has not been consistently found.

- The most common causes of hypercalcemia are primary hyperparathyroidism in outpatients, and malignant hypercalcemia (eg, caused by squamous cell cancers, breast cancer, myeloma, and lymphoma) in the inpatient setting.

- There is little evidence of long-term clinical benefit from supplementation with dehydroepiandrosterone (DHEA) or testosterone in older adults.

Impaired homeostatic regulation, a hallmark of aging, occurs in many endocrine systems but may become manifest only during stress. For example, fasting blood glucose concentrations change little with normal aging, increasing 1–2 mg/dL per decade of life. In contrast, glucose concentrations after glucose challenge (eg, postprandially) increase much more in healthy older adults than in young adults. In some cases, a loss of function in one aspect of endocrine function can result in a compensatory change in endocrine regulation and be associated with changes in catabolism to maintain homeostasis. For example, decreased testosterone production by the testes, which is seen in many older men, may be partially compensated for by an increase in secretion of pituitary luteinizing hormone and offset by a decrease in metabolism of testosterone. In other instances, compensatory changes or changes in hormone catabolism do not fully offset age-related impairment in endocrine functions, as illustrated by the age-related decline in basal serum aldosterone concentrations. In this case, a decline in aldosterone clearance fails to offset the decrease in aldosterone secretion.

As with diseases in other organ systems, endocrine disorders in older adults often display nonspecific, muted, or atypical symptoms and signs. Some of these presentations are well-defined syndromes that are seen almost exclusively in older adults, such as apathetic thyrotoxicosis or hyperosmolar nonketotic state in patients with type 2 diabetes mellitus. However, more commonly, endocrine disorders present with subtle, nonspecific symptoms, such as cognitive impairment or reduced functional status; some patients may have no complaints. Indeed, the diagnosis of endocrinopathies such as primary hyperparathyroidism, type 2 diabetes mellitus, hypothyroidism, and hyperthyroidism in older adults commonly results from abnormalities found on routine laboratory testing. Finally, nodules are more common with aging in all glands and are often detected incidentally on imaging studies. The presence of a nodule per se is not necessarily an indication of a disease needing treatment in older adults.

Laboratory evaluation of older adults for endocrine disorders can be complicated by coexisting medical illnesses and medications. For example, the presence of serious acute or chronic nonthyroidal illness can lead to the mistaken impression of a thyroid disorder because of an increase or decrease in T_4 concentrations and sometimes increased or decreased TSH concentrations in sick but euthyroid older adults. As a result of biological and assay variability, hormone concentrations may vary considerably in the short term. Therefore, abnormal hormone measurements should always be repeated to confirm endocrine dysfunction, and a stimulatory or suppression test may be required to firmly establish a diagnosis of endocrine hypofunction or hyperfunction, respectively. Furthermore, ranges of normal laboratory values for endocrine testing are commonly established in younger adults, and even age-adjusted norms for

Table 64.1—Circulating Hormone Levels in Normal Aging, Hypothyroidism, and Hyperthyroidism

Circulating Hormone	Normal Aging	Subclinical Primary Hypothyroidism	Overt Primary Hypothyroidism	Secondary Hypothyroidism	Subclinical Hyperthyroidism	Overt Hyperthyroidism
T_4	NL	NL	↓	↓	NL	↑(may be NL in T_3 toxicosis)
T_3	↓ or NL	Not useful to measure*	Not useful to measure*	↓	NL	NL or ↑(↑ in T_3 toxicosis)
TSH	NL or ↑	↑	↑	NL or ↓	↓	↓

T_4=thyroxine, T_3=triiodothyronine, TSH=thyroid-stimulating hormone
↓ = decreased, ↑= increased, NL = within normal limits
*T_3 is within normal limits in about 1/3 of overtly hypothyroid patients and does not fall below normal range until free T_4 is already low.

laboratory tests may be confounded by the inclusion of older adults who are ill. Consequently, normal ranges for healthy older adults are not available for many laboratory tests.

THYROID DISORDERS

With aging, a decrease in T_4 secretion is balanced by a decrease in T_4 clearance, resulting in unchanged circulating T_4 concentrations (Table 64.1). T_3 concentrations are unchanged until extreme old age, when they decrease slightly, possibly reflecting a decrease in 5′-deiodinase activity with aging. T_3 concentrations are also commonly decreased in nonthyroidal illness because of decreased peripheral conversion of T_4 to T_3. The distribution of TSH concentrations shifts toward a higher level with increasing age, with the 97.5th percentile of TSH distribution of 6.3–7.5 mIU/L in adults ≥80 years old, contributing to the higher prevalence of biochemical hypothyroidism. This shift toward higher TSH concentrations with age appears also to apply to extremely long-lived individuals. Nonspecific, atypical, or asymptomatic presentations of thyroid disease are common in older adults. Laboratory testing in stable outpatients using TSH measurements is the most reliable way to identify hypothyroidism or hyperthyroidism in older adults who are not acutely ill. There is no consensus regarding screening asymptomatic older adults for hypo- and hyperthyroidism. However, the prevalence of hypothyroidism and hyperthyroidism is sufficiently high to warrant TSH testing in all older adults with a recent decline in clinical, cognitive, or functional status, or on admission to a nursing home. However, the results of thyroid function testing can be confusing in euthyroid patients with significant concurrent illnesses (discussed below).

Hypothyroidism

Most prevalence estimates of hypothyroidism in older adults range from 0.5% to 5% for overt disease, depending on the population studied. As in younger people, most cases of hypothyroidism in older adults are due to chronic autoimmune thyroiditis (Hashimoto disease). Symptoms of hypothyroidism are often atypical in older adults. Some clinical features of hypothyroidism (eg, dry skin, decreased skin turgor, slowed mentation, weakness, constipation, anemia, hyponatremia, arthritis, paresthesias, peripheral neuropathy, gait disturbances, edema, and increased myocardial fraction of creatine kinase) can misleadingly suggest other diseases. Furthermore, these symptoms usually have an insidious onset and a slow rate of progression. Consequently, the diagnosis of hypothyroidism is rarely made based on clinical examination in older adults, and laboratory testing for a serum TSH level is necessary to detect most cases of hypothyroidism in this population. In addition, older adults with mild hypothyroidism who develop serious nonthyroidal illness may rapidly become severely hypothyroid, a situation that increases susceptibility to myxedema coma. Demented older adults with hypothyroidism rarely recover normal cognitive function with thyroid replacement, but cognition, functional status, and mood may improve with treatment of the hypothyroidism.

Subclinical hypothyroidism is characterized by increased serum TSH (>4.5 mIU/L) and normal free T_4 concentrations and is defined biochemically without regard to the presence or absence of clinical symptoms (Table 64.1). Subclinical hypothyroidism has been reported in up to 15% of people ≥65 years old and is more common in women. However, up to 70% of these individuals have values within their age-specific 97.5th percentile limits, and those with exceptional longevity have higher TSH levels than those 70 years old. Furthermore, TSH levels increased over a 13-year longitudinal follow-up of an aging cohort (mean age 85 years at final assessment). These findings suggest that using an age-specific TSH reference range would reduce the risk of mislabeling many older adults as having subclinical hypothyroidism. Epidemiologic studies in older adults have not found a consistent association between subclinical hypothyroidism and risk of coronary heart disease mortality or total mortality. Overall, meta-analyses in patients with subclinical hypothyroidism have reported a clearer association between increased risk of cardiovascular disease events in persons younger than 65 years of age and in older adults with TSH levels ≥10 mIU/L.

In observational studies of patients with subclinical hypothyroidism, a lower risk of ischemic heart disease and heart failure events has been reported, as well as all-cause mortality, in patients treated with levothyroxine than in untreated patients. However, the lower risk of ischemic heart disease events associated with treatment over a 7.6-year period occurred only in patients <70 years old, not in patients ≥70 years old. In randomized controlled trials (RCTs) of T_4 supplementation in older adults, those with subclinical hypothyroidism did not show a consistent improvement in symptoms, although those with TSH concentrations >10–12 mIU/L and those with greater symptom burden may derive symptomatic benefit. Other studies found that levothyroxine may improve surrogate markers of cardiovascular risk (eg, serum cholesterol levels) and lessen the effects of some comorbidities in older adults, eg, reduced rate of decline in renal function with levothyroxine treatment in patients with chronic kidney disease (mean age 63.2 years, mean TSH 8.86 mIU/L, in study participants).

Potentially confusing scenarios in the diagnosis of hypothyroidism may occur in *nonthyroidal illness*. By itself, an increased TSH concentration is usually due to primary hypothyroidism, but TSH levels may be low during acute nonthyroidal illness and then transiently increase during the recovery phase. Importantly, TSH levels normalize within 12 months in up to 50% of older adults with a single increased TSH level >5.5 mIU/L. Therefore, the diagnosis of hypothyroidism should be confirmed by the combination of a persistently increased TSH concentration and a decreased free T_4 level. The most common alteration in thyroid hormone levels in nonthyroidal illness is a decrease in serum T_3 levels (*low T_3 syndrome*) with normal TSH levels, occurring even in mild nonthyroidal illnesses. In severe nonthyroidal illnesses, circulating total T_4 levels decrease (*low T_4 syndrome*) without increased TSH concentrations. Free T_4 concentrations are usually normal in the low T_4 syndrome. Thyroid hormone supplementation has not been shown to be beneficial in these patients, and it may be harmful. An inappropriately normal or low TSH concentration found in conjunction with a low free T_4 concentration suggests *secondary hypothyroidism*, which is also characterized by the presence of hypopituitarism (deficiencies in other pituitary hormones) (Table 64.1). To minimize confusion between thyroid disease and the nonthyroidal illness syndrome, thyroid function testing in seriously ill patients should be performed only if thyroid dysfunction is strongly suspected, with repeat testing performed after recovery from acute illnesses. Endocrinology referral is indicated to guide testing and management in many of these situations.

T_4 replacement is usually started at a low dosage in older adults (eg, 25 mcg/d, or 50 mcg/d in those without evidence of coronary heart disease), increasing the dosage every 4–6 weeks until TSH concentrations reach the normal range. However, in patients with severe cardiac disease, it may be prudent to begin replacement therapy at even lower dosages (eg, 12.5 mcg/d) if patients have minimal symptoms of hypothyroidism (SOE=D). In these patients, thyroid replacement should not be withheld for fear of exacerbating cardiac disease; instead, the goal is to reduce or eliminate symptoms of hypothyroidism while minimizing the potential for exacerbating cardiac symptoms, such as angina. Adverse effects may occur more commonly in patients taking thyroid extract than with levothyroxine, and there is insufficient information about the safety and benefits of free triiodothyronine surges occurring shortly after ingestion of thyroid extracts; therefore, the use of thyroid extract cannot be recommended. Furthermore, combination therapy with levothyroxine plus L-triiodothyronine is not recommended in older adults because of an increased risk of cardiovascular complications.

Older adults who are severely hypothyroid at presentation should receive higher initial T_4 replacement doses of 50–100 mcg orally, or as high as 200 mcg IV followed by 100 mcg IV daily until oral intake is possible for those with myxedema stupor or coma, even if there is preexisting heart disease (SOE=D). Older adults with severe hypothyroidism or myxedema stupor or coma should also be tested to exclude concomitant adrenal insufficiency and should be given stress doses of glucocorticoids before T_4 to avoid precipitating an adrenal crisis with T_4 replacement.

Thyroid hormone requirements decrease with age because of a decreased clearance rate; T_4 replacement dosages are as much as a third lower in older than in younger adults. The average T_4 replacement dosage in older adults is approximately 110 mcg/d. However, in many older hypothyroid patients, low T_4 doses (25–50 mcg/d) are sufficient to normalize serum TSH levels. Thyroid hormone is best taken fasting to avoid reduced absorption related to food and other medications (eg, calcium, iron, or soy). The target TSH level should be higher in older than in younger adults (4–7 mIU/L [SOE=D]). Over-replacement of thyroid hormone should be avoided, because osteopenia and exacerbation of heart disease may occur. With correction of the hypothyroid state, the clearance rate of medications such as antiepileptics, digoxin, and opioid analgesic agents may be affected, necessitating dosage adjustments.

Hyperthyroidism

Hyperthyroidism develops in 0.5%–2.3% of older adults, and 15%–25% of all cases of thyrotoxicosis are in adults ≥60 years old. In the United States, most cases in older adults are due to Graves disease, but toxic multinodular goiter and autonomously functioning adenomas are more common in older than in younger adults, especially in populations with low iodine intake.

Hyperthyroidism often presents with vague, atypical, or nonspecific symptoms in frail older adults. Many findings that are common in younger adults (eg, tremor, hyperkinesis, heat intolerance, tachycardia, frequent bowel movements, ophthalmopathy, increased perspiration, goiter, brisk reflexes) are less common or absent in older adults, whereas other manifestations, such as atrial fibrillation, heart failure, weight loss, muscle atrophy, and weakness, are more common in older adults. Older adults more often present with a paucity of symptoms than young adults, which may lead to delays in treatment and poorer outcomes. Older adults can present with *apathetic thyrotoxicosis*, a well-known clinical presentation of hyperthyroidism that is rarely seen in younger adults, in which the usual hyperkinetic presentation is replaced by depression, inactivity, lethargy, or withdrawn behavior, often in association with symptoms such as anorexia, weight loss, constipation, muscle weakness, or cardiac symptoms. A low TSH concentration is associated with a 3-fold higher risk of developing atrial fibrillation within 10 years, and hyperthyroidism is present in 13%–30% of older adults with atrial fibrillation. Hyperthyroidism is a cause of secondary osteoporosis and should be considered in the evaluation of patients with decreased bone mass.

A highly sensitive TSH test is adequate as an initial test for hyperthyroidism in relatively healthy older adults, but the diagnosis should be confirmed with free T_4 and T_3 tests (Table 64.1). Most asymptomatic older adults with low serum TSH concentrations are clinically euthyroid; they have normal T_4 and T_3 concentrations, and normal TSH on repeat testing 4–6 weeks later. T_3 *toxicosis*, with increased T_3 but normal T_4 concentrations (Table 64.1), is seen in a minority of hyperthyroid patients, but it is more common with aging, especially in older adults with toxic adenomas or toxic multinodular goiter. T_4 *toxicosis*, with a low serum TSH level together with high serum T_4 and normal to low T_3 levels, may be seen in hyperthyroid older patients with decreased conversion of T_4 to T_3 associated with aging and concomitant nonthyroidal illness. Diagnostic confusion can occasionally occur in euthyroid patients with nonthyroidal illness or medications causing increased T_4 concentrations (*high T_4 syndrome*). Finally, serum TSH levels may be low in euthyroid patients with severe nonthyroidal illnesses (eg, associated with glucocorticoid and dopamine treatment and prolonged fasting).

Radioactive iodine (RAI) uptake and scanning may be useful in determining the etiology of hyperthyroidism. Increased RAI uptake in one or more nodules may occur in toxic multinodular goiter or toxic adenomas, whereas diffusely increased uptake may be seen in Graves disease. Decreased RAI uptake is consistent with thyroiditis, exogenous thyroid supplementation, or iodine-induced hyperthyroidism. Endocrinology consultation may be helpful to assist in the interpretation of thyroid function tests.

Subclinical hyperthyroidism is defined biochemically as a low or undetectable serum TSH level with normal free T_4 and T_3 levels (Table 64.1), with or without signs and symptoms (despite the "subclinical" label) consistent with thyroid hormone excess. Its prevalence increases with age, ranging from <1% to as high as 10%, depending on the population studied. However, exogenous subclinical hyperthyroidism is present in 20%–40% of older patients on levothyroxine supplementation. Overt hyperthyroidism (Table 64.1) develops in 1%–2% of patients per year with a TSH concentration of <0.1 mIU/L but is uncommon in those with TSH concentrations of 0.1–0.45 mIU/L. TSH concentrations normalize over time in many of these patients, although in those with undetectable TSH levels, persistence of subclinical hyperthyroidism is the most common outcome.

There is good evidence for an association between subclinical hyperthyroidism and atrial fibrillation in those with TSH concentrations <0.45 mIU/L, especially when concentrations are <0.1 mIU/L. Furthermore, a meta-analysis of individual level data from 10 prospective cohort studies concluded that there is an increased risk of cardiovascular (HR 1.29; 95% CI, 1.02–1.62) and total mortality (HR 1.24; 95% CI, 1.06–1.46) in patients with subclinical hyperthyroidism. The risk of cardiovascular mortality was higher in those with TSH levels <0.1 mIU/L than in those with levels of 0.1–0.45 mIU/L. Observational data strongly suggest that subclinical hyperthyroidism accelerates bone mineral density (BMD) loss and increases fracture risk, especially in people with a TSH concentration <0.1 mIU/L, but even thyroid function within the high-normal range is associated with reduced BMD and increased risk of hip and other nonvertebral fractures. In postmenopausal women, ongoing bone losses associated with TSH concentrations <0.1–0.2 mIU/L are stabilized by treating the hyperthyroidism. Data on the association between subclinical hyperthyroidism and cognitive impairment and the development of dementia are conflicting.

Treatment of hyperthyroidism should be strongly considered (and endocrinology consultation is strongly advised) in all adults >60 years old with persistently low TSH concentrations <0.1 mIU/L, based on the increased risk of atrial fibrillation, congestive heart failure, osteoporosis, and evidence of progressively increased mortality risk with age in these individuals (SOE=C). Current guidelines suggest treatment of older adults with milder subclinical hyperthyroidism (persistently suppressed TSH levels 0.1–0.4 mIU/L); the presence of symptoms or comorbidities, including heart disease and osteoporosis, may weigh in favor of treatment. Of note, a prospective observational study in women >65 years old found that symptoms, incidence of atrial fibrillation, BMD, and bone turnover markers were similar in people with TSH levels between 0.1–0.4 mIU/L compared to age-matched euthyroid controls. While the duration of mild subclinical hyperthyroidism in these participants was unknown and adverse skeletal and cardiac effects are possible during long-term follow-up, these findings suggest that immediate treatment of mild subclinical hyperthyroidism may be unwarranted in some older adults (eg, those without skeletal and heart comorbidities). In such cases, it may be appropriate to consider treatment if these problems arise during follow-up.

RAI therapy under the supervision of an endocrinologist is the treatment of choice for most older adults with hyperthyroidism caused by Graves disease or toxic nodular thyroid disease, although antithyroid thiourea drugs (methimazole or propylthiouracil) are commonly used as well. RAI treatment is usually curative in patients with toxic adenoma, but higher or repeated doses are often necessary for patients with toxic multinodular goiter. Thiourea treatment should be considered before RAI (SOE=B), but some experts believe the risk of exacerbating thyrotoxicosis is sufficiently low that the risks of these drugs may outweigh the anticipated benefit. β-Blocking agents are helpful to manage symptoms such as tachycardia, tremor, and anxiety[OL] (SOE=B), and should be considered even in asymptomatic older patients to lessen the increased risk of complications due to worsening of hyperthyroidism (SOE=C). Patients receiving β-blocking agents should be monitored for changes in cardiopulmonary function. Older adults with thyrotoxicosis may also require treatment of coexisting congestive heart failure, myocardial ischemia, and atrial arrhythmias, including atrial fibrillation. Treatment with β-blocking agents may be sufficient to manage cardiovascular morbidity due to subclinical hyperthyroidism, notably atrial fibrillation.

After RAI therapy, patients should be monitored by serial measurements of TSH concentration for eventual development of hypothyroidism and for persistent or recurrent hyperthyroidism. With resolution of hyperthyroidism, the clearance rate of other medications may decrease, necessitating dosage adjustments to avoid excessive drug concentrations.

Nodular Thyroid Disease and Thyroid Cancer

The incidence of multinodular goiter increases with age. Multinodular goiters often have autonomously functioning areas, and administration of exogenous thyroid hormone to suppress these goiters can cause iatrogenic hyperthyroidism. Older adults with multinodular goiter can develop iodine-induced thyrotoxicosis after receiving radiocontrast or amiodarone.

Approximately 90% of women ≥70 years old and 60% of men ≥80 years old have thyroid nodules. Most of these nodules are nonpalpable and are detected incidentally on highly sensitive ultrasound or imaging studies done for other reasons (eg, carotid duplex ultrasound). Thyroid cancer is present in 4%–6.5% of thyroid nodules, and the prevalence of cancer is higher in adults >60 years old with nodules, especially men. Incidentally discovered nonpalpable nodules are as likely to be malignant as palpable nodules. The reported incidence of thyroid cancer has increased markedly in recent decades while thyroid cancer mortality rates have remained stable, reflecting increased detection of low-risk cases of papillary thyroid cancer. In 2017, the U.S. Preventive Services Task Force (USPSTF) recommended against screening for thyroid cancer after determining that the harms exceed the benefits. Of note, studies reviewed by the USPSTF involved primarily younger and middle-aged adults, and the increase in thyroid cancer incidence is much less evident in older than in middle-aged adults. Although the incidence of differentiated thyroid cancers is similar in older and younger adults, thyroid lymphomas are more common in older adults and anaplastic thyroid carcinomas are found almost exclusively in this population. Additionally, even well-differentiated papillary and follicular carcinomas are more aggressive and are associated with increased mortality in older adults. Based on the foregoing, the risk of thyroid cancer over-diagnosis and over-treatment may be higher in younger and middle-aged people than in older adults.

Ultrasound of the thyroid is the most sensitive test to detect thyroid nodules. Screening ultrasonography of the thyroid is not indicated in the general population, but ultrasonography and a serum TSH level are indicated in all older adults with known or suspected thyroid nodules or multinodular goiter (SOE=A) (Table 64.2). Autonomously functioning thyroid nodules are rarely malignant, so no further evaluation for cancer is generally required in patients with low TSH concentrations and a "hot" (increased RAI uptake) nodule on radionuclide thyroid scanning that corresponds to a palpable nodule. Radionuclide thyroid scanning is not indicated in individuals with normal or increased TSH levels; these scans cannot conclusively distinguish whether a "cold"

Table 64.2—Indications for Thyroid Ultrasonography

Screening
- History of head and neck irradiation
- Multiple endocrine neoplasia type 2
- Family history of thyroid cancer*

Diagnosis
- Unexplained cervical lymphadenopathy
- All patients with known or suspected thyroid nodules or multinodular goiter
- Selection of thyroid nodule(s) for biopsy
- Guidance for fine-needle aspiration of single or multiple thyroid nodules
- Identification of nodular characteristics suspicious for cancer
- Thyroid nodule discovered incidentally on CT, MRI, or PET scanning

*Current guidelines do not recommend for or against screening ultrasonography in people with familial follicular cell–derived differentiated thyroid cancer because of lack of evidence that this would lead to reduced morbidity or mortality.

(nonfunctioning) nodule is benign or malignant, and fine-needle aspiration (FNA) is needed to exclude malignancy (SOE=A). Endocrinology referral is generally indicated for further diagnostic evaluation and management.

In current guidelines, risk stratification and decisions to pursue FNA are based both on ultrasound characteristics and size of the nodule. In general, in people without known thyroid cancer risk factors, only nodules >1 cm require evaluation for malignancy because of their potential to be clinically significant cancers. Nodules that are purely cystic do not require FNA. Benign thyroid nodules on FNA should be followed with ultrasonography within 12 to ≥24 months after the initial procedure, as determined by risk stratification based on ultrasonography pattern (SOE=D). FNA should be repeated when the results are nondiagnostic. If FNA cytology is diagnostic of or suspicious for a malignancy, surgery should be performed (SOE=A). Lobectomy may be considered for some low-risk differentiated thyroid cancers (DTC), eg, lesions <4 cm. Molecular testing may help to reduce the number of diagnostic thyroid surgeries in patients ultimately found to have benign thyroid nodules. Postoperative RAI should be administered to patients with high-risk DTC and some with intermediate-risk DTC but not to low-risk patients (SOE=B). Levothyroxine suppressive therapy may be indicated to reduce the risk of cancer recurrence and mortality for patients with thyroid cancer after near-total or total thyroidectomy, but adverse cardiac effects and osteoporosis can occur with long-term thyroid suppression. Current guidelines propose ongoing risk stratification to determine the degree of optimal TSH suppression (SOE=C). β-Blocking agents[OL] and bone antiresorptive agents[OL] can help minimize these untoward effects (SOE=D).

Table 64.3—Causes of Age-Related Changes in Calcium Homeostasis

Decreased concentrations of 25(OH)D and 1,25(OH)$_2$D
Decreased renal 1α-hydroxylase activity
Decreased vitamin D synthesis by the skin
Decreased sunlight exposure (housebound and institutionalized older adults)
Decreased intestinal absorption of dietary calcium
Inadequate dietary calcium and vitamin D intake
Decreased intestinal responsiveness to 1,25(OH)$_2$D
Decreased gastric acid secretion
Lactase deficiency (causing avoidance of dairy products)
Increase in serum parathyroid hormone concentrations
Slight decrease in serum calcium concentrations
Decreased renal clearance of parathyroid hormone
Decreased parathyroid hormone responsiveness

Importantly, in a nomenclature revision, encapsulated papillary neoplasms now known as noninvasive follicular thyroid neoplasms with papillary-like nuclear features (NIFTP) behave in a highly indolent fashion and are no longer considered malignant. Although thyroid lobectomy is still required to diagnose NIFTP, more extensive completion thyroidectomy and postoperative RAI are not indicated for this condition.

DISORDERS OF PARATHYROID AND CALCIUM METABOLISM

Important changes occur with aging in several systems that regulate calcium homeostasis, ultimately leading to decreased bone mass and, in some cases, osteoporosis in older adults (Table 64.3). The net effect of these changes is to increase circulating concentrations of parathyroid hormone (PTH), which increases 30% between 30 and 80 years of age. Serum calcium concentrations remain normal with the increase in PTH, but the balance between bone resorption and bone formation is changed in favor of resorption, resulting in decreased bone mass and increased risk of osteoporosis with aging.

Vitamin D Deficiency

Vitamin D deficiency, defined as a circulating 25(OH)D level <20 ng/mL, is very common. In the National Health and Nutrition Examination Survey (NHANES) 2000–2004, 26.6% of men and 33.6% of women of all races >70 years old had serum 25(OH)D levels <20 ng/mL. Increased bone turnover and bone loss, especially of cortical bone, is a major consequence of the secondary hyperparathyroidism that arises in vitamin D–deficient older adults. Beyond its skeletal effects, vitamin D deficiency is associated with muscle weakness and can contribute to fall risk in some individuals.

Table 64.4—Typical Laboratory Results in the Differential Diagnosis of Hypercalcemia

Laboratory Test	Primary Hyperparathyroidism	Humoral Hypercalcemia of Malignancy	Local Osteolytic Hypercalcemia
Serum calcium	↑	↑ or ↑↑	↑ or ↑↑
Serum phosphate	↓ or low-normal	↓	↑
Urine calcium	↑	↑	↑
Parathyroid hormone	↑	↓↓	↓↓
Parathyroid hormone-related peptide	0	↑	0

NOTE: The diagnosis of malignancy-related hypercalcemia is normally straightforward, and extensive diagnostic testing is rarely required.
↑ = increased, ↑↑ = markedly increased, ↓ = decreased, ↓↓ = markedly decreased, 0 = undetectable

Patients with severe vitamin D deficiency (25[OH]D levels <10 ng/mL) are commonly treated with 50,000 IU/week of vitamin D_2 or D_3 orally for 8–12 weeks followed by vitamin D_3 at 800 IU/d thereafter, but the comparative efficacy of this practice versus other dosing regimens is unknown. The dose above which vitamin D becomes toxic is unclear, but high-dose vitamin D supplementation, eg, doses well above the IOM-recommended safe upper limit of 4,000 IU/d for prolonged periods, may cause vitamin D intoxication with hypercalciuria (the initial manifestation of toxicity), hypercalcemia, impaired kidney function, and bone loss. Exceptions include individuals with malabsorption (eg, celiac disease) or severe obesity, who may require vitamin D supplementation in very large doses to maintain vitamin D sufficiency.

Although current data are insufficient to determine the optimal dose, a dose adequate to maintain 25(OH)D levels >30 ng/mL is prudent and safe. Maintaining adequate calcium intake (1,000–1,500 mg/d from the diet and supplements) is also important for bone health and prevention of secondary hyperparathyroidism. Daily dietary intake of calcium (mainly in dairy products) should be factored in, which in some people may obviate the need for calcium supplements. Obese people are at high risk of vitamin D deficiency, likely because vitamin D is fat soluble and sequestered in body fat. Consequently, the increment in 25(OH)D levels after either sunlight exposure or oral vitamin D supplementation is less in obese adults than in nonobese adults, and longer periods of vitamin D supplementation may be required to normalize 25(OH)D levels in obese vitamin D–deficient individuals. Obese individuals (BMI >30 kg/m^2), people taking medications that accelerate vitamin D metabolism such as phenytoin and phenobarbital, and those with malabsorption syndromes who are vitamin D–deficient often require vitamin D dosages much higher than 1,000 IU/d to normalize 25(OH)D levels.

The main form of vitamin D in circulation, 25(OH)D, is measured in serum to evaluate vitamin D status. Measurement of 1,25(OH)$_2$D$_3$, the active metabolite of vitamin D, is not useful to assess in most individuals, because levels are normal or increased in vitamin D–deficient individuals with secondary hyperparathyroidism. Levels of 1,25(OH)$_2$D$_3$ are mostly used clinically in patients with late-stage chronic kidney disease.

Importantly, despite having lower total 25(OH)D levels, black Americans have higher BMD and lower fracture risk than white Americans; the concentration of bioavailable 25(OH)D may in fact be similar to that of white Americans when vitamin D–binding protein is considered. Black Americans have higher intestinal calcium absorption efficiency and lower urinary calcium excretion than white Americans and may have skeletal resistance to secondary hyperparathyroidism. Consequently, modestly low 25(OH)D levels in black Americans may not necessarily indicate true vitamin D deficiency, and vitamin D deficiency may be overdiagnosed in this population.

Hypercalcemia

Primary hyperparathyroidism (PHPT) and malignancy are the most common causes of hypercalcemia in older adults. The annual incidence of PHPT is approximately 1 per 1,000, and the disease is 3-fold more prevalent in women than in men. Most patients with PHPT are asymptomatic, and the diagnosis is made after an incidental finding of hypercalcemia on a chemistry battery. When the disease is symptomatic, older adults are more likely than younger adults to present with neuropsychiatric symptoms that may be subtle, such as depression and cognitive impairment, or with neuromuscular problems such as proximal muscle weakness and osteoporosis. Typical laboratory findings in PHPT and other common causes of hypercalcemia are shown in Table 64.4. The diagnosis of PHPT is confirmed with an increased or high normal PTH concentration, using an assay for intact PTH, in the presence of hypercalcemia. A low 24-hour urinary calcium excretion distinguishes familial hypocalciuric hypercalcemia from PHPT. Familial hypocalciuric hypercalcemia is associated with longstanding mild hypercalcemia, does not respond to parathyroidectomy, and is generally not associated with complications. Normocalcemic PHPT may be identified during the evaluation of older adults with reduced BMD. Causes of secondary hyperparathyroidism should be excluded in these patients, including renal failure, vitamin D deficiency, calcium malabsorption (eg, from celiac disease), and urinary calcium loss due to the use of loop diuretics.

Indications for parathyroid surgery are shown in Table 64.5. In RCTs evaluating parathyroidectomy in patients with mild, apparently asymptomatic disease, BMD and other measures that may be relevant to quality of life improved after parathyroidectomy. Asymptomatic patients can safely be followed without surgery at least for several years; many of these patients remain stable without deterioration of biochemical indices or BMD for up to 10 years. However, after 8–10 years, about 25% of these patients develop progressive disease, including worsening hypercalcemia, hypercalciuria, and reductions in BMD. Bone density eventually declines in most patients after 10–15 years, especially at cortical sites such as the femoral neck or forearm. Parathyroidectomy can be performed safely in older adults, even those >80 years old, who may experience improvements in symptoms comparable to those in younger adults, as well as improvements in function (SOE=B). Although most people with PHPT are older adults, only 1 in 4 patients >70 years old who meet surgical criteria undergo parathyroidectomy. In general, surgery should be offered to all older adults meeting criteria who have minimal perioperative risk and sufficient life expectancy. The best outcomes are achieved by surgeons who have extensive experience with the procedure.

Asymptomatic patients who are managed conservatively should avoid lithium carbonate, thiazide diuretics, volume depletion, and immobilization. Baseline assessment in these patients should include blood pressure; serum calcium, phosphate, and creatinine; creatinine clearance; and bone densitometry. Follow-up assessments should include serum calcium and creatinine every 12 months and bone densitometry (at 3 sites) every 12–24 months (SOE=C). Some manifestations of PHPT such as reduced BMD and fracture risk are exacerbated by vitamin D deficiency and improve with vitamin D repletion. Moderate calcium (eg, 1,200 mg/d [SOE=C]) and vitamin D supplementation (eg, starting dose of 600–1,000 IU/d with a goal of 25(OH)D level ≥20–30 ng/mL [SOE=C]) should be maintained. In addition, these patients should be followed clinically for development of nephrolithiasis, fractures caused by minimal trauma, and neuropsychiatric or neuromuscular symptoms.

Medical management of PHPT may be appropriate in nonsurgical candidates when it is desirable to lower the serum calcium level, increase BMD, or

Table 64.5—Indications for Parathyroid Surgery in Primary Hyperparathyroidism

Symptomatic primary hyperparathyroidism

Asymptomatic primary hyperparathyroidism in the following situations:
- Total serum calcium concentrations >1 mg/dL above the normal range
- Creatinine clearance <60 mL/min
- Markedly decreased BMD (T score below −2.5 at lumbar spine, hip, or distal ⅓ of radius on bone densitometry)
- Vertebral fracture
- Nephrolithiasis or nephrocalcinosis on imaging
- 24-hour urine calcium >400 mg/d, together with increased stone risk by biochemical stone risk analysis
- Neurocognitive and neuropsychiatric symptoms attributable to primary hyperparathyroidism (endorsed by some but not all guidelines)
- Consider in some patients with cardiovascular disease on a case-by-case basis to mitigate cardiovascular sequelae (endorsed by some but not all guidelines)*

BMD=bone mineral density
*Available data linking primary hyperparathyroidism and cardiovascular disease are observational.

both. Options for patients with low BMD include the bisphosphonate alendronate[OL], which improves BMD in patients with PHPT without consistently affecting calcium or PTH concentrations (SOE=A). However, it is unknown whether alendronate or other bisphosphonates reduce fracture risk in these patients. Cinacalcet, a calcimimetic agent that inhibits parathyroid cell function, reduces or normalizes serum calcium concentrations and reduces PTH concentrations during long-term treatment of PHPT, but BMD is not increased. Accordingly, the role of cinacalcet is limited to management of symptomatic or severe hypercalcemia in patients who cannot undergo parathyroid surgery (SOE=C). Limited data suggest that combined therapy with cinacalcet and a bisphosphonate may accomplish both calcium lowering and improvement in BMD in people who have both low BMD and severe hypercalcemia (SOE=B). Estrogen–progestin therapy increases BMD in postmenopausal women with PHPT but without consistent effects on serum calcium or PTH levels. Estrogen–progestin therapy may be a useful option for women who are not surgical candidates, especially those with menopausal symptoms, but the benefits and risks must be considered in light of contraindications to this therapy.

In hospitalized patients, the most common cause of hypercalcemia is a malignancy that produces PTH-related peptide (PTHrp) (Table 64.4), often referred to as humoral hypercalcemia of malignancy, with hypercalcemia resulting primarily from increased net bone resorption. The presence of an underlying cancer is usually evident on examination and routine diagnostic testing. These patients are often managed primarily by consulting oncologists, and treatment of the underlying cancer may improve and prevent recurrence of hypercalcemia. Squamous cell cancers of the lung or head and neck are common causes of hypercalcemia due to PTHrp production. Other common malignancies associated with hypercalcemia include breast cancer, lymphoma, and myeloma, although the mechanisms of the hypercalcemia associated with these malignancies are usually not PTHrp-mediated and may be responsive to glucocorticoid treatment. Acute treatment for hypercalcemia of malignancy includes volume replacement with intravenous saline. A parenteral bisphosphonate such as pamidronate or zoledronic acid should be given, along with treatment for the underlying malignancy, if possible. In addition to their usefulness in treatment of hypercalcemia, high-potency bisphosphonates such as zoledronic acid may decrease bone pain and the risk of pathologic fractures in patients with osteolytic bone metastases from a variety of cancers (SOE=A). Potential nephrotoxicity associated with these agents may be minimized by adhering to recommended dosages and infusion times, but these agents should be used cautiously, if at all, in people with a creatinine clearance of ≤30 mL/min. Cancer patients receiving repetitive dosing of parenteral bisphosphonates who have had recent dental extractions, dental implants, poorly fitting dentures, or preexisting mandibular disease, or receiving high-dosage glucocorticoid treatment are at increased risk of osteonecrosis of the jaw. Denosumab is an approved alternative to bisphosphonates for treatment of hypercalcemia of malignancy refractory to bisphosphonates. It may also prevent skeletal-related events (eg, fractures, pain from bone metastases) in people with bone metastases from solid tumors but not for patients with multiple myeloma, and it may be useful for patients in whom bisphosphonates are contraindicated because of severe renal impairment. Hypercalcemic patients with vitamin D deficiency may become hypocalcemic after receiving bisphosphonates or denosumab.

Paget Disease of Bone

Paget disease is characterized by localized areas of increased bone remodeling, resulting in a change in bone architecture and an increased tendency to deformity and fracture. Its prevalence increases with aging, affecting 2%–5% of people ≥50 years old. Paget disease is usually asymptomatic and localized and is often diagnosed as an incidental finding on radiographs or during evaluation for an unexplained increase in serum alkaline phosphatase. The most commonly affected sites are the pelvis, spine, femur, tibia, and skull. When Paget disease is symptomatic, pain is the most common presenting symptom, either localized to the affected bones or resulting from secondary osteoarthritic changes, often in the hips, knees, and vertebrae. When bone deformities occur, the long bones of the legs are usually affected, often with bowing. Skull involvement may result in sensorineural hearing loss, thought to be due to cochlear damage rather than to compression of the eighth cranial nerve. Paraplegia or quadriplegia occurs rarely as a consequence of spinal stenosis from vertebral involvement or as vascular steal from spinal cord adjacent to vascular pagetic bone; it may be reversible with timely treatment. The most devastating complication of Paget disease is malignant transformation of affected bone, particularly osteosarcoma.

When Paget disease is suspected, plain radiographs should be obtained of areas of suspected involvement. After the diagnosis is made, a radionuclide bone scan is useful to determine the extent of the disease, along with serum alkaline phosphatase (SAP) or bone-specific alkaline phosphatase (BSAP) to determine the level of metabolic activity. The primary indication for treatment in asymptomatic patients is active disease in areas where complications may occur, including the skull, weight-bearing bones, and bone adjacent to major joints, which may increase the risk of secondary osteoarthritis (SOE=C). Bisphosphonates suppress the accelerated bone turnover and bone remodeling characteristic of Paget disease and are the treatment of choice for most patients with active disease who are at risk of complications (SOE=A). Increasing evidence indicates that a single dose of zoledronic acid 5 mg IV is superior to other bisphosphonates for patients without contraindications (such as glomerular filtration rate <35 mL/min). Zoledronic acid is more likely to achieve a complete and sustained response to therapy, including improved pain and quality of life, than other bisphosphonates (SOE=A). Bisphosphonates may help to prevent or slow the development of hearing loss and osteoarthritis in joints adjacent to those affected with Paget disease (SOE=C), although joint replacement may be necessary in some individuals to restore function and relieve joint pain. Pretreatment with an aminobisphosphonate (eg, zoledronic acid or alendronate) may be advisable 1–4 months before elective total joint replacement to minimize the risks of intraoperative bleeding due to increased blood flow to pagetic bone and postoperative loosening of the prosthesis (SOE=B).

Calcium and vitamin D should be administered concomitantly with bisphosphonates to prevent hypocalcemia[OL]. NSAIDs may be useful in treating secondary osteoarthritis for short periods (eg, several weeks), although even short courses of treatment with

Table 64.6—Regulation of Anterior Pituitary Hormones

Synthetic Cells in Anterior Pituitary	Hormone	Factors Promoting Secretion	Factors Inhibiting Secretion	Comments
Somatotrophs	Growth hormone	GHRH	Somatostatin, IGF-1	GHRH and somatostatin are produced by the hypothalamus, IGF-1 primarily by the liver.
Mammotrophs	Prolactin	TRH	Dopamine	TRH and dopamine are produced by the hypothalamus. Antipsychotic and opiate drugs inhibit dopamine activity.
Thyrotrophs	TSH	TRH	Dopamine	TRH and dopamine are produced by the hypothalamus. Antipsychotic and opiate drugs inhibit dopamine activity.
Corticotrophs	ACTH	Corticotropin-releasing hormone	Cortisol	Systemic corticosteroid drugs inhibit ACTH release.
Gonadotrophs	LH, FSH	GnRH	Estradiol, testosterone	GnRH is produced by the hypothalamus. Prolactin and opiate drugs inhibit GnRH release.

GHRH=growth hormone–releasing hormone, TRH=thyrotropin-releasing hormone, TSH=thyroid-stimulating hormone, ACTH=adrenocorticotropic-releasing hormone, LH=leutinizing hormone, FSH=follicle-stimulating hormone, GnRH=gonadotropin-releasing hormone

NSAIDs expose older adults to known risks, including increased risk of GI bleeding, renal dysfunction, heart attack and stroke, and other adverse effects. During treatment, patients should be monitored clinically for changes in bone pain, joint function, and neurologic status. SAP or BSAP levels should be monitored to assess the initial and ongoing response to bisphosphonate therapy.

DISORDERS OF THE ANTERIOR PITUITARY

Secondary hypothyroidism results from undersecretion of TSH by the anterior pituitary. Patients with suspected secondary hypothyroidism (Table 64.1) require neuroimaging of the hypothalamus and pituitary as well as measurement of other pituitary hormones, with special attention to exclude secondary adrenal insufficiency before T_4 administration that could result in adrenal crisis.

For major hormones produced by the anterior pituitary and the factors influencing their secretion or action, see Table 64.6. Hypothalamic-pituitary-adrenal (HPA) axis function changes little with age. Basal adrenocorticotropic hormone (ACTH) levels are unchanged in later life, but the effects of aging on the ACTH response to stress can vary, depending on the stressor. Increases in cortisol and ACTH levels in response to metyrapone, ovine corticotropin-releasing hormone (CRH), and insulin-induced hypoglycemia are normal or slightly prolonged with aging. Inhibition of ACTH secretion by cortisol is unchanged with aging, indicating that feedback sensitivity to cortisol is unchanged. The dose-dependent suppression of CRH-induced ACTH release by dexamethasone is blunted with aging.

Hyperprolactinemia and Pituitary Adenomas

Some older adults develop mild hyperprolactinemia due to causes such as renal failure, primary hypothyroidism, hypothalamic diseases that interfere with synthesis of dopamine (prolactin-inhibitory factor), and medications that inhibit dopamine activity (eg, antipsychotics, opioids, and metoclopramide). The clinical manifestations of hyperprolactinemia often go unrecognized in older adults and are usually subtle, including sexual dysfunction, gynecomastia, and rarely galactorrhea. Hyperprolactinemia should be considered in evaluation of secondary causes of osteoporosis in older men, because the antigonadotropic actions of prolactin may cause hypogonadism and accelerated bone loss.

Endocrinology consultation may help to ensure appropriate diagnosis and management of patients with hyperprolactinemia and pituitary tumors. When hyperprolactinemia is detected in asymptomatic patients, macroprolactinemia due to less bioactive dimeric and polymeric forms of prolactin should be excluded to avoid further unnecessary evaluation and management in these patients. In patients with true hyperprolactinemia, treatment of underlying secondary causes of hyperprolactinemia or discontinuation of medications such as antipsychotics often resolve the problem. MRI of the hypothalamus and pituitary is generally indicated to exclude a tumor or other lesion after investigation of secondary causes of hyperprolactinemia. Nonfunctioning pituitary adenomas can cause hyperprolactinemia by compressing the pituitary stalk or hypothalamus, thereby interfering with dopamine inhibition of prolactin secretion. Failure to recognize this possibility may lead to a misdiagnosis of prolactinoma and ineffective treatment with dopamine agonists rather than surgical treatment for tumors other than prolactinomas. However, prolactin levels >200 ng/mL nearly always indicate the presence of a prolactinoma, with higher prolactin levels predicting larger tumor mass.

Hyperprolactinemia due to a pituitary microprolactinoma (defined as <10 mm in size) may be managed with observation if the patient is asymptomatic, or with a dopamine agonist if secondary osteoporosis or symptoms such as sexual dysfunction are present. Dopamine agonists are first-line treatment for hyperprolactinemia from any cause and are effective in reducing prolactin concentrations. Older adults are at risk of adverse effects of these agents, including hallucinations and GI symptoms, so dopamine agonists should be started at low doses and the dose increased slowly. Cabergoline is the preferred dopamine agonist for its efficacy in decreasing prolactin levels, the size of pituitary macroadenomas (ie, ≥10 mm), and the likelihood of causing adverse effects. Compulsive behaviors, including hypersexuality and excessive gambling, may occur with dopamine agonists. Dosing should be titrated to normalize prolactin levels, with MRI repeated in 1 year or sooner if hyperprolactinemia or symptoms worsen despite treatment. Serial visual field testing is indicated for patients with macroadenomas near the optic chiasm. Trans-sphenoidal surgery or radiation therapy is occasionally necessary in patients with macroprolactinomas and persistent visual field defects or in those who cannot tolerate dopamine agonists.

Although the incidence of pituitary adenomas increases with age, most of these tumors remain asymptomatic. The majority of pituitary adenomas are nonfunctioning, followed by smaller numbers of prolactinomas and GH-secreting tumors. Nonsecreting and gonadotropin- or α-subunit-secreting adenomas are typically large at the time of diagnosis because of the absence of symptoms associated with hormone excess. Symptoms in these patients are generally due to mass effect, eg, headache, visual field abnormalities due to pressure on the optic chiasm, and panhypopituitarism.

Increasingly, pituitary incidentalomas are found on imaging studies ordered to evaluate comorbid illnesses in older adults. When these lesions are identified, careful clinical evaluation and measurement of pituitary and end-organ hormones should be performed to exclude hypopituitarism and hormone hypersecretion. A visual field examination is required when the tumor is adjacent to the optic chiasm or optic nerves. Pituitary microadenomas may be managed expectantly. Patients with macroadenomas other than prolactinomas should be referred for trans-sphenoidal surgery if there are visual field abnormalities due to compression of the optic chiasm or optic nerves; if there is hypersecretion of TSH, ACTH, or GH; or if other neurologic symptoms are present. Hypopituitarism (if present) may persist after pituitary adenomas are surgically removed, so hypopituitarism by itself is not an indication for surgery. The risks of trans-sphenoidal surgery have been reported to increase with age, but postoperative hypopituitarism and other complications are less likely and outcomes are similar to those in younger adults when these surgeries are performed at specialized centers by surgeons with extensive experience.

Hypopituitarism and the Empty Sella Syndrome

Hypopituitarism has been reported to develop in ⅓ to ½ of older adults with diagnosed pituitary tumors. Other causes of hypopituitarism in older adults include traumatic brain injury (TBI), infections such as tuberculosis, metastatic cancer, prior irradiation or surgery for pituitary tumors, and vascular disorders such as pituitary infarction or carotid artery aneurysms. An increasing number of cases of hypophysitis with impaired anterior pituitary function have been reported in melanoma patients treated with ipilimumab; older men appear especially at risk. Manifestations of *panhypopituitarism* include fatigue, hypogonadism and loss of libido, hypotension, weight loss, hypoglycemia, and hyponatremia. When the diagnosis is suspected, concurrent measurement of hormone levels in the pituitary and target organ(s) is indicated to determine whether hormonal axis responses are appropriate, typically with endocrinology referral. Dynamic testing of the HPA axis with ACTH stimulation testing is also indicated to evaluate for secondary adrenal insufficiency.

After even minor falls or trauma with head injury, acute hypopituitarism occurs commonly in older adults. In the acute phase (first 7–10 days), potentially life-threatening glucocorticoid insufficiency may develop, and serial morning cortisol measurements should be obtained, especially when hypotension, hypoglycemia, or hyponatremia are present. Acute diabetes insipidus may also occur. Evaluation of GH, thyroid, and gonadal axis function is unnecessary in the acute phase. After the acute phase of TBI, some hormonal deficiencies that were manifest initially may resolve and others may develop. Although the natural history of hypopituitarism after TBI is not well described, it is appropriate (in consultation with an endocrinologist) to monitor for signs and symptoms and to obtain hormone measurements 3–6 months and at 1 year after the TBI, and to reevaluate hormonal status whenever concerning symptoms develop.

Cases of empty sella syndrome are increasingly being detected as neuroimaging procedures performed for other indications have increased. Pituitary height and volume tend to diminish with aging in healthy adults, and empty sella has been observed in 19% of older study participants. Most cases of *primary empty sella syndrome* (ie, not associated with pituitary tumors or their treatment) occur in obese, middle-aged women with hypertension. In contrast to men, most women with this condition do not have significant pituitary hormone hypofunction. It is unknown whether an incidental finding of empty sella in otherwise healthy older adults has any functional significance. These patients are typically managed with visual field testing and pituitary and target organ hormone measurements to detect abnormalities in pituitary hormones.

DISORDERS OF THE ADRENAL CORTEX

Basal serum cortisol concentrations do not change with aging, because decreased cortisol secretion is balanced by a decrease in clearance. Clinically, acute cortisol responses to stress may be higher and more prolonged in older than in younger adults, possibly because cortisol clearance is reduced. Accordingly, in nonemergent situations, adrenal function testing should be deferred at least 48 hours after major stressors, such as surgery or trauma. In older adults with a normal ACTH stimulation test in whom adrenal insufficiency is suspected, endocrinology consultation is recommended to assist with further testing.

Hypoadrenocorticoidism

Chronic glucocorticoid therapy is the most common cause of adrenal failure in older adults because of chronic suppression of adrenal function. Recovery of adrenal axis function is variable and may take several months to a year. Autoimmune-mediated adrenal failure is less common in older than in younger adults; in contrast, tuberculosis, adrenal metastases, and adrenal hemorrhage in anticoagulated patients are more common. Additionally, prolonged use of megestrol acetate (eg, as an appetite stimulant) may cause ACTH suppression and hypoadrenocorticoidism.

Older adults with chronic adrenal insufficiency may present with nonspecific symptoms such as anorexia, nausea, weight loss, abdominal pain, weakness, hypotension, or impaired functional status, and hyponatremia and hyperkalemia may not always be present. Accordingly, a high index of suspicion is required to make the diagnosis. When adrenocortical insufficiency is suspected, the ACTH stimulation test should be performed (SOE=A), and therapy initiated (SOE=B). A normal serum cortisol (basal or 30–60 minutes after administration of 250 mcg of ACTH [cosyntropin]) is ≥18-20 mcg/dL. A serum ACTH concentration should be obtained before administration of cosyntropin to distinguish secondary adrenal insufficiency (decreased pituitary ACTH secretion), which is characterized by a low or normal ACTH concentration, from primary adrenal insufficiency (PAI), which is associated with a high ACTH concentration. Patients with suspected PAI should have simultaneous measurements of plasma renin and aldosterone to detect mineralocorticoid deficiency. In older adults instructed to stop chronic glucocorticoid therapy, the drug should be tapered gradually (SOE=D), and stress dose coverage given for major surgery and other acute physiologic stresses until adrenocortical function has returned to normal (SOE=D). Recovery of the HPA axis may take >9 months.

Acute adrenal insufficiency is a potentially life-threatening emergency. Patients in suspected adrenal crisis should, after blood draw for diagnosis, receive IV hydrocortisone at stress doses (hydrocortisone 100–200 mg over 24 hours continuously or in divided doses every 6 hours [SOE=A]) without waiting for laboratory confirmation, along with intravenous volume resuscitation with careful monitoring of volume status and electrolytes. The underlying cause of the adrenal crisis (eg, infection) should be determined and treated. Hydrocortisone replacement may provide sufficient mineralocorticoid activity in PAI, unless mineralocorticoid deficiency is severe. In chronic adrenal insufficiency, older adults should receive the minimum glucocorticoid and, in PAI, mineralocorticoid replacement doses needed to relieve symptoms and to avoid long-term complications of glucocorticoid excess, volume overload, hypertension, and electrolyte disturbances. Typical replacement doses of glucocorticoid are hydrocortisone 15–25 mg daily in two or three divided doses (SOE=B), or prednisone or prednisolone 3–5 mg daily in one or two divided doses (SOE=D). Mineralocorticoid replacement in PAI is fludrocortisone 50–100 mcg daily (SOE=A). During minor illnesses, patients should take 2–3 times the usual maintenance dose of glucocorticoid for 3 days (SOE=B). These patients should wear a medical alert bracelet or necklace indicating adrenal insufficiency and should be given parenteral stress dose glucocorticoids in the event of major illnesses, trauma, or major surgery (SOE=D).

Hyperadrenocorticoidism

Exogenous glucocorticoids are the most common cause of hyperadrenocorticoidism in older adults, often causing adverse events, including psychiatric and cognitive symptoms, osteoporosis, myopathy, and glucose intolerance. Notably, the use of 10 mg/d of prednisone continuously for >90 days is associated with a 7-fold increase in hip fractures and a 17-fold increased risk

Table 64.7—Diagnostic Evaluation of Hormone Hypersecretion in Patients with Adrenal Incidentalomas

Indications	Potential Diagnosis	Test to Order	Result Supporting the Diagnosis
All patients with incidentaloma and Cushing syndrome manifestations, before major surgery	Functional adrenocortical adenoma	1-mg overnight dexamethasone suppression test	Failure to suppress serum cortisol
All patients with incidentaloma	Pheochromocytoma	24-hour urine for fractionated metanephrines or plasma-free metanephrines	Increased
Before major surgery	Pheochromocytoma	Plasma-free metanephrines	Increased
Hypertension with or without hypokalemia	Primary aldosteronism	Ratio of morning plasma aldosterone concentration to plasma renin activity	Increased

of vertebral fractures. For patients beginning long-term glucocorticoid therapy, baseline and follow-up bone densitometry measurements are indicated; and calcium and vitamin D (SOE=B) and antiresorptive agents, such as bisphosphonates, should be started as appropriate in patients at high risk of fractures for prevention or treatment of glucocorticoid-induced osteoporosis (SOE=A or B, depending on risk group). Teriparatide may be used in cases of severe bone loss (SOE=A). To counteract corticosteroid-induced suppression of sex hormones, hormone replacement therapy may also be appropriate in some cases.

Adrenal Neoplasms

In radiographic studies, the prevalence of clinically inapparent adrenal masses (adrenal incidentalomas) is estimated to be 3%–4% in middle-aged adults, rising to ≥10% in older adults. Most of these are benign adrenocortical adenomas, although pheochromocytomas and adrenocortical carcinomas are also found. When an incidentaloma is discovered, it is important to exclude pheochromocytoma, because these are not uncommon and potentially life threatening.

The goals of assessment are to determine whether the tumor is functional (hormone-secreting) (Table 64.7) and malignant. Endocrinology referral is appropriate when evidence of hormone excess is present. Many adrenocortical adenomas have a degree of functional autonomy, and subclinical glucocorticoid hypersecretion is present in 5%–24% of cases of adrenal incidentalomas. An overnight low-dose (1 mg) dexamethasone suppression test together with measurement of a morning serum ACTH level are appropriate to exclude subclinical Cushing syndrome. Although some of these patients may be at increased risk of new vertebral fractures, hypertension, insulin resistance, and other metabolic derangements, it is unclear whether the long-term outcomes of adrenalectomy are superior to those of medical management. Moreover, screening all older adults with adrenal incidentalomas for glucocorticoid hypersecretion would yield a high proportion of false-positive results. Accordingly, it may be best to limit testing for hyperadrenocorticoidism to younger individuals, those with a symptom complex suggesting hyperadrenocorticoidism, and patients scheduled for major surgery who are at risk of postoperative adrenal crisis due to diminished HPA axis reserve from chronic glucocorticoid excess (SOE=D). Similarly, the merits of screening for primary aldosteronism (PA) in hypertensive older adults are uncertain, and the long-term outcomes of medical versus surgical management of PA are unclear. The risks and benefits of unilateral adrenalectomy for hypertensive older patients with PA due to unilateral adenoma or adrenal hyperplasia should be assessed on a case-by-case basis. Older patients with PA who are unable or unwilling to undergo surgery, or who have bilateral adrenal disease, should be treated with a mineralocorticoid receptor antagonist (SOE=B).

The most helpful indicator in initial assessment of malignancy risk in patients with adrenal incidentaloma is the attenuation coefficient in Hounsfield units (HU) on noncontrast CT imaging. Lesions with attenuation values of ≤10 HU are probably benign. Adrenal masses with values >10 HU but smaller than 4 cm are also likely to be benign adenomas. Interdisciplinary case review and consideration of surgical resection may be appropriate for masses ≥4 cm, especially for lesions >6 cm, and with imaging characteristics suggesting malignancy, such as irregular shape, unilaterality, tumor calcification, and rapid growth rate (SOE=B). In patients with masses >2 cm without clearly benign features who are followed expectantly, imaging should be repeated in 6–12 months to identify rapidly growing tumors, because they are more likely to be malignant (SOE=B).

Adrenal Androgens

Adrenal production of dehydroepiandrosterone (DHEA) and its sulfate (DHEA-S) is the main source of androgens in women; in men the adrenals contribute little to overall androgen production. DHEA and DHEA-S are prohormones that are converted to more active androgens and estrogens in the adrenal glands and peripheral tissues. While trials of oral DHEA have not shown health benefits in postmenopausal women, vaginal low-dose DHEA administration is an approved treatment for the genitourinary syndrome of menopause (see Estrogen Therapy, below). In the vagina, DHEA is converted locally into estrogens and androgens, and daily vaginal administration of DHEA 6.5 mg was found to improve menopausal vaginal atrophy without changing serum levels of estrogenic or androgenic metabolites.

Oral DHEA is available in the United States only as a dietary supplement. The potency and purity of these preparations is unreliable, and the long-term safety of oral DHEA supplementation has not been established.

TESTOSTERONE

Total and free testosterone (T) levels gradually and progressively decline with age and are lower in healthy older men than in younger men; older men commonly have T levels below the normal range for young men. Aging may be associated with nonspecific complaints, such as decreased libido and potency, reduced energy, depressed mood, weakness, decreased muscle mass, osteopenia, and memory loss. Because these manifestations are also consistent with those of T deficiency, the possibility arises that declining T with aging might contribute to their development, and that T treatment might prevent or treat them. Whether declining T levels in older men are simply a biomarker of poor health or a deficiency state in need of treatment is not yet known.

Older men may exhibit varying degrees of combined primary and secondary testicular dysfunction. In advanced old age, testicular production of T decreases, associated with increased gonadotropin levels (primary hypogonadism). Comorbidities and medications may also lead to suppression of gonadotropin levels so that they are not increased but inappropriately normal (secondary hypogonadism). Overt secondary testicular failure is common in chronically ill and debilitated older men and in men receiving chronic opioids or glucocorticoids. These men have severely low T levels and manifestations suggesting T deficiency, such as decreased libido, hair loss, and muscle weakness. T replacement therapy may be warranted in these severely clinically and biochemically T-deficient patients, as it is in hypogonadal young men, but adequate studies of the benefits and risks of T treatment in these patient populations have not been performed.

In the United States, the use of T supplementation by older men has increased nearly 10-fold in the past two decades, driven at least in part by direct-to-consumer advertising campaigns and the availability of transdermal T gel and patch formulations. Many men who are started on T supplementation have not had recent measurement of serum T concentrations, indicating that inappropriate prescribing is common.

Until recently, trials of T treatment in older men have had methodologic limitations. The most consistent findings in early studies were increased muscle mass and decreased fat mass. Effects on physical performance, BMD, sexual function, and energy were inconsistent.

The carefully designed Testosterone Trials (TTrials) were a group of 7 coordinated double-blind, placebo-controlled trials in men ≥65 years old with symptoms and objective evidence of low libido, low vitality, and walking difficulty, and with morning total T levels <275 ng/dL on two occasions. Men were treated with testosterone gel for 1 year at dosages adjusted to maintain normal T levels. Outcomes thought to be related to T deficiency, including sexual function, vitality, physical function, cognitive function, anemia, BMD, and cardiovascular health were assessed. Results showed modest improvements in sexual function; small improvements in walking distance, mood, and depression symptoms; and no change in vitality. BMD increased in amounts comparable to those achieved with standard osteoporosis therapies, and estimated bone strength improved. However, BMD was not low in study participants, and the study was not designed to assess changes in fracture risk. T treatment did not improve memory or other cognitive functions in men with age-associated memory impairment but did increase hemoglobin levels in men with anemia as well as those without anemia. In a cardiovascular sub-study using CT to measure coronary artery plaque volume, compared with placebo, T treatment was associated with a greater increase in total and noncalcified plaque volume but not in calcified plaque or in the number of cardiovascular events.

The TEAAM Trial was a randomized, controlled trial of T supplementation for 3 years in healthy men ≥60 years old with total T levels of 100–400 ng/dL or free T levels <50 pg/mL. Modest improvements in stair-climbing power, muscle mass, and power were found in the group receiving supplement, but the clinical significance of these findings is uncertain. Results of ultrasonography and CT did not show an effect of T on the rates of change in coronary artery calcium or common carotid artery intima-media thickness. Meta-analyses of trials of T treatment have reported conflicting results of the risk of cardiovascular events in participants receiving T. Taken together, the TTrials and the TEAAM Trial provide evidence only for short-term benefits of T treatment but do not allay concerns about possible long-term risks of cardiovascular, prostate, or other adverse events.

Men with clinical manifestations of T deficiency should be evaluated initially with a morning, preferably

Table 64.8—Testosterone Preparations Available in the United States for Hypogonadal Older Men

Preparation	Initial Treatment Dosage
Testosterone enanthate or cypionate	75 mg IM every week, or 150 mg IM every 2 weeks
Testosterone undecanoate	750 mg IM initially, followed by 750 mg IM 4 weeks later, then 750 mg every 10 weeks thereafter
Nonscrotal transdermal patch	2 or 4 mg transdermal every night
Gel	1% gel: 25–100 mg transdermal every day 1.62% gel: 20.25–81 mg every day 2% gel: 10–70 mg every day
Solution	30–120 mg applied to axilla once daily
Intranasal gel	5.5 mg (1 actuation) each nostril 3 times daily
Buccal tablet	30 mg applied to buccal mucosa every 12 hours
Testosterone pellets	150–450 mg SC every 3–6 months

fasting, serum total T level using an accurate and reliable assay. The diagnosis should be confirmed with a repeat morning total T, or, ideally, with a morning serum free T level, measured by equilibrium dialysis or calculated from measurements of total T and sex hormone–binding globulin (SHBG). Alternatively, a bioavailable (non–sex hormone–binding globulin-bound) T level may be determined. Direct "analogue" immunoassays for free T are widely used but are inaccurate and not recommended. If abnormally low T levels are confirmed, luteinizing hormone and follicle-stimulating hormone levels should be obtained to determine whether low T is due to a disorder of the testes (primary hypogonadism) or a hypothalamic-pituitary disorder (secondary hypogonadism). Medications that can suppress gonadotropins (eg, glucocorticoids, opioids, and other medications with CNS activity) should be discontinued if possible, and a prolactin level obtained if gonadotropins are low or inappropriately normal in the presence of low T levels. High prolactin concentrations inhibit gonadotropin secretion and could be due to a pituitary adenoma, a hypothalamic disorder, or medications. Further studies (eg, MRI of the pituitary fossa, assessment of other pituitary functions) may be warranted in such patients with guidance from an endocrinologist. Baseline BMD measurements should be obtained in older men with decreased T levels to exclude osteoporosis.

T supplementation should be considered only after potentially reversible functional causes of hypogonadism are addressed. Based on the uncertainties described above, the FDA cautions that T replacement therapy may be associated with increased cardiovascular risk. Accordingly, caution is suggested when using T treatment in frail older men with established cardiovascular disease or cardiovascular risk factors. After explicit discussion of the uncertain risks and benefits of T therapy, including potential increased cardiovascular and prostate cancer risk, a trial of T supplementation may be appropriate in older men with unequivocally and repeatedly severely low serum total and free (or bioavailable) T levels (eg, <200 ng/dL), and clinical features suggesting hypogonadism (eg, loss of libido, muscle wasting or weakness, osteoporosis or mild anemia of unclear cause)[OL] (SOE=C). Clinicians should aim to achieve total T levels in the lower part of the normal range for young men (eg, 400–500 ng/dL). Androgen replacement therapy is inappropriate in asymptomatic older men with low-normal total and free T levels who do not have clinical manifestations consistent with T deficiency. Older men with mildly reduced T levels and nonspecific symptoms will benefit most from other approaches, including lifestyle interventions, for problems such as obesity, muscle weakness, erectile dysfunction, depression, and osteoporosis. T administration is contraindicated in patients with prostate cancer and breast cancer and should be avoided in men with the following: undiagnosed prostate nodule or induration on digital rectal examination, consistently increased prostate-specific antigen (PSA) levels, erythrocytosis, severe lower urinary tract symptoms due to benign prostatic hyperplasia, or uncontrolled severe heart failure (SOE=C). For available preparations of T, see Table 64.8.

Men should be monitored closely for efficacy as well as for adverse events of T treatment, including new or worsening snoring, observed apnea during sleep, or excessive daytime sleepiness that may suggest obstructive sleep apnea. Routine monitoring for efficacy and potential adverse effects should be performed within the first year after initiation and then annually thereafter (SOE=C). Monitoring should include measurement of serum hematocrit to check for erythrocytosis, and inquiry about lower urinary tract symptoms and gynecomastia at 3–6 months after starting T treatment. Prostate cancer screening should be offered with a discussion of risks and benefits of screening to men with a remaining life expectancy of >10 years, particularly in men at high risk for prostate cancer (black Americans or men who have a first-degree relative with prostate cancer). If desired by the patient, serum PSA and digital rectal examination should be performed before and 3–12 months after starting T treatment (to detect the presence of prostate cancer at baseline or shortly after starting therapy). Serum T levels should be monitored to assess the adequacy of delivery, especially in men receiving transdermal T formulations (patch or gel). After T treatment has begun, a PSA concentration >4 ng/mL (or >3 ng/mL in men with a high risk of prostate cancer), or a palpable prostate nodule or induration, can indicate the presence of previously undetected prostate cancer. In these circumstances, T treatment should be discontinued until the prostate has been fully evaluated by a urologist (SOE=C). Despite this guidance, there is as yet no direct evidence that T treatment increases risk of prostate cancer or symptomatic benign prostatic hyperplasia.

RESOURCES

- Snyder PJ, Bhasin S, Cunningham GR, et al. Lessons From the Testosterone Trials. *Endocr Rev*. 2018;39(3):369–386.

- Stott DJ, Rodondi N, Kearney PM, et al; TRUST Study Group. Thyroid hormone therapy for older adults with subclinical hypothyroidism. *N Engl J Med*. 2017;376(26):2534–2544.

CHAPTER 65—DIABETES MELLITUS

KEY POINTS

- Diabetes mellitus, one of the most common chronic conditions in older adults, results in decreased life expectancy, numerous complications and comorbidities, a higher risk of other common geriatric conditions (eg, polypharmacy, urinary incontinence, falls, cognitive impairment, depression, chronic pain), and disability.

- Lifestyle modifications, such as exercise and weight loss, have been demonstrated to prevent diabetes in high-risk patients and can help in management of hyperglycemia in patients with diabetes.

- Because of the great heterogeneity in the older population, treatment goals for older diabetic patients must be carefully individualized.

- Although the target blood pressure is debated, attempts to lower blood pressure are important for older hypertensive diabetic patients.

- Diabetes self-management is an important part of diabetes care, and annual self-management training is a covered benefit under Medicare Part B.

Diabetes mellitus (DM), which is a group of metabolic disorders characterized by hyperglycemia due to abnormalities in insulin secretion, insulin action, or both, is one of the most common chronic diseases affecting older adults. Because the general population is aging and rates of obesity are increasing among middle-aged adults, people ≥65 years old will constitute the majority of diabetic adults in the United States and in other developed countries in the coming decades. The age-adjusted prevalence of DM is higher among black Americans and Hispanic Americans than white Americans. Further, black Americans suffer from complications of diabetes at disproportionately higher rates than white Americans. Research is only starting to decipher the effects of race on diabetes development and outcomes.

DM in older adults leads to higher rates of vascular complications and geriatric syndromes, which in turn lead to increased morbidity and mortality. Older adults with diabetes can expect a 10-year reduction in life expectancy and a mortality rate nearly twice that of people without diabetes. In addition, older adults disproportionately experience the vascular complications of diabetes such as atherosclerosis, neuropathies, visual impairment, and renal insufficiency. Mobility problems are about 2–3 times more likely, and disability in activities of daily living is about 1.5 times more likely, in older adults with diabetes than in those without.

PATHOPHYSIOLOGY OF DIABETES

More than 90% of older adults with diabetes have type 2 DM, which is generally characterized by insulin resistance, increased insulin requirements to maintain euglycemia, and ultimately relative insulin deficiency when the pancreatic beta cells are unable to meet the higher insulin requirements. The prevalence of type 2 DM increases with age.

Less than 10% of older adults with diabetes have type 1 DM, which is characterized by autoimmune destruction of pancreatic beta cells, resulting in an absolute insulin deficiency. Unlike most patients with type 2 DM, all patients with type 1 DM require exogenous insulin.

DIAGNOSIS AND EVALUATION

In 2009, an international group of diabetes experts recommended using a hemoglobin A_{1c} (HbA_{1c}) level of ≥6.5% to diagnose diabetes; the American Diabetes Association (ADA) participated in that decision and formally adopted this recommendation in 2010. This decision was based on the ease of performing the HbA_{1c} test, which can facilitate diagnosis of more people with diabetes. None of the diagnostic criteria include any adjustments for age. The 4 ways to establish the diagnosis of diabetes mellitus are summarized below; each must be confirmed, on a subsequent day, preferably by the same method.

- HbA_{1c} ≥6.5% using an assay standardized to the national glycohemoglobin standardization program

- Symptoms of polyuria, polydipsia, and unexplained weight loss, plus a random plasma glucose concentration of ≥200 mg/dL (11.1 mmol/L)

- A plasma glucose concentration after an 8-hour fast of ≥126 mg/dL (7 mmol/L)

- A plasma glucose concentration of ≥200 mg/dL (11.1 mmol/L) measured 2 hours after ingestion of 75 g of glucose in 300 mL of water administered after an overnight fast

PREVENTION

Several diabetes prevention trials demonstrated that in people with impaired glucose tolerance at high risk of developing type 2 DM, lifestyle modification that focuses on diet, exercise, and weight loss can delay or prevent progression to diabetes (SOE=A). The largest of these studies was the Diabetes Prevention Program, which tested whether metformin or lifestyle modification decreased progression to diabetes in high-risk adults. Among older adults (>60 years), lifestyle modification was especially powerful, decreasing the incidence of diabetes by 71% compared with usual care in 2.8 years of follow-up. Metformin, however, decreased the incidence of diabetes by only 11% in older adults, compared with 44% in younger adults (25–44 years old). Thus, for obese older adults at high risk of diabetes, the preferred approach to diabetes prevention should involve lifestyle modification (diet, exercise, and weight loss) and not initiation of metformin.

MANAGEMENT

General Principles

Older adults with diabetes require a comprehensive evaluation, which in the primary care setting may be done over several patient visits. For patients with significant functional impairments and comorbidities, including those with psychosocial problems and caregiver requirements, a formal, comprehensive geriatric assessment may be needed. Regardless of how the comprehensive evaluation of an older adult with DM is handled, 3 issues deserve special attention.

First, the history and physical examination must include evaluation of risk factors for atherosclerotic disease and the presence of all comorbid diseases. Diabetes is a well-established risk factor for atherosclerotic cardiovascular disease (ASCVD), so other risk factors such as smoking, family history, hypertension, and hyperlipidemia should also be explored. Diabetes is also associated with multiple vascular complications that may be subclinical or clinical. The presence of coronary artery disease, peripheral vascular disease, neuropathy, foot problems, and medical eye disease must be determined. In many cases, subspecialty consultation (such as for retinopathy) and laboratory or diagnostic testing is indicated. In addition, older adults with diabetes are also likely to have prevalent chronic diseases that are not necessarily associated with their diabetes, such as osteoarthritis, which may affect DM management.

Second, obtaining a thorough medication history is important. Certain medications, such as glucocorticoids, can contribute to hyperglycemia. More often, older adults may be prescribed multiple drugs for multiple comorbidities and may experience adverse drug events, trouble with medication management, or difficulty affording medications for their diabetes. A medication review will help to minimize polypharmacy and to formulate optimal and individualized treatment plans.

Third, assessments of common geriatric syndromes and psychosocial domains are critical. Multiple studies have shown that functional impairment, urinary incontinence, falls, pain, cognitive impairment, and depression are all more common in older adults with diabetes (SOE=B). An assessment of geriatric syndromes will help identify important factors that affect treatment plans. For example, a functional assessment will help identify a patient's ability to increase physical activity. A cognitive and depression assessment will help identify a patient's ability to self-manage his or her diabetes. Psychosocial assessment may help to identify important elements that support the patient's DM management (such as involved family members) and barriers that may limit the patient's ability to adhere to treatment plans.

Goals of Diabetes Care

The clinician should develop goals for management and individualized clinical targets with each older adult with diabetes, involving the caregiver when appropriate. The goals of DM management in older adults include the following:

- Control of hyperglycemia and its symptoms

- Evaluation and treatment of associated risks for atherosclerotic and microvascular disease

- Evaluation and treatment of diabetes complications

- Avoiding hypoglycemia

Although these goals are similar for older and younger people with diabetes, the management of older patients is complicated by the medical and functional heterogeneity of this group. In fact, this heterogeneity is a key consideration in developing individualized diabetes management interventions and clinical targets for older patients with diabetes. Some may have developed diabetes in middle age and have developed multiple related comorbidities. Others may have just converted from impaired glucose tolerance to diabetes and have few complications or comorbidities. In addition to medical heterogeneity, older adults with diabetes are heterogeneous in their functional status. Many are active with excellent function. Others are disabled and frail, with advanced cognitive impairment, multiple comorbidities and complications, and significant functional limitations. Still others are in between, with mild or early functional limitations, several related comorbidities, and multiple risks for worsening morbidity.

An important consideration in treating older adults with diabetes is life expectancy, in the context of the time needed for clinical benefit from a specific intervention. Clinical trials have demonstrated that >8 years are needed before the benefits of glycemic control are reflected in reduced microvascular complications such as diabetic retinopathy or kidney disease but that only 2–3 years are required to see benefits from better control of blood pressure and lipids (SOE=A). Attempting tight glycemic control in a patient with limited life expectancy often leads to increased risk of hypoglycemia with little chance that the patient will survive to benefit from the long-term lower risk of vascular complications. Conversely, it is important to remember that the median remaining life expectancy for a 70-year-old woman is 17 years, which allows plenty of time for diabetes complications to develop. Therefore, for a person in his or her early 70s who is newly diagnosed or highly functional, diabetes management is similar to that of a younger person, but with consideration of slightly relaxing the glycemic target to 7%–7.5%. In general, glycemic control should be tighter in healthier older patients with an extended life expectancy, and less stringent in sicker older patients with limited life expectancy.

Patient preferences must be elicited and considered, because the patient is the one who will ultimately manage his or her diabetes and comorbid conditions. Some patients do not want to follow some management recommendations. Some fear dependency and the need for assistance more than death. Some find certain medications or monitoring activities burdensome.

Therefore, it is important to establish individual goals for diabetes management and clinical targets with patients; to reevaluate the patient's clinical, functional, and social status if these goals and targets are not being met; and to determine if caregiver support or specialty input is needed. A practical clinical method of individualizing and prioritizing diabetes care is to assess goals and preferences, assess patient longevity and functional status, consider the time needed for treatment impact, screen for geriatric syndromes, and assist patients with decision making and prioritization of treatment strategies.

The American Geriatrics Society developed guidelines for improving the care of older adults with diabetes mellitus in 2003 and published an update in 2013. The ADA annually updates its guidelines for the medical care of patients with diabetes. Both guidelines stress that older adults with diabetes are remarkably heterogeneous, requiring clinicians to individualize both treatment goals and therapies to achieve optimal patient outcomes.

INTERVENTIONS

Evidence supports the effectiveness of several components of diabetes care, including control of lipids and blood pressure, smoking cessation, appropriate eye and foot care, diabetes education and self-management support for medication adherence, appropriate nutrition, weight loss if indicated, and increased physical activity (SOE=A). Studies suggest that these interventions decrease vascular complications, including myocardial infarctions and strokes (macrovascular outcomes) and nephropathy and retinopathy (microvascular outcomes). Home monitoring of blood glucose has not been found to be cost-effective (SOE=A). Very few of the data supporting these interventions were obtained from research studies of older adults, adding uncertainty to whether these conclusions are appropriate for geriatric patients. In addition, debates continue about the targets for glycemic and blood pressure control. It is likely that many management guidelines can be generalized to the care of many older adults with diabetes, particularly those who are healthy and functional. But for some older patients, particularly those with severe comorbidities and disabilities, aggressive management is not likely to provide benefit and may even result in harm, such as hypoglycemia with aggressive glycemic control or hypotension with aggressive blood pressure control.

Older adults with diabetes should undergo age-appropriate prevention interventions such as influenza and pneumococcal vaccinations. In addition, because lower extremity infections and amputations are more common in older adults with diabetes than in those without diabetes, careful annual foot examination is recommended. To screen for kidney disease, a test for the presence of albuminuria should be performed at diagnosis and annually (SOE=C). If a patient is taking an ACE inhibitor or angiotensin-receptor blocker, there is no need for continued screening for albuminuria (SOE=D).

Diabetes Education and Self-Management Support

Because diabetes is a disease for which the patient and/or caregivers bear the primary responsibility for management and ultimate control, it is imperative that the patient and/or caregiver(s) are wholly engaged in diabetes self-management. Therefore, education about diabetes, and particularly diabetes self-management, are key components of effective care. Often, basic education can be accomplished in the primary care setting. Patients with diabetes and other comorbidities may need referral to a diabetes educator for one-on-one counseling or group classes, enrollment in a comprehensive diabetes disease management program, or specialty physician care. Annual diabetes self-management training is a covered benefit under Medicare Part B. Education programs for DM may be particularly important in older adults with diabetes who are members of minority groups, particularly black Americans or Hispanic Americans. For patients who are cognitively impaired, significantly disabled or frail, or have communication issues (eg, limited English proficiency), caregivers must be highly involved and educated about diabetes and its management.

Diabetes self-management and support must encompass several important areas. The older patient, and caregiver if appropriate, must be educated about hypo- and hyperglycemia, including precipitating factors, prevention, symptoms, monitoring, treatment, and indications for notifying the clinician. For patients requiring insulin, the patient and caregiver should be taught blood glucose self-monitoring, with periodic reassessment and reinforcement of technique as needed. Finally, every older adult with diabetes and the caregiver(s) should be educated about risk factors for foot ulcers and amputation. Ability to care for the feet (including trimming toenails and inspection for sores) should be emphasized.

Diet and physical activity remain important components of the initial and ongoing management of patients with diabetes. Specific dietary recommendations must be tailored for each individual and include assessment of cholesterol intake and weight management. Physical activity programs should also be individualized. The patient should be assessed regularly for level of physical activity and informed about the benefits of exercise and available resources for becoming more active.

Smoking Cessation

Meta-analyses of studies suggest that smoking cessation reduces cardiovascular events 3- to 5-fold among patients with diabetes compared with patients without diabetes. Further, smoking cessation leads to greater reductions in mortality than control of blood pressure or lipids. Thus, smoking cessation counseling and pharmacologic intervention should be offered to any older adult with diabetes who smokes.

Aspirin for Primary Prevention of Cardiovascular Disease

It is unclear whether older adults with diabetes but no other history of cardiovascular disease would benefit from aspirin. The American Diabetes Association suggests that low-dose aspirin (75–162 mg daily) may be beneficial in adults with diabetes if they have a 10-year risk of cardiovascular events of at least 10%, *and* they are without an increased risk of bleeding (SOE=C). In contrast, the 2016 European Guidelines on Cardiovascular Disease Prevention recommends against aspirin use for primary prevention.

Blood Pressure Management

A number of randomized controlled trials provide strong evidence that management of hypertension in adults with diabetes reduces cardiovascular events and mortality; some of these studies included substantial numbers of older adults with diabetes (SOE=A). The most appropriate target blood pressure for older diabetic patients is unclear. The Eighth Joint National Committee (JNC-8) guideline recommended a target blood pressure of <140/90 mmHg, and the preponderance of evidence suggests that for healthier patients with fewer comorbidities, few functional limitations, and longer life expectancy, a blood pressure target of 120–140 systolic and 70–80 diastolic may be ideal. In the international ADVANCE trial, with 11,140 people having a mean age of 66 years, a mean blood pressure of 136/73 mmHg was achieved in the intensive treatment group, in which the relative risk of cardiovascular death decreased 18% and the relative risk of all-cause death decreased 14% (ARR=1.3%, NNT=79 for all-cause mortality over 5 years) (SOE=A). In contrast, in the ACCORD study, a blood pressure of <119/70 mmHg was achieved in the intensive treatment arm (versus 140/70 mmHg in the standard treatment arm), and no significant benefit of intensive blood pressure on cardiovascular outcomes was observed (SOE=A).

Some older adults may not be able to tolerate intensive blood pressure lowering; thus, hypertension treatment should be advanced gradually. Recent studies demonstrated that the use of multiple antihypertensive drugs was associated with increased serious adverse effects, such as hypotension, syncope, and worsening renal function. If a patient develops orthostasis, then falls, fractures, and functional limitations may result. For patients with orthostatic hypotension, the harms of treatment may outweigh the benefits, and relaxing the blood pressure target may be most appropriate. Evidence for the choice of antihypertensive medication in older adults with diabetes suggests that most classes chosen (diuretics, ACE inhibitors, β-blockers, and calcium channel blockers) have comparable effectiveness in reducing cardiovascular disease and mortality. ACE inhibitors (SOE=A) and angiotensin II receptor blockers (SOE=B) have additional renal benefit for people with diabetic nephropathy as compared with other classes of antihypertensive medication.

Lipid Management

Randomized controlled trials and a meta-analysis have confirmed the benefit of the statin drugs, particularly for secondary prevention of cardiovascular events (SOE=A). In general, most studies with statin management suggest that patients with diabetes benefit more from cholesterol lowering than those without diabetes, and secondary prevention is particularly beneficial. Analyses have calculated NNTs of 14 to 46 for secondary prevention of one major cardiovascular event over 5 years of lipid-lowering treatment in diabetic patients.

In contrast to secondary prevention, there is conflicting data on whether primary prevention of hyperlipidemia decreases cardiovascular events in patients with diabetes. In 2013, the American Heart Association, American College of Cardiology, and the National Heart, Lung and Blood Institute published new guidelines for cholesterol treatment to decrease atherosclerotic disease. They suggested that although LDL levels are beneficial in risk-stratifying patients, there is little evidence that treating to a specific LDL target is beneficial. For adults with diabetes age 40–75 and LDL between 70–189 mg/dL, high-dose statins are recommended for those with 10-year ASCVD risk ≥7.5%. Moderate-dose statins are recommended for those with ASCVD risk <7.5%. Further, the 2017 ADA guidelines suggest that although continuation of statins beyond age 75 is reasonable, it is important to routinely evaluate the risk-benefit profile for this age group to determine the appropriateness of high-intensity statin use. It is unclear whether starting statins for primary prevention is beneficial for those >75 years old.

Lipid panel and alanine aminotransferase concentration should be measured within 12 weeks of starting or changing the dosage of a statin or niacin to assess adherence and response to the drug. Routine monitoring of liver function tests is unnecessary in patients who have been taking statins. Statins can cause a range of muscle injury, ranging from rhabdomyolysis (<0.5% of patients) to myalgias (9.3% among healthy, young volunteers). More potent statins at higher doses appear to increase the risk of adverse effects.

There have been concerns about statin use and its possible effects on cognitive dysfunction and diabetes incidence. A systematic review in 2013 that evaluated cognition in patients receiving statins found no adverse effect of these drugs on cognition; therefore, the concerns about cognitive dysfunction should not deter the use of statins in adults at high risk of ASCVD. Several studies have suggested increased risk of diabetes with statin use, but it is important to consider risk-benefit profile. A meta-analysis of 13 randomized controlled trials of 91,140 participants showed an odds ratio of 1.09 for a new diagnosis of diabetes, so that, on average, treatment with statin for 255 participants over 4 years resulted in one additional case of diabetes while preventing 5.4 vascular events.

Glycemic Control

Control of hyperglycemia in diabetes is important to prevent the symptoms of uncontrolled hyperglycemia, such as weight loss, fatigue, and polyuria and polydipsia. Improved glucose control may reduce infection risk as well. The benefit of treatment of hyperglycemia in type 2 DM to prevent vascular complications is more controversial. Control of hyperglycemia to near-normal levels may prevent retinal and renal complications, but the effects are modest and lead to a 1.5- to 3-fold increase in the risk of serious hypoglycemia (SOE=A). Three large, randomized trials of intensive versus moderate control of hyperglycemia, VADT, ADVANCE, and ACCORD, did not demonstrate any benefit of intensive control (targeting HbA_{1c} to <6.5%) on cardiovascular outcomes (SOE=A). The glycemic control arm of ACCORD was terminated early because of excess mortality in the intensively controlled group (1.41% versus 1.14% per year; hazard ratio 1.22 [95% CI, 1.01–1.46]). All three studies investigated patients with long-standing diabetes and included older patients with comorbidities (mean ages were 60 ± 6 years in VADT, 62 ± 6 years in ACCORD, and 66 ± 6 years in ADVANCE; <1% of enrolled patients were ≥80 years old at baseline). Long-term follow-up (10–20 years) of the UK Prospective Diabetes Study (UKPDS) suggested an effect of more intensive control on cardiovascular outcomes, but UKPDS targeted younger adults (mean age 54) with newly diagnosed diabetes.

The VADT and ADVANCE trials found that control of hyperglycemia to a target HbA_{1c} <7% in patients with long-standing diabetes reduced microalbuminuria, and analyses of ACCORD also showed lower rates of microvascular complications (SOE=A). Given the benefits of tighter glycemic control on microvascular complications and the associated harms of tighter glycemic control on hypoglycemic risks and mortality, glycemic targets for all patients with diabetes are unclear and continue to be debated. Most guidelines and experts strongly recommend individualizing glycemic targets, with a HbA_{1c} target near 7% appropriate for healthier older adults with excellent self-management skills and closer to 8.5%–9% for more frail patients.

Pharmacologic Interventions for Diabetes

In addition to the biguanide, sulfonylurea, thiazolidinediones, α-glucosidase inhibitors for oral agents and insulin for injectable agent, newer classes of medications both in oral and injectable forms have been developed to treat diabetes. There are several classes of medications (Table 65.1 and Table 65.2) for treatment of diabetes with the goals of glycemic control and reduction of long-term complications. The medications can be used alone or in combination in a stepwise approach. The regimen should be reassessed and adjusted over time as goals change, the disease progresses, or complications develop.

Metformin is the first-line therapy for diabetes because of its high efficacy on glycemic control, low hypoglycemia risk, and strong evidence of improved clinical outcomes. It can contribute to GI adverse effects, such as dyspepsia, change in bowel habits, or abdominal discomfort. Although lactic acidosis has historically been a concern with metformin use, a Cochrane review found no significantly increased risk of this metabolic complication. In older adults taking metformin, renal function should be monitored at least annually and with any increase in dosage. For those ≥80 years old or suspected to have reduced muscle mass, renal function can be monitored by using a formula that accounts for age, or through a timed urine collection, which can be cumbersome to perform. Sulfonylureas are also very effective in glycemic control; however, they carry a moderate risk of hypoglycemia; these medications must be used cautiously in older adults with significant hepatic and renal insufficiency, because the primary site of metabolism is the liver and excretion is via the kidneys. Meglitinides are similar to sulfonylureas in terms of mechanism of action but may have a slightly lower risk of hypoglycemia. α-Glucosidase inhibitors impair the breakdown of carbohydrates in the gut and limit absorption; the residual carbohydrates in the intestinal lumen are responsible for diarrhea observed in about 25% of older adults who use these medications. The thiazolidinediones, although apparently well tolerated by most patients, carry black box warnings because of a risk of worsening of heart failure; they should be avoided in patients with NYHA Class III or IV heart failure. Because of the concern about increased cardiovascular events, access to rosiglitazone was restricted from 2010 to 2014. However, subsequent analysis of data from the Rosiglitazone Evaluated for Cardiovascular Outcomes and Regulation of Glycemia in Diabetes (RECORD) trial suggested that rates of cardiovascular events were not different between participants taking rosiglitazone versus other classes of medications for diabetes. The RECORD study results led the FDA to lift the restrictions on rosiglitazone prescription. Pioglitazone should be avoided in those with bladder cancer. Sodium glucose cotransporter 2 (SGLT2) inhibitors promote renal excretion of glucose to reduce blood glucose levels. Hypoglycemia risk is low, and SGLT2 inhibitors may decrease weight and blood pressure through osmotic diuresis. However, SGLT2 inhibitors may lead to dehydration and orthostatic hypotension as well as an increased risk of vulvovaginal candidiasis and urinary tract infections. The DPP-4 enzyme inhibitors and newer injectable agents, the glucagon-like peptide 1-receptor agonists (GLP-1-RA) such as exenatide, are effective in lowering glucose levels. DPP-4 enzyme inhibitors are generally well tolerated and weight neutral, but GLP-1-RA can have GI adverse effects, which may contribute to weight loss. GLP-1-RA should be avoided in patients with significant chronic kidney disease, gastroparesis, history of pancreatitis, and family or personal history of medullary thyroid cancer.

The GLP-1-RA have a limited role in routine care of older adults with diabetes, because they are costly and require injection, but liraglutide should be considered for its additional benefit of reducing cardiovascular risk among the subpopulation of older adults approximately 60–70 years old, who have type 2 diabetes and also one or more cardiovascular risk factor(s).

In caring for older adults with type 2 DM, insulin is generally used as part of dual therapy with metformin, or in the transition from oral to injectable therapy. The appropriate HbA_{1c} goal should be determined before starting insulin therapy, reassessed every 3 months during initial treatment, and monitored every 6 months once at target. Adequate glycemic control can often be achieved with a once daily long-acting insulin preparation or two injections daily of an intermediate-acting insulin preparation for older diabetic patients who are not candidates for oral medications and/or who have difficulty with adherence to multiple oral or injectable agents.

Hypoglycemia is increasingly recognized as an important issue among older adults with diabetes. Longer-acting sulfonylureas (such as glyburide) more commonly cause hypoglycemia than shorter-acting sulfonylureas (such as glipizide). The greatest risk of insulin therapy is hypoglycemia; frail older adults are at higher risk of serious hypoglycemia than healthier, more functional individuals. In patients with a history of hypoglycemia, or those with multiple comorbidities and poor functional status who are at risk of hypoglycemia, short-acting sulfonylureas or oral antidiabetics that do not cause hypoglycemia should be used. Psychosocial reasons for hypoglycemia must be investigated and treated, such as an inability to understand self-management because of cognitive problems, inadequate diabetes knowledge, difficulty in implementing therapy because of disability, cost, or lack of caregiver support. The management plan for an older adult with diabetes who experiences severe or frequent hypoglycemia should be modified, and the clinician should consider increasing the glycemic target.

MANAGEMENT OF DIABETES ACROSS THE CONTINUUM OF CARE

Older adults living with diabetes may transition through different levels of care, including home and/or assisted living, hospital, skilled-nursing facility and/or nursing home, and hospice. Management of diabetes may differ in different settings, depending on the level of support available at each site.

For those who are independent and living in the community or in assisted living, it is reasonable to manage diabetes in a step-wise fashion. In addition to involving family members or caregivers for adults living at home, it is important to consider the support available

Table 65.1—Pharmacologic Agents for Treating Diabetes Mellitus

Medication Class Individual Agent(s)	HbA_{1c} Lowering (percent)	Mechanism of Action	Risk of Hypoglycemia	Weight	Other Adverse Effects
Oral Agents					
Biguanide Metformin	1–2	Inhibit hepatic gluconeogenesis, increase insulin sensitivity, decrease intestinal glucose absorption	Low	Neutral/loss	GI, lactic acidosis
2nd-Generation sulfonylureas Glimepiride Glipizide Glyburide	1–2	Increase insulin secretion	Moderate	Gain	GI, skin reaction, abnormal liver function tests
α-Glucosidase inhibitors Acarbose Miglitol	0.5–1	Delay glucose absorption	Moderate	Gain	GI
DPP-4 enzyme inhibitors Alogliptin Linagliptin Sitagliptin Saxagliptin	0.5–1	Inhibit degradation of endogenous incretin hormones	Low	Neutral	Rare
Meglitinides Nateglinide Repaglinide	1–2	Increase insulin secretion	Moderate	Gain	Hypoglycemia
Thiazolidinediones Pioglitazone Rosiglitazone	0.5–1.5	Increase insulin sensitivity	Low	Gain	Edema, risk of heart failure, fracture
SGLT2 inhibitors Canagliflozin Dapagliflozin Empagliflozin	0.5–1.5	Promote renal excretion of glucose	Low	Loss	Genitourinary infection, dehydration, hypotension, fracture
Other Bromocriptine Colesevelam	0.5	Unknown Bile acid sequestrant			GI GI
Injectable Agents					
GLP-1 receptor agonists Exenatide Liraglutide Lixisenatide Albiglutide Dulaglutide	0.7–1	Increase insulin secretion, slow gastric emptying, reduce postprandial glucagon, reduce food intake	Low	Loss	GI
Amylin analogue Pramlintide	0.4–0.7	Slow gastric emptying, promote satiety, reduce abnormal postprandial rise of glucagon	Low	Loss	GI
Insulin	Unlimited		High	Gain	Hypoglycemia

from facility staff at assisted living when choosing the appropriate regimen for glycemic control. Importantly, assisted living facilities often have few or no staff with medical training. Tradeoffs are common between glycemic control and preferred residential arrangements.

When older adults with diabetes are hospitalized, blood glucose levels can fluctuate in the setting of acute illness, altered oral intake, or prescribed hospital diet. In the NICE-SUGAR trial, the risk of severe hypoglycemia and mortality was increased when blood glucose

Table 65.2—Insulin Preparations

Preparations	Onset	Peak (hours)	Duration (hours)	Number of Injections or Inhalations/day
Rapid-acting				
Insulin glulisine (Apidra)	20 min	0.5–1.5	3–4	3
Insulin lispro (Humalog)	15 min	0.5–1.5	3–4	3
Insulin aspart (NovoLog)	30 min	1–3	3–5	3
Inhaled (Afrezza)[a]	15 min	1	3–4	3
Regular (eg, Humulin R, Humulin R U-500, Novolin R)[b]	0.5–1 h	2–3	5–8	1–3
Intermediate or long-acting				
NPH (eg, Humulin, Novolin)[b]	1–1.5 h	4–12	24	1–2
Insulin detemir (Levemir)	3–4 h	6–8	6–24 depending on dose	1–2
Insulin glargine (Lantus, Toujeo, Basaglar)[c]	2–4 h	—	24	1
Insulin degludec (Tresiba)	1 h	12	>24	1
Combinations				
Isophane insulin and regular insulin injectable (Novolin 70/30)	See individual drugs	2–12	24	1–2
Insulin lispro protamine suspension and insulin lispro (Humalog mix 50/50; 75/25)	See individual drugs	1–6.5	14–24	1–2
Insulin degludec and insulin aspart (Ryzodeg 70/30)	See individual drugs	1	>24	1–2

NOTE: NPH = neutral protamine Hagedorn (insulin)
[a] Available as 4-unit and 8-unit single-use cartridges administered by inhalation.
[b] Also available as mixtures of NPH and regular in 50:50 proportions.
[c] To convert from NPH dosing, give same number of units once a day. For patients taking NPH q12h, decrease the total daily units by 20% and titrate on basis of response. Starting dosage in insulin-naive patients is 10 U once daily at bedtime.
SOURCE: Adapted with permission from Reuben DB, Herr KA, Pacala JT, et al. *Geriatrics At Your Fingertips*, 20th ed. New York: American Geriatrics Society; 2018:107–108.

levels were tightly controlled in ICU patients. It is reasonable to hold non-insulin therapies while a patient is hospitalized. Insulin therapy should be initiated for patients with persistent hyperglycemia ≥180 mg/dL and adjusted to a target of 140–180 mg/dL for both critically ill and non-critically ill patients. These targets can be achieved with basal insulin, or basal insulin plus bolus correction ("sliding scale") insulin regimen for patients with poor oral intake or nothing by mouth status. An insulin regimen with basal, nutritional, and correction components is preferred for patients with adequate nutritional intake. Intravenous insulin is preferred in critically ill patients who experience diabetic ketoacidosis or hyperosmolar hyperglycemia with mental obtundation. Basal/bolus insulin with or without correction regimens lead to better glycemic control and reduced hospital complications than sliding scale insulin alone. Hypoglycemia protocols should be implemented when blood glucose is ≤70 mg/dL. When a patient is ready to be discharged, it is important to consider the support for diabetes care available in the discharge setting and adjust the treatment for diabetes accordingly, based on the type and severity of diabetes, the effects of the acute illness on the patient's glucose, the patient's goals, and the ability to attain glycemic control. Communication with the outpatient provider about diabetes management can facilitate safe transitions of care in this regard.

Older adults who reside transiently in skilled-nursing facilities are often recovering from an acute illness with rehabilitation needs, or have significant functional decline and frailty. As demonstrated in a retrospective study, one-third of these older adults living with diabetes had documented hypoglycemia. They often rely completely on the care plan and nursing support to receive their medications. Furthermore, they may have less regular food intake due to their other comorbidities or symptoms, such as anoxia, dysphagia, cognitive impairment, and renal dysfunction. Medical providers are also not required to evaluate patients daily in skilled-nursing facilities or in long-term care nursing home settings. In this case, it is reasonable to establish protocols to alert medical providers so that management of diabetes can be assessed and adjusted as necessary. For example, it could be established that medical providers should be notified for blood glucose measurements <60 mg/dL within 1 hour, and >300 mg/dL in 24 hours.

A much less stringent approach to glycemic control is appropriate for those receiving palliative and/or hospice care, given prognosis and the prominence of comfort as a goal of care. Such a patient (or surrogate) may opt to decline blood glucose monitoring and treatment of diabetes altogether, or reducing the frequency of fingerstick blood testing. In a stable patient, the goal is to prevent hypoglycemia and symptomatic hyperglycemia (which may lead to dehydration). If insulin is used in a patient with organ failure, it is reasonable to titrate down the insulin dosage as oral intake of food and fluid declines. In a patient who is dying, it is reasonable to stop all diabetic agents in those with type 2 DM. A small amount of insulin may be used for dying patients who have type 1 DM to prevent acute hyperglycemic complications.

CHOOSING WISELY® RECOMMENDATIONS

Diabetes Mellitus

- Avoid using medications to achieve hemoglobin A_{1c} <7.5% in most adults ≥65 years old; moderate control is generally better.

- There is no evidence that using medications to achieve tight glycemic control in most older adults with type 2 diabetes is beneficial. Among non-older adults, except for long-term reductions in myocardial infarction and mortality with metformin, using medications to achieve glycated hemoglobin levels less than 7% is associated with harms, including higher mortality rates. Tight control has been consistently shown to produce higher rates of hypoglycemia in older adults. Given the long timeframe to achieve theorized microvascular benefits of tight control, glycemic targets should reflect patient goals, health status, and life expectancy. Reasonable glycemic targets would be 7%–7.5% in healthy older adults with long life expectancy, 7.5%–8% in those with moderate comorbidity and a life expectancy <10 years, and 8%–9% in those with multiple morbidities and shorter life expectancy.

RESOURCES

- American Diabetes Association Standards of Medical Care in Diabetes 2017. *Diabetes Care.* 2017;40(Suppl 1):S1–S135.

- Coke L, Dennison Himmelfarb C. Type 2 diabetes in the older adult: the need for assessment of frailty. *J Cardiovasc Nurs.* 2017;32(6):511–513.

- Pogach L, Colburn J, Lugo A, et al. VA/DoD Clinical Practice Guideline for the Management of Type 2 Diabetes Mellitus in Primary Care. 2017; Version 5.0: https://www.healthquality.va.gov/guidelines/CD/diabetes/ (accessed Feb 2019).

CHAPTER 66—HEMATOLOGY

KEY POINTS

- The hematopoietic reserve capacity of the bone marrow diminishes with advancing age.

- Anemia of chronic disease is commonly multifactorial.

- Data from the National Health and Nutrition Examination Survey III (NHANES III) indicate that about 35% of all anemias among older adults in the United States result from nutrient deficiencies (iron, vitamin B_{12}, and/or folate), 45% are attributable to chronic disease(s), and 20% are unexplained despite an exhaustive evaluation.

- Molecular assays may help in the diagnosis of unknown anemia if standard evaluation is unrevealing.

- The aging bone marrow has a propensity to develop myeloid clones; 10% of the general population >70 years old carry mutations in genes associated with myeloid neoplasms.

- Coagulation enzyme activity increases with advancing age. This biochemical hypercoagulability can lead to increased thrombotic events in older adults.

HEMATOPOIETIC STEM CELLS AND AGING

The hematopoietic system derives from a pool of hematopoietic stem cells (HSCs) that can self-renew and/or differentiate along one of several lineages to form mature RBCs, WBCs, or platelets. HSCs differentiate into mature cells through an intermediate set of progenitors and precursors, each with decreasing self-renewal potential and increasing lineage commitment. Hematopoiesis is thereby tightly regulated by a complex series of interactions among HSCs, their stromal microenvironment, and regulatory molecules, including hematopoietic growth factors (HGFs). The orderly development of the hematopoietic system in vivo and the maintenance of homeostasis require a strict balance between self-renewal, differentiation, maturation, and cell loss.

An important question with regard to the aging hematopoietic system is whether the pluripotent HSC has a finite replicative capacity. Bone marrow culture studies show that maintenance of hematopoiesis varies inversely with donor age. Mouse studies demonstrate a decreased ability to regenerate the hematopoietic system and to generate mature lymphocytes, and an increased propensity for myeloid differentiation with age. This skewed pattern of myeloid-lymphoid differentiation is thought to be an inherent attribute of the aging HSC. Thus, it has been postulated that the myeloid dominance of adult human leukemia may in part be driven by an age-related deficient lymphopoiesis and development of myeloid clones. The myeloid clones contain genetic and epigenetic changes that are associated with an increased risk of developing age-associated hematopoietic disease, such as leukemia or myeloproliferative and myelodysplastic neoplasms. In the general population, 10% of those >70 years old carry mutations in genes associated with myeloid neoplasms. Changes in the aging bone marrow microenvironment contribute as well and allow for this clonal development and genetic changes.

ANEMIA

Anemia is the most common age-related hematologic abnormality. According to World Health Organization criteria, anemia is diagnosed if hemoglobin concentration is <13 g/dL in men and <12 g/dL in women.

Older adults, especially those seen during acute hospitalization or in geriatric clinics or long-term care facilities, have a higher prevalence of anemia. Results from NHANES III in the United States indicated that the prevalence of anemia in community-dwelling adults >65 years old was 11% in men and 10.2% in women. In several studies, the prevalence of anemia in the population >80 years old is reported as 18%–22% in men and 12%–16% in women. The exact etiology of anemia often remains unexplained, despite appropriate evaluation.

The importance of anemia in older adults relates not only to its underlying cause but also to its clinical manifestations. It is postulated that anemia in older adults leads to decreases in cardiac output, local tissue hypoxia, aggravation of comorbidities, and functional decline. Along these lines, anemia in older adults is associated with impaired performance-based mobility function such as walking speed or ability to rise from a chair, impaired balance, falls, frailty, cognitive decline, the occurrence of depressive symptoms, and a decrease in quality of life. Women >65 years old with hemoglobin concentrations <11 g/dL have a higher risk of all-cause mortality than those whose hemoglobin concentrations are ≥12 g/dL. This increased risk of mortality is independent of the presence of other comorbidities.

Evaluation of Anemia

The presence of multiple pathologies in older adults can make evaluation of anemia challenging. Attempting to determine the cause of anemia when the hemoglobin concentration is 12–13 g/dL may not be helpful, and decisions about how aggressively to evaluate these patients depend on clinical judgment. Once a decision has been made to investigate a low hemoglobin concentration, the principles involved in assessment and evaluation do not depend on patient age. The differential diagnostic considerations include blood loss, destruction, production deficit, or a combination of these. Morphology and red cell indices, such as the mean corpuscular volume (MCV), can help in the evaluation. For a summary of the causes of the various anemias seen in older adults, see Table 66.1. The sequence of workup should be guided by the most probable and clinically relevant cause. The consideration of the platelet and white blood counts will help to identify a red blood cell lineage problem versus a broader underlying bone marrow process. Bone marrow biopsy is generally indicated after exhaustion of morphologic and laboratory workup in the setting of at least 2 or more abnormal cell lines. Molecular testing can assess for underlying mutations. A referral to a hematologist is advised when biopsy or molecular testing is contemplated.

The manufacture of RBCs follows a well-established sequence. Thyroid-stimulating hormone, testosterone, and erythropoietin all stimulate stem cells to undergo 4 rounds of cell division over a period of 6–7 days. During the final step, the nucleus is extruded, forming a reticulocyte. The reticulocytes enter the peripheral circulation for approximately 24 hours. Mature RBCs remain in the peripheral circulation for about 120 days until removal by the reticuloendothelial system. An absolute reticulocyte count helps confirm the presence of an appropriate bone marrow response. A lack of reticulocytes, after hormonal, toxic or infectious etiologies have been excluded, should trigger review of a peripheral smear to assess for morphologic features suggesting a bone marrow replacement process (see marrow failure, below).

Hemoglobinopathies are conditions of faulty RBC assembly and are usually inherited but sometimes remain unrecognized until older age. They are divided into qualitative (sickle cell trait/disease) versus quantitative (thalassemias) etiologies. Indications of impaired hemoglobin synthesis are an abnormal MCV or alterations in the morphology of RBCs on the peripheral smear. The diagnosis is generally established with the help of a hemoglobin electrophoresis. (Hemoglobin electrophoresis will not identify a sickle cell trait; this requires genetic testing.)

Acquired assembly defects includes toxins, such as lead poisoning, or lack of iron (see iron deficiency anemia), Vitamin B_{12}, folic acid or copper, and it is important to differentiate between a deficit of intake and a deficit of absorption. Acute illness, medications and/or

Table 66.1—Physiologic Classification of Anemia

Classification	Possible Causes
Hypoproliferative	Iron-deficient erythropoiesis (iron deficiency, chronic) Erythropoietin lack (renal, endocrine) Stem-cell dysfunction Aplastic anemia
Ineffective erythropoiesis	Macrocytic (vitamin B_{12}, folate, myelodysplastic syndrome [refractory anemia]) Microcytic (thalassemia, sideroblastic) Normocytic (myelodysplastic syndrome)
Hemolytic	Immunologic (idiopathic, secondary) Intrinsic (abnormal hemoglobin, metabolic) Extrinsic (mechanical)

SOURCE: Data from Chatta GS, Lipschitz DA. Aging and hematopoiesis. In: Hazzard WR, Blass JP, Ettinger WH Jr., et al., eds. *Principles of Geriatric Medicine and Gerontology*. 5th ed. New York: McGraw-Hill Health Professions Division; 2003:763–770.

toxins can alter these processes and cause interruptions in red cell assembly, resulting in the clinical and laboratory picture of an anemia of chronic disease.

Iron-Deficiency Anemia

Iron is the only nutrient that limits the rate of erythropoiesis alone. An inadequate iron supply for erythropoiesis is the most common cause of anemia in older adults, resulting in a hypoproliferative and microcytic anemia. This iron restriction is diagnosed by the presence of a decreased serum iron, a decreased transferrin saturation (serum iron concentration divided by the serum total iron binding capacity or serum transferrin concentration, expressed as a percentage), and a normal or decreased serum ferritin concentration. Serum iron levels and transferrin saturation are regulated by the release of iron from its storage sites (macrophages in the reticuloendothelial system [RES]). Iron deficiency may trigger evaluation for blood loss from the GI or female reproductive tracts.

Iron deficiency can be treated with either parenteral or oral iron preparations. Intravenous administration is indicated in patients receiving an erythrocyte-stimulating agent during dialysis, or if the use of oral iron preparations is untenable. Multiple intravenous iron products are available, with similar efficacy and a reasonable safety profile. The choice of agent is based on the patient's allergy history and the length of infusion course desired.

As first-line, the oral route is preferred for iron supplementation. Ferrous sulfate 325 mg, given 1 hour before or 2 hours after a meal, will provide 195 mg of elemental iron. Ferrous gluconate, another option, provides less elemental iron per dose. There is no significant difference among the oral iron preparations

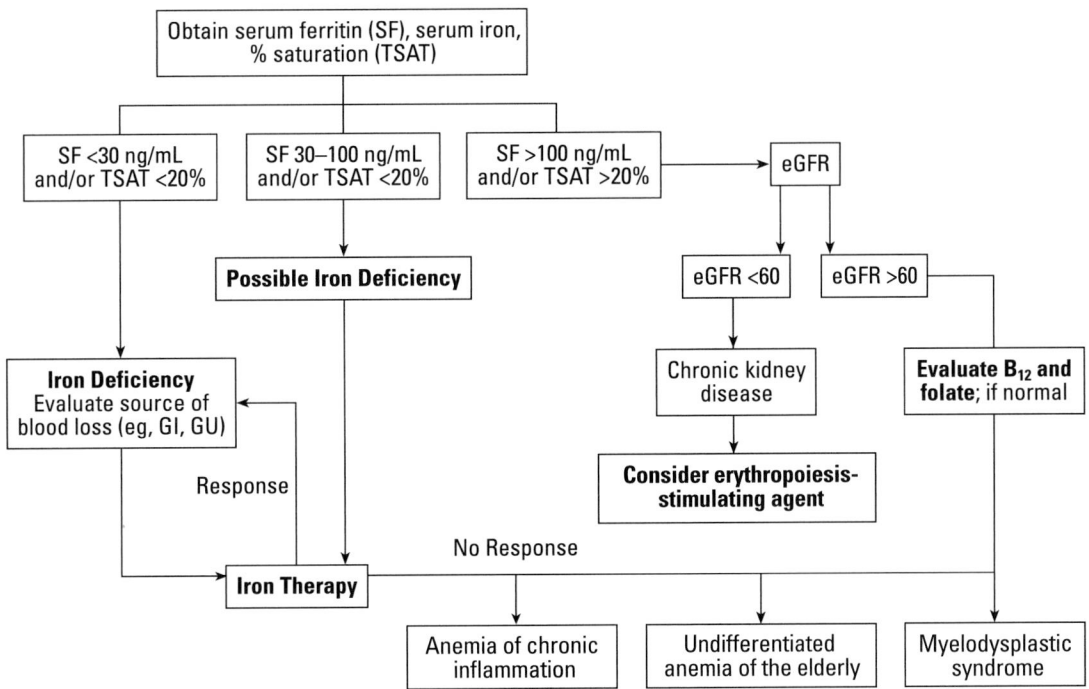

Figure 66.1—Evaluation of Possible Undifferentiated Anemia

SOURCE: Adapted with permission from Reuben DB, Herr K, Pacala JT, et al. *Geriatrics At Your Fingertips*. 20th ed. New York: American Geriatrics Society; 2018:149.

in regard to either efficacy or adverse-event profile. Optimal dosing frequency of oral iron is an area of active research, and some studies suggest that alternate-day dosing may yield better absorption than daily dosing. Multiple daily doses of oral iron supplements are commonly prescribed, but many patients are unable to tolerate more than a single tablet per day. The incidence of constipation is higher if oral iron is administered at 3 times a day, and absorption in the intestines is limited at higher doses. Oral iron absorption requires that the upper portion of the small bowel be intact and appropriately acidified by gastric secretions. In the presence of achlorhydria from gastric resection, atrophic gastritis, or pharmacologic suppression, iron absorption may be impaired. Supplementation with oral vitamin C (500 mg with each oral dose of iron) or vitamin C–containing products, such as orange juice, will correct this malabsorption defect. Celiac disease, which is characteristically associated with iron malabsorption, is an unusual cause of iron deficiency in the older population.

Common dose-related adverse events of oral iron preparations include mild nausea and constipation. For this reason, the frequency and dosage of administration may require adjustment to ensure compliance. Tablets containing a lower elemental dose of iron (15–20 mg), such as ferric gluconate, may be better tolerated than higher dose preparations. Iron elixir and liquid iron drops may be better absorbed; however, the adverse-event profile is similar to that for tablet preparations.

Treatment may need to continue for ≥6 months to adequately replace iron stores.

For a useful algorithm for evaluation and treatment of a patient with possible iron-deficiency anemia, see Figure 66.1.

Anemia of Inflammation/Anemia of Chronic Disease

Anemia of inflammation, or anemia of chronic disease, is defined by a constellation of morphologic, laboratory, and clinical features reflecting the presence of some other major disease process. Iron abnormalities, including a normal to increased ferritin in the setting of decreased serum iron, transferrin levels, and iron saturation, are a hallmark. The bone marrow shows normal erythroid precursors with increased storage iron. When considering the disorder, measurement of erythrocyte sedimentation rate or C-reactive protein level may be helpful. Pathophysiology of the anemia of chronic disease is complex and appears to result from an immunologic response and imbalance. Cytokines adversely impact iron homeostasis and erythropoiesis. Patients' symptoms are typically more attributable to their underlying disease than to the resulting anemia.

Hepcidin, a 25-amino acid peptide produced in the liver, is involved in the pathogenesis of anemia of chronic inflammation. Hepcidin functions as a direct mediator of iron homeostasis, reducing both intestinal iron absorption as well as release of RES macrophage iron to erythroid progenitors. Although hepcidin levels have been reported to be increased nearly 100-fold in association with anemia of chronic inflammation, studies on the clinical utility of hepcidin measurement remain limited by the availability of a suitable clinical assay.

The possibility of a multifactorial causation, including blood loss, malnutrition, or hemolysis, should always be considered when anemia of chronic disease is associated with a hemoglobin concentration of <10 g/dL. In this circumstance, laboratory investigations commonly have equivocal results; hence, a bone marrow examination may be required. Clinical judgment is important in deciding how aggressive the evaluation for anemia ought to be. Treatment is directed toward the underlying disease, although there is some evidence that patients with profound fatigue may benefit transiently from iron infusions. Sometimes, patients respond to erythropoietin replacement therapy; however, this is often not the case, because increased inflammatory cytokines render bone marrow erythroid precursors resistant to the effect of erythropoietin. Patients with endogenous erythropoietin levels >500 mU/mL are unlikely to respond.

Marrow Failure

Marrow failure is generally associated with suppression of all 3 cell lines and with peripheral cytopenias. Common causes include medications, immune damage to the stem-cell population, infections, and marrow replacement by malignant cells or fibrous tissue. The latter is usually associated with a myelophthisic blood picture (tear drop, nucleated RBCs, giant platelets, and metamyelocytes) as a reflection of the disruption of marrow stromal architecture. Multiple myeloma, a plasma cell dyscrasia, is included in the differential diagnosis and is commonly found in older patients. An increased protein gap (serum total protein minus albumin concentrations), M-spike (paraprotein), and abnormal free light chain ratio in the setting of renal insufficiency, hypercalcemia, and anemia are highly suggestive of this diagnosis.

An isolated suppression of erythropoiesis is referred to as pure red cell aplasia. This disorder can be related to medication or caused by benign or malignant abnormalities of lymphocytes, including thymoma or viral infections (eg, parvovirus B19). Patients have an isolated anemia, an increased serum iron, and an absence of erythroid precursors on bone marrow examination. Patients with parvovirus infection typically have reduced red cell precursors, which, if present, may have peculiar intranuclear inclusion bodies. Treatment is usually supportive.

Differential Diagnosis of Anemia

Macrocytic versus Microcytic Anemias

Ineffective erythropoiesis (Table 66.1) describes the process of premature intramedullary death of abnormal red cells, with decreased release of red cells into the circulation. The MCV is helpful in differentiating among anemias. Macrocytic anemias are subdivided into those with a normal red cell distribution width (RDW), caused by marrow failure (aplastic anemia, myelodysplasia, and others), and those with high RDW, caused by autoimmune hemolysis, cold agglutinins, and folate or vitamin B_{12} deficiency.

Pernicious anemia is an example of a macrocytic anemia. Pernicious anemia results from malabsorption of vitamin B_{12} as a consequence of antibodies against gastric parietal cells and intrinsic factor. Chronic pancreatitis and diseases of the distal ileum can also cause vitamin B_{12} deficiency. An increased prevalence of B_{12} deficiency has also been reported in patients with diabetes taking metformin, chronic use of proton-pump inhibitors, and those on strict vegetarian diets. In contrast, folate deficiency is rare in older adults. Alcohol and various drugs (eg, metformin, valproic acid) can interfere with folate absorption and metabolism. Vulnerability to folate deficiency is significantly greater in conditions that result in increased folate demand, such as inflammation, neoplasia, or hemolytic anemia.

The most common causes of microcytic anemias are iron-deficiency anemia, anemia of chronic disease, and thalassemia minor. Sideroblastic anemias can also present with microcytosis. This heterogeneous group of disorders is characterized by the presence of iron deposits in the mitochondria of normoblasts. The underlying pathophysiology is a defect involving iron incorporation into the heme molecule. This defect can be secondary to an intrinsic marrow lesion, or can be triggered by inflammation, neoplasia, nutritional deficiencies (eg, of copper or vitamin B_6), or medications (eg, antibiotics, chelators, antituberculous drugs). A common finding is the presence of a dimorphic (hypochromic and normochromic) RBC population. The diagnosis is made by demonstration of ringed sideroblasts and by the presence of myeloid and erythroid maturation abnormalities in the bone marrow.

Hemolysis

Accelerated RBC destruction may arise from acquired or inherited disorders. A low haptoglobin, increased bilirubin, and increased LDH are diagnostic. Hemolysis is differentiated into intravascular versus extravascular categories. Hereditary disorders include membrane or enzyme defects, such as hereditary spherocytosis, G6PD deficiency, and hemoglobin synthesis abnormalities. Acquired disorders include immune related from red cell infections (eg, malaria and others), alloantibodies (eg, transfusions and others), or autoantibodies (collagen vascular disease and others), and non-immune related, including mechanical damage from heart valves, burns, or membrane abnormalities (paroxysmal nocturnal hemoglobinuria).

Autoimmune hemolysis is the most common kind of hemolytic anemia in older adults. It is frequently associated with a lymphoproliferative disorder (non-Hodgkin lymphoma or chronic lymphocytic leukemia), collagen vascular disease, or drug ingestion. Corticosteroids and splenectomy are effective treatment options in patients with IgG red cell antibodies that cause a warm autoimmune hemolysis. Patients with IgM red cell antibodies usually have cold reactive antibodies and are typically refractory to splenectomy and corticosteroids. These patients can be treated by keeping them warm and administering warmed blood products. In the case of refractory cold disease, plasmapheresis may be indicated.

Blood Loss

Anemia in older adults should generally trigger consideration of blood loss from the GI or genitourinary tracts. Typical findings in anemia from blood loss are low iron, low serum ferritin, and high total iron binding capacity, reflecting absent iron stores. Medication-related gastritis, angiodysplasia, and benign tumors are common causes and should be considered as well as malignancy. Frail patients with contraindications to an invasive procedure might benefit from advanced imaging modalities.

PLATELETS AND COAGULATION DISORDERS

Bleeding diatheses are uncommon in older adults but may pose a serious threat. Mucocutaneous bleeding is usually associated with a quantitative or qualitative platelet-related abnormality. Bleeding into tissue or joints is more typical of coagulation disorders.

Thrombocytopenia and Thrombocytosis

Platelets play an important role both in hemostasis and thrombosis.

Thrombocytopenia is common and usually multifactorial in older patients. When evaluating a patient with a low platelet count, clinicians should include in the differential life-threatening microangiopathic hemolytic anemias such as disseminated intravascular coagulation (DIC), thrombotic thrombocytopenic purpura (TTP), hemolytic uremic syndrome (HUS), and heparin-induced thrombocytopenia. If platelet clumping is seen in blood samples drawn in EDTA tubes, blood should be redrawn in either a heparin or citrate blood tube to determine if the clumping is benign.

DIC is commonly associated with severe infections or disseminated cancer and presents with intravascular hemolysis and a consumptive coagulopathy. The presence of red cell fragmentation, thrombocytopenia, hemosiderinuria, and prolonged prothrombin and partial thromboplastin times are suggestive of this diagnosis. Treatment of DIC entails treating the underlying disorder as well as providing blood product support, including fresh frozen plasma and cryoprecipitate (if fibrinogen is <100 ng).

TTP and HUS are characterized by microangiopathic hemolysis and thrombocytopenia. Neurologic symptoms and renal dysfunction are seen in patients with TTP, whereas HUS is characterized by renal involvement. TTP is triggered by a markedly decreased plasma ADAMTS13, an enzyme responsible for cleavage of large molecular weight von Willebrand factor. HUS may be preceded by an episode of diarrhea and is commonly associated with the presence of Shiga toxin–producing *E coli* or pneumococcal infection. In adults, it is often difficult to distinguish between TTP and HUS at presentation, and the initial treatment is the same with supportive care and fresh frozen plasma or cryoprecipitate. TTP responds to treatment with plasma exchange, whereas HUS is relatively unresponsive to this therapeutic option. TTP is thought to be idiopathic in about 40% of the patients, with the remaining cases thought to be due to autoimmune causes, infection, or cancer (27%), drug-induced (12%), pregnancy (7%), or hematopoietic stem cell transplantation (6%).

Heparin-induced thrombocytopenia develops after exposure to heparin products. Antibodies bind to heparin–platelet factor 4 complexes, and subsequently to FC receptors on platelets, triggering an escalated platelet activation. Patients require prompt treatment with direct thrombin inhibitors. The diagnostic gold standard is the serotonin-release assay.

ITP is a diagnosis of exclusion. Symptomatic patients are treated with intravenous immune globulin (IVIG) and steroid taper. Unsuccessful treatment attempts can be managed with splenectomy, chemotherapy (danazol, rituximab), and/or thrombopoietin-receptor agonists.

Thrombocytosis is most commonly reactive but may be triggered by an underlying bone marrow mutation. Essential thrombocythemia (described further below), a myeloid proliferative neoplasm, is triggered by acquired driver mutations in JAK2, CALR, or MPL. The diagnosis is established through a bone marrow biopsy. Depending on age and clinical presentation, patients may need treatment with cytoreductive drug therapy in addition to aspirin, to reduce the risk of thrombotic events.

Qualitative Platelet Problems

Platelet function disorders, although uncommon, can cause bleeding in older adults. They can be classified into hereditary, such as Bernard-Soulier syndrome or

Glanzmann thrombasthenia, or acquired disorders. By far the most common acquired disorders are secondary to medications (aspirin or non-aspirin NSAIDs). Platelet function testing can help to differentiate the underlying etiology.

Clotting Disorders

Clotting disorders can be divided into inherited and acquired disorders. Most thrombotic events in older adults are provoked and require a limited period of anticoagulation. The CHEST Antithrombotic Therapy for VTE Disease guideline and expert panel report is a sound reference for length of treatment and choice of agent. Common acquired prothrombotic conditions include antiphospholipid syndrome, cancer, trauma, and surgery. Inherited clotting disorders include prothrombin gene mutation, protein C and S deficiency, and factor V Leiden. In older patients with unprovoked or unexplained recurrent thromboembolic events, it is reasonable to perform laboratory testing for inherited clotting disorders. Up to 10% of selected octogenarians with recurrent clots have mutations.

Prothrombin gene mutation is the second most common inherited thrombophilia in the United States. It is caused by a mutation in the prothrombin (factor II) gene. Patients have increased prothrombin levels that may trigger thrombosis. Proteins C and S are vitamin K–dependent anticoagulants. Protein C is converted to activated protein C and inactivates factors Va and VIIIa, whereas protein S acts as a non-enzymatic cofactor to activate protein C. Deficiencies in proteins C and S predispose to inappropriate clotting. Factor V Leiden results from a point mutation in the factor V gene. The mutation renders factor V resistant to inactivation by activated protein C and increased risk of venous thromboembolism.

Antithrombin deficiency results from a defect in inhibiting thrombin and activated factors X and IX. Antithrombin deficiency results in a hypercoagulable condition.

Bleeding Disorders

Bleeding disorders in older adults are commonly acquired and usually found in patients with liver disease or clotting factor deficiencies. Von Willebrand disease (vWD) is one of the most common bleeding disorders and categorized into quantitative, qualitative, or a combination of both defects. Type 1 vWD, characterized by a quantitative deficiency, is the most common type in older adults.

Older adults may also acquire circulating clotting factor inhibitors and even present with the clinical picture of hemophilia. The most common such disorder is caused by an inhibitor to factor VIII. Its onset is often sudden, and patients present with significant bleeding into soft tissue, including muscle, because titers of factor VIII antibodies can be very high. These soft-tissue bleeds differ from the hemarthrosis events commonly seen with congenital hemophilia. Treatment involves factor replacement.

Deficiency of the vitamin K–dependent clotting factors tends to occur in older adults with major illnesses. Disorders of the hepatobiliary tree, antibiotics that neutralize bowel bacteria (a major source of vitamin K), malabsorption, and severe malnutrition are the common causes. The deficits are readily treated with oral or intravenous vitamin K. All patients who need warfarin reversal should receive vitamin K replacement. The subcutaneous administration of vitamin K is discouraged because of a slower time to correction of prolonged INR and variable absorption. In patients receiving warfarin who have severe bleeding and who are unable to receive fresh frozen plasma or in those in need of urgent reversal, a 4-factor prothrombin complex concentrate or 3-factor prothrombin complex concentrate plus recombinant activated factor VIIa may be administered.

MYELOID HEMATOLOGIC MALIGNANCIES

Myeloid hematologic malignancies are among the most common malignancies in older adults. They include the group of acute myeloid leukemias, myelodysplastic syndromes (MDS), myeloproliferative neoplasms (MPN), and combined myelodysplastic and myeloproliferative disorders.

Myelodysplastic Syndromes

The myelodysplastic syndromes (MDS) are a group of stem-cell disorders characterized by disordered hematopoiesis, occurring primarily in the older age group. This very heterogeneous collection of disorders is characterized by cytopenia, and treatment requires a risk-adapted approach. They are classified according to the 2016 WHO myelodysplastic syndrome subtypes classification as MDS with single or multilineage dysplasia, MDS with ring sideroblasts, isolated del(5q), excess blasts, or unclassified.

Cytogenetic abnormalities are relatively common in MDS, and one of particular interest in older adults is deletion of the long arm of chromosome 5 (5q–). The median age at presentation is 66 years, and the 5q– syndrome is characterized by macrocytic anemia, modest leukopenia, normal or increased platelet counts, and marrow erythroid hypoplasia or hyperplasia; it is also more common in women.

Treatment of MDS depends on symptoms, cytogenetics, and comorbid conditions. A referral to a hematologist is indicated to discuss treatment options, which include chemotherapy and, in selected individuals, transplantation. The concern in every myelodysplastic disorder is risk of transitioning into an acute leukemia.

Chronic Myeloproliferative Neoplasms

Chronic myeloproliferative neoplasms (MPNs) are a heterogeneous group of myeloid disorders. Cytogenetic abnormalities in cell clones drive these malignant processes associated with extramedullary hematopoiesis, resulting in organomegaly and increased blood counts. Historically, MPNs included CML, polycythemia vera (PV), essential thrombocythemia (ET), and idiopathic myelofibrosis (IMF), but MPNs also include an abundance of other stem cell mutations. MPNs are commonly seen in older adults and are characterized by involvement of multipotent hematopoietic progenitor cells. Their hallmark is marrow hypercellularity with overproduction of usually more than one bone marrow lineage, with thrombotic and hemorrhagic diatheses. The risk of all MPNs is spontaneous transformation to acute leukemia. The diagnostic criteria for PV, ET, and IMF adopted by WHO include the identification of clonal markers. JAK2 V617F is present in about 95% of patients with PV and in about half of patients with ET and IMF. For more detailed information on mutations, readers may consult the current WHO classification of myeloid neoplasms and acute leukemia (most recent is the 2016 update).

CML is commonly treated with tyrosine kinase inhibitors. PV is symptomatically treated with serial phlebotomy. ET is treated with aspirin and, based on further risk stratification, with cytoreductive hydroxyurea.

Ruxolitinib, a JAK1 and JAK2 inhibitor, has been approved for treatment of symptomatic patients with IMF or myelofibrosis developing as a result of ET, or PV. Ruxolitinib is not curative but considerably reduces spleen size and untoward symptoms in selected patients.

RESOURCES

- Spivak JL. Myelodysplastic neoplasms: contemporary review and how we treat. *N Engl J Med*. 2017;376(22):2168–2181.

- Steensma DP. New challenges in evaluating anemia in older persons in the era of molecular testing. *Hematology Am Soc Hematol Euc Program*. 2016 Dec 2;2016(1):67–73.

CHAPTER 67—ONCOLOGY AND HEMATOLOGIC MALIGNANCIES

KEY POINTS

- Older adults and black Americans of all ages are more likely to develop cancer and present with more advanced disease.

- Older age has a variable association with the aggressiveness and growth rate of malignant tumors.

- Surgery, radiation therapy, chemotherapy, and biologic therapies, including immunotherapy, are safe and effective treatment interventions for older cancer patients when appropriate precautions are taken based on the patient's comorbidities, vital organ functions, and medications.

- No demonstrated age-associated resistance to chemotherapy has been demonstrated.

- Although some acute toxicities (eg, nausea, vomiting, and hair loss) of chemotherapy are less prominent in older adults, other toxicities such as myelosuppression, diarrhea, and neuropathy are more common.

- Geriatric assessment can help determine which older patients are more likely to benefit from more intensive cancer treatment and which are most likely to experience toxicity.

Cancer is a disease associated with aging—most cancer diagnoses and deaths occur in people >65 years old. Currently, the median age of patients with a new cancer diagnosis is 70 years. On the basis of the aging of the U.S. population and the known association between cancer and aging, a dramatic increase in the number of new cancer diagnoses is projected for the next 20 years. It is anticipated that patients ≥65 years old will account for 70% of all cancer diagnoses by the year 2030.

According to the National Cancer Institute's Surveillance, Epidemiology and End Results data, over 70% of cancer deaths are in people >65 years old. One in four deaths in the United States is caused by cancer. Overall cancer incidence rates decreased in the most recent time period in both men (1.7% per year from 2004 to 2013) and women (0.2% per year from 2004 to 2013), largely due to decreases in the 3 major cancer sites in men (lung, prostate, and colorectum) and 2 major cancer sites in women (breast and colorectum). Among men, cancer death rates combined decreased by approximately 16% during this time-period; among women, overall cancer death rates decreased by approximately 13%. Although progress has been made in reducing incidence and mortality rates and improving survival, cancer still accounts for more deaths than heart disease in people <85 years old. After age 85, heart disease becomes the number one killer, and the risk of cancer declines for reasons that are not well defined. Because of the paucity of older adults in cancer clinical trials, it is not clear how much of the improvement in cancer treatment has translated to the benefit of older patients. However, when such data have been evaluated (eg, for colon cancer, breast cancer) within clinical trials, it appears that treatments shown to be effective in younger patients are also effective in select older patients (SOE=A). The older patients in clinical trials, however, tend to be healthy (ie, not multimorbid and without significant functional impairment)), and thus not always reflective of patients routinely seen in clinical practice.

Although cancer has long been recognized as a disease of older people, emphasis on the interactions of cancer and aging is a recent development. Experimental data and clinical experience have indicated that tumors are not resistant to treatment by virtue of age alone. However, age is associated with reductions in certain organ functions, and these deficiencies in physiologic reserve might be magnified by comorbid conditions. Cancer treatments can therefore be associated with an increase in adverse events, and treatment should be tailored to the older individual, taking into consideration potential increased toxicities and balancing this with expectations of survival in the context of comorbidities. Although we have much to learn about providing optimal management of cancer in older adults, especially those who are vulnerable or frail, some research has shown that geriatric assessment can help to identify those older patients who are more likely to benefit from aggressive treatment and those who are at greater risk of toxicities from therapy.

Four questions form the basis of this new emphasis: Why are tumors more common in older adults? Is there a difference in tumor aggressiveness with advancing age? Should cancer treatment be different for older patients? How can cancer treatment be best individualized for older patients?

Ethnic Differences in Cancer Incidence and Mortality

As the demographics of the U.S. population changes, additional information is needed on incidence and on natural history differences in cancers that develop in different ethnic and racial groups. There is a lack of basic data about aging minority populations. This is largely because of small sample sizes of these populations and to language barriers that prevent certain racial and ethnic groups from participating in survey research. The U.S. Census Bureau estimates that by 2050, Hispanic individuals will account for nearly 25% of the population, and African Americans, Asian individuals, and Native Americans combined will total another 25%. By the year 2050, under current projections, U.S. numbers in minority populations are expected to outpace the number of white individuals. Although the number of older white individuals is anticipated to double to 62 million, the number of African American individuals will nearly quadruple to over 9 million. Older Hispanic individuals will total about 12 million, 11 times as many as in 1990. The number of American Indian and Alaska Natives will grow to 562,000, and the number of older Asian and Pacific Islanders will approach 7 million.

Cancer incidence and death rates are lower in other racial and ethnic groups than in white and black populations for all cancer sites combined and for the four most common cancer sites. Overall, black Americans have the highest cancer incidence and mortality rates. Cancer incidence among black Americans is 10% higher than among white Americans, 50%–60% higher than among Hispanic Americans and Asian Americans, and more than twice as high as among Native Americans. Black Americans with cancer have shorter survival times than white Americans at all stages of diagnosis. Relative 5-year survival rates are higher among people diagnosed at younger ages (52% among black Americans diagnosed before age 45) than in those diagnosed at older ages (43% among those diagnosed after age 75). The cancer death rate for black Americans is about 30% higher than for white Americans and more than twice as high as for Hispanic Americans, Asian Americans, and Native Americans.

The factors contributing to the ethnic differences are not defined. However, certain data suggest that when the quality of the health care delivered to white and black Americans is similar, disease outcomes in the two groups are comparable (SOE=B).

CANCER BIOLOGY AND AGING

Numerous explanations have been offered for the biologic connection between cancer and aging, including extended exposure to carcinogens, increased DNA instability resulting in a higher mutation potential, telomere shortening, immune dysregulation, and increased susceptibility to oxidative stress. Although these explanations for the link between cancer and aging are plausible, they do not pinpoint the reason why one older adult is more susceptible to cancer than another. Furthermore, the association between cancer and aging is complex. Population-based studies demonstrate a steady rise in the probability of developing cancer across the strata of age, but few studies have examined cancer prevalence and mortality in the highest age groups.

Explaining the Increased Prevalence of Cancer with Age

The prevalence of cancer increases with age for at least three reasons. First, cancers, particularly those that occur in people >65 years old, are thought to develop over a long period, perhaps decades. This is best exemplified by the current understanding of colon cancer, which has been shown to develop because of an accumulation of several damaging genetic events occurring in a stochastic manner over time. Colon cancer, which occurs via an intermediate precursor (the adenomatous polyp), is an example of the multi-step genetic changes required over time for cancer development. In colon cancer, mutations in tumor suppressor genes such as inactivation of the *APC* and *DCC* genes and subsequent additional genetic defects in oncogenes such as *KRAS* promote the accumulation of mutations that lead to carcinogenesis. If mutations are acquired at a constant rate, older people are more likely to have lived long enough to develop the 8 to 10 genetic lesions it takes to develop a malignancy. In contrast, lymphomas are just as likely to occur in younger as in older people. Lymphocytes normally undergo gene rearrangements and mutations to generate antigen receptors, and these processes appear to be particularly vulnerable to errors that can lead to lymphoma at any age.

A second reason for the greater prevalence of cancer with advancing age is that DNA repair mechanisms are thought to decline with age. As a consequence, cells can accumulate damage. Normally, a dividing cell pauses in G1 (the gap after mitosis [M] and before DNA replication [S]) and in G2 (the gap after S and before M) to take inventory and repair any damage before proceeding to the next phase. These are the G1 and G2 checkpoints. Older cells may fail to detect and/or repair damage and fail to accurately control DNA replication. This leads to aneuploidy and uncontrolled proliferation. In younger people, these aberrations can trigger the death of the cell (ie, apoptosis); in older people, the errors may be tolerated and fail to signal cell death. Cells without functioning checkpoints are vulnerable to loss of growth control. Telomere dysfunction and increased epigenetic gene silencing have also been implicated in the pathogenesis of cancers. Telomeres are essential for chromosomal stability; with aging, their length progressively shortens, which interferes with cell division. This instability at the cellular level increases the rate of somatic mutations that predispose to cancer and other disorders like aplastic anemia. Paradoxically, human cancers have developed mechanisms to maintain telomere length for survival. Autophagy is interrupted with aging, which leads to the accumulation of damaged proteins and mitochondria, which in turn are a source of reactive oxygen species and contribute to cancer.

Finally, a third contribution to increased cancer incidence in older people may be a decline in the function of the immune system, particularly in cellular immunity. A number of findings suggest that the immune system can recognize and control certain cancers. A decline in immune function may lead to the emergence of a cancer in an older adult that was controlled when that person was younger.

The Different Characteristics of Cancer with Age

A long-held but incompletely documented clinical notion that cancers in older people are less aggressive or slower growing has not been consistently supported by epidemiologic data from tumor registries or large clinical trials. Such data can be confounded by geriatric problems that shorten survival independently of the cancer (eg, comorbidity, multiple medications, clinician or family bias regarding diagnosis and treatment in older adults, and age-associated life stresses). These factors may counter any primary influence that aging might have on tumor aggressiveness. Despite these uncertainties, however, there is experimental support for the contention that tumor aggressiveness declines with age. Data obtained from laboratory animals with a wide range of tumors under highly controlled circumstances demonstrate slower tumor growth, fewer experimental metastases, and longer survival in old mice. Tumor growth involves several levels of interaction between the tumor and the host. It may be that tumor angiogenesis is impaired in older people, thereby impeding the rate of tumor growth. The clinical applicability of this work is limited, inasmuch as it is difficult to know in any given individual whether the course of the disease will be characterized by an indolent or aggressive pattern of growth.

Breast cancer is the most notable clinical example of an age-associated decline in tumor aggressiveness. Older patients are more likely to have more favorable histologic types, higher levels of estrogen- and progesterone-receptor expression, lower growth fraction, and less frequent metastases. In a published series on breast cancer patients with primary tumors ≤1 cm in diameter, the single most important predictor of metastasis to axillary nodes has consistently been found to be patient age: patients <50 years old have the highest likelihood of spread, whereas those >70 years old have the lowest likelihood of spread. Stage for stage in breast cancer, older patients seem to have longer survival times than younger patients (SOE=A).

By contrast, Hodgkin lymphoma seems to be a more aggressive disease in older patients. The most likely reason for the age-associated differences in prognosis is that Hodgkin lymphoma is a different disease in patients ≥45 years old than in younger patients. Incidence data demonstrate two distinct peak incidence rates, one at age 32 years and one at age 84 years. The frequency of particular histologic subtypes of Hodgkin lymphoma is different in younger and older patients: nodular sclerosis is the most common subtype in younger patients, whereas mixed cellularity is the most common in older patients. In all reported treatment series, older age is an independent prognostic factor. Additional study is necessary to document age-associated differences in tumor cell biology.

Acute leukemias, like Hodgkin lymphoma, biologically appear to be a different disease in older people; the MDR1 drug resistance pump (which eliminates toxins, including certain cancer chemotherapy agents, from the cell) is more commonly expressed, thus conferring relative treatment resistance and shorter overall survival time compared with younger patients. However, for most cancer types, the molecular biology and clinical behavior of the tumor can appear similar across the aging spectrum.

PRINCIPLES OF CANCER MANAGEMENT

Randomized clinical trials are the most reliable method of studying medical intervention, and treatment decisions are best founded on their results. However, despite efforts from the cooperative oncology groups, patients entered into trials are by and large younger and presumably healthier than the typical older patient with the same cancer type. Only 3% of older patients with cancer are enrolled in cancer treatment–based clinical trials. There is little evidence of efficacy and tolerability of cancer treatment in older patients, especially those who are >75 years old and/or vulnerable because of comorbidities. Furthermore, common endpoints of these trials are overall survival (for therapeutic interventions) or disease-specific mortality (for prevention studies), which are not always the most appropriate outcomes for older patients (because of their inherently limited remaining life expectancies on the basis of age alone). More and more, clinical researchers are addressing issues of geriatric oncology. New, geriatrics-oriented trials are focusing more on symptom reduction and quality-of-life outcomes rather than on life expectancy exclusively. Surveys have indicated that many older adults, when fully informed, most often choose life-extending treatments, even at the risk of toxicity. Because of physiologic changes in older adults, there is potential for an increase in adverse events associated with standard chemotherapy and other cancer management options. However, acute toxicities (eg, nausea, vomiting, hair loss) may actually be less prominent in this population (SOE=B). In any case, although quality of life remains a primary treatment consideration, older adults should not be denied efforts at extending life on the basis of chronologic age alone.

Oncologists are often faced with the challenge of making cancer treatment decisions in older adults in the absence of evidence-based guidelines. Aging is associated with a multitude of physiologic changes, which in turn are magnified by medical comorbidities and related issues such as polypharmacy and functional impairments. Appropriate treatment for cancer can be safe and effective in older adults if an adequate assessment is done and appropriate precautions are undertaken (eg, augmenting supportive care resources and interventions). Unfortunately, the fear of treatment-related adverse events and lack of evidence-based data can lead to the undertreatment of cancer and decreased survival in this population. Life expectancy based on chronologic age is heterogeneous, with comorbidities, functional impairment/disability, and geriatric syndromes all influencing the range. After estimating a patient's life expectancy, it should be determined whether the benefit of a suggested treatment is likely to be realized in the remaining life span. This consideration is important as well when making treatment decisions about adjuvant cancer therapy. Assessment of underlying health status is particularly important for older patients with advanced cancer, for whom, relatively speaking, the benefits of treatment may be low and the toxicity of treatment high. Full geriatric assessment is the gold standard for evaluation of the older patient; it provides an assessment of the global health of the patient, including an evaluation of functional status, comorbid medical conditions, cognition, nutrition, polypharmacy, psychological status, social support, and geriatric syndromes. Each domain is an independent predictor of morbidity and mortality in older patients.

Guidelines for both the assessment of the older patient with cancer and treatment algorithms are in progress. The National Comprehensive Cancer Network's Older Adult Oncology guidelines are the most well developed (www.nccn.org/professionals/physician_gls/f_guidelines.asp [accessed Feb 2019]).

Assessment of the Older Cancer Patient

The database regarding the application of the geriatric assessment to patients with cancer and the use of it to determine the capacity of patients to tolerate treatment are growing. Several abbreviated versions of geriatric assessment are being evaluated for their ability to predict treatment tolerability (eg, VES-13, G8), but even these tools need to be applied and interpreted with good clinical judgment. For example, knowing only an individual patient's current level of physical activity could be misleading. Two patients of similar chronologic age may have the same assessment score. However, an 85-year-old who was mowing his lawn last month but now presents with a cancer-related decline in function is much more likely to tolerate cancer treatment than a similarly aged patient whose baseline level of physical activity has remained poor.

Although the commonly used Karnofsky Performance Status and Eastern Cooperative Oncology Group (ECOG) performance measures do correlate with treatment toxicity, these tools alone do not predict outcomes as well as geriatric assessment in older adults.

Although data are evolving, few oncology trials that have provided evidence for cancer treatment in older adults have included any formulation of a geriatric assessment. Geriatric assessment can detect issues pertinent to cancer management that could otherwise go unrecognized. Dependence on caregivers for assistance with basic activities and instrumental activities of daily living (ADLs, IADLs) has been shown to be predictive of mortality in geriatric oncology patients, and it has been observed that older patients with cancer have a higher incidence of basic ADL and IADL deficiencies than age-matched controls. The prevalence of comorbidity increases with age and can affect survival of patients with advanced cancer. Polypharmacy, another target of interest of geriatric assessment, can complicate cancer treatment and increase the risk of adverse events from chemotherapy; further, it may increase the risk of nonadherence to cancer treatments given by mouth. Weight loss, particularly sarcopenia, is a marker of declining nutritional status commonly observed in the geriatric population, particularly in those who are or become frail. Studies of community-dwelling geriatric patients without cancer found a 2-fold increased risk of mortality in those patients with weight loss of 5% of body weight.

Approximately 20% of community-dwelling older adults screen positive for some degree of cognitive impairment. The presence of cognitive disorders, particularly more advanced forms of dementia, may limit life expectancy and influence the decision-making for cancer-related treatment, as well as providing informed consent for such treatments.

Additionally, patients with cognitive impairment may have more difficulty reporting treatment-related adverse effects without the involvement of a dedicated caregiver. Geriatric assessment also entails an assessment of mood, and studies have identified depression as a significant prognostic factor in patients (of any age) undergoing treatment for cancer. In both the geriatrics and oncology literature, social isolation has been associated with increased risk of mortality. Older cancer patients, in general, may often require considerable support from a caregiver. Researchers have found that social support, such as marital status, can independently affect cancer outcomes.

In studies that have evaluated the impact of geriatric assessment on survival in older cancer patients, factors that were independently associated with worse overall survival have included low albumin, ECOG performance status ≥2, positive geriatric depression screen, advanced stage disease, malnutrition, and advanced age.

In addition to prognosis, geriatric assessment can also help estimate the risk of clinically significant toxicity from chemotherapy. In one study of 500 patients, several geriatric assessment factors were associated with experiencing a Grade 3–5 toxicity, with Grade 5 signaling death attributable to treatment. Patients ≥65 years old with cancer (and from seven institutions) completed a pre-chemotherapy geriatric assessment. Grade 3–5 toxicity occurred in 53% of these patients (39% Grade 3, 12% Grade 4, 2% Grade 5). Risk factors for Grade 3–5 toxicity included age ≥73 years, cancer type (gastrointestinal or genitourinary), standard dosing of chemotherapy, use of >1 chemotherapy agent concurrently, falls in last 6 months, assistance with IADLs, and decreased social activity. In a second study, which developed The Chemotherapy Risk Assessment Scale for High-Age Patients (CRASH) Score, over 500 patients ≥70 years old initiating chemotherapy completed a baseline geriatric assessment. Severe toxicity was observed in 64% of patients. The best model for hematologic toxicity included IADL score, LDH level, diastolic blood pressure, and chemotherapy regimen. The best predictive model for nonhematologic toxicity included performance status, Mini–Mental score (cognition), Mini-Nutritional Assessment score, and chemotherapy regimen. Overall, these predictive risk stratification schemes allow clinicians to better identify which patients are at highest risk of chemotherapy toxicity, and thus could be used in further research to identify and apply interventions to reduce development of such toxicities in more vulnerable older patients with cancer.

Geriatric assessment requires a multidisciplinary approach and analysis of the data to create a personalized plan. Incorporation of a geriatric assessment into care of older adults improves outcomes by preventing disability and reducing hospitalizations, and it may prove beneficial for older cancer patients. Recent studies have shown that geriatric assessment is feasible in oncology clinical assessment and cooperative group clinical trials, and that factors within geriatric assessment can predict toxicity from chemotherapy. Geriatric assessment permits stratification of patients into "fit," "vulnerable," and "frail" subgroups, and such a scheme may help to identify patients more likely to benefit from standard treatments and those at highest risk of toxicity. More data are necessary to examine whether geriatric assessment and related interventions can improve outcomes, and how best to use this resource-intensive approach to care. It is likely that support drawing from multidisciplinary expertise, including social work, physical therapy, occupational therapy, pharmacy, and nutrition, can help develop geriatric assessment–guided interventions for an at-risk older adult with cancer. For example, studies among older adults with cancer have shown review of medication usage by a pharmacist can decrease suboptimal prescribing and potentially lead to a decrease of adverse drug events.

Treatment Options for Older Patients with Cancer

Current forms of cancer treatment include surgery, radiation, chemotherapy, hormone manipulation, and biologic therapy. Some cancer types and stages require multi-modality treatment incorporating several of these approaches. Age alone does not preclude any of these approaches, but because of aging-related physiologic changes in certain organ systems and the prevalence of age-associated conditions (eg, multimorbidity, functional and cognitive impairment), special considerations are warranted when formulating a treatment plan for this population.

Cancer Screening

Screening for breast, colon, lung, and (in some cases) cervical cancer can be considered for selected subsets of the population. Prostate cancer screening is controversial at any age and is unlikely to benefit someone with <10 years of remaining life expectancy. Both the American Society of Clinical Oncology and the American Board of Internal Medicine's Choosing Wisely® campaign recommend considering life expectancy and the risks of testing, overdiagnosis, and overtreatment when recommending cancer screening for older adults. Assessing remaining life expectancy should involve a comprehensive evaluation of health status and include functional impairment/disability, comorbidities, and geriatric syndromes. The trajectory

Table 67.1—Chemotherapy Issues in Geriatric Oncology

Issue	Comments
General	■ Comorbidities and multiple medications add complexity.
Pharmacokinetic changes	■ A progressive delay with age in the elimination of renally excreted medications, due to a reduction in glomerular filtration rate, can contribute to more severe toxicity.
Pharmacodynamic changes	■ Possible enhanced resistance with age to antitumor agents. ■ Increased expression of the multidrug resistance gene has been reported in some older adults. ■ Increased tumor hypoxia with age has been observed in a murine model.
Toxicity	■ Generally, mucositis, cardiotoxicity, and peripheral and central neurotoxicity become more common and more severe with aging (SOE=B). ■ Cardiotoxicity is a complication of anthracyclines and anthraquinones, mitomycin C, and high-dose cyclophosphamide, and its incidence increases with age. ■ Peripheral neurotoxicity with vincristine is more common and more severe in older adults. ■ The incidence of cerebellar toxicity from high-dose cytosine arabinoside increases with age.
Myelotoxicity	■ Chemotherapy-related myelotoxicity can become more severe and more prolonged with aging. Nevertheless, moderately toxic treatment regimens, such as CMF (cyclophosphamide, methotrexate, fluorouracil), cisplatin and fluorouracil, and cisplatin and etoposide are tolerated by many patients ≥70 years old without life-threatening neutropenia or thrombocytopenia (SOE=A). ■ The frequency of infections is markedly increased among older patients with acute leukemia who undergo intensive induction treatment.
Recent advances	■ Granulocyte colony-stimulating factor and granulocyte-macrophage colony-stimulating factor have reduced the incidence of neutropenic infections in patients receiving intensive treatment, and their effectiveness does not appear to be diminished with advancing patient age. ■ Certain new medications or new formulations may be particularly suitable for older patients, eg, oral etoposide, gemcitabine, vinorelbine, nab-paclitaxel, subcutaneous bortezomib, and liposomal doxorubicin.

and expected survival from cancer should be balanced with other health status issues to identify the patients most likely to benefit from cancer screening.

Chemotherapy

Aging can be associated with changes in key pharmacologic parameters of antineoplastic agents and in the susceptibility to end-organ toxicity (Table 67.1). Understanding the physiologic aspects of aging is important, because these changes have implications for efficacy of and tolerance to systemic cancer therapy. Anatomical and structural changes accompanying aging can adversely impact physiologic reserve in all organ systems. Cancer treatment should be tailored to take into account toxicity, and the loss of physiologic reserve is variable across patients of the same chronologic age. Several changes are important to consider. Older patients have decreased cardiac reserve. Both conventional chemotherapies like doxorubicin and targeted agents like trastuzumab can potentiate heart failure. Older adults are more susceptible to chemotherapy-related mucositis secondary to changes in the mucosal protective mechanism. Intestinal motility, absorptive surface area, and GI blood flow are also decreased and may increase risk of nausea, vomiting, and diarrhea. A decrease in the vital capacity of the lungs, along with impaired gas exchange can exacerbate the toxicity of radiation.

The time to recovery from physiologic compromise is also prolonged for older adults undergoing cancer treatment and is particularly relevant in tissues such as the bone marrow. A dysregulated bone marrow in the context of a treated older patient increases the risk of chemotherapy-induced neutropenia (and thus infection), anemia, and thrombocytopenia, all of which can adversely impact prognosis. Finally, older adults are especially susceptible to confusion, syncope, and falls because of common changes in blood pressure, carotid baroreflex sensitivity, cerebral blood flow, and dysequilibrium.

One of the most consistent pharmacokinetic changes of aging is a delay in the elimination of renally excreted medications because of a reduced glomerular filtration rate. The prolonged half-life of these agents can account in part for more severe toxicity. Several chemotherapy agents (eg, cisplatin, lenalidomide, and capecitabine) are contraindicated or need dose adjustment in renal impairment. It is possible to reduce toxicity with appropriate dosing. For example, in a study of women ≥65 years old with metastatic breast cancer, dosages of methotrexate and cyclophosphamide were modified according to creatinine clearance. As a consequence, myelosuppression was markedly reduced without compromise in efficacy.

Owing to differences in their pharmacokinetics and pharmacodynamics, certain chemotherapy agents can be particularly suitable for treating older patients. Oral etoposide provides valuable palliation for small-cell cancer of the lung with a potentially lower risk of complications. Weekly administered vinorelbine, gemcitabine, and taxanes are agents that are active against lung and breast cancer and can be well tolerated and effective in older adults.

Some chemotherapy-related toxicities occur in higher frequencies in older patients. Toxicities that occur with commonly used chemotherapy agents include neuropathy, GI adverse events such as diarrhea and mucositis, and fatigue. Chemotherapy toxicity can have significant functional consequences in older adults. Chemotherapy-induced peripheral neuropathy (from such agents as paclitaxel, bortezomib, brentuximab, or oxaliplatin) may have significant consequences for older patients who have other physical performance problems and may increase the risk of falls. Diarrhea can lead to dehydration and delirium. Because older patients may have less resilience in returning to baseline physiologic status after chemotherapy toxicity, "starting low and going slow" is a reasonable approach with chemotherapy, especially for those with metastatic disease for whom chemotherapy has only palliative benefit. In other words, starting therapy with a single agent versus combination agents, choosing weekly lower-dose administration versus every-3-week dosing for certain agents, or beginning with an empirically reduced dose may allow for decreased toxicity. More data are needed regarding the balance of efficacy and toxicity with these approaches. Other supportive care practices should be undertaken for an older patient on chemotherapy, including scheduling of frequent visits, close attention to medications (including supportive care medications such as benzodiazepines and psychotropics routinely used in mitigating chemotherapy-induced nausea), evaluation for appropriate social support and caregiver involvement, and consideration for growth factor use (eg, filgrastim) when appropriate.

Hormonal Therapy

Hormonal treatment is effective in cancers of the breast, prostate, and endometrium. Most of these approaches are well tolerated by older adults and commonly are the treatment of choice in this age group. However, adverse events of hormonal therapies should be considered in older patients. Tamoxifen, a selective estrogen-receptor modulator, has antagonistic and partial agonistic effects. It is a useful therapy in adjuvant treatment of breast cancer and also has estrogen-like positive effects on cardiovascular risk factors and bone disease in the postmenopausal setting. Aromatase inhibitors are oral medications that have been proved to be more efficacious than tamoxifen in adjuvant treatment of breast cancer, as well as for treatment of metastatic disease. Although the drugs are generally well tolerated, osteoporosis and fractures are more common in patients on aromatase inhibitors. Treatment with aromatase inhibitor therapy does not negatively affect cognitive function.

Hormonal therapies are the first-line of treatment for patients with systemic prostate cancer. The most commonly used hormonal therapies significantly decrease testosterone levels. Because prostate cancer can be an indolent and chronic disease, older men can be subjected to adverse events of hormonal therapies for many years. Growing evidence shows that hormonal therapy is associated with metabolic syndrome, cardiovascular disease, osteoporosis/fractures, and physical performance decrements in older men. The decision to start hormonal treatment should be thoughtfully considered and should take into account life expectancy, prostate cancer severity, and overall health status.

Biologic, Targeted, and Immunotherapies

Over the last decade, the options for biologic and targeted therapies for cancer have grown significantly. These options have significantly changed the field of oncology. Immunotherapy, or modulation of immune response, is a particularly attractive option in treating older adults, whose natural defenses against cancer can be impaired by immune senescence. Several immunotherapy agents, alone or in combination with other agents, have become approved for many tumor types in the advanced setting. These agents are still clearly inadequate to restore a normal immune response in older adults. Targeted therapies involve options that influence the activity of a specific receptor involved in cancer signaling. These options, including monoclonal antibodies or small molecule inhibitors, are used with chemotherapy or as a single agent, depending on the stage and type of cancer. Adverse-event profiles tend to be different for these agents than for traditional chemotherapy agents, given their more targeted mechanism of action. For example, many agents (such as the monoclonal antibody bevacizumab and the oral agents sunitinib and sorafenib) target the vascular endothelial growth factor (VEGF) receptor, thereby limiting tumor-related angiogenesis. These agents are associated with vascular adverse events given their mechanism of action, such as hypertension and thromboembolism, which can be a significant issue in patients who already have a history of these conditions. Hypertension can be particularly difficult to control, and close interdisciplinary care and communication are necessary to prevent treatment-related complications.

Several immunotherapy options have been available for selected cancers. Recombinant α-interferon has been used in melanoma, renal cell carcinoma, and several hematologic malignancies. High-dose interleukin-2 (IL-2) has been used with potential curative intent for advanced melanoma and renal cell carcinoma, but typically in younger patients. These agents have been supplanted mostly by newer immunotherapy agents. In melanoma, ipilimumab, a monoclonal antibody directed at cytotoxic T lymphocyte–associated antigen-4 (CTLA-4), as well as nivolumab and pembrolizumab, monoclonal antibodies directed against the programmed death receptor-1 (PD-1), which are found mainly on T cell surfaces, are now used. These immunologic agents have unusual and significant adverse-event profiles, such as autoimmune-mediated colitis and endocrinopathies, particularly when ipilimumab is used in combination with a PD-1 or programmed death ligand-1 (PDL-1) inhibitor. PD-1 and PD-L1 inhibitors are now used in treatment of a wide variety of cancers, including non-small-cell and small-cell lung cancer, renal cell carcinoma, bladder cancer, Hodgkin lymphoma, head/neck squamous cell carcinoma, certain colorectal and breast cancers, hepatocellular carcinoma, glioblastoma, and esophageal cancer. Limited data exist regarding their safety and efficacy in older patients, particularly those >70–75 years old and with worse functional status; however, small studies suggest that in fit older patients, the safety and efficacy of these agents appear similar to that encountered in their younger counterparts.

Monoclonal antibodies directed against CD20 (rituximab) expressed on B-cell lymphomas and against HER-2/*neu* (trastuzumab) expressed on breast cancer and other epithelial malignancies are effective treatments. These humanized antibodies generally show mild toxicity. Patients can develop hypotension or shortness of breath with the first infusion because of complement fixation. Symptoms abate when the infusion rate is slowed, and such symptoms rarely recur. Although monoclonal antibodies and targeted therapies are thought to be safer than chemotherapy because of decreased risk of myelosuppression, adverse events do occur and supportive mechanisms, such as more frequent follow-up visits to ensure tolerability, should be considered for older patients. Of note, many of the newer agents are administered as oral agents. Nonadherence is linked to adverse cancer outcomes, and therefore close monitoring of compliance is important.

Antibody-drug conjugates have also been developed in cancer therapeutics. These agents combine a monoclonal antibody directed at a specific cancer target with a cytotoxic agent. An example of this is ado-trastuzumab emtansine (TDM-1), which combines trastuzumab, a monoclonal antibody targeting the her-2/*neu* receptor in breast cancer, with DM-1, a cytotoxic chemotherapeutic agent. These therapies provide more directed anticancer therapy. Although they can still elicit systemic adverse events, these effects are generally deemed more manageable than those arising from non-targeted systemic chemotherapeutic agents.

Health care providers should be cognizant of specific or unique toxicities that may be seen in older patients with cancer who are receiving chemotherapy, biologic or immunotherapy agents. Because these drugs can affect multiple organs, it is not uncommon for these toxicities to manifest during routine health visits. For some key systemic adverse events from these agents, see Table 67.2.

Radiation Therapy

Radiation therapy provides palliation for virtually all cancers, and it may be part of a treatment plan for lymphomas and cancers of the prostate, bladder, cervix, esophagus, breast, brain, and lung. In combination with cytotoxic chemotherapy, radiation therapy has allowed organ preservation in cancers of the anus, bladder, head and neck, and in extremity sarcomas. A central issue for radiation therapy in older adults is safety. There has been a trend for almost five decades to use radiation therapy as an alternative to surgery in poor surgical candidates, mainly patients ≥65 years old, tacitly assuming that such an approach is less toxic. In fact, published reports have indicated that radiation therapy is both safe and effective in older patients (SOE=A). However, concern remains when treatment involves irradiation of the whole brain (fear of neurologic sequelae, including dementia) or pelvis (fear of marrow aplasia, myelodysplasia, or radiation enteritis), but no systematic investigation has categorically substantiated these concerns.

Advances in radiation therapy include techniques that allow less impact by radiation fields on normal tissues adjacent to tumor (eg, intensity-modulated radiation therapy [IMRT]); new applications of brachytherapy (insertion of radiation sources into the tumor bed mainly for breast, prostate, and gynecologic cancers); and development of radiosurgical approaches (a precisely focused external beam of radiation at relatively high doses) that allow destruction of small lesions (usually ≤4 cm in diameter and usually fewer than 5 lesions) of the brain, lung, and liver.

Surgery

Concerns related to cancer surgery in older adults are safety and rehabilitative potential. Several reports indicate that age itself is not a risk factor for elective

Table 67.2—Select Toxicities of Cancer Treatment Agents

Adverse Effect	Agents
Hypertension	VEGFR TKIs: sorafenib, sunitinib, pazopanib, axitinib, cabozantinib, lenvatinib, vandetanib, regorafenib VEGFR mAbs: bevacizumab, aflibercept, ramucirumab
QT_c prolongation	*Higher risk:* Vandetanib, lenvatinib bcr-abl/KIT TKIs: nilotinib Arsenic trioxide *Lower risk:* Osimertinib bcr-abl/KIT TKIs: imatinib, dasatinib, ponatinib, bosutinib BRAF inhibitors in combination with MEK inhibitors: vemurafenib + cobimetinib, dabrafenib + tremetinib Ibrutinib
Acneiform rash	EGFR TKIs: afatinib > erlotinib, gefitinib > osimertinib EGFR mAbs: cetuximab, panitumumab
Maculopapular rash	VEGFR TKIs bcr-abl/KIT TKIs BRAF inhibitors Anti-PD-L1 antibodies: nivolumab, pembrolizumab, avelumab, atezolizumab Anti-CTLA-4 antibodies: ipilimumab Ibrutinib Idelalisib
Hand-foot syndrome	Capecitabine > 5-fluorouracil VEGFR TKIs Liposomal doxorubicin
Keratoacanthomas, other cutaneous squamous cell carcinomas	BRAF inhibitors
Cardiotoxicity: decreased LVEF	*Higher risk:* Anti-HER2 therapy: trastuzumab, pertuzumab, lapatinib, ado-trastuzumab (TDM-1) Osimertinib BRAF inhibitors in combination with MEK inhibitors *Lower risk:* VEGFR TKIs bcr-abl/KIT TKIs
Myocarditis, pericarditis (can lead to decreased LVEF)	Anti-PD-L1 antibodies (immunotherapy)
Peripheral neuropathy	Platinum: oxaliplatin > carboplatin, cisplatin Vinca alkaloids: vincristine > vinorelbine, vinblastine Taxanes: paclitaxel > nab-paclitaxel > docetaxel > cabazitaxel Epothilones: ixabepilone > eribulin Proteasome inhibitors: bortezomib (less common with subcutaneous administration) > carfilozomib, ixasomib Brentuximab vedotin Immunomodulatory drugs: thalidomide > lenalidomide, pomalidomide
Myelosuppression (targeted therapies)	CDK inhibitors: palbociclib, ribociclib
Thyroid dysfunction	Anti-PD-L1 antibodies +/- Anti-CTLA4 antibodies (ipilimumab) VEGFR TKIs VEGFR mAbs bcr-abl/KIT TKIs Idelalisib > ibrutinib, venetoclax
Proteinuria, arterial thromboembolic disease	VEGFR TKIs VEGFR mAbs
Electrolyte disturbances	
Potassium	Venetoclax Abiraterone
Magnesium	Cisplatin EGFR mAbs: cetuximab, panitumumab
Fluid retention	Abiraterone > enzalutamide Venetoclax Ibrutinib
Dyslipidemia	mTOR inhibitors: everolimus, temsirolimus Abiraterone

Note: VEGFR = vascular endothelial growth factor receptor, TKI = tyrosine kinase inhibitors, mAbs = monoclonal antibodies, EGFR = epidermal growth factor receptor, CTLA-4 = cytotoxic T lymphocyte–associated antigen-4, HER2 = human epidermal growth factor receptor 2, CDK = cyclin-dependent kinase, mTOR = mammalian target of rapamycin cancer surgery, but the length of hospital stay and the time to full recovery become longer with advancing age. Similar results have been reported both from referral centers and community hospitals.

Advances in anesthesia and surgery have benefited older patients. Included among these are endoscopic procedures that provide valuable palliation for the many tumors of the GI tract, and the greater use of spinal anesthesia for major abdominal interventions, with a substantial decline in perioperative complications and mortality. More widespread use of laparoscopic surgical techniques and application of laser and photodynamic therapy is also broadening the surgical armamentarium and providing a larger proportion of older patients with treatment options that confer a lower risk of complications.

The trend to manage cancer without deforming surgery can preclude the need for complex rehabilitation and can be of special value for older adults. Organ preservation without compromise of treatment outcome is obtainable for certain cancers such as those of the head and neck that involve radiation with or without chemotherapy. Also, the use of initial (neoadjuvant) chemotherapy before primary surgery has been effective in patients with large primary breast and lung cancers. Such an approach can result in less extensive and potentially more curative surgical procedures.

Quality-of-Life Issues

Several studies have determined that the perception of quality of life is highly subjective and poorly assessed by external observers, even by those who have close relationships with the patient. Furthermore, there is considerable discrepancy between the physician's determination of the patient's quality of life and the patient's own assessment, with physicians tending to underestimate the patient's quality of life (SOE=B).

Early assessments of quality of life focused on functional status and freedom from pain, but these factors, although important, are inadequate for evaluating far-reaching consequences of serious diseases on all domains of life. In the past decade, several instruments for measuring quality of life have been validated and used successfully to study specific problems, such as the effects on quality of life of intensive care, the consequences of limb amputation or of partial and total mastectomy, and iatrogenic erectile dysfunction. These instruments are questionnaires querying an individual to rate his or her own well-being in several dimensions with a categorical or a visual analog scale. Several scales have been used and validated for older patients with cancer (eg, Functional Assessment of Cancer Therapy and EORTC Quality of Life Questionnaire Core). Unfortunately, these instruments have not been modified to account for the special needs of older adults, and the relationship between geriatric assessment and quality-of-life measurement tools remains unclear. Although it is reasonable to assume that the importance of some factors, such as professional or job satisfaction, may decline with age, the importance of others, including social support and perception of family burden, can become more prominent.

Other problems related to assessing quality of life include the length and/or complexity of some questionnaires; some older adults can be overwhelmed and require assistance. In addition, little progress has been made in assessment of quality of life in cognitively impaired individuals. Studies of pain in individuals with dementia have demonstrated the reliability of repetitive behavioral testing in assessing discomfort, even in patients with cognitive impairment. It is credible but unproved that the same principles can be applied to assessing quality of life in dementia patients.

At present, the main application of quality-of-life assessment in clinical decision-making concerns the choice between interventions yielding comparable survival. An area of potential use is in medical decisions involving limited survival benefits but at the price of a decline in quality of life. At present, the value of this trade-off is evaluated with measures known as "quality-of-life adjusted survival" or "quality-adjusted time without symptoms or toxicity," both of which may be important to consider for adults ≥70 years old. Again, further research is needed in the melding of geriatric assessment and quality-of-life instruments to address these specific knowledge gaps.

SPECIFIC CANCERS

Among women, the three most commonly diagnosed types of cancer are cancers of the breast, lung and bronchus, and colorectum, accounting for 50% of estimated cancer cases. Breast cancer alone is expected to account for 29% of all new cancer cases among women. Among men, cancers of the prostate, lung and bronchus, and colorectum account for 48% of all newly diagnosed cancers. Prostate cancer alone accounts for 26% of incident cases in men. Based on cases diagnosed between 1999 and 2005, an estimated 92% of these new cases of prostate cancer are expected to be diagnosed at local or regional stages, for which the 5-year relative survival approaches 100%.

Breast Cancer

Worldwide, nearly a third of breast cancer cases are seen in patients >65 years old; in more developed countries, this proportion rises to more than 40%. Advanced age at diagnosis of breast cancer is associated with more favorable tumor biology as indicated by increased hormone sensitivity and lower grades and proliferative indices. However, older patients are more likely to present with larger and more advanced tumors. Overall, there seem to be no major differences in outcomes in stage-matched patients as age increases. Nevertheless, older patients are less likely to be treated according to accepted treatment guidelines, and undertreatment can have an adverse impact on overall outcome. The explanation for these age-related differences in approach to treatment is complex and includes provider and patient bias, psychosocial issues, cost, and proximity to treatment centers. Heterogeneity in overall health status also influences decision-making for treatment. Despite the fact that breast cancer occurs mainly in older patients, this population is under-represented in clinical trials. Less than 5% of participants included in clinical trials that evaluate adjuvant chemotherapy are ≥75 years old. Age is a significant predictor of whether older patients with breast cancer are offered entry into clinical trials, despite the fact that older patients are just as likely as younger patients to participate if given the opportunity. Because comorbidities and functional status significantly affect prognosis and treatment choice, thorough consideration must be given to the overall health of older patients.

For patients with localized cancer, the evidence supports surgical treatment versus primary hormonal treatment. Breast conservation treatment, consisting of breast-conserving surgery (lumpectomy or partial mastectomy) and postoperative radiotherapy, is now recommended as the standard of care for patients of all ages with early disease. As in younger patients, total mastectomy remains a surgical option for older patients who prefer it over breast conservation treatment and for those who decline or are not candidates for postoperative breast radiotherapy. Mastectomy is considered in patients with large primary lesions. Axillary lymph node dissection should be done in patients with clinical evidence of axillary lymph node involvement. However, for those without clinical lymph node involvement, sentinel lymph node dissection has been introduced as an alternative to axillary lymph node dissection. Sentinel lymph node biopsy has been shown to be a safe and accurate method of predicting axillary status in patients with breast cancer, including those ≥70 years old. It is now widely considered an acceptable treatment option in patients of all ages with no clinical evidence of axillary involvement. Findings from sentinel biopsies in older patients with breast cancer could significantly affect subsequent treatment decisions, including adjuvant systemic treatment. Data suggest that sentinel node sampling is just as accurate as axillary dissection but considerably less toxic (SOE=A).

Postoperative Irradiation after Lumpectomy

Although irradiation after lumpectomy is safe in women ≥65 years old, it may be a source of significant inconvenience and cost. The value of postoperative irradiation has been questioned because the local recurrence rate of breast cancer may decrease with age, and the inconvenience of daily radiation treatment protocols may outweigh the limited benefits for some. In patients ≥70 years old who receive breast-conserving therapy followed by adjuvant hormonal therapy, omission of adjuvant radiation therapy can be considered for patients with certain lower risk features. Individuals without adjuvant radiation therapy experience higher rates of local/regional recurrence, but overall survival appears not to be significantly different.

Hormonal Treatment

Adjuvant hormonal therapy is recommended for estrogen receptor–positive breast cancer. Aromatase inhibitors are used as first-line treatment in women with estrogen receptor–positive tumors, and the medication is given for at least 5 years although emerging data suggests 10 years duration may be superior. Aromatase inhibitors are both more effective and less toxic than tamoxifen (SOE=A). Evidence suggests that even frail, older women tolerate aromatase inhibitor therapy well, although this treatment is less likely to be offered by oncologists to this group of patients.

Initial Management of Metastatic Breast Cancer

Women ≥65 years old with metastatic, hormone receptor–positive breast cancer who are not significantly symptomatic from their disease are likely to experience effective palliation with hormonal therapy. Chemotherapy has also been shown to be safe and effective in this group of patients and is preferred first-line treatment in patients who are in visceral crisis (eg, having pain or high symptom burden due to metastatic disease in visceral organs such as lungs or liver). Generally, single agents are used, and treatment is begun at full dosage for fit older adults with modifications based on any toxicities that develop. In vulnerable older adults, treatment can usually begin safely at 75% of the recommended dosage.

Lung Cancer

Lung cancer is the leading cause of cancer-related death in Western countries for both men and women. More than half of patients diagnosed with lung cancer are ≥70 years old. Management options for lung cancer are based on the cell type. Non–small-cell lung cancer (NSCLC) constitutes at least 80% of all lung cancers, with small-cell cancer making up the remaining. Most patients with lung cancer present with advanced-stage disease, in which the goal of therapy is generally palliative. Lung cancer staging runs from Stage 1 to 4, taking into account tumor size and location of involvement, nodal status, and whether or not there are distant metastases. Lung cancer is becoming increasingly common in older women for reasons that are not completely understood. The increase may be due to higher smoking rates among women. In addition, some data suggest that women are at greater risk (than men) of developing lung cancer per unit of tobacco exposure. Early recognition and surgical resection remain the best chance for cure for early-stage disease. However, stereotactic radiation is a nonsurgical alternative for patients with inoperable stage 1 and some stage 2 NSCLC, or for those who elect not to have surgery. Over the past decade, chemotherapy has produced clinical responses and provided effective palliation for a portion of patients with metastatic disease. A meta-analysis of more than 50 trials comparing chemotherapy to best supportive care indicated that chemotherapy is not associated with a worse outcome in older adults and thus paved the way for exploration of better suited regimens.

Stage 3 NSCLC among older adults is more difficult to address because many patients may not be fit to undergo definitive concurrent chemoradiation, and often sequential approaches, or radiation therapy alone, are used. Supportive care and interdisciplinary team management is even more critical for these patients undergoing combined modality therapy. In potentially resectable stage 3a disease, neoadjuvant approaches followed by surgical resection are considered on a case-by-case basis with multidisciplinary input from thoracic surgery, radiation, and medical oncology.

Combination chemotherapy with a platinum doublet is the standard of care for treatment of most cases of advanced NSCLC. Historically, oncologists have been concerned about tolerability of platinum-based doublets in older lung cancer patients. A randomized phase III study evaluated patients ≥70 years old with advanced lung cancer and determined that this population still benefited from doublet chemotherapy regimens (median overall survival 10.3 months for doublet chemotherapy versus 6.2 months for monotherapy, $P<.0001$) (SOE=A). However, toxic adverse events were noted more frequently in the doublet chemotherapy arm, and most patients enrolled in the study had excellent performance status. First-line immunotherapy is also an option for patients with advanced NSCLC whose tumors overexpress PD-L1 with improved cancer-related outcomes over chemotherapy and generally less toxicity. Longer-term functional and other outcomes in older adults receiving immunotherapy remain less clear.

Small-cell lung cancer remains a diagnosis exclusive to patients with heavy smoking exposure and is often treated with chemotherapy and/or radiation therapy without surgery, depending on the stage of disease. Brain metastatic relapse is common and has paved way for the consideration of prophylactic cranial irradiation, but the longer-term neurocognitive effects of this treatment on older adults are less well understood. Newer radiation techniques are being developed to minimize these effects through the evaluation of hippocampal-sparing treatment planning and the use of memantine after whole brain irradiation. This cancer remains clinically aggressive, and the benefits and toxicities of second- and third-line therapies have to be carefully weighed along with goals of care and quality-of-life considerations.

Colon Cancer

Colonoscopy has become the mainstay of prevention of colon cancer, primarily because it enables direct visualization of the entire colon and biopsy of encountered lesions. Polyps do not usually cause symptoms, but they may bleed or predispose to cancer. Colonic polyps are usually classified as neoplastic (adenomas) or non-neoplastic (hyperplastic). Approximately 40% of the U.S. population ≥50 years old have one or more adenomas. Detection and removal of adenomas significantly decrease the morbidity and mortality associated with colorectal cancer. Old age and male gender are major risk factors. First-degree relatives of patients with adenomas are also at increased risk of colorectal cancer and should undergo screening. Adenomas are most often detected by colon cancer screening tests, primarily sigmoidoscopy. Because adenomas do not typically bleed, the fecal occult blood test is an insensitive screening method. Fecal DNA testing is a more sensitive option in screening for colon cancer and needs to be repeated only every 3 years if initially negative. Older age, villous histology, and size >1 cm are independent risk factors for malignancy within an adenoma. The risk of colon cancer also increases with the number of high-risk adenomas present.

Colonoscopy with endoscopic polypectomy remains the ideal examination for the detection and removal of adenomatous polyps. The examination should be meticulous, with emphasis to mucosal detail to not miss flat or depressed adenomatous lesions. In addition, a minimum of 6 minutes of colonoscopic withdrawal time is associated with increased polyp yield. Large adenomas that cannot be safely or completely resected endoscopically should generally be removed by segmental colectomy. If a polyp is detected by barium enema, colonoscopy is recommended to establish the histology, remove the polyp, and search for other lesions. If a single polyp is detected by sigmoidoscopy, it should be biopsied. If the polyp is hyperplastic, colonoscopy is not required. If the polyp is adenomatous, full colonoscopy is warranted. In patients with a known history of polyps, discontinuation of surveillance should be considered in those >75 years old in whom a follow-up examination is normal or shows only small tubular adenomas.

A 3-year interval for surveillance colonoscopy is safe and cost-effective for most patients with adenomas. If only a small tubular adenoma is found, the interval may be extended to 5 years; in contrast, after removal of a large villous adenoma, a 1-year follow-up is recommended. After a negative screening or surveillance colonoscopy, an examination interval of 5 years appears to be sufficient. Patients with colorectal cancer should also have regular colonoscopic surveillance for adenomas starting 1 year after surgery, because these patients have adenoma or cancer recurrence rates of 25%–30% at 3 years.

Colorectal cancer is the third leading cause of cancer in the United States and the second leading cause of cancer death. The risk of colorectal cancer increases dramatically with age, with >90% of cases occurring in people >50 years old. Two-thirds of patients with colorectal cancer are ≥65 years old. Women are more likely than men to harbor right-sided colonic adenomas. The risk of colorectal cancer in patients with rectal bleeding is age related and may reach 25% in patients ≥80 years old. Up to 40% of colorectal cancer arises proximal to the splenic flexure, and <10% is within reach of digital rectal examination. Because it is impossible to identify the source of bleeding by clinical criteria, a colonoscopy should be performed in all cases of hematochezia, occult GI bleeding, iron-deficiency anemia, or even melena after a negative upper endoscopy (SOE=C). Other symptoms, such as abdominal pain, altered bowel habits, or pencil-thin feces are less predictive of colorectal cancer but still require thorough investigation, starting with a colonoscopy. Typically, right-sided cancers present with iron-deficiency anemia and occult GI bleeding, whereas left-sided cancers lead to obstructive symptoms, changes in bowel habits, and overt hematochezia.

Surgical excision may be adequate for lesions confined to the colon, but if regional nodes are involved, postoperative adjuvant chemotherapy (usually 5-fluorouracil plus leucovorin) has reduced recurrence by 40%–50% (SOE=A). The addition of oxaliplatin to 5-fluorouracil for adjuvant chemotherapy has improved outcomes for younger patients with regional nodes after resection (ie, stage 3 disease). Trials that have evaluated this regimen included very few older patients, so more data are necessary. Oxaliplatin may not have the same safety and efficacy profile in the adjuvant setting in older patients with colon cancer than it does in younger patients. For patients with localized rectal cancer, the standard of care involves a multidisciplinary approach, including medical oncology, radiation oncology, and surgery, because treatment involves a multimodal approach.

The standard of care in patients with stage 4 (metastatic) colorectal cancer is systemic chemotherapy with or without antibody therapy and surgical intervention when appropriate for curative intent or symptom management. There is a subset of patients with metastatic colorectal cancer with <5 metastatic sites involving liver and/or lung ("oligometastatic disease") for whom surgery, stereotactic radiotherapy, and/or ablative strategies can be implemented with curative intent, but this requires multimodal treatment and rigorous multidisciplinary evaluation. Age per se should not be considered a contraindication for surgery to treat colorectal cancer. In patients with hepatic metastasis only, hepatic resection can offer a chance of long-term survival. In selected older patients, this procedure is safe and feasible with a survival benefit similar to that of younger people (SOE=B). However, older patients who undergo this procedure are not routinely offered perioperative chemotherapy, which is often necessary to achieve longer-term disease control.

Overall, survival of patients with metastatic disease in the liver or other organs has improved significantly because of new medications, such as irinotecan and oxaliplatin, that have induced partial remissions in a subset of patients. Survival has increased from 6 months on average to >2 years for patients who can tolerate treatment. Active debate continues on the use of combination therapy versus monotherapy in the management of older patients with metastatic colon cancer because of a similar overall survival benefit noted in several trials. Capecitabine, an oral 5-fluorouracil pro-drug, is an option for older patients, especially those who are wary of infusional regimens, but it may have an impact on quality of life that is worse than that of infusional 5-fluorouracil. New medications that target a tyrosine kinase (an integral enzyme for cellular proliferation) within tumor cells and neutralize VEGF (thought to promote angiogenesis) have improved outcomes. Bevacuzimab, a VEGF antibody, has been shown to improve overall survival of older adults when used in combination with standard chemotherapy (SOE=A). The incidence of arterial thromboembolic events increases with age, and caution must be used when prescribing this agent in older adults. For patients whose colorectal cancer is *RAS* wild-type, adding monoclonal antibodies (ie, cetuximab, panitumumab) to the epidermal growth factor receptor can improve survival. Several other options have evolved beyond 5-fluorouracil–based chemotherapy, including immunotherapy for microsatellite instability-high tumors, as well as the oral drugs regorafenib and trifluridine/tipiracil for patients in whom multiple lines of prior therapy have not been effective.

Gastric and Esophageal Cancers

Cancers originating in the lower esophagus, gastroesophageal junction, and gastric area are treated similarly, because they share a common pathogenesis, regardless of histology. Approximately 60% of esophageal and gastric cancers arise in patients ≥65 years old. Fit older patients with resectable disease should be considered for preoperative chemotherapy with radiation or perioperative chemotherapy in conjunction with surgery. A multidisciplinary approach, including medical oncology, radiation oncology, and surgery, is very important from the beginning of the decision-making process. Often definitive chemoradiation is offered for locally advanced disease in inoperable patients or for those who forgo esophagectomy. In older patients with recurrent and metastatic disease, palliative chemotherapy not only improves overall survival but also improves quality of life. The efficacy and tolerability of a platinum-containing regimen in patients ≥70 years old has been established and is comparable to that in younger patients. The major drawback of combination chemotherapy regimens is the likely need for a central venous line for administration and high incidence of line-related complications. Similar outcomes have been shown when capecitabine (oral pro-drug of 5-fluorouracil) was substituted for infusional 5-fluorouracil, and when oxaliplatin is substituted for cisplatin (similar to treatment results for colorectal cancer). In older patients who cannot tolerate combination chemotherapy, single agent 5-fluorouracil or capecitabine are reasonable initial options.

Esophageal cancer is commonly diagnosed at an advanced, incurable stage in older patients who are not candidates for tumor resection. These patients are plagued by symptoms of esophageal obstruction or fistula formation, dysphagia, aspiration, and weight loss. In such instances, endoscopic palliation can be achieved with either laser therapy or placement of a single, permanent, metal stent. Laser therapy with neodymium-yttrium-aluminum-garnet (Nd:YAG) fulgurates the malignant obstructing tissue and restores luminal patency in >90% of cases, with a 5% risk of perforation. Relief can last for up to several months; treatments may be repeated. Photodynamic therapy uses a photosensitizing agent in combination with endoscopic laser exposure. It is more effective than Nd:YAG laser for palliation and has fewer complications, but it can cause skin photosensitivity. Treatment with self-expanding metal stents is preferable for patients with a malignant stricture or an esophagobronchial fistula, because it relieves dysphagia and aspiration in up to 95% of patients and has a low complication rate (SOE=B). The disadvantages of stents include their high cost, tumor ingrowth, and stent migration. Alternatively, palliative radiation to the primary tumor can provide symptomatic relief in two-thirds or more of patients with more advanced disease.

Prostate Cancer

Prostate cancer affects older men disproportionately. In the United States, it is estimated that over 1 million men ≥75 years old have the disease, with more than 60% of all new cases diagnosed in men >65 years old. Because of the long natural history of the disease, the case fatality rate is low in the young. It is notable, however, that 70% of men who die of prostate cancer are ≥75 years old. Advanced prostate cancer cannot be cured and affects patients whose disease has spread beyond the prostate and/or are symptomatic, as well as patients with biochemical recurrence only (a rise in prostate-specific antigen with no evidence of disease). Androgen-deprivation therapy (ADT) is used in the initial management of these patients and is associated with a multitude of adverse events, including hot flashes, sexual dysfunction, osteoporosis, and metabolic syndrome. ADT consists of gonadotropin releasing–hormone agonist or antagonist as well as an antiandrogen, and their effects lie in their ability to lower the testosterone levels available to the cancer cells. Given the significant consequence of ADT in older men, serious discussion must be undertaken with the patient regarding risks versus benefits before beginning therapy. For older patients with indolent cancer characteristics and no clinical symptoms, active surveillance should be considered. The addition of chemotherapy (ie, docetaxel) or complementary drugs that impair androgen synthesis (ie, abiraterone) to ADT have shown improved survival over ADT alone, particularly in those with high disease burden. However, such combination strategies may augment the adverse events of ADT and introduce new toxicities that may be challenging for older adults, particularly those with significant cardiovascular comorbidity, because fluid retention and hypertension may be exacerbated.

In older men, when the disease has progressed on ADT alone (castrate-resistant prostate cancer), standard-dose chemotherapy is docetaxel given every 3 weeks. Subset analysis of the index trials has established that men >75 years old had an equivalent response to that of the younger population but with a predictable increase in toxicity, especially myelosuppression. A lower weekly dosage of docetaxel has been studied in an attempt to address the issue of myelosuppression and other adverse events seen with standard-dose chemotherapy. Results from these studies indicate that this schedule has a modest effect on the progression-free survival but does not impact overall survival. Several new regimens have been approved for treatment of castrate-resistant prostate cancer. Abiraterone and enzalutamide, inhibitors of the androgen receptor, have both been shown to improve overall survival in this setting, even without prior docetaxel use. Key trials of both drugs included patients ≥75 years old (>25% of study population) and clinical benefit was seen across age subgroups. Overall survival was also improved with sipuleucel-T, an autologous active cellular-based immunotherapy, when compared with placebo in a trial in which the median age was 72 years old (SOE=A).

Bladder Cancer

Age is an independent risk factor for development of transitional cell cancer of the bladder. The median age at diagnosis is 69 years for men and 71 years for women, with the peak incidence at 85 years. With advanced age, there is an increased risk of detecting higher stage and higher grade cancers. Treatment is based on whether the disease is muscle invasive and metastatic or not.

Neoadjuvant chemotherapy with cisplatin-based chemotherapy followed by radical cystectomy with pelvic lymph node dissection and urinary diversion remains the standard of care in patients with clinically localized muscle invasive cancer. However, most older patients do not undergo this procedure for a multitude of reasons, including concerns about high perioperative morbidity. The patients who do undergo this procedure can still have poor oncologic outcomes because of inadequate pelvic lymph node dissection and inadequate use of chemotherapy in the neoadjuvant or adjuvant setting. Alternative approaches like extensive transurethral resection and radiation therapy with chemotherapy are at best only palliative. Bladder-sparing approaches with chemoradiation can be considered in patients who are high risk for surgery but are associated with worse overall and cancer-specific survival.

Cisplatin-based therapy is the most effective regimen for patients with this cancer in both the localized and metastatic setting but is associated with various toxicities, including renal insufficiency, nausea and vomiting, myelosuppression and neuropathy. Because of the high prevalence of impaired renal function and other comorbidities, >40% of the population is ineligible for a cisplatin-based regimen. In patients who are not eligible for cisplatin, several other regimens have been studied and include single agent gemcitabine, paclitaxel, combination regimens of gemcitabine/paclitaxel and gemcitabine/carboplatin; these have all demonstrated modest activity with good tolerance. Immunotherapy with agents such as nivolumab, atezolizumab, avelumab, and durvalumab are now part of the treatment options for second-line advanced bladder cancer and will likely become first-line options for patients who cannot safely receive cisplatin-based chemotherapy.

Renal Cell Cancer

The average age at presentation of renal cell cancer is 64 years in both sexes. Currently, >60% of cases are diagnosed incidentally compared with the 1970s when only 10% of cancers were found by chance. As a result, more patients are diagnosed with early stage disease. The treatment for local disease can be surgery (radical or partial nephrectomy) or ablative therapies (radiofrequency, cryotherapy). Although in most cases surgery is safe, complications such as alteration of renal function may occur, especially in older adults, with physiologic renal impairment at baseline. Given that the growth rate of small renal cell cancer is low and that the capacity to induce dissemination of metastases is limited, active surveillance can be proposed for asymptomatic patients and for those who are frail with a limited remaining life expectancy. The average growth rate is approximately 0.30 cm per year, and 1% of patients develop metastatic disease.

In advanced disease, the role of cytoreductive nephrectomy to significantly prolong survival, delay time to progression, and enhance the response to systemic biologic therapy in the postoperative period is well established in select young patients with metastatic renal cell cancer. Patients ≥75 years old have a higher risk of perioperative mortality. In spite of this increased early death, the median survival is similar in older versus younger patients. Because of the high perioperative mortality, until more data is available in the targeted agent era, it is perhaps reasonable to consider these agents alone.

In contrast to other malignancies, renal cell cancer is not treated with chemotherapy. For a long time, interleukin-2 and interferon were the only available systemic options for management of renal cell cancer. The toxicities of these cytokines (fatigue, edema, depression, cardiovascular adverse events) were an obstacle to treatment in both the young and old. Agents (eg, sunitinib, pazopanib) targeting tumor angiogenesis (VEGF inhibitor) and intracellular pathways mediating proliferation and growth (mammalian target of rapamycin, an mTOR inhibitor) (eg, everolimus) have demonstrated improved efficacy with a favorable toxicity profile in phase III trials and have largely replaced cytokine treatments. The median age of patients in most of these trials was 62 years, and in all of these studies >30% of the study population was older than 65 years.

These targeted agents have unique adverse events that can adversely impact outcome in older adults, including diarrhea, hand/foot syndrome, hypertension, cardiovascular toxicity (both ischemia and heart failure), mucositis, skin toxicities, and fatigue. Retrospective subgroup analysis of trials suggests a similar benefit in patients of all age groups, with similar toxicity and a beneficial effect on quality of life. In the absence of prospective controlled comparison between different agents, when selecting an agent, the toxicity profile and implications of specific comorbid conditions should be taken into account. Co-management with geriatrics and primary care is necessary to manage hypertension and other cardiovascular toxicities.

HEMATOLOGIC MALIGNANCIES, LYMPHOMAS, AND MULTIPLE MYELOMA

Leukemias

Acute myeloid leukemia (AML) in older adults is more likely to be refractory to treatment and to have a smoldering course, for which only supportive care is administered. Older age is a poor prognostic factor for AML, independent of cytogenetics. What is not clear is whether the prevalence of unfavorable cytogenetic abnormalities and of multilineage neoplastic involvement increases with age in de novo AML. The subset of patients with myelodysplasia who do not have excess blasts or overt leukemia but are neutropenic and have recurrent infections may benefit from intermittent treatment with granulocyte colony-stimulating factor.

In a trial with older patients with AML, delayed treatment was much less effective than immediate treatment. Although this study established the value of timely chemotherapy, the choice of treatment (whether full-dose induction or low-dose cytarabine) remains controversial. Low-intensity therapy with agents such as 5-azacytadine or decitabine may be considered for older patients, particularly those who are unfit or have significant comorbidities.

Chronic lymphocytic leukemia (CLL) is the most common form of leukemia in the Western world; about 12,500 cases are diagnosed each year in the United States. The incidence is declining for unknown reasons. The median age at diagnosis is 61 years. The diagnosis is most often made incidentally when a peripheral WBC count reveals leukocytosis with a small-lymphocyte count >4,000/µL. Treatment is generally instituted only to control a life-threatening or symptomatic complication. The major complications are infection and marrow failure. Because about 25% of patients develop autoimmune anemia or thrombocytopenia sometime in the course of the disease, it is important to investigate the mechanism of any decline in peripheral blood cell counts. Autoimmune mechanisms can be treated with glucocorticoids or splenectomy, whereas marrow infiltration by tumor cells requires antitumor therapy. The treatment options for CLL have expanded beyond chlorambucil and fludarabine-based regimens. Ibrutinib, a novel oral inhibitor of Bruton's tyrosine kinase, was shown to be more effective than chlorambucil in a trial specific to older adults, with a favorable toxicity and adherence profile. Idelalisib, an oral PI3K inhibitor approved for relapsed CLL in combination with rituximab, is now being evaluated as a first-line option for older adults as well. More novel anti-CD20 antibodies (ie, ofatumumab, obinutuzumab) beyond rituximab (ie, targeting B cells) have also been developed for use in CLL and other indolent lymphomas. These antibodies have led to improved response and progression-free survival rates when combined with chlorambucil versus chlorambucil plus rituximab or chlorambucil alone.

Non-Hodgkin Lymphoma

Although there are about 38 named varieties of lymphoma, the two most common forms (diffuse large B-cell lymphoma and follicular lymphoma) account for about 75% of cases. The prognosis of non-Hodgkin lymphoma worsens with age, but the explanation remains unclear. It is likely that older adults are more susceptible to the complications of intensive treatment.

The treatment of older adults with diffuse large B-cell lymphoma has improved in recent years. In this group, 60%–70% of patients obtain a durable complete remission with combination chemotherapy (eg, cyclophosphamide, doxorubicin, vincristine, prednisone [CHOP]) plus rituximab (R-CHOP). Administration of lower-than-normal dosages results in a poorer outcome. Hematopoietic growth factors can lessen the hematopoietic toxicity of treatment. R-mini-CHOP (ie, R-CHOP using attenuated doses of only the chemotherapeutic agents) and R-bendamustine may be alternatives to standard-dosing CHOP for patients ≥80 years old or those younger with significant multimorbidity.

The treatment of follicular lymphoma is more controversial. Localized forms of the disease (seen in 15% of patients) are curable with radiation therapy. In the 85% of patients with more advanced disease, single agent and combination chemotherapy can sometimes induce long, complete remissions (median duration 6–7 years). However, in patients with other serious morbidities and a remaining life expectancy of <5 years, treatment may not be needed because of the indolent nature of the disease progression.

Hodgkin Lymphoma

Hodgkin disease exhibits a curious bimodal age-incidence curve, with a second peak late in life. Compared with younger patients, older patients with advanced disease may respond less well to therapy and have lower survival rates (SOE=C). Several factors can contribute to this poorer prognosis: more extensive disease at presentation, biologic variations from true Hodgkin lymphoma, greater toxicity with standard treatment regimens, and less aggressive treatment. Older adults can usually tolerate full doses of doxorubicin, bleomycin, vinblastine, and dacarbazine (ABVD) without life-threatening bone-marrow toxicity. However, many older patients have underlying cardiac and/or pulmonary disease that precludes the safe use of ABVD.

Multiple Myeloma and Monoclonal Gammopathy of Uncertain Significance (MGUS)

Multiple myeloma is diagnosed in almost 20,000 people each year in the United States. The median age at diagnosis is 68 years; it is rare in people <40 years old. The incidence in black Americans is twice that in white Americans. The classic triad of myeloma is marrow plasmacytosis (>10%), lytic bone lesions, and a serum or urine (or both) monoclonal gammopathy.

Monoclonal gammopathy is common in older adults, estimated at 6% of those ≥70 years old. When an abnormal paraprotein is discovered on serum immunoelectrophoresis, the best diagnostic test to distinguish myeloma from MGUS is a skeletal survey. If the skeletal survey is normal, a bone marrow biopsy is still indicated to determine the presence of marrow plasmacytosis. Patients with MGUS have marrow plasma cells constituting <10% of the total cell number; do not have lytic bone lesions; and usually do not have other features of myeloma, including hypercalcemia, renal failure, anemia, or susceptibility to infection. MGUS progresses to multiple myeloma or lymphoma at a rate of 1% per year (SOE=B).

Patients with myeloma require treatment when the lytic bone lesions become symptomatic or progressive, infections are recurrent, or the serum paraprotein level increases. Standard treatment consists of multiagent combination regimens (eg, bortezomib plus lenalidomide plus dexamethasone [VRD]), especially for those who have high-risk disease and for those who will go on to receive high-dose therapy plus an autologous stem-cell transplant. Many older, frail patients receive reduced-dose lenalidomide plus dexamethasone. Comorbidities and renal function may impact selection, dosing, and intensity of treatment. A frailty index has been developed by the International Myeloma Working Group to better gauge prognosis and toxicities from treatment in older adults. Newer, more targeted antimyeloma drugs, including daratumumab and elotuzumab, have emerged for relapsed disease. Supportive care includes bisphosphonates to decrease bone turnover, erythropoietin and other hematinics for related anemia, intravenous immunoglobulin for recurrent infections, radiation therapy for symptomatic bone lesions, maintenance of hydration to preserve renal function, adequate analgesia, and multidisciplinary management of functional status.

PRINCIPLES OF MANAGEMENT

Both the incidence and prevalence of cancer increase with age, and older adults more often present with advanced-stage disease. Screening older populations with appropriate life expectancies for certain cancer types can lead to early detection of more curable lesions. Older patients can have less physiologic reserve than younger patients, but unless a specific comorbid illness is influencing baseline organ function, cancer treatments with curative or palliative potential should be offered to most patients in most settings, regardless of age. However, treatment intensity, availability of caregiver and/or social support, and supportive care plans must all be considered. Curative surgical procedures may require more prolonged convalescence, but recovery from most procedures is expected. Radiation therapy alone is safe and effective in the same settings in which it is used in younger patients. Chemotherapy may need to be adjusted to the individual patient's level of tolerance of the adverse events, but usually the changes should be made in the face of toxicities that actually develop rather than on toxicities anticipated to develop. Biologic therapies also are generally safe for older patients. Combined modality treatment strategies for advanced cancers require careful multidisciplinary evaluation, communication, and management.

CHOOSING WISELY® RECOMMENDATIONS

Oncology

- Do not recommend screening for breast cancer, colorectal cancer, or prostate cancer (with the PSA test) without considering life expectancy and the risks of testing, overdiagnosis, and overtreatment.

- Assessing remaining life expectancy should involve a comprehensive evaluation of health status and include disability, comorbidity, and geriatric syndromes.

RESOURCES

- Hurria A, Mohile S, Gajra A, et al. Validation of a prediction tool for chemotherapy toxicity in older adults with cancer. *J Clin Oncol.* 2016;34(20):2366–2371.

- Hurria A, Wildes T, Blair SL, et al. Senior adult oncology, version 2.2014: clinical practice guidelines in oncology. *J Natl Compr Canc Netw.* 2014;12(1):82–126.

NORMAL LABORATORY VALUES*
Referenced in the Questions and Critiques

BLOOD, PLASMA, SERUM CHEMISTRIES

Alanine aminotransferase (ALT)   0–35 U/L

Aspartate aminotransferase (AST)   0–35 U/L

Bicarbonate (CO_2)   21–30 mEq/L

Blood gas studies:

  PO_2 83–108 mmHg

  PCO_2 Women: 32–45 mmHg; Men: 35–48 mmHg

  pH   7.35–7.45

  Oxygen saturation   95%–98%

Blood urea nitrogen (BUN)   8–20 mg/dL

Calcium   8.8–10.3 mg/dL

Calcium, ionized   4.5–5.6 mEq/L

Carcinoembryonic antigen   <2.5 ng/mL

Chloride   98–106 mEq/L

Cholesterol:

  Total   Desirable: 200 mg/dL

  High-density lipoprotein (HDL)   Desirable: >39 mg/dL

  Low-density lipoprotein (LDL)   Recommended: <130 mg/dL, lower for those with CHD risk factors or vascular disease

  Moderate risk: 130–159 mg/dL

  High risk: ≥160 mg/dL

Creatinine   0.7–1.5 mg/dL

Creatine kinase   Women: 26–140 U/L; Men: 38–174 U/L

Digoxin (therapeutic level)   0.8–2.0 ng/mL for rate control; 0.6–0.8 for heart failure

Ferritin   20–250 ng/mL

Folate   2.2–17.3 ng/mL

Glucose   Fasting: 70–105 mg/dL
  2-hour postprandial: <140 mg/dL

Hemoglobin A_{1c} 4.0%–6.0%

Homocysteine   5–15 μmol/L

Iron   50–150 mcg/dL; iron saturation ([iron/iron-binding capacity] × 100) ≤10% abnormal

Iron-binding capacity, total   250–450 mcg/dL

Lactate dehydrogenase   60–100 U/L

Methylmalonic acid (MMA)   0.08–0.56 μmol/L

Magnesium   1.8–3.0 mg/dL

Parathyroid hormone   10–65 pg/mL

Phosphatase, acid   0.5–5.5 U/L

Phosphatase, alkaline   20–135 U/L

Phosphorus (≥60 yr old)   Women: 2.8–4.1 mg/dL
  Men: 2.3–3.7 mg/dL

Potassium   3.5–5 mEq/L

Prostate-specific antigen (PSA)   <4 ng/mL

Protein, total   6.4–8.3 g/dL

  Albumin 3.5–5.5 g/dL

  Globulin 2.0–3.5 g/dL

Rheumatoid factor, latest test   >1:80 is abnormal

Sodium   136–145 mEq/L

Testosterone:

  Women <3.5 nmol/L (<100 ng.dL)

  Men 10–35 nmol/L (300–1,000 ng/dL)

Thyrotropin (TSH)   0.5–5.0 μU/mL

Thyroxine (T_4)   Total: 5–12 mcg/dL; Free: 0.9–2.4 ng/dL

Triglycerides   Recommended: <150 mg/dL

Uric acid   2.5–8.0 mg/dL

Vitamin B_{12} 200–950 pg/mL

25(OH) vitamin D (total)   30–75 mcg/L

HEMATOLOGY

RBC count   Women: 4.2–5.4 × 10^6/μL; Men: 4.7–6.1 × 10^6/μL

Erythrocyte sedimentation rate (Westergren)   0–35 mm/h

Hematocrit   Women: 33%–43%; Men: 39%–49%

Hemoglobin   Women: 11.5–15.5 g/dL; Men: 14–18 g/dL

WBC count and differential   4,800–10,800/μL

  Segmented neutrophils 54%–62%

  Band forms 3%–5%

  Lymphocytes 23%–33%

  Monocytes 3%–7%

  Eosinophils 1%–3%

  Basophils <1%

Mean corpuscular hemoglobin   28–32 pg

Mean corpuscular volume   86–98 fL (86–98 mm^3)

Platelet count   150,000–450,000/μL

URINE

Creatinine clearance   90–140 mL/min

Creatinine, urine   Women: 11–20 mg/kg/24 h
  Men: 14–26 mg/kg/24 h

Urine, postvoid residual volume   <50 mL, normal; >200 mL, abnormal; 50–200 mL, equivocal

---

*Note: Because normal ranges vary among laboratories, data in this table may not conform with that of all laboratories.

INDEX OF QUESTION NUMBERS BY PRIMARY TOPIC

Addictions 78, 112
Anxiety Disorders 19, 113
Assessment 23, 27

Behavioral Disturbances in Dementia 32, 34
Biology 55, 103

Cardiovascular Diseases 76, 124
Caregiving 41, 77
Cerebrovascular Disease—see Stroke and Cerebrovascular Disease
Community-Based Care 95, 101
Complementary and Integrative Medicine 81, 123
Cultural Aspects of Care 65, 83

Delirium 58, 60
Dementia 53, 72
Demography 8, 118
Dentistry and Oral Health 29, 74
Depression and Other Mood Disorders 33, 36
Dermatology 3, 30
Diabetes Mellitus 31, 61
Disorders of the Foot 50, 82
Dizziness 99, 121

Endocrinology 87, 102
Ethics and Law 17, 126

Falls 63, 108
Financing, Coverage, and Costs of Health Care 20, 79
Frailty 88, 109

Gait Impairment 46, 62
Gastroenterology 56, 116
Gynecology 1, 4

Hearing Loss 13, 66
Heart Failure 14, 104
Hematology 6, 73
Hospital Care 12, 70
Hypertension 16, 37

Infectious Diseases 18, 77
Intellectual and Developmental Disabilities 51, 94

Lesbian Gay Bisexual Transgender Health 90, 124

Mistreatment 25, 105
Multimorbidity 56, 119
Musculoskeletal Pain 38, 92

Nephrology 48, 69
Neurology 71, 75
Nursing-Home Care 11, 93
Nutrition and Weight 39, 84

Oncology and Hematologic Malignancies 74, 125
Osteoporosis 2, 98
Outpatient Care Systems 22, 115

Pain Management 80, 96
Palliative Care 42, 52
Perioperative Care 91, 114
Personality and Somatic Symptom Disorders 28, 57
Pharmacotherapy 9, 120
Physical Activity 24, 40
Podiatry—see Disorders of the Foot
Pressure Injuries and Wound Care 45, 70
Prevention—see Screening and Prevention
Prognostication 14, 26
Prostate Disease and Cancer 86, 89
Pulmonology 21, 114

Rehabilitation 5, 47
Rheumatology 110, 122

Schizophrenia Spectrum and Other Psychotic Disorders 54, 67
Screening and Prevention 7, 64
Sexuality 34, 107
Sleep Issues 43, 68
Stroke and Cerebrovascular Disease 100, 106
Swallowing and Feeding 49, 59
Syncope 71, 111

Transitions of Care 35, 85

Urinary Incontinence 4, 15

Visual Loss and Other Eye Conditions 10, 117

QUESTIONS

Note: The table of Normal Laboratory Values on the inside cover may be consulted for any of the questions in this book.

1. An 82-year-old woman comes to the office because she has had vaginal discharge and light-pink spotting intermittently for at least 2 years. She is not sexually active and has no pain. She underwent a hysterectomy and a "bladder lift," which included mesh, approximately 10 years ago. She has been treated for *Candida* and bacterial vaginosis in the past without resolution of discharge and spotting.

   On examination, the external vulva is normal, without lesions or ulcerations. On speculum examination, there is a normal vaginal cuff with no evidence of recurrent vaginal prolapse. A small area (<0.5 cm) of granulation tissue is noted in the anterior vagina, and a bristly material is felt at that location. A saline wet mount shows normal epithelial cells and vaginal pH of 7.0.

   Which one of the following would be the best treatment plan?

   (A) Referral for surgical management
   (B) Metronidazole vaginal gel
   (C) Oral fluconazole
   (D) Estradiol vaginal cream

2. A 78-year-old woman comes to the office for evaluation because she slipped off the bed when she was getting dressed. The fall caused a small abrasion on her buttocks but no acute pain. She had a bone density test 1.5 years ago; T-score at that time was −1.5. She describes a diet high in calcium and vitamin D (calcium 1,200 mg/d from dairy products and vitamin D 800 mg/d from fish, eggs, and dairy, plus a vitamin D supplement, 400 IU/d).

   Which one of the following is the most appropriate next step for this patient?

   (A) Radiography to exclude pelvic fracture
   (B) Measurement of vitamin D level
   (C) Completion of the Fracture Risk Assessment tool (FRAX®)
   (D) Repeat bone densitometry

3. A 76-year-old man comes to the office because he has constant itching all over his body that began 6 months ago. The itching is worse on his back and extremities. OTC moisturizers provide only modest relief. He can identify no alleviating or exacerbating factors, including no weather or temperature variation.

   On physical examination, the patient is in no distress. Sclera are anicteric. There are linear erosions on the back, with sparing of areas that the patient cannot reach. Dryness and xerotic scale are diffuse. There is no evidence of a primary eruption.

   Which one of the following medications is the likely cause of this patient's sebostatic and xerotic pruritus?

   (A) Atenolol
   (B) Acetaminophen
   (C) Tramadol
   (D) Trimethoprim-sulfamethoxazole

4. A 76-year-old woman comes to the office because for the past 4 months she has had urge urinary incontinence. Before then, she had frequent incontinence episodes associated with bending at the waist or coughing. Onset of urge incontinence was gradual, but she now has episodes several times each week. She has had no vaginal discharge or hematuria. She has a monogamous relationship with her spouse of 48 years. History includes hypertension, osteoarthritis of the knees, hypothyroidism, and vaginal hysterectomy for uterine fibroids at age 53 years.

   On physical examination, there is grade 1 pelvic organ prolapse. She is able to perform isolated contraction of pelvic floor muscles. Vaginal epithelium is thin, with mild irritation. She reports a burning sensation during the manual vaginal examination with petroleum jelly lubricant. Ultrasonography of the bladder shows 40 mL residual urine after she voids. Urinalysis shows no leukocyte esterase, no nitrates, and no hemoglobin; there are 5–10 white blood cells and 0 red blood cells per high-power field. Culture reveals *Escherichia coli* (<10,000 colony-forming units) that is sensitive to all tested antibiotics.

Which one of the following is the most appropriate initial treatment for this patient's urinary leakage?

(A) Fesoterodine 4 mg/d
(B) Percutaneous stimulation of the tibial nerve
(C) Cystoscopy with intradetrusor injection of onabotulinumtoxinA
(D) Behavioral therapy with pelvic floor muscle exercises

5. A 79-year-old woman undergoes evaluation related to a stage 2 pressure injury. She had surgery and short-term rehabilitation after she fractured her right hip and is now being cared for in her daughter's home with the assistance of home care services. She is reluctant to ambulate. She prefers to lie on her back at all times in a regular bed and has not wanted to reposition.

Which one of the following would be most effective in preventing the stage 2 pressure injury from increasing in size and severity?

(A) Apply a transparent film dressing.
(B) Recommend use of a reactive support surface.
(C) Recommend nutritional supplementation.
(D) Encourage ambulation.

6. A 79-year-old woman is admitted to the hospital because she fractured her hip. History includes hypertension and type 2 diabetes mellitus. On examination, vital signs are normal and Confusion Assessment Method (CAM) screen is negative for delirium. Hemoglobin is 8.5 mg/dL.

Which one of the following interventions is most likely to prevent incident delirium?

(A) Blood transfusion to goal hemoglobin level of 10 mg/dL
(B) Preoperative geriatric consultation
(C) Strict avoidance of opiate medication
(D) Low-dose haloperidol prophylaxis

7. A 69-year-old woman comes to the office for her annual wellness examination. She was hospitalized 3 times in the past year because of exacerbation of chronic obstructive pulmonary disease (COPD) and overdose of benzodiazepines and opioids. In addition to COPD and substance abuse, history includes hepatitis C, obstructive sleep apnea, and osteoarthritis. She does not adhere to medication regimens because of their cost. She smokes cigarettes, 1 pack/d for the last 30 years. She uses a wheelchair regularly because severe osteoarthritis makes walking difficult. Since she moved to subsidized housing from a homeless shelter, she has more reliable transportation for medical care, and someone helps her with daily chores. She is up-to-date with influenza and pneumonia vaccines. She has never had screening for breast, cervical, or colorectal cancer.

On examination, blood pressure is 127/80 mmHg, heart rate is 80 beats per minute, and BMI is 30 kg/m^2. Heart and lung sounds are distant; no crackles, wheezes, or rhonchi are heard. There are mild, bilateral knee effusions and crepitus.

Which one of the following screening tests would be most useful at this time?

(A) Colonoscopy
(B) Lipid panel
(C) Computed tomography of the chest
(D) Depression screen

8. Compared with older adults in metropolitan communities, older adults in rural communities are more likely to have which one of the following?

(A) Higher income levels
(B) Lower all-cause mortality rates
(C) Higher rates of using public transportation
(D) Less access to health care services

9. An 86-year-old man comes to the emergency department because he has had dizziness, abdominal pain, and black stool for 1 day. He lives alone; his family and neighbors check on him daily. He describes an episode of "food poisoning" approximately 3 days ago, during which he had multiple bouts of vomiting and diarrhea. For the past 2 days he has been using bismuth subsalicylate 2–3 times daily, as an OTC remedy for his gastrointestinal symptoms. History includes anemia, atrial fibrillation, and hypertension. Current medications are dabigatran 150 mg orally twice daily (for 2 years), fosinopril 10 mg/d (for 20 years), hydrochlorothiazide 12.5 mg/d orally (for 20 years), ferrous sulfate 325 mg twice daily, and a daily multivitamin.

On examination, blood pressure is 110/68 mmHg (baseline, 148/82 mmHg), heart rate is 104 beats per minute, and respiratory rate is 18 breaths per minute.

Laboratory findings:
Hemoglobin	9.0 g/dL (baseline, 12 g)
Hematocrit	28% (baseline, 36%)
Platelet count	281 × 10^9/L
BUN	28 mg/dL
Serum creatinine	1.9 mg/dL (baseline 1.4 mg/dL)
Estimated creatinine clearance	22 mL/min (baseline, 58 mL/min)

Which one of the following is the most likely cause of his presenting symptoms?

(A) Dabigatran overdose
(B) Drug interaction between dabigatran and bismuth subsalicylate
(C) Salicylate overdose from bismuth subsalicylate
(D) Drug interaction between hydrochlorothiazide and bismuth subsalicylate

10. A 75-year-old man comes to the office for routine follow-up. He recently had surgery to remove a cataract in his right eye, and he mentions that his eye doctor told him that his visual acuity is now 20/25 in both eyes. Yet he is puzzled, because there are times when he cannot see well, such as when he drives at dusk or in the rain. His eye doctor mentioned no other ocular pathology.

Which one of the following age-related changes is the most likely cause of his difficulty driving at dusk or in the rain?

(A) Reduced accommodation
(B) Decreased contrast sensitivity
(C) Increased glare sensitivity
(D) Reduced upgaze

11. A 78-year-old woman is admitted to a long-term care facility after lengthy hospitalization for stroke. Nursing staff document 3 pressure injuries in various locations and note that she will require wound evaluation and numerous dressing changes. No measurements or photographs are taken of the pressure injuries. A wound care provider examines the patient 48 hours after admission.

On physical examination, there is a stage 4, clean, granulating sacral pressure injury, measuring 9 × 6 × 0.5 cm; an unstageable pressure injury on the right trochanter, measuring 2 × 5 cm, with dry, hard necrotic eschar and no drainage; and a skin tear (not pressure injury) measuring 4 × 3 cm, with a partial skin flap/pedicle. There is no evidence of infection.

Which one of the following should have been done on admission to the long-term care facility?

(A) Debridement of sacral wound
(B) Assessment and documentation of wound, with measurements
(C) Application of a nonadherent dressing to all wounds
(D) Application of gauze to pack the pressure injury

12. An 82-year-old woman is brought to the emergency department because she is coughing and has shortness of breath. She is lethargic, confused, and easily distracted, and she is trying to pull out intravenous lines. History includes systolic heart failure, coronary artery disease, hypertension, and renal insufficiency. Heart failure is diagnosed, and Confusion Assessment Method (CAM) is positive for delirium.

Which one of the following is the best initial treatment for managing this patient's delirium?

(A) Administer haloperidol.
(B) Administer lorazepam.
(C) Encourage family to spend time at bedside.
(D) Apply soft wrist restraints.

13. A 78-year-old woman comes to the office because she has difficulty understanding conversations in noisy environments. She is referred for audiology evaluation. Audiometry demonstrates mild hearing loss at low frequencies, sloping to profound loss at high frequencies; hearing thresholds for air and bone conduction overlap. Speech discrimination is 83% in the right ear and 85% in the left.

Which one of the following is the most likely cause of this patient's hearing loss?

(A) Conductive hearing loss
(B) Central auditory processing disorder
(C) Sensorineural hearing loss
(D) Ménière disease

14. The family of a 74-year-old woman comes to the office to discuss goals of care. The patient resides in a nursing home and has Alzheimer disease. She is oriented only to self and recognizes family and close friends. She participates in activities in the facility with assistance, but she does not maintain any personal hobbies. Within the last 2 years she has had increasing lower-extremity edema, managed with furosemide 20 mg/d and compression stockings. Within the last year, she has had increasing dyspnea with regular activities, and nursing home staff has noted some dyspnea at rest. She has been hospitalized twice because of increasing dyspnea accompanied by orthopnea, labored breathing, low oxygen saturation on room air, and edema that does not improve with diuretics, stockings, or elevation.

At the last hospital admission, N-terminal prohormone of brain natriuretic peptide (NT-ProBNP) was 2,000 pg/mL, BUN was 22 mg/dL, and creatinine level was 1.5 mg/dL. BMI was 22 kg/m^2. Transthoracic echocardiography showed an ejection fraction of 55% without any significant valvular abnormalities or pulmonary pressure elevation.

At discharge, carvedilol, furosemide, and lisinopril were added to her medication regimen.

Which one of the following factors is most predictive of her poor long-term survival?

(A) Ejection fraction of 55%
(B) Estimated glomerular filtration (eGFR) of 34 mL/min/1.73 m^2
(C) NT-ProBNP value of 2,000 pg/mL
(D) New York Heart Association (NYHA) Class III

15. A 90-year-old woman comes to the office accompanied by her daughter, who serves as her primary caregiver. The patient started donepezil for Alzheimer disease 6 months ago. The dosage was titrated from 5 mg/d to 10 mg/d at 1 month but was decreased back to 5 mg/d 3 months ago because of increasing gastrointestinal adverse effects (diarrhea and fecal urgency, with occasional fecal incontinence). The patient's daughter reports that, overall, her mother's cognitive function has stabilized since starting the acetylcholinesterase inhibitor, and she would like to continue it. Over the past few weeks, however, the mother asks to void up to 10 times daily. After consultation with their local pharmacist, they were informed that urinary frequency is an adverse drug event associated with donepezil. The daughter asks about strategies to manage the urinary frequency; she is open to additional drug therapy. The mother's history includes hypertension; her blood pressure has been maintained at goal with amlodipine 10 mg/d.

On physical examination, blood pressure is 124/76 mmHg. There is no evidence of pelvic organ prolapse or atrophic vaginitis. Ultrasonography of the bladder shows postvoid residual of 45 mL within 15 minutes of a void.

Which one of the following medications would be appropriate to consider for her urinary symptoms?

(A) Immediate-release oxybutynin
(B) Oral memantine
(C) Mirabegron
(D) Immediate-release tolterodine

16. An 88-year-old woman comes to the office for a 6-month follow-up examination. She resides in an assisted-living facility and is independent in all basic and instrumental activities of daily living. She mentions occasional dizziness on standing, but she has never fainted. History includes hypertension; she had a myocardial infarction 10 years ago. Current medications are hydrochlorothiazide, lisinopril, and aspirin.

    On physical examination, blood pressure is 160/70 mmHg sitting and 135/60 mmHg standing. A soft carotid bruit is heard on the left. A soft grade 2/6 systolic murmur is heard over the left side of the chest. Electrocardiography shows left ventricular enlargement.

    Laboratory findings:
Creatinine	1.2 mg/dL
Sodium	136 mEq/L
Potassium	4.5 mEq/L
Calcium	9.5 mg/dL

    Which one of the following is the most appropriate recommendation?

    (A) Replace hydrochlorothiazide with amlodipine.
    (B) Replace hydrochlorothiazide with diltiazem.
    (C) Replace lisinopril with losartan.
    (D) Replace lisinopril with metoprolol succinate.

17. An 85-year-old woman comes to the office with her son, who requested an urgent appointment over concerns regarding her finances. The son says that several of her checks have been cashed without her knowledge, and several credit card transactions on her account seem suspicious (eg, purchases at convenience stores that she has never visited). The patient does not recall these transactions. The son, who has joint ownership on the accounts, notified her bank and credit card company of fraudulent activity. The patient lives with her son and attends an adult day health center. Other than her son, an assistant at the center is her only close personal contact; occasionally, the assistant takes her purse to run errands on her behalf. History includes mild to moderate Alzheimer disease and depression. Current medications are sertraline, donepezil, and calcium and vitamin D supplements.

    On examination, there are deficits in short-term recall and abnormal clock drawing; both findings are unchanged from prior visits.

    Which one of the following is the most appropriate next step?

    (A) Advise the patient not to lend her purse to the assistant.
    (B) Initiate the process for a court-appointed conservator of finances.
    (C) Contact the adult day health center to inquire about the assistant.
    (D) Report the case to adult protective services.

18. An 82-year-old woman with a bioprosthetic mitral valve has new fevers of uncertain etiology.

    After obtaining blood cultures, which one of the following is the next best step in the management for possible bacterial endocarditis in this patient?

    (A) Observe and monitor.
    (B) Request a transesophageal echocardiography.
    (C) Start empiric antibiotic therapy.
    (D) Confirm the presence of Janeway lesions or Osler nodes.

19. A 79-year-old woman is brought to the emergency department with a history of anxiety of 2–3 weeks. Her family reports worsening confusion and disorientation as well as behavior problems, including agitation and suicidal ideation. Her symptoms were initially attributed to worsening of her dementia but then accelerated. History includes dementia and hypertension. Current medications are donepezil, memantine, lisinopril, and paroxetine, which was prescribed for anxiety 2 months ago.

    On examination, the patient is combative and disoriented. Laboratory findings include low serum sodium level and low plasma osmolarity. Urine sodium level and osmolarity are increased.

    Which one of the following medications is the most likely cause of her hyponatremia?

    (A) Donepezil
    (B) Paroxetine
    (C) Memantine
    (D) Lisinopril

20. An 84-year-old woman with dementia comes to the office for a transitional care visit. She is unaccompanied. She was recently discharged from the hospital after admission for fluid overload. Over the past 6 months, she has been admitted 4 times: twice for fluid overload (she often forgets to take her medications), once for a fall, and once for dehydration. She has lost approximately 4.5 kg (10 lb) over the last 6 months. She typically eats one big meal each day. A family friend brings meals 3 times each week and she heats up TV dinners for her other meals. Her daughter oversees her finances and has encouraged her to look at nursing facilities, but she is adamant about remaining in her own home. She uses a front-wheeled walker for ambulation, and she no longer drives.

On physical examination, she appears thin and disheveled but in no acute distress. Blood pressure is 132/87 mmHg sitting and 105/72 mmHg standing. Heart rate is 72 beats per minute, and respiratory rate is 18 breaths per minute. There is 1+ edema bilaterally. Score on the Montreal Cognitive Assessment is 22/30. All other findings are normal.

Which one of the following is the most appropriate referral to make at this time?

(A) Program of All-Inclusive Care for the Elderly (PACE)
(B) Assisted-living facility
(C) Nursing facility for rehabilitation
(D) Home health services for nursing care

21. An 84-year-old woman comes to the clinic for routine follow-up. She describes a gradual decrease in exercise tolerance over the last year, especially when she guides tours in the museum where she volunteers. The year before, her volunteer activities were interrupted by back-to-back hospitalizations to treat dyspnea. History includes chronic obstructive pulmonary disease, hypertension, hypercholesterolemia, and stroke. Current medications are albuterol, fluticasone/salmeterol, tiotropium, clopidogrel, aspirin, labetalol, lisinopril, and rosuvastatin.

On examination, blood pressure is 122/58 mmHg, heart rate is 50 beats per minute, and respiratory rate is 16 breaths per minute. Lungs are clear, and there is no lower-extremity edema or increased jugular venous pressures.

Echocardiography shows concentric left ventricular hypertrophy, normal left ventricular function, and diastolic dysfunction. Pulmonary function tests show a moderate obstructive defect without significant improvement after administration of aerosolized bronchodilators.

Which one of the following interventions is most likely to improve this patient's functional exercise capacity?

(A) Nocturnal oxygen therapy
(B) Diuretic therapy
(C) Aerobic exercise training
(D) Placement of implantable cardioverter-defibrillator (ICD)

22. A 58-year-old woman comes to the office because she has difficulty caring for her parents, both of whom receive care at the same practice. Her parents' income is low, and they are dual-eligible for Medicare and Medicaid. She has moved into her parents' home to take care of her father, who has Alzheimer disease, while her mother is in the hospital recovering from hip surgery. She is in danger of losing her full-time job as a school cafeteria worker, because she missed work once and was late twice this week because of her father's agitation. In addition, her work schedule prevents her from meeting with the hospitalist to discuss her mother's care. She believes she has no choice but to quit her job so that she can take care of her parents.

Which one of the following is the most appropriate recommendation for the daughter?

(A) Request funds from the local Alzheimer's Association.
(B) Participate in a Medicaid self-direction program.
(C) Regularly attend an Alzheimer's Association support group.
(D) Request visiting nurse services provided by the Department of Health.

23. An 85-year-old man comes to the office with his daughter, who is concerned about his driving. He lives alone in a rural community and drives to the grocery store, office visits, and occasionally to her home. Two days ago, he was in a minor car accident after he turned into a one-way street in the wrong direction. History includes hypertension, for which he takes amlodipine 5 mg/d, and gastroesophageal reflux disease, for which he takes omeprazole 40 mg/d.

    Which one of the following is the most appropriate next step?

    (A) Recommend that his daughter take away his keys.
    (B) Refer him for driving assessment.
    (C) Perform a cognitive evaluation.
    (D) File a report with the Department of Motor Vehicles.

24. An 80-year-old woman comes to the urgent care center because she slipped on wet steps yesterday evening while she was watering her plants. She scraped the back of her leg but did not hit her head. She has fallen 3 other times in the last year. Her last fall was 3 months ago. On that occasion, she went to the emergency department because she struck her head on the bathroom vanity. Noncontrast computed tomography of the head showed nonspecific microvascular ischemic changes and no acute bleeding. History includes hypertension, well-controlled diabetes mellitus, and atrial fibrillation. Current medications are lisinopril, carvedilol, metformin, and warfarin.

    On physical examination, blood pressure is 132/86 mmHg, with no postural changes, and heart rate is 80 beats per minute and irregularly irregular. Neurologic findings are normal. International normalized ratio (INR) is 3.0. The posterior surface of her right leg has a superficial abrasion with surrounding ecchymoses; there are no other injuries. She walks slowly, with a shortened stride length on a slightly wide base, and turns en bloc.

    Which one of the following is the best next step?

    (A) Discontinue warfarin.
    (B) Refer to a community exercise program.
    (C) Begin cholecalciferol 50,000 IU weekly.
    (D) Provide educational materials about fall risk.

25. A 75-year-old woman who lives alone requires a home visit for medical care. It is winter, and her home is cold. She states that her furnace does not work but that her son brought over a new kerosene heater last night. The heater has not been filled or started. She cannot afford repairs to her furnace, and she declines help from the Area Agency on Aging for home repair. The telephone numbers she provides for her family contacts are disconnected. She refuses to leave her home. History includes moderate dementia, hypertension, arthritis, and chronic obstructive lung disease. Current medications are acetaminophen 500 mg twice daily, hydrochlorothiazide 25 mg/d, and tiotropium inhaler 5 mcg/d. She smokes 1 pack of cigarettes daily and refuses to stop; she does not drink alcohol.

    On physical examination, temperature is 37°C (98.6°F), blood pressure is 135/78 mmHg, heart rate is 68 beats per minute, respiratory rate is 12 breaths per minute, and oxygen saturation is 95% on room air. Her extremities are cool. Breath sounds are distant. There is mild bilateral pedal edema. Score on Mini–Mental State Examination is 22 of 30, which is unchanged from her score 3 months ago.

    Which one of the following organizations can assist in ensuring the safety of this patient?

    (A) Adult protective services
    (B) Visiting nurse agency
    (C) Police department
    (D) Fire department

26. An 82-year-old man comes to the office because he feels poorly. Over the past 2 months he has become short of breath, has gradually gained weight, and has had swelling in his legs. He can no longer shower on his own or walk >1 block because of his dyspnea. History includes hyperlipidemia, hypertension, mild cognitive impairment, and type 2 diabetes mellitus. He has never smoked. His wife confirms his adherence to a low-sodium diet and to medications. His last hospitalization was 2 years ago, and he worries that he will need to go to the hospital soon.

    On physical examination, blood pressure is 114/60 mmHg, heart rate is 70 beats per minute and irregularly irregular, and oxygen saturation is 94% on room air. BMI is 26.9 kg/m². Jugular veins are distended and there are bibasilar crackles.

There is 1+ pitting edema at the mid-shins bilaterally. Laboratory results include creatinine of 2.2 mg/dL and hemoglobin A_{1c} of 8.2%.

Which one of the following prognostic tools is most appropriate for estimating his all-cause mortality?

(A) Advanced Dementia Prognostic Tool
(B) BODE Index (BMI, airflow obstruction, dyspnea, exercise)
(C) ePrognosis calculator
(D) Palliative prognostic score

27. A 72-year-old man comes to the office accompanied by his son. He lives independently and says that he has no issues to discuss. The son, however, is concerned that he has uncharacteristically been giving a lot of money to solicitors. He is also concerned because his father has been expressing anger about the children in the neighborhood. This too is uncharacteristic of him. The patient explains that the children's loudness sometimes upsets him. He does not feel depressed, and says that he is sleeping well. He admits that his memory is "not as good as it used to be," with trouble remembering names and dates of appointments, but he ascribes this to normal aging. On further questioning, he mentions that he fell a few weeks ago, when he tripped as he stepped onto a curb. He was not injured.

Which one of the following would be the most appropriate referral to make at this time?

(A) Comprehensive geriatric assessment
(B) Program of All-Inclusive Care for the Elderly (PACE)
(C) Assisted-living facility
(D) Home health for physical therapy

28. An 83-year-old woman comes to the office accompanied by her husband. He states that his wife has not spoken for 1 month, since their daughter announced that her son was gay. The patient communicates via notes and gestures and can attract attention through sound signals, such as coughing. When directly addressed today, she uses a notepad or turns to her husband so that he can answer for her. Oral and written comprehension is maintained. The patient seems unconcerned about the burden her mutism places on others and is clear that she wishes to be taken seriously.

Her husband says that she continues daily activities, such as reading and cooking, and that her appetite and sleep patterns have not changed. When she is asked directly whether she feels sad, she looks surprised and shakes her head, indicating "no." Her husband says that she had a similar response at the time of her father's death; that episode lasted 2 weeks and resolved completely. Last week her husband took her to the emergency department, where computed tomography of the head, electroencephalography, and otolaryngology evaluation disclosed no abnormality.

On physical examination, all findings are normal.

Which one of the following is the most likely diagnosis?

(A) Somatic symptom disorder
(B) Delirium
(C) Conversion disorder
(D) Depressive disorder

29. A 66-year-old man comes to the office because he has a swelling in the buccal gingiva of tooth #20. Five months ago, a small mass developed in the buccal aspects of teeth #18 and #19 that was diagnosed as squamous cell carcinoma. That lesion was removed in conjunction with extraction of teeth #18 and #19 and excision of the alveolar bone in the area, along with 27 regional lymph nodes, all of which were clear, with no evidence of cancer. He did not undergo radiation therapy.

History includes infection with human immunodeficiency virus (HIV) for 22 years and type 2 diabetes mellitus for 10 years. He had osteomyelitis in his femur after radiation treatment for disseminated Kaposi sarcoma

>20 years ago, and he has had recurrent anal intraepithelial neoplasia for the past 6 years, treated with localized excision and laser ablation. Current medications are insulin, metformin, atazanavir, ritonavir, and raltegravir.

On physical examination, there is a firm, nontender enlargement in the buccal aspect of tooth #20, wrapping around and extending into the edentulous space behind the tooth. The lesion has a mixed appearance of erythema and increased vascularity. Periodontal probing shows a deep pocket in the distal aspect of tooth #20; the probe causes bleeding.

Which one of the following is the most likely diagnosis?

(A) Diabetes-related periodontal abscess
(B) Recurrent squamous cell carcinoma
(C) Recurrent Kaposi sarcoma
(D) Osteonecrosis of the jaw

30. An 80-year-old man comes to the office because he has a brown patch on his face that started changing about 1 month ago. History includes several basal cell carcinomas, as well as squamous cell carcinomas removed by surgery. He grew up in Arizona, where he had extensive sun exposure. He continues to spend time in the sun and uses sun protection intermittently.

On examination, there is a 2-cm brown patch on the right cheek. Most of the lesion is a homogenous brown; there is a focus of darker brown with red coloration. There is no texture to the lesion and no tenderness. Surgical scars appear well healed, with no evidence of recurrence. The remainder of the skin examination is unremarkable.

Which one of the following is the most likely diagnosis?

(A) Severely atypical nevus
(B) Nodular melanoma
(C) Metastatic melanoma
(D) Lentigo maligna

31. A 65-year-old woman comes to the office for her Welcome to Medicare preventive visit. History includes diabetes mellitus (diagnosed 3 years ago), hypertension, and osteoarthritis of the knee and hip. Current medications are acetaminophen 1,000 mg three times daily, tramadol 50 mg three times daily as needed, metformin 1,000 mg twice daily, and lisinopril 40 mg/d. She uses a 4-wheeled walker to assist with ambulation.

On examination, BMI is 30 kg/m². Cardiovascular and pulmonary findings are unremarkable. There is bilateral knee crepitus with extension, with no focal pain. With the walker, gait is stable but slightly wide based with decreased knee flexion. Hemoglobin A_{1c} level is 8.5%.

Which one of the following is the most appropriate recommendation?

(A) Weight loss to achieve normal BMI
(B) Diabetes self-management education program
(C) Prescription for glipizide
(D) Exercise prescription for walking 150 min/week at moderate intensity

32. An 82-year-old woman is brought to the emergency department by her family because she has increased agitation. She has been hitting her adult daughter and trying to run away from home because she believes that her daughter has been poisoning her. The daughter first noticed her mother's memory decline 5 years ago. The patient has lived with her daughter for the past 3 years and is now unable to manage finances, drive, or cook alone. History includes Alzheimer disease, for which she began taking donepezil 1 year ago.

Which one of the following is the most appropriate pharmacotherapy?

(A) Risperidone[OL]
(B) Bupropion[OL]
(C) Clozapine[OL]
(D) Divalproex sodium[OL]

33. A 72-year-old woman comes to the office because she has symptoms of depression. History includes presently untreated bipolar disorder, hypothyroidism, and hypertension. Current medications are levothyroxine and chlorthalidone.

Which one of the following medications is considered first-line treatment for bipolar depression?

(A) Bupropion
(B) Lamotrigine
(C) Valproate
(D) Risperidone

34. A 74-year-old man comes to the office because he has erectile dysfunction. His wife died 1 year ago; they had been married 50 years. He is in a new relationship, and his partner has expressed a strong desire for sexual activity. For the past 10 years he has had progressive difficulty with achieving an erection; the difficulty has worsened in the last 6 months. History includes myocardial infarction, angina, and type 2 diabetes mellitus, with occasional episodes of hypoglycemia. The myocardial infarction occurred 2 months ago, and he has recovered well. Current medications are insulin, rosuvastatin 10 mg/d, atenolol 50 mg twice daily, aspirin 81 mg/d, and nitroglycerin as needed.

On physical examination, there is a soft systolic murmur and trace edema of the lower extremities. The remainder of the examination is normal.

Laboratory findings include hemoglobin A_{1c} of 7.2% and total testosterone level of 350 ng/dL.

Which one of the following factors is the most likely primary cause of his erectile dysfunction?

(A) Neurologic
(B) Psychogenic
(C) Vascular
(D) Endocrine

35. A 79-year-old woman comes to the office 6 days after discharge from hospitalization for heart failure. It was her third hospital admission for heart failure within the past year. History also includes type 2 diabetes mellitus, obesity, hypertension, and hyperlipidemia. Current medications are aspirin 81 mg/d, furosemide 40 mg/d, metformin 500 mg/d, lisinopril 10 mg/d, and atorvastatin 40 mg/d. She has dyspnea on exertion.

On physical examination, she has gained 1.6 kg (3.5 lb) since discharge. Blood pressure is 142/86 mmHg and heart rate is 72 beats per minute. Bilateral crackles are heard at both lung bases, and there is lower-extremity edema.

At the time of discharge, which one of the following would most significantly help prevent readmission?

(A) Home visit nursing to provide self-care education and clinical evaluations
(B) Telemonitoring of vital signs and weight reported to providers
(C) Medication reconciliation, patient education, and medication optimization by pharmacist
(D) Heart failure education provided by a nurse before discharge

36. Which one of the following is associated with the highest risk of suicide in older adults?

(A) Depression
(B) Terminal illness
(C) Prior suicide attempt
(D) Chronic pain

37. An 82-year-old woman comes to the office for her annual visit. She asks whether she could stop taking any of her medications, explaining that she "is tired of taking so many." History includes heart failure with reduced ejection fraction, ischemic heart disease, hyperlipidemia, hypertension, hypothyroidism, and osteoporosis. Current medications are amlodipine 5 mg/d, enalapril 5 mg twice daily, furosemide 10 mg/d, vitamin D 2,000 IU/d, levothyroxine 100 mcg/d, metoprolol extended release 50 mg/d, and rosuvastatin 10 mg/d.

On examination, heart rate is 72 beats per minute sitting and 74 beats per minute standing. Blood pressure is 112/70 mmHg sitting (right arm, regular cuff) and 109/65 mmHg standing. Over the past 6 months, systolic blood pressure taken when sitting has ranged from 105 mmHg to 113 mmHg; diastolic blood pressure has ranged from 68 mmHg to 72 mmHg. Estimated creatinine clearance is 50 mL/min.

Which one of the following medications can be safely discontinued at this time?

(A) Amlodipine
(B) Metoprolol
(C) Enalapril
(D) Furosemide

38. A 75-year-old woman comes to the office because she has right-sided medial knee pain. The pain began 2 years ago and has slowly progressed. She currently takes acetaminophen and duloxetine for the pain. She is interested in nonpharmacologic interventions to reduce pain and improve her function.

On examination, vital signs are normal. BMI is 24.7 kg/m². There is mild crepitus on extension and mild tenderness along the medial joint line in the right knee. The rest of the musculoskeletal examination is unremarkable except for small, asymptomatic Heberden nodes in 2 fingers of the right hand. Standing bilateral radiography demonstrates mild osteoarthritis (Kellgren and Lawrence system grade 1–2) of the left knee and moderate osteoarthritis (Kellgren and Lawrence system grade 3) affecting primarily the medial compartment of the right knee joint.

Which one of the following nonpharmacologic approaches is the best recommendation for this patient?

(A) Dieting to achieve 5% weight loss
(B) Neoprene brace for the right knee
(C) Lateral patella taping to the right knee
(D) Aerobic, land-based exercise

39. A 75-year-old man comes to the office for routine follow-up. History includes diabetes mellitus, hypertension, and hypercholesterolemia. Current medications are aspirin 81 mg/d, glipizide 10 mg/d, lisinopril 10 mg/d, simvastatin 40 mg/d, and a daily multivitamin. His friend takes omega-3 fatty acids 500 mg/d, and he asks whether he would also benefit from the supplement.

Which one of the following is true regarding omega-3 fatty acid supplementation?

(A) Increases risk of hypoglycemia
(B) Reduces risk of sudden coronary death
(C) Increases risk of hypercoagulability
(D) Worsens cognitive decline

40. An 86-year-old woman comes to the office accompanied by her daughter, who is concerned because her mother has fallen twice in the past 6 months, each time without injury. The patient states that, each time, she tripped and lost her balance. There is no history of dizziness, syncope, or arrhythmia. Her medical history includes hypertension, hyperlipidemia, right hip replacement, and cataract surgery. Current medications are lisinopril, atorvastatin, and aspirin.

On examination, blood pressure is 136/86 mmHg with no orthostatic changes, and heart rate is 72 beats per minute and regular. Heart sounds are regular, with no murmurs, and lungs are clear. There is no edema. Neurologic findings indicate normal proprioception, reflexes, and sensation to touch. Muscle strength is normal.

Which one of the following is the most appropriate recommendation for this patient?

(A) Encourage her to be more physically active.
(B) Recommend a strength, endurance, and balance program.
(C) Recommend any form of exercise as long as it is ongoing.
(D) Recommend a progressive strengthening program.

41. An 82-year-old man is brought to the office by his daughter because she is exhausted by caring for him. He and his wife immigrated to the United States from Venezuela 40 years ago, and the couple shares an apartment with their daughter and her children. History includes Alzheimer disease and glaucoma. Current medications are prednisolone and dorzolamide eye drops. He rarely uses his walker and has fallen 3 times in the last year. He needs assistance with dressing and bathing. He often becomes disoriented and aggressive in the evening, especially when his daughter tries to convince him to shower or change clothes.

On physical examination, he has a hunched posture on ambulation, with small steps and poor foot lift. He has an unsteady gait.

Which one of the following increases his risk of nursing home placement?

(A) Hispanic heritage
(B) Daughter's exhaustion
(C) His marital status
(D) His living arrangements

42. An 86-year-old woman is brought to the office for a follow-up visit, accompanied by her daughter (her durable power of attorney) and her caregiver. History includes Alzheimer disease, stage 4 lung cancer, and recent right lower-extremity deep-vein thrombosis. The caregiver states that the patient spends most of the day asleep, often difficult to arouse. Her appetite has decreased notably in the last 6 weeks; at her visit to the oncologist 1 month ago, weight was down by 2.3 kg (5 lb). At that visit, the option of hospice was discussed with the patient's daughter. The daughter is not ready for her mother to start hospice care and asks what can be done to improve her caloric intake.

On examination, weight has decreased further by 4.6 kg (10 lb).

Which one of the following is the most appropriate initial recommendation for this patient?

(A) Oral dronabinol 2.5 mg twice daily
(B) Oral megestrol acetate 400 mg/d
(C) Placement of gastrostomy tube for enteral feedings
(D) Small meals of the patient's favorite foods

43. A 66-year-old woman comes to the office because for 6 months she has had increasing difficulty staying asleep. She falls asleep after about an hour but wakes up 3–4 hours later almost every night. About 2 or 3 nights per week she can fall back to light, interrupted sleep after 30–60 minutes; other times, she is up for the rest of the night. She states that she does not snore and the awakenings are not breathing related. Her schedule for the past 20 years has been to go to bed at 10 PM and wake up at 6:30 AM. She was diagnosed with insomnia in her 40s and was treated with cognitive-behavioral therapy (CBT) and intermittently with zolpidem.

She does not feel depressed and there have been no changes in her lifestyle. She sees a therapist who has been working with her on CBT for insomnia for the past 3 months. She asks for medication to help her stay asleep. History includes hypertension and mild depression.

On physical examination, blood pressure is 132/89 mmHg.

Which one of the following medications would be the most appropriate initial recommendation?

(A) Zaleplon
(B) Zolpidem
(C) Trazodone
(D) Suvorexant

44. A 78-year-old man is brought to the office by his family because he is agitated and aggressive, such that they feel threatened by his behavior. He has a neurocognitive disorder. The family asks about pharmacologic options that could mitigate his behavior. If drug therapy is unsuccessful, they will seek institutionalization.

Which one of the following is the most appropriate pharmacologic treatment for this patient?

(A) Quetiapine[OL]
(B) Lorazepam[OL]
(C) Citalopram[OL]
(D) Combination therapy with dextromethorphan[OL] and quinidine[OL]

45. An 86-year-old man undergoes evaluation because he has several pressure injuries. He has end-stage cancer with bone metastasis and is on home hospice; he does not want further cancer treatment or hospitalization. He has lost 27.2 kg (60 lb) over several months and refuses food. Liquid intake is minimal, and urinary catheter yields minimal output.

On physical examination, there is a stage 3, necrotic, draining pressure injury measuring 8.5 × 3 × 0.4 cm, on the left great trochanter. A breakdown is starting on the left shoulder, and there are skin tears on the arms. A large butterfly discoloration on the sacral area, measuring 9 × 10 cm, appears to be new, within the past week according to his wife.

The patient and family understand that maintenance wound care is the treatment of choice. No other aggressive treatments are being done. The family has removed the specialty mattress from the patient's bed at his request. He does not want to be turned and wants to be left to just rest.

Which one of the following is the best approach for this patient's multiple skin injuries?

(A) Perform negative-pressure wound treatment.
(B) Debride the necrotic pressure ulcer.
(C) Provide comfort wound care.
(D) Order specialty bed.

46. An 89-year-old woman is admitted to the hospital because she has complications associated with pneumonia. At baseline, the patient lives in her own home, is independent in basic activities of daily living, and walks with no assistive device. During the hospital stay, physical therapy assessment records her gait speed as 0.30 m/s.

    Which one of the following best describes the significance of this patient's gait speed?

    (A) It is within the normal range for hospitalized oldest-old adults.
    (B) It indicates mild impairment and should be monitored closely for further decline.
    (C) It indicates dysmobility and increased fall risk.
    (D) It indicates increased risk of discharge to institutional setting.

47. A 78-year-old man comes to the office because he fell at home. History includes Parkinson disease. He adheres to his current medication regimen of carbidopa/levodopa (25/100) three times daily. The medication has not changed recently. He uses a standard 4-point walker to facilitate ambulation. There has been no change in his vision and hearing.

    On physical examination, there is no orthostatic hypotension. Core strength is preserved. There is bruising over his left shoulder, with no evidence of head trauma or focalized neurologic weakness. Resting tremor is more obvious in the right upper extremity than the left. He has some difficulty maneuvering the walker through the door of the examination room. Gait speed is slow, and he demonstrates freezing. Overall, the findings are similar to those from the last examination 6 months ago.

    Which one of the following is the most appropriate intervention?

    (A) Admit to nursing facility for physical therapy.
    (B) Recommend use of a 4-wheeled walker.
    (C) Recommend around-the-clock home aide and use of a 1-point cane.
    (D) Recommend use of a front-wheeled walker.

48. A 78-year-old woman comes to the office for a scheduled yearly visit. She has generally been well and has no acute medical concerns. She lives independently with her husband. She is active and walks approximately 1.5 miles, 4–5 days each week. There is no history of diabetes mellitus, hypertension, or coronary artery disease. Current medications are aspirin 81 mg/d, calcium 500 mg/d, and vitamin D 1,000 IU/d.

    On physical examination, blood pressure is 130/70 mmHg, and heart rate is 76 beats per minute. Heart and lung findings are normal. A comparison of current and previous laboratory findings shows an increase in serum creatinine level, from 0.9 mg/dL to 1.3 mg/dL, and a decrease in glomerular filtration rate (GFR), from 70 mL/min to 40 mL/min.

    Which one of the following is the most likely cause of the change in this patient's renal function?

    (A) Glomerulosclerosis, tubular atrophy, and interstitial fibrosis
    (B) Microinfarctions of the cortical glomeruli and decreased medullary volume
    (C) Glomerular basement membrane thinning and pericapsular fibrosis
    (D) Interstitial eosinophilic infiltration and glomerular atrophy

49. A 67-year-old man comes to the office because he has had difficulty swallowing for the past week. He describes an uncomfortable sensation of food sticking in his chest. The sensation does not occur when he drinks liquids. History includes hypertension, gastroesophageal reflux disease (GERD), cirrhosis secondary to hepatitis C, and osteoarthritis; he is HIV positive. Current medications are antiretroviral therapy, proton pump inhibitor, and acetaminophen; attempts to swallow pills produce pain over the midsternum.

On physical examination, his weight is down 1.4 kg (3 lb).

Which one of the following is the most appropriate initial step in evaluation?

(A) Modified barium swallow
(B) Barium esophagography
(C) Upper endoscopy
(D) Esophageal manometry

50. An 85-year-old man comes to the office for routine follow-up. History includes coronary artery disease, diabetes mellitus, fatty liver disease, and osteoarthritis. He had coronary bypass surgery 6 years ago. He is independent in all activities of daily living.

    On physical examination, several toe nails, including those of the first toe of both feet, are significantly deformed. The nail plate is thickened with subungual debris and has a brown-yellow hue. The skin of both feet shows diffuse scale on the base of the feet and between the toes. All other physical findings are unchanged from previous visits.

    On further questioning, the patient says that he has no personal or family history of psoriasis. He does not know when his nails began to change, nor does he recall specific trauma to the involved digits. He has not used any treatment.

    Which one of the following is the most important risk factor for this patient's nail condition?

    (A) Diabetes mellitus
    (B) Peripheral vascular disease
    (C) Advanced age
    (D) Poor foot care

51. A 57-year-old man is brought to the office by staff from his group home. He received a diagnosis of autistic spectrum disorder (formerly, autism) in childhood and schizophrenia in his 20s. He has been on antipsychotic medication since then. He is currently on quetiapine. He has not had any blood work in at least 7 years and has not had a colonoscopy. Staff reports he dislikes going to see doctors, at least partly because he does not like being touched. He allows only a cursory examination today. Poor dentition and obesity (BMI 35 kg/m^2) are noted. There is a family history of diabetes and heart disease.

    Which one of the following is the best next step in providing care for this patient?

    (A) Refill medications and arrange follow-up in 3 months.
    (B) Have nurse draw blood while he is in the office today.
    (C) Provide education on healthy lifestyle changes and follow up in 2 weeks.
    (D) Schedule dental work and colonoscopy under general anesthesia.

52. A 71-year-old black American man comes to the office for an annual wellness check-up. History includes coronary artery disease, chronic obstructive pulmonary disease (COPD), benign prostatic hyperplasia, and stage 3 chronic kidney disease. He has had a stent placement and is on home oxygen. He was admitted to the ICU last year for exacerbation of COPD, and doctors and nurses discussed code status preferences with him. He has no documented advance directives and becomes visibly uncomfortable when asked about them.

    Which one of the following factors is most likely to be a barrier to his completion of advance directives?

    (A) Mistrust of the health care system
    (B) Higher socioeconomic status
    (C) Number of comorbidities
    (D) History of ICU care

53. A 63-year-old man comes to the office accompanied by his wife, who is concerned about changes she has seen in his behavior over the past year. He is a retired army major. He has become messy and unpredictable; for example, last week she found him cutting up all the curtains in the house. He gorges on food and is no longer quiet and polite; instead, he has become abusive and now uses coarse language. During the interview, the patient is oblivious to his wife's statements. History includes hypertension.

    On examination, the patient appears unkempt. Hypertension is under control, and all other findings are normal, except for the Mini–Mental State Examination on which he scores 23.

Which one of the following is the most likely diagnosis?

(A) Delirium
(B) Frontotemporal lobar degeneration
(C) Adjustment disorder following retirement
(D) Substance use disorder

54. A 70-year-old woman comes to the office to establish care because her previous clinician retired. She is a retired nursing supervisor. Her main concern is that for the past year, her neighbors have been trying to get her to move by purposefully damaging the steps leading up to her doorway. She does not know why her neighbors wish her harm. She produces several photographs to illustrate the damage; the steps appear to be intact. Her daughter lives with her, but she has asked the daughter to leave because she believes her daughter has damaged the interior steps that lead to the second floor. The patient says that her daughter "has her reasons but she's secretive, can't be trusted." The patient is active in her church and manages her household, shopping, and finances without assistance.

During the interview, the patient is alert and courteous. She is well dressed. She denies any history of abuse. Laboratory findings from 6 months ago confirm that she is in good health. She consents to cognitive assessment and mentions that her previous clinician also performed an assessment, the results of which were normal. Findings from today's assessment are normal.

Which one of the following is the most likely diagnosis?

(A) Mild frontotemporal neurocognitive disorder (dementia)
(B) Delusional disorder
(C) Schizophreniform disorder
(D) Paranoid personality disorder

55. Which one of the following reflects the approximate prevalence of centenarians in developed countries?

(A) 1 per 1,000
(B) 1 per 5,000
(C) 1 per 10,000
(D) 1 per 50,000

56. A 78-year-old man comes to the office for routine follow-up. History includes coronary artery disease, hypertension, diabetes mellitus, and chronic obstructive pulmonary disease. He had 3-vessel bypass surgery 7 years ago. His most recent colonoscopy was 10 years ago; results were normal. There is no family history of colorectal cancer. He asks whether he should have a repeat colorectal cancer screen.

Which one of the following is the most appropriate recommendation?

(A) Home testing for blood in stool
(B) Sigmoidoscopy
(C) Colonoscopy
(D) No screening

57. A 70-year-old woman comes to the office because she has a self-inflicted wound to her left forearm. She tried to treat herself but decided that a clinician should evaluate the wound. History includes type 2 diabetes mellitus, which has been difficult to stabilize; she has a distant history of anorexia, depression, and alcohol abuse. At today's appointment, she describes herself as lonely, irritable, and anxious.

On examination, the bandage around her wound is elaborate, but the wound is superficial.

Which one of the following is the most appropriate intervention?

(A) Hypnosis
(B) Mood stabilizer
(C) Anxiolytic (benzodiazepine) and cognitive-behavioral psychotherapy
(D) Antidepressant and cognitive-behavioral psychotherapy

58. An 84-year-old man is brought to the emergency department by his family. His daughter is concerned that he has mouth pain. She has noticed that he has not wanted to open his mouth and grimaces when others try to open it. His daughter states that he usually eats well, but he has accepted only some liquids for the last 7 days. He has been more lethargic and less interactive with his family over the past 5 days. History includes coronary artery disease, coronary artery bypass graft, prostate cancer, moderate cognitive impairment, osteoarthritis, and bilateral knee replacement.

Which one of the following is the most likely diagnosis?

(A) Worsening of dementia
(B) Delirium
(C) Depression
(D) Acute stroke

59. An 85-year-old woman with dementia undergoes evaluation because she has lost 3.6 kg (8 lb) in 3 months. She lives in a long-term care facility and is dependent for all activities of daily living. She is minimally verbal. She is hand fed by staff; they have recently noted that she pockets food during meals.

If enteral feeding with a gastrostomy tube were initiated in this patient, which one of the following would be most likely?

(A) Decreased contact time with nursing and support staff
(B) Improved survival
(C) Decreased likelihood of pressure ulcers
(D) Improved functional status

60. An 80-year-old woman is admitted to the hospital because of worsening agitation that began a few days ago. History includes moderate Parkinson disease. She refuses physical examination; laboratory tests indicate urinary tract infection, and computed tomography of the head shows a new subdural hematoma. She is trying to leave and cannot be redirected. Her family is at bedside. At 1:00 AM the agitation worsens, and the patient tries to hit the nursing staff. She has been receiving her routine medications.

Which one of the following should be started to lessen the patient's agitation?

(A) Lorazepam
(B) Haloperidol
(C) Quetiapine
(D) Citalopram

61. An 85-year-old man comes to the office to review laboratory results after his Medicare Annual Wellness visit. Initial fasting blood glucose level was 140 mg/dL; on repeat testing, the level is 135 mg/dL. The patient is a life-long runner, has never smoked, and has maintained a BMI of 21 kg/m² throughout adulthood. He asks what other factors may have contributed to the development of diabetes.

Which one of the following is the most likely mechanism to have caused diabetes in this patient?

(A) Decreased cytokine production
(B) Low basal insulin levels
(C) Impaired pancreatic β-cell function
(D) Increased β-cell mass

62. A 78-year-old man comes to the office accompanied by his daughter, who is concerned about his frequent falls. She says that he tends to fall when he is away from home; he does not fall often in his house. The patient is unconcerned about the falls.

On examination, blood pressure and heart rate are normal, including postural responses. Visual, vestibular, and peripheral sensations are normal. Muscle strength, motion, and endurance are normal, and there is no rigidity or abnormal resistance to passive motion of the joints. Gait speed is 1.18 m/s, and he steps over an obstacle placed in his path with no difficulty, with a few small steps on approach. He does not make appropriate adjustments to maneuver past the furniture in the examination room or past other people in the hallway.

Which one of the following is most likely to be a factor in his falls?

(A) Cognitive dysfunction
(B) Cerebellar disorder
(C) Parkinson disease or parkinsonian syndrome
(D) Spinal stenosis

63. A 78-year-old man comes to the office because he would like advice on how to reduce his risk of falling. He nearly fell last week on icy sidewalk while getting out of a car, and he is afraid that he will break a hip. History includes hypertension, benign prostatic hyperplasia, and bilateral knee osteoarthritis. Current medications are hydrochlorothiazide, amlodipine, terazosin, and topical diclofenac as needed for knee pain.

On physical examination, blood pressure is 128/68 mmHg and heart rate is 64 beats per minute after sitting for 5 minutes, and 118/62 mmHg and 70 beats per minute after standing for 3 minutes. He completes the Timed Up and Go test in 15 seconds. He steadies himself with his arm on the examination table when he performs a semi-tandem stance. The remainder of the neurologic and cardiovascular examination is normal.

Which one of the following is the best intervention to reduce risk of a fall and subsequent fracture?

(A) Tai chi
(B) Calcium supplement
(C) Discontinue terazosin
(D) Hip protectors

64. A 65-year-old woman comes to the office for routine follow-up. She does not take any medication regularly, and she remains active. She mentions that she is expecting her first grandchild in a few months and will help take care of the newborn on a daily basis.

Vaccination against which one of the following infections should be recommended at this time?

(A) *Haemophilus influenzae* type B
(B) Rotavirus
(C) *Bordetella pertussis*
(D) Hepatitis B virus

65. An 87-year-old woman discusses her goals and preferences for end-of-life care. She describes herself as a very spiritual member of the Buddhist Zen community and wants her spiritual community to support her through end-of-life decision-making. She has advanced coronary artery disease, New York Heart Association class 4 heart failure, and stage 4 chronic kidney disease. She has been admitted to the hospital 3 times in the past 6 months.

Regarding the patient's health care, which one of the following is a tenet of her spiritual community?

(A) Blood transfusions cannot be given.
(B) Artificial feeding cannot be given.
(C) A family member is the preferred surrogate.
(D) No specific health care directive has been developed.

66. A 72-year-old man comes to the office because he has difficulty hearing, dating back about 5 years. He is accompanied by his daughter, who states that he sets the television volume to be excessively loud, often does not understand conversations on the telephone, and has difficulty participating in conversations in noisy environments. They are concerned about what is causing the hearing loss. The patient has no tinnitus, vertigo, otalgia, or discharge from the ears, and has had no ear infections or trauma.

Which one of the following is the most appropriate initial step in evaluating the patient's hearing loss?

(A) Audiogram
(B) Tuning fork test (Weber and Rinne tests)
(C) Pneumatic otoscopy
(D) *Hearing Handicap Inventory for the Elderly-Screening* questionnaire

67. An 82-year-old man undergoes evaluation because he has become increasingly disruptive in the dining room at his nursing home. He accuses staff and other residents of conspiring to poison his food. His tablemates have moved away, and staff has ceased efforts to reassure him or correct his perceptions. He will eat food that his family brings, but they cannot visit daily; when they leave meals for staff to serve him, he again complains of contamination. History includes Alzheimer disease. His family describes him as having always been overly cautious. They state that it was suspiciousness toward caregivers, rather than Alzheimer disease, that necessitated entry into long-term care. They ask about the risks and benefits of initiating medical therapy to address his behavior.

    He has lost 1.8 kg (4 lb) in the last 60 days and his BMI is now 20 kg/m^2; physical examination and laboratory findings do not identify a cause for the weight loss.

    Which one of the following is true for this patient?

    (A) A second-generation antipsychotic agent would double his mortality rate compared with placebo.
    (B) Citalopram at a dose of 40 mg would be the best choice for his symptoms.
    (C) Control of symptoms with a second-generation antipsychotic agent would carry a higher risk of mortality than use of a first-generation agent.
    (D) His symptoms justify use of a second-generation antipsychotic agent.

68. A 72-year old man comes to the office because for the past 2 years he has had episodes in which he yells and behaves violently during sleep. The frequency and intensity of these episodes have increased over the past 6 months, to 3 or 4 nights per week. His wife states that he moves his arms as if he is punching or kicking, and speaks loudly and sometimes swears. He has fallen out of bed but has not sustained any injuries. He recalls sometimes dreaming that he is fighting or fending off an attack. His regular sleep time is 10 PM and wake time is 6 AM. He does not take any medications regularly.

    On physical examination, neurologic findings are normal for his age.

    Which one of the following disorders is most likely to develop in this patient?

    (A) Alzheimer disease
    (B) Parkinson disease
    (C) Wernicke-Korsakoff syndrome
    (D) Frontotemporal dementia

69. A 78-year-old man is brought to the office by his son, who is concerned about his unsteady gait and mild confusion in the past week. The patient had fallen at home that morning, with no consequent injury. The patient lives alone. He had mild dyspnea with accompanying cough 2 days ago; pneumonia was diagnosed, and he is currently on antibiotic therapy. History includes hypertension, depression, osteoarthritis, and mild gastritis. Current medications are duloxetine, hydrochlorothiazide, azithromycin, omeprazole, and naproxen. The patient's eating and drinking habits have not changed. He does not have any more dyspnea or cough. He never smoked.

    On physical examination, blood pressure is 130/90 mmHg, heart rate is 78 beats per minute, respiratory rate is 12 breaths per minute, and temperature is normal. He is cognitively intact. Lung fields have clear breath sounds, and the rest of the examination is unremarkable.

    Which one of the following diagnostic studies will reveal the most likely reason for this patient's symptoms?

    (A) Complete blood count
    (B) Chest radiography
    (C) Serum electrolytes
    (D) Plasma osmolality

70. A 75-year-old man is admitted to the orthopedic unit after surgery to repair a fractured right femur. He fell off a 6′ ladder, and approximately 6 hours passed before he was found, lying on his back in the yard. He had surgery 3 hours after arrival at the emergency department. The admitting nurse on the orthopedic unit documents a 7 × 10 cm purple-maroon discoloration at the sacral-coccygeal area; skin is intact. The discoloration is nonblanching and symmetric. It is documented as ecchymosis from a traumatic fall.

Which one of the following pressure injury designations describes the ecchymotic area?

(A) Deep-tissue injury
(B) Stage 1
(C) Stage 2
(D) Stage 3

71. A 72-year-old man comes to the office because he has fallen several times. In the past year, he has felt increasingly less steady when he walks, and he now infrequently leaves the house. He has lost consciousness 7 times in the past 2 months. According to his wife, in each episode, he rose from bed after taking a nap and then suddenly collapsed to the floor unconscious. He remained unconscious and still for 10 seconds before regaining consciousness and full control of his body. The patient has no prodrome before losing consciousness. History includes advanced Parkinson disease, transient ischemic attacks, hypertension, and diabetes mellitus. Current medications are aspirin, carbidopa/levodopa, metformin, and lisinopril. There have been no recent dosage changes.

On physical examination, supine blood pressure is 110/80 mmHg and standing blood pressure is 100/80 mmHg, without any changes in heart rate. Mental status, cranial nerve function, and strength are normal. There is masking of facies, mild cogwheel rigidity in the wrists, bradykinesia, and loss of vibratory sensation in the feet. Ankle deep tendon reflexes are absent. Gait is slow. Electrocardiography and echocardiography findings are unremarkable.

Which one of the following is the most likely cause of his loss of consciousness?

(A) Insufficient dosage of carbidopa/levodopa
(B) Dysfunction of the autonomic nervous system
(C) Critical stenosis of the basilar artery
(D) Focal dysplasia of the right temporal lobe

72. A 73-year-old man comes to the office because he is concerned about his risk of Alzheimer disease. His father was diagnosed with Alzheimer disease at age 73; there is no other family history of Alzheimer disease or other dementias. The patient has no cognitive symptoms and is in good health. He had a mild traumatic brain injury last year after a fall, but symptoms and signs resolved. He drinks alcohol, 1 or 2 standard drinks 3 days each week, but there is no evidence of alcohol abuse.

Which one of the following increases this patient's long-term risk of Alzheimer disease, compared with other older adults?

(A) His age
(B) Parent with Alzheimer disease
(C) Head injury without loss of consciousness
(D) Excess alcohol intake

73. An 85-year-old man comes to the office because he has had lower energy levels and increased fatigue with his usual activities. History includes longstanding stable chronic kidney disease, stage 4.

Laboratory findings indicate stable renal function. Hemoglobin is 8.5 g/dL, with evidence of microcytosis. There is iron deficiency, with iron saturation at 8% and ferritin level at 85 ng/mL.

Which one of the following is the most appropriate next step for managing this patient's anemia secondary to chronic kidney disease?

(A) Course of intravenous iron
(B) Initiation of oral iron supplements
(C) Blood transfusion
(D) Initiation of erythropoietin

74. An 82-year-old man comes to the office because he has pain at the site of a maxillary posterior tooth extracted 3 months ago by his dentist. History includes prostate cancer with bone metastasis, for which he has been treated with zoledronic acid infusion for the past 12 months. He has a 60 pack-year history of cigarette smoking.

On examination, the extraction socket has not healed, and the gingival tissue is open, with bone protruding from the site. The area is erythematous, with some purulent drainage and foul odor emanating from his mouth.

Which one of the following is the most likely diagnosis?

(A) Metastatic prostate cancer
(B) Osteonecrosis of the jaw
(C) Oral squamous cell carcinoma
(D) Incomplete tooth extraction with residual root

75. A 70-year-old man undergoes evaluation as part of admission to a long-term care facility. He has lived alone in an apartment with home health services and family support, independently eating, ambulating, and managing his own medications, but he required help for most instrumental activities of daily living. However, over the past 3 months, he has had increasing fatigue, worsening ambulation, new urinary and fecal incontinence, and decreasing cognitive function. One of his daughters who lives nearby and visits daily initially resisted his relocation to a facility, noting that on some days "he is almost normal." Still, the changes prompted the decision to transition to long-term care. History includes mild dementia, myocardial infarction 1 year ago, benign prostatic hyperplasia, and osteoporosis. Current medications are donepezil, aspirin, metoprolol, rosuvastatin, losartan, furosemide, tamsulosin, calcium, and vitamin D.

On physical examination, vital signs are normal. He is alert and fully oriented, but he does not recognize family and is unable to follow simple commands. There are no convulsions. Muscle tone is normal. He is in a wheelchair wearing incontinence pads. There is 1+ pitting edema to the mid-shin bilaterally. The remainder of the examination is unremarkable. Echocardiography 1 year ago showed an ejection fraction of 38%.

Which one of the following is the best next step in evaluating this patient's functional decline?

(A) Standardized cognitive assessment
(B) Depression screen
(C) Electroencephalography (EEG)
(D) Lumbar puncture

76. An 82-year-old woman had a syncopal event while vacationing on Cape Cod with her family. It was a hot day, and she sat in the sun for about 2 hours. She passed out as she stood to go to the bathroom. History includes moderate aortic stenosis, hypertension, and mild Parkinson disease; there is a distant history of non–ST-elevation myocardial infarction (NSTEMI). She has been taking metoprolol for years for coronary heart disease and hypertension. She also takes chlorthalidone, selegiline, carbidopa/levodopa, atorvastatin, and aspirin. Echocardiography performed 6 months ago showed a 1.2-cm^2 aortic valve diameter and a 32-mm peak gradient. Systolic function was normal, but diastolic filling was mildly impaired.

Which one of the following is the most likely explanation for her syncope?

(A) Multifactorial etiology
(B) Cardiac ischemia
(C) Aortic stenosis
(D) Autonomic dysfunction

77. A 75-year-old woman comes to the office for routine follow-up. On examination, blood pressure is 160/90 mmHg; the patient explains that she ran out of her medications a few days ago. She is increasingly exhausted by caring for her husband, who has Alzheimer disease. She has assumed responsibility for all driving. She manages his medications in addition to her own; their various refills are due asynchronously, so she goes to the pharmacy almost weekly. Last week she was delayed at the pharmacy; she came back to find that her husband left the house looking for her, and a neighbor had brought him back. She is now worried about leaving him alone.

At this visit, her and her husband's medications are reviewed, and the regimens simplified. The pharmacy is contacted and asked to synchronize dispensing so that she can pick up all prescriptions monthly, rather than weekly. The patient is reminded that she and her husband should avoid OTC agents, particularly antihistamines, because of their potential to cause delirium. The appointment runs significantly behind schedule.

Which one of the following would reduce her burden?

(A) Psychologic support and caregiver training
(B) Chronic care management services
(C) Nursing home placement
(D) Medication simplification

78. A 70-year-old man comes to the office for a routine health visit. History includes hypertension, benign prostatic hyperplasia, hyperlipidemia, and type 2 diabetes mellitus, controlled by diet. He lives alone and has no specific health concerns. In response to review of substance history, he states that he does not use tobacco and consumes alcohol occasionally. When questioned further, he reports that he drinks three 12-oz beers daily and never has >4 drinks on a single occasion. He has no desire to cut down on alcohol use, does not crave alcohol when he does not drink, has not had a change in his drinking habits, and has never withdrawn from alcohol.

Which one of the following would best define his drinking pattern?

(A) Low-risk drinking
(B) At-risk drinking
(C) Alcohol abuse
(D) Alcohol use disorder

79. An 87-year-old woman comes to the office accompanied by her daughter, who has been caring for her at home. History includes Alzheimer disease. The daughter reports that the patient's condition has progressively declined over the past year. The patient is now fully incontinent, resists showering, does not sleep at night, and tends to wander out the door. The daughter cannot continue to take care of her mother and would like to move her to a facility that specializes in dementia care. She was told by a friend that Medicare will pay for the facility if the doctor signs an order. Neither the mother nor the daughter has financial resources.

Which one of the following is true regarding the role of Medicare in post-acute and long-term care services?

(A) Medicare will pay for skilled care at a nursing facility for 100 days; family is responsible for copayment after the first 20 days.
(B) The patient should apply for Medicaid, which will pay for her nursing home care.
(C) Medicare will pay for a part-time aide to help with basic activities of daily living in the patient's home.
(D) Medicare hospice services will pay for her room and board at a hospice facility.

80. A 75-year-old white woman resides in a nursing home. She has moderate vascular dementia and chronic pain related to rheumatoid arthritis. She has an 11th grade education.

Which one of the following is associated with the greatest likelihood that her pain will be undertreated?

(A) Her age
(B) Her race
(C) Cognitive impairment
(D) Education level

81. A 75-year-old woman comes to the office because she has trouble sleeping. She goes to bed at 8 PM, sleeps about 3 hours, and tosses and turns for the rest of the night, getting up at 8 AM. She does not have nocturia, and she is not depressed. She exercises about 45 min/d by walking. She has tried OTC Tylenol® PM, but it leaves her groggy.

Which one of the following should be recommended first?

(A) Sleep restriction therapy
(B) Relaxation therapy
(C) Cognitive-behavioral therapy for insomnia
(D) Referral for sleep study

82. A 78-year-old man comes to the office for follow-up related to gout in the right first metatarsophalangeal (MTP) joint. He has not had gout pain for 2 weeks. He fell in his home twice in the last 2 weeks when doing his regular activities. He did not lose consciousness and does not know why he fell. He was not injured. In addition to gout, history includes hypertension, bronchitis, and osteoarthritis. He walks barefoot at home to avoid pressure on his right first MTP joint, and he is wearing sandals today.

On physical examination, when he is supine, blood pressure is 146/78 mmHg, heart rate is 85 beats per minute, and oxygen saturation is 95%. After he stands for 3 minutes, blood pressure is 135/76 mmHg, heart rate is 90 beats per minute, and oxygen saturation is 96%. Cognition and sensation are intact. Visual acuity is corrected with bifocal lenses, and visual field is intact. Dix-Hallpike maneuver is negative for dizziness or nystagmus. Range of motion is normal, except the patient reports stiffness at end range for hip flexion. Strength is 5/5 for all lower-extremity major muscle groups. There is bilateral hallux valgus, with no redness, swelling, or tenderness of the right first MTP joint. Gait speed is 1.1 m/s.

Which one of the following interventions is most likely to decrease his overall risk of falls?

(A) Prisms to improve peripheral vision
(B) Treatment of orthostatic hypotension
(C) Referral to a community-based exercise program
(D) Footwear modification

83. A 76-year-old black man comes to the emergency department because he has back pain that started after he fell from a ladder. He is a widower who lives alone. History includes heart failure. He does not have paresthesias, and the pain does not radiate; there have been no changes in bowel or bladder habits. Comprehensive neurologic examination shows no deficits.

Which one of the following is most likely to affect whether he will receive an opioid?

(A) His race
(B) His age
(C) Presence of heart failure
(D) His marital status

84. A 74-year-old woman comes to the office for routine follow-up. She works 3 days each week in a library, shelving books and doing activities with children. History includes hypertension, for which she takes amlodipine 5 mg/d. She asks whether she should take a multivitamin.

Which one of the following is the most appropriate recommendation?

(A) Take a generic multivitamin.
(B) Take a multivitamin specifically formulated for older women.
(C) Defer discussion until routine laboratory tests are completed.
(D) Eat a well-balanced diet instead of taking a multivitamin.

85. A 79-year-old woman is hospitalized for pneumonia. History includes chronic obstructive pulmonary disease (COPD), hypertension, hyperlipidemia, heart failure, and atrial fibrillation. This is her second admission in 6 months. The hospital team is ready to discharge her to home.

Which one of the following is most likely to help this patient avoid readmission to the hospital?

(A) Follow-up appointment with her provider
(B) Availability of community resources
(C) Involvement of a transitional care program
(D) Comprehensive discharge summary and medication reconciliation

86. An 82-year-old man comes to the office for routine follow-up. He states that he is not sure he empties his bladder completely when he voids. He has had gradual onset of urgency with the need to void, and occasionally he experiences incontinence on the way to the bathroom. On average, he voids 8 times daily and twice overnight. He occasionally experiences hesitancy when initiating a void, and the stream is interrupted and weak. He describes post-void dribbling and staining on his undergarments. History includes hypertension, hypercholesterolemia, and stroke 2 years ago, with no residual weakness. Current medications are amlodipine, hydrochlorothiazide, rosuvastatin, and aspirin.

On physical examination, blood pressure is 118/64 mmHg. The suprapubic area is slightly tender and dull to percussion. Genitalia are normal. The prostate is moderately enlarged and nontender, without nodularity or other abnormality. Bladder ultrasonography after attempted void shows postvoid residual of 175 mL. Urinalysis reveals no evidence of infection. Creatinine level is 1.1 mg/dL.

Which one of the following is the most appropriate next step?

(A) Stop hydrochlorothiazide.
(B) Start oxybutynin.
(C) Start tamsulosin.
(D) Refer for urodynamic evaluation.

87. A 78-year-old man comes to the office because he recently started a relationship with a new partner and he worries about his inability to maintain an erection. He is divorced and has 3 children from a previous marriage. He has had no memory loss, changes in mood, weight loss or gain, heat intolerances, skin or hair changes, reduced libido, or muscle weakness. History includes diabetes, hypertension, chronic obstructive pulmonary disease, depression, and obesity. Current medications are metformin 1,000 mg twice daily, lisinopril 10 mg/d, tiotropium 18 mcg/d, fluticasone/salmeterol 250/50, NPH insulin 15 U twice daily, aspirin 81 mg/d, and paroxetine 60 mg/d.

On examination, temperature is 36.1°C (97°F), heart rate is 72 beats per minute, respiratory rate is 16 breaths per minute, and blood pressure is 136/64 mmHg. BMI is 35 kg/m². The prostate is slightly enlarged, with no nodules. Right testis is 11 cc and left testis is 12.5 cc.

Laboratory findings:

Complete blood count	Normal
Hemoglobin A_{1c}	8.2%
Thyrotropin	1.24 mIU/mL
Total testosterone	200 ng/dL
Sex-hormone-binding globulin	8 nmol/L
Testosterone	
Free (calc)	5 ng/dL
Free and weakly bound	120 ng/dL

Which one of the following is the most appropriate initial step for managing this patient's erectile dysfunction?

(A) Start intramuscular testosterone cypionate, 150 mg every 2 weeks.
(B) Change paroxetine to mirtazapine.
(C) Start sildenafil, 100 mg one hour before sexual activity.
(D) Increase metformin to 1,500 mg twice daily.

88. Which one of the following interventions is *not* endorsed by a consensus of experts regarding treatment for physical frailty?

(A) Calorie and protein supplementation
(B) Hormone supplementation
(C) Vitamin D supplementation
(D) Reduction in polypharmacy

89. A 78-year-old man comes to the office because he is bothered by frequent nighttime urination. He gets up 2–4 times each night to urinate, and he urinates every 2–3 hours during the day. There is no discomfort or hematuria. History includes diabetes mellitus and hypertension. Current medications are hydrochlorothiazide 12.5 mg/d, losartan 100 mg/d, and extended-release metformin 500 mg/d. There is no history of heart disease, stroke, or other significant illness. Recent electrocardiography and laboratory findings (including urinalysis and prostate-specific antigen level) were normal. His hemoglobin A_{1c} was 7.8%.

On examination, blood pressure is 145/75 mmHg sitting and 137/68 mmHg standing. Heart rate is 73 beats per minute. His home blood pressure measurements are consistent with the office measurements. Prostate is 3+ enlarged, smooth, and nontender.

Which one of the following is the best choice to replace hydrochlorothiazide in this patient?

(A) Aliskiren
(B) Doxazosin
(C) Nebivolol
(D) Amlodipine

90. A 62-year-old man comes to the office to discuss whether he should hire formal caregivers to help him care for his partner. His partner is 75 years old, has been HIV positive for 20 years, and has had progressive cognitive decline over the past 5 years. They have been together for 30 years and have combined finances. In the past few months, his partner has wandered out of the home in the middle of the night, and he almost started a fire by leaving a gas burner on. The patient telecommutes from home but is having trouble completing work projects because the partner is requiring more supervision.

For this couple, which one of the following is more likely to be a concern, compared with a heterosexual couple?

(A) Financial limitations
(B) Fear of discrimination by professional caregivers
(C) Caregiver burnout
(D) Loss of health insurance

91. A 74-year-old woman comes to the office because she believes that her ability to organize family activities and to remember appointments has declined. She cannot recall a specific point at which the decline began. History includes diabetes, hypertension, and coronary disease. She had right aortofemoral bypass for leg claudication 3 months ago.

On examination, vital signs are normal, and she appears well. She cannot spell "WORLD" backward and gets frustrated when attempting to do so. Pulses are normal, and there are no motor or sensory deficits.

Which one of the following is the most likely diagnosis?

(A) Parkinson disease
(B) Stroke
(C) Postoperative cognitive dysfunction
(D) Vascular dementia

92. An 80-year-old man comes to the office because he has had intermittent low back pain since he tripped and fell on an uneven walkway 8 weeks ago. He had no other injuries. He takes acetaminophen for the pain. Stretching and physical therapy have been helpful but have not eliminated the pain.

Which one of the following nonpharmacologic treatments has an effect on subacute low back pain?

(A) Bed rest for 2 weeks
(B) Massage
(C) Ice packs
(D) Lumbar support

93. A 70-year-old man is being discharged after a hospital stay for a lower-extremity open, draining wound. He will need intravenous antibiotic therapy for 6 weeks, and the wound requires irrigation, packing, and dressing twice daily. He lives alone and does not have family or friends who live close by to assist in his care. He would like to go home, but he is willing to consider placement if necessary.

Which one of the following is the most appropriate location for discharge for this patient?

(A) Acute rehabilitation facility
(B) Skilled nursing facility
(C) Home, with home care
(D) Continued inpatient stay

94. A 55-year-old woman with Down syndrome is brought in by her parents, with whom she has lived her entire life. They are concerned because she has had a change in her ability to perform previously mastered tasks, as well as a change in behavior, becoming more easily agitated and more difficult to calm than previously. They cannot give a clear idea of when the changes began, but report that their son visited recently and noticed a difference compared with when he last saw his sister 1 year ago.

Which one of the following is the best pharmacologic treatment for this patient?

(A) Memantine 5 mg/d
(B) Memantine 10 mg/d
(C) Donepezil 5 mg/d
(D) Donepezil 10 mg/d

95. An 88-year-old man requires a home visit for medical care. His wife called this morning to report that a new pressure injury developed on his right leg over the past 48 hours. He is homebound because he has severe lumbosacral spinal stenosis, with partial paralysis of his lower limbs. His wife is his full-time caregiver. History also includes coronary artery disease, peripheral vascular disease, and type 2 diabetes mellitus with peripheral neuropathy. He has an indwelling Foley catheter. He has no pain, fever, or chills. He reports increased drainage over the past 24 hours.

   On examination, there is a 2 × 3 pressure injury on his right lower leg. The injury is eroding into the muscle layer and has a necrotic base. The patient's cognition is intact. Permission is obtained to photograph the lesion and transmit the image to a consulting dermatologist for advice.

   The patient's insurance coverage is through Medicare Part C fee-for-service.

   In addition to the patient's county of residence, which one of the following will affect payment for the dermatology consultation?

   (A) Real-time communication with the consultant
   (B) Consultant's county of practice
   (C) Severity of the illness under review
   (D) Physician–physician nature of the communication

96. A 79-year-old woman comes to the office because she has chronic, severe, persistent pain in multiple joints. History includes osteoarthritis, hypertension, and chronic kidney disease. Medications include acetaminophen 650 mg every 8 hours. She does physical therapy–prescribed exercises daily, with minimal relief. The pain prevents her from such activities as grocery shopping and cleaning. Injection of corticosteroids into the joints no longer provides relief. The patient agrees to try low-dose oxycodone. She states that in the past she felt unwell when taking narcotic analgesics and is worried about adverse effects.

   Which one of the following should be prescribed for this patient to treat the most common adverse effect of oxycodone?

   (A) Methylphenidate
   (B) Naloxone
   (C) Prochlorperazine
   (D) Senna

97. An 84-year-old nursing home resident recently completed a course of antibiotics for urinary tract infection (UTI). She had a previous UTI approximately 6 months ago. She has occasional stress incontinence, which is unchanged from baseline, but otherwise has no urinary symptoms. History includes mild Alzheimer disease and distant breast cancer. Her daughter asks how UTIs can be prevented in the future. Examination shows no palpable bladder. She has atrophic vaginitis.

   Which one of the following options should be considered in this patient?

   (A) Oral cranberry capsules
   (B) Oral ciprofloxacin
   (C) Intravaginal metronidazole
   (D) Intravaginal estrogen

98. A 69-year-old postmenopausal woman comes to the office because she is concerned about her bone health. She does not have a personal history of fragility fracture; her mother sustained a left hip fracture after a fall at age 68. Bone densitometry screen (DXA) done 4 years ago showed osteopenia. She is at low risk of fracture based on her Fracture Risk Assessment (FRAX®) score. History includes type 2 diabetes mellitus, which has been well controlled for 15 years, previously with a thiazolidinedione and currently with a sodium/glucose cotransportor-2 (SGLT-2) inhibitor. Recent hemoglobin A_{1c} was 7.2%. She quit smoking 10 years ago and rarely drinks alcohol. Arrangements are made for repeat DXA scan, including trabecular bone score.

Which one of the following is true about this patient's trabecular bone score?

(A) It is associated with an increased risk of osteoporotic fracture in postmenopausal women with type 2 diabetes mellitus.
(B) It entails additional images and radiation exposure for the patient.
(C) It can be used to monitor response to osteoporosis treatment.
(D) Her low score is correlated with lower fracture risk.

99. A 72-year-old man comes to the emergency department because he had sudden onset of vertigo, nausea, blurry vision, and left facial numbness while watching television. The symptoms lasted a few minutes before resolving completely. He had 2 similar episodes over the previous 3 days. History includes hypertension and hyperlipidemia. He has a 50 pack-year history of cigarette smoking.

On examination, blood pressure is 153/90 mmHg, heart rate is 78 beats per minute and regular, respiratory rate is 14 breaths per minute, and oxygen saturation is 98% on room air. Neurologic and all other findings are normal. Computed tomography (CT) of the head is normal.

Which one of the following would most likely establish the diagnosis for this patient?

(A) Dix-Hallpike test
(B) CT angiography of the head and neck
(C) Doppler ultrasonography of the carotid arteries
(D) Magnetic resonance imaging (MRI) of the brain

100. A 65-year-old man with a history of atrial fibrillation is admitted to a skilled-nursing facility because he had a middle cerebral artery stroke. He has unilateral weakness and dysarthria. In his work with occupational therapy, he has difficulty with recent memory but no difficulty with word-finding. After 2 weeks of rehabilitation, his cognition remains impaired, and improvement in overall functional status is less than expected. Score on the Patient Health Questionnaire-9 (PHQ-9) is 15; Montreal Cognitive Assessment score is 21/30. Laboratory findings are normal.

Which one of the following is the best next step in management?

(A) Start oral donepezil 5 mg/d and titrate.
(B) Start oral memantine 5 mg/d and titrate.
(C) Order computed tomography of the head.
(D) Start sertraline 50 mg/d and titrate.

101. A 90-year-old woman comes to the office for a routine visit. She lives alone in a 2-story house and no longer drives. She is accompanied by her daughter, who is visiting from out of town. She is enrolled in both Medicare and Medicaid. History includes lumbosacral spinal stenosis, osteoporosis (old T12 compression fracture), chronic low back pain, and macular degeneration. Current medications are acetaminophen and alendronate. The daughter mentions that the house is less clean than in the past, and the patient admits that she finds cleaning, shopping, and laundry increasingly burdensome. No family members live locally, and she does not want people whom she does not know in her home. She would consider relocating to preserve her independence.

On physical examination, height is 1.5 m (5 ft) and weight is 37 kg (82 lb), a 2.7-kg (6-lb) loss over 6 months. There is kyphosis with bilateral lumbosacral paravertebral spasm. There is no midline tenderness. Lower-extremity reflexes are normal.

Laboratory findings are normal except for hemoglobin level of 11.8 mg/dL and albumin level of 2.8. Urinalysis is normal.

Which one of the following community supports is most appropriate for this patient?

(A) Assisted-living facility
(B) Senior apartment
(C) Continuing-care retirement community
(D) Adult day care

102. An 88-year-old man is brought to the emergency department because he is confused. His daughters accompany him; over the past several weeks, they had noticed that he was becoming more forgetful and confused, forgetting information he knows well, such as his daughters' phone numbers and even his birthday. They report that he has had no recent illness, but that he was started on citalopram and ranitidine 3 weeks ago by his primary care clinician. History includes gout, osteoarthritis, peripheral vascular disease, heart failure, gastroesophageal reflux disorder, and mild cognitive impairment. Current medications are aspirin 81 mg/d, metoprolol 50 mg twice daily, simvastatin 40 mg/d, ranitidine 150 mg twice daily, allopurinol 100 mg/d, acetaminophen 650 mg three times daily, and citalopram 20 mg/d.

On physical examination, temperature is 36.1°C (97°F), heart rate is 72 beats per minute, respiratory rate is 16 breaths per minute, and blood pressure is 126/64 mmHg sitting and 119/62 mmHg standing. BMI is 21 kg/m². The patient is pleasant and in no distress; he is alert and oriented to place but not to year, month, or day. There are lung crackles but no rhonchi or wheezing. The prostate is slightly enlarged. There is 1+ nonpitting edema and reduced muscle tone and bulk. Score on the Mini-Cog™ is 1/5. All other findings are normal.

Laboratory findings:

Complete blood count	Normal
Glucose	91 mg/dL
Sodium	121 mEq/L
Potassium	5 mEq/L
Chloride	86 mEq/L
Serum bicarbonate	25.0 mEq/L
Creatinine	0.57 mg/dL
Serum osmolality	268 mOsm/kg
Urine osmolarity	590 mOsm/kg
Urine sodium	132 mEq/L
Urine creatinine	93 mg/dL
Thyrotropin	1.24 mIU/mL
Cortisol (AM)	17 mcg/dL

In addition to restricting free water to normalize the patient's sodium levels, which one of the following is the most appropriate initial step in managing his confusion?

(A) Start furosemide 40 mg IV daily.
(B) Start normal saline at 150 mL/hr.
(C) Taper off citalopram.
(D) Stop ranitidine.

103. Which one of the following is true regarding male compared with female centenarians?

(A) There are half as many men as women.
(B) Men are more likely to be functionally independent.
(C) Men have a higher prevalence of chronic cardiovascular disease.
(D) Men are more likely to be taking medications.

104. A 67-year-old man comes to the office for follow-up after discharge from a nursing facility where he recovered from below-the-knee amputation of his left leg. While in the nursing home, he has been gaining weight and developing mild ankle swelling. The medical staff added bumetanide to his medication regimen for this excess fluid. Since returning home 1 week ago, he has noticed increasing dyspnea with activity and orthopnea, and the edema has progressed further in his lower extremities, with possible dehiscence at the surgical amputation site. History includes ischemic cardiomyopathy (ejection fraction of 42%), coronary artery disease, diabetes mellitus, and peripheral vascular disease. Ten years ago, he had coronary artery bypass of 4 vessels. Current medications are aspirin, hydralazine, isosorbide dinitrate, insulin glargine, insulin aspart, lisinopril, bumetanide, and carvedilol. He adheres to the medication regimen as well as to a 2 g sodium diet and 1.5 L of fluid per day restriction. He has followed up with his vascular surgery and wound care team, who found no sign of infection. He remains worried about whether the swelling will affect healing of the amputation.

On examination, blood pressure is 129/70 mmHg, heart rate is 77 beats per minute, and respiratory rate is 18 breaths per minute. He has bilateral edema in his lower extremities.

Which one of the following is the most appropriate next step for managing the patient's congestive symptoms?

(A) Intensify fluid restriction.
(B) Limit sodium intake further.
(C) Double the bumetanide dose.
(D) Add metolazone.

105. A 72-year-old woman comes to the office for her annual wellness visit. She is an established patient who lived alone until recently, when her grandson and great-grandchild moved in with her. History includes hypertension, which is managed well with medication; she has a remote history of breast cancer, treated with mastectomy and chemotherapy.

    On physical examination, blood pressure is 166/90 mmHg. All other findings are normal, and cognition is intact. When asked about her adherence to the medication regimen, she starts to cry. She states that she can no longer afford her antihypertensive medication, because her grandson constantly asks for money, threatening to leave and not let her see her great-granddaughter if she does not comply.

    Which one of the following aspects of the grandson's behavior could be considered an example of financial exploitation?

    (A) Moving in with his grandmother
    (B) Asking her to give him money
    (C) Threatening to keep her from seeing her great-grandchild
    (D) No financial exploitation because she was not forced to sign any documents

106. An 83-year-old man comes to the office because 2 days ago he had an episode of garbled speech that lasted ≤1 minute. He is accompanied by his wife, who describes the sudden onset of word-finding difficulty, during which he substituted the word "juice" with the word "fuse" and was unable to follow her instruction to sit down in the kitchen chair. There were no other signs before or since the event. History includes a lacunar stroke 6 years ago, hypertension, diabetes mellitus, and hyperlipidemia. Current medications are atorvastatin, lisinopril, hydrochlorothiazide, metformin, and aspirin (81 mg/d); he has not missed any doses.

    On examination, blood pressure is normal, and heart rate is 78 beats per minute. There are no carotid bruits, and cardiac auscultation is normal. There is a left facial palsy, which has been present since his stroke 6 years ago. Speech and language findings are normal, and there are no new focal neurologic deficits.

    Which one of the following should be done first?

    (A) Begin warfarin.
    (B) Order electroencephalography (EEG).
    (C) Increase aspirin dosage to 325 mg/d.
    (D) Order carotid Doppler ultrasound.

107. A 78-year-old woman who lives in Miami comes to the office because she wants to confirm that she has not acquired a sexually transmitted infection (STI). She began a relationship with a new partner 3 months ago. She feels well, and she has had no genital ulcers, vaginal discharge, dyspareunia, dysuria, abdominal or pelvic pain, or fevers. History includes depression, the onset of which coincided with the death of her husband 4 years ago. All of her health maintenance is up to date.

    Screening for which one of the following should be offered as part of routine STI testing for this patient?

    (A) Human papillomavirus (HPV)
    (B) Zika virus
    (C) Human immunodeficiency virus (HIV)
    (D) *Mycoplasma genitalium*

108. An 82-year-old woman who lives in a nursing home is evaluated because she fell while getting out of bed to go to the bathroom. She slipped on a blanket that had slid to the floor. She is unable to recount more detail about her fall. The nurse reports that she said she had no pain after the fall and was able to walk to the bathroom with her walker. Immediately after the fall, seated blood pressure was 144/78 mmHg and heart rate was 86 beats per minute. History includes moderate-stage Alzheimer disease; her most recent score on the Mini–Mental Status Examination was 18 of 30.

Which one of the following is the best intervention to reduce this patient's risk of another fall?

(A) Use of a bed alarm
(B) Nursing education about fall prevention
(C) Raised bed rails at night
(D) Multifactorial intervention

109. Which one of the following is the most effective frailty screen for use in clinical practice?

(A) Self-reported health
(B) Gait speed
(C) Polypharmacy
(D) Assessment by general practitioner

110. An 80-year-old woman comes to the office because she has increasing shoulder pain, profound fatigue, and new, left-sided headache. She describes 2 recent episodes, each lasting a few minutes, of a "veil" falling over her left eye. History includes polymyalgia rheumatica, first diagnosed 3 months ago. Initial treatment was prednisone 15 mg/d; the dosage was reduced 4 weeks ago, to 12.5 mg/d.

On examination, there is no tenderness over the left temporal artery. Funduscopic examination reveals pallor of the optic nerve.

Which one of the following is the most appropriate next step?

(A) Resume prednisone 15 mg/d.
(B) Begin methylprednisolone 1,000 mg/d IV for 3 days.
(C) Obtain biopsy of the temporal artery.
(D) Obtain color Doppler ultrasonography of the temporal artery.

111. A 70-year-old man comes to the emergency department because he lost consciousness earlier in the day. He states that, the previous evening, he was at a social gathering where he drank more alcohol than usual for him. When he woke up this morning he went to the bathroom and, while urinating, collapsed onto the bathroom floor. His spouse witnessed the event and did not notice any abnormal movements. He regained consciousness after 10 seconds, without alteration of mental status. He did not suffer a head injury. He had no prodromal symptoms and currently feels well. History includes hypertension and diabetes mellitus. Current medications are lisinopril 40 mg/d and metformin 1 g twice daily.

On physical examination, temperature, blood pressure, and neurologic findings are normal.

Which one of the following is the best recommendation for this patient?

(A) Drink extra fluids.
(B) Reduce the dosage of lisinopril.
(C) Sit during urination.
(D) Avoid alcohol altogether.

112. A 75-year-old man comes to the office for a routine health check. His spouse died 2 months ago. He expresses sadness at her passing and feels that life has lost meaning. He has some difficulty falling asleep. He states that there has been no change in his energy level or appetite and that he has no feelings of guilt or suicidal or homicidal ideation. Before his wife's death, he drank 2–4 beers each night; during his monthly poker game with friends, he drinks 6–8 beers. Since her death, he drinks 6 beers each night because he thinks it helps him sleep, but he worries that he may have an issue with drinking. He asks for help cutting back. History includes essential hypertension, hyperlipidemia, and stage 2 chronic kidney disease.

Which one of the following treatments should be tried first for this patient?

(A) Citalopram
(B) Naltrexone
(C) Disulfiram
(D) Cognitive-behavioral therapy

113. An 82-year-old woman comes to the office because she has had worsening anxiety and worry for the last 8 months. She describes sleeping poorly, being tired, and having generalized aches for several weeks. She is accompanied by her daughter, who states that she consistently worries about her grandchildren as well as her husband, who has well-controlled diabetes mellitus and hypertension. Generalized anxiety disorder is diagnosed.

    Which one of the following is the best treatment option for this patient?

    (A) Benzodiazepines and cognitive-behavioral therapy (CBT)
    (B) CBT only
    (C) Selective serotonin reuptake inhibitor (SSRI) and CBT
    (D) SSRI only

114. A 76-year-old woman with coronary artery disease comes to the office for preoperative medical evaluation before coronary bypass graft surgery (CABG) in 3 weeks. She is an active smoker.

    Which one of the following interventions will decrease her risk of postoperative pulmonary complications?

    (A) Preoperative inspiratory muscle training
    (B) Preoperative smoking cessation
    (C) Preoperative inhaled β-agonist
    (D) Postoperative use of incentive spirometry

115. A bedbound 94-year-old woman requires a home visit for medical care. She lives in her own home, supported by her children and their families. She is nonverbal and incontinent. She does chew and swallow. History includes Alzheimer disease without behavior disturbance, osteoarthritis of several joints, and essential hypertension. Current medications are acetaminophen and hydrochlorothiazide. Her family is present, and disease trajectory is discussed with them.

    On physical examination, blood pressure is 143/78 mmHg, heart rate is 73 beats per minute, and respiratory rate is 12 breaths per minute. Skin is intact. Muscle tone is increased in all extremities. She responds to voice and touch with eye tracking but does not speak during the visit.

    Which one of the following will determine the level of reimbursement for this visit?

    (A) Documentation of complexity of the visit
    (B) Distance traveled to visit
    (C) Number of family members involved in the summary discussion
    (D) Skilled service referrals generated by visit

116. An 82-year-old man comes to the office because he has been coughing during meals. He almost choked once. He has no pain with swallowing and no sensation of food stuck in his throat. The cough developed gradually over the past month. History includes Parkinson disease, hypertension, and hyperlipidemia. Current medications are carbidopa/levodopa, lisinopril, and atorvastatin.

    Which one of the following is the most appropriate next step to establish the diagnosis in this patient?

    (A) Esophageal manometry
    (B) Barium swallow test
    (C) Videofluoroscopy
    (D) Upper endoscopy

117. An 84-year-old man is brought to the office because his right eye is red. There is moderate watery discharge. He says that the eye feels gritty but does not itch, and he has no eye pain or light sensitivity. There is no baseline information on visual acuity, but he thinks his vision is unchanged, and nursing home staff confirm that there has been no evidence of a change in vision. History includes Alzheimer disease. He seems to have a cold and is sneezing.

    On examination, eye movements are intact. There is moderate bulbar conjunctival injection of the right eye. Conjunctival hemorrhage extends from 6 o'clock to 9 o'clock positions. Right preauricular lymph node is slightly tender.

    Which one of the following is the most appropriate management of the red eye?

    (A) Antibiotic eye drops
    (B) Referral to an ophthalmologist
    (C) Artificial tears as needed
    (D) Antihistamine eye drops

118. Which one of the following is most likely to be a characteristic of older adults living in poverty in the United States?

    (A) Male sex
    (B) Non-Hispanic white ethnicity
    (C) Living alone
    (D) Age between 65 and 74 years old

119. An 80-year-old woman comes to the office to discuss her oncologist's recommendation that she consider adjuvant chemotherapy. She recently had surgery for an obstructing colon cancer; regional lymph nodes were positive for metastatic adenocarcinoma. Her recovery from surgery was prolonged because of difficulty with ambulation and increased weakness. History includes heart failure (ejection fraction of 19%) and chronic obstructive pulmonary disease. In the past year, she has had 3 episodes of respiratory failure requiring ventilator therapy. She is concerned about the potential adverse effects of adjuvant chemotherapy.

    Which one of the following would provide the most useful information to help with her decision?

    (A) Clinical practice guidelines related to her diseases
    (B) Number of patients who would need to be treated for 1 patient to benefit from the chemotherapy
    (C) Chance of harm from treatment
    (D) Lag time between treatment and benefit

120. A 70-year-old man comes to the office for a follow-up visit. History includes hyperlipidemia, trigeminal neuralgia, benign prostatic hyperplasia, and Parkinson disease. Current medications include carbamazepine, rosuvastatin, selegilene, and tamsulosin. Hypovitaminosis D was diagnosed 3 months ago, and he began treatment with vitamin D_3 2,000 IU/d by mouth. At today's visit, the vitamin D concentration is unchanged from 3 months ago.

    Which one of his medications is most likely affecting his vitamin D concentration?

    (A) Carbamazepine
    (B) Rosuvastatin
    (C) Selegiline
    (D) Tamsulosin

121. An 83-year-old woman comes to the office because she has had episodes of dizziness in the past month. She has continual unsteadiness that is unchanged by position; there is no new numbness or weakness. She has not fallen, but the unsteadiness has caused her to turn down invitations and stop going to her weekly bridge game. She has not been sleeping well. Her husband died 1 year ago. History includes hypertension, osteoarthritis, and glaucoma.

    On examination, she appears thin but in no distress. She has lost 2.3 kg (5 lb) since her last visit. Orthostatic vital signs are normal. Visual acuity and hearing are grossly intact. She has full strength. Sensory examination is normal to pinprick and vibratory sensation in all extremities. Reflexes are 2+ throughout. Gait is slow and hesitant but narrow based and steady.

    Which one of the following is the best next step?

    (A) Obtain magnetic resonance imaging (MRI) of the cervical spine.
    (B) Perform Dix-Hallpike test.
    (C) Screen for depression.
    (D) Conduct tilt-table test.

122. An 80-year-old man comes to the office because he has new onset of right elbow pain after a weekend of gardening. He recalls no specific trauma. History includes type 2 diabetes mellitus, osteoarthritis, hypertension, end-stage renal disease, and gout. The diabetes is controlled by diet, and he is on hemodialysis. Current medications are quinapril 20 mg/d, acetaminophen 650 mg three times daily, and allopurinol 200 mg/d.

    On physical examination, blood pressure is 155/85 mmHg, heart rate is 90 beats per minute, and temperature is 37.5°C (99.5°F). He appears to be in moderate distress and is holding his right elbow. The elbow is diffusely red and edematous, especially the extensor aspect, with +2 edema. Elbow extension is possible to 165 degrees; the last 10 degrees is limited by pain. Radial pulses are normal. Monofilament examination reveals mild distal peripheral neuropathy in both feet. Hands are normal except for the presence of Heberden nodes in multiple distal interphalangeal joints.

Laboratory findings:
Hemoglobin	12 mg/dL
White blood cell count	11,000/μL (80% neutrophils)
Hemoglobin A_{1c}	8%
Serum creatinine	1.9 mg/dL
Serum uric acid	6 mg/dL
Erythrocyte sedimentation rate	50 mm/hr

Radiography of the right elbow shows diffuse soft-tissue swelling.

Which one of the following is the most appropriate next step?

(A) Ultrasonography-guided aspiration of the elbow joint
(B) Cephalexin 250 mg four times daily for 7 days
(C) Needle aspiration of the olecranon bursa
(D) Colchicine 1.2 mg now, then 0.6 mg tomorrow

123. An 80-year-old woman comes to the office for routine follow-up. She lives in a nursing home. History includes diabetes, hypertension, hypercholesterolemia, and recurrent urinary tract infections. Current medications are aspirin 81 mg/d daily, sitagliptin 50 mg/d, lisinopril 20 mg/d, simvastatin 40 mg/d, and 2 cranberry capsules daily. She has not had any recent infections.

Which one of the following statements is true regarding the role of cranberry products in preventing urinary tract infections for older women in nursing homes?

(A) Cranberry products can prevent urinary tract infections.
(B) Cranberry juice is the only cranberry product that prevents urinary tract infections.
(C) Cranberry juice is more effective than capsules in preventing urinary tract infections.
(D) Data do not support use of cranberry products to prevent urinary tract infections.

124. A 68-year-old woman comes to the office to establish care. She is lesbian and has recently retired to the area. History includes hypertension and chronic kidney disease. She smokes tobacco and is moderately obese.

She is at increased risk for which one of the following, compared with risks for a heterosexual woman?

(A) Cervical cancer
(B) Cardiovascular disease
(C) Colon cancer
(D) Kidney cancer

125. An 88-year-old woman is brought to the emergency department because she has had generalized weakness and confusion for the past 2 days. History includes breast cancer, hypertension, mild cognitive impairment, and gait disorder. Her daughter reports that the patient had been doing well at home, with improving strength, since her mastectomy and radiation treatment 6 months ago.

On physical examination, vital signs are stable. Her eyes remain closed and she is difficult to arouse. General physical findings are normal; musculoskeletal and neurologic examinations are difficult to perform because of her altered mental status. Laboratory findings, including urinalysis, are normal. Magnetic resonance imaging of the brain without contrast shows multiple lesions consistent with metastatic disease, likely related to her breast cancer.

A meeting is held with the patient, her husband and children, and the medical team. The family is informed that the change in mental status is due to multiple metastatic lesions in the brain. The patient's husband states that his wife had repeatedly said that she would decline further treatment if her breast cancer ever returned, including no surgery, radiation, or chemotherapy. He asks whether hospice is an option.

Which one of the following is required for this patient to qualify for the Medicare hospice benefit?

(A) "Do not resuscitate" (DNR) code status
(B) Estimated life expectancy <6 months
(C) Uncontrolled symptoms
(D) Diagnosis of metastatic cancer

126. An 80-year-old man of Chinese descent is admitted to the hospital because he has abdominal pain, nausea, vomiting, and jaundice. Pancreatic cancer was recently diagnosed. His family members ask doctors and nurses not to tell him about the recent diagnosis.

Which one of the following is the most appropriate next step in responding to the family's request?

(A) Disclose the diagnosis to the patient.
(B) Ask the patient about his interest in learning about his medical condition.
(C) Honor the family's request.
(D) Defer to the oncologist to discuss with the family.

QUESTIONS, ANSWERS AND CRITIQUES

Note: The Strength of Evidence (SOE) classification and definitions are found on the inside front cover, and the table of Normal Laboratory Values on the inside back cover may be consulted for any of the questions in this book.

1. An 82-year-old woman comes to the office because she has had vaginal discharge and light-pink spotting intermittently for at least 2 years. She is not sexually active and has no pain. She underwent a hysterectomy and a "bladder lift," which included mesh, approximately 10 years ago. She has been treated for *Candida* and bacterial vaginosis in the past without resolution of discharge and spotting.

    On examination, the external vulva is normal, without lesions or ulcerations. On speculum examination, there is a normal vaginal cuff with no evidence of recurrent vaginal prolapse. A small area (<0.5 cm) of granulation tissue is noted in the anterior vagina, and a bristly material is felt at that location. A saline wet mount shows normal epithelial cells and vaginal pH of 7.0.

    Which one of the following would be the best treatment plan?

    (A) Referral for surgical management
    (B) Metronidazole vaginal gel
    (C) Oral fluconazole
    (D) Estradiol vaginal cream

    ANSWER: D

    The most common presenting symptoms of mesh exposure are vaginal discharge, vaginal bleeding or spotting, dyspareunia, and partner report of pain with coitus (SOE=B). Exposed vaginal mesh can often be seen on speculum examination or palpated on bimanual examination as a bristly plastic.

    In women who are relatively asymptomatic (eg, because they are not sexually active) and who have a small area of exposed type 1 macroporous polypropylene mesh, conservative management with topical vaginal estrogen may provide treatment without necessitating surgical removal (SOE=C). This is the best option for this patient. In women who have more troublesome symptoms (eg, interference with sexual activity, or discomfort from discharge, bleeding, or pain), referral for surgical management is appropriate (SOE=C).

    Vaginal mesh exposure can occur after the following procedures: placement of a midurethral sling with polypropylene mesh material for correction of stress urinary incontinence, sacrocolpopexy with permanent mesh material for pelvic organ prolapse, or vaginal prolapse surgery with mesh augmentation (with or without a commercial vaginal mesh kit). Recent warnings from the U.S. Food and Drug Administration have intensified public awareness of mesh complications after surgery for incontinence or prolapse.

    The incidence of vaginal mesh exposure after placement of type 1 macroporous polypropylene mesh for pelvic floor disorders varies by the type of surgery: midurethral sling procedures, 2%–3%; abdominal sacrocolpopexy with hysterectomy, 3%–6%; and sacrocolpopexy without hysterectomy, 1%–3%. The highest rates are seen with transvaginal prolapse surgery (3%–15%).

    Exposure of mesh depends not only on the type of surgery performed but also on intrinsic properties of the mesh, patient factors, and surgeon experience. Nonwoven type 1 macroporous polypropylene mesh is associated with the lowest occurrence of mesh erosion in incontinence and prolapse surgery (SOE=A). Patient factors that increase risk of mesh exposure are diabetes mellitus, smoking, vaginal atrophy, and concomitant hysterectomy at time of prolapse repair.

    Treatment for bacterial vaginosis with metronidazole or for candidiasis with fluconazole would not be appropriate in this patient, because she has been treated for these conditions in the past without resolution of symptoms and the vaginal discharge is most likely caused by the vaginal mesh exposure.

2. A 78-year-old woman comes to the office for evaluation because she slipped off the bed when she was getting dressed. The fall caused a small abrasion on her buttocks but no acute pain. She had a bone density test 1.5 years ago; T-score at that time was −1.5. She describes a diet high in calcium and vitamin D (calcium 1,200 mg/d from dairy products and vitamin D 800 mg/d from fish, eggs, and dairy, plus a vitamin D supplement, 400 IU/d).

Which one of the following is the most appropriate next step for this patient?

(A) Radiography to exclude pelvic fracture
(B) Measurement of vitamin D level
(C) Completion of the Fracture Risk Assessment tool (FRAX®)
(D) Repeat bone densitometry

ANSWER: C

The FRAX® tool is the most appropriate assessment option for this patient. Its algorithms integrate clinical risk factors with bone mineral density (BMD) at the femoral neck to evaluate 10-year probability of hip or other osteoporotic fracture. Derived from cohorts in Europe, North America, Asia, and Australia, FRAX® relies on the following data: age, sex, weight, height, prior fracture history, parent with hip fracture, current smoker, corticosteroid use, and history of rheumatoid arthritis.

    Baseline measurement of BMD using bone densitometry is recommended for women ≥65 years old and for men and women at risk of fracture (SOE=A). Retesting should be done every ≥2 years to assess changes in BMD (SOE=C). For individuals with a low risk of fracture who do not appear to be at risk of rapid bone loss, intervals of 5–10 years may be sufficient (SOE=C). Repeat testing at intervals of <2 years adds little to the predictive value of baseline testing with regard to future risk of falls. For this patient, repeat bone densitometry is unnecessary because her previous scan was within the past 2 years.

    Radiography is not sufficient for diagnosis of osteoporosis or assessment of risk from future fracture. It is inappropriate for this patient, because there is no indication of fracture.

    According to the U.S. Preventive Services Task Force (USPSTF), there is insufficient evidence 1) to evaluate the balance of benefit and harm of combined vitamin D and calcium supplementation for primary prevention of fractures in premenopausal women, and 2) to balance the benefit and harm of daily supplementation with >400 IU of vitamin D and >1,000 mg of calcium for primary prevention of fractures in noninstitutionalized postmenopausal women. This patient is taking in adequate amounts of calcium and vitamin D through her diet based on USPSTF and Institute of Medicine recommendations (1,200 mg of calcium and 800 IU of vitamin D for persons >70 years old). The USPSTF has concluded there is insufficient evidence to support screening for vitamin D levels.

3. A 76-year-old man comes to the office because he has constant itching all over his body that began 6 months ago. The itching is worse on his back and extremities. OTC moisturizers provide only modest relief. He can identify no alleviating or exacerbating factors, including no weather or temperature variation.

On physical examination, the patient is in no distress. Sclera are anicteric. There are linear erosions on the back, with sparing of areas that the patient cannot reach. Dryness and xerotic scale are diffuse. There is no evidence of a primary eruption.

Which one of the following medications is the likely cause of this patient's sebostatic and xerotic pruritus?

(A) Atenolol
(B) Acetaminophen
(C) Tramadol
(D) Trimethoprim-sulfamethoxazole

ANSWER: A

Pruritus is the most common skin concern in older patients; the extent of symptoms varies. It affects quality of life and can contribute to significant morbidity if left unmanaged. The causes are diverse, ranging from normal physiologic changes to occult malignancy. One common cause is adverse effect of medications.

    Atenolol, acetaminophen, tramadol, and trimethoprim-sulfamethoxazole each cause or exacerbate pruritus, through different pathophysiologic mechanisms. The different mechanisms present differently.

Atenolol and other β-blockers are common causes of the distressing xerotic-type pruritus seen in this patient (SOE=B). The pruritus does not cause end-organ damage, and management should focus on skin hydration. Acetaminophen can damage the hepatobiliary system, leading to hyperbilirubinemia and increased bile acid levels that cause pruritus. For this patient, the presence of anicteric sclera makes acetaminophen a very unlikely cause of pruritus. Tramadol causes pruritus through neurologic or histamine-release mechanisms; this is a less likely cause in the presence of severe xerosis, as seen in this patient. Trimethoprim-sulfamethoxazole commonly causes a morbilliform skin rash, which this patient does not have. It may also cause pruritus that is related to hypersensitivity reactions, such as Stevens-Johnson syndrome.

4. A 76-year-old woman comes to the office because for the past 4 months she has had urge urinary incontinence. Before then, she had frequent incontinence episodes associated with bending at the waist or coughing. Onset of urge incontinence was gradual, but she now has episodes several times each week. She has had no vaginal discharge or hematuria. She has a monogamous relationship with her spouse of 48 years. History includes hypertension, osteoarthritis of the knees, hypothyroidism, and vaginal hysterectomy for uterine fibroids at age 53 years.

On physical examination, there is grade 1 pelvic organ prolapse. She is able to perform isolated contraction of pelvic floor muscles. Vaginal epithelium is thin, with mild irritation. She reports a burning sensation during the manual vaginal examination with petroleum jelly lubricant. Ultrasonography of the bladder shows 40 mL residual urine after she voids. Urinalysis shows no leukocyte esterase, no nitrates, and no hemoglobin; there are 5–10 white blood cells and 0 red blood cells per high-power field. Culture reveals *Escherichia coli* (<10,000 colony-forming units) that is sensitive to all tested antibiotics.

Which one of the following is the most appropriate initial treatment for this patient's urinary leakage?

(A) Fesoterodine 4 mg/d
(B) Percutaneous stimulation of the tibial nerve
(C) Cystoscopy with intradetrusor injection of onabotulinumtoxinA
(D) Behavioral therapy with pelvic floor muscle exercises

ANSWER: D

This patient has mixed stress and urge urinary incontinence. A positive standing cough test is a highly specific sign for stress incontinence (SOE=A), and her history of difficulty holding urine supports a diagnosis of urge urinary incontinence. Guidelines recommend behavioral therapy as an appropriate first management strategy for urinary incontinence in older adults (SOE=A). In a Cochrane review that included only randomized trials, pelvic floor muscle therapy improved outcomes for women with stress or mixed urinary incontinence (SOE=A). This patient is a strong candidate for behaviorally based therapy with pelvic floor muscle (Kegel) exercises. In addition, she should be taught to contract her pelvic floor muscles just before activities that usually induce stress leakage (eg, coughing, sneezing, lifting), as well as to manage urgency by staying still and repeatedly contracting the pelvic floor muscles until the urgency is gone, and only then proceeding to the bathroom; if the urgency returns on the way to the bathroom, she should again "freeze and squeeze."

Fesoterodine would treat urge symptoms and urgency incontinence but likely would not help stress symptoms. Percutaneous tibial nerve stimulation involves neuromodulation for overactive bladder symptoms such as urgency, frequency, and urge incontinence for patients in whom conservative therapy (with behavioral and drug-based approaches) has failed. It is approved by the U.S. Food and Drug Administration (FDA). Cystoscopic intradetrusor injection of onabotulinumtoxinA is also approved by the FDA for refractory symptoms secondary to overactive bladder. These treatment modalities would not be expected to address her symptoms of stress incontinence.

5. A 79-year-old woman undergoes evaluation related to a stage 2 pressure injury. She had surgery and short-term rehabilitation after she fractured her right hip and is now being cared for in her daughter's home with the assistance of home care services. She is reluctant to ambulate. She prefers to lie on her back at all times in a regular bed and has not wanted to reposition.

Which one of the following would be most effective in preventing the stage 2 pressure injury from increasing in size and severity?

(A) Apply a transparent film dressing.
(B) Recommend use of a reactive support surface.
(C) Recommend nutritional supplementation.
(D) Encourage ambulation.

ANSWER: D

This patient's immobility and inactivity can lead to development of a more serious pressure injury. The best management strategy would be to educate the patient and her daughter about the importance of ambulation and getting out of bed (SOE=C). The family should be encouraged to follow up with a physical therapist for gait training to assist with balance and improve ambulation. Getting out of bed and ambulating is the best measure for preventing further deterioration of the pressure injury.

A preventive protocol, based on assessment of this patient and her home environment, is needed to decrease potential for another fall. In addition, her reasons for avoiding ambulation need to be ascertained; she may be afraid of hurting her fractured leg, or pain control measures may be inadequate. She may be depressed or anxious, in which case she may benefit from psychologic support.

A turning schedule would also be good for prevention and healing, but the patient resists being turned or repositioned. A reactive support surface is a specialized mattress or bed designed to redistribute pressure, manage microclimate, and decrease risk of pressure injury (SOE=C). Although a reactive (powered or non-powered) support surface may also benefit the patient, if she is not getting out of bed or turning, she will still be at risk of further skin breakdown.

While a wound dressing will be needed, more specific information is needed about the wound to determine the appropriate treatment plan.

Nutrition is also an important component of pressure injury management. In general, the caloric requirement for wound healing is 30–35 Kcal/kg/day (SOE=B). Protein is required for wound healing, but the exact amount has not been established. The current recommendation for protein is 1–1.5 g/kg/day, but more may be required depending on the patient's clinical condition.

6. A 79-year-old woman is admitted to the hospital because she fractured her hip. History includes hypertension and type 2 diabetes mellitus. On examination, vital signs are normal and Confusion Assessment Method (CAM) screen is negative for delirium. Hemoglobin is 8.5 mg/dL.

Which one of the following interventions is most likely to prevent incident delirium?

(A) Blood transfusion to goal hemoglobin level of 10 mg/dL
(B) Preoperative geriatric consultation
(C) Strict avoidance of opiate medication
(D) Low-dose haloperidol prophylaxis

ANSWER: B

In a trial of patients with hip fracture receiving standard care in an orthopedic ward, 126 patients were randomly assigned to a proactive (initiated preoperatively) or a reactive (within 24 hours after surgery) geriatric consultation. The consultant visited daily and provided structured recommendations addressing 10 domains (including central nervous system, oxygen delivery, fluid and electrolyte levels, and pain management). The intervention group (proactive consultation) had 36% fewer cases of incident delirium; number needed to treat (NNT) to prevent 1 case of delirium was 5.6. A meta-analysis of randomized trials of team-based and ward-based comprehensive geriatric assessment for preventing delirium in hip-fracture patients (which included the aforementioned trial) reported significant reduction in delirium in the groups that received team-based interventions.

Undertreated pain and inadequate analgesia were identified as risk factors for delirium in a prospective cohort study in which 541 patients with hip fracture were enrolled. Postoperative delirium occurred in 16% of the cohort. Patients who received parenteral morphine sulfate equivalents at <10 mg/d were more likely to develop delirium than patients who received more analgesia. In cognitively intact patients, delirium was 9 times more likely to develop in patients with undertreated pain than in patients with adequately treated pain.

To determine whether maintenance of hemoglobin >10 g/dL in postoperative hip-fracture patients reduces the incidence and severity of delirium, a study was conducted (ancillary to the *Transfusion Trigger Trial for Functional Outcomes in Cardiovascular Patients Undergoing Surgical Hip Fracture Repair* ([FOCUS]). In the ancillary study, 139 hip-fracture patients (mean age 81.5 years) with cardiovascular disease (or risk factors for cardiovascular disease) and hemoglobin <10 g/dL postoperatively were randomly assigned to liberal transfusion to maintain hemoglobin >10 g/dL or to restrictive transfusion, limited to cases of symptomatic anemia or hemoglobin <8 g/dL. There was no significant difference in presence or severity of delirium as identified by CAM in the 2 groups.

Perioperative use of haloperidol has not been shown to reduce the incidence of postoperative delirium in hip-fracture patients. In a systematic review and meta-analysis of 19 randomized or cohort studies of use of antipsychotics to prevent or treat delirium, 7 studies (n=1,970 patients) compared efficacy of antipsychotics with placebo in preventing postoperative delirium, and 4 studies specifically evaluated haloperidol. Antipsychotics did not significantly reduce the incidence, duration, or severity of delirium.

7. A 69-year-old woman comes to the office for her annual wellness examination. She was hospitalized 3 times in the past year because of exacerbation of chronic obstructive pulmonary disease (COPD) and overdose of benzodiazepines and opioids. In addition to COPD and substance abuse, history includes hepatitis C, obstructive sleep apnea, and osteoarthritis. She does not adhere to medication regimens because of their cost. She smokes cigarettes, 1 pack/d for the last 30 years. She uses a wheelchair regularly because severe osteoarthritis makes walking difficult. Since she moved to subsidized housing from a homeless shelter, she has more reliable transportation for medical care, and someone helps her with daily chores. She is up-to-date with influenza and pneumonia vaccines. She has never had screening for breast, cervical, or colorectal cancer.

On examination, blood pressure is 127/80 mmHg, heart rate is 80 beats per minute, and BMI is 30 kg/m². Heart and lung sounds are distant; no crackles, wheezes, or rhonchi are heard. There are mild, bilateral knee effusions and crepitus.

Which one of the following screening tests would be most useful at this time?

(A) Colonoscopy
(B) Lipid panel
(C) Computed tomography of the chest
(D) Depression screen

ANSWER: D

Lag time to benefit—the time between a preventive intervention and an improved health outcome—is an important factor when assessing the usefulness of preventive screening tests. It is important to consider the time to benefit in relation to the patient's overall prognosis.

The Medicare Annual Wellness Examination covers screening for cardiovascular disease, colorectal cancer, depression, and lung cancer. This patient's multimorbidities place her at relatively high risk of mortality (~43%) in the next 5 years, according to the Schonberg Index (SOE=A). Screening for depression can improve clinical outcomes. If the screen is positive, treatment with antidepressants, psychotherapy, or both can decrease clinical morbidity. The lag time to benefit for depression screening and treatment can be as short as 6–8 weeks.

A lipid panel is easy to perform, and improvement in cholesterol levels may take only a few months to achieve, yet the lag time between screening and prevention of a cardiovascular event may be 1–2 years, which is longer than the lag time to benefit interval for depression. Based on her age, the guidelines for cancer screening are applicable. However, for this patient, screening for colorectal or lung cancer may yield less benefit than screening for depression, because the lag time between screening and benefit is about 10 years for both colorectal and lung cancer.

8. Compared with older adults in metropolitan communities, older adults in rural communities are more likely to have which one of the following?

   (A) Higher income levels
   (B) Lower all-cause mortality rates
   (C) Higher rates of using public transportation
   (D) Less access to health care services

ANSWER: D

In data from 2010, adults ≥65 years old made up 12% of the population in large central metropolitan communities and 18% in rural communities. The growth in population of older adults in rural communities may herald a unique public health challenge. The mortality rate for older adults in large, metropolitan communities is about 4,900 per 100,000, whereas the mortality rate is 5,600 per 100,000 in non-metropolitan communities. The higher mortality rate is likely due to a combination of factors. Older adults in rural communities tend to be poorer and sicker. Rural communities often have a limited infrastructure; some areas lack even basic amenities, such as running water or central heat. Furthermore, access to health care is a challenge. Rural areas generally lack public transportation and have fewer health care providers serving those geographic areas. Consequently, even when transportation is available, older adults in rural areas tend to travel longer distances for health care services, particularly for specialty care.

9. An 86-year-old man comes to the emergency department because he has had dizziness, abdominal pain, and black stool for 1 day. He lives alone; his family and neighbors check on him daily. He describes an episode of "food poisoning" approximately 3 days ago, during which he had multiple bouts of vomiting and diarrhea. For the past 2 days he has been using bismuth subsalicylate 2–3 times daily, as an OTC remedy for his gastrointestinal symptoms. History includes anemia, atrial fibrillation, and hypertension. Current medications are dabigatran 150 mg orally twice daily (for 2 years), fosinopril 10 mg/d (for 20 years), hydrochlorothiazide 12.5 mg/d orally (for 20 years), ferrous sulfate 325 mg twice daily, and a daily multivitamin.

On examination, blood pressure is 110/68 mmHg (baseline, 148/82 mmHg), heart rate is 104 beats per minute, and respiratory rate is 18 breaths per minute.

Laboratory findings:

Hemoglobin	9.0 g/dL (baseline, 12 g)
Hematocrit	28% (baseline, 36%)
Platelet count	281 × 10^9/L
BUN	28 mg/dL
Serum creatinine	1.9 mg/dL (baseline 1.4 mg/dL)
Estimated creatinine clearance	22 mL/min (baseline, 58 mL/min)

Which one of the following is the most likely cause of his presenting symptoms?

(A) Dabigatran overdose
(B) Drug interaction between dabigatran and bismuth subsalicylate
(C) Salicylate overdose from bismuth subsalicylate
(D) Drug interaction between hydrochlorothiazide and bismuth subsalicylate

ANSWER: A

This patient is experiencing gastrointestinal bleeding caused by an accidental overdose of dabigatran. Dabigatran is a direct thrombin inhibitor that is primarily eliminated in the urine. The dosage of dabigatran for this patient was appropriate for his baseline renal function; however, his recent gastrointestinal illness likely caused him to become dehydrated and sustain acute kidney injury, as evidenced by his relative hypotension, tachycardia, increased BUN and serum creatinine levels, and decreased creatinine clearance. The acute decline in renal function has reduced the renal clearance of dabigatran, increasing his systemic exposure and leading to overdose. Dabigatran should be discontinued while the acute bleeding is managed. A specific reversal agent for dabigatran (idarucizumab) has been approved by the U.S. Food and Drug Administration.

Once the bleeding episode is resolved, the patient should be reassessed before restarting oral anticoagulants. The risk of gastrointestinal bleeding increases in older adults and is associated with significant morbidity, but this must be considered along with risk of stroke from untreated atrial fibrillation. If he is considered a candidate for restarting anticoagulation, the dosage should be adjusted for renal function. The dosage of dabigatran should be reduced to 75 mg twice daily for creatinine clearance between 15 mL/min and 30 mL/min; dabigatran should generally be avoided in patients with creatinine clearance <15 mL/min. Apixaban may confer less risk of gastrointestinal bleeding than other direct oral anticoagulants. Doses of apixaban should be reduced to 2.5 mg twice daily for patients with 2 or 3 of the following: age ≥80 years old, weight <60 kg, or serum creatinine ≥1.5 mg/dL. Renal function should be assessed periodically in patients who continue on long-term therapy, particularly older adults. Alternatively, warfarin may be considered a better option because it does not depend on renal function for clearance, but does require regular, frequent monitoring of the international normalized ratio (INR).

No pharmacokinetic drug interactions have been reported between dabigatran or hydrochlorothiazide and bismuth subsalicylate. There is a possibility that the salicylate component may have an additive effect when combined with dabigatran. However, the more likely explanation for bleeding in this patient is unintended overdose with dabigatran. Bismuth subsalicylate should also be discontinued in the event of bleeding.

Bismuth subsalicylate undergoes dissociation in the gastrointestinal tract. The bismuth portion is not absorbed and is eliminated in the feces. The absorption of the salicylate component of bismuth subsalicylate is >90%; based on the dosage the patient reports taking, salicylate ingestion was approximately 1.5 g/d (500 mg per dose), which is within an acceptable range for therapeutic dose.

Black tongue and black stools are common adverse effects of bismuth subsalicylate. This discoloration is caused by a reaction between the bismuth and trace amounts of sulfur in saliva in the gastrointestinal tract, forming bismuth sulfide. The change in color is temporary and harmless; it can last for several days after the last dose. The report of black stool fits within the time course to be considered an adverse effect of bismuth subsalicylate. However, this temporary harmless discoloration of stool does not explain his dizziness, anemia, and relative hypotension.

10. A 75-year-old man comes to the office for routine follow-up. He recently had surgery to remove a cataract in his right eye, and he mentions that his eye doctor told him that his visual acuity is now 20/25 in both eyes. Yet he is puzzled, because there are times when he cannot see well, such as when he drives at dusk or in the rain. His eye doctor mentioned no other ocular pathology.

Which one of the following age-related changes is the most likely cause of his difficulty driving at dusk or in the rain?

(A) Reduced accommodation
(B) Decreased contrast sensitivity
(C) Increased glare sensitivity
(D) Reduced upgaze

ANSWER: B

Standard visual acuity is not an accurate predictor of visual function as a person ages. Standard visual acuity is tested under high-contrast, ideal conditions that rarely exist outside the eye doctor's office. Better predictors are contrast sensitivity, glare sensitivity, and acuity performance under reduced illumination (mesopic acuity). Performance in each of these areas decreases for older adults, with or without other causes of impaired visual acuity.

Contrast sensitivity is the ability to see an object as different from its background. The black-on-white eye chart offers high-contrast sensitivity with low camouflage. Dusk, cloudiness, and rain reduce contrast sensitivity and impair visual function, even in the presence of good standard visual acuity. Reduced contrast sensitivity makes it much more difficult to differentiate objects (including pedestrians) from the low-light background. Decreased contrast sensitivity best explains this patient's concern for night driving (SOE B). Another contributor to his concern is the reduced ability of aging eyes to detect motion in low-light conditions.

The age-related reduction in upgaze may affect the older driver by reducing the ability to recognize street and traffic signs (SOE=C), but it does not affect ability to discriminate visually at dusk or when it rains.

Increased glare sensitivity also occurs with aging but does not relate to this patient's concern about driving at dusk or in the rain. Increased glare sensitivity is a factor in such situations as driving out of a dark parking garage into bright sunlight, presence of bright roadside lights, and oncoming headlights.

Reduced accommodation of the lens is nearly universal by age 50 years, accounting for the fact that by age 50, most people need glasses for reading. It does not affect night driving.

11. A 78-year-old woman is admitted to a long-term care facility after lengthy hospitalization for stroke. Nursing staff document 3 pressure injuries in various locations and note that she will require wound evaluation and numerous dressing changes. No measurements or photographs are taken of the pressure injuries. A wound care provider examines the patient 48 hours after admission.

On physical examination, there is a stage 4, clean, granulating sacral pressure injury, measuring 9 × 6 × 0.5 cm; an unstageable pressure injury on the right trochanter, measuring 2 × 5 cm, with dry, hard necrotic eschar and no drainage; and a skin tear (not pressure injury) measuring 4 × 3 cm, with a partial skin flap/pedicle. There is no evidence of infection.

Which one of the following should have been done on admission to the long-term care facility?

(A) Debridement of sacral wound
(B) Assessment and documentation of wound, with measurements
(C) Application of a nonadherent dressing to all wounds
(D) Application of gauze to pack the pressure injury

ANSWER: B

Pressure injuries can deteriorate rapidly. Assessment and documentation of the etiology of all wounds is crucial. All wounds should be evaluated by the clinician within 8 hours of admission, according to the National Pressure Ulcer Advisory Panel, and weekly thereafter. Pressure injuries are a reportable condition in the long-term care setting, so documentation of correct etiology is important (per federal regulation).

Skin tears are not pressure ulcers; they should be documented as a separate wound. A skin tear is an acute wound caused by shear, friction, or blunt force, resulting in separation of skin layers. A skin tear can be partial thickness (separation of the epidermis from the dermis) or full thickness (separation of both the epidermis and dermis from underlying structures).

There are multiple debridement options. A clean, granulating pressure injury does not need debridement. Unstageable pressure injuries are usually debrided per clinician orders. Moist wound therapy is the standard of care for pressure injuries. Packing may be required after a debridement. A nonadherent dressing is standard for management of skin tears.

A key component to prevent pressure injuries and skin tears is to recognize fragile, thin, vulnerable skin and pressure points and to modify care accordingly.

12. An 82-year-old woman is brought to the emergency department because she is coughing and has shortness of breath. She is lethargic, confused, and easily distracted, and she is trying to pull out intravenous lines. History includes systolic heart failure, coronary artery disease, hypertension, and renal insufficiency. Heart failure is diagnosed, and Confusion Assessment Method (CAM) is positive for delirium.

Which one of the following is the best initial treatment for managing this patient's delirium?

(A) Administer haloperidol.
(B) Administer lorazepam.
(C) Encourage family to spend time at bedside.
(D) Apply soft wrist restraints.

ANSWER: C

Nonpharmacologic intervention is the best approach for management of delirium. A number of simple approaches are helpful in reducing the risk of incident delirium and may be helpful in management. These include clocks and calendars to help a person stay oriented; a calm and comfortable environment with family at the bedside; regular verbal reminders of current location and what is happening around the patient; avoidance of change in surroundings and caregivers; avoidance of intravenous lines and Foley catheters; uninterrupted periods of sleep at night, with low levels of noise and minimal light during sleep; avoidance of physical restraints and tubes; opportunities to get out of bed, walk, and perform self-care activities; and provision of eyeglasses, hearing aids, and other adaptive equipment as needed.

In patients receiving palliative care, individualized management of delirium precipitants and supportive strategies are more effective than administration of risperidone or haloperidol in reducing signs and shortening the duration of delirium.

If nonpharmacologic approaches are insufficient, haloperidol can be prescribed at a low dose (0.25–0.5 mg). For patients with Parkinson disease or parkinsonian features, quetiapine 12.5 mg would be preferred over haloperidol because it has a lower incidence of extrapyramidal adverse effects. Benzodiazepines such as lorazepam should be avoided, because they may worsen confusion and sedation and can prolong delirium (SOE=A); the exception is cases in which delirium is caused by withdrawal from alcohol or benzodiazepines, in which case lorazepam is the drug of choice.

13. A 78-year-old woman comes to the office because she has difficulty understanding conversations in noisy environments. She is referred for audiology evaluation. Audiometry demonstrates mild hearing loss at low frequencies, sloping to profound loss at high frequencies; hearing thresholds for air and bone conduction overlap. Speech discrimination is 83% in the right ear and 85% in the left.

Which one of the following is the most likely cause of this patient's hearing loss?

(A) Conductive hearing loss
(B) Central auditory processing disorder
(C) Sensorineural hearing loss
(D) Ménière disease

ANSWER: C

The audiometry results describe sensorineural hearing loss, specifically presbycusis. Presbycusis, the most common cause of hearing loss in older adults, is a symmetric hearing loss resulting from changes in the sensory hair cells in the cochlea. The characteristic audiogram displays mild to moderate hearing loss at lower frequencies, sloping to a moderate, severe, or even profound hearing loss at higher frequencies. The audiogram of Ménière disease is asymmetric, affecting one ear, and at least initially would show hearing loss at low frequencies.

The audiogram is used to determine whether hearing loss is sensorineural or conductive, or a mixture of the two, and whether the loss is symmetric (ie, the pattern of hearing is the same in both ears). Patients who have asymmetric hearing loss should be referred to an otolaryngologist for further evaluation.

The audiogram quantifies the degree of hearing loss. On every audiogram, the x-axis represents the frequency tested (Hz) and the y-axis indicates the lowest decibel at which the patient hears a sound at the given frequency. Hearing the frequency at decibels ≤25 is considered within the range of normal hearing; 25–40 dB indicates mild hearing loss, 41–55 dB indicates moderate hearing loss, 56–80 dB represents severe hearing loss, and >81 dB indicates profound hearing loss. Often, the hearing for an individual patient spans different degrees of loss at different frequencies. The patient in this case has mild hearing loss at lower frequencies, sloping to profound loss (requiring higher decibels) at higher frequencies.

Air and bone conduction is tested to differentiate between sensorineural (pathology in the cochlea or brain) and conductive (pathology in the external or middle ear) hearing loss. Air conduction tests, during which the patient listens to a sound via a headphone, cover the entirety of the auditory system, from external ear to brain. Bone conduction is tested by placing a vibrating mechanism (tuning fork) on the mastoid process, thereby bypassing the external ear and ossicles of the middle ear. The tuning fork directly vibrates the cochlea, which, based on the frequency and intensity of vibration, is interpreted as sound. Sensorineural hearing loss is diagnosed if a patient has hearing loss and the bone conduction line and air conduction line are the same, as is seen in this patient. This means that the hearing loss is at a common pathway of the two testing mechanisms—either the cochlea or the brain; no component of the hearing loss is due to the external or middle ear. If the bone and air conduction lines differ, then the loss is conductive. The difference between the air conduction and bone conduction lines is often referred to as the *air-bone gap*. In the case described here, because the air and bone conduction measures overlap, there is no conductive hearing loss. Many patients have mixed hearing loss with both conductive and sensorineural components.

Patients with conductive hearing loss should be referred to an otolaryngologist for evaluation and discussion of options; in some cases, conductive hearing loss may be surgically treated. The type of amplification used can range from assistive listening devices to hearing aids, and the best options can be determined by a trained audiologist.

Audiometry has limited value in detection of central auditory processing disorders. Speech discrimination (done during audiometry) is sometimes used as a surrogate but has limitations. For a person with poor speech discrimination, normal findings on audiogram support a central processing disorder. Relatively good speech discrimination in the presence of hearing loss essentially excludes this diagnosis.

14. The family of a 74-year-old woman comes to the office to discuss goals of care. The patient resides in a nursing home and has Alzheimer disease. She is oriented only to self and recognizes family and close friends. She participates in activities in the facility with assistance, but she does not maintain any personal hobbies. Within the last 2 years she has had increasing lower-extremity edema, managed with furosemide 20 mg/d and compression stockings. Within the last year, she has had increasing dyspnea with regular activities, and nursing home staff has noted some dyspnea at rest. She has been hospitalized twice because of increasing dyspnea accompanied by orthopnea, labored breathing, low oxygen saturation on room air, and edema that does not improve with diuretics, stockings, or elevation.

At the last hospital admission, N-terminal prohormone of brain natriuretic peptide (NT-ProBNP) was 2,000 pg/mL, BUN was 22 mg/dL, and creatinine level was 1.5 mg/dL. BMI was 22 kg/m^2. Transthoracic echocardiography showed an ejection fraction of 55% without any significant valvular abnormalities or pulmonary pressure elevation. At discharge, carvedilol, furosemide, and lisinopril were added to her medication regimen.

Which one of the following factors is most predictive of her poor long-term survival?

(A) Ejection fraction of 55%
(B) Estimated glomerular filtration (eGFR) of 34 mL/min/1.73 m^2
(C) NT-ProBNP value of 2,000 pg/mL
(D) New York Heart Association (NYHA) Class III

ANSWER: C

N-terminal prohormone of brain natriuretic peptide (NT-ProBNP) is the most powerful short- and long-term predictor of mortality risk in older adults hospitalized with acute decompensation due to heart failure. In the Copenhagen Hospital Heart Failure study, on multivariate analysis, NT-proBNP level was predictive of 1-year mortality in patients with heart failure, but left ventricular ejection fraction and NYHA class were not.

Discussions regarding goals of care and prognosis are important in older adults with acute decompensation and decline due to heart failure, especially for patients with significant comorbidities. Predictive models used for advanced heart failure provide accurate 1-, 2-, and 3-year survival rates. In a retrospective study of patients >75 years old with decompensated heart failure, overall long-term survival was poor at 5 years. NT-proBNP was the most powerful short- and long-term predictor of risk of death at 2 months and at 1 year (SOE=B). Other variables independently associated with prognosis include eGFR, hemoglobin level, presence of diabetes, systolic blood pressure, and moderate to severe tricuspid regurgitation.

Other measures that appear to also have consistent independent prognostic value include NYHA symptom class, left ventricle dimensions on echocardiography, radionuclide ejection fraction, and ischemic basis of heart failure.

The cutoff for the predictive ability of ejection fraction is not completely clear beyond recommendations for implantation of a cardioverter-defibrillator when ejection fraction is ≤30%. Some studies have shown that in patients hospitalized for heart failure, left ventricular ejection fraction ≤45% indicates increased risk of short- and long-term mortality. Most studies agree that once the ejection fraction is ≤20%, it does not add to predictive value (SOE=B).

Renal failure as evidenced by eGFR is a predictor of mortality in patients with heart failure: >40% of patients with heart failure have chronic kidney disease, and the close relationship between chronic kidney disease and heart failure worsens the prognosis (SOE=B). However, a single NT-proBNP cutoff provided relevant prognostic information irrespective of eGFR value.

15. A 90-year-old woman comes to the office accompanied by her daughter, who serves as her primary caregiver. The patient started donepezil for Alzheimer disease 6 months ago. The dosage was titrated from 5 mg/d to 10 mg/d at 1 month but was decreased back to 5 mg/d 3 months ago because of increasing gastrointestinal adverse effects (diarrhea and fecal urgency, with occasional fecal incontinence). The patient's daughter reports that, overall, her mother's cognitive function has stabilized since starting the acetylcholinesterase inhibitor, and she would like to continue it. Over the past few weeks, however, the mother asks to void up to 10 times daily. After consultation with their local pharmacist, they were informed that urinary frequency is an adverse drug event associated with donepezil. The daughter asks about strategies to manage the urinary frequency; she is open to additional drug therapy. The mother's history includes hypertension; her blood pressure has been maintained at goal with amlodipine 10 mg/d.

On physical examination, blood pressure is 124/76 mmHg. There is no evidence of pelvic organ prolapse or atrophic vaginitis. Ultrasonography of the bladder shows postvoid residual of 45 mL within 15 minutes of a void.

Which one of the following medications would be appropriate to consider for her urinary symptoms?

(A) Immediate-release oxybutynin
(B) Oral memantine
(C) Mirabegron
(D) Immediate-release tolterodine

ANSWER: C

In general, prescribing cascades—starting a medication to manage the adverse effects of another medication—should be avoided. However, in this case, the patient and family have voiced a preference to continue the medication for memory and would like to consider drug therapy for the urinary symptoms.

The mainstay drug therapy for Alzheimer disease is an acetylcholinesterase inhibitor (pro-cholinergic therapy), while urgency symptoms and urge urinary incontinence are treated with antimuscarinic anticholinergic medications. The potential for development of bladder and bowel symptoms once patients start acetylcholinesterase drugs for dementia has been demonstrated in population-based studies, and urinary frequency and diarrhea are listed as potential adverse reactions. Mirabegron, a β-3-adrenoreceptor agonist, represents a relatively new class of bladder relaxant with a mechanism of action different from that of anticholinergic bladder relaxants. As a noradrenergic agonist, adverse effects include an increase in blood pressure (mean increase of 5 mmHg) and arrhythmias. For patients in whom total anticholinergic burden is a concern, which may be increased with older anticholinergics such as tolterodine, a β-3-agonist bladder relaxant should be considered as an alternative.

Although most individuals prescribed anticholinergic bladder relaxant therapy have no discernible cognitive decline, some individuals will have precipitous, identifiable cognitive adverse effects (SOE=B). The cognitive adverse effects of oxybutynin have been shown to be related to peak drug levels (SOE=A). Immediate-release medication with the same total dosage could potentially worsen this effect. Starting memantine is unlikely to address the current urinary and bowel symptoms.

16. An 88-year-old woman comes to the office for a 6-month follow-up examination. She resides in an assisted-living facility and is independent in all basic and instrumental activities of daily living. She mentions occasional dizziness on standing, but she has never fainted. History includes hypertension; she had a myocardial infarction 10 years ago. Current medications are hydrochlorothiazide, lisinopril, and aspirin.

On physical examination, blood pressure is 160/70 mmHg sitting and 135/60 mmHg standing. A soft carotid bruit is heard on the left. A soft grade 2/6 systolic murmur is heard over the left side of the chest. Electrocardiography shows left ventricular enlargement.

Laboratory findings:
Creatinine	1.2 mg/dL
Sodium	136 mEq/L
Potassium	4.5 mEq/L
Calcium	9.5 mg/dL

Which one of the following is the most appropriate recommendation?

(A) Replace hydrochlorothiazide with amlodipine.
(B) Replace hydrochlorothiazide with diltiazem.
(C) Replace lisinopril with losartan.
(D) Replace lisinopril with metoprolol succinate.

ANSWER: A

Symptomatic orthostatic hypotension in older hypertensive patients (decrease of ≥20 mmHg systolic or ≥10 mmHg diastolic pressure) is a common risk factor for cardiovascular disease (including atrial fibrillation), syncope, falls, and fractures (SOE=B). Reducing the intensity of antihypertensive medication may reduce orthostatic hypotension. Diuretic drugs are known to cause orthostatic hypotension and should be avoided or used at low doses. Amlodipine is less likely to contribute to orthostatic hypotension and is probably safer in this patient.

Switching an angiotensin receptor blocker for an angiotensin-converting enzyme inhibitor has no effect on orthostatic hypotension. β-Blockers would not be first- or second-line treatment for hypertension in the absence of symptomatic coronary disease. Replacing hydrochlorothiazide with a high-dose calcium channel blocker would not prevent the orthostatic hypotension.

17. An 85-year-old woman comes to the office with her son, who requested an urgent appointment over concerns regarding her finances. The son says that several of her checks have been cashed without her knowledge, and several credit card transactions on her account seem suspicious (eg, purchases at convenience stores that she has never visited). The patient does not recall these transactions. The son, who has joint ownership on the accounts, notified her bank and credit card company of fraudulent activity. The patient lives with her son and attends an adult day health center. Other than her son, an assistant at the center is her only close personal contact; occasionally, the assistant takes her purse to run errands on her behalf. History includes mild to moderate Alzheimer disease and depression. Current medications are sertraline, donepezil, and calcium and vitamin D supplements.

    On examination, there are deficits in short-term recall and abnormal clock drawing; both findings are unchanged from prior visits.

    Which one of the following is the most appropriate next step?

    (A) Advise the patient not to lend her purse to the assistant.
    (B) Initiate the process for a court-appointed conservator of finances.
    (C) Contact the adult day health center to inquire about the assistant.
    (D) Report the case to adult protective services.

    ANSWER: D

    Financial exploitation is the illegal or improper use of a vulnerable person's funds, property, or assets. Most likely, this patient is a victim. *Age-associated financial vulnerability* refers to a change in financial behavior that places an older adult at risk of loss of resources and is inconsistent with their prior behavior. A financially vulnerable older adult is at risk of financial exploitation in the form of scams, theft, and fraudulent activity on the part of individuals who are in direct contact with the patient. The lifetime prevalence of financial exploitation is estimated at 4.7%; most perpetrators are family members, friends, or personal care aides (SOE=B). In addition to its impact on a person's estate, financial exploitation can affect the victim's mental health, risk of hospitalization, risk of institutionalization, and survival (SOE=B). It is therefore important to detect financial vulnerability early, to protect older adults when vulnerability is identified (eg, with a durable power of attorney for finances), and to act quickly when financial exploitation is suspected.

    This patient is financially vulnerable given her deficits in memory and executive function, which can affect her decision-making and ability to recall specific financial transactions. Depression also puts her at risk of financial vulnerability (SOE=B). Although her credit card information could have been stolen electronically, the fact that her checks are being cashed suggests that someone close to her is repeatedly financially exploiting her. Reporting the case to adult protective services is the best initial step, because financial exploitation is a form of elder abuse. In many states, the physician is mandated to report the exploitation. Adult protective services can investigate the source of exploitation, intervene to protect the adult from further exploitation, and assist with legal action to recover damages (SOE=D).

    Advising the patient not to lend her purse to the assistant may not be effective, given her dementia and memory deficits. Adult protective services will likely contact the adult day health center as part of its investigation. A conservator of finances is a court-appointed surrogate who manages the finances of an adult who cannot manage them. A conservator is not necessary at this time because the son, as a joint account owner, can cancel the current credit card and initiate a fraud investigation through the company and bank.

18. An 82-year-old woman with a bioprosthetic mitral valve has new fevers of uncertain etiology.

    After obtaining blood cultures, which one of the following is the next best step in the management for possible bacterial endocarditis in this patient?

    (A) Observe and monitor.
    (B) Request a transesophageal echocardiography.
    (C) Start empiric antibiotic therapy.
    (D) Confirm the presence of Janeway lesions or Osler nodes.

ANSWER: C

A high index of suspicion with aggressive diagnostic and therapeutic approaches is indicated to ensure timely diagnosis and appropriate therapy for possible bacterial endocarditis. Prompt intravenous administration of bactericidal antibiotics is indicated. After appropriate samples are obtained for culture, empiric antibiotic therapy should be initiated.

The most common pathogen in older adults is *Staphylococcus aureus*, which is often methicillin resistant. Coagulase-negative *Staphylococcus*, *Enterococcus*, and *Streptococcus bovis* are also common. *Streptococcus viridans* is found less often than in younger populations. Morbidity and mortality from endocarditis are higher in older adults, due in part to comorbidities and lower cardiopulmonary reserves.

Valvular prostheses, degenerative valve disease, mitral annular calcification, and mitral valve prolapse all tend to increase susceptibility of older adults to bacterial endocarditis. The high prevalence of diabetes, genitourinary and gastrointestinal cancer, chronic illness, hemodialysis, indwelling vascular catheters, pacemakers and implantable cardioverter defibrillators, and prosthetic implants adds to risks.

In older adults with endocarditis, there are fewer vegetations and emboli, and abscesses are more common. Transesophageal echocardiography is more sensitive than transthoracic echocardiography for detecting lesions. Nonetheless, the common presence of valvular calcifications and the shadowing associated with prosthetic valves both still confound transesophageal as well as transthoracic echocardiographic assessments.

Clinical signs of endocarditis are less reliable in older adults. Vascular- and immune-mediated phenomena, such as embolic events, splenomegaly, Osler nodes (tender subcutaneous violaceous nodules mostly on the pads of the fingers and toes), and Janeway lesions (nontender erythematous macules on the palms and soles) are less common than in younger adults.

19. A 79-year-old woman is brought to the emergency department with a history of anxiety of 2–3 weeks. Her family reports worsening confusion and disorientation as well as behavior problems, including agitation and suicidal ideation. Her symptoms were initially attributed to worsening of her dementia but then accelerated. History includes dementia and hypertension. Current medications are donepezil, memantine, lisinopril, and paroxetine, which was prescribed for anxiety 2 months ago.

On examination, the patient is combative and disoriented. Laboratory findings include low serum sodium level and low plasma osmolarity. Urine sodium level and osmolarity are increased.

Which one of the following medications is the most likely cause of her hyponatremia?

(A) Donepezil
(B) Paroxetine
(C) Memantine
(D) Lisinopril

ANSWER: B

This patient has delirium likely due to medication-induced hyponatremia, most likely from paroxetine, a selective serotonin reuptake inhibitor (SSRI). Older adults are at risk for SSRI-induced hyponatremia and syndrome of inappropriate antidiuretic hormone secretion (SIADH). The increase in antidiuretic hormone causes reabsorption of free water by the kidney, with compensatory reduction in the activity of the renin-aldosterone pathway and an increase in urine sodium. The incidence of SIADH does not appear to be dose dependent and can occur as early as 2 weeks after starting the SSRI. Risk factors include baseline low sodium levels and low BMI.

The first step in management would be to hold the SSRI and restrict free water intake. Although antipsychotic agents are sometimes used to manage behavior disturbance in delirium, addressing an identifiable and correctable cause should come first. The use of sedative hypnotics should be avoided in delirium.

Donepezil, memantine, and lisinopril are not associated with hyponatremia.

20. An 84-year-old woman with dementia comes to the office for a transitional care visit. She is unaccompanied. She was recently discharged from the hospital after admission for fluid overload. Over the past 6 months, she has been admitted 4 times: twice for fluid overload (she often forgets to take her medications), once for a fall, and once for dehydration. She has lost approximately 4.5 kg (10 lb) over the last 6 months. She typically eats one big meal each day. A family friend brings meals 3 times each week and she heats up TV dinners for her other meals. Her daughter oversees her finances and has encouraged her to look at nursing facilities, but she is adamant about remaining in her own home. She uses a front-wheeled walker for ambulation, and she no longer drives.

On physical examination, she appears thin and disheveled but in no acute distress. Blood pressure is 132/87 mmHg sitting and 105/72 mmHg standing. Heart rate is 72 beats per minute, and respiratory rate is 18 breaths per minute. There is 1+ edema bilaterally. Score on the Montreal Cognitive Assessment is 22/30. All other findings are normal.

Which one of the following is the most appropriate referral to make at this time?

(A) Program of All-Inclusive Care for the Elderly (PACE)
(B) Assisted-living facility
(C) Nursing facility for rehabilitation
(D) Home health services for nursing care

ANSWER: A

PACE is the best option for the ongoing care of this patient, who wishes to remain in her home despite her need for nursing home level of care (SOE=C). Within its catchment area, PACE provides integrated care for patients ≥55 years old who are eligible for nursing home placement. A multidisciplinary team delivers services in the enrollee's home, in the program's adult day centers, or in the inpatient setting. PACE is financed through capitated payments from Medicare and Medicaid; the program assumes full financial responsibility for all medical costs of the enrollee. Persons not Medicaid eligible may enroll and pay the equivalent of Medicaid share out of pocket.

Given her frequent hospital admissions, suspected dementia, weight loss, and falls, this patient needs more care than can be provided by home health care services. While these services would certainly be beneficial, this patient's safety would remain at risk when workers were not in the home with her. Nursing home admission is a viable option for this patient, yet she insists on her independence and is unlikely to be amenable to moving. A nursing facility is a short-term option after hospitalization but will not provide for her long-term need for daily supervision. By referring her to PACE, she would receive the increased supervision that would allow her to remain at home at night. A referral for an assisted-living facility might be an option, but she declines relocation, and she likely requires more assistance than could be provided in assisted living.

A referral to PACE should be considered, when available, in medically complicated patients who qualify for nursing-home level of care but maintain a desire to remain in the community. PACE enrollment improves quality of care and is associated with decreased mortality, preservation of function, improved caregiver and enrollee satisfaction, fewer hospital and nursing home days, and lower costs to Medicare and Medicaid (SOE=A). PACE is a high-quality community-based alternative to institutional settings.

21. An 84-year-old woman comes to the clinic for routine follow-up. She describes a gradual decrease in exercise tolerance over the last year, especially when she guides tours in the museum where she volunteers. The year before, her volunteer activities were interrupted by back-to-back hospitalizations to treat dyspnea. History includes chronic obstructive pulmonary disease, hypertension, hypercholesterolemia, and stroke. Current medications are albuterol, fluticasone/salmeterol, tiotropium, clopidogrel, aspirin, labetalol, lisinopril, and rosuvastatin.

On examination, blood pressure is 122/58 mmHg, heart rate is 50 beats per minute, and respiratory rate is 16 breaths per minute. Lungs are clear, and there is no lower-extremity edema or increased jugular venous pressures. Echocardiography shows concentric left ventricular hypertrophy, normal left ventricular function, and diastolic dysfunction. Pulmonary function tests show a moderate obstructive defect without significant improvement after administration of aerosolized bronchodilators.

Which one of the following interventions is most likely to improve this patient's functional exercise capacity?

(A) Nocturnal oxygen therapy
(B) Diuretic therapy
(C) Aerobic exercise training
(D) Placement of implantable cardioverter-defibrillator (ICD)

ANSWER: C

Aerobic exercise will improve this patient's symptoms and her quality of life. Aerobic exercise in healthy older adults increases peak VO_2, which represents cardiac output and arteriovenous oxygen difference. An increase in peak VO_2 would cause marked improvement in ventilator and lactate thresholds, augmentation of blunted endothelium-mediated flow-dependent vasodilation, and improvement in autonomic and neurohumoral changes in heart failure. These changes are reflected in improved quality of life, likely because of improved exercise tolerance, improved 6-minute walk tests, and reduced rates of hospital admissions (SOE=B).

Diuretic therapy is a key component in treatment of heart failure. Treatment of volume overload improves symptoms of dyspnea and exercise tolerance. However, no randomized controlled trials have assessed the effects of loop diuretics on symptoms, and care must be used because of the effects of loop diuretics on renal function and hypercalciuria (SOE=D). This patient has no evidence of volume overload.

Although small randomized trials of short duration have demonstrated that nocturnal oxygen improves sleep quality in patients with heart failure, there is no consistent evidence that oxygen therapy improves cardiac function, quality of life, or clinical outcome of these patients (SOE=C). In addition, supplemental oxygen has been suggested to cause hyperoxia, which can adversely affect myocardial function because of the generation of oxygen-free radicals.

ICDs reduce mortality in treatment of ventricular arrhythmias and sudden cardiac death (SOE=B). However, there is no known impact on functional exercise capacity. In addition, ICD firing is associated with significant anxiety and depression. The Heart Rhythm Society does not recommend use of ICDs for prevention of sudden cardiac death in persons with New York Heart Association Class IV (SOE=B) unless the person is also a candidate for a left ventricular assist device as destination therapy, cardiac transplantation, or cardiac resynchronization.

22. A 58-year-old woman comes to the office because she has difficulty caring for her parents, both of whom receive care at the same practice. Her parents' income is low, and they are dual-eligible for Medicare and Medicaid. She has moved into her parents' home to take care of her father, who has Alzheimer disease, while her mother is in the hospital recovering from hip surgery. She is in danger of losing her full-time job as a school cafeteria worker, because she missed work once and was late twice this week because of her father's agitation. In addition, her work schedule prevents her from meeting with the hospitalist to discuss her mother's care. She believes she has no choice but to quit her job so that she can take care of her parents.

Which one of the following is the most appropriate recommendation for the daughter?

(A) Request funds from the local Alzheimer's Association.
(B) Participate in a Medicaid self-direction program.
(C) Regularly attend an Alzheimer's Association support group.
(D) Request visiting nurse services provided by the Department of Health.

ANSWER: B

Informal care is mainly provided by working-age adults, who bear most of the economic burden in "opportunity costs"—the economic value of activities forgone because of providing care. National estimates indicate that it costs less to pay informal (family) caregivers than formal caregivers. Half of all older Medicaid beneficiaries who use long-term care receive services at home or in the community, rather than in institutional settings (SOE=A). This family may be eligible for a Medicaid self-direction program, under which the Medicaid beneficiary (rather than an agency) hires, trains, supervises, and manages the workers who provide personal care and related services for the beneficiary (SOE=B). In most cases, a family member, friend, or other person known to the beneficiary is paid to provide direct personal care to the beneficiary. States are required to arrange for a system of supports to help the Medicaid beneficiary develop a service and budget plan, manage the services and service providers, and perform the responsibilities of an employer. The Medicaid beneficiary is supported by a broker (counselor or consultant) who acts as the beneficiary's agent in identifying the services and service providers (usually an informal caregiver, such as a family member). The Medicaid beneficiary is also supported by financial management services and access to an independent advocacy system available in the state. The amount and frequency of support vary by beneficiary and by circumstance.

The Alzheimer's Association does not usually have funds to help caregivers directly. It provides information regarding potential sources of support, including where to look for financial support, and caregivers of those with Alzheimer disease should be encouraged to use the Alzheimer's Association website (www.alz.org). Caregivers also benefit from participating in Alzheimer's Association support groups by receiving emotional support and encouragement (not financial), and they should be encouraged to participate.

Intermittent nurse visits or limited daily aides, although helpful, cannot address all the caregiving needs. In the long term, the father will need increasing support, and the daughter will have to plan with the mother and other family members how best to address this.

23. An 85-year-old man comes to the office with his daughter, who is concerned about his driving. He lives alone in a rural community and drives to the grocery store, office visits, and occasionally to her home. Two days ago, he was in a minor car accident after he turned into a one-way street in the wrong direction. History includes hypertension, for which he takes amlodipine 5 mg/d, and gastroesophageal reflux disease, for which he takes omeprazole 40 mg/d.

Which one of the following is the most appropriate next step?

(A) Recommend that his daughter take away his keys.
(B) Refer him for driving assessment.
(C) Perform a cognitive evaluation.
(D) File a report with the Department of Motor Vehicles.

ANSWER: C

Older drivers have higher rates of motor vehicle collisions per mile driven than younger drivers (SOE=A). Specific risk factors include impairments in hearing, vision, cognition, and function (SOE=A). Sedating or anticholinergic medications can also impair driving. Initial screening tests may be done in the office setting. These should include functional and cognitive assessment and hearing and vision evaluations. The first priority, before reporting this patient or asking his daughter to take away his keys, is to identify any medical problems that might affect his driving. A family member's report of an accident or moving violation should also trigger a medical evaluation for impairments that may interfere with safe driving.

Patients who demonstrate deficits in function, cognition, hearing, or vision, or demonstrate a pattern of unsafe driving, can be referred for a formal driving evaluation. A comprehensive driving evaluation by a trained professional, usually an occupational therapist, is an objective process. Formal driving evaluations generally take 2–3 hours. They usually consist of a clinical evaluation (including a variety of cognitive, visual, and physical assessments) and an on-the-road test with oral feedback or a written report on the results. Some of these assessments may have associated fees. Occupational therapists may identify deficits amenable to vehicle modification or rehabilitation so that the older adult can continue to drive safely.

Requirements for reporting accidents or unsafe driving vary by state.

24. An 80-year-old woman comes to the urgent care center because she slipped on wet steps yesterday evening while she was watering her plants. She scraped the back of her leg but did not hit her head. She has fallen 3 other times in the last year. Her last fall was 3 months ago. On that occasion, she went to the emergency department because she struck her head on the bathroom vanity. Noncontrast computed tomography of the head showed nonspecific microvascular ischemic changes and no acute bleeding. History includes hypertension, well-controlled diabetes mellitus, and atrial fibrillation. Current medications are lisinopril, carvedilol, metformin, and warfarin.

On physical examination, blood pressure is 132/86 mmHg, with no postural changes, and heart rate is 80 beats per minute and irregularly irregular. Neurologic findings are normal. International normalized ratio (INR) is 3.0. The posterior surface of her right leg has a superficial abrasion with surrounding ecchymoses; there are no other injuries. She walks slowly, with a shortened stride length on a slightly wide base, and turns en bloc.

Which one of the following is the best next step?

(A) Discontinue warfarin.
(B) Refer to a community exercise program.
(C) Begin cholecalciferol 50,000 IU weekly.
(D) Provide educational materials about fall risk.

ANSWER: B

Meta-analyses of randomized trials show that exercise reduces both the risk of falls and injuries related to falls in community-dwelling older adults (SOE=A). The U.S. Preventive Services Task Force (USPSTF) recommends exercise or physical therapy to prevent falls in community-dwelling adults ≥65 years old who are at increased risk of falls (grade B recommendation). Multifactorial and exercise interventions were associated with fall-related benefit. Vitamin D supplementation interventions have had mixed results.

Predisposition to falls with potential head trauma is rarely a contraindication to use of anticoagulants in older adults with atrial fibrillation. The risk of fall-related intracranial hemorrhage is often surpassed by the benefit of stroke prevention (SOE=B). A Markov decision analysis model showed that persons with an average risk of stroke from atrial fibrillation (6% per year in the absence of anticoagulation) would need to fall approximately 295 times in 1 year for the risks of intracranial hemorrhage associated with anticoagulation to outweigh its benefits of reduction in stroke risk. This patient has a $CHADS_2$* score of 3, placing her at high risk of stroke.

Vitamin D supplementation may improve bone mineral density and muscle function, and several meta-analyses have shown benefit of vitamin D in reducing fall risk in community-dwelling older adults (SOE=B.) However, not all meta-analyses and clinical trials have shown benefit, perhaps because of different inclusion criteria, different baseline vitamin D levels, and differences in dosing schedules. The USPSTF currently recommends 600–800 IU of vitamin D daily to prevent falls in community-dwelling older adults at increased risk of falls (grade B recommendation). Higher doses of vitamin D administered at less-frequent intervals have not been shown to reduce fall risk and may increase the risk of falls and fractures. For patients with moderate to severe vitamin D deficiency (25[OH]D <20 ng/mL) or malabsorption, higher doses may be appropriate. This patient does not have known deficiency or malabsorption, and thus there is no indication for high-dose vitamin D. Furthermore, vitamin D doses >4,000 IU/d (or its equivalent) can be associated with acute toxicity.

Educational materials on prevention of falls as a stand-alone intervention have not reduced the rate of falls or risk of falling (SOE=B).

*$CHADS_2$: congestive heart failure, hypertension, age ≥75 years, diabetes mellitus, stroke (double weight)

25. A 75-year-old woman who lives alone requires a home visit for medical care. It is winter, and her home is cold. She states that her furnace does not work but that her son brought over a new kerosene heater last night. The heater has not been filled or started. She cannot afford repairs to her furnace, and she declines help from the Area Agency on Aging for home repair. The telephone numbers she provides for her family contacts are disconnected. She refuses to leave her home. History includes moderate dementia, hypertension, arthritis, and chronic obstructive lung disease. Current medications are acetaminophen 500 mg twice daily, hydrochlorothiazide 25 mg/d, and tiotropium inhaler 5 mcg/d. She smokes 1 pack of cigarettes daily and refuses to stop; she does not drink alcohol.

On physical examination, temperature is 37°C (98.6°F), blood pressure is 135/78 mmHg, heart rate is 68 beats per minute, respiratory rate is 12 breaths per minute, and oxygen saturation is 95% on room air. Her extremities are cool. Breath sounds are distant. There is mild bilateral pedal edema. Score on Mini–Mental State Examination is 22 of 30, which is unchanged from her score 3 months ago.

Which one of the following organizations can assist in ensuring the safety of this patient?

(A) Adult protective services
(B) Visiting nurse agency
(C) Police department
(D) Fire department

ANSWER: A

This patient is at risk to herself and others because of her smoking and kerosene heater. She has no safe strategy for heating, and no one to assist her. It is not clear whether her lack of insight is a change from her baseline personality or is a sign of a newly developed cognitive impairment or psychiatric disorder. She is not willing to relocate for safety.

When the actions of an adult affect his or her safety and infringe on the safety of others, adult protective service agencies are empowered to investigate the safety issues and assess the adult's decision-making capacity and can act to ensure safety without the adult's consent. All information generated in these evaluations remains confidential. Mandatory reporting rules by health care professionals vary by state, so providers should know their state regulations.

Visiting nurses are often among the first to recognize safety issues but cannot act without consent. Police and fire responders are frequently called by neighbors or friends who are concerned about safety. In the absence of criminal aspects of danger, they are not authorized to proceed without consent.

26. An 82-year-old man comes to the office because he feels poorly. Over the past 2 months he has become short of breath, has gradually gained weight, and has had swelling in his legs. He can no longer shower on his own or walk >1 block because of his dyspnea. History includes hyperlipidemia, hypertension, mild cognitive impairment, and type 2 diabetes mellitus. He has never smoked. His wife confirms his adherence to a low-sodium diet and to medications. His last hospitalization was 2 years ago, and he worries that he will need to go to the hospital soon.

On physical examination, blood pressure is 114/60 mmHg, heart rate is 70 beats per minute and irregularly irregular, and oxygen saturation is 94% on room air. BMI is 26.9 kg/m². Jugular veins are distended and there are bibasilar crackles. There is 1+ pitting edema at the mid-shins bilaterally. Laboratory results include creatinine of 2.2 mg/dL and hemoglobin A_{1c} of 8.2%.

Which one of the following prognostic tools is most appropriate for estimating his all-cause mortality?

(A) Advanced Dementia Prognostic Tool
(B) BODE Index (BMI, airflow obstruction, dyspnea, exercise)
(C) ePrognosis calculator
(D) Palliative prognostic score

ANSWER: C

This patient has new-onset atrial fibrillation with symptoms of acute heart failure. The ePrognosis calculators (http://eprognosis.ucsf.edu/calculators/#) identify the appropriate prognostic index for clinicians to use to estimate mortality for older adults who do not have a dominant terminal illness. ePrognosis incorporates patient setting (home, nursing home, hospital, or hospice), patient's country of residence, and time frame for the clinical issue (1 year or 4–10 years) with patient age, comorbid conditions, functional status, and presence of any illness that limits life expectancy. Prognostication allows the clinician to work with the patient and family to identify realistic, achievable goals of care, based on the likelihood that an intervention will achieve a desired outcome, or that the patient will live long enough to benefit from the intervention (lag time to benefit). Prognostication also facilitates discussion about alternatives, such as hospice. Older adults are often interested in outcomes other than life expectancy, such as level of independence or need for nursing home placement.

The other options listed are disease-specific prognostic tools. Single, disease-specific prognostic indices may not apply to older adults, because they often have multiple chronic progressive diseases and functional impairment. The Advanced Dementia Prognostic Tool is appropriate only for nursing home residents with advanced dementia. The BODE Index is designed for ambulatory patients with chronic obstructive pulmonary disease. The Palliative Prognostic Score is intended for patients with advanced solid tumors who are participating in home hospice.

27. A 72-year-old man comes to the office accompanied by his son. He lives independently and says that he has no issues to discuss. The son, however, is concerned that he has uncharacteristically been giving a lot of money to solicitors. He is also concerned because his father has been expressing anger about the children in the neighborhood. This too is uncharacteristic of him. The patient explains that the children's loudness sometimes upsets him. He does not feel depressed, and says that he is sleeping well. He admits that his memory is "not as good as it used to be," with trouble remembering names and dates of appointments, but he ascribes this to normal aging. On further questioning, he mentions that he fell a few weeks ago, when he tripped as he stepped onto a curb. He was not injured.

Which one of the following would be the most appropriate referral to make at this time?

(A) Comprehensive geriatric assessment
(B) Program of All-Inclusive Care for the Elderly (PACE)
(C) Assisted-living facility
(D) Home health for physical therapy

ANSWER: A

Given the concerns regarding this patient's cognition, changes in personality, and recent fall, he would be best served by a comprehensive geriatric assessment—the multidisciplinary process that allows for identification of medical, functional, cognitive, and psychosocial problems of an older adult (SOE=C). The goal of the assessment is to formulate a coordinated plan to maximize the patient's overall health and independence while minimizing disability. Indications for referral for comprehensive geriatric assessment include advanced age, medical comorbidities, psychosocial disorders, specific geriatric conditions (eg, falls, cognitive decline, functional disability), predicted high utilization of health care, or potential change in living conditions (ie, change in the level of care needed). At its core, the assessment team comprises a physician, nurse, and social worker. An extended team of physical and occupational therapists, pharmacists, psychologists, psychiatrists, nutritionists, dentists, opticians, podiatrists, and audiologists is accessed when appropriate. Some of the major components of the assessment include functional capacity, cognition, polypharmacy, gait and balance (fall risk), social support, and goals of care. Comprehensive geriatric assessment differs from standard medical evaluation in that it includes nonmedical domains and involves a multidisciplinary team that focuses on quality of life. The assessment programs that address adherence to recommendations have been associated with improved outcomes.

The Program of All-Inclusive Care for the Elderly (PACE) is a valuable service for patients and their families who qualify for nursing home care yet prefer to remain in their communities. This patient, however, lacks a diagnosis for his cognitive disorder. Comprehensive geriatric assessment covers diagnostic testing and then follows up with planning for the patient's medical conditions and social situation.

Home health services might be helpful for this patient in the future, but now a more comprehensive evaluation is necessary to understand his medical comorbidities and his needs for safety at home. It is unlikely that he needs around-the-clock nursing care at this time. Careful assessment of his medical conditions and social situation is warranted before considering placement in an assisted-living facility. A more thorough cognitive evaluation will also assist in this regard.

28. An 83-year-old woman comes to the office accompanied by her husband. He states that his wife has not spoken for 1 month, since their daughter announced that her son was gay. The patient communicates via notes and gestures and can attract attention through sound signals, such as coughing. When directly addressed today, she uses a notepad or turns to her husband so that he can answer for her. Oral and written comprehension is maintained. The patient seems unconcerned about the burden her mutism places on others and is clear that she wishes to be taken seriously.

Her husband says that she continues daily activities, such as reading and cooking, and that her appetite and sleep patterns have not changed. When she is asked directly whether she feels sad, she looks surprised and shakes her head, indicating "no." Her husband says that she had a similar response at the time of her father's death; that episode lasted 2 weeks and resolved completely. Last week her husband took her to the emergency department, where computed tomography of the head, electroencephalography, and otolaryngology evaluation disclosed no abnormality.

On physical examination, all findings are normal.

Which one of the following is the most likely diagnosis?

(A) Somatic symptom disorder
(B) Delirium
(C) Conversion disorder
(D) Depressive disorder

ANSWER: C

The most likely diagnosis is conversion disorder. According to the *Diagnostic and Statistical Manual of Mental Disorders, Fifth Edition* (DSM-5), this disorder is related to somatic symptom and related disorders, a group of 5 heterogeneous diagnoses that have in common the presence of distressing physical symptoms and abnormal thoughts, behaviors, and feelings associated with the physical symptoms.

This patient has impaired phonation, without physical impairment. Diagnosis of conversion disorder is based on the following: the symptoms concern altered voluntary motor control, there is incompatibility between the symptom and recognized medical conditions, the deficit causes clinically significant impairment in social areas, and the deficit is not better explained by another medical or mental disorder. Other factors supporting the diagnosis are the history of similar symptoms and the likelihood that onset is associated with stress. In this case, the potential stressor relates to the announcement that her grandson is gay.

Breaking with earlier editions, the DSM-5 does not require that the symptoms be feigned or confabulated. Neither *la belle indifférence* nor motivation for secondary gain is considered critical to the diagnosis. Personality traits are not predisposing factors for development of medically unexplained symptoms in later life (SOE=C).

Psychogenic aphonia is considered a functional voice disorder. In the field of psychiatric symptomatology, mutism can be part of a melancholic syndrome, delirium, psychotic disorder, or, as in this case, a conversion syndrome (SOE=C). Major depressive episode is less likely, because core depressive symptoms are absent.

A diagnosis of somatic symptom disorder requires that the patient have a distressing or disruptive somatic symptom accompanied by concerns about the seriousness of the medical symptom or by a high level of anxiety about the symptom. The assessment of somatic symptom disorder in older adults is challenging because of the prevalence of somatic multimorbidity (SOE=C).

Delirium is not likely in this case, because there are no alterations or fluctuations in cognition, consciousness, or attention, which are the central diagnostic criteria.

29. A 66-year-old man comes to the office because he has a swelling in the buccal gingiva of tooth #20. Five months ago, a small mass developed in the buccal aspects of teeth #18 and #19 that was diagnosed as squamous cell carcinoma. That lesion was removed in conjunction with extraction of teeth #18 and #19 and excision of the alveolar bone in the area, along with 27 regional lymph nodes, all of which were clear, with no evidence of cancer. He did not undergo radiation therapy.

History includes infection with human immunodeficiency virus (HIV) for 22 years and type 2 diabetes mellitus for 10 years. He had osteomyelitis in his femur after radiation treatment for disseminated Kaposi sarcoma >20 years ago, and he has had recurrent anal intraepithelial neoplasia for the past 6 years, treated with localized excision and laser ablation. Current medications are insulin, metformin, atazanavir, ritonavir, and raltegravir.

On physical examination, there is a firm, nontender enlargement in the buccal aspect of tooth #20, wrapping around and extending into the edentulous space behind the tooth. The lesion has a mixed appearance of erythema and increased vascularity. Periodontal probing shows a deep pocket in the distal aspect of tooth #20; the probe causes bleeding.

Which one of the following is the most likely diagnosis?

(A) Diabetes-related periodontal abscess
(B) Recurrent squamous cell carcinoma
(C) Recurrent Kaposi sarcoma
(D) Osteonecrosis of the jaw

ANSWER: B

The case described here represents recurrent squamous cell carcinoma in an HIV-positive patient. Management includes biopsy of the lesion to establish the diagnosis, HPV typing, and referral for surgical excision and radiation therapy. Current trends in oral cancer epidemiology in the United States show a reduction in rates among older male smokers (the traditional at-risk group) and a dramatic increase in incidence rates among middle-aged white men who are often nonsmokers. This phenomenon is attributed to reduction in the rates of tobacco and alcohol use and an increase in infection with HPV (SOE=A). About 7% of the adult population in the United States is estimated to have oral HPV; 1.0% carry HPV type 16. Among HIV-seropositive patients, the HPV carriage rate is >12% (SOE=B). In the case of this patient, biopsy results are likely to indicate that the tumor is HPV positive. The higher rate of oral HPV infection may be responsible, in part, for the higher rate of oropharyngeal squamous cell carcinoma among HIV-positive patients, a rate estimated to be 3 times higher than that of the general population. Other factors include tobacco and alcohol use, other infections, immunosuppression, and long-term use of antiretroviral drugs.

HPV-positive squamous cell carcinoma is a genetically, clinically, and epidemiologically distinct subtype of head and neck cancer; it has a predilection for the posterior part of the oral cavity and the oropharynx, a more indolent clinical course, and a lower rate of metastasis. HPV-positive oropharyngeal cancers have a better clinical prognosis, both in terms of progression rates and response to treatment (SOE=B). At the molecular level, HPV infection of keratinocytes appears to activate tumor suppressor genes and induce P53 dysfunction and better apoptotic response of cancer cells to radiation and chemotherapy, thereby improving the overall cancer prognosis. For HPV-positive tumors, HIV infection may negatively affect locoregional control (recurrence or second primary tumors), a possibility that helps explain the recurrence of squamous cell carcinoma in this patient within a short period.

There is good evidence that diabetes and periodontal disease have a bidirectional relationship (SOE=B). Data from the U.S. National Health and Nutrition Examination Survey (NHANES) III show that adults with diabetes have a significantly higher prevalence of severe periodontitis than those without diabetes. Conversely, a recent large prospective study showed a greater increase in hemoglobin A_{1c} among participants with advanced periodontitis than among those without periodontitis, and several meta-analyses have confirmed that effective periodontal therapy can result in reduced hemoglobin A_{1c} among patients with diabetes. Periodontitis is a disease caused by anaerobic bacteria from the biofilm within the periodontal pocket, where infection leads to a complex cascade of tissue-destructive pathways triggered by bacterial products and fueled by inflammatory mediators. A number of inflammatory mediators associated with periodontitis are involved in impaired intracellular insulin signaling and insulin resistance, suggesting common molecular mechanisms between the two. The clinical presentation of periodontitis is that of inflammation in the gingiva and destruction of the supporting connective tissue and bone. When there is acute infection in the periodontal pocket (periodontal abscess), purulence is present on periodontal probing. In this case, the nontender and firm enlargement of tissues beyond the periodontal structures is not consistent with a periodontal abscess.

Osteonecrosis of the jaw presents as exposed and necrotic bone, a feature not seen in this patient. It is a disease associated with cancer and its therapy. Dental extractions, therapy with high-dose bisphosphonates or denosumab (SOE=A), and radiation are all risk factors for osteonecrosis of the jaw.

The patient in this scenario was treated for Kaposi sarcoma 20 years ago. Combination antiretroviral therapy, as this patient is receiving, has resulted in a dramatic decline in new and recurrent disease. Therefore, it is unlikely that recurrent Kaposi sarcoma accounts for the patient's new oral lesion.

30. An 80-year-old man comes to the office because he has a brown patch on his face that started changing about 1 month ago. History includes several basal cell carcinomas, as well as squamous cell carcinomas removed by surgery. He grew up in Arizona, where he had extensive sun exposure. He continues to spend time in the sun and uses sun protection intermittently.

On examination, there is a 2-cm brown patch on the right cheek. Most of the lesion is a homogenous brown; there is a focus of darker brown with red coloration. There is no texture to the lesion and no tenderness. Surgical scars appear well healed, with no evidence of recurrence. The remainder of the skin examination is unremarkable.

Which one of the following is the most likely diagnosis?

(A) Severely atypical nevus
(B) Nodular melanoma
(C) Metastatic melanoma
(D) Lentigo maligna

ANSWER: D

Lentigo maligna is a type of melanoma that typically presents in sun-exposed areas in older patients (SOE=A). It is most common on the head and neck. Lesions can develop from a prior lentiginous lesion or de novo. They are usually asymptomatic, pigmented macules or patches with variable pigment, or localized variation in an otherwise homogenous color distribution. The color variation described in the patient's new lesion makes this diagnosis very likely. On pathology, the lesions are an in-situ form of melanoma. Lesions can grow vertically but are thought to initially grow slowly in a linear, radial fashion.

Atypical nevus refers to a nevus with irregular borders and coloration. These are stable lesions, unlike the rapidly changing lesion described in this patient. Atypical nevi are seen across age groups. Nodular melanoma is seen predominantly in persons 40–60 years old, yet it remains an important consideration in older adults. The macular, flat lesion described in this case is not typical of nodular melanoma. Metastatic melanoma commonly presents on the skin, near a primary lesion, but it can appear on the skin at distant sites. Most commonly, metastatic lesions appear in other organs, such as the lung, brain, or liver.

31. A 65-year-old woman comes to the office for her Welcome to Medicare preventive visit. History includes diabetes mellitus (diagnosed 3 years ago), hypertension, and osteoarthritis of the knee and hip. Current medications are acetaminophen 1,000 mg three times daily, tramadol 50 mg three times daily as needed, metformin 1,000 mg twice daily, and lisinopril 40 mg/d. She uses a 4-wheeled walker to assist with ambulation.

On examination, BMI is 30 kg/m². Cardiovascular and pulmonary findings are unremarkable. There is bilateral knee crepitus with extension, with no focal pain. With the walker, gait is stable but slightly wide based with decreased knee flexion. Hemoglobin A_{1c} level is 8.5%.

Which one of the following is the most appropriate recommendation?

(A) Weight loss to achieve normal BMI
(B) Diabetes self-management education program
(C) Prescription for glipizide
(D) Exercise prescription for walking 150 min/week at moderate intensity

ANSWER: B

All adults with diabetes should receive education that will allow for ongoing diabetes self-care (SOE=B). Diabetes self-management education should be provided at the time of diagnosis, annually, during transitions in care, and when new health conditions develop (SOE=C). Studies have found that education on self-management is associated with improved diabetes knowledge and self-care behaviors, lower hemoglobin A_{1c} levels, lower self-reported weight, improved quality of life, healthy coping, and reduced health care costs (SOE=B). Medicare Part B provides reimbursement for education or support when it is provided by a program that meets national standards and is recognized by the American Diabetes Association or other approval bodies.

This patient is taking the maximum dosage of metformin. Her diabetes is not under control. While she likely will need an additional agent, self-management along with lifestyle changes should be the next step. Sulfonylurea medications such as glipizide should be used with caution in older patients because of the risk of hypoglycemia.

In addition to individualized nutrition counseling, an individualized program for physical activity is a key component of support. Weight loss, even modest amounts, will improve glucose control. Physical activity training is particularly important in improving and maintaining physical functioning among older adults with diabetes (SOE=A). The patient in this case uses a 4-wheeled walker and has symptomatic knee and hip osteoarthritis that limits her ability to walk. The generic recommendation to walk 150 min/week is inappropriate, because the patient would likely not perform the activity. As recommended by the American College of Sports Medicine, an effective exercise prescription should tailor the intensity, frequency, duration, and type of activity for each individual.

32. An 82-year-old woman is brought to the emergency department by her family because she has increased agitation. She has been hitting her adult daughter and trying to run away from home because she believes that her daughter has been poisoning her. The daughter first noticed her mother's memory decline 5 years ago. The patient has lived with her daughter for the past 3 years and is now unable to manage finances, drive, or cook alone. History includes Alzheimer disease, for which she began taking donepezil 1 year ago.

Which one of the following is the most appropriate pharmacotherapy?

(A) Risperidone[OL]
(B) Bupropion[OL]
(C) Clozapine[OL]
(D) Divalproex sodium[OL]

ANSWER: A

Behavioral and psychologic signs in dementia are considered noncognitive disturbances and are often difficult to manage, increasing caregiver burden and leading to earlier nursing home placement. The disturbances are present in about 60%–98% of patients with dementia and can occur at all disease stages. Symptoms include depression, psychosis, apathy, agitation, aggression, anxiety, delusions, hallucinations, sleep disturbances, repetitive vocalizations, resistance to care, and wandering. No medications have been approved by the U.S. Food and Drug Administration (FDA) for the treatment of agitation or psychosis in dementia. Off-label use of medications is common but requires clear justification in individual patients.

Several second-generation antipsychotic medications have a modest effect of lessening neuropsychiatric symptoms in dementia. However, there are risks, as emphasized by the FDA black-box warning regarding increased mortality and cardiovascular events in patients with dementia. Other potential adverse effects include stroke, extrapyramidal symptoms, and QT_c prolongation. Risperidone[OL] is the most appropriate choice for this patient. She has a delusion (false fixed belief) that her daughter is poisoning her and is acting on that belief by threatening her daughter, which compromises her ability to remain in the community. Antipsychotic medications can be effective in individuals with dangerous agitation or psychosis; the potential risks should be weighed against the benefits and discussed with the family. Risperidone^{OL} may be more effective than placebo for symptoms such as aggression and paranoid ideation in patients with dementia (SOE=B).

Bupropion^{OL} is an antidepressant and has no evidence of efficacy in Alzheimer disease with psychosis. Clozapine^{OL} may be effective in treating psychosis in dementia, but it is not a good first choice because it requires weekly blood counts to monitor for agranulocytosis. Divalproex sodium^{OL} is a mood stabilizer that may be effective for mania-like behavioral symptoms in patients with dementia (SOE=C) but also is less effective for psychosis.

33. A 72-year-old woman comes to the office because she has symptoms of depression. History includes presently untreated bipolar disorder, hypothyroidism, and hypertension. Current medications are levothyroxine and chlorthalidone.

Which one of the following medications is considered first-line treatment for bipolar depression?

(A) Bupropion
(B) Lamotrigine
(C) Valproate
(D) Risperidone

ANSWER: B

Mood stabilizers are preferable to antidepressants for acute and maintenance treatment of bipolar depression. On the basis of drug interactions and adverse effect profile, lamotrigine is preferable to valproate, carbamazepine, and lithium for treatment in older adults. In patients with bipolar disorder type I and type II who present with depressive symptoms and a relatively rare history of manic episodes, bupropion is a reasonable adjuvant to lamotrigine. If the presentation is characterized by mixed symptoms or frequent episodes of mania, it is preferable to use a second mood stabilizer or a second-generation antipsychotic, such as risperidone, as an adjuvant.

34. A 74-year-old man comes to the office because he has erectile dysfunction. His wife died 1 year ago; they had been married 50 years. He is in a new relationship, and his partner has expressed a strong desire for sexual activity. For the past 10 years he has had progressive difficulty with achieving an erection; the difficulty has worsened in the last 6 months. History includes myocardial infarction, angina, and type 2 diabetes mellitus, with occasional episodes of hypoglycemia. The myocardial infarction occurred 2 months ago, and he has recovered well. Current medications are insulin, rosuvastatin 10 mg/d, atenolol 50 mg twice daily, aspirin 81 mg/d, and nitroglycerin as needed.

On physical examination, there is a soft systolic murmur and trace edema of the lower extremities. The remainder of the examination is normal.

Laboratory findings include hemoglobin A$_{1c}$ of 7.2% and total testosterone level of 350 ng/dL.

Which one of the following factors is the most likely primary cause of his erectile dysfunction?

(A) Neurologic
(B) Psychogenic
(C) Vascular
(D) Endocrine

ANSWER: C

For this patient, as in most cases, a vascular disorder is the most likely cause of erectile dysfunction. Atherosclerosis affects the penile arteries, often well before cardiovascular disease manifests (SOE=A). Erectile dysfunction of vascular etiology can predict the occurrence of myocardial infarction and stroke. If the patient achieves an erection, venous rapid release of blood or incompetent valves may lead to an inability to maintain the erection.

The lack of any deficits on examination makes a neurologic cause unlikely. Performance anxiety with a new partner is an important cause to consider, but given that the difficulty dates back a number of years, occurring with his wife, a psychogenic source is not likely to be the primary problem for this patient. His testosterone level is within the normal range; thus, the erectile dysfunction is unlikely to have an endocrine etiology.

35. A 79-year-old woman comes to the office 6 days after discharge from hospitalization for heart failure. It was her third hospital admission for heart failure within the past year. History also includes type 2 diabetes mellitus, obesity, hypertension, and hyperlipidemia. Current medications are aspirin 81 mg/d, furosemide 40 mg/d, metformin 500 mg/d, lisinopril 10 mg/d, and atorvastatin 40 mg/d. She has dyspnea on exertion.

On physical examination, she has gained 1.6 kg (3.5 lb) since discharge. Blood pressure is 142/86 mmHg and heart rate is 72 beats per minute. Bilateral crackles are heard at both lung bases, and there is lower-extremity edema.

At the time of discharge, which one of the following would most significantly help prevent readmission?

(A) Home visit nursing to provide self-care education and clinical evaluations
(B) Telemonitoring of vital signs and weight reported to providers
(C) Medication reconciliation, patient education, and medication optimization by pharmacist
(D) Heart failure education provided by a nurse before discharge

ANSWER: A

Heart failure is the most common discharge diagnosis in patients >65 years old, and 1 in 4 patients admitted with heart failure will have an unplanned readmission within 30 days of discharge. Vigilant follow-up after hospital discharge can improve outcomes for this high-risk population.

Home nursing most reliably reduces hospital readmission rates for patients with heart failure (SOE=A). Home nursing provides intermittent care focused on monitoring symptoms and signs (such as changes in blood pressure and weight), providing education (including information about medications), and providing other services, such as wound care and management of intravenous medication. Other services include physical, occupational, and speech and language therapy. A 2017 analysis of Medicare claims data suggests that intensive home health nursing and early provider follow-up were more effective in reducing readmission rates than less intensive home care and later post-acute follow-up. A 2017 systematic review and network meta-analysis compared the effectiveness of transitional care services for patients with heart failure in both readmission rates and mortality. Nurse home visits were most effective, followed by nurse case management and disease management clinics. For mortality reduction, nurse home visits were most effective, followed by disease management clinics. In this analysis, telephone, telemonitoring, pharmacist services, and education interventions did not influence clinical outcomes.

36. Which one of the following is associated with the highest risk of suicide in older adults?

(A) Depression
(B) Terminal illness
(C) Prior suicide attempt
(D) Chronic pain

ANSWER: A

Depression confers the highest risk of suicide in older adults. Older adults are less likely to report suicidal thoughts and more likely to die from suicide attempts than younger adults. The ratio of attempted suicide to completed suicide is 200:1 among younger persons and 4:1 among older adults. Depression is the factor associated with the highest population-attributable risk for suicide in later life according to psychological autopsy studies.

Terminal illness, prior suicide attempt, and chronic pain also carry an increased risk of suicide but to a lesser degree than depression. Other psychiatric illnesses, such as nonaffective psychoses, anxiety disorders, and substance use disorders, have also been linked to suicide in older adults. Additional factors that place older adults at increased risk of suicide include personality traits such as neuroticism, some physical illnesses (cardiovascular disease, malignancy, chronic pain), functional impairment, and life stressors. Most suicides in older adults involve white men, and the most common method is a firearm.

37. An 82-year-old woman comes to the office for her annual visit. She asks whether she could stop taking any of her medications, explaining that she "is tired of taking so many." History includes heart failure with reduced ejection fraction, ischemic heart disease, hyperlipidemia, hypertension, hypothyroidism, and osteoporosis. Current medications are amlodipine 5 mg/d, enalapril 5 mg twice daily, furosemide 10 mg/d, vitamin D 2,000 IU/d, levothyroxine 100 mcg/d, metoprolol extended release 50 mg/d, and rosuvastatin 10 mg/d.

On examination, heart rate is 72 beats per minute sitting and 74 beats per minute standing. Blood pressure is 112/70 mmHg sitting (right arm, regular cuff) and 109/65 mmHg standing. Over the past 6 months, systolic blood pressure taken when sitting has ranged from 105 mmHg to 113 mmHg; diastolic blood pressure has ranged from 68 mmHg to 72 mmHg. Estimated creatinine clearance is 50 mL/min.

Which one of the following medications can be safely discontinued at this time?

(A) Amlodipine
(B) Metoprolol
(C) Enalapril
(D) Furosemide

ANSWER: A

In accordance with guidelines from JNC-8,* the blood pressure goal for this patient is <150/90 mmHg. However, there is controversy regarding blood pressure goals in light of the ACCORD* and SPRINT* studies, which have been published since the JNC-8 guidelines were issued. These newer studies suggest that more intensive blood pressure goals might reduce mortality and cardiovascular disease (CVD) outcomes. In the SPRINT trial, participants >50 years old without diabetes or history of stroke were randomly assigned to the standard blood pressure target (systolic pressure <140 mmHg) or to an intensive target (systolic pressure <120 mmHg). Compared with the standard target group, the group randomly assigned to the intensive blood pressure target had a 25% lower relative incidence of CVD (absolute rates, 6.8% vs 5.2%) and a 43% lower relative CVD-related mortality rate (absolute rates, 1.4% vs 0.8%). The benefits of achieving intensive blood pressure targets were observed in persons >75 years old and in frail persons. As with most randomized clinical trials, the individuals in this study were healthier than the general population, and it is not clear how these results will be incorporated into the next JNC guideline update. In 2017, the American College of Physicians and the American Academy of Family Physicians published clinical guidelines for adults ≥60 years old, recommending initiation of treatment for persons with systolic blood pressure persistently ≥150 mmHg to achieve a target systolic pressure <150 mmHg. The expectation is that systolic pressure <150 mmHg would reduce the risk of mortality, stroke, and cardiac events (SOE=A). Individual assessment of benefit and harm is particularly important in older adults who have multiple chronic conditions and take many medications; they may be more susceptible to serious harm from falls, syncope, and hypotension, as has been observed in some trials.

In clinic today and during past visits, this patient's blood pressure is well below goal. Given her multiple comorbidities and medications and her stated desire to reduce her pill burden, she would benefit from discontinuation of one of her antihypertensive agents. Before discontinuing any drug, it is important to ascertain its role in the patient's other comorbidities. Amlodipine was likely added to this patient's regimen as an additional agent to help control blood pressure. Because there is no other clear indication for amlodipine, it would be reasonable to start by discontinuing amlodipine. The other antihypertensive agents that she takes—an angiotensin-converting enzyme inhibitor and a β-blocker—have mortality benefits in heart failure with reduced ejection fraction (SOE=A); thus, they should be continued at this time. Furosemide contributes to lowering blood pressure. In addition, it is used for symptomatic treatment for heart failure, so it should also be continued.

*JNC-8: Eighth Joint National Committee; ACCORD: Action to Control Cardiovascular Risk in Diabetes; SPRINT: Systolic Blood Pressure Intervention Trial

38. A 75-year-old woman comes to the office because she has right-sided medial knee pain. The pain began 2 years ago and has slowly progressed. She currently takes acetaminophen and duloxetine for the pain. She is interested in nonpharmacologic interventions to reduce pain and improve her function.

On examination, vital signs are normal. BMI is 24.7 kg/m². There is mild crepitus on extension and mild tenderness along the medial joint line in the right knee. The rest of the musculoskeletal examination is unremarkable except for small, asymptomatic Heberden nodes in 2 fingers of the right hand. Standing bilateral radiography demonstrates mild osteoarthritis (Kellgren and Lawrence system grade 1–2) of the left knee and moderate osteoarthritis (Kellgren and Lawrence system grade 3) affecting primarily the medial compartment of the right knee joint.

Which one of the following nonpharmacologic approaches is the best recommendation for this patient?

(A) Dieting to achieve 5% weight loss
(B) Neoprene brace for the right knee
(C) Lateral patella taping to the right knee
(D) Aerobic, land-based exercise

ANSWER: D

A 2015 Cochrane review found high-quality evidence for improvement in pain and moderate-quality evidence for improvement in function for land-based aerobic exercise in individuals with knee osteoarthritis (SOE=A, B). The effects seen were comparable to those of NSAIDs.

Weight loss in obese persons with knee osteoarthritis improves pain and quality of life. Excessive weight increases the load placed on lower extremity joints, increasing the stress, and could worsen breakdown of cartilage. Despite some clear limitations, BMI is often used as a surrogate marker to determine whether a patient has a normal, healthy weight (BMI 18.5–24.9 kg/m²), is overweight (BMI 25–29.9 kg/m²), or is obese (BMI ≥30 kg/m²). This patient has a BMI within the normal range, and there is no evidence that weight loss will improve her symptoms or quality of life (SOE=C).

A 2012 Cochrane review found inconclusive evidence regarding the utility of bracing or orthotics in management of medial compartment knee arthritis, with low-quality evidence showing no difference in pain or function after 12 months of bracing (SOE=C). The American College of Rheumatology 2012 guidelines for nonpharmacologic and pharmacologic therapies in osteoarthritis conditionally recommend medially directed patellar taping; the guidelines do not make any recommendation for laterally directed patellar taping (SOE=C).

39. A 75-year-old man comes to the office for routine follow-up. History includes diabetes mellitus, hypertension, and hypercholesterolemia. Current medications are aspirin 81 mg/d, glipizide 10 mg/d, lisinopril 10 mg/d, simvastatin 40 mg/d, and a daily multivitamin. His friend takes omega-3 fatty acids 500 mg/d, and he asks whether he would also benefit from the supplement.

Which one of the following is true regarding omega-3 fatty acid supplementation?

(A) Increases risk of hypoglycemia
(B) Reduces risk of sudden coronary death
(C) Increases risk of hypercoagulability
(D) Worsens cognitive decline

ANSWER: B

Eicosapentaenoic acid (EPA) and docosahexaenoic acid (DHA) are essential long-chain omega-3 fatty acids. There is a third, short-chain omega-3 fatty acid, α-linolenic acid, which is found more in plant oils. EPA and DHA—but not α-linolenic acid—have been shown to reduce cardiovascular risk.

For persons with known cardiovascular disease, the American Heart Association recommends EPA/DHA 1 g/d. In the GISSI Prevention trial, heart attack survivors who took omega-3 fatty acids 1 g/d for 3 years had a lower incidence of repeat heart attack, stroke, or sudden death (SOE=B). For persons without known cardiovascular disease, the American Heart Association recommends servings of oily fish twice each week, or EPA/DHA 500 mg/d. The recommendation for lowering triglycerides is EPA/DHA 2–4 g/d.

In a study comparing use of EPA supplementation and statin with statin alone, the combination of EPA supplementation and statin was associated with a 19% relative reduction in major coronary events after 5 years for persons who had a history of coronary artery disease.

The combination reduced major coronary events by 18% among participants with no history of coronary events, but the results were not significant (SOE=B).

Omega-3 fatty acids have also been shown to increase anticoagulant effects. In 1 study of patients with stable coronary artery disease, the combination of aspirin 81 mg/d and EPA plus DHA supplementation was similar to aspirin 325 mg/d in terms of anticoagulation benefits (SOE=B). Omega-3 fatty acids have no effect on glucose regulation.

Observational studies seem to suggest that omega-3 fatty acids may protect people from cognitive decline. However, results of several randomized controlled trials did not show benefit of supplementation with omega-3 fatty acids on cognitive decline in healthy older adults. It is possible that these studies were not long enough to discern a potential effect of omega-3 fatty acids (SOE=B).

40. An 86-year-old woman comes to the office accompanied by her daughter, who is concerned because her mother has fallen twice in the past 6 months, each time without injury. The patient states that, each time, she tripped and lost her balance. There is no history of dizziness, syncope, or arrhythmia. Her medical history includes hypertension, hyperlipidemia, right hip replacement, and cataract surgery. Current medications are lisinopril, atorvastatin, and aspirin.

On examination, blood pressure is 136/86 mmHg with no orthostatic changes, and heart rate is 72 beats per minute and regular. Heart sounds are regular, with no murmurs, and lungs are clear. There is no edema. Neurologic findings indicate normal proprioception, reflexes, and sensation to touch. Muscle strength is normal.

Which one of the following is the most appropriate recommendation for this patient?

(A) Encourage her to be more physically active.
(B) Recommend a strength, endurance, and balance program.
(C) Recommend any form of exercise as long as it is ongoing.
(D) Recommend a progressive strengthening program.

ANSWER: B

Although persons who are more active have fewer falls, it does not appear that falls can be prevented by simply encouraging older people to be more active. Ongoing, balance-challenging exercise on a regular basis for a sustained period is essential to significantly reduce fall risk.

The U.S. Preventive Services Task Force found convincing evidence that exercise or physical therapy has moderate benefit in preventing falls in older adults. A multicomponent exercise intervention that consists of strength, endurance, and balance training appears to be the best strategy for improving gait, balance, and strength, as well as reducing the rate of falls in older individuals (SOE=A). A benefit of a reduction in falls is that adults can maintain their functional capacity as they age. Most of the studies demonstrating improvement in gait, balance, and fall risk have used multicomponent exercise training.

Exercise programs that challenge balance are more effective in preventing falls than programs that do not. Additionally, effects on fall prevention are greater with more exercise. Fall prevention programs should offer ongoing exercise or encourage people to continue exercising after the formal program ends.

41. An 82-year-old man is brought to the office by his daughter because she is exhausted by caring for him. He and his wife immigrated to the United States from Venezuela 40 years ago, and the couple shares an apartment with their daughter and her children. History includes Alzheimer disease and glaucoma. Current medications are prednisolone and dorzolamide eye drops. He rarely uses his walker and has fallen 3 times in the last year. He needs assistance with dressing and bathing. He often becomes disoriented and aggressive in the evening, especially when his daughter tries to convince him to shower or change clothes.

On physical examination, he has a hunched posture on ambulation, with small steps and poor foot lift. He has an unsteady gait.

Which one of the following increases his risk of nursing home placement?

(A) Hispanic heritage
(B) Daughter's exhaustion
(C) His marital status
(D) His living arrangements

ANSWER: B

Numerous studies have examined risk factors for nursing home placement among patients with dementia. White patients, as compared with patients of other ethnicities, are more likely to be placed in nursing homes (SOE=A). Older age, greater dementia severity, and the presence of behavioral and psychological symptoms of dementia (as present in this scenario) are also risk factors. The type of dementia does not affect long-term placement. Living with a family caregiver and being married are associated with significantly lower risk. However, caregiver burden, as is present in this scenario, significantly increases the risk of placement (SOE=A). Dependency in ≥3 activities of daily living also increases the likelihood of nursing home placement.

It is important for clinicians to screen for caregiver burden and fatigue at every encounter, because burden not only increases the likelihood of nursing home placement but also has adverse health outcomes for the caregivers. This patient's daughter is caring for her children and her father, who has Alzheimer disease complicated by multiple deficits in activities of daily living (gait impairment, assistance needed for shower and dressing) and behavioral disturbances. She admits to being exhausted. Not all caregivers will report this, however, and screening for caregiver burden can help identify those at risk or hesitant to admit to this common problem.

42. An 86-year-old woman is brought to the office for a follow-up visit, accompanied by her daughter (her durable power of attorney) and her caregiver. History includes Alzheimer disease, stage 4 lung cancer, and recent right lower-extremity deep-vein thrombosis. The caregiver states that the patient spends most of the day asleep, often difficult to arouse. Her appetite has decreased notably in the last 6 weeks; at her visit to the oncologist 1 month ago, weight was down by 2.3 kg (5 lb). At that visit, the option of hospice was discussed with the patient's daughter. The daughter is not ready for her mother to start hospice care and asks what can be done to improve her caloric intake.

On examination, weight has decreased further by 4.6 kg (10 lb).

Which one of the following is the most appropriate initial recommendation for this patient?

(A) Oral dronabinol 2.5 mg twice daily
(B) Oral megestrol acetate 400 mg/d
(C) Placement of gastrostomy tube for enteral feedings
(D) Small meals of the patient's favorite foods

ANSWER: D

Loss of appetite is almost universal at the end of life, and it is usually more distressing to the family than to the patient. This patient has advanced cancer with a poor prognosis. An increase in appetite and weight is unlikely to improve her quality of life or clinical outcome. Patient and family education on the effects of terminal cancer on appetite and weight is essential. Any uncontrolled symptoms that may contribute to the patient's anorexia, such as constipation and nausea, should be addressed. Finally, her diet should be liberalized to include calorically dense food, particularly those that are her favorites.

Other interventions for anorexia have limited benefit and potential risks for patients with advanced cancer. Neither enteral nor total parenteral nutrition has been shown to improve life expectancy or quality of life for patients with end-stage cancer and is not recommended for this patient. Although pharmacologic appetite stimulants such as dronabinol and megestrol acetate have been shown to increase appetite and even weight in some studies, their use does not improve survival or clinical outcome (SOE=C). Dronabinol can affect mental status and should be used in caution with this patient with dementia. Megestrol acetate is associated with an increased risk of thromboembolism and would be inappropriate for this patient, given her recent history of deep-vein thrombosis.

43. A 66-year-old woman comes to the office because for 6 months she has had increasing difficulty staying asleep. She falls asleep after about an hour but wakes up 3–4 hours later almost every night. About 2 or 3 nights per week she can fall back to light, interrupted sleep after 30–60 minutes; other times, she is up for the rest of the night. She states that she does not snore and the awakenings are not breathing related. Her schedule for the past 20 years has been to go to bed at 10 PM and wake up at 6:30 AM. She was diagnosed with insomnia in her 40s and was treated with cognitive-behavioral therapy (CBT) and intermittently with zolpidem.

She does not feel depressed and there have been no changes in her lifestyle. She sees a therapist who has been working with her on CBT for insomnia for the past 3 months. She asks for medication to help her stay asleep. History includes hypertension and mild depression.

On physical examination, blood pressure is 132/89 mmHg.

Which one of the following medications would be the most appropriate initial recommendation?

(A) Zaleplon
(B) Zolpidem
(C) Trazodone
(D) Suvorexant

ANSWER: D

The first-line approach for treatment of insomnia is to promote healthy sleep habits with cognitive-behavioral therapy for insomnia (CBT-I) (SOE=A). The American College of Physicians recommends that all adult patients receive CBT-I as the initial treatment for chronic insomnia disorder. For adults in whom CBT-I alone is unsuccessful, clinicians should discuss with the patient the benefits, harms, and cost of pharmacologic therapy.

Although CBT-I improved sleep-onset insomnia symptoms in this patient, she continues to have difficulty maintaining sleep. The best choice is a medication that improves both sleep onset and sleep maintenance. Particularly in an older adult, the risk of falls, cognitive impairment, and next day sedation are important considerations. Zaleplon, zolpidem, and suvorexant—but not trazodone—are approved by the U.S. Food and Drug Administration for treatment of insomnia disorder and have been studied in older adults (SOE=B). Suvorexant is an orexin receptor antagonist that has been shown to be effective for improving sleep onset and continuity and short-term sleep outcomes for adults with insomnia disorder (SOE=A). Short-term use is generally recommended.

Zaleplon has a short half-life and is not approved for sleep-maintenance insomnia. Zolpidem may be effective but it is primarily indicated for sleep initiation. In older adults, trazodone can increase daytime sedation and impair daytime function.

Although open-label trials have been performed for >6 months, comparative effectiveness and long-term efficacy of most pharmacotherapies for insomnia are generally lacking.

44. A 78-year-old man is brought to the office by his family because he is agitated and aggressive, such that they feel threatened by his behavior. He has a neurocognitive disorder. The family asks about pharmacologic options that could mitigate his behavior. If drug therapy is unsuccessful, they will seek institutionalization.

Which one of the following is the most appropriate pharmacologic treatment for this patient?

(A) Quetiapine[OL]
(B) Lorazepam[OL]
(C) Citalopram[OL]
(D) Combination therapy with dextromethorphan[OL] and quinidine[OL]

ANSWER: C

Citalopram^{OL} is the most appropriate option, although it may worsen cognition, and its dose range is limited by risk of prolongation of the QT$_c$ interval. Citalopram is a selective serotonin reuptake inhibitor (SSRI) that has been shown to be as effective as risperidone in treating agitation and psychosis in patients with Alzheimer disease. It can also treat co-occurring depression and anxiety. The U.S. Food and Drug Administration (FDA) has issued an advisory for use of citalopram because of the dose-dependent risk of QT$_c$ prolongation. Although 30 mg/d was found to reduce agitation (SOE=A), the FDA recommends a maximum dosage of 20 mg/d for patients >60 years old (SOE=B).

The combination of dextromethorphan^{OL} and quinidine^{OL} has been shown to reduce agitation, with few adverse effects, in patients with Alzheimer disease, but the data are limited to 1 study (SOE=C). The combination is approved by the FDA for treatment of pseudobulbar affect. Dextromethorphan is a low-affinity N-methyl-D-aspartate receptor antagonist, serotonin and norepinephrine reuptake inhibitor, and nicotinic $\alpha_3\beta_4$ receptor antagonist. Quetiapine^{OL} can be effective for dementia-related agitation and has a wider dose range than citalopram, but it is associated with a small but statistically significant increase in mortality (SOE=B). Lorazepam^{OL} is a sedative that can increase confusion, risk of falls, and paradoxical agitation in older patients. It has been used as rescue medication for agitation in pharmacologic trials.

45. An 86-year-old man undergoes evaluation because he has several pressure injuries. He has end-stage cancer with bone metastasis and is on home hospice; he does not want further cancer treatment or hospitalization. He has lost 27.2 kg (60 lb) over several months and refuses food. Liquid intake is minimal, and urinary catheter yields minimal output.

On physical examination, there is a stage 3, necrotic, draining pressure injury measuring 8.5 × 3 × 0.4 cm, on the left great trochanter. A breakdown is starting on the left shoulder, and there are skin tears on the arms. A large butterfly discoloration on the sacral area, measuring 9 × 10 cm, appears to be new, within the past week according to his wife.

The patient and family understand that maintenance wound care is the treatment of choice. No other aggressive treatments are being done. The family has removed the specialty mattress from the patient's bed at his request. He does not want to be turned and wants to be left to just rest.

Which one of the following is the best approach for this patient's multiple skin injuries?

(A) Perform negative-pressure wound treatment.
(B) Debride the necrotic pressure ulcer.
(C) Provide comfort wound care.
(D) Order specialty bed.

ANSWER: C

A palliative care approach to pressure injuries begins with educating the patient and family regarding realistic treatments and providing emotional support. Palliative care involves managing care to enhance individual comfort, well-being, and quality of life, while respecting the patient's wishes (SOE=C). It is important to reduce suffering and keep the patient comfortable by eliminating painful dressing changes and unnecessary turning or repositioning. Comfort measures are appropriate when there is no realistic goal of healing and the patient has requested no further treatment. Factors leading to designating a wound as palliative include unmodifiable risk factors or medical conditions such as poor nutrition, inadequate perfusion, multisystem organ failure, immune compromise, irreversible anasarca, a terminal prognosis that prevents the normal healing process, and presence of artificial life support. The acronym SCALE (skin changes at life's end) refers to the clinical phenomena (skin failure) that occur when the dying process compromises homeostasis. Skin failure is the localized death of skin and underlying tissues due to decreased blood flow secondary to dysfunction of other body systems, often multiple system organ failure.

Like other vital body systems, the skin can become dysfunctional at the end of life, with loss of integrity and reduced ability to use nutrients and to sustain normal skin function. The changes can be classified as acute, chronic, or end-stage.

Numerous dressings are available for maintenance care, including foams, silicone, and alginate dressings. The dressing should absorb and wick drainage, control odor, and allow painless removal; it should be changed every 3–5 days (SOE=B). Wound odor can be minimized with charcoal- or chlorophyll-containing dressings, or metronidazole gel[OL]. Any pain related to the wound should also be addressed. A good frame of reference is to keep the patient clean, dry, pain free, and comfortable.

Negative pressure wound therapy, debridement, and other ancillary treatments are generally used when the goal is healing.

46. An 89-year-old woman is admitted to the hospital because she has complications associated with pneumonia. At baseline, the patient lives in her own home, is independent in basic activities of daily living, and walks with no assistive device. During the hospital stay, physical therapy assessment records her gait speed as 0.30 m/s.

Which one of the following best describes the significance of this patient's gait speed?

(A) It is within the normal range for hospitalized oldest-old adults.
(B) It indicates mild impairment and should be monitored closely for further decline.
(C) It indicates dysmobility and increased fall risk.
(D) It indicates increased risk of discharge to institutional setting.

ANSWER: C

This patient walked without an assistive device before her illness. Her current gait speed is 0.30 m/s, which is lower than the cut-off of 0.56 m/s for increased fall risk. Gait speed is a strong indicator of health and function and is proposed as the sixth vital sign. Like blood pressure or body temperature, gait speed may be a nonspecific indicator, with normal and abnormal values. Persistently abnormal values are indicators of poor health. This patient's speed is considered seriously abnormal and should be interpreted as an indicator of dysmobility. She would likely benefit from further assessment to determine whether an intervention is warranted.

Gait speed is a significant predictor of disability, cognitive decline, falls, hospitalization, nursing home admission, and mortality (SOE=A). Walking is a complex task that places demands on multiple systems. Gait speed may represent the integrated performance of the nervous, musculoskeletal, and cardiopulmonary systems; as such, it may have a role in estimating the overall burden of disease and predict an array of outcomes.

In adults, normal self-selected gait speed is 1.2–1.3 m/s. The mean gait speed in a hospital setting is 0.50 m/s; speed <0.15 m/s is associated with discharge to an institutional setting. Researchers have estimated that gait speed of 0.74–1.2 m/s is generally required to safely cross a street. Gait speed cut-points have been proposed: superior gate speed is ≥1.4 m/s; normal, 1.0–1.4 m/s; mildly abnormal, 0.6–1.0 m/s; and seriously abnormal, <0.60 m/s.

47. A 78-year-old man comes to the office because he fell at home. History includes Parkinson disease. He adheres to his current medication regimen of carbidopa/levodopa (25/100) three times daily. The medication has not changed recently. He uses a standard 4-point walker to facilitate ambulation. There has been no change in his vision and hearing.

On physical examination, there is no orthostatic hypotension. Core strength is preserved. There is bruising over his left shoulder, with no evidence of head trauma or focalized neurologic weakness. Resting tremor is more obvious in the right upper extremity than the left. He has some difficulty maneuvering the walker through the door of the examination room. Gait speed is slow, and he demonstrates freezing. Overall, the findings are similar to those from the last examination 6 months ago.

Which one of the following is the most appropriate intervention?

(A) Admit to nursing facility for physical therapy.
(B) Recommend use of a 4-wheeled walker.
(C) Recommend around-the-clock home aide and use of a 1-point cane.
(D) Recommend use of a front-wheeled walker.

ANSWER: D

Over time, most patients with Parkinson disease have progressive problems with gait and balance.

This patient has difficulty maneuvering his assistive device. For most patients with Parkinson disease, the use of a standard walker (without wheels) increases freezing. For these patients, the use of a front-wheeled walker results in less variability in gait and decreases freezing (SOE=B). However, the use of a 4-wheeled walker may increase the risk of falling because of the festinating gait pattern and difficulty stopping associated with Parkinson disease.

Use of a 4-point cane—not a 1-point cane—may be appropriate for some patients who do not need or want a walker. The benefit of admission to a nursing facility for physical therapy may be limited for this patient, given that his core strength is preserved.

48. A 78-year-old woman comes to the office for a scheduled yearly visit. She has generally been well and has no acute medical concerns. She lives independently with her husband. She is active and walks approximately 1.5 miles, 4–5 days each week. There is no history of diabetes mellitus, hypertension, or coronary artery disease. Current medications are aspirin 81 mg/d, calcium 500 mg/d, and vitamin D 1,000 IU/d.

On physical examination, blood pressure is 130/70 mmHg, and heart rate is 76 beats per minute. Heart and lung findings are normal. A comparison of current and previous laboratory findings shows an increase in serum creatinine level, from 0.9 mg/dL to 1.3 mg/dL, and a decrease in glomerular filtration rate (GFR), from 70 mL/min to 40 mL/min.

Which one of the following is the most likely cause of the change in this patient's renal function?

(A) Glomerulosclerosis, tubular atrophy, and interstitial fibrosis
(B) Microinfarctions of the cortical glomeruli and decreased medullary volume
(C) Glomerular basement membrane thinning and pericapsular fibrosis
(D) Interstitial eosinophilic infiltration and glomerular atrophy

ANSWER: A

In most people, renal function declines after age 40 at a mean rate of 1% per year, with some acceleration in later years. This age-related change is distinct from kidney diseases that are common in older adults, such as diabetic nephropathy. Microscopically, the changes include an increased prevalence of nephrosclerosis consisting of arteriosclerosis, glomerulosclerosis, and tubular atrophy with interstitial fibrosis. These changes ultimately lead to a decreased number of functional glomeruli as well as some hypertrophy of the remaining functional glomeruli.

The prevalence of atherosclerosis of the renal arteries increases with age. Infarctions of the kidney are not age-related changes; however, arteriosclerosis of the small arteries of the kidney is believed to cause ischemia of the nephron. This ischemia leads to glomerulosclerosis and tubular atrophy. Specifically, there is pericapsular fibrosis, wrinkling of the capillary tufts, and gradually progressive thickening (not thinning) of the basement membranes of the glomeruli. Additionally, hyaline material deposits within Bowman's space. As a result of these changes, there is collapse of the glomeruli tufts with resultant sclerosis. The tubules atrophy with fibrosis as well. There is progressive accumulation of lymphocytes and macrophages but not eosinophils within the renal interstitium.

With age, overall renal mass decreases by 25%–30%. This change in mass occurs gradually, beginning in the third or fourth decade. Macroscopically, the renal cortical volume decreases and the medullary volume increases. With further aging, the decrease in cortical volume becomes more prominent, and renal cysts increase in number and size. The cysts typically are benign.

Because of these changes, older adults have less renal functional reserve, which places them at greater risk of acute kidney injury if kidney disease develops. It had been thought that after an episode of acute kidney injury, renal function in older adults would return to premorbid levels. However, more recent evidence has shown that acute kidney injury may precipitate worsening renal function and development of more severe chronic kidney disease.

These micro- and macro-anatomic changes of the renal system lead to an overall decrease in kidney function as measured by GFR, with resultant impairment of sodium conservation and excretion and decreased concentrating and diluting capacity and filtration. Depending on the degree of renal impairment, dosages of medications cleared by the kidney may need to be adjusted. Nephrotoxic medications and NSAIDs need to be used with caution or avoided. When estimating renal function for dosage adjustment of renally excreted drugs, creatinine clearance based on the Cockcroft-Gault equation is preferred over estimated GFR reported by the laboratory.

Age-related functional decline of kidneys is believed to have little effect on overall life expectancy.

49. A 67-year-old man comes to the office because he has had difficulty swallowing for the past week. He describes an uncomfortable sensation of food sticking in his chest. The sensation does not occur when he drinks liquids. History includes hypertension, gastroesophageal reflux disease (GERD), cirrhosis secondary to hepatitis C, and osteoarthritis; he is HIV positive. Current medications are antiretroviral therapy, proton pump inhibitor, and acetaminophen; attempts to swallow pills produce pain over the midsternum.

On physical examination, his weight is down 1.4 kg (3 lb).

Which one of the following is the most appropriate initial step in evaluation?

(A) Modified barium swallow
(B) Barium esophagography
(C) Upper endoscopy
(D) Esophageal manometry

ANSWER: C

This patient's sensation of food sticking in his chest points to an esophageal cause for dysphagia. Impacted food bolus is the most common cause of acute-onset dysphagia; patients present generally within hours after eating meat, with total inability to swallow even saliva. Endoscopy is used to clear food impaction. There is general agreement that the initial evaluation of esophageal dysphagia should be with upper endoscopy (SOE=B). The procedure is diagnostic and often also allows immediate treatment for peptic strictures, esophageal rings, and similar conditions, as well as biopsy of abnormal tissue.

The modified barium swallow is helpful in diagnosis of oropharyngeal but not esophageal causes of dysphagia. Barium esophagography may allow detection of structural changes, such as stricture, cancer, or esophageal rings, and may suggest a motility disorder (delayed clearance of barium from the esophagus), but will miss conditions such as candidiasis and esophagitis from reflux. Esophageal manometry is useful in detection or confirmation of motility disorders.

This patient's history of HIV puts him at risk of esophageal candidiasis, a condition that presents with odynophagia and is generally diagnosed during endoscopy. Characteristic changes are white, mucosal plaque-like lesions; the diagnosis is confirmed by biopsy. His history of GERD puts him at risk of an esophageal stricture that would be diagnosed and likely treated during endoscopy. Esophageal carcinoma can present with progressive esophageal dysphagia, usually for solids first and then for liquids.

50. An 85-year-old man comes to the office for routine follow-up. History includes coronary artery disease, diabetes mellitus, fatty liver disease, and osteoarthritis. He had coronary bypass surgery 6 years ago. He is independent in all activities of daily living.

On physical examination, several toe nails, including those of the first toe of both feet, are significantly deformed. The nail plate is thickened with subungual debris and has a brown-yellow hue. The skin of both feet shows diffuse scale on the base of the feet and between the toes. All other physical findings are unchanged from previous visits.

On further questioning, the patient says that he has no personal or family history of psoriasis. He does not know when his nails began to change, nor does he recall specific trauma to the involved digits. He has not used any treatment.

Which one of the following is the most important risk factor for this patient's nail condition?

(A) Diabetes mellitus
(B) Peripheral vascular disease
(C) Advanced age
(D) Poor foot care

ANSWER: C

Onychomycosis is a fungal infection of the nail that typically presents with dystrophy and discoloration of the toe nails. It is usually chronic; treatment is difficult, and infections are often asymptomatic. The prevalence of onychomycosis increases with age. It is estimated to occur in 20% of adults >60 and 50% of adults >70 years old (SOE=C). Thus, advanced age results in a 5-fold increase in risk of onychomycosis. The reason for the increased risk is thought to be related to slower nail plate growth, relative immunosuppression, difficulty performing foot care, and increased fungal exposure. Although the infection is indolent, it can lead to breaks in the skin if skin care is not maintained. The skin breaks increase the risk of cellulitis.

Age is the strongest but not the only risk factor for onychomycosis. Patients with diabetes are 2–3 times more likely to have the infection. Poor foot care in itself is not a major risk factor, although it may be a contributor in older adults. Peripheral vascular disease increases the risk of cellulitis but not the risk for development of onychomycosis.

Treatment is notably challenging, because regrowth of the nail can take >1 year in older adults. The treatment plan should include maintenance of the nails to prevent skin breakdown. Cure rates for topical agents, such as ciclopirox, are estimated at only 25%. Oral agents, such as fluconazole, terbinafine, and itraconazole, are more effective (41%, 66%, and 70% cure rates, respectively). The decision to treat with a systemic agent should be made on a case-by-case basis, with thorough evaluation of comorbidities as well as risk–benefit analysis.

51. A 57-year-old man is brought to the office by staff from his group home. He received a diagnosis of autistic spectrum disorder (formerly, autism) in childhood and schizophrenia in his 20s. He has been on antipsychotic medication since then. He is currently on quetiapine. He has not had any blood work in at least 7 years and has not had a colonoscopy. Staff reports he dislikes going to see doctors, at least partly because he does not like being touched. He allows only a cursory examination today. Poor dentition and obesity (BMI 35 kg/m^2) are noted. There is a family history of diabetes and heart disease.

Which one of the following is the best next step in providing care for this patient?

(A) Refill medications and arrange follow-up in 3 months.
(B) Have nurse draw blood while he is in the office today.
(C) Provide education on healthy lifestyle changes and follow up in 2 weeks.
(D) Schedule dental work and colonoscopy under general anesthesia.

ANSWER: C

Patients with intellectual and developmental disabilities are living longer but still have a shorter life span than an age-matched cohort without disability. Overall life expectancy is 65 years, varying somewhat depending on specific diagnoses. In patients with chronic physical symptoms associated with their disability, illnesses typically related to aging (eg, heart disease, diabetes, arthritis, dementia) develop earlier, irrespective of whether there is an associated intellectual disability. Reasons for this include poorer access to health care (due to finances and lack of providers experienced in or comfortable with this population), poor diet (due to finances or lack of knowledge regarding healthy eating habits), more sedentary lifestyle (due to physical limitations [including vision problems], social limitations, and knowledge deficits), and physical manifestations of the underlying disorder (eg, cerebral palsy, muscular dystrophies).

In persons with developmental and intellectual disabilities, major mental illnesses, such as schizophrenia, develop at the same rate as in the general population.

The best next step is to provide information on a healthy lifestyle and arrange for follow-up in 2 weeks. Studies have shown that providing education on diet and exercise can have a positive effect on lifestyle choices (SOE=C). Following up soon after the initial visit may allow the provider to develop a rapport and begin to address other health concerns, without overwhelming the patient at the initial visit.

Simply refilling prescriptions does not address the need for health screening or obvious concerns about metabolic syndrome. Waiting 3 months to follow up makes it difficult for the provider to develop rapport with the patient. If the patient has metabolic syndrome, changing medication may be beneficial if tolerated and effective, and waiting 3 months does not address the concern in a timely manner.

Although there is a need for screening blood work, doing it in the office at the first visit, when staff already has difficulty getting the patient to attend appointments, may make it more difficult at future visits. Ordering blood work at a site other than the office may interfere less with the doctor-patient relationship, because the patient may not directly connect the blood work with the visits.

Sometimes it is necessary to do some procedures under anesthesia, especially if the degree of disability is more severe. However, every effort should be made to do as many procedures as possible in the usual fashion. If it is necessary to do procedures under anesthesia, the patient should be informed beforehand about what to expect.

52. A 71-year-old black American man comes to the office for an annual wellness check-up. History includes coronary artery disease, chronic obstructive pulmonary disease (COPD), benign prostatic hyperplasia, and stage 3 chronic kidney disease. He has had a stent placement and is on home oxygen. He was admitted to the ICU last year for exacerbation of COPD, and doctors and nurses discussed code status preferences with him. He has no documented advance directives and becomes visibly uncomfortable when asked about them.

Which one of the following factors is most likely to be a barrier to his completion of advance directives?

(A) Mistrust of the health care system
(B) Higher socioeconomic status
(C) Number of comorbidities
(D) History of ICU care

ANSWER: A

Consistent evidence suggests that black Americans have disproportionately poor end-of-life care and are less likely to participate in advance care planning than non-black Americans. Among Medicare recipients, black Americans are also more likely to receive life-sustaining interventions, which may be both a cause of poor end-of-life care and a consequence of lower participation in advance care planning. Interactions among barriers and facilitators to advance care planning in black American populations are complex.

Noncompletion of advance directives among black Americans is attributed in many studies to a preference for life-sustaining treatments, or to religiosity or poor health literacy. Factors that contribute to the differences between black Americans' and white Americans' attitudes about advance care planning include discomfort discussing death, greater preference for life-sustaining treatment, mistrust of the medical system, and religiosity (SOE=B). Factors that positively predict or facilitate completion of advance directives include higher income level, knowledge about the directives, and history of ICU care (SOE=B).

A review of the literature highlights the complex interactions that affect advance care planning among black Americans. As a group, black Americans appear more likely to engage in discussion about end-of-life care than to complete formal documentation. Because strategies to improve completion of advance directives among black Americans remain unsuccessful after >20 years of effort, the review suggests that future approaches must engage faith and family in discussions on advance care planning (SOE=B).

53. A 63-year-old man comes to the office accompanied by his wife, who is concerned about changes she has seen in his behavior over the past year. He is a retired army major. He has become messy and unpredictable; for example, last week she found him cutting up all the curtains in the house. He gorges on food and is no longer quiet and polite; instead, he has become abusive and now uses coarse language. During the interview, the patient is oblivious to his wife's statements. History includes hypertension.

On examination, the patient appears unkempt. Hypertension is under control, and all other findings are normal, except for the Mini–Mental State Examination on which he scores 23.

Which one of the following is the most likely diagnosis?

(A) Delirium
(B) Frontotemporal lobar degeneration
(C) Adjustment disorder following retirement
(D) Substance use disorder

ANSWER: B

This patient's personality change is most likely due to frontotemporal lobar degeneration. He manifests a significant, persistent change from baseline, causing clinically significant distress or impairment in social, occupational, or other important areas of functioning. Inappropriate social behavior is an early symptom of frontotemporal lobar degeneration; it includes behavioral disinhibition, apathy, loss of sympathy and empathy, perseveration and stereotyped or compulsive rituals, and hyperorality, including changes in food choice and orientation (SOE=B). His score on the neurocognitive screen is consistent with this diagnosis, as is the progression of illness over a long interval.

In delirium, the disturbance develops over a short period (usually hours to a few days), and tends to fluctuate in severity during the course of a day. Personality changes may also occur in the context of substance use disorders, especially if the disorder is longstanding. The clinician should inquire carefully about the nature and extent of substance use. In this case, the wife's statement relates no substance abuse.

Personality change due to another medical condition can be distinguished from personality disorder by the requirement of a clinically significant change from baseline personality functioning and the presence of a specific etiologic medical condition. In this case, adjustment disorder due to retirement would be plausible were the changes in behavior not so extraordinary.

54. A 70-year-old woman comes to the office to establish care because her previous clinician retired. She is a retired nursing supervisor. Her main concern is that for the past year, her neighbors have been trying to get her to move by purposefully damaging the steps leading up to her doorway. She does not know why her neighbors wish her harm. She produces several photographs to illustrate the damage; the steps appear to be intact. Her daughter lives with her, but she has asked the daughter to leave because she believes her daughter has damaged the interior steps that lead to the second floor. The patient says that her daughter "has her reasons but she's secretive, can't be trusted." The patient is active in her church and manages her household, shopping, and finances without assistance.

During the interview, the patient is alert and courteous. She is well dressed. She denies any history of abuse. Laboratory findings from 6 months ago confirm that she is in good health. She consents to cognitive assessment and mentions that her previous clinician also performed an assessment, the results of which were normal. Findings from today's assessment are normal.

Which one of the following is the most likely diagnosis?

(A) Mild frontotemporal neurocognitive disorder (dementia)
(B) Delusional disorder
(C) Schizophreniform disorder
(D) Paranoid personality disorder

ANSWER: B

The patient in this case has a fixed belief (delusion) that is possible but not credible and that has persisted for >6 months, making delusional disorder the most likely presumptive diagnosis. Although she is suspicious of both her neighbors and her daughter, it is not clear that she has the pervasive distrust of others' motivation and belief in their harmful intent that would be consistent with paranoid personality disorder. She does not exhibit the disorganized speech, behavior, or loss of interest that is consistent with schizophreniform disorder. Similarly, frontotemporal neurocognitive disorders typically distort personality and promote disinhibition early in the course of illness rather than present with delusion.

55. Which one of the following reflects the approximate prevalence of centenarians in developed countries?

(A) 1 per 1,000
(B) 1 per 5,000
(C) 1 per 10,000
(D) 1 per 50,000

ANSWER: B

Centenarians are among the fastest-growing age groups in developed countries. In the early 1990s, centenarian prevalence in the United Kingdom and the United States was about 1 per 10,000 people; that prevalence has since doubled, to 1 per 5,000. According to the U.S. Census Bureau, in 2000, there were approximately 50,000 centenarians; in 2014, that number grew to about 72,000.

56. A 78-year-old man comes to the office for routine follow-up. History includes coronary artery disease, hypertension, diabetes mellitus, and chronic obstructive pulmonary disease. He had 3-vessel bypass surgery 7 years ago. His most recent colonoscopy was 10 years ago; results were normal. There is no family history of colorectal cancer. He asks whether he should have a repeat colorectal cancer screen.

Which one of the following is the most appropriate recommendation?

(A) Home testing for blood in stool
(B) Sigmoidoscopy
(C) Colonoscopy
(D) No screening

ANSWER: D

Because this patient has underlying comorbidities and no family history of colorectal cancer, he should not have further colorectal cancer screening. The U.S. Preventive Services Task Force recommends against colorectal cancer screening in adults between 76 and 85 years old, unless there is increased risk of colorectal cancer (SOE=B). Further, this patient's life expectancy is <10 years, and the American Cancer Society and the U.S. Multi-Society Task Force on Colorectal Cancer have advised no colorectal cancer screening for patients with life expectancy <10 years (SOE=C).

Sigmoidoscopy and colonoscopy are equally effective in screening for colorectal cancer (SOE=B); however, this patient should not undergo either procedure. Potential harm from either procedure outweighs the limited reduction in mortality from diagnosing possible colorectal cancer. Home tests for blood in stool are an effective tool for colorectal cancer screening (SOE=B). If the test is positive, then further evaluation may be necessary. Nonetheless, home screening is not appropriate for this patient, given his life expectancy.

57. A 70-year-old woman comes to the office because she has a self-inflicted wound to her left forearm. She tried to treat herself but decided that a clinician should evaluate the wound. History includes type 2 diabetes mellitus, which has been difficult to stabilize; she has a distant history of anorexia, depression, and alcohol abuse. At today's appointment, she describes herself as lonely, irritable, and anxious.

On examination, the bandage around her wound is elaborate, but the wound is superficial.

Which one of the following is the most appropriate intervention?

(A) Hypnosis
(B) Mood stabilizer
(C) Anxiolytic (benzodiazepine) and cognitive-behavioral psychotherapy
(D) Antidepressant and cognitive-behavioral psychotherapy

ANSWER: D

Treatment of personality disorders in older adults involves the same basic approaches as with younger patients but should incorporate a much broader understanding of the impact of age-related stressors and comorbidities. The rigid, pervasive patterns in cognition, affectivity, interpersonal functioning, and impulse control can jeopardize the course of treatment (SOE=C). For example, it is harder to medicate people with personality disorders; they have higher rates of attrition with pharmacologic treatments (SOE=B). Pharmacologic interventions can also be thwarted by the patient's tendency to exaggerate medication adverse effects, or by drug abuse.

In this case, the best intervention would be cognitive-behavioral psychotherapy and antidepressants. Current research shows the efficacy of psychotherapy for patients with a personality disorder. The goal is to increase adaptive coping strategies while mitigating the impact of maladaptive behaviors. Treatment targets should be selected hierarchically, based on the severity and the degree with which they interfere with the patient's quality of life. Suicidal behaviors are the first target.

Two types of psychotherapy seem appropriate: either dialectical behavior therapy focused on acceptance and self-awareness, or techniques of schema therapy. Schema therapy focuses on the dysfunctional constructs built throughout the patient's life to modify life perspectives, adjust role investments, and reconcile intergenerational linkage (SOE=C).

Because this patient has histrionic personality disorder associated with an exaggerated sense of self-importance, psychotherapy could focus on emotional regulation, while validating her importance as a person and increasing her awareness of the consequences of her behavior on other people. Hypnosis would not be the primary technique for these aims.

Simultaneous with psychotherapy, an antidepressant could also be introduced to target symptoms of depression and anxiety (SOE=B).

Benzodiazepines should be avoided, particularly considering her history of substance abuse. There is no evidence that a mood stabilizer benefits a person with personality disorder, absent bipolar disease.

58. An 84-year-old man is brought to the emergency department by his family. His daughter is concerned that he has mouth pain. She has noticed that he has not wanted to open his mouth and grimaces when others try to open it. His daughter states that he usually eats well, but he has accepted only some liquids for the last 7 days. He has been more lethargic and less interactive with his family over the past 5 days. History includes coronary artery disease, coronary artery bypass graft, prostate cancer, moderate cognitive impairment, osteoarthritis, and bilateral knee replacement.

Which one of the following is the most likely diagnosis?

(A) Worsening of dementia
(B) Delirium
(C) Depression
(D) Acute stroke

ANSWER: B

Delirium is a serious disturbance in a person's mental abilities that results in a decreased awareness of his or her environment and confused thinking. The onset of delirium is usually sudden, often within hours or a few days.

Acute change in mental status is a required feature for diagnosis of delirium. For this patient, the change in cognition is acute in onset, and other underlying symptoms suggest possible delirium. Further evaluation is needed to ascertain the primary reason for the cause of delirium, such as uncontrolled pain or dehydration.

Delirium, especially prolonged or persistent, may lead to worsening of underlying dementia. This would be apparent only if impairment persists after delirium clears.

This patient shows no specific signs that suggest depression. The poor oral intake appears to be secondary to oral pain. He does not have any focal deficit that would suggest acute stroke.

Besides uncontrolled pain, other risk factors for delirium include dementia, advanced age, male gender, acute cardiac or pulmonary events, prolonged bed rest, drug withdrawal (sedatives, alcohol), fecal impaction, fluid or electrolyte disturbance, indwelling devices (eg, catheters), infections (especially respiratory or urinary tract), adverse drug event, use of restraints, severe anemia, and urinary retention (SOE=A).

59. An 85-year-old woman with dementia undergoes evaluation because she has lost 3.6 kg (8 lb) in 3 months. She lives in a long-term care facility and is dependent for all activities of daily living. She is minimally verbal. She is hand fed by staff; they have recently noted that she pockets food during meals.

If enteral feeding with a gastrostomy tube were initiated in this patient, which one of the following would be most likely?

(A) Decreased contact time with nursing and support staff
(B) Improved survival
(C) Decreased likelihood of pressure ulcers
(D) Improved functional status

ANSWER: A

Careful hand feeding is recommended for providing nutritional support to persons with advanced dementia to avoid risks associated with tube feeding (American Geriatrics Society, *Choosing Wisely*). Compared with tube feeding, careful hand feeding requires much more staff time and resident contact by nursing and support staff (SOE=C).

For patients with advanced dementia, insertion of feeding tubes and the timing of insertion have no effect on mortality, nor is there evidence of increased survival by initiating feeding via gastrostomy tube (SOE=B).

Feeding tubes are not associated with prevention or improved healing of pressure ulcers. Rather, there is some evidence that use of percutaneous endoscopic gastrostomy tubes is associated with increased risk of pressure ulcers among nursing home residents with advanced cognitive impairment (SOE=C).

Enteral tube feeding was widely adopted in the United States, and to a greater degree in other countries, under the assumption that consistent delivery of calories would improve nutrition and function in persons with dementia. While data are limited, expert opinion is that this is not the case. There are good data that nursing home residents who are tube fed have increased hospitalization rates. Hospital stays are associated with more rapid cognitive decline in persons with dementia (SOE=C).

60. An 80-year-old woman is admitted to the hospital because of worsening agitation that began a few days ago. History includes moderate Parkinson disease. She refuses physical examination; laboratory tests indicate urinary tract infection, and computed tomography of the head shows a new subdural hematoma. She is trying to leave and cannot be redirected. Her family is at bedside. At 1:00 AM the agitation worsens, and the patient tries to hit the nursing staff. She has been receiving her routine medications.

Which one of the following should be started to lessen the patient's agitation?

(A) Lorazepam
(B) Haloperidol
(C) Quetiapine
(D) Citalopram

ANSWER: C

If nonpharmacologic interventions alone are not successful in managing delirium, and if prompt symptom control is needed, as in this patient, pharmacologic treatment can be added to the nonpharmacologic methods. The goal is to use as small a dose as possible, and for the shortest duration. The focus should be on identifying and managing the underlying cause of delirium to help minimize use of psychotropic medications. Quetiapine is the preferred agent for the treatment of delirium for patients with Parkinson disease or Lewy body dementia because it has fewer extrapyramidal adverse effects than other agents (SOE=A). The dosage is 12.5 mg every 12 hours as needed for mild agitation, or 25 mg every 12 hours for moderate to severe agitation.

High-potency antipsychotic agents such as haloperidol[OL] may be used in low doses (0.5–1 mg by mouth, intravenously, or intramuscularly once, and then repeated every 1–2 hours as needed) for management of agitation or psychotic symptoms in patients with delirium without Parkinson disease. Patients should be monitored for extrapyramidal adverse effects, prolonged QT_c interval, neuroleptic malignant syndrome, torsade de pointes, and withdrawal dyskinesia. Haloperidol should be avoided in patients with Parkinson disease or parkinsonian features (SOE=A).

The selective serotonin reuptake inhibitor citalopram is used for management of mood (depression or anxiety) in older adults. It is not indicated for management of behavioral symptoms in delirium.

Lorazepam is the drug of choice only when delirium is caused by withdrawal from alcohol or benzodiazepines. Otherwise, benzodiazepines should be avoided, because they worsen confusion and sedation (SOE=A). For patients with delirium from alcohol intoxication or withdrawal, replacement of nutritional and electrolyte deficiencies should be addressed as well.

The cholinergic system has a key role in cognition and attention, and there is extensive evidence to support cholinergic deficiency in the pathophysiology of delirium. Among the various hypotheses proposed for development of delirium, the most commonly implicated are increased level of dopamine and reduced level of acetylcholine (causing increased neural excitability) (SOE=A). This may explain the effectiveness of antipsychotic agents in managing delirium behavior.

61. An 85-year-old man comes to the office to review laboratory results after his Medicare Annual Wellness visit. Initial fasting blood glucose level was 140 mg/dL; on repeat testing, the level is 135 mg/dL. The patient is a life-long runner, has never smoked, and has maintained a BMI of 21 kg/m² throughout adulthood. He asks what other factors may have contributed to the development of diabetes.

Which one of the following is the most likely mechanism to have caused diabetes in this patient?

(A) Decreased cytokine production
(B) Low basal insulin levels
(C) Impaired pancreatic β-cell function
(D) Increased β-cell mass

ANSWER: C

Aging has direct effects on β-cell proliferation and function and contributes indirectly to impaired insulin sensitivity (or increased insulin resistance) through lifestyle- and comorbidity-related risk factors. β-Cell mass declines with age. Insulin resistance in turn may contribute to further impairment of β-cell function.

Studies in age-matched cohorts found that aging contributes to development of type 2 diabetes through impaired β-cell function and impaired β-cell adaptation to insulin resistance, leading to impaired insulin secretion (SOE=B).

Although aging per se has minimal direct effect on insulin action, insulin resistance may develop because of diminished physical activity, obesity, and loss of lean body mass, particularly in adults with disproportional loss of skeletal muscle over adipose tissue. An absolute or relative increase of body adiposity (particularly in the central body), often associated with advancing age, appears to account in large part for the age-related increase in insulin resistance. Among adults without diabetes, intra-abdominal fat mass correlates with insulin resistance and age after controlling for obesity. However, insulin resistance is more closely associated with abdominal adiposity than with age.

Impaired pancreatic β-cell adaptation to insulin resistance appears to be an important contributing factor to age-related glucose intolerance and risk of diabetes. Age has no independent effect on insulin sensitivity when controlled for obesity (SOE=B); age-related reductions in insulin sensitivity are likely due to an age-related increase in adiposity rather than a consequence of advanced chronologic age. Increasing physical activity in older adults reduces both insulin resistance and risk of diabetes.

Additional factors that contribute to age-associated insulin resistance include visceral adiposity and associated adipokines and inflammation, oxidative stress, mitochondrial dysfunction, and possibly an intrinsic decline in insulin sensitivity in muscle fibers. Animal and observational studies in people found associations between low-grade inflammation and increased risk of diabetes, and pro-inflammatory cytokines such as C-reactive protein, interleukin-6, and tumor necrosis factor-α have been found to inhibit insulin signaling, thereby increasing insulin resistance and risk of type 2 diabetes mellitus (SOE=C). The role of mitochondrial function in aging and type 2 diabetes mellitus remains unclear.

62. A 78-year-old man comes to the office accompanied by his daughter, who is concerned about his frequent falls. She says that he tends to fall when he is away from home; he does not fall often in his house. The patient is unconcerned about the falls.

On examination, blood pressure and heart rate are normal, including postural responses. Visual, vestibular, and peripheral sensations are normal. Muscle strength, motion, and endurance are normal, and there is no rigidity or abnormal resistance to passive motion of the joints. Gait speed is 1.18 m/s, and he steps over an obstacle placed in his path with no difficulty, with a few small steps on approach. He does not make appropriate adjustments to maneuver past the furniture in the examination room or past other people in the hallway.

Which one of the following is most likely to be a factor in his falls?

(A) Cognitive dysfunction
(B) Cerebellar disorder
(C) Parkinson disease or parkinsonian syndrome
(D) Spinal stenosis

ANSWER: A

This patient has difficulties related to motor planning: he does not navigate around furniture or adapt to changing conditions in the environment (eg, others along his path). His inability to adapt or adjust his movements as needed suggests that cognitive dysfunction may be a factor in his falls. That he is more likely to fall away from home, in less familiar places, and his lack of concern about the falls are common features of a mild cognitive impairment. He has little insight into his cognitive difficulties, and thus walks freely, falls frequently, and yet remains unafraid of falling again.

He has no deficits in muscle force, motion, or endurance in relation to walking. A problem of cerebellar origin is unlikely, given normal findings on sensory examination and his postural responses to perturbation. The lack of sensory changes, muscle strength deficits, and pain or altered posture (eg, forward flexed trunk) argue against spinal stenosis as a contributor to the frequent falls.

Walking is complex: multiple limbs move in different directions while the body progresses forward in the direction of intent, using a rhythmic pattern of stepping integrated with posture of the trunk and various phases of gait, all of which happen in an environment that may include changing conditions and barriers. The factors characteristic of motor control include muscle actions in walking; use of energy for walking, force to propel the body, stability, and maneuvering; neural control to use movement-related feedback and to integrate components; and environmental challenges (ice, wind, distractions) that require appropriate gait adjustment while the walker remains mindful of his or her intent. Most of these factors occur without the person's direct focus.

Because gait can be affected by changes in any of the involved body systems, assessment includes an examination of the effector systems (muscles, motion, force, and fuel), information about the environment and moving within the world (somatosensory, vision, and vestibular), and brain use of the information available (processing, adaptation, planning). Gait changes, speed, step-width abnormalities, stance time variability, step length and width variability, and cadence are associated with risk of falls and mobility-related disability. Cognitive function (with lack of consensus of threshold) has been associated with falls (SOE=B). Gait and cognitive problems are independently associated with an increased fall risk for older adults.

63. A 78-year-old man comes to the office because he would like advice on how to reduce his risk of falling. He nearly fell last week on icy sidewalk while getting out of a car, and he is afraid that he will break a hip. History includes hypertension, benign prostatic hyperplasia, and bilateral knee osteoarthritis. Current medications are hydrochlorothiazide, amlodipine, terazosin, and topical diclofenac as needed for knee pain.

On physical examination, blood pressure is 128/68 mmHg and heart rate is 64 beats per minute after sitting for 5 minutes, and 118/62 mmHg and 70 beats per minute after standing for 3 minutes. He completes the Timed Up and Go test in 15 seconds. He steadies himself with his arm on the examination table when he performs a semi-tandem stance. The remainder of the neurologic and cardiovascular examination is normal.

Which one of the following is the best intervention to reduce risk of a fall and subsequent fracture?

(A) Tai chi
(B) Calcium supplement
(C) Discontinue terazosin
(D) Hip protectors

ANSWER: A

Several meta-analyses of randomized trials in community-dwelling older adults show that exercise reduces the risk of falls, including injurious falls, and exercise programs incorporating balance components are most effective. Tai chi, which includes strength and balance training, was effective at reducing the rate of falls and injurious falls at 12 months by 43% and 50%, respectively, in a recent meta-analysis of 10 trials (SOE=A).

Calcium supplementation alone has not been shown to reduce fall risk. Supplementation as part of a combined, multifactorial approach to fall risk reduction did reduce falls in a recent meta-analysis of 238 randomized, controlled trials of fall prevention (SOE=A). Trials and meta-analyses of calcium supplementation alone have shown mixed results for reduction of fracture risk in community-dwelling older adults. In meta-analyses, calcium combined with vitamin D and another pharmacologic treatment for osteoporosis did reduce fracture risk, including hip fracture risk, in patients with osteoporosis (SOE=A). This patient does not have known osteoporosis. Bone density screening for osteoporosis would be appropriate for him, given that he is >70 years old and at risk of falls.

Although findings have been inconsistent, treatment of orthostatic hypotension may reduce fall risk (SOE=B). However, this patient does not meet diagnostic criteria for orthostatic hypotension (≥20 mmHg decrease in systolic pressure or ≥10 mmHg decrease in diastolic pressure within 3 minutes of standing). Also, stopping treatment with terazosin may exacerbate lower urinary tract symptoms associated with prostatic hyperplasia.

A meta-analysis pooling data from 5 trials of >5,000 community-dwelling older adults found no evidence that hip protectors reduce the incidence of hip fracture. Hip protectors may fail to prevent injury because they are not worn consistently, particularly over the long-term, or because injury occurs in circumstances that preclude their use (SOE=C).

64. A 65-year-old woman comes to the office for routine follow-up. She does not take any medication regularly, and she remains active. She mentions that she is expecting her first grandchild in a few months and will help take care of the newborn on a daily basis.

Vaccination against which one of the following infections should be recommended at this time?

(A) *Haemophilus influenzae* type B
(B) Rotavirus
(C) *Bordetella pertussis*
(D) Hepatitis B virus

ANSWER: C

Adults ≥65 years old should receive a single booster dose of tetanus, diphtheria, and pertussis (Tdap) vaccine to prevent *Bordetella pertussis* infection, particularly if they will have close contact with infants <12 months old (SOE=A).

Over the past few decades, there has been a resurgence of *B pertussis*. Although pertussis in older adults can range from mild, cold-like symptoms to severe respiratory infections, infants <12 months old carry the biggest burden of morbidity and mortality. Household contacts transmit pertussis to infants in 50%–75% of cases. There is not yet an effective neonatal vaccine for pertussis. To protect infants and decrease their risk of pertussis exposure, the U.S. Centers for Disease Control and Prevention recommends a strategy termed *cocooning*, in which infants' close contacts (parents, grandparents, siblings, and caretakers) are vaccinated. The Tdap vaccine should be administered to prevent pertussis in older adults as well as their contacts.

The safety of the Tdap vaccine in adults ≥65 years old has been demonstrated. Either Tdap formulation (Boostrix® or Adacel®) can be administered. While Boostrix® is preferred, providers should not miss an opportunity to vaccinate an individual ≥65 years old, so whichever Tdap vaccine is available should be administered. Tdap should be administered regardless of the interval since the last Td booster. Subsequent tetanus booster doses, in the form of Td, should be given at 10-year intervals throughout adulthood. If it is not possible to determine whether an adult has had a Tdap vaccine, it is reasonable to proceed with administration and documentation of Tdap.

Vaccines to prevent rotavirus, hepatitis B virus, and *Haemophilus influenzae* type B infection will presumably be administered to the infant in this case, rather than to the grandmother, in accordance with recommendations from the Advisory Committee on Immunization Practices.

65. An 87-year-old woman discusses her goals and preferences for end-of-life care. She describes herself as a very spiritual member of the Buddhist Zen community and wants her spiritual community to support her through end-of-life decision-making. She has advanced coronary artery disease, New York Heart Association class 4 heart failure, and stage 4 chronic kidney disease. She has been admitted to the hospital 3 times in the past 6 months.

Regarding the patient's health care, which one of the following is a tenet of her spiritual community?

(A) Blood transfusions cannot be given.
(B) Artificial feeding cannot be given.
(C) A family member is the preferred surrogate.
(D) No specific health care directive has been developed.

ANSWER: D

Spirituality and religion play an important role in patient and family decision-making. Specific religious concerns about death and dying have led to religious advance directives. Formal religious bodies have made efforts to relate advance health care directives to their own religious perspectives.

Case studies involving religion and medicine fall along a continuum. At one end, some religious communities have tried to remain outside the secular legal system. At the other end, some religious communities have recognized the authority of secular law and try to work within the system to obtain legally sanctioned exemptions or protection for specific religious tenets. Some closed religious groups that do not believe in medicine remain insulated and reject medical care. Other, more open, religious groups choose to interact with the secular world but do not seek medical care for themselves.

Most religious communities have formalized, specific advance health care directives for their congregation members except for the Buddhist community. Because there are no specific health care directives, options A, B, and C are incorrect.

Agudath Israel of America, a religious body representing a group of Orthodox Jews, has developed its own Jewish Health Care Proxy and Halachic Living Will. This document affirms the following: "I am Jewish. It is my desire, and I hereby direct, that all health care decisions for me be made pursuant to Jewish law and custom as determined in accordance with strict Orthodox interpretation and tradition."

Jehovah's Witnesses take a firm stance on blood transfusions. They regularly update their no-blood medical treatment directives to include no transfusion of whole blood, red cells, white cells, platelets, or plasma. These directives help medical and legal personnel understand the choices Jehovah's Witnesses make regarding their medical treatment. Jehovah's Witnesses have accepted medical care for themselves and their children but do not consent to receiving blood or blood products. Although the courts have upheld the right of adults to refuse blood for themselves, the courts have not allowed parents to refuse blood products on behalf of their children.

Christian Scientists generally believe in not providing medical care for themselves and their children. Their advance health care directive includes language such as: "I am a member of the Church of Christ, Scientist, also known as the Christian Science denomination. The tenets and practices of Christian Science include healing entirely by prayer or spiritual means. Therefore, in lieu of any and all forms of medical treatment, including those thought necessary to sustain my life, I authorize and direct my agent to arrange for my health care by spiritual means through prayer, exclusively, in accordance with the tenets and practices of Christian Science." The directive also contains other options, such as: "My agent may, if my agent determines it appropriate, cause me to receive assistance from a medical doctor or a dentist, as the case may be, where such assistance consists of a more or less mechanical nature, such as the pulling of a tooth, setting of a broken bone, or the taking of stitches. Such assistance is consistent with the tenets and practices of Christian Science."

66. A 72-year-old man comes to the office because he has difficulty hearing, dating back about 5 years. He is accompanied by his daughter, who states that he sets the television volume to be excessively loud, often does not understand conversations on the telephone, and has difficulty participating in conversations in noisy environments. They are concerned about what is causing the hearing loss. The patient has no tinnitus, vertigo, otalgia, or discharge from the ears, and has had no ear infections or trauma.

Which one of the following is the most appropriate initial step in evaluating the patient's hearing loss?

(A) Audiogram
(B) Tuning fork test (Weber and Rinne tests)
(C) Pneumatic otoscopy
(D) *Hearing Handicap Inventory for the Elderly-Screening* questionnaire

ANSWER: C

The initial step in evaluating this patient's hearing loss would be to perform pneumatic otoscopy. Although he likely has presbycusis, hearing loss should be evaluated using a systematic approach. Hearing loss can occur anywhere along the tract from the external ear to the central processing of sound in the brain. Problems can arise in 4 main areas: from the external ear canal to the tympanic membrane, the middle ear space with the ossicular chain, the inner ear and cochlea, and the central processing centers in the brain.

The external ear canal and tympanic membrane (ear drum) should be examined first for causes of hearing loss. This is easily accomplished with an otoscope. Otoscopy is used to exclude an obstruction along the ear canal and to examine the tympanic membrane, which provides information about the status of the middle-ear space. The external canal should be evaluated to ensure there is no cerumen impaction or foreign material (eg, cotton lint). The tympanic membrane should be evaluated for perforations, air-fluid levels, and bulges. Pneumatic otoscopy (a puff of air pushed through the otoscope) is used to assess the mobility of the tympanic membrane. An immobile ear drum can be a sign of otitis media, chronic effusion, or other pathology in the middle ear space, each of which can contribute to hearing loss.

If otoscopy findings are normal, the next step would be examination with a 512-Hz tuning fork. The 512-Hz frequency provides the best combination of sensitivity and specificity for denoting hearing loss. The tuning fork is used to conduct the Weber and Rinne tests, which assess whether the patient has sensorineural hearing loss (cochlear or brain pathology) or conductive hearing loss (external or middle ear pathology). Any cerumen impaction should be removed before performing these maneuvers. For the Weber test, the vibrating tuning fork is placed on the midline of the face—on the forehead, bridge of the nose (nasion), or front teeth (not dentures)—and the patient is asked where he or she hears the sound. The normal response is midline or "everywhere." If the sound lateralizes to one ear, there may be conductive loss in that ear, or sensorineural loss in the other ear. For the Rinne test, a vibrating tuning fork is placed on the mastoid process (to generate sound #1) and then in front of the external auditory meatus (to generate sound #2). If the patient perceives that sound #2 is louder than sound #1, there is either normal hearing or sensorineural hearing loss in that ear. The perception that sound #1 is louder indicates conductive hearing loss in that ear.

Once otoscopy and tuning fork examinations have been performed, the patient may be referred for an audiogram to identify the type and extent of hearing loss and determine the optimal treatment. Any impacted cerumen should be removed before audiogram for the test to be valid.

The *Hearing Handicap Inventory for the Elderly-Screening* (HHIE-S) is a validated questionnaire used to detect hearing impairment and assess its impact on quality of life. HHIE-S has been translated into and validated in several languages. Because this patient is aware of hearing loss and how it affects his quality of life, such screening is not necessary.

67. An 82-year-old man undergoes evaluation because he has become increasingly disruptive in the dining room at his nursing home. He accuses staff and other residents of conspiring to poison his food. His tablemates have moved away, and staff has ceased efforts to reassure him or correct his perceptions. He will eat food that his family brings, but they cannot visit daily; when they leave meals for staff to serve him, he again complains of contamination. History includes Alzheimer disease. His family describes him as having always been overly cautious. They state that it was suspiciousness toward caregivers, rather than Alzheimer disease, that necessitated entry into long-term care. They ask about the risks and benefits of initiating medical therapy to address his behavior.

He has lost 1.8 kg (4 lb) in the last 60 days and his BMI is now 20 kg/m², physical examination and laboratory findings do not identify a cause for the weight loss.

Which one of the following is true for this patient?

(A) A second-generation antipsychotic agent would double his mortality rate compared with placebo.
(B) Citalopram at a dose of 40 mg would be the best choice for his symptoms.
(C) Control of symptoms with a second-generation antipsychotic agent would carry a higher risk of mortality than use of a first-generation agent.
(D) His symptoms justify use of a second-generation antipsychotic agent.

ANSWER: D

Second-generation antipsychotic agents carry a "black-box" warning because they are associated with an increased risk of mortality and stroke for persons with neurocognitive disorders. However, the risk of mortality expressed as the number of exposed individuals needed to demonstrate harm ranges from 50 to 100, not a doubling of the risk (SOE=A). Moreover, continued weight loss in this frail older adult is an imminent rather than potential threat, such that an intervention—even one with associated risks—is justified. Nonetheless, the effectiveness of second-generation antipsychotics is modest at best. First-generation antipsychotic agents do not exhibit lower risk and, depending on the agent, are more likely to prolong QT_c interval and increase the risk of an arrhythmia (SOE=A). Citalopram is often the first choice to combat agitation and psychosis (SOE=B), but doses >20 mg are associated with prolonged QT_c intervals. However, effectiveness was dose dependent with doses >20 mg considerably more beneficial.

68. A 72-year old man comes to the office because for the past 2 years he has had episodes in which he yells and behaves violently during sleep. The frequency and intensity of these episodes have increased over the past 6 months, to 3 or 4 nights per week. His wife states that he moves his arms as if he is punching or kicking, and speaks loudly and sometimes swears. He has fallen out of bed but has not sustained any injuries. He recalls sometimes dreaming that he is fighting or fending off an attack. His regular sleep time is 10 PM and wake time is 6 AM. He does not take any medications regularly.

On physical examination, neurologic findings are normal for his age.

Which one of the following disorders is most likely to develop in this patient?

(A) Alzheimer disease
(B) Parkinson disease
(C) Wernicke-Korsakoff syndrome
(D) Frontotemporal dementia

ANSWER: B

Vocalization or aggressive motor behavior, or both, occurring during sleep and associated with dream mentation and dream enactment is typical of rapid eye movement (REM) sleep behavior disorder (RBD). Persons with RBD have a loss of the normal muscle atonia that occurs in REM sleep. Diagnosis is based on history and polysomnography findings that demonstrate increased motor activity in REM sleep (REM sleep without atonia). Diagnosis also requires history or video evidence (from polysomnography) of dream enactment behavior. RBD is common in patients with Parkinson disease and is also associated with other synucleinopathies, such as dementia with Lewy bodies and multiple system atrophy. Longitudinal studies have shown that idiopathic RBD is a precursor of Parkinson disease and other synucleinopathies. The conversion rate can be as high as 80% over several decades (SOE=A).

Alzheimer disease and frontotemporal dementia are not typically associated with RBD, and RBD has not been shown to be a precursor or risk factor for these disorders. In some cases of RBD in patients with Alzheimer disease and other tauopathies, RBD may have been due to medications that alter REM sleep (SOE=C). There is no known association between Wernicke encephalopathy and RBD.

69. A 78-year-old man is brought to the office by his son, who is concerned about his unsteady gait and mild confusion in the past week. The patient had fallen at home that morning, with no consequent injury. The patient lives alone. He had mild dyspnea with accompanying cough 2 days ago; pneumonia was diagnosed, and he is currently on antibiotic therapy. History includes hypertension, depression, osteoarthritis, and mild gastritis. Current medications are duloxetine, hydrochlorothiazide, azithromycin, omeprazole, and naproxen. The patient's eating and drinking habits have not changed. He does not have any more dyspnea or cough. He never smoked.

On physical examination, blood pressure is 130/90 mmHg, heart rate is 78 beats per minute, respiratory rate is 12 breaths per minute, and temperature is normal. He is cognitively intact. Lung fields have clear breath sounds, and the rest of the examination is unremarkable.

Which one of the following diagnostic studies will reveal the most likely reason for this patient's symptoms?

(A) Complete blood count
(B) Chest radiography
(C) Serum electrolytes
(D) Plasma osmolality

ANSWER: C

Hyponatremia is the most common sodium disorder among older adults. The clinical manifestations of mild hyponatremia in this population include cognitive impairment, gait instability, and falls. This patient's use of the selective serotonin and norepinephrine reuptake inhibitor duloxetine, hydrochlorothiazide, and NSAIDs, along with the new onset of a pulmonary process, makes hyponatremia secondary to inappropriate antidiuretic hormone release (SIADH) the most likely diagnosis. Besides these common causes of SIADH, older adults are also known to have increased secretion of basal antidiuretic hormone, resulting in decreased ability to excrete free water.

Older guidelines recommended routine follow-up chest radiography at about 6 weeks after episodes of community-acquired pneumonia, presumably to screen for malignancy after an acute infiltrate has cleared. More recent guidelines recommend this practice only for patients with persistent symptoms or those at higher risk of underlying malignancy (especially smokers and those >50 years old). Repeat chest radiography will unlikely reveal any new lesions that can cause the patient's symptoms. The serum or plasma osmolality is a measure of the different solutes in plasma. Serum osmolality is indicated to evaluate the etiology only after a patient has been determined to be hyponatremic. It is unlikely that an anemia from a possible gastritis or upper gastrointestinal bleeding could produce this clinical picture.

70. A 75-year-old man is admitted to the orthopedic unit after surgery to repair a fractured right femur. He fell off a 6′ ladder, and approximately 6 hours passed before he was found, lying on his back in the yard. He had surgery 3 hours after arrival at the emergency department. The admitting nurse on the orthopedic unit documents a 7 × 10 cm purple-maroon discoloration at the sacral-coccygeal area; skin is intact. The discoloration is nonblanching and symmetric. It is documented as ecchymosis from a traumatic fall.

Which one of the following pressure injury designations describes the ecchymotic area?

(A) Deep-tissue injury
(B) Stage 1
(C) Stage 2
(D) Stage 3

ANSWER: A

This patient lay on hard ground for 6 hours, then was in the emergency department for an additional 3 hours, followed by surgery and recovery for another 3 hours. He was on his back for the entire time, until after the surgical procedure stabilized the fracture. The ecchymotic area is most likely a pressure injury, from sustained or prolonged pressure of laying on his back without repositioning.

According to the National Pressure Ulcer Advisory Panel, deep-tissue pressure injury refers to:

…Intact or non-intact skin with localized area of persistent non-blanchable deep red, maroon, purple discoloration or epidermal separation revealing a dark wound bed or blood-filled blister. Pain and temperature change often precede skin color changes. Discoloration may appear differently in darkly pigmented skin. This injury results from intense and/or prolonged pressure and shear forces at the bone-muscle interface. The wound may evolve rapidly to reveal the actual extent of tissue injury, or may resolve without tissue loss. If necrotic tissue, subcutaneous tissue, granulation tissue, fascia, muscle or other underlying structures are visible, this indicates a full-thickness pressure injury (unstageable, stage 3 or stage 4).... [The term *deep-tissue pressure injury* should not be used] to describe vascular, traumatic, neuropathic, or dermatologic conditions (SOE=C).

Sustained compression of tissue can cause a deep-tissue injury to develop rapidly. The first surface indicator may be deep purple discoloration that resembles a bruise. Deep-tissue pressure injuries can evolve into more extensive full-thickness loss. Research on pressure ulcers has focused on determining the minimal degree of loading (pressure) that will consistently lead to tissue damage. Evidence to date indicates that pressure-related damage may occur within a short period (minutes to hours), and the specific time frame and pressure intensity varies from person to person, depending on their clinical condition.

71. A 72-year-old man comes to the office because he has fallen several times. In the past year, he has felt increasingly less steady when he walks, and he now infrequently leaves the house. He has lost consciousness 7 times in the past 2 months. According to his wife, in each episode, he rose from bed after taking a nap and then suddenly collapsed to the floor unconscious. He remained unconscious and still for 10 seconds before regaining consciousness and full control of his body. The patient has no prodrome before losing consciousness. History includes advanced Parkinson disease, transient ischemic attacks, hypertension, and diabetes mellitus. Current medications are aspirin, carbidopa/levodopa, metformin, and lisinopril. There have been no recent dosage changes.

On physical examination, supine blood pressure is 110/80 mmHg and standing blood pressure is 100/80 mmHg, without any changes in heart rate. Mental status, cranial nerve function, and strength are normal. There is masking of facies, mild cogwheel rigidity in the wrists, bradykinesia, and loss of vibratory sensation in the feet. Ankle deep tendon reflexes are absent. Gait is slow. Electrocardiography and echocardiography findings are unremarkable.

Which one of the following is the most likely cause of his loss of consciousness?

(A) Insufficient dosage of carbidopa/levodopa
(B) Dysfunction of the autonomic nervous system
(C) Critical stenosis of the basilar artery
(D) Focal dysplasia of the right temporal lobe

ANSWER: B

Autonomic nervous system dysfunction can cause neurogenic orthostatic hypotension that presents as recurrent syncope. Patients with neurogenic orthostatic hypotension often report that syncope occurs within seconds of standing up. This patient's presentation is nonspecific for neurogenic orthostatic hypotension, and other causes should be excluded, such as volume status and medication adverse effects. Common causes of autonomic dysfunction are advanced Parkinson disease and diabetic neuropathy, the latter suggested by the patient's loss of vibratory sensation in the feet and lack of ankle deep tendon reflexes.

Carbidopa/levodopa may worsen orthostatic hypotension, and patients with a history of hypotension should be counseled on this potential adverse effect before starting or during upward titration of this medication. An insufficient dosage of carbidopa/levodopa is not likely the cause of this patient's recurrent syncope.

Symptomatic critical stenosis of the basilar artery (vertebrobasilar syndrome) can produce loss of consciousness, but it generally would be accompanied by other focal neurologic signs localizing to the brain stem and cerebellum, with deficits in cranial nerve, coordination, motor, and sensory systems. The patient's normal neurologic examination and lack of focal neurologic complaints, such as persistent vertigo and double vision, are not consistent with this diagnosis.

Focal dysplasia of the temporal lobe is a common cause of seizure. Seizures can cause loss of consciousness but generally do not follow an orthostatic pattern; more classically, they present with focal or generalized convulsive activity, which this patient does not have.

72. A 73-year-old man comes to the office because he is concerned about his risk of Alzheimer disease. His father was diagnosed with Alzheimer disease at age 73; there is no other family history of Alzheimer disease or other dementias. The patient has no cognitive symptoms and is in good health. He had a mild traumatic brain injury last year after a fall, but symptoms and signs resolved. He drinks alcohol, 1 or 2 standard drinks 3 days each week, but there is no evidence of alcohol abuse.

Which one of the following increases this patient's long-term risk of Alzheimer disease, compared with other older adults?

(A) His age
(B) Parent with Alzheimer disease
(C) Head injury without loss of consciousness
(D) Excess alcohol intake

ANSWER: B

As both the prevalence and awareness of dementia increase worldwide, questions regarding risk become more common. In addition to medical risk factors (hypertension, diabetes, smoking), a variety of other factors are associated with risk. This patient is at increased risk compared with the general population because of his age, his father's age at diagnosis, and his history of traumatic brain injury (SOE=A).

Family history is a significant risk factor: A history of 1 parent with Alzheimer disease confers a 2-fold higher risk for offspring, after controlling for education, smoking, presence of *APOE* genotype, and other vascular and known genetic risk factors. The parent's age at diagnosis is crucial; risk is increased primarily for those whose parent was <80 years old at time of diagnosis. Maternal and paternal dementia are associated with similar levels of risk (SOE=A).

Increasing age is a significant risk factor for both incident and prevalent Alzheimer disease. Approximately 19% of persons with Alzheimer disease are <75 years old, and risk increases substantially after age 65. In 2016, there were an estimated 63,000 new cases of Alzheimer disease among adults 65–74 years old in the United States (approximately 2 per 1,000 persons in this age group).

Compared with abstinence, light to moderate consumption of alcohol may have a protective effect on risk of Alzheimer disease. Although definition of "light to moderate" consumption varies by study, this patient is well within the range—his drinking does not place him at increased risk (SOE=B). It is not known what effect heavy consumption of alcohol has on risk of Alzheimer disease, in the absence of other factors.

Traumatic brain injury is a disruption in brain function due to an external mechanical force. Most typically, the injury is considered mild if it was of short duration (often <30 min), if Glasgow Coma Scale score was >12, and if there was no need for prolonged hospitalization. Mild traumatic brain injury is associated with increased risk of later neurologic disease; more severe head injury is associated with a higher risk. Persons who have had multiple traumatic brain injuries have a higher risk of dementia than those who have a single injury (SOE=A).

73. An 85-year-old man comes to the office because he has had lower energy levels and increased fatigue with his usual activities. History includes longstanding stable chronic kidney disease, stage 4.

Laboratory findings indicate stable renal function. Hemoglobin is 8.5 g/dL, with evidence of microcytosis. There is iron deficiency, with iron saturation at 8% and ferritin level at 85 ng/mL.

Which one of the following is the most appropriate next step for managing this patient's anemia secondary to chronic kidney disease?

(A) Course of intravenous iron
(B) Initiation of oral iron supplements
(C) Blood transfusion
(D) Initiation of erythropoietin

ANSWER: A

Anemia is common among patients with chronic kidney disease, and correction of hemoglobin measures improves both symptoms and quality of life. The anemia is mainly caused by a decrease in erythropoietin production in the kidneys; it can be partially corrected with administration of erythropoiesis-stimulating agents (ESAs). However, underlying treatable conditions, such as iron or vitamin deficiencies, must be excluded before beginning treatment with ESAs. Patients with chronic kidney disease often have concurrent iron deficiency, which must be corrected with intravenous administration of iron before administration of ESAs. Oral iron supplements are unlikely to correct the anemia of chronic kidney disease. Blood transfusion is not recommended; the goal of administration of ESAs is to limit blood transfusions and their associated complications. For erythropoietin to be effective, iron stores need to be repleted before treatment.

Studies looking at correction of anemia have found no benefit in higher hemoglobin targets; rather, there is evidence of harm in patients randomly assigned to higher targets. Higher hemoglobin targets (>13 g/dL) were associated with significant adverse effects, such as access-site thrombosis, strokes, and possibly cardiovascular events. In light of this, the KDIGO guidelines recommend that, in all adult patients, ESAs should be used to maintain hemoglobin levels at around 11.5 g/dL, not to increase levels to >13 g/dL.

74. An 82-year-old man comes to the office because he has pain at the site of a maxillary posterior tooth extracted 3 months ago by his dentist. History includes prostate cancer with bone metastasis, for which he has been treated with zoledronic acid infusion for the past 12 months. He has a 60 pack-year history of cigarette smoking.

On examination, the extraction socket has not healed, and the gingival tissue is open, with bone protruding from the site. The area is erythematous, with some purulent drainage and foul odor emanating from his mouth.

Which one of the following is the most likely diagnosis?

(A) Metastatic prostate cancer
(B) Osteonecrosis of the jaw
(C) Oral squamous cell carcinoma
(D) Incomplete tooth extraction with residual root

ANSWER: B

According to the American Association of Oral and Maxillofacial Surgeons, medication-related osteonecrosis of the jaw presents clinically as exposed bone that has not healed after at least 8 weeks in a patient who has not had radiation to the head and neck and who has no evidence of metastatic disease at the jaw. Its prevalence is up to 0.01% in patients receiving oral bisphosphonates, 12% in patients receiving intravenous bisphosphonates, and 16% in patients receiving a combination of bisphosphonates and bone-modifying agents such as denosumab or antiangiogenic agents. The increased dosages of antiresorptive therapy that are typically prescribed for cancer indications places patients with cancer at substantially higher risk for osteonecrosis of the jaw.

Osteonecrosis most commonly occurs after tooth extraction but can also occur with periodontal disease or trauma to the oral cavity, or spontaneously. The tendency of osteonecrosis to affect the maxillary bones can be explained by the greater concentration of bisphosphonates in these structures, which are subject to constant functional trauma from chewing and consequent constant bone remodeling. Clinical manifestations, such as intense pain, paresthesias, mucosal ulcerations, exposed underlying bone, fistula, and sometimes jaw fracture are characteristics of advanced medication-related osteonecrosis of the jaw. In early stages there are often no symptoms, and radiographic manifestations may not be detected (SOE=A). Although the lesion has signs of secondary infection, the underlying pathophysiology is necrotic bone rather than infection. In cases of infected bisphosphonate-related osteonecrosis of the jaw, oral antibiotics and antibacterial mouth rinses are usually adequate to treat the infection, without biopsy (SOE=B).

Prostate cancer is unlikely to metastasize to the maxilla. Tumors from distant organs and tissues infrequently metastasize to the oral cavity; according to the literature, metastatic tumors comprise only about 1% of all oral malignancies. The most common primary sites that metastasize to the oral cavity are lung for men and breast for women (SOE=B). Prostate cancer metastasizes most frequently to the spine before lung and liver in most patients.

Oral squamous cell carcinoma is more common in older than in younger adults, especially among smokers. It is generally asymptomatic until later stages, when it presents as an exophytic mass protruding from a nonhealing socket. It is usually not accompanied by infection (SOE= B).

Incomplete tooth extraction with residual root is unlikely because it does not usually present with bone extruding from the socket. Residual root can be easily excluded with radiography (SOE=C). Normal healing of the extraction socket produces soft-tissue healing within 1 month and bony healing by 6 months. Although healing may be slower in older patients, especially if they have diabetes, an extraction socket would not remain open for >6 months, unless there is underlying pathology (SOE=C).

75. A 70-year-old man undergoes evaluation as part of admission to a long-term care facility. He has lived alone in an apartment with home health services and family support, independently eating, ambulating, and managing his own medications, but he required help for most instrumental activities of daily living. However, over the past 3 months, he has had increasing fatigue, worsening ambulation, new urinary and fecal incontinence, and decreasing cognitive function. One of his daughters who lives nearby and visits daily initially resisted his relocation to a facility, noting that on some days "he is almost normal." Still, the changes prompted the decision to transition to long-term care. History includes mild dementia, myocardial infarction 1 year ago, benign prostatic hyperplasia, and osteoporosis. Current medications are donepezil, aspirin, metoprolol, rosuvastatin, losartan, furosemide, tamsulosin, calcium, and vitamin D.

On physical examination, vital signs are normal. He is alert and fully oriented, but he does not recognize family and is unable to follow simple commands. There are no convulsions. Muscle tone is normal. He is in a wheelchair wearing incontinence pads. There is 1+ pitting edema to the mid-shin bilaterally. The remainder of the examination is unremarkable. Echocardiography 1 year ago showed an ejection fraction of 38%.

Which one of the following is the best next step in evaluating this patient's functional decline?

(A) Standardized cognitive assessment
(B) Depression screen
(C) Electroencephalography (EEG)
(D) Lumbar puncture

ANSWER: C

For this patient with subacute decline in function and cognition and new urinary and fecal incontinence, new-onset seizure disorder must be excluded with an EEG. If the EEG is suggestive of seizure activity, the patient should be referred to neurology for further evaluation and treatment. Seizure disorder has a bimodal age distribution, with onset most common in children and older adults. New-onset seizures in older adults should raise suspicion for an underlying cause, such as anoxic or traumatic brain injury, ischemic or hemorrhagic stroke, or presence of a mass.

The incidence and prevalence of epilepsy in older adults is much higher than previously estimated, and average annual prevalence and incidence increases with age. Patients with Alzheimer disease and psychiatric disease have an increased incidence of new-onset seizures. This patient has mild dementia of unknown etiology, and he had a myocardial infarction 1 year ago, during which he could have experienced anoxia. He has no focal neurologic deficits to suggest the presence of a tumor or mass; the subacute onset and decline and the lack of focal neurologic deficits make ischemic or hemorrhagic stroke less likely. Nonetheless, neuroimaging should be performed alongside or after EEG to exclude these possibilities.

Standardized cognitive assessment should be performed on admission to a long-term care facility, particularly in the setting of mild dementia. However, given his subacute decline and history suggesting that his current cognitive status is far below his prior baseline, standardized cognitive assessment will not reveal the underlying cause of his cognitive decline. Furthermore, cognitive assessment is not reliable in the setting of ongoing seizure activity. Performing a standardized screen for depression, such as the Geriatric Depression Scale, would delay diagnosis of likely new-onset seizures; in addition, the standardized screen would be less effective in detecting depression in the setting of ongoing seizures. Depression can cause subacute cognitive decline in patients with dementia, or it can masquerade as dementia. This patient may be depressed, but depression would not explain more worrisome signs such as urinary and fecal incontinence, decreased ambulation, and inability to recognize family. Increasing the dosage of donepezil is inappropriate because the patient's subacute decline cannot be explained by the natural course of dementia. In addition, donepezil may slow the rate of cognitive decline, but it has not been shown to improve cognitive function.

Lumbar puncture is incorrect because there are no focal neurologic signs or any indication of infection.

76. An 82-year-old woman had a syncopal event while vacationing on Cape Cod with her family. It was a hot day, and she sat in the sun for about 2 hours. She passed out as she stood to go to the bathroom. History includes moderate aortic stenosis, hypertension, and mild Parkinson disease; there is a distant history of non–ST-elevation myocardial infarction (NSTEMI). She has been taking metoprolol for years for coronary heart disease and hypertension. She also takes chlorthalidone, selegiline, carbidopa/levodopa, atorvastatin, and aspirin. Echocardiography performed 6 months ago showed a 1.2-cm² aortic valve diameter and a 32-mm peak gradient. Systolic function was normal, but diastolic filling was mildly impaired.

Which one of the following is the most likely explanation for her syncope?

(A) Multifactorial etiology
(B) Cardiac ischemia
(C) Aortic stenosis
(D) Autonomic dysfunction

ANSWER: A

Although structural diseases such as aortic stenosis, conduction disease, ischemia, pulmonary hypertension, or their treatments (such as β-blockers or selegiline) may each cause syncope in older adults, a multifactorial etiology for syncope is relatively more common (SOE=B).

Orthostasis is a particularly common aspect of syncope in older adults when impairment of baroreceptors is compounded by poor hydration and excessive vasodilating medications or alcohol. Postprandial hypotension and diminished thirst with aging commonly exacerbate these susceptibilities.

Cardiovascular diseases (valvular heart disease, conduction disease, atrial fibrillation, pulmonary hypertension, amyloidosis) may contribute to syncopal risks, as do many noncardiovascular diseases (diabetes, Parkinson disease presenting with autonomic dysfunction, dementia, dehydration) and medications (including α- and β-blockers, calcium channel blockers, angiotensin-converting enzyme inhibitors, diuretics, and cholinergic medications).

Aortic stenosis is a common cause of effort syncope, when cardiac output cannot increase to meet demands. Pulmonary hypertension, atrial myxoma, hypertrophic cardiomyopathy, aortic dissection, and pulmonary emboli are less common abnormalities that can also predispose to syncope.

Bradyarrhythmia and tachyarrhythmia may potentially undercut cardiac output and increase risks of syncope. Bradycardia in older adults often results from medications (such as β-blockers) and from conduction disease and sick sinus syndrome. Atrial and ventricular tachycardias are also highly prevalent with age, and predispose to impaired cardiac output, particularly in combination with ventricular diastolic filling abnormalities.

Reflex-mediated etiologies of syncope, such as vasovagal syncope and carotid sinus syndrome, are common in older adults. Vasovagal syncope typically occurs from either unopposed vagal tone (cardioinhibitory) or from peripheral and splanchnic pooling (vasodepressor). In adults with carotid sinus hypersensitivity, pressure on the neck can trigger the carotid sinus and provoke decreased sympathetic tone, with excessive vasodilation, bradycardia, and diminished cardiac output.

77. A 75-year-old woman comes to the office for routine follow-up. On examination, blood pressure is 160/90 mmHg; the patient explains that she ran out of her medications a few days ago. She is increasingly exhausted by caring for her husband, who has Alzheimer disease. She has assumed responsibility for all driving. She manages his medications in addition to her own; their various refills are due asynchronously, so she goes to the pharmacy almost weekly. Last week she was delayed at the pharmacy; she came back to find that her husband left the house looking for her, and a neighbor had brought him back. She is now worried about leaving him alone.

At this visit, her and her husband's medications are reviewed, and the regimens simplified. The pharmacy is contacted and asked to synchronize dispensing so that she can pick up all prescriptions monthly, rather than weekly. The patient is reminded that she and her husband should avoid OTC agents, particularly antihistamines, because of their potential to cause delirium. The appointment runs significantly behind schedule.

Which one of the following would reduce her burden?

(A) Psychologic support and caregiver training
(B) Chronic care management services
(C) Nursing home placement
(D) Medication simplification

ANSWER: A

Several clinician-supported (versus medically focused) interventions have been shown to help caregivers cope, reduce their stress, and improve their confidence in responding effectively to a patient's needs. A meta-analysis of interventions found that evidence supports targeting caregiver psychologic well-being and education (SOE=A). Longer, more intense programs that incorporated caregiver education were associated with greater effects.

Models of this type of intervention include REACH,* REACH II, and REACH VA*, a randomized controlled trial and a propensity-score matched, retrospective cohort study, respectively, and the MIND at Home* pilot study, a randomized controlled trial. In REACH II and REACH VA, nonclinical counselors were trained to role-play, to discuss techniques to manage common caregiver situations, and to use a dyad-specific resource book, in both Spanish and English. The counselors then provided a 6-month multicomponent intervention for caregivers, comprising education, stress management, problem-solving, skills training, and telephone support (SOE=A).

The MIND at Home pilot (SOE=A) compared a needs-based intervention, specific to individual patients and caregivers, with augmented care as usual. Nonclinical memory care coordinators were trained to develop a care plan and implement a multidimensional 18-month intervention based on a multidomain-focused needs assessment of both the person with dementia and the caregiver. Caregivers were offered education regarding dementia and management of dementia-related behavioral symptoms, resource referral, and attention to general and mental healthcare.

Other models that are being tested include the ABC Program at Eskenazi Health in Indiana, which provides comprehensive medical home care that includes dementia care and support, and COACH, a Veterans Affairs program. These programs may not cost more to deliver, and the quality of care provided may be superior to that of traditional medical care alone.

Caregivers themselves recognize and identify the areas in which they need help. In a systematic review of 12 qualitative studies examining self-perceived needs of family caregivers of community-dwelling older adults, education and support were identified as broad themes: Sub-themes included information on basic and instrumental activities of daily living and neuropsychiatric symptoms, need for help with their own physical and psychologic well-being, and help managing their own lives (SOE=A). Most multicomponent interventions address these needs but are not widely available. Obstacles to widespread implementation include the heterogeneity of the target population and lack of societal agreement both on boundaries between personal autonomy and safety and on allocation of resources. However, it is widely accepted that clinicians should anticipate the emergence of cognitive and executive impairment in aging patients and recognize that dementia care involves a focus on two people—the person with dementia and the caregiver. Office staff should maintain an updated supply of information regarding resources for caregivers. The information available on the Internet can be overwhelming and inaccurate.

Besides their medical needs, the couple described in this case have needs that may be addressed by staff other than the clinician. The Centers for Medicare & Medicaid Services management fee codes for chronic care cover services overseen, but not directly provided, by the clinician. Whether chronic care management services would be effective at reducing caregiver burden is uncertain.

Given the demands on the caregiver, and the escalating nature of demands associated with dementia, many clinicians may suggest nursing home placement to reduce the caregiver's stress. However, stress and burden often persist after placement. Also, most people prefer to stay in their own home as long as possible. Respite may be an option, either through an adult day program or through an extended break, which many residential care facilities offer.

Simplification of the medication regimen is not known to reduce caregiver burden.

*REACH: Resources for Enhancing Alzheimer's Caregivers Health; VA: Veterans Affairs; MIND at Home: Maximizing Independence at Home; ABC: Aging Brain Care; COACH: Caring for Older Adults and Caregivers at Home

78. A 70-year-old man comes to the office for a routine health visit. History includes hypertension, benign prostatic hyperplasia, hyperlipidemia, and type 2 diabetes mellitus, controlled by diet. He lives alone and has no specific health concerns. In response to review of substance history, he states that he does not use tobacco and consumes alcohol occasionally. When questioned further, he reports that he drinks three 12-oz beers daily and never has >4 drinks on a single occasion. He has no desire to cut down on alcohol use, does not crave alcohol when he does not drink, has not had a change in his drinking habits, and has never withdrawn from alcohol.

Which one of the following would best define his drinking pattern?

(A) Low-risk drinking
(B) At-risk drinking
(C) Alcohol abuse
(D) Alcohol use disorder

ANSWER: B

For healthy adults ≥65 years old, at-risk drinking is defined as more than 1 standard drink per day (or more than 7 drinks per week) and no more than 2 episodes of binge drinking (≥4 drinks in 1 day) during a 3-month period. Low-risk drinking would be defined as intake below this standard. At-risk drinking is anything above this standard. Distinguishing at-risk from low-risk drinking is essential, because numerous health problems have been linked to at-risk drinking, including impaired driving, increased risk of stroke caused by bleeding, and increased risk of falls and fractures (SOE=A).

Alcohol use disorder is the term used by the *Diagnostic and Statistical Manual of Mental Disorders, Fifth Edition* (DSM-5) for problem alcohol use. Previously, in DSM-4, alcohol use disorder comprised 2 different diagnoses: *alcohol abuse* and *alcohol dependence*; the DSM-5 combination of these diagnoses into a single term indicates that the diagnoses lie along a spectrum of illness. Persons with at-risk drinking should be assessed for alcohol use disorder. The disorder is diagnosed when a person meets 2 of 11 criteria within a 12-month period. The severity of the disorder is based on the number of criteria present: mild disease, 2 or 3 criteria present; moderate, 4 or 5 criteria; and severe, ≥6 criteria. The criteria for diagnosis of alcohol use disorder follow:

- Consuming alcohol in larger amounts or over a longer period than intended
- Persistent desire or unsuccessful efforts to cut down on alcohol use
- Inordinate amount of time spent in activities necessary to obtain, use, or recover from alcohol
- Craving alcohol
- Recurrent alcohol use resulting in failure to fulfill major obligations at work, school, or home
- Continued alcohol use despite persistent social or interpersonal problems caused by such use
- Forgoing or reducing important social, occupational, or recreational activities to use alcohol
- Recurrent alcohol use in hazardous situations
- Use despite acknowledgement of persistent or recurrent physical or psychological problem related to alcohol
- Tolerance to alcohol (need for increased amounts to achieve desired effect, or markedly diminished effect with continued use of the same amount of alcohol)
- Withdrawal from alcohol, manifested by symptoms of withdrawal or use of alcohol or related substances to relieve or avoid withdrawal symptoms

Older adults who consume ≥4 drinks daily or who have alcohol use disorder are at greatest risk of physical disability and illness related to drinking. Identifying and reducing rates of alcohol use in this population has been linked to improvement in physical disability (SOE=B).

79. An 87-year-old woman comes to the office accompanied by her daughter, who has been caring for her at home. History includes Alzheimer disease. The daughter reports that the patient's condition has progressively declined over the past year. The patient is now fully incontinent, resists showering, does not sleep at night, and tends to wander out the door. The daughter cannot continue to take care of her mother and would like to move her to a facility that specializes in dementia care. She was told by a friend that Medicare will pay for the facility if the doctor signs an order. Neither the mother nor the daughter has financial resources.

Which one of the following is true regarding the role of Medicare in post-acute and long-term care services?

(A) Medicare will pay for skilled care at a nursing facility for 100 days; family is responsible for copayment after the first 20 days.
(B) The patient should apply for Medicaid, which will pay for her nursing home care.
(C) Medicare will pay for a part-time aide to help with basic activities of daily living in the patient's home.
(D) Medicare hospice services will pay for her room and board at a hospice facility.

ANSWER: B

Medicare Part A covers nursing care and subacute rehabilitation in a nursing facility under certain conditions for up to 100 days. A person with Medicare Part A is eligible to receive services for a condition requiring nursing or rehabilitation after a qualifying inpatient hospital stay (comprising 3 midnights), as determined by a physician. Outpatient emergency visits or observation stays do not count toward the qualifying days. Once a person meets criteria for a stay at a nursing facility, Medicare will cover 100% of the cost for days 1–20. For days 21–100, the patient is responsible for the copayment. This patient does not qualify for skilled services because she does not have an acute condition or a qualifying hospital stay. Some patients request hospitalization for 3 midnights to get coverage for the initial placement in a nursing facility. However, a person must meet hospital inpatient criteria to satisfy this rule, or otherwise would be engaging in Medicare fraud.

Nursing facilities can provide long-term care for patients with a mental or physical condition that requires regular health-related care and services, above the level of room and board, that are not available in the community. The long-term care is covered privately by the patient, by long-term care insurance arranged by the patient, or by Medicaid. Medicaid is a joint federal and state government program that helps people with low income and assets pay for some or all of their health care bills. Unlike Medicare, Medicaid pays for custodial care in nursing homes and at home. In addition to long-term care in a nursing home, Medicaid covers doctor visits, hospital costs, and long-term care services provided at home. Overall program rules for eligibility and covered services are based on federal requirements, but states have considerable leeway in how they operate their programs.

Medicare Parts A and B cover eligible home-health services, including intermittent nursing and other services, for homebound patients. The benefits do not require a preceding qualifying hospital stay, but the patient must have a face-to-face visit with a physician to determine eligibility. Medicare home-health services do not cover round-the-clock care at home, homemaker services, or help with activities of daily living.

Hospice care is covered by Medicare Part A. It is reserved for persons with a terminal condition who have a prognosis of ≤6 months, as determined by 2 physicians. Persons who choose hospice care forgo any treatment with curative intent, and instead focus their goals on comfort care. Medicare does not cover room and board in a nursing home except for short respite stays. Additionally, this patient does not yet appear to meet criteria for end-stage Alzheimer disease, so she would not qualify to receive hospice services as this time.

80. A 75-year-old white woman resides in a nursing home. She has moderate vascular dementia and chronic pain related to rheumatoid arthritis. She has an 11th grade education.

    Which one of the following is associated with the greatest likelihood that her pain will be undertreated?

    (A) Her age
    (B) Her race
    (C) Cognitive impairment
    (D) Education level

    ANSWER: C

    A recent cross-sectional study examined factors related to prescribing of opioids or NSAIDs within 30 days of pain onset for nursing home residents in the United States. Residents were ≥65 years old and had persistent, noncancer pain; patients with terminal illness, Alzheimer disease, or severe cognitive impairment were excluded. The study found that pain was undertreated in nursing home residents: 16.7% of residents with persistent pain received no prescription analgesics. After adjustment for potential confounding covariates, results showed that residents who are ≥95 years old, more cognitively impaired, or black or Asian are less likely to receive a prescription analgesic.

    Patients with dementia may not be able to report or localize their pain. Clinicians may also hesitate to prescribe pain medications, despite the presence of pain. In patients with cognitive impairment, the more significant the degree of impairment, the higher the odds of not receiving a prescription pain medication. For example, as compared with a patient with a Cognitive Performance Scale score of 0, a patient with a score of 4 (moderately severe impairment) had an odds ratio (OR) of 2.12 (95% confidence interval [CI], 1.71–2.62, $P<.001$). It is important to assess for common pain behaviors in cognitively impaired older adults. These include changes in facial expressions, verbalizations, body movements, interpersonal interactions and activities, and mental status (SOE=B).

    The odds of not receiving a prescription pain medication increases with increasing age. There was a small increased risk with patients 75–84 years old (OR 1.30; CI, 1.16–1.47, $P<.001$) and a significant age-associated risk with patients ≥95 years old (OR 2.06; CI, 1.70–2.49, $P<.001$) compared with patients 65–74 years old. Thus, this patient is at much greater risk of not receiving a prescription pain medication because of her cognitive impairment rather than her age.

    Black and Asian races were associated with a small increased risk of not receiving a prescription pain medication as compared with white race (black race: OR 1.20; CI, 1.03–1.39, $P=.02$; Asian race: OR 1.97; CI, 1.22–3.20, $P=.006$). Thus, this patient's white race would not be associated with an increased risk of pain undertreatment.

    Higher education level was associated with a small increased risk of not receiving a pain prescription. Compared with adults who did not graduate from high school, high school graduates had an OR of 1.10 (CI, 1.01–1.21, $P=.04$) and college graduates had an OR of 1.22 (CI, 1.02–1.46, $P=.03$).

81. A 75-year-old woman comes to the office because she has trouble sleeping. She goes to bed at 8 PM, sleeps about 3 hours, and tosses and turns for the rest of the night, getting up at 8 AM. She does not have nocturia, and she is not depressed. She exercises about 45 min/d by walking. She has tried OTC Tylenol® PM, but it leaves her groggy.

    Which one of the following should be recommended first?

    (A) Sleep restriction therapy
    (B) Relaxation therapy
    (C) Cognitive-behavioral therapy for insomnia
    (D) Referral for sleep study

    ANSWER: A

    The American Academy of Sleep Medicine, British Association for Psychopharmacology, and the American College of Physicians recommend use of behavioral therapies over medications as initial therapy for insomnia. Behavioral therapies can include sleep restriction therapy, relaxation therapy, cognitive therapy, and cognitive-behavioral therapy. Sleep restriction therapy involves limiting the total time spent in bed. Initially, patients keep a sleep log to help them determine the average number of hours they actually sleep each night. This average becomes the baseline for how long they may stay in bed. Once they are able to sleep for that amount of time, they may progressively increase the length of time they stay (ie, sleep) in bed. A systematic review showed a medium to large effect of this technique on subjective sleep variables, comparable to effects achieved with cognitive-behavioral interventions (SOE=B). Sleep restriction therapy has the advantage of allowing patients to improve quality of sleep on their own; this may be particularly useful when access to providers trained in cognitive-behavioral therapy for insomnia is limited.

Cognitive-behavioral therapy for insomnia is the most comprehensive approach (SOE=B). It combines several approaches over several weeks. Therapy may include sleep hygiene training, sleep restriction, and working with a therapist on issues related to anxiety and intrusive thoughts. Cognitive-behavioral therapy for insomnia has been shown to have moderate- to high-quality effectiveness in randomized trials, including improvement in sleep onset latency, wake time after sleep onset, and sleep efficiency (SOE=B). The benefits seem to last beyond the therapy course.

Relaxation therapy comprises progressive muscle relaxation, during which the patient relaxes 1 muscle at a time until the whole body is relaxed. One trial showed that progressive relaxation improved measures of sleep but not daytime function. Another randomized trial showed modest improvement in sleep measures but not as much as with cognitive-behavioral therapy (SOE=B).

Referral for a sleep study is inappropriate for this patient because she has no symptoms that suggest sleep apnea.

82. A 78-year-old man comes to the office for follow-up related to gout in the right first metatarsophalangeal (MTP) joint. He has not had gout pain for 2 weeks. He fell in his home twice in the last 2 weeks when doing his regular activities. He did not lose consciousness and does not know why he fell. He was not injured. In addition to gout, history includes hypertension, bronchitis, and osteoarthritis. He walks barefoot at home to avoid pressure on his right first MTP joint, and he is wearing sandals today.

On physical examination, when he is supine, blood pressure is 146/78 mmHg, heart rate is 85 beats per minute, and oxygen saturation is 95%. After he stands for 3 minutes, blood pressure is 135/76 mmHg, heart rate is 90 beats per minute, and oxygen saturation is 96%. Cognition and sensation are intact. Visual acuity is corrected with bifocal lenses, and visual field is intact. Dix-Hallpike maneuver is negative for dizziness or nystagmus. Range of motion is normal, except the patient reports stiffness at end range for hip flexion. Strength is 5/5 for all lower-extremity major muscle groups. There is bilateral hallux valgus, with no redness, swelling, or tenderness of the right first MTP joint. Gait speed is 1.1 m/s.

Which one of the following interventions is most likely to decrease his overall risk of falls?

(A) Prisms to improve peripheral vision
(B) Treatment of orthostatic hypotension
(C) Referral to a community-based exercise program
(D) Footwear modification

ANSWER: D

Improper footwear is associated with falls in older adults (SOE=C). Studies show that older adults often wear slippers or socks or walk barefoot in the home. Sandals generally offer little support and may be similar to walking barefoot.

Prisms are used to improve peripheral vision, particularly for persons with homonymous hemianopsia, a condition that results in visual field cuts on the right or left side. Affected persons may bump into people or objects on the side of the deficit, which may lead to increased accidental falls. This patient's visual fields are intact, and the history and examination findings do not support this cause.

Orthostatic hypotension is defined as a 20/10 mmHg drop in blood pressure when moving from supine to standing positions. Ideally, the second blood pressure measurement should be taken 2 minutes after the patient stands. Although this patient's blood pressure drops when he stands, the change does not meet the criteria for orthostatic hypotension. Additionally, the patient's history does not include lightheadedness, dizziness, or loss of consciousness, and his falls do not occur when he stands.

A community-based exercise program may benefit this patient for fall prevention, but the first intervention would still be to modify his footwear.

83. A 76-year-old black man comes to the emergency department because he has back pain that started after he fell from a ladder. He is a widower who lives alone. History includes heart failure. He does not have paresthesias, and the pain does not radiate; there have been no changes in bowel or bladder habits. Comprehensive neurologic examination shows no deficits.

Which one of the following is most likely to affect whether he will receive an opioid?

(A) His race
(B) His age
(C) Presence of heart failure
(D) His marital status

ANSWER: A

Disparities persist in prescribing of opioids for minorities. A 2008 study found that white patients with pain were more likely to receive an opioid than patients of other races; opioid prescribing rates were 40% for white patients and 32% for all other patients. In that study, differential prescribing by race or ethnicity was evident for all types of pain visits, and was more pronounced with increasing pain severity. Statistical adjustment for pain severity and other factors did not substantially attenuate these differences, with white patients remaining significantly more likely to receive an opioid prescription than black patients.

In a more recent study, differential prescribing by race or ethnicity was not found for all types of pain visits. However, compared with non-Hispanic whites, non-Hispanic blacks were less likely to receive an opioid prescription at discharge from the emergency department for back pain and abdominal pain, but not for toothache, fractures and kidney stones, after adjusting for other covariates.

Racial or ethnic minority patients with pain should be encouraged to accurately report pain intensity, and clinicians need to acknowledge their own belief systems regarding pain and to develop strategies to overcome unconscious, potentially harmful, negative stereotyping of minority patients.

The presence of heart failure and marital status has not been shown to affect the prescribing of opioids.

84. A 74-year-old woman comes to the office for routine follow-up. She works 3 days each week in a library, shelving books and doing activities with children. History includes hypertension, for which she takes amlodipine 5 mg/d. She asks whether she should take a multivitamin.

Which one of the following is the most appropriate recommendation?

(A) Take a generic multivitamin.
(B) Take a multivitamin specifically formulated for older women.
(C) Defer discussion until routine laboratory tests are completed.
(D) Eat a well-balanced diet instead of taking a multivitamin.

ANSWER: D

Vitamins are not synthesized in adequate amounts in human beings but are obtained through a regular, balanced diet. Recommended dietary amounts or allowances are the daily nutrient intake that meets requirements for most individuals. Deficiencies in vitamins may or may not have associated symptoms.

Despite lack of evidence, many older adults believe vitamin supplementation is necessary for overall health and well-being, including bone, joint, and heart health. Reviewing use of supplemental vitamins, the U.S. Preventive Services Task Force concluded that current evidence is insufficient to assess the balance of benefits and harms of single- or multivitamin use, specifically for reduction of cardiovascular or cancer risk. Further, the findings noted that β-carotene and vitamin E did not reduce the risk of either lung cancer or dementia. It is possible that the oxidative stress from supplementation might cause harm in some individuals.

Conversely, healthy diets have demonstrated benefits for prevention of disease and overall health. The Mediterranean, heart-healthy, and Nordic diets have all demonstrated benefits for the metabolic syndrome (SOE=A). These diets are low in sodium and contain fruits, vegetables, whole grains, dairy components, monounsaturated fatty acids, and omega-3 fatty acids. The Mediterranean diet has been noted to improve cardiovascular risk factors, reduce blood pressure, and improve overall quality of life (SOE=A). No adverse events are associated with any of these diets.

Many older adults do not eat a healthy diet. Routine laboratory tests may help to identify vitamin deficiencies, and when there are known deficiencies, supplementation of vitamins is appropriate. However, a multivitamin would not be sufficient for supplementation of specific vitamin deficiencies. Inappropriate use or overuse of some vitamins can result in adverse effects, such as diarrhea or nausea.

85. A 79-year-old woman is hospitalized for pneumonia. History includes chronic obstructive pulmonary disease (COPD), hypertension, hyperlipidemia, heart failure, and atrial fibrillation. This is her second admission in 6 months. The hospital team is ready to discharge her to home.

Which one of the following is most likely to help this patient avoid readmission to the hospital?

(A) Follow-up appointment with her provider
(B) Availability of community resources
(C) Involvement of a transitional care program
(D) Comprehensive discharge summary and medication reconciliation

ANSWER: C

Transitional care programs for home care after hospitalization, using directed discharge planning and follow-up protocols, reduce early repeat hospitalizations. For example, the Care Transitions Intervention®, a patient-centered self-management program coordinated by a health coach, reduces repeat hospitalizations. The Re-Engineered Discharge intervention, in which a nurse discharge advocate and a clinical pharmacist work together to coordinate hospital discharge, educate patients, and reconcile medications, was found to decrease emergency department and hospital use within 30 days of discharge. The Transitional Care Model uses an advanced-practice nurse to assist with the transition of frail older adults with complex medical needs; this model reduces rehospitalizations, length of time between discharge and rehospitalization, and costs of care.

Other interventions, such as medication reconciliation, comprehensive discharge summary review, assessment of community resources, and provider follow-up, also have been shown to impact readmission, and also are important to be addressed individually or, more effectively, as part of an overall transitions discharge program.

As outlined by the Joint Commission (and endorsed by several medical associations), each hospital discharge summary should contain the following key components: reason for hospitalization, significant findings, procedures and treatments provided, patient's discharge condition, patient and family instructions, and attending physician's signature.

In addition to reviewing the discharge summary, contact with the patient's caregiver may be essential in determining the patient's needs. Early follow-up should be arranged with the patient's primary care provider after hospital discharge. Several studies based on Medicare claims data indicate decreased rates of readmission with early follow-up, especially for patients at higher risk of hospital readmission.

Determination of community resources for this patient would be helpful, but it is not the first step for a patient who may be unsafe at home (SOE=D). Community services may provide additional support for patients who chose to reside in the home but require additional supervision or support. Community services vary by geographic location, and providers should be knowledgeable about access to local services. Referrals to social work services and the local Area Agency on Aging can also assist patients and families in identifying resources.

Caregiver support in this patient's home is also important to her ability to stay out of the hospital. Patients who require close supervision over a prolonged period require additional care by formal or informal caregivers. Special attention should be focused on the availability of the caregiver and the functional, social, and environmental barriers for patients. Functional limitations and difficulty with mobility and self-care tasks, social isolation and lack of support from family and friends, economic challenges, and the physical home environment also have all been shown to lead to readmission (SOE=B).

86. An 82-year-old man comes to the office for routine follow-up. He states that he is not sure he empties his bladder completely when he voids. He has had gradual onset of urgency with the need to void, and occasionally he experiences incontinence on the way to the bathroom. On average, he voids 8 times daily and twice overnight. He occasionally experiences hesitancy when initiating a void, and the stream is interrupted and weak. He describes post-void dribbling and staining on his undergarments. History includes hypertension, hypercholesterolemia, and stroke 2 years ago, with no residual weakness. Current medications are amlodipine, hydrochlorothiazide, rosuvastatin, and aspirin.

    On physical examination, blood pressure is 118/64 mmHg. The suprapubic area is slightly tender and dull to percussion. Genitalia are normal. The prostate is moderately enlarged and nontender, without nodularity or other abnormality. Bladder ultrasonography after attempted void shows postvoid residual of 175 mL. Urinalysis reveals no evidence of infection. Creatinine level is 1.1 mg/dL.

    Which one of the following is the most appropriate next step?

    (A) Stop hydrochlorothiazide.
    (B) Start oxybutynin.
    (C) Start tamsulosin.
    (D) Refer for urodynamic evaluation.

    ANSWER: C

    Tamsulosin, like many agents used to treat benign prostatic hyperplasia, acts via a mechanism of α-adrenergic antagonism (α-blockade) that reduces the dynamic resistance of the bladder outlet (SOE=A). Benign prostatic hyperplasia may cause both obstructive (pushing to begin void, starting and stopping stream, sense of incomplete emptying, weak stream) and irritative (frequency, urgency, nocturia) symptoms. Not all men with hyperplasia have symptoms. Men with benign prostatic hyperplasia may have symptoms of overactive bladder (urgency, urge urinary incontinence, nocturia, and frequency), but overactive bladder does not cause some of the severe obstructive-type symptoms that this patient experiences. Referral to a urologist is recommended for persistent urinary retention >300 mL after initiation of the α-blocker.

    Hydrochlorothiazide, a first-line therapy for hypertension, has a weak diuretic effect that generally wanes after the first month of therapy. It is unlikely to be a significant contributor to this patient's urinary symptoms.

    Most drug studies of bladder relaxants exclude persons with postvoid residual ≥150 mL. This patient would be at risk of worsened urinary retention if a bladder relaxant such as oxybutynin were started at this time. Urodynamic assessment would not be appropriate now but could be considered in the future if the patient is interested in a surgical approach. Urodynamic studies would confirm whether bladder outlet obstruction is contributing to the urinary retention.

87. A 78-year-old man comes to the office because he recently started a relationship with a new partner and he worries about his inability to maintain an erection. He is divorced and has 3 children from a previous marriage. He has had no memory loss, changes in mood, weight loss or gain, heat intolerances, skin or hair changes, reduced libido, or muscle weakness. History includes diabetes, hypertension, chronic obstructive pulmonary disease, depression, and obesity. Current medications are metformin 1,000 mg twice daily, lisinopril 10 mg/d, tiotropium 18 mcg/d, fluticasone/salmeterol 250/50, NPH insulin 15 U twice daily, aspirin 81 mg/d, and paroxetine 60 mg/d.

    On examination, temperature is 36.1°C (97°F), heart rate is 72 beats per minute, respiratory rate is 16 breaths per minute, and blood pressure is 136/64 mmHg. BMI is 35 kg/m². The prostate is slightly enlarged, with no nodules. Right testis is 11 cc and left testis is 12.5 cc.

    Laboratory findings:

Complete blood count	Normal
Hemoglobin A_{1c}	8.2%
Thyrotropin	1.24 mIU/mL
Total testosterone	200 ng/dL
Sex-hormone-binding globulin	8 nmol/L
Testosterone	
Free (calc)	5 ng/dL
Free and weakly bound	120 ng/dL

Which one of the following is the most appropriate initial step for managing this patient's erectile dysfunction?

(A) Start intramuscular testosterone cypionate, 150 mg every 2 weeks.
(B) Change paroxetine to mirtazapine.
(C) Start sildenafil, 100 mg one hour before sexual activity.
(D) Increase metformin to 1,500 mg twice daily.

ANSWER: B

Hypogonadism results in failure of the testes to produce testosterone, either because of primary failure of the testes (primary hypogonadism) or disruptions in the hypothalamic-pituitary-testicular (HPT) axis. Androgen deficiency should be diagnosed only when symptoms and signs of hypogonadism are supported by unequivocal low serum testosterone levels. In patients with an abnormal total testosterone level, especially when the level is near the lower limit of normal and when alterations in sex-hormone-binding globulin (SHBG) are suspected, free or bioavailable testosterone should be measured.

Obesity is one of several health conditions that can affect testosterone and SHBG levels. Although the exact mechanism is unclear, epidemiologic studies have shown that low testosterone and SHBG levels are associated with increased central adiposity.

All selective serotonin reuptake inhibitors (SSRIs) can cause delayed ejaculation, reduced libido, and erectile dysfunction. Some studies may suggest higher rates of sexual dysfunction with one SSRI over another, yet generally the differences between individual SSRIs are not clinically meaningful. Some studies have reported a prevalence of sexual dysfunction with paroxetine as high as 70%. Few studies suggest that either a dose reduction or change from SSRIs or serotonin-norepinephrine reuptake inhibitors (SNRIs) to alternatives such as bupropion or mirtazapine can improve sexual dysfunction (SOE=B).

Testosterone therapy is indicated in symptomatic men with classic androgen deficiency syndromes and unequivocal low serum levels, with the goal of maintaining secondary sex characteristics and improving sexual functioning. Testosterone therapy is contraindicated in men with a history of breast or prostate cancer and should be used with caution in men with a hematocrit >50%, untreated severe sleep apnea, severe lower urinary tract symptoms, or uncontrolled heart failure. Testosterone therapy can improve sexual function in men >65 years old, even in those with moderately low total concentration levels (SOE=A). However, given the association of SSRIs with erectile dysfunction and the likelihood that obesity is affecting this patient's total testosterone levels (note his free and weakly bound levels are normal), as well as the lack of other hypogonadal symptoms, it would be best to change the antidepressant before initiating hormonal therapy.

Sildenafil may be an appropriate next step in treatment of this condition, but it should not be the initial step. If sildenafil is considered, the lowest possible dosage (25 mg) should be used.

Better control of this patient's diabetes is indicated but will likely have little effect on his erectile dysfunction. However, he is taking the maximum dosage of metformin, so insulin dosage would need to be adjusted. Dosage adjustment of metformin is important in patients with impaired renal function. The target hemoglobin A_{1c} should be around 8% for patients in this age group.

88. Which one of the following interventions is *not* endorsed by a consensus of experts regarding treatment for physical frailty?

(A) Calorie and protein supplementation
(B) Hormone supplementation
(C) Vitamin D supplementation
(D) Reduction in polypharmacy

ANSWER: B

Most studies have been small or lack evidence that hormone therapy is associated with improvement in overall frailty (SOE=C).

There is some evidence to support the following as having some efficacy in the treatment of frailty (SOE=C).
- Exercise (resistance and aerobic)
- Caloric and protein support
- Vitamin D supplementation
- Reduction of polypharmacy

A systematic review found that 45–60 minutes of exercise 3 times each week seems to have positive effects on frail older adults and may be used for management of frailty.

Exercise in frail individuals increases functional performance, walking speed, number of chair stands per minute, stair climbing, and balance, and decreases depression and fear of falling.

According to the Cochrane Collaboration, calorie supplementation enhances weight gain and reduces mortality and complications in undernourished older adults.

In older adults who have a deficiency of 25(OH)D, there is evidence that vitamin D supplementation will reduce falls and hip fractures.

Polypharmacy is recognized as a possible major contributor to the pathogenesis of frailty. Hence, reduction in inappropriate medicines may decrease adverse effects in frail populations.

89. A 78-year-old man comes to the office because he is bothered by frequent nighttime urination. He gets up 2–4 times each night to urinate, and he urinates every 2–3 hours during the day. There is no discomfort or hematuria. History includes diabetes mellitus and hypertension. Current medications are hydrochlorothiazide 12.5 mg/d, losartan 100 mg/d, and extended-release metformin 500 mg/d. There is no history of heart disease, stroke, or other significant illness. Recent electrocardiography and laboratory findings (including urinalysis and prostate-specific antigen level) were normal. His hemoglobin A_{1c} was 7.8%.

On examination, blood pressure is 145/75 mmHg sitting and 137/68 mmHg standing. Heart rate is 73 beats per minute. His home blood pressure measurements are consistent with the office measurements. Prostate is 3+ enlarged, smooth, and nontender.

Which one of the following is the best choice to replace hydrochlorothiazide in this patient?

(A) Aliskiren
(B) Doxazosin
(C) Nebivolol
(D) Amlodipine

ANSWER: B

Doxazosin is an α-receptor blocker that can be an effective antihypertensive agent. Like other α-blockers, it reduces symptoms of prostatism by its effect on smooth muscle. For this patient, it offers a "2-for-1" therapeutic benefit.

Orthostatic hypotension is a known potential adverse effect; patients should be warned about the possibility of dizziness on standing. It is for this reason that doxazosin is on the American Geriatrics Society Beers Criteria® list of medications to use with caution in older adults. In this case, the benefit of treating both this patient's hypertension and benign prostatic hypertrophy may outweigh the risks associated with the adverse effects of doxazosin.

Aliskiren is the only direct renin antagonist approved by the U.S. Food and Drug Administration for treatment of hypertension. Because of its potential to impair renal function, aliskiren is contraindicated in patients taking an angiotensin-converting enzyme inhibitor (lisinopril) or angiotensin receptor blocker (losartan).

Nebivolol is a β-receptor blocker with vasodilator action. It is not indicated in the absence of coronary disease (angina, after myocardial infarction) or heart failure. It has no reported benefit for prostatism. β-Blockers are no longer indicated as first-line therapy for hypertension. Amlodipine, a dihydropyridine calcium channel blocker, is an effective antihypertensive drug, but has no benefit with regard to symptoms of prostatism.

90. A 62-year-old man comes to the office to discuss whether he should hire formal caregivers to help him care for his partner. His partner is 75 years old, has been HIV positive for 20 years, and has had progressive cognitive decline over the past 5 years. They have been together for 30 years and have combined finances. In the past few months, his partner has wandered out of the home in the middle of the night, and he almost started a fire by leaving a gas burner on. The patient telecommutes from home but is having trouble completing work projects because the partner is requiring more supervision.

For this couple, which one of the following is more likely to be a concern, compared with a heterosexual couple?

(A) Financial limitations
(B) Fear of discrimination by professional caregivers
(C) Caregiver burnout
(D) Loss of health insurance

ANSWER: B

There is longstanding, often justifiable, concern regarding involvement of formal caregivers and their attitudes toward lesbian, gay, bisexual, transgender (LGBT) persons. Fear of having to dissemble or hide ("re-enter the closet" or "straighten up the home") in anticipation of a professional caregiving arrangement can cause additional distress (SOE=B).

Financial constraints can affect all older patients regardless of sexuality. The cost of providing care services in the home can be considerable, even prohibitive. Incomes of older gay couples are similar to those of the general older adult population.

Caregiving for patients with dementia can increase risk of burnout regardless of sexuality. Further, among older LGBT persons, the potential absence of a caregiver can weigh more heavily (SOE=A). Many gay men anticipate that they will become caregivers to someone else, but 20% are unsure about who would eventually care for them. For un-partnered LGBT persons, 33% are unsure about care.

Like heterosexual couples, unmarried LGBT couples may not be able to provide health care insurance to their partners through their employers. With the Supreme Court decision allowing same-sex marriage, government and employers who offer health insurance to married heterosexual couples must offer the same benefits to same-sex couples. We do not know if the couple described above is married. Married same-sex couples with health insurance do not face any different challenges to maintaining that coverage than heterosexual couples.

91. A 74-year-old woman comes to the office because she believes that her ability to organize family activities and to remember appointments has declined. She cannot recall a specific point at which the decline began. History includes diabetes, hypertension, and coronary disease. She had right aortofemoral bypass for leg claudication 3 months ago.

On examination, vital signs are normal, and she appears well. She cannot spell "WORLD" backward and gets frustrated when attempting to do so. Pulses are normal, and there are no motor or sensory deficits.

Which one of the following is the most likely diagnosis?

(A) Parkinson disease
(B) Stroke
(C) Postoperative cognitive dysfunction
(D) Vascular dementia

ANSWER: C

Significant cognitive dysfunction sometimes occurs in the postoperative period, possibly manifested as an inability to perform executive tasks. The incidence of postoperative cognitive decline is not known, most likely because the entity is ill defined, and it is unclear how long the syndrome may last. Most patients return to their preoperative baseline within 3 months of surgery, though the dysfunction has been reported to last up to 5 years in patients who undergo cardiac surgery (SOE=C). The most common method of identifying postoperative cognitive decline is with neurocognitive testing, such as the Montreal Cognitive Assessment. Postoperative cognitive decline can lead to impairment in patients' quality of life, unintended exit from the workforce, and increased mortality (SOE=C). Although no strong data exist, a potentially modifiable risk factor for postoperative cognitive decline is to use lower doses of anesthetic agents. However, several meta-analyses found no difference between the incidence of postoperative cognitive decline in patients who received general versus regional anesthesia (SOE=A). In a large cohort of older adults undergoing inhalational versus intravenous anesthesia, patients who received inhalational anesthesia were more likely to have postoperative cognitive impairment, as evidenced by decreasing scores on the Mini–Mental State Examination (SOE=B); the reason for the difference is unclear. Few data exist as to the causes of postoperative cognitive decline, and there has yet to be any meaningful therapeutic intervention. Further studies are needed to elucidate the natural history of postoperative cognitive dysfunction.

Cognitive decline can be a sign of Parkinson disease, but this patient does not have rigidity, a resting tremor, or bradykinesia to support this diagnosis. Although stroke can also cause cognitive dysfunction, her specific neurocognitive abnormalities are not localizable. Infarction of a single area of the brain would not be expected to produce cognitive dysfunction without other abnormalities, such as aphasia, hemiparesis, or difficulty with coordination. Repeated small neurologic insults can result in cognitive decline, as evidenced in vascular dementia, but there is usually a stepwise progression of deficits that is identifiable either to the patient or to his or her caregivers.

92. An 80-year-old man comes to the office because he has had intermittent low back pain since he tripped and fell on an uneven walkway 8 weeks ago. He had no other injuries. He takes acetaminophen for the pain. Stretching and physical therapy have been helpful but have not eliminated the pain.

Which one of the following nonpharmacologic treatments has an effect on subacute low back pain?

(A) Bed rest for 2 weeks
(B) Massage
(C) Ice packs
(D) Lumbar support

ANSWER: B

For subacute low back pain, superficial heat, acupuncture, and massage can be helpful. Acupuncture involves placing small needles at specific points on the body meridians.

According to traditional Chinese medical theory, energy runs through the meridians; pain is a manifestation of energy that is "stuck." Studies show a small reduction in pain with acupuncture compared with NSAIDs (SOE=B). Massage involves manual manipulation of soft tissue. In the short term, it moderately improves subacute back pain (SOE=B). Superficial heat wraps are used to increase cutaneous blood flow to the area and have been shown to moderately improve subacute back pain (SOE=B). Ice packs do not reduce subacute low back pain.

Short periods of bed rest may be helpful, but prolonged bed rest is associated with deconditioning and longer rehabilitation.

Lumbar supports have not been shown in studies to be beneficial (SOE=B).

93. A 70-year-old man is being discharged after a hospital stay for a lower-extremity open, draining wound. He will need intravenous antibiotic therapy for 6 weeks, and the wound requires irrigation, packing, and dressing twice daily. He lives alone and does not have family or friends who live close by to assist in his care. He would like to go home, but he is willing to consider placement if necessary.

Which one of the following is the most appropriate location for discharge for this patient?

(A) Acute rehabilitation facility
(B) Skilled nursing facility
(C) Home, with home care
(D) Continued inpatient stay

ANSWER: B

The decision of where to discharge is often one of the most challenging recommendations to make during discharge planning. There are no standardized tools to assist providers in these decisions. Discharge planning should begin when the patient is admitted to the hospital and should be considered throughout the hospital stay. Because of the variability in a patient's hospital course, it can be difficult for providers to track the various elements that need to be considered when choosing appropriate postacute care. The electronic health record (EHR) and specialized algorithms, such as the Decision Support and Discharge Screening (D2S2) tool that can be embedded into the EHR, can calculate readmission risk and recommend potential sites for postacute care. Thorough assessment and documentation within the EHR can help the health care team make the appropriate recommendation for postacute care (SOE=A).

Many patients have informal caregivers who can provide most of the needed care. However, at times the care required can exceed the capabilities or availability of the caregiver. Patients who are discharged from the hospital often have impaired function that contributes to an increase in needs. Selecting the appropriate postacute discharge location can reduce readmissions and limit adverse events.

A skilled nursing facility is the most appropriate choice for this patient, given the lack of home support and his need for intravenous administration of antibiotics and twice-daily wound care. If indicated, the patient can obtain physical therapy while at the nursing facility. The frequency of therapy has been associated with a decrease in length of stay for Medicare-eligible patients. Before recommending placement in a skilled nursing facility, the patient's eligibility should be determined. The person must need skilled care (in this case, because of the use of parenteral antibiotics and twice-daily wound care) to be covered by Medicare. Medicare covers a stay in a skilled nursing facility for up to 100 days, with co-payment after 20 days.

A thorough discharge plan is imperative for care coordination with providers at the next site of care. Discharge instructions for both the patient and the postacute care team require detailed accounts, especially when there is no common EHR. The discharge summary should include medication reconciliation, test results, and pending tests, in addition to summary of hospital course, list of primary diagnosis and comorbidities, advance directives, and plan of treatment.

The information provided for this patient does not include evidence of deconditioning or limitations with functional status; discharge to acute rehabilitation cannot be recommended without such information. The recommendation to discharge a patient to acute rehabilitation is made collaboratively by an interdisciplinary team. During hospitalization, a thorough assessment from a physical or occupational therapist, or both, is required to determine whether the patient meets eligibility requirements. Referral to acute rehabilitation requires that the patient be able to participate in ≥3 hours of intensive therapy daily. The patient would be able to receive intravenous therapy, but the primary focus in a rehabilitation facility is to restore functional capabilities.

When there is appropriate home care and transitional care services are in place, patient discharge to the home is most beneficial in terms of health outcomes. For this patient, home would not be the best location for postacute care because of the lack of caregiver support and the need for nursing attention.

Delaying hospital discharge is also not the best option for many reasons, including lack of insurance reimbursement for non-medically needed hospital days, high risk of hospital-acquired infections, and increased risk of delirium for older adults with prolonged hospital stays.

94. A 55-year-old woman with Down syndrome is brought in by her parents, with whom she has lived her entire life. They are concerned because she has had a change in her ability to perform previously mastered tasks, as well as a change in behavior, becoming more easily agitated and more difficult to calm than previously. They cannot give a clear idea of when the changes began, but report that their son visited recently and noticed a difference compared with when he last saw his sister 1 year ago.

Which one of the following is the best pharmacologic treatment for this patient?

(A) Memantine 5 mg/d
(B) Memantine 10 mg/d
(C) Donepezil 5 mg/d
(D) Donepezil 10 mg/d

ANSWER: C

Diagnosing and treating dementia in any patient can be challenging, even more so in patients with intellectual disabilities. Because of the underlying cognitive deficits in patients with Down syndrome (as well as those with other intellectual disabilities), the earliest signs of dementia often go unnoticed, and they tend to receive a diagnosis of dementia later in the disease process. The increased risk of Alzheimer disease is significant in Down syndrome: neuropathologic changes develop in essentially all patients by age 40, and up to 75% of patients are clinically affected by age 60. The gene for amyloid precursor protein is located on chromosome 21;

this may account for the extremely high incidence of Alzheimer disease in patients with Down syndrome. The time between diagnosis and death is shorter than in other populations and is likely multifactorial—diagnosis at a later stage, lower premorbid functioning, and perhaps other factors not yet identified.

Treatment recommendations for dementia in patients with Down syndrome are identical to those for Alzheimer disease in the general population. A cholinesterase inhibitor is considered first-line treatment (SOE=A). Galantamine is indicated in mild to moderate disease, and donepezil or rivastigmine is indicated in mild to severe disease. Memantine is used in moderate to severe disease; it is not indicated for monotherapy and is generally added to treatment with a cholinesterase inhibitor.

Any medication should always be used at the lowest effective dosage; because persons with Down syndrome are often sensitive to medication adverse effects, it is especially important to start at the lowest dosage possible. This is particularly prudent for donepezil, which carries a risk of seizures, which are fairly common in Down syndrome.

95. An 88-year-old man requires a home visit for medical care. His wife called this morning to report that a new pressure injury developed on his right leg over the past 48 hours. He is homebound because he has severe lumbosacral spinal stenosis, with partial paralysis of his lower limbs. His wife is his full-time caregiver. History also includes coronary artery disease, peripheral vascular disease, and type 2 diabetes mellitus with peripheral neuropathy. He has an indwelling Foley catheter. He has no pain, fever, or chills. He reports increased drainage over the past 24 hours.

On examination, there is a 2 × 3 pressure injury on his right lower leg. The injury is eroding into the muscle layer and has a necrotic base. The patient's cognition is intact. Permission is obtained to photograph the lesion and transmit the image to a consulting dermatologist for advice.

The patient's insurance coverage is through Medicare Part C fee-for-service.

In addition to the patient's county of residence, which one of the following will affect payment for the dermatology consultation?

(A) Real-time communication with the consultant
(B) Consultant's county of practice
(C) Severity of the illness under review
(D) Physician–physician nature of the communication

ANSWER: A

Telemedicine modalities for diagnosis and management of homebound patients continue to increase. Early examples included scales for monitoring weight of patients with heart failure; current technologies can include monitoring of cardiac rhythm, transmission of images, and therapeutic interviewing, such as behavioral health intervention.

Reimbursement has been a primary barrier to use of these modalities (internet access technology may also be a limiting factor in some homes or areas). The Centers for Medicare & Medicaid Services is developing reimbursement strategies. As of 2018, Medicare compensates for telemedicine services for patients who reside in a county outside a metropolitan statistical area, or in a Health Professional Shortage Area located in a rural census tract. Also as of 2018, Medicare requires that the audio/visual communication system allow real-time communication between providers. Stored information that is reviewed at a later time is compensated only in demonstration project settings.

A wide variety of health professionals are covered for reimbursement, in addition to physicians.

There is no minimum standard of severity of diagnosis or illness that is required for telemedicine consultation.

96. A 79-year-old woman comes to the office because she has chronic, severe, persistent pain in multiple joints. History includes osteoarthritis, hypertension, and chronic kidney disease. Medications include acetaminophen 650 mg every 8 hours. She does physical therapy–prescribed exercises daily, with minimal relief. The pain prevents her from such activities as grocery shopping and cleaning. Injection of corticosteroids into the joints no longer provides relief. The patient agrees to try low-dose oxycodone. She states that in the past she felt unwell when taking narcotic analgesics and is worried about adverse effects.

Which one of the following should be prescribed for this patient to treat the most common adverse effect of oxycodone?

(A) Methylphenidate
(B) Naloxone
(C) Prochlorperazine
(D) Senna

ANSWER: D

The most common adverse effect of opioid therapy is constipation, which results from many factors, including decreased gastrointestinal secretions, decreased intestinal motility, and dehydration. Tolerance does not develop to this adverse effect. Senna is a stimulant laxative that is helpful in opioid-induced constipation. Stimulant laxatives should not be prescribed to patients with signs or symptoms of bowel obstruction. Stool softeners do not stimulate the bowels and are often insufficient for opioid-induced constipation. Bulking agents, such as fiber and psyllium, should be avoided in frail, older, inactive adults who have poor fluid intake because they pose a risk of fecal impaction and obstruction.

Other potential adverse effects of opioids are sedation, respiratory depression, and nausea and vomiting. Patients usually overcome the sedation from opioids within days to weeks as tolerance develops. Patients should be warned about the increased risk of falls and should be counseled not to drive or operate heavy equipment after starting opioids. A small number of patients experience excessive sedation, limiting their function; for these patients, a short course of low-dose methylphenidate may be useful (SOE=D).

Respiratory depression, the most serious potential adverse effect of opioids, is an adverse effect to which tolerance usually develops rapidly. Naloxone can reverse opioid-induced respiratory depression. However, because naloxone can precipitate a pain crisis and acute withdrawal symptoms, treatment should be delayed as long as possible, with careful observation of respiratory rate and oxygen saturation.

Nausea and vomiting are common and often resolve after the first few doses of opioids. In patients with persistent nausea, reversible causes (such as constipation) should be excluded, and it may be worthwhile to switch to an alternative opioid (SOE=D). Antiemetic agents, such as prochlorperazine, can be used, with close attention paid to potential adverse effects.

97. An 84-year-old nursing home resident recently completed a course of antibiotics for urinary tract infection (UTI). She had a previous UTI approximately 6 months ago. She has occasional stress incontinence, which is unchanged from baseline, but otherwise has no urinary symptoms. History includes mild Alzheimer disease and distant breast cancer. Her daughter asks how UTIs can be prevented in the future. Examination shows no palpable bladder. She has atrophic vaginitis.

Which one of the following options should be considered in this patient?

(A) Oral cranberry capsules
(B) Oral ciprofloxacin
(C) Intravaginal metronidazole
(D) Intravaginal estrogen

ANSWER: D

A few small studies support use of intravaginal estrogen to reduce recurrence of UTI in postmenopausal women, particularly with the presence of atrophic vaginitis/urethritis.

Several studies have shown no effect of cranberry (either juice or capsules) in preventing recurrent UTIs. The most recent study evaluated 185 older women in a randomized, double-blind study. After 1 year, there was no significant difference between the two groups in the presence of bacteriuria with pyuria (SOE=A). Prophylactic antibiotics have some efficacy in preventing UTI recurrences, but there is a significant risk of *Clostridium difficile* infection and the emergence of drug-resistant bacteria. Thus, oral antibiotics should not be offered as part of a first-line approach to prevent UTIs. Further, ciprofloxacin has the potential to cause confusion and arrhythmias in older adults.

There is no role for intravaginal metronidazole in the prevention of UTIs.

98. A 69-year-old postmenopausal woman comes to the office because she is concerned about her bone health. She does not have a personal history of fragility fracture; her mother sustained a left hip fracture after a fall at age 68. Bone densitometry screen (DXA) done 4 years ago showed osteopenia. She is at low risk of fracture based on her Fracture Risk Assessment (FRAX®) score. History includes type 2 diabetes mellitus, which has been well controlled for 15 years, previously with a thiazolidinedione and currently with a sodium/glucose cotransportor-2 (SGLT-2) inhibitor. Recent hemoglobin A_{1c} was 7.2%. She quit smoking 10 years ago and rarely drinks alcohol. Arrangements are made for repeat DXA scan, including trabecular bone score.

Which one of the following is true about this patient's trabecular bone score?

(A) It is associated with an increased risk of osteoporotic fracture in postmenopausal women with type 2 diabetes mellitus.
(B) It entails additional images and radiation exposure for the patient.
(C) It can be used to monitor response to osteoporosis treatment.
(D) Her low score is correlated with lower fracture risk.

ANSWER: A

Postmenopausal women with diabetes have higher bone mineral density but lower trabecular bone score than women who do not have diabetes. Trabecular bone score helps predict fracture in this group of patients and may be particularly useful in other patient groups for whom bone mineral density may be high, but fracture risk is increased (SOE=C).

Trabecular bone score is a gray-level textural measurement that uses the 2-dimensional images already obtained by DXA scan; it does not require additional images or radiation. A high score indicates better bone microarchitecture and lower fracture risk. The use of changes in trabecular bone score has not been validated for monitoring efficacy of therapy.

99. A 72-year-old man comes to the emergency department because he had sudden onset of vertigo, nausea, blurry vision, and left facial numbness while watching television. The symptoms lasted a few minutes before resolving completely. He had 2 similar episodes over the previous 3 days. History includes hypertension and hyperlipidemia. He has a 50 pack-year history of cigarette smoking.

On examination, blood pressure is 153/90 mmHg, heart rate is 78 beats per minute and regular, respiratory rate is 14 breaths per minute, and oxygen saturation is 98% on room air. Neurologic and all other findings are normal. Computed tomography (CT) of the head is normal.

Which one of the following would most likely establish the diagnosis for this patient?

(A) Dix-Hallpike test
(B) CT angiography of the head and neck
(C) Doppler ultrasonography of the carotid arteries
(D) Magnetic resonance imaging (MRI) of the brain

ANSWER: B

When a patient presents with dizziness, it is important to determine whether he or she is referring to vertigo, presyncope, dysequilibrium, or a psychogenic incident. Patients should be asked to describe their symptoms without using the word "dizzy." Vertigo refers to the perception that the world is spinning around the person, or that the person is spinning in a stationary world.

This patient reports episodic vertigo in addition to other neurologic symptoms. Both his history of vascular risk factors and the localization of his symptoms to the brain stem are highly concerning for transient ischemic attacks (TIAs) in the vertebrobasilar distribution. Patients who have TIAs because of vertebrobasilar insufficiency commonly describe vertigo with associated brain-stem symptoms such as diplopia, numbness (which may be crossed on the face and body), ataxia, nausea and vomiting, and weakness. Therefore, urgent imaging of the vessels is indicated. CT angiography offers a quick, accurate method to assess for cerebrovascular stenosis. If cerebrovascular stenosis is present, pharmacologic or neurointerventional management may be undertaken to prevent progression to a posterior circulation stroke.

Benign paroxysmal positional vertigo (BPPV) is a common cause of episodic vertigo and its incidence increases with age. Patients often describe brief episodes (lasting seconds) of vertigo when they roll over in bed or turn their head. BPPV is thought to be caused by disordered endolymph movement related to dislodged otoconia in the semicircular canal. It is most easily diagnosed with a consistent history and a positive finding on Dix-Hallpike test. Because BPPV is a peripheral process, there are no accompanying brain-stem signs. Because this patient has symptoms of brain-stem pathology, the Dix-Hallpike test would not establish the diagnosis.

Doppler ultrasonography of the carotid arteries is commonly performed in the evaluation of TIA. However, it assesses only large-vessel anterior circulation, and would not identify posterior circulation stenosis.

Because this patient's symptoms are transient and findings are normal on the neurologic examination, it is unlikely that an infarct will be found on MRI. Further, the evaluation for TIA focuses on finding potential areas of intervention. Thus, CT angiography is preferred over an MRI as the next step.

100. A 65-year-old man with a history of atrial fibrillation is admitted to a skilled-nursing facility because he had a middle cerebral artery stroke. He has unilateral weakness and dysarthria. In his work with occupational therapy, he has difficulty with recent memory but no difficulty with word-finding. After 2 weeks of rehabilitation, his cognition remains impaired, and improvement in overall functional status is less than expected. Score on the Patient Health Questionnaire-9 (PHQ-9) is 15; Montreal Cognitive Assessment score is 21/30. Laboratory findings are normal.

Which one of the following is the best next step in management?

(A) Start oral donepezil 5 mg/d and titrate.
(B) Start oral memantine 5 mg/d and titrate.
(C) Order computed tomography of the head.
(D) Start sertraline 50 mg/d and titrate.

ANSWER: D

The most likely cause of this patient's lagging improvement is depression. Although depression develops in nearly 30% of stroke patients, the association between the two continues to be under-recognized. Untreated, depression can affect functional recovery and manifest in signs of cognitive impairment (SOE=B). A PHQ-9 score of 15 indicates moderate to severe depression. Treatment with a selective serotonin reuptake inhibitor may help his depression and result in improved cognition, with the possibility of improving his rehabilitation potential (SOE=A).

Donepezil and memantine are acceptable treatment options for patients with a diagnosis of dementia but might not significantly benefit this patient with untreated depression.

Unless there are significant changes in his mental status or new, focalized neurologic deficits are present, computed tomography of the head will not modify the treatment plan.

101. A 90-year-old woman comes to the office for a routine visit. She lives alone in a 2-story house and no longer drives. She is accompanied by her daughter, who is visiting from out of town. She is enrolled in both Medicare and Medicaid. History includes lumbosacral spinal stenosis, osteoporosis (old T12 compression fracture), chronic low back pain, and macular degeneration. Current medications are acetaminophen and alendronate. The daughter mentions that the house is less clean than in the past, and the patient admits that she finds cleaning, shopping, and laundry increasingly burdensome. No family members live locally, and she does not want people whom she does not know in her home. She would consider relocating to preserve her independence.

On physical examination, height is 1.5 m (5 ft) and weight is 37 kg (82 lb), a 2.7-kg (6-lb) loss over 6 months. There is kyphosis with bilateral lumbosacral paravertebral spasm. There is no midline tenderness. Lower-extremity reflexes are normal.

Laboratory findings are normal except for hemoglobin level of 11.8 mg/dL and albumin level of 2.8. Urinalysis is normal.

Which one of the following community supports is most appropriate for this patient?

(A) Assisted-living facility
(B) Senior apartment
(C) Continuing-care retirement community
(D) Adult day care

ANSWER: A

This patient is not maintaining her weight, and she is having difficulty managing her home environment. She has no family locally, and she prefers to move rather than have aides or other workers in her home. She would benefit from an environment that offers meals and supports instrumental activities of daily living. This combination of services is available in assisted-living facilities. Services vary by ownership and location but always include meals, cleaning and laundry services, social activities, transportation, and medication oversight. Although options are more limited, there are facilities that will accept Medicaid at admission. The patients or family members pay most costs of care. Many facilities provide additional services at added cost.

Senior housing is usually in apartment settings in a building with security and maintenance. Residents must be able to live independently in their apartments; meals are not provided. Individual residents may arrange for community support services, such as home health aides to assist with social activities and basic and instrumental activities of daily living. Larger buildings may have consulting arrangements with social workers or visiting nurses to assist residents. The patient in this case needs help with shopping, cleaning, laundry, and preparing meals. A senior housing unit would not reduce the burdens she currently has.

Continuing-care retirement communities offer a range of settings under a single management entity and often on a single campus. While payment models vary, most require a substantial fee up front to enter the community. In some, a resident must enter the community in the "independent living" area of the community. Home care support, assisted-living facilities, and nursing home facilities are available as the resident's needs increase. The community usually provides care management during transitions. All charge monthly fees, depending on location and services. This patient has limited resources and would be unable to afford a continuing-care retirement community.

Adult day care offers lunch, social activities, and exercise. Many also offer custodial care and more advanced services. This patient would remain alone in the morning and at night, and be responsible for meals, medications, and home maintenance. While paid caregivers could be hired to come to her home, she does not want strangers in her home and she needs more support than day care can offer.

102. An 88-year-old man is brought to the emergency department because he is confused. His daughters accompany him; over the past several weeks, they had noticed that he was becoming more forgetful and confused, forgetting information he knows well, such as his daughters' phone numbers and even his birthday. They report that he has had no recent illness, but that he was started on citalopram and ranitidine 3 weeks ago by his primary care clinician. History includes gout, osteoarthritis, peripheral vascular disease, heart failure, gastroesophageal reflux disorder, and mild cognitive impairment. Current medications are aspirin 81 mg/d, metoprolol 50 mg twice daily, simvastatin 40 mg/d, ranitidine 150 mg twice daily, allopurinol 100 mg/d, acetaminophen 650 mg three times daily, and citalopram 20 mg/d.

On physical examination, temperature is 36.1°C (97°F), heart rate is 72 beats per minute, respiratory rate is 16 breaths per minute, and blood pressure is 126/64 mmHg sitting and 119/62 mmHg standing. BMI is 21 kg/m². The patient is pleasant and in no distress; he is alert and oriented to place but not to year, month, or day. There are lung crackles but no rhonchi or wheezing. The prostate is slightly enlarged. There is 1+ nonpitting edema and reduced muscle tone and bulk. Score on the Mini-Cog™ is 1/5. All other findings are normal.

Laboratory findings:

Complete blood count	Normal
Glucose	91 mg/dL
Sodium	121 mEq/L
Potassium	5 mEq/L
Chloride	86 mEq/L
Serum bicarbonate	25.0 mEq/L
Creatinine	0.57 mg/dL
Serum osmolality	268 mOsm/kg
Urine osmolarity	590 mOsm/kg
Urine sodium	132 mEq/L
Urine creatinine	93 mg/dL
Thyrotropin	1.24 mIU/mL
Cortisol (AM)	17 mcg/dL

In addition to restricting free water to normalize the patient's sodium levels, which one of the following is the most appropriate initial step in managing his confusion?

(A) Start furosemide 40 mg IV daily.
(B) Start normal saline at 150 mL/hr.
(C) Taper off citalopram.
(D) Stop ranitidine.

ANSWER: C

The combination of low serum osmolality and high urine osmolarity, along with normal thyrotropin and morning cortisol readings, suggests that this patient has syndrome of inappropriate antidiuretic hormone secretion (SIADH). Selective serotonin reuptake inhibitors (SSRIs) such as citalopram, along with sulfonylureas, antiepileptic agents, and tricyclic antidepressants, have been associated with SIADH. In a retrospective study in Canada of >100,000 patients, SSRI use was associated with a higher 30-day hospitalization risk with hyponatremia (relative risk 5.46 [95% confidence interval, 4.32–6.91]) and hyponatremia and delirium (relative risk 4.00 [95% confidence interval, 1.75–9.16]). Therefore, it is most reasonable to taper the dosage of citalopram, in addition to restricting free water (SOE=B).

Because older adults are at risk of water and electrolyte imbalances, acute or chronic hyponatremia is a common cause of delirium. Urine-concentrating ability, osmoreceptor and baroreceptor systems, and thirst sensation—all regulators of antidiuretic hormone (ADH)—are blunted in older adults, thereby creating an excess of ADH and predisposing to hyponatremia. Even a mild decrease in sodium can result in a clinically meaningful event. In addition to its ability to cause cognitive impairment, hyponatremia is an independent risk factor for falls and fractures because it is associated with changes in gait and balance and increased risk of osteoporosis.

The patient's volume status can help identify the cause of hyponatremia. Hypervolemic hyponatremia is generally caused by volume-excess disorders such as cirrhosis, heart failure, or occasionally kidney failure. This patient has a history of heart failure, but examination findings suggest that he is not volume overloaded. Therefore, a loop diuretic is not indicated. Hypovolemic hyponatremia is characterized by low total body volume, but that is not supported in this case, given the patient's relatively normal blood pressures and absent orthostatic changes.

Ranitidine and other H_2 blockers have been associated with delirium (SOE=B). Although it would be reasonable to discontinue the ranitidine, tapering the citalopram is more likely to address the delirium.

103. Which one of the following is true regarding male compared with female centenarians?

(A) There are half as many men as women.
(B) Men are more likely to be functionally independent.
(C) Men have a higher prevalence of chronic cardiovascular disease.
(D) Men are more likely to be taking medications.

ANSWER: B

Female centenarians outnumber male centenarians 9 to 1 (SOE=A). However, centenarian men are much more likely to be functionally independent than their female counterparts (SOE=A). Male centenarians are also more likely than female centenarians to escape or delay age-related diseases. In their 80s and 90s, men generally have higher mortality rates associated with age-related diseases, such as heart disease, stroke, chronic obstructive pulmonary disease, and diabetes. Relatively more men than women die of these diseases, but the women who survive incur attendant chronic disabilities. Surviving male centenarians have fewer diseases and take fewer medications (SOE=A). Men who survive age-

104. A 67-year-old man comes to the office for follow-up after discharge from a nursing facility where he recovered from below-the-knee amputation of his left leg. While in the nursing home, he has been gaining weight and developing mild ankle swelling. The medical staff added bumetanide to his medication regimen for this excess fluid. Since returning home 1 week ago, he has noticed increasing dyspnea with activity and orthopnea, and the edema has progressed further in his lower extremities, with possible dehiscence at the surgical amputation site. History includes ischemic cardiomyopathy (ejection fraction of 42%), coronary artery disease, diabetes mellitus, and peripheral vascular disease. Ten years ago, he had coronary artery bypass of 4 vessels. Current medications are aspirin, hydralazine, isosorbide dinitrate, insulin glargine, insulin aspart, lisinopril, bumetanide, and carvedilol. He adheres to the medication regimen as well as to a 2 g sodium diet and 1.5 L of fluid per day restriction. He has followed up with his vascular surgery and wound care team, who found no sign of infection. He remains worried about whether the swelling will affect healing of the amputation.

On examination, blood pressure is 129/70 mmHg, heart rate is 77 beats per minute, and respiratory rate is 18 breaths per minute. He has bilateral edema in his lower extremities.

Which one of the following is the most appropriate next step for managing the patient's congestive symptoms?

(A) Intensify fluid restriction.
(B) Limit sodium intake further.
(C) Double the bumetanide dose.
(D) Add metolazone.

ANSWER: D

In advanced stages of heart failure, diuretics may fail to control salt and water retention despite appropriate dosages. This phenomenon—*diuretic resistance*—may be caused by decreased renal function and reduced and delayed peak concentrations of loop diuretics in the tubular fluid but may also be observed in the absence of these pharmacokinetic abnormalities. The prevalence of diuretic resistance among patients with heart failure is unknown.

Diuretic resistance can be addressed by treatment with diuretics with different mechanisms of action. Metolazone, a thiazide-like diuretic, works by a different mechanism than loop diuretics. It indirectly decreases the amount of water reabsorbed into the bloodstream by the kidneys. The addition of metolazone may ease the patient's congestive symptoms. Serum electrolyte levels should be measured at appropriate intervals, and the patient should be observed for clinical signs of fluid or electrolyte imbalance (or both): namely, hyponatremia, hypochloremic alkalosis, and hypokalemia.

Chronic administration of loop diuretics results in a diminished natriuretic effect (braking phenomenon, or *postdiuretic sodium retention*). This phenomenon refers to stimulation of sodium and water reabsorption in the downstream nephron segments. Increasing the dosage of the loop diuretic bumetanide will accentuate the phenomenon and worsen this patient's symptoms.

The first step in management of diuretic resistance is ascertaining adherence to salt and fluid restriction and to the medication regimen, which this patient states he does. Intensifying fluid and diet restriction may cause malnutrition, which is a common problem among older patients with heart failure and most likely decreases quality of life.

105. A 72-year-old woman comes to the office for her annual wellness visit. She is an established patient who lived alone until recently, when her grandson and great-grandchild moved in with her. History includes hypertension, which is managed well with medication; she has a remote history of breast cancer, treated with mastectomy and chemotherapy.

On physical examination, blood pressure is 166/90 mmHg. All other findings are normal, and cognition is intact. When asked about her adherence to the medication regimen, she starts to cry. She states that she can no longer afford her antihypertensive medication, because her grandson constantly asks for money, threatening to leave and not let her see her great-granddaughter if she does not comply.

Which one of the following aspects of the grandson's behavior could be considered an example of financial exploitation?

(A) Moving in with his grandmother
(B) Asking her to give him money
(C) Threatening to keep her from seeing her great-grandchild
(D) No financial exploitation because she was not forced to sign any documents

ANSWER: C

Threatening to keep the patient from her great-grandchild or abandon her is an example of coercion and represents financial exploitation.

Although the exchange of money or resources is a necessary aspect of financial exploitation, it is not in itself wrong for a family member to ask another family member for money. The exploitation comes when the grandson pressures his grandmother for the money by threatening to abandon her or keep the great-grandchild from her (SOE=A).

A family member's dependence on another family member is not in itself abuse. However, the perpetrator's dependence on the victim (in this case, the grandson moving into his grandmother's house) is a risk factor for elder mistreatment but is not in itself abuse (SOE=A).

Asking patients whether they have been forced to sign documents or checks is a specific screen for financial exploitation. Assessment tools used to identify financial exploitation vary in their inclusion of this item.

Financial exploitation is characterized by the misappropriation of a person's money or property, usually by a family member. The prevalence varies from 1% to 16%, depending on the study population and research methods. Black older adults may be at 3 times the risk as other older adults. Victim risk factors include social isolation, diminished capacity, and increased functional dependence on caregivers. Perpetrator risk factors include mental illness, substance abuse, and significant dependence on the older adult. If there is a concern related to abuse by the power of attorney, the treatment team should request copies of relevant documents to ensure that the assumption of fiduciary responsibilities is authorized; authorities should be notified if there are concerns. In cases like the scenario described above, appropriate responses include multidisciplinary initiatives, such as mobilizing other family members and involving community agencies to assist the older adult and the perpetrator (SOE=A).

106. An 83-year-old man comes to the office because 2 days ago he had an episode of garbled speech that lasted ≤1 minute. He is accompanied by his wife, who describes the sudden onset of word-finding difficulty, during which he substituted the word "juice" with the word "fuse" and was unable to follow her instruction to sit down in the kitchen chair. There were no other signs before or since the event. History includes a lacunar stroke 6 years ago, hypertension, diabetes mellitus, and hyperlipidemia. Current medications are atorvastatin, lisinopril, hydrochlorothiazide, metformin, and aspirin (81 mg/d); he has not missed any doses.

On examination, blood pressure is normal, and heart rate is 78 beats per minute. There are no carotid bruits, and cardiac auscultation is normal. There is a left facial palsy, which has been present since his stroke 6 years ago. Speech and language findings are normal, and there are no new focal neurologic deficits.

Which one of the following should be done first?

(A) Begin warfarin.
(B) Order electroencephalography (EEG).
(C) Increase aspirin dosage to 325 mg/d.
(D) Order carotid Doppler ultrasound.

ANSWER: D

This patient may have had a transient ischemic attack (TIA). The combination of sudden onset and short duration, as well as the specific descriptors of the event, suggests a reversible aphasia. The history of stroke and presence of stroke risk factors further suggest TIA. Electrocardiography and Doppler ultrasonography of the carotid arteries should be expedited to identify the cause of the TIA and to assess risk of recurrent TIA or stroke. Studies should include head and neck vascular imaging, possibly magnetic resonance imaging of the brain or screening computed tomography of the head. Screening carotid Doppler study and electrocardiography and/or monitoring are appropriate tests to start the expedited evaluation. Given the patient's age, atrial fibrillation may be the mechanism of the TIA. Transthoracic echocardiography may also be appropriate.

There is no evidence that adding an anticoagulant such as warfarin to daily aspirin or increasing the dosage of aspirin, in the absence of a known thrombotic or embolic source, is effective for secondary stroke prevention. Dual agents may in fact increase the risk of systemic bleeding (SOE=A). Notably, there are limited clinical situations in which it is appropriate to prescribe both aspirin as a cardioprotective agent and an anticoagulant to prevent a thrombotic or embolic event, but it is not appropriate in the case described here.

EEG is not indicated in the absence of seizure activity and postictal state.

107. A 78-year-old woman who lives in Miami comes to the office because she wants to confirm that she has not acquired a sexually transmitted infection (STI). She began a relationship with a new partner 3 months ago. She feels well, and she has had no genital ulcers, vaginal discharge, dyspareunia, dysuria, abdominal or pelvic pain, or fevers. History includes depression, the onset of which coincided with the death of her husband 4 years ago. All of her health maintenance is up to date.

Screening for which one of the following should be offered as part of routine STI testing for this patient?

(A) Human papillomavirus (HPV)
(B) Zika virus
(C) Human immunodeficiency virus (HIV)
(D) *Mycoplasma genitalium*

ANSWER: C

All persons who seek evaluation or treatment for STIs should be screened for HIV infection. Although this patient has no specific symptoms, she is requesting screening. According to 2015 guidelines from the Centers for Disease Control and Prevention, screening for HIV infection should be part of routine testing for STIs (SOE=A). The guidelines recommend that, in the absence of symptoms, testing for HIV, gonorrhea, chlamydia, syphilis, trichomoniasis, hepatitis B virus, and hepatitis C virus infection should be offered to all adults who seek evaluation and treatment for STIs, regardless of age.

This question addresses a significant issue in geriatrics, ie, the importance of appropriate STI counseling and testing in older adults. The number of sexually active older adults is increasing, as is the number of persons living with HIV. Some studies suggest that, over the past 20 years, rates of STIs have more than doubled in older adults. Older black women constitute the fastest growing group of new cases of HIV in the United States, with heterosexual sex as the primary mode of transmission in this group.

Despite the importance of this issue, providers are less likely to take a sexual history from an older adult, less likely to offer counseling on safer sex practices, and less likely to offer testing for HIV infection. Consequently, older adults who acquire HIV infection often present with more advanced disease than younger individuals, and their disease is more likely to progress to acquired immunodeficiency syndrome (AIDS).

If there is a concern for acute retroviral syndrome in this patient, a plasma RNA test should be used in conjunction with an HIV antibody test.

Tests for HPV are available to detect oncogenic strains of HPV infection and are used in the context of cervical cancer screening and management or follow-up of abnormal cervical cytology or histology. Routine cervical screening should begin at 21 years of age and continue through age 65 to prevent invasive cervical cancer.

Zika virus, an emerging infection, is mainly a concern for pregnant women. Testing for Zika virus infection might be considered if the patient had recently experienced symptoms, because some cases of Zika virus have been reported in Miami. However, routine screening is not recommended for asymptomatic, nonpregnant women.

Mycoplasma genitalium, an emerging STI, is a recognized cause of nongonococcal urethritis. *M genitalium* should be suspected in cases of persistent or recurrent urethritis and may be considered in persistent or recurrent cases of cervicitis and pelvic inflammatory disease. This patient has no signs or symptoms to suggest infection. No diagnostic test for *M genitalium* has been approved by the U.S. Food and Drug Administration.

108. An 82-year-old woman who lives in a nursing home is evaluated because she fell while getting out of bed to go to the bathroom. She slipped on a blanket that had slid to the floor. She is unable to recount more detail about her fall. The nurse reports that she said she had no pain after the fall and was able to walk to the bathroom with her walker. Immediately after the fall, seated blood pressure was 144/78 mmHg and heart rate was 86 beats per minute. History includes moderate-stage Alzheimer disease; her most recent score on the Mini–Mental Status Examination was 18 of 30.

Which one of the following is the best intervention to reduce this patient's risk of another fall?

(A) Use of a bed alarm
(B) Nursing education about fall prevention
(C) Raised bed rails at night
(D) Multifactorial intervention

ANSWER: D

A meta-analysis of 13 studies of interventions to prevent falls in nursing homes found that multifactorial interventions tailored to the patient, which can include medication review, environmental changes, exercise interventions, and education for patient and families, reduced falls, whereas single interventions did not. Similarly, a systematic review of 60 randomized controlled trials of fall prevention found that multifactorial interventions reduced falls in hospitals and found possible benefit in nursing facilities (SOE=B).

Bed and chair alarms have not been shown to reduce falls in the nursing-home setting despite widespread use. Repeated triggering of an alarm can be bothersome to patients and hard for staff to interpret. Trials examining bed alarm use in nursing facilities and hospitals have not demonstrated reduction in falls. Multicomponent interventions, including alarms, have shown mixed results (SOE=C).

Raising the bed rails is a type of physical restraint, because bed rails restrict voluntary movement out of bed. In observational studies, physical restraints, including bed rails, have not been shown to reduce fall risk and have been associated with an increase in falls in nursing facilities (SOE=C).

There is limited evidence that nursing staff education about fall prevention reduces falls in nursing facilities. Trial data have been negative or shown fall reduction only for patients with mild or no cognitive impairment when staff education is combined with patient education. This patient has moderate Alzheimer disease; thus, educational interventions directed at staff about fall risk reduction may not be effective (SOE=C).

109. Which one of the following is the most effective frailty screen for use in clinical practice?

(A) Self-reported health
(B) Gait speed
(C) Polypharmacy
(D) Assessment by general practitioner

ANSWER: B

Neither of the established models of frailty—the Cardiovascular Health Study phenotype model or the Canadian Study of Health and Aging cumulative deficit model—are suitable for use in an office setting. In an effort to identify a simple, easily interpreted test for frailty, with high sensitivity and specificity in an office setting, the diagnostic accuracy of 7 screening models was compared against the established models. The models were self-reported health, gait speed, polypharmacy, general practitioner assessment, PRISMA* 7 (7-item self-completion questionnaire), the Timed Up and Go test, and the Groningen Frailty Indicator (GFI).

Gait speed, the PRISMA 7 tool, and the Timed Up and Go test demonstrate high sensitivity and moderate specificity for identifying frailty, whereas self-reported health, clinical assessment by general practitioner, polypharmacy, and GFI are notably less accurate.

Gait speed of ≤0.8 m/s (taking longer than 5 seconds to walk 4 meters) has a sensitivity of 0.99 for identifying frailty; virtually all older adults with frailty would be expected to have a positive test (SOE=B). Further, the high negative predictive value of 0.99 indicates that older adults with gait speed >0.8 m/s are extremely unlikely to be frail.

However, the corresponding sensitivity of 0.64 and positive predictive value of 0.26 indicate that only 1 person in 4 with a gait speed ≤0.8 m/s will be frail on the basis of a reference standard. Applying these rules to the other instruments identifies a relatively high proportion of error rates, but particularly so for self-reported health, clinical assessment by general practitioner, polypharmacy, and GFI. This means that the utility of any of these instruments as a single test is limited for identifying frailty in routine care.

It is possible to improve diagnostic accuracy through two approaches. First, predictive values are proportionate to population prevalence, so applying the test in an older population, in which the prevalence of frailty is likely to be higher, will potentially improve accuracy. Second, a 2-stage assessment process could be used, whereby a test with high sensitivity is followed by a reference standard test or by a second index test with high specificity, to identify frailty with greater accuracy. However, how this might be achieved reliably in routine care would need to be investigated.

*PRISMA: Program of Research to Integrate Services for the Maintenance of Autonomy.

110. An 80-year-old woman comes to the office because she has increasing shoulder pain, profound fatigue, and new, left-sided headache. She describes 2 recent episodes, each lasting a few minutes, of a "veil" falling over her left eye. History includes polymyalgia rheumatica, first diagnosed 3 months ago. Initial treatment was prednisone 15 mg/d; the dosage was reduced 4 weeks ago, to 12.5 mg/d.

On examination, there is no tenderness over the left temporal artery. Funduscopic examination reveals pallor of the optic nerve.

Which one of the following is the most appropriate next step?

(A) Resume prednisone 15 mg/d.
(B) Begin methylprednisolone 1,000 mg/d IV for 3 days.
(C) Obtain biopsy of the temporal artery.
(D) Obtain color Doppler ultrasonography of the temporal artery.

ANSWER: B

This patient, like 10%–20% of patients with polymyalgia rheumatica, has giant cell arteritis (GCA), a large-vessel vasculitis affecting vessels in the cranial and carotid circulations and the aorta and its branches. The presence of amaurosis fugax and optic nerve pallor suggests ischemic optic neuropathy, which typically leads to permanent loss of vision if untreated. Administration of pulse-dose methylprednisolone is indicated to decrease edema and prevent further tissue damage and necrosis. Other presentations of suspected GCA that warrant pulse-dose corticosteroid therapy include transient ischemic attack, stroke, and angina. At completion of pulse-dose therapy, oral prednisone 1 mg/kg/d should be started. The dosage can be reduced by 10%–20% every 2–4 weeks; once a dosage of 10 mg/d is reached, reduction can be by 1-mg increments monthly. The patient should begin therapy to prevent corticosteroid-induced osteoporosis, and consideration should be given to prophylaxis for *Pneumocystis jiroveci* pneumonia (SOE=C).

Patients who have a relapse of polymyalgia rheumatica symptoms after prednisone taper should resume the last dosage that provided symptom control, with a slower taper thereafter. However, because this patient has GCA with impending loss of vision, moderate-dose prednisone is insufficient.

Temporal artery biopsy is the gold standard for diagnosis of GCA. Because vasculitis can have a segmental distribution, biopsy specimens should be ≥1.5–2 cm long; biopsy of the contralateral artery has been reported to increase diagnostic yield. GCA is characterized by a vasculitis predominated by mononuclear cell infiltration and granulomatous inflammation, often with giant cells. Temporal artery biopsy, which may not be immediately available, retains its sensitivity for 2–4 weeks after initiation of high-dose corticosteroid therapy (SOE=A). Therefore, in this patient with high clinical suspicion of GCA and at high risk of permanent complications, anticipated biopsy should not delay initiation of therapy.

Color Doppler ultrasonography can be used to visualize superficial arteries. Homogeneous wall thickening (*halo sign*) signifies vessel edema and has a sensitivity and specificity of 75% and 83%, respectively, for predicting positive results from temporal artery biopsy. Ultrasonography is not routinely used for diagnosis of GCA. Other imaging modalities have some utility in assessing the extent of disease in biopsy-proven GCA; in particular, magnetic resonance angiography has been used to define involvement of the aorta and its branches.

111. A 70-year-old man comes to the emergency department because he lost consciousness earlier in the day. He states that, the previous evening, he was at a social gathering where he drank more alcohol than usual for him. When he woke up this morning he went to the bathroom and, while urinating, collapsed onto the bathroom floor. His spouse witnessed the event and did not notice any abnormal movements. He regained consciousness after 10 seconds, without alteration of mental status. He did not suffer a head injury. He had no prodromal symptoms and currently feels well. History includes hypertension and diabetes mellitus. Current medications are lisinopril 40 mg/d and metformin 1 g twice daily.

On physical examination, temperature, blood pressure, and neurologic findings are normal.

Which one of the following is the best recommendation for this patient?

(A) Drink extra fluids.
(B) Reduce the dosage of lisinopril.
(C) Sit during urination.
(D) Avoid alcohol altogether.

ANSWER: C

Micturition syncope is a common cause of neurally mediated syncope in older adults. The best management is to advise the patient to sit while he urinates, to avoid the possibility of falling. Micturition syncope is characterized by syncope or presyncopal symptoms after urination. In general, patients do not recall any premonitory symptoms. Patients are at higher risk of these events after taking vasodilators and after drinking alcohol. There generally is no intracranial pathology, and patients do not require neurologic evaluation.

Syncope from an underlying infection would imply hypovolemia secondary to insensible fluid losses from fever. This patient, however, has normal vital signs, so drinking extra fluids will not be effective for this etiology. The patient appears to be on an appropriate dosage of his blood pressure medication, and there are no recent changes in his requirement or his volume of distribution that call for a change in dosage. Although his previous night's ingestion of alcohol may have contributed to his symptoms, the temporal relationship of his micturition and the resultant syncope makes micturition-related syncope more likely.

112. A 75-year-old man comes to the office for a routine health check. His spouse died 2 months ago. He expresses sadness at her passing and feels that life has lost meaning. He has some difficulty falling asleep. He states that there has been no change in his energy level or appetite and that he has no feelings of guilt or suicidal or homicidal ideation. Before his wife's death, he drank 2–4 beers each night; during his monthly poker game with friends, he drinks 6–8 beers. Since her death, he drinks 6 beers each night because he thinks it helps him sleep, but he worries that he may have an issue with drinking. He asks for help cutting back. History includes essential hypertension, hyperlipidemia, and stage 2 chronic kidney disease.

Which one of the following treatments should be tried first for this patient?

(A) Citalopram
(B) Naltrexone
(C) Disulfiram
(D) Cognitive-behavioral therapy

ANSWER: D

In persons with intact cognition, cognitive-behavioral therapy is associated with increased rates of remission of alcohol use disorder, especially when combined with participation in groups such as Alcoholics Anonymous (SOE=C). Further, the patient in this case shows signs of bereavement disorder beyond his alcohol use disorder, and he would benefit from psychotherapy.

Although pharmacotherapy can be offered for alcohol use disorder, most agents have not been studied in older adults. The most studied medication for treatment of alcohol use disorder is naltrexone, which is generally well tolerated; however, evidence of its efficacy in older adults stems largely from post-hoc analysis (SOE=B).

The evidence is less consistent for other agents such as disulfiram, which is known to have greater risk of harm for older adults with comorbid medical conditions than for younger adults, in the event of a reaction (SOE=C).

Antidepressants, including the selective serotonin reuptake inhibitor (SSRI) citalopram, have been used for treatment of alcohol use disorder, but evidence is inconsistent as to their utility (SOE=D).

113. An 82-year-old woman comes to the office because she has had worsening anxiety and worry for the last 8 months. She describes sleeping poorly, being tired, and having generalized aches for several weeks. She is accompanied by her daughter, who states that she consistently worries about her grandchildren as well as her husband, who has well-controlled diabetes mellitus and hypertension. Generalized anxiety disorder is diagnosed.

Which one of the following is the best treatment option for this patient?

(A) Benzodiazepines and cognitive-behavioral therapy (CBT)
(B) CBT only
(C) Selective serotonin reuptake inhibitor (SSRI) and CBT
(D) SSRI only

ANSWER: C

The ideal treatment for anxiety disorders in older adults is the same as in younger adults: combination of an antidepressant, such as an SSRI, and CBT. There is ample evidence that older adults can learn new skills in CBT and use them effectively over time (SOE=A).

Pharmacotherapy is often used as first-line treatment for anxiety disorders in late life, yet augmenting the pharmacotherapy with behavioral therapy improves worry symptoms and reduces relapse rates in older adults (SOE=A). Indeed, for some patients, starting a new medication that will require time and dose titration to bring about remission is anxiety provoking. Because therapists trained in the full array of CBT interventions are not always easily accessible, the practitioner should, at a minimum, advise behavioral activation, ie, increased physical, social, and mental activity for distraction and positive reinforcement.

Benzodiazepines are the most commonly prescribed anxiolytic agent for adult patients. Although they immediately reduce anxiety symptoms, their use, especially in older adults, is strongly discouraged because they increase the risk of falls and cognitive impairment. In addition, concern is increasing regarding benzodiazepine dependence in both younger and older patients.

114. A 76-year-old woman with coronary artery disease comes to the office for preoperative medical evaluation before coronary bypass graft surgery (CABG) in 3 weeks. She is an active smoker.

Which one of the following interventions will decrease her risk of postoperative pulmonary complications?

(A) Preoperative inspiratory muscle training
(B) Preoperative smoking cessation
(C) Preoperative inhaled β-agonist
(D) Postoperative use of incentive spirometry

ANSWER: A

Postoperative pulmonary complications such as atelectasis, pneumonia, and respiratory failure are common. Risk factors for these complications include advanced age, chronic obstructive pulmonary disease, heart failure, current smoking, obstructive sleep apnea, obesity, and functional dependence. Smokers with chronic heart or lung disease have a 2- to 5-fold increased risk of perioperative complications.

Patients with weaker respiratory muscles are at increased risk of clinically significant inspiratory muscle fatigue postoperatively, with collapse of alveoli, poor clearance of secretions, pneumonia, and respiratory failure. Inspiratory muscle training comprises exercises, led by a respiratory therapist, designed to increase respiratory muscle strength or muscle endurance, or both. Typical programs include 5 to 7 sessions per week for >2 weeks before surgery. A meta-analysis of 11 trials, comprising 675 participants after coronary artery bypass graft (CABG) or abdominal surgery, found that inspiratory muscle training was associated with a relative risk of pneumonia of 0.45 (95% confidence interval, 0.26–0.77) compared with usual care, and the training reduced length of hospital stay by 1.3 days (SOE=B).

A systematic review found no benefit for postoperative incentive spirometry compared with usual care for prevention of pulmonary complications after abdominal surgery. However, the review included trials that were small and considered of low quality. An older systematic review in post-CABG patients also showed no benefit from incentive spirometry (SOE=B).

Intensive interventions for smoking cessation, starting 1–2 months before surgery with serial counseling visits and use of nicotine replacement therapy, have been shown to reduce postoperative complications. Brief interventions have a smaller impact on smoking cessation and do not reduce postoperative complications. This patient will be undergoing surgery in 2 weeks and is therefore less likely to benefit from preoperative smoking cessation.

Preoperative use of inhaled β-agonists has shown no benefit in reducing risk of postoperative pulmonary complications.

115. A bedbound 94-year-old woman requires a home visit for medical care. She lives in her own home, supported by her children and their families. She is nonverbal and incontinent. She does chew and swallow. History includes Alzheimer disease without behavior disturbance, osteoarthritis of several joints, and essential hypertension. Current medications are acetaminophen and hydrochlorothiazide. Her family is present, and disease trajectory is discussed with them.

On physical examination, blood pressure is 143/78 mmHg, heart rate is 73 beats per minute, and respiratory rate is 12 breaths per minute. Skin is intact. Muscle tone is increased in all extremities. She responds to voice and touch with eye tracking but does not speak during the visit.

Which one of the following will determine the level of reimbursement for this visit?

(A) Documentation of complexity of the visit
(B) Distance traveled to visit
(C) Number of family members involved in the summary discussion
(D) Skilled service referrals generated by visit

ANSWER: A

Medicare reimbursement for house calls is determined by the complexity of the visit, as it is in any health care setting. The complexity is primarily determined by the number of encounter diagnoses. Identification of the appropriate level of complexity will facilitate reimbursement of the health care provider for the cognitive skills used in providing care for this patient. For example, for a patient with dementia, the encounter diagnosis could be memory loss, or late-onset dementia, or late-onset dementia with behavioral manifestations. Other factors that affect billing include the comprehensiveness of the history, physical examination, and review of outside records, as well as the number of active problems reflected in the care plan. Documentation of the amount of time spent in the encounter may also influence reimbursement.

Medicare does not consider travel time in determining reimbursement. Many practices that engage in house calls cluster visits geographically to minimize the effect of travel time on productivity.

Caregivers of homebound patients are often actively involved in the house call and anticipate the opportunity to interact with the visiting provider. Documentation of time spent counseling—not the number of individuals who participate in the counseling—may contribute to reimbursement.

The number of referrals made to licensed professionals, such as visiting nurses, or rehabilitation therapists, does not affect reimbursement for primary care visits. Medicare forbids any financial benefit from referrals to home care agencies.

116. An 82-year-old man comes to the office because he has been coughing during meals. He almost choked once. He has no pain with swallowing and no sensation of food stuck in his throat. The cough developed gradually over the past month. History includes Parkinson disease, hypertension, and hyperlipidemia. Current medications are carbidopa/levodopa, lisinopril, and atorvastatin.

Which one of the following is the most appropriate next step to establish the diagnosis in this patient?

(A) Esophageal manometry
(B) Barium swallow test
(C) Videofluoroscopy
(D) Upper endoscopy

ANSWER: C

Oropharyngeal or esophageal dysphagia occurs in 60% of patients >65 years old in the outpatient setting. Patients with oropharyngeal dysphagia usually choke, cough after they eat, or retain food in the mouth after they attempt to swallow. Any new onset requires thorough evaluation. The dysphagia should be evaluated with videofluoroscopy to assess the swallowing mechanism and detect aspiration.

Parkinson disease, which this patient has, can cause oropharyngeal dysphagia.

Adjusting the dosage of carbidopa/levodopa may not improve his dysphagia (SOE=C); the effectiveness of carbidopa/levodopa in treatment of dysphagia is controversial (SOE=B). Studies have shown that use of rotigotine transdermal patch improves swallowing in patients with Parkinson disease and dysphagia (SOE=B), but videofluoroscopy should be done first to exclude other potential causes of dysphagia, such as stroke, Alzheimer disease, myasthenia gravis, and malignancies of the oropharynx.

This patient's symptoms are more consistent with oropharyngeal than esophageal dysphagia. Esophageal dysphagia often presents with the sensation of food stuck in the throat. It is best evaluated by upper endoscopy. Barium swallow is an alternative to endoscopy. Advantages of upper endoscopy include direct visualization of pathology, biopsy of lesions, and even therapy (eg, dilation of strictures). Esophageal manometry may be helpful in diagnosis of achalasia or esophageal spasm but is not indicated in this case.

117. An 84-year-old man is brought to the office because his right eye is red. There is moderate watery discharge. He says that the eye feels gritty but does not itch, and he has no eye pain or light sensitivity. There is no baseline information on visual acuity, but he thinks his vision is unchanged, and nursing home staff confirm that there has been no evidence of a change in vision. History includes Alzheimer disease. He seems to have a cold and is sneezing.

On examination, eye movements are intact. There is moderate bulbar conjunctival injection of the right eye. Conjunctival hemorrhage extends from 6 o'clock to 9 o'clock positions. Right preauricular lymph node is slightly tender.

Which one of the following is the most appropriate management of the red eye?

(A) Antibiotic eye drops
(B) Referral to an ophthalmologist
(C) Artificial tears as needed
(D) Antihistamine eye drops

ANSWER: C

Vascular congestion in an eye ("red eye") is usually due to an allergic response or to viral or bacterial infection. This patient has signs of a cold, which suggests that an adenovirus is the likely cause of his red eye. Viruses cause nearly 80% of all cases of acute conjunctivitis; between 65% and 90% of cases of viral conjunctivitis are due to adenoviruses. The eye discharge in viral conjunctivitis is typically watery; another characteristic finding is ipsilateral preauricular adenopathy. In addition to acute viral conjunctivitis, this patient has a subconjunctival hemorrhage, likely due to rubbing his right eye. Artificial tears are appropriate to reduce the eye irritation in viral conjunctivitis.

Viral conjunctivitis is a contagious condition. Nursing home staff need to glove and wash hands after caring for this patient and administering any eye drops. Viral conjunctivitis resolves in approximately 1 week, and the hemorrhage resolves in 2–3 weeks.

Warning signs that the patient needs prompt referral to an ophthalmologist include change in visual acuity, swelling of the lid or lacrimal sac, severe pain, and abnormal eye movements (ophthalmoplegia). The lack of these symptoms or signs in this patient makes referral unnecessary.

Allergic conjunctivitis is generally bilateral, is chronic or recurrent, and most commonly causes itching, none of which are present in this patient. Therapy for allergic conjunctivitis often includes a topical antihistamine, which is not indicated for this patient.

The nature of the eye discharge and the slightly tender preauricular lymph nodes help to differentiate viral from bacterial conjunctivitis. Bacterial conjunctivitis is usually purulent. Patients may simply awaken with discharge (mattering) and stuck eyelids. Generally, there is no preauricular adenopathy unless conjunctivitis is severe and hyperacute. Use of antibiotics speeds resolution of symptoms, but many cases of bacterial conjunctivitis will resolve without topical antibiotics (SOE=A). Immunocompromised patients (eg, patients receiving corticosteroids) and patients with copious purulent drainage should receive antibiotics. The patient in this case does not have signs of bacterial conjunctivitis and does not need topical antibiotics.

118. Which one of the following is most likely to be a characteristic of older adults living in poverty in the United States?

(A) Male sex
(B) Non-Hispanic white ethnicity
(C) Living alone
(D) Age between 65 and 74 years old

ANSWER: C

Although >25 million older Americans live at or below the federal poverty level ($29,425 per year for a single person), the percentage decreased steadily between 1966 and 2014, from about 29% to 10%. Reasons for the decline include improvements in Social Security, the adoption of Medicare, increased participation in the labor force among older adults, and higher levels of education among more recent cohorts of older adults. Rates of older adults living in poverty are consistently higher for those who live alone than for those who are married, and this holds across sex and racial groups.

Among adults ≥65 years old, a higher percentage of women than men live in poverty (12.1% versus 7.4%), regardless of race. Within race/ethnic groups, the poverty is more than twice as large among Hispanic and black adults ≥65 years old than among older white adults (17.4%, 18.8%, and 7.1%, respectively).

Among older adults, rates of poverty increase with age. In 2014, rates of poverty were 8.7% for persons 65–74 years old, 11.3% for those 75–84 years old, and 12.7% for those ≥85 years old.

119. An 80-year-old woman comes to the office to discuss her oncologist's recommendation that she consider adjuvant chemotherapy. She recently had surgery for an obstructing colon cancer; regional lymph nodes were positive for metastatic adenocarcinoma. Her recovery from surgery was prolonged because of difficulty with ambulation and increased weakness. History includes heart failure (ejection fraction of 19%) and chronic obstructive pulmonary disease. In the past year, she has had 3 episodes of respiratory failure requiring ventilator therapy. She is concerned about the potential adverse effects of adjuvant chemotherapy.

Which one of the following would provide the most useful information to help with her decision?

(A) Clinical practice guidelines related to her diseases
(B) Number of patients who would need to be treated for 1 patient to benefit from the chemotherapy
(C) Chance of harm from treatment
(D) Lag time between treatment and benefit

ANSWER: D

For a patient with multiple morbidities, an important consideration is the estimated length of time needed to benefit from treatment. Information on lag time between treatment and benefit would help the patient decide on her best course. Most likely, she would die from heart failure or chronic obstructive pulmonary disease before she would die of colon cancer.

The amount of reduction of mortality from the cancer, or the number of patients needed to treat for 1 patient to benefit, is less important if she is more likely to die of competing morbidities. Clinical practice guidelines rarely address management related to multiple morbidities. Knowing likelihood of harm would be helpful only if there is a chance of long-term survival, in which the potential for benefit would outweigh the potential for harm.

120. A 70-year-old man comes to the office for a follow-up visit. History includes hyperlipidemia, trigeminal neuralgia, benign prostatic hyperplasia, and Parkinson disease. Current medications include carbamazepine, rosuvastatin, selegilene, and tamsulosin. Hypovitaminosis D was diagnosed 3 months ago, and he began treatment with vitamin D_3 2,000 IU/d by mouth. At today's visit, the vitamin D concentration is unchanged from 3 months ago.

Which one of his medications is most likely affecting his vitamin D concentration?

(A) Carbamazepine
(B) Rosuvastatin
(C) Selegiline
(D) Tamsulosin

ANSWER: A

Vitamin D is essential for the regulation of calcium and phosphorus homeostasis. Calcidiol, or 25(OH)D, is the primary form of vitamin D stored and transported by the body. It is activated to $1,25(OH)_2D_3$ in the kidney and some target tissues. However, 25(OH)D is also deactivated by CYP3A4 enzyme. Therefore, induction of CYP3A4 enzyme can decrease the total amount of vitamin D available in the body.

Many reports in the literature link CYP3A4-inducing medications (eg, phenytoin, rifampin) and osteomalacia that has been attributed to vitamin D deficiency. This suggests that the vitamin D requirement may be increased in patients taking CYP3A4 inducers.

Carbamazepine is a potent inducer of CYP3A4 enzyme, and the magnitude of induction is both dose- and time-dependent. Patients receiving chronic carbamazepine therapy have higher CYP3A4 activity and thus are more likely to have increased catabolism of vitamin D, leading to vitamin D deficiency. These patients often require long-term, high-dose vitamin D supplementation to prevent vitamin D deficiency.

Rosuvastatin is partially metabolized through CYP2C9 enzyme and does not induce or inhibit CYP3A4 enzymes. Selegiline and tamsulosin are substrates, but not inducers, of CYP3A4. Rosuvastatin, selegiline, and tamsulosin would likely not be responsible for this patient's unchanged vitamin D concentration.

121. An 83-year-old woman comes to the office because she has had episodes of dizziness in the past month. She has continual unsteadiness that is unchanged by position; there is no new numbness or weakness. She has not fallen, but the unsteadiness has caused her to turn down invitations and stop going to her weekly bridge game. She has not been sleeping well. Her husband died 1 year ago. History includes hypertension, osteoarthritis, and glaucoma.

On examination, she appears thin but in no distress. She has lost 2.3 kg (5 lb) since her last visit. Orthostatic vital signs are normal. Visual acuity and hearing are grossly intact. She has full strength. Sensory examination is normal to pinprick and vibratory sensation in all extremities. Reflexes are 2+ throughout. Gait is slow and hesitant but narrow based and steady.

Which one of the following is the best next step?

(A) Obtain magnetic resonance imaging (MRI) of the cervical spine.
(B) Perform Dix-Hallpike test.
(C) Screen for depression.
(D) Conduct tilt-table test.

ANSWER: C

Functional dizziness refers to a feeling of dizziness, vertigo, or imbalance that has a somatoform or psychogenic origin. It is estimated to account for 8%–10% of cases of dizziness in a neuro-otology office (SOE=C). The dizziness is often difficult for the patient to describe; it might include a sense of floating or imbalance. There are no clinical characteristics that suggest a more definite etiology for the symptoms. Patients with chronic vestibular issues may become depressed; similarly, patients who are depressed may report dizziness, as well as other somatic symptoms that do not have a pathological correlate. In this patient, questioning reveals that she is at high risk of depression: she reports social withdrawal, she has lost weight, she has insomnia, and her husband recently died. Thus, a more formal depression screen would be the best next diagnostic test.

Despite indications that depression might be the cause of her symptoms, it is important to consider other etiologies. Vision and hearing dysfunction, autonomic dysfunction, and cervical myelopathy all could prompt a report of dizziness, and the examination findings would likely point toward one of these causes. Patients with cervicogenic dizziness also commonly describe neck pain, weakness, and numbness. Hyperreflexia is a common examination finding.

A tilt-table test is indicated if autonomic dysfunction is suspected. For this patient, the test is likely to have a low yield, given the lack of a positional component to her symptoms and the normal orthostatic findings.

The Dix-Hallpike test is the most common clinical maneuver used to diagnose benign paroxysmal positional vertigo. However, this patient does not describe symptoms that are specific to benign paroxysmal positional vertigo, and thus this test is unlikely to be helpful.

122. An 80-year-old man comes to the office because he has new onset of right elbow pain after a weekend of gardening. He recalls no specific trauma. History includes type 2 diabetes mellitus, osteoarthritis, hypertension, end-stage renal disease, and gout. The diabetes is controlled by diet, and he is on hemodialysis. Current medications are quinapril 20 mg/d, acetaminophen 650 mg three times daily, and allopurinol 200 mg/d.

On physical examination, blood pressure is 155/85 mmHg, heart rate is 90 beats per minute, and temperature is 37.5° C (99.5° F). He appears to be in moderate distress and is holding his right elbow. The elbow is diffusely red and edematous, especially the extensor aspect, with +2 edema. Elbow extension is possible to 165 degrees; the last 10 degrees is limited by pain. Radial pulses are normal. Monofilament examination reveals mild distal peripheral neuropathy in both feet. Hands are normal except for the presence of Heberden nodes in multiple distal interphalangeal joints.

Laboratory findings:

Hemoglobin	12 mg/dL
White blood cell count	11,000/μL (80% neutrophils)
Hemoglobin A$_{1c}$	8%
Serum creatinine	1.9 mg/dL
Serum uric acid	6 mg/dL
Erythrocyte sedimentation rate	50 mm/hr

Radiography of the right elbow shows diffuse soft-tissue swelling.

Which one of the following is the most appropriate next step?

(A) Ultrasonography-guided aspiration of the elbow joint
(B) Cephalexin 250 mg four times daily for 7 days
(C) Needle aspiration of the olecranon bursa
(D) Colchicine 1.2 mg now, then 0.6 mg tomorrow

ANSWER: C

In this patient, the physical examination findings—particularly, the relatively free movement of his elbow joint—are most consistent with acute olecranon bursitis. The etiology is most likely infection, even if there is no visible skin break. Patients on hemodialysis are at high risk of soft-tissue and joint infections. Acute gout flare is also possible and needs to be excluded. The best option is to aspirate fluid from the infected olecranon bursa, preferably guided by ultrasonography or computed tomography (SOE=D). In some cases, a surgical drain may be placed to ensure good drainage of the tissue. Hemorrhagic bursitis is also possible, given the impaired platelet function and the use of anticoagulants during hemodialysis. Patients on hemodialysis have a lower risk of gout flare than patients receiving peritoneal dialysis. However, because there are many reported cases of coexisting gout and musculoskeletal infection, tissue samples should be obtained whenever possible for culture and crystal examinations before starting treatment (SOE=D). However, empiric therapy with colchicine is not indicated.

Aspiration of the elbow joint should be avoided, because the procedure may introduce pathogens from the surrounding soft tissue into the joint, causing an iatrogenic septic arthritis. The most common pathogen for septic olecranon bursitis is *Staphylococcus aureus,* followed by *Streptococcus* species. The initial antibiotic regimen depends on local infection epidemiology. When septic bursitis is suspected in an immunocompromised patient, many clinicians choose to assume the presence of resistant organisms until culture results are available (SOE=D). Therapy with cephalexin is not appropriate.

123. An 80-year-old woman comes to the office for routine follow-up. She lives in a nursing home. History includes diabetes, hypertension, hypercholesterolemia, and recurrent urinary tract infections. Current medications are aspirin 81 mg/d daily, sitagliptin 50 mg/d, lisinopril 20 mg/d, simvastatin 40 mg/d, and 2 cranberry capsules daily. She has not had any recent infections.

Which one of the following statements is true regarding the role of cranberry products in preventing urinary tract infections for older women in nursing homes?

(A) Cranberry products can prevent urinary tract infections.
(B) Cranberry juice is the only cranberry product that prevents urinary tract infections.
(C) Cranberry juice is more effective than capsules in preventing urinary tract infections.
(D) Data do not support use of cranberry products to prevent urinary tract infections.

ANSWER: D

Proanthocyanidins, a class of polyphenols found in plants, are powerful antioxidants that remove harmful free oxygen radicals from cells. Some are also cytotoxic to tumor cells. Although cranberry has high concentrations of proanthocyanidins that inhibit *Escherichia coli* adhesion in vitro and are responsible for the berry's antiseptic effects, studies have failed to support use of cranberry products as urinary antiseptics (SOE=C). Cranberry has not been shown to be effective in prevention or treatment of urinary tract infections. Studies also have not shown that either cranberry juice or capsule forms taken for >1 year either prevent or treat urinary tract infections in older women in nursing homes (SOE=B).

124. A 68-year-old woman comes to the office to establish care. She is lesbian and has recently retired to the area. History includes hypertension and chronic kidney disease. She smokes tobacco and is moderately obese.

She is at increased risk for which one of the following, compared with risks for a heterosexual woman?

(A) Cervical cancer
(B) Cardiovascular disease
(C) Colon cancer
(D) Kidney cancer

ANSWER: B

Lesbian and bisexual women are at increased risk of obesity and hypercholesterolemia, and thereby at increased risk of cardiovascular disease. On average, lesbian and bisexual women have a higher BMI than heterosexual women. Older lesbian women are twice as likely as heterosexual women to report being heavy smokers (SOE=B).

Lesbian and bisexual women are, on average, at decreased risk of cervical cancer. Bisexual women, as well as lesbian women who have ever had sexual intercourse with a male partner, remain at some risk of cervical cancer (SOE=B). There are no data to suggest that the risk of colon cancer is different between lesbian, bisexual women and heterosexual women, independent of obesity (SOE=B). On average, lesbian women are at increased risk of arthritis (SOE=B). LGBT persons are not at any increased risk of kidney cancer.

125. An 88-year-old woman is brought to the emergency department because she has had generalized weakness and confusion for the past 2 days. History includes breast cancer, hypertension, mild cognitive impairment, and gait disorder. Her daughter reports that the patient had been doing well at home, with improving strength, since her mastectomy and radiation treatment 6 months ago.

On physical examination, vital signs are stable. Her eyes remain closed and she is difficult to arouse. General physical findings are normal; musculoskeletal and neurologic examinations are difficult to perform because of her altered mental status. Laboratory findings, including urinalysis, are normal. Magnetic resonance imaging of the brain without contrast shows multiple lesions consistent with metastatic disease, likely related to her breast cancer.

A meeting is held with the patient, her husband and children, and the medical team. The family is informed that the change in mental status is due to multiple metastatic lesions in the brain. The patient's husband states that his wife had repeatedly said that she would decline further treatment if her breast cancer ever returned, including no surgery, radiation, or chemotherapy. He asks whether hospice is an option.

Which one of the following is required for this patient to qualify for the Medicare hospice benefit?

(A) "Do not resuscitate" (DNR) code status
(B) Estimated life expectancy <6 months
(C) Uncontrolled symptoms
(D) Diagnosis of metastatic cancer

ANSWER: B

This patient has metastatic breast cancer. Given her current condition and the decision not to pursue further interventions, her life expectancy can be estimated to be ≤6 months, which makes her a candidate for hospice.

Hospice is supported through Medicare, Medicaid, the Veterans Health Administration, and most commercial insurance policies. Patients with Medicare Part A are eligible for the Medicare hospice benefit if they have a chronic or terminal illness with life expectancy ≤6 months if the disease runs its expected course, as certified by 2 physicians (typically, the primary medical doctor and the hospice medical director). Once a patient with Medicare coverage decides to pursue hospice care, he or she signs off of Medicare Part A and signs up for the Medicare hospice benefit. This benefit covers a variety of services, including care by a multidisciplinary team, durable medical equipment, medical supplies, and medications related to the terminal diagnosis.

A diagnosis of cancer is not required, nor must a patient sign a DNR order to qualify for hospice. However, most hospice agencies require or at least recommend DNR code status for their patients, because it reflects the goals of hospice care. Uncontrolled symptoms are not a requirement for hospice. Symptoms, such as pain and dyspnea, are primary targets of the hospice team and will be addressed in the goals of care and treatment plan for the patient.

126. An 80-year-old man of Chinese descent is admitted to the hospital because he has abdominal pain, nausea, vomiting, and jaundice. Pancreatic cancer was recently diagnosed. His family members ask doctors and nurses not to tell him about the recent diagnosis.

Which one of the following is the most appropriate next step in responding to the family's request?

(A) Disclose the diagnosis to the patient.
(B) Ask the patient about his interest in learning about his medical condition.
(C) Honor the family's request.
(D) Defer to the oncologist to discuss with the family.

ANSWER: B

In some cultures, it is commonly believed that telling patients about a serious or terminal diagnosis may be injurious to the patient's health or hasten death. There is no consensus in bioethics or ethnogeriatrics concerning the rigorous application of full clinical disclosure in every situation. Bioethical frameworks vary across countries and cultures. In the United States, the 1990 Patient Self-Determination Act affirms the individual's right to make medical decisions. It is generally agreed that it is important to incorporate the patient's beliefs concerning disclosure and truth telling into clinical planning whenever possible. Some patients may prefer not to know if they are terminally ill and may ask that family members or other caregivers receive all diagnostic information and make all treatment decisions. Other patients may want to be directly involved in all aspects of diagnosis and treatment. Still other patients may wish to listen to discussions but delegate decision-making to family surrogates.

Optimally, each patient's preferences regarding disclosure of serious clinical findings should be ascertained early in the clinical relationship and reconfirmed at intervals. If the patient does not wish to know his diagnosis, he has the right to choose not to be informed. Asking the patient about whether he wants to receive information about diagnosis and treatment, and to participate in medical decisions, is the most appropriate next step (SOE=C).

Exploring the family's concerns is important but does not supplant the need to have a direct conversation with the patient. Telling the patient before ascertaining his interest is not appropriate. Asking his oncologist to speak with him is also not ideal, because there is no clear indication or guarantee what the oncologist will discuss with the patient.

Recent studies refute the common perception that many Asian patients do not wish to participate in medical decisions related to serious illness. A survey conducted in China, comprising 150 pairs of hospitalized patients with cancer and their family members, found that more patients than families believed that patients should be informed of their illnesses (98% versus 67%), that patients should be informed of their condition completely (69% versus 19%), and that patients should be informed by doctors (55% versus 11%), all $P<.001$. A similar survey of 520 adult patients with cancer was conducted in Pakistan: 60% of respondents wanted a health care provider to give them detailed information about their prognosis and life expectancy. Patients who wanted information withheld were significantly more likely to be female, to have a lower socioeconomic status, or to have lung cancer; age did not play a significant role.

A survey in Taiwan of patients with advanced cancer found that truth telling significantly reduced their uncertainty and anxiety and did not affect their state of spiritual well-being; before hospice referral, patients aware of their prognosis were more likely to sign a "do not resuscitate" consent. Similarly, in a United States study of 590 patients with advanced cancer (median survival, 5.4 months), 71% wanted to be told their life expectancy. Prognostic disclosure was not associated with worse patient-clinician relationships, sadness, or anxiety.

GRS10 EDITORIAL BOARD

CO-CHIEF EDITORS, SYLLABUS

G. Michael Harper, MD, AGSF
Professor of Medicine
University of California San Francisco
Staff Physician, San Francisco Veteran Affairs Medical Center
San Francisco, CA

William L. Lyons, MD, AGSF
Professor
Division of Geriatrics, Gerontology, and Palliative Medicine
Department of Internal Medicine
University of Nebraska Medical Center
Omaha, NE

EDITORS

Jessica L. Colburn, MD
Assistant Professor of Medicine
Johns Hopkins University School of Medicine
Division of Geriatric Medicine and Gerontology
Baltimore, MD

Timothy W. Farrell, MD, AGSF
Associate Professor of Medicine (Division of Geriatrics)
Adjunct Associate Professor of Family Medicine
University of Utah School of Medicine
Physician Investigator, VA SLC Geriatric Research, Education, and Clinical Center
Director, University of Utah Health Sciences Interprofessional Education Program
Salt Lake City, UT

Jonathan M. Flacker, MD, AGSF
Chief Medical Officer
JenCare Georgia
Atlanta, GA

Lisa J. Granville, MD, FACP, AGSF
Professor and Associate Chair
Department of Geriatrics
Florida State University College of Medicine
Tallahassee, FL

Melinda S. Lantz, MD
Vice Chair
Chief of Geriatric Psychiatry
Mount Sinai Beth Israel
Associate Professor of Psychiatry
Icahn School of Medicine at Mount Sinai
New York, NY

Amy M. Westcott, MD, MHPE, CMD, AGSF
Associate Professor of Medicine in Geriatrics and Palliative Medicine
Penn State College of Medicine, Hershey, PA
Medical Director for Pennsylvania and Delaware, Optum
Horsham, PA

CHIEF EDITOR, QUESTIONS

Jane F. Potter, MD, FACP, AGSF
Professor of Medicine
Division of Geriatrics, Gerontology and Palliative Care
Department of Internal Medicine
University of Nebraska Medical Center
Home Instead Center for Successful Aging
Omaha, NE

QUESTION EDITORS

Jonathan S. Appelbaum, MD, FACP, AAHIVS
Laurie L. Dozier Jr., MD, Education Director and Professor of Internal Medicine
Chair, Department of Clinical Sciences
Florida State University College of Medicine
Tallahassee, FL

Ian M. Deutchki, MD
Assistant Professor
Departments of Family Medicine and Geriatrics
University of Rochester
Rochester, NY

Rachel K. Miller, MD, MsED
Associate Professor
Division of Geriatrics
Perelman School of Medicine
University of Pennsylvania
Crescenz VA Medical Center
Philadelphia VA Home Based Primary Care
Philadelphia, PA

Gary J. Kennedy, MD
Professor and Vice Chair for Education
Director, Division of Geriatric Psychiatry and Fellowship Program
Department of Psychiatry and Behavioral Sciences
Montefiore Medical Center
Albert Einstein College of Medicine
Bronx, NY

Rainier Patrick Soriano, MD
Associate Professor, Medicine, Medical Education, Geriatrics
Director of Curriculum and Director of Educational Technology
Department of Medical Education
Icahn School of Medicine at Mount Sinai
New York, NY

CONSULTING EDITOR FOR PHARMACOTHERAPY

Judith L. Beizer, PharmD, BCGP, FASCP, AGSF
 Clinical Professor
 College of Pharmacy and Health Sciences
 St. John's University
 Queens, NY

CONSULTING EDITOR FOR ETHNOGERIATRICS

Sharon A. Brangman, MD, FACP, AGSF
 Distinguished Service Professor
 Inaugural Chair, Department of Geriatrics
 Director, Nappi Longevity Institute
 SUNY Upstate Medical University
 Syracuse, NY

SPECIAL ADVISORS

Kevin T. Foley, MD, FACP, AGSF
 Associate Professor
 Department of Family Medicine
 Director of Education and Clinical Operations
 Division of Geriatrics and Gerontology
 Michigan State University - Clinical Center
 East Lansing, MI

Matthew K. McNabney, MD, AGSF
 Associate Professor of Medicine
 Johns Hopkins University
 Fellowship Program Director - Geriatrics
 Medical Director - Hopkins ElderPlus
 Baltimore, MD

NURSING ADVISOR

Elizabeth Galik, PhD, CRNP, FAAN, FAANP
 Professor
 University of Maryland School of Nursing
 Baltimore, MD

STUDENT ADVISOR

Laura K. Byerly, MD
 Assistant Professor of Medicine
 Division of General Internal Medicine & Geriatrics
 Oregon Health & Science University
 Portland, OR
 (Dr. Byerly was a geriatric medicine fellow at UCSF during her term as Student Advisor.)

CONTRIBUTING *GRS10* CHAPTER AUTHORS

Melinda Gail Abernethy, MD, MPH
Associate Director
Female Pelvic Medicine and Reconstructive Surgery Fellowship
Assistant Professor of Gynecology and Obstetrics
Johns Hopkins University School of Medicine
Baltimore, MD

Kathleen M. Akgün, MD, MS
Director, VA MICU
VA Connecticut Healthcare System
West Haven, CT
Associate Professor
Yale University School of Medicine
Department of Internal Medicine
Section of Pulmonary, Critical Care and Sleep Medicine
New Haven, CT

Cathy A. Alessi, MD, AGSF
Director, Geriatric Research, Education and Clinical Center
Veterans Administration Greater Los Angeles Healthcare System
Professor, David Geffen School of Medicine at UCLA
Los Angeles, CA

Neil B. Alexander, MD
Director, Mobility Research Center
Ivan P. Duff Collegiate Professor
Division of Geriatric and Palliative Medicine
Department of Internal Medicine
Research Professor, Institute of Gerontology, University of Michigan
Director, VA Ann Arbor Health Care System GRECC
Ann Arbor, MI

Naomi B. Anker, MD
Assistant Professor
Department of Medicine, Division of Nephrology
San Francisco VA Healthcare System
University of California San Francisco
San Francisco, CA

Alicia I. Arbaje, MD, MPH, PhD
Associate Professor of Medicine
Director of Transitional Care Research
Division of Geriatric Medicine and Gerontology
Johns Hopkins University School of Medicine
Baltimore, MD

Priscilla F. Bade, MD, FACP, CMD
Professor of Internal Medicine
Sanford School of Medicine
University of South Dakota
Rapid City, SD

Judith L. Beizer, PharmD, BCGP, FASCP, AGSF
Clinical Professor
College of Pharmacy and Health Sciences
St. John's University
Queens, NY

Sarah D. Berry, MD, MPH
Associate Professor of Medicine
Harvard Medical School
Beth Israel Deaconess Medical Center and Hebrew SeniorLife
Boston, MA

Kecia-Ann Blissett, DO
Director of Geriatric Psychiatry Outpatient Services
Associate Geriatric Psychiatry Fellowship Training Director
Assistant Professor
Icahn School of Medicine at Mount Sinai
New York, NY

Emily Bowen, MD
Geriatrics Fellow
Division of Geriatric Medicine
UT Southwestern Medical Center
Dallas, TX

Cynthia M. Boyd, MD, MPH
Professor
Division of Geriatric Medicine and Gerontology
Department of Medicine
Johns Hopkins University School of Medicine
Baltimore, MD

Cynthia J. Brown, MD, MSPH, AGSF
Professor and Director, Division of Gerontology, Geriatrics, and Palliative Care
University of Alabama at Birmingham
Birmingham/Atlanta GRECC
Birmingham, AL

Maciej S. Bukowski, PhD, FACN, FTOS
Research Professor of Medicine and Pediatrics
Department of Medicine
Division of Gastroenterology, Hepatology and Nutrition
Vanderbilt University Medical Center
Nashville, TN

Johanna A. Cabassa, MD
Geriatric Psychiatrist
Department of Psychiatry and Behavioral Sciences
Montefiore Medical Center
The University Hospital of The Albert Einstein College of Medicine
Bronx, NY

Thomas V. Caprio, MD, MPH, MS, AGSF
Associate Professor of Medicine/Geriatrics
Program Director, Geriatric Medicine Fellowship
Project Director, Finger Lakes Geriatric Workforce Enhancement Program
Chief Medical Officer, UR Medicine Home Care
University of Rochester Medical Center
Rochester, NY

Jarrod A. Carrol, MD
Associate Physician
Department of Geriatrics, Palliative and Continuing Care
Kaiser Permanente, West Los Angeles Medical Center
Los Angeles, CA

Sujana S. Chandrasekhar, MD, FACS
Past President, American Academy of Otolaryngology-Head and Neck Surgery
Partner, ENT and Allergy Associates, LLP
Director of Neurotology, James J Peters VA Medical Center
Clinical Professor of Otolaryngology
Zucker School of Medicine at Hofstra-Northwell
Clinical Associate Professor of Otolaryngology
Icahn School of Medicine at Mount Sinai
New York, NY

Pei Chen, MD
Assistant Professor
Division of Geriatrics, Department of Medicine
University of California, San Francisco
Associate Medical Director
UCSF Center for Geriatric Care
San Francisco, CA

Colleen Christmas, MD, FACP
Associate Professor of Medicine
Director, Primary Care Track
Johns Hopkins University School of Medicine
Baltimore, MD

Leo M. Cooney, Jr, MD
Humana Foundation Professor of Geriatric Medicine
Yale University School of Medicine
New Haven, CT

Grace A. Cordts, MD, MPH, MS
Medical Director
Optum Complex Population Management
Pittsburgh, PA

Jason Costa, MD
Fellow in Cardiovascular Disease
New York University School of Medicine
New York, NY

Kumar Dharmarajan, MD, MBA
Chief Scientific Officer
Clover Health
Jersey City, NJ

Danielle J. Doberman, MD, MPH, HMDC
Medical Director, Palliative Medicine Program
Assistant Professor, Department of Medicine
Associate Program Director, Palliative Medicine Fellowship
Johns Hopkins Hospital
Baltimore, MD

John A. Dodson, MD, MPH, FACC
Assistant Professor of Medicine and Population Health
Director, Geriatric Cardiology Program
Leon H. Charney Division of Cardiology
New York University School of Medicine
New York, NY

Catherine E. Dubeau, MD
Professor of Medicine – Geriatrics
Dartmouth Geisel School of Medicine
Lebanon, NH

Robert Eckles, DPM, MPH
Dean, Clinical and Graduate Medical Education
New York College of Podiatric Medicine
New York, NY

Manuel A. Eskildsen, MD, MPH, CMD, AGSF
Associate Clinical Professor
David Geffen School of Medicine at UCLA
Los Angeles, CA

Neal S. Fedarko, PhD
Professor, Division of Geriatric Medicine and Gerontology, Department of Medicine
Director, Institute for Clinical and Translational Research Clinical Research Core Laboratory
Co-director, Biology of Healthy Aging Program
Johns Hopkins University School of Medicine
Baltimore, MD

Luigi Ferrucci, MD, PhD
Senior Investigator
NIA Scientific Director
Chief, Longitudinal Studies Section
National Institute on Aging
Bethesda, MD

Kathleen T. Foley, PhD, OTR/L, FAOTA
Associate Professor and Director, School of Occupational Therapy
Ivester College of Health Sciences
Brenau University
Norcross, GA

Elizabeth Galik, PhD, CRNP, FAAN, FAANP
Professor
University of Maryland School of Nursing
Baltimore, MD

Angela Gentili, MD
Professor of Internal Medicine
Associate Director, Geriatrics Fellowship Training Program
VAMC/Virginia Commonwealth University
Richmond, VA

JoAnn A. Giaconi, MD
Associate Professor of Clinical Ophthalmology
David Geffen School of Medicine at UCLA
Stein Eye Institute
Chief of Ophthalmology, Veterans Administration Los Angeles
Los Angeles, CA

Michael Godschalk, MD
Staff Physician
McGuire VA Medical Center
Professor of Internal Medicine
Virginia Commonwealth University School of Medicine
Richmond, VA

Thomas M. Gill, MD
Professor of Medicine, Epidemiology, and Investigative Medicine
Humana Foundation Professor of Geriatric Medicine
Yale University
New Haven, CT

Suzanne M. Gillespie, MD, RD, CMD, AGSF
Associate Chief of Staff
Geriatrics Extended Care
Canandaigua VA Medical Center
Canandaigua, NY
Associate Professor of Medicine
Division of Geriatrics/Aging
University of Rochester
Rochester, NY

Jane M. Grant-Kels, MD, FAAD
Professor of Dermatology, Pathology and Pediatrics
University of Connecticut Health Center
Founding Director of the Cutaneous Oncology Center and Melanoma Program
Vice Chair, Department of Dermatology
Founding Chair Emeritus, Department of Dermatology
Founding Director Emeritus, Dermatology Residency and Dermatopathology Laboratory
Farmington, CT

Lisa J. Granville, MD, FACP, AGSF
Professor and Associate Chair
Department of Geriatrics
Florida State University College of Medicine
Tallahassee, FL

David A. Gruenewald, MD, FACP
Associate Professor of Medicine
Division of Gerontology and Geriatric Medicine
Department of Medicine
University of Washington School of Medicine
Medical Director, Palliative Care and Hospice Service
Geriatrics and Extended Care Service
Department of Veterans Affairs Puget Sound Health Care System
Seattle, WA

Ihab Hajjar, MD, MS, FACP
Associate Professor of Medicine and Neurology
Division of Geriatrics and General Internal Medicine
Department of Medicine and Neurology
Emory University
Atlanta, GA

Scott Hebert, MD
Department of Internal Medicine
Section of Hematology and Oncology
Louisiana State University
New Orleans, LA

Kevin T. Hendler, DDS, FASGD, DABSCD, FICD
Associate Professor, Medicine and Geriatrics
Emory University School of Medicine
Director, Geriatric Dentistry
Ina T. Allen Dental Center, Emory Healthcare
Atlanta, GA

Timothy Holahan DO, CMD
Assistant Professor of Medicine
Geriatric Medicine and Palliative Care
University of Rochester Medical Center
Rochester, NY

Manisha Juthani-Mehta, MD
Associate Professor of Medicine
Infectious Diseases Fellowship Program Director
Associate Program Director, Internal Medicine Residency Program
Director of Internal Medicine Fellowship Programs
Department of Internal Medicine
Section of Infectious Diseases
Yale University School of Medicine
New Haven, CT

Sarah H. Kagan, PhD, RN
Lucy Walker Honorary Term Professor of Gerontological Nursing
School of Nursing
Gerontological Clinical Nurse Specialist
Abramson Cancer Center at Pennsylvania Hospital
University of Pennsylvania
Philadelphia, PA

Philip O. Katz, MD
Professor of Medicine
Director, Motility Laboratories
Jay Monahan Center for Gastrointestinal Health
Weill Cornell Medical College
New York, NY

Gary J. Kennedy, MD
Professor and Vice Chair for Education
Director, Division of Geriatric Psychiatry and Fellowship Program
Department of Psychiatry and Behavioral Sciences
Montefiore Medical Center
Albert Einstein College of Medicine
Bronx, NY

Douglas P. Kiel, MD, MPH
Director, Musculoskeletal Research Center
Institute for Aging Research
Hebrew SeniorLife and Professor of Medicine
Department of Medicine
Beth Israel Deaconess Medical Center and Harvard Medical School
Boston, MA

Michael Krol, MD
Attending Physician
Austin Geriatric Specialists
Austin, TX

Mark Lachs, MD, MPH
Professor of Medicine and Co-Chief
Division of Geriatrics and Gerontology
Cornell Weill Medical College
New York, NY

Melinda S. Lantz, MD
Vice Chair
Chief of Geriatric Psychiatry
Mount Sinai Beth Israel
Associate Professor of Psychiatry
Icahn School of Medicine at Mount Sinai
New York, NY

Paul LaStayo, PT, PhD, CHT
Professor
Department of Physical Therapy and Athletic Training
University of Utah
Salt Lake City, UT

Helen Lavretsky, MD, MS
Division of Psychiatry
Professor of Psychiatry In-Residence
Director, Late-life Mood, Stress, and Wellness Research Program
Semel Institute for Neuroscience and Human Behavior
David Geffen School of Medicine at UCLA
Los Angeles, CA

Sei J. Lee, MD, MAS
Associate Professor
Division of Geriatrics
University of California, San Francisco
Senior Scholar, San Francisco VA Quality Scholars Fellowship
San Francisco, CA

Susan W. Lehmann, MD
Clinical Director, Division of Geriatric Psychiatry and Neuropsychiatry
Director, Geriatric Psychiatry Day Hospital
Psychiatry Clerkship Director
Associate Professor, Department of Psychiatry and Behavioral Sciences
Member, Miller-Coulson Academy of Clinical Excellence
Baltimore, MD

Jeffrey M. Levine, MD, AGSF, CWSP
Associate Clinical Professor of Geriatrics and Palliative Care
Icahn School of Medicine at Mount Sinai
New York, NY

Daphne Lo, MD, MAEd
Assistant Clinical Professor
Division of Geriatrics
University of California San Francisco
Medical Director
Home Based Primary Care
San Francisco Veterans Affairs Health Care System
San Francisco, CA

Kenneth W. Lyles, MD, AGSF
Professor of Medicine
Duke University School of Medicine
Durham VA Medical Center
Durham, NC

Allison Magnuson, DO
Assistant Professor of Medicine
Geriatric Oncology
University of Rochester Medical Center
Rochester, NY

Ronald J. Maggiore, MD
Assistant Professor of Medicine
Department of Medicine
Division of Hematology/Oncology
University of Rochester
Rochester, NY

Una E. Makris, MD, MCS
Associate Professor, Department of Internal Medicine
Division of Rheumatic Diseases
UT Southwestern Medical Center and Dallas VAMC
Dallas, TX

Edward R. Marcantonio, MD, SM
Professor of Medicine
Harvard Medical School
Section Chief for Research
Director, Aging Research Program
Division of General Medicine and Primary Care
Beth Israel Deaconess Medical Center
Boston, MA

Robin Marcus, PT, PhD, OCS
Professor and Chief Wellness Officer
Associate Dean for Clinical Affairs, College of Health
Department of Physical Therapy and Athletic Training
Salt Lake City, UT

Alvin M. Matsumoto, MD
Associate Director
Geriatric Research, Education and Clinical Center
VA Puget Sound Health Care System
Professor, Division of Gerontology and Geriatric Medicine
Department of Medicine
University of Washington School of Medicine
Seattle, WA

Daniel McGovern, MD
Attending Psychiatrist
Inpatient Unit Chief
Department of Psychiatry
Mount Sinai Beth Israel
New York, NY

Matthew K. McNabney, MD
Associate Professor of Medicine
Johns Hopkins University
Fellowship Program Director, Geriatrics
Medical Director, Hopkins ElderPlus
Baltimore, MD

Brianna Morgan, MSN, AGPCNP-BC
Palliative and Geriatric Nurse Practitioner
Abramson Cancer Center at Pennsylvania Hospital
Philadelphia, PA

Daniel L. Murman, MD, MS, FAAN
Director, Behavioral and Geriatric Neurology Program
Professor, Department of Neurological Sciences
University of Nebraska Medical Center
Omaha, NE

Aman Nanda, MD, AGSF, CMD
Associate Professor of Medicine
Program Director
Geriatric Medicine Fellowship Program
The Warren Alpert Medical School of Brown University
Providence, RI

Judith Neugroschl, MD
Medical Director
Mount Sinai School of Medicine
Alzheimer's Disease Research Center Clinical Core
Co-Director, ADRC Education and Information Transfer Core
New York, NY

James T. Pacala, MD, MS, AGSF
Professor and Head
Department of Family Medicine and Community Health
University of Minnesota Medical School
Minneapolis, MN

Vyjeyanthi S. Periyakoil, MD
Associate Professor
Director, Palliative Care Education and Training
Director, eCampus Geriatrics
VA Palo Alto Health Care System and Stanford University School of Medicine
Stanford, CA

Edgar Pierluissi, MD
Professor of Medicine, University of California at San Francisco
Medical Director, Acute Care for Elders (ACE) Unit
San Francisco General Hospital
San Francisco, CA

Margaret Pisani, MD, MPH
Associate Professor
Yale University School of Medicine
Pulmonary and Critical Care Medicine
New Haven, CT

James S. Powers, MD, AGSF
Professor of Medicine
Vanderbilt University Medical Center
Associate Clinical Director, TVHS GRECC
Nashville, TN

Pradeep S. Prasad, MD, MBA
Associate Clinical Professor of Ophthalmology
Stein Eye Institute
David Geffen School of Medicine at UCLA
Chief, Division of Ophthalmology
Harbor-UCLA Medical Center
LA County Department of Health Services
Los Angeles, CA

Thomas M. Reske, MD, PhD, FACP, CMD
Assistant Clinical Professor
Section of Hematology, Oncology and Geriatric Medicine
Louisiana State University HSC New Orleans
New Orleans, LA

Michael W. Rich, MD, AGSF, FACC
Professor of Medicine
Washington University School of Medicine
St. Louis, MO

Josette A. Rivera, MD
Associate Professor of Medicine
Division of Geriatrics
University of California San Francisco
San Francisco, CA

Tony Rosen, MD, MPH
Assistant Professor of Emergency Medicine
Department of Emergency Medicine
Weill Cornell Medical College/New York-Presbyterian Hospital
New York, NY

Theresa A. Rowe, DO, MS
Assistant Professor
Division of General Internal Medicine and Geriatrics
Northwestern University
Feinberg School of Medicine
Chicago, IL

Paul Scalzo, BS
Research Technologist
Clinical Pharmacology Analytical Laboratory
Division of Clinical Pharmacology
Johns Hopkins University School of Medicine
Baltimore, MD

J. William Schleifer, MD
Assistant Professor of Medicine
Department of Internal Medicine, Division of Cardiology
University of Nebraska Medical Center
Omaha, NE

Mara A. Schonberg, MD, MPH
Director of Research in Shared Decision Making
Associate Professor of Medicine
Beth Israel Deaconess Medical Center
Harvard Medical School
Boston, MA

Priya Sharma, MD, FRCPC
Psychiatrist
Hotel Dieu Grace Hospital
Windsor, ON, Canada

Win-Kuang Shen, MD
Professor of Medicine
Mayo Clinic College of Medicine
Chair, Department of Cardiovascular Diseases
Mayo Clinic Arizona
Phoenix, AZ

Mark J. Simone, MD, AGSF
Assistant Professor of Medicine
Harvard Medical School
Associate Program Director-Primary Care
Mt Auburn Internal Medicine Residency Program
Geriatrician, Quimby Center for Geriatric Care
Mount Auburn Hospital
Cambridge, MA

Richard G. Stefanacci, DO, MGH, MBA, AGSF, CMD
Faculty, Thomas Jefferson University, Jefferson College of Population Health
Philadelphia, PA
Chief Medical Director, The Access Group
Berkeley Heights, NJ
Medical Director, Population Health, AtlantiCare/Geisinger
Atlantic City, NJ

Margarita Sotelo, MD
Associate Clinical Professor
Divisions of Geriatrics and Hospital Medicine
University of California San Francisco
San Francisco, CA

Amir E. Soumekh, MD
Assistant Professor of Clinical Medicine
Jay Monahan Center for Gastrointestinal Health
Weill Cornell Medical College
New York, NY

Amy Swift, MD
Attending Psychiatrist
Dual Diagnosis Team
Assistant Director Addiction Psychiatry Fellowship
Mount Sinai Beth Israel
New York, NY

Ayman Samman Tahhan, MD
Cardiovascular Disease Fellow
Emory University School of Medicine
Atlanta, GA

Zaldy S. Tan, MD, MPH
Medical Director, UCLA Alzheimer's and Dementia Care Program
Philo Van Wagoner Professor of Medicine
Assistant Dean for Curricular Affairs
David Geffen School of Medicine at UCLA
Los Angeles, CA

Kristen Thornton, MD, FAAFP, AGSF, CWSP
Clinical Assistant Professor of Family Medicine
University of Rochester School of Medicine and Dentistry
Rochester, NY

Taya Varteresian, DO, MSMD
MH Psychiatrist
Los Angeles County Department of Mental Health
Assistant Clinical Professor of Psychiatry and Human Behavior
University of California Irvine
Irvine, CA

Elizabeth K. Vig, MD, MPH
Associate Professor, Department of Medicine
Division of Gerontology and Geriatric Medicine
University of Washington
Staff Physician, Geriatrics and Extended Care
VA Puget Sound Health Care System
Seattle, WA

Jeremy D. Walston, MD
Raymond and Anna Lublin Professor of Geriatric Medicine
Johns Hopkins Asthma and Allergy Center
Baltimore, MD

Andrew Warren, MB, BS, DPhil
Psychiatrist
Sheppard Pratt Physicians Association
Baltimore, MD

Michael R. Wasserman, MD, CMD
Chief Executive Officer
Rockport Healthcare Services
Los Angeles, CA

Eric Widera, MD
Professor of Clinical Medicine
Division of Geriatrics
Program Director, Geriatric Medicine Fellowship
University of California San Francisco
Director, Hospice and Palliative Care
San Francisco VA Medical Center
San Francisco, CA

CONTRIBUTING *GRS10* QUESTION AUTHORS

Emaad Abdel-Rahman, MD, PhD, FASN
Professor, Internal Medicine/Nephrology
Director, Kidney Center Clinic and Dialysis Unit
Director, Therapeutic Extra-Corporeal Unit
Head, Section of Geriatric Nephrology
Interim Director, Nephrology Transplant
University of Virginia
Charlottesville, VA

Jonathan S. Appelbaum, MD, FACP, AAHIVS
Laurie L. Dozier, Jr., MD, Education Director and Professor of Internal Medicine
Florida State University College of Medicine
Tallahassee, FL

Michele C. Balas, PhD, RN, APRN-NP, FCCM
Associate Professor
Center of Excellence in Critical and Complex Care
The Ohio State University College of Nursing
Columbus, OH

Matthew Barrett, MD
Assistant Professor
Department of Neurology
Charlottesville, VA

Lisa C. Barry, PhD, MPH
Assistant Professor of Psychiatry
UConn Center on Aging
Farmington, CT

Rachelle Bernacki, MD, MS, AGSF
Director of Quality Initiatives
Adult Palliative Care
Dana Farber Cancer Institute
Division of Aging
Brigham and Women's Hospital
Boston, MA

Michael Bogaisky, MD
Assistant Professor
Division of Geriatrics
Albert Einstein College of Medicine
Bronx, NY

Kenneth Brummel-Smith, MD, AGSF
Health and Aging Policy Fellow
Charlotte Edwards Maguire Professor and Chair,
Department of Geriatrics
Florida State University College of Medicine
Tallahassee, FL

Morgan Carlson, PhD
Research Investigator, Drug Discovery
Genomics Institute of the Novartis Research Foundation
San Diego, CA

Susan Charette, MD
Clinical Professor
Division of Geriatrics
Department of Medicine
Los Angeles, CA

Carl I. Cohen, MD
SUNY Distinguished Service Professor
Professor and Director
Division of Geriatric Psychiatry
SUNY Downstate Medical Center
Brooklyn, NY

Leo M. Cooney, Jr, MD
Humana Foundation Professor of Geriatric Medicine
Yale University School of Medicine
New Haven, CT

Mary Ellen Csuka, MD
Professor
Division of Rheumatology
Department of Medicine
Medical College of Wisconsin
Milwaukee, WI

Della E. Dillard, MD, MBA
Assistant Professor
Donald W. Reynolds Department of Geriatric Medicine
Department of Medicine
University of Oklahoma
Oklahoma City, OK

Ian M. Deutchki, MD
University of Rochester Medical Center
School of Medicine and Dentistry
Assistant Professor
Department of Family Medicine and Department of Medicine
Division of Geriatrics
Rochester, NY

Justin Endo, MD, FAAD
Assistant Professor of Dermatology
University of Wisconsin
Madison, WI

Jerome Epplin, MD, AGSF
Clinical Professor
Southern Illinois School of Medicine
Litchfield Family Practice Center
Litchfield, IL

Daniel E. Forman, MD, FACC, FAHA
Chair, Section of Geriatric Cardiology
University of Pittsburgh Medical Center
Pittsburgh, PA

Susan M. Friedman, MD, MPH, AGSF
Associate Professor of Medicine
Research Director, Geriatric Fracture Center
University of Rochester School of Medicine and Dentistry
Rochester, NY

Shelly L. Gray, PharmD, MS, AGSF
Professor and Vice Chair, Pharmacy
Director, Geriatrics Pharmacy Program
School of Pharmacy
University of Washington
Seattle, WA

Asaff Harel, MD
Department of Neurology
Mount Sinai Medical Center
New York, NY

Elizabeth N. Harlow, MD
Assistant Professor
Geriatrics, Internal Medicine
Omaha, NE

Holly B. Hindman, MD, MPH
Associate Professor of Ophthalmology and Visual Science
Flaum Eye Institute
University of Rochester
Rochester, NY

Lianne Hirano, MD
Acting Assistant Professor
Division of Gerontology & Geriatric Medicine
Harborview Medical Center
Seattle, WA

Ted Johnson, MD, MPH, AGSF
Professor of Medicine and Epidemiology, Emory University
Division Chief, General Medicine & Geriatrics
Atlanta Site Director, Birmingham/Atlanta VA GRECC
Decatur, GA

Fran E. Kaiser, MD, AGSF, FGSA
Adjunct Professor of Medicine
St. Louis University School of Medicine
St Louis, MO
Executive Medical Director
Region Medical Director Program
Merck and Co., Inc
Upper Gwynedd, PA

Helen Kao, MD
University of California, San Francisco
Division of Geriatrics
San Francisco, CA

Anne Kenny, MD
Professor of Medicine
Department of Medicine
University of Connecticut Health Center
Farmington, CT

Tia Kostas, MD
Assistant Professor of Medicine
Section of Geriatrics and Palliative Medicine
University of Chicago
Chicago, IL

Lawrence R. Krakoff, MD
Professor of Medicine
Center for Cardiovascular Health
Mount Sinai Medical Center
New York, NY

Stephen Krieger, MD
Associate Professor of Neurology
Corinne Goldsmith Dickinson Center for MS
Director, Neurology Residency Program
Icahn School of Medicine at Mount Sinai
New York, NY

Lorand Kristof, MD, MSc
Assistant Clinical Professor
McMaster University
Department of Family Medicine
Wise Elephant Family Health Team
Brampton Civic Hospital
William Osler Health System
Brampton, Ontario

Chandrika Kumar, MD, FACP
Director of Resident Geriatric Medical Education
Associate Fellowship Director
Yale University School of Medicine
New Haven, CT
Geriatric Consult Service
West Haven Veterans Administration
West Haven, CT

Mark S. Lachs, MD, MPH
Irene F. and I. Roy Psaty Distinguished Professor of Medicine
Co-chief, Division of Geriatrics and Palliative Medicine
Director of Geriatrics
The New York-Presbyterian Health Care System
New York, NY

Sei J. Lee, MD, MAS
Associate Professor
University of California, San Francisco
Senior Scholar, SF VA Quality Scholars Fellowship
Division of Geriatrics
San Francisco, CA

Michael C. Lindberg, MD, FACP
Chief Medical Officer
Monadnock Community Hospital
Peterborough, NH

Hannah I. Lipman, MD, MS
Associate Director, Montefiore-Einstein Center for Bioethics
Chief, Bioethics Consultation Service
Associate Professor of Medicine
Divisions of Geriatrics and Cardiology
Bronx, NY

Hao Liu, PT, PhD, MD
Associate Professor of Physical Therapy
University of North Texas Health Science Center
Fort Worth, TX

Vera P. Luther, MD, FACP
Associate Professor of Medicine
Director, Infectious Diseases Fellowship
Associate Program Director, Internal Medicine Residency
Department of Internal Medicine
Section on Infectious Diseases
Wake Forest School of Medicine
Winston-Salem, NC

Bryan C. Markinson, DPM
Associate Professor of Orthopedic Surgery
Chief, Podiatric Medicine and Surgery
The Leni and Peter W. May Department of Orthopedic Surgery
Icahn School of Medicine at Mount Sinai
New York, NY

Diana V. Messadi, DDS, MMSc, DMSc
Professor of Dentistry
Associate Dean for Education and Faculty Development
Chair, Section of Oral Medicine and Orofacial Pain
UCLA School of Dentistry
Los Angeles, CA

Leigh Ann Mike, PharmD, BCPS, CGP
Clinical Assistant Professor
Coordinator, Plein Certificate in Geriatric Pharmacy
University of Washington School of Pharmacy
Consultant Pharmacist, UW Pharmacy Cares
Seattle, WA

Karen L. Miller, MD
Adjunct Associate Professor
Department of Obstetrics and Gynecology
University of Utah
Salt Lake City, UT

Irene Moore, MSW, LISW-S, AGSF
Professor, Department of Family & Community Medicine
Assistant Director, Geriatric Medicine Program
University of Cincinnati Geriatric Medicine Program
Cincinnati, OH

Alison A. Moore, MD, MPH
Professor, Departments of Medicine and Psychiatry
David Geffen School of Medicine at UCLA
Division of Geriatric Medicine
Los Angeles, CA

Cynthia X. Pan, MD, FACP, AGSF
Chief, Division of Geriatrics and Palliative Care Medicine
New York Presbyterian Queens
Associate Professor of Clinical Medicine
Weill Cornell Medical College
Flushing, NY

Kourosh Parham, MD, PhD, FACS
Associate Professor of Surgery
Director of Research, Division of Otolaryngology
Department of Surgery
UConn Health
Farmington, CT

Barbara Resnick, PhD, CRNP, FAAN, FAANP, AGSF
Professor
Sonya Ziporkin Gershowitz Chair in Gerontology
University of Maryland School of Nursing
Baltimore, MD

Miriam Rodin, MD, PhD
Professor of Geriatric Medicine
Department of Internal Medicine
St. Louis University School of Medicine
St. Louis, MO

Laurence Z. Rubenstein, MD, MPH, FACP, AGSF
Professor and Chairman
Reynolds Department of Geriatric Medicine
The Donald W. Reynolds Chair in Geriatric Medicine
The University of Oklahoma, Health Sciences Center
Oklahoma City, OK

Alessandra Scalmati, MD, PhD
Department of Psychiatry and Behavioral Sciences
Montefiore Medical Center
The University Hospital of The Albert Einstein College of Medicine
Outpatient Department of Psychiatry
Bronx, NY

Krupa Shah, MD, MPH, AGSF
Assistant Professor
University of Rochester School of Medicine & Dentistry
Division of Geriatrics and Aging
Department of Medicine
Rochester, NY

Nina J. Solenski, MD
Associate Professor in Neurology
Department of Neurology
University of Virginia
Charlottesville, VA

Margarita Sotelo, MD
Associate Clinical Professor
Divisions of Geriatrics and Hospital Medicine
University of California San Francisco
San Francisco, CA

Richard G. Stefanacci, DO, MGH, MBA, AGSF, CMD
Thomas Jefferson University
College of Population Health
Philadelphia, PA
Chief Medical Officer
The Access Group
Berkeley Heights, NJ

Martin Steinberg, MD
Assistant Professor of Psychiatry and Behavioral Sciences
Johns Hopkins Bayview Medical Center
Baltimore, MD

Winnie Suen, MD, AGSF
Medical Director of Geriatrics
Section Chief of Geriatrics
Inova Fairfax Hospital
Falls Church, VA

Dennis H. Sullivan, MD, AGSF
Director, Geriatric Research Education and Clinical Center
Central Arkansas Veterans Healthcare System
Professor and Vice-Chair
Donald W Reynolds Department of Geriatrics
University of Arkansas for Medical Sciences
Little Rock, AR

George E. Taffet, MD, FACP
Professor in Medicine
Chief, Geriatrics
Geriatrics and Cardiovascular Sciences
Robert J. Luchi, MD Chair in Geriatric Medicine
Baylor College of Medicine
Head of the Division of Geriatrics
The Methodist Hospital
Houston, TX

George Taler, MD
Director, Long Term Care
Washington Hospital Center
Professor, Clinical Medicine, Geriatrics and Long Term Care
Georgetown University School of Medicine
Washington, DC

John A. Taylor, III, MD, MS
Associate Professor of Surgery
Division of Urology
Chairman, Cancer Committee
University of Connecticut Health Center
Farmington, CT

Ipsit V. Vahia, MD
Assistant Professor of Psychiatry
Director of Research, Senior Behavioral Health
Stein Institute for Research on Aging
University of California, San Diego
La Jolla, CA

Camille P. Vaughan, MD, MS
Assistant Professor of Medicine, Emory University
Associate Section Chief for Research, Geriatrics and Gerontology
Investigator, Birmingham/Atlanta VA GRECC
Decatur, GA

Fran Valle, DNP, CRNP
Assistant Professor of Nursing
Director of the Post Master's Doctor of Nursing Practice Program
University of Maryland School of Nursing
Baltimore, MD

Dennis T. Villareal, MD, FACP, FACE
Professor, Baylor College of Medicine
Michael E. DeBakey VA Medical Center
Houston, TX

Barbara E. Weinstein, PhD
Professor and Founding Executive Officer
Health Sciences Doctoral Programs and AuD Program
Professor Speech Language Hearing Sciences
The Graduate Center
The City University of New York
New York, NY

Julie Wetherell, MD
Staff Psychologist
VA San Diego Healthcare System
Professor of Psychiatry
University of California San Diego
La Jolla, CA

G. Darryl Wieland, PhD, MPH, AGSF
Senior Research Scientist
Center for Population Health and Aging
Social Science Research Institute
Duke University
Durham, NC

Rebecca Wysoske, MD
Assistant Professor
College of Medicine
Department of Psychiatry
University of Nebraska Medical Center
Omaha, NE

Fariba S. Younai, DDS
Professor of Clinical Dentistry
Oral Medicine and Orofacial Pain
Vice Chair, Division of Oral Biology and Medicine
UCLA School of Dentistry
Los Angeles, CA

Michi Yukawa MD, MPH
Professor of Medicine
Medical Director of Community Living Center
San Francisco VA Medical Center
University of California, San Francisco
San Francisco, CA

Raymond Yung, MD
Professor of Internal Medicine
Chief, Division of Geriatric and Palliative Medicine
University of Michigan
Ann Arbor, MI

Valerie Zamudio, MD
Longterm Care Physician and Faculty
Geriatrics, Palliative Medicine, and Continuing Care Services
Kaiser Permanente Los Angeles Medical Center
Los Angeles, CA

Phyllis C. Zee, MD, PhD
Professor of Neurology
Department of Neurobiology and Physiology
Director Sleep Disorders Center
Chicago, IL

Richard A. Zweig, PhD
Director, Ferkauf Older Adult Program
Associate Professor of Psychology
Ferkauf Graduate School of Yeshiva University
Assistant Professor of Psychiatry
Albert Einstein College of Medicine
Bronx, NY

Jessica L. Zwerling, MD, MS
Assistant Professor
The Saul R. Korey Department of Neurology
Albert Einstein College of Medicine/Montefiore Medical Center
Neurologist and Director of the Memory Disorders Center
Associate Director of the Center for the Aging Brain
Program Director, Geriatric Neurology Fellowship
Montefiore Medical Center
Bronx, NY

DISCLOSURES OF FINANCIAL INTERESTS

As an accredited provider of Continuing Medical Education, the American Geriatrics Society continually strives to ensure that the education activities planned and conducted by our faculty meet generally accepted ethical standards as codified by the ACCME, the Food and Drug Administration, and the American Medical Association. To this end, we have implemented a process wherein everyone who is in a position to control the content of an educational activity has disclosed all relevant financial relationships with any commercial interests within the past 12 months as related to the content of their presentations and under which we work to resolve any real or apparent conflicts of interest. Conflicts of interest in this particular CME activity have been resolved by having the presentation content independently peer reviewed before publication by the Editorial Board and Question Review Committee.

The following contributors (and/or their spouses/partners) have reported real or apparent conflicts of interest that have been resolved through a peer review content validation process:

Jonathan S. Appelbaum, MD, FACP, AAHIVS
Dr. Appelbaum is on the advisory board for Merck and Viiv Healthcare.

Ihab Hajjar, MD, MS, FACP, AGSF
Dr. Hajjar is a recipient of a research grant from Alzamed.

Theodore M. Johnson II, MD, MPH, AGSF
Dr. Johnson was a paid consultant for Vantia (2015) and Medtronic (2016).

Helen Lavretsky, MD, MS
Dr. Lavretsky received a research grant from Allergan.

Pearl G. Lee, MD, MS
Dr. Lee is on the research advisory committee of T1D Exchange of Unitio, Inc. and received writing and editorial support from Sanofi US, Inc.

Kenneth W. Lyles, MD, AGSF
Dr. Lyles is a paid consultant for Health Decisions, Durham, NC. He is Cofounder and Equity Owner: BisCardia, Inc.; Faculty Connection, LLC. He is Co-Inventor of US Patent Application: "Methods for preventing or reducing secondary fractures after hip fracture" #20050272707; Inventor of US Patent Application: "Medication Kits and Formulations for Preventing, Treating or Reducing Secondary Fractures After Previous Fracture" #12532285; Co-Inventor of US Patent: "Bisphosphonate Compositions and Methods for Treating Heart Failure" 15/864,327; and Co-Inventor of US Patent: "Bisphophonate Compositions and Methods for Treating and/or Reducing Cardiac Dysfunction" 14/358,468.

Alvin M. Matsumoto, MD
Dr. Matsumoto is a paid consultant for Aytu Biosciences and AbbVie.

James T. Pacala, MD, MS, AGSF
Dr. Pacala is a paid board member of UCare Minnesota.

Richard G. Stefanacci, DO, MGH, MBA, AGSF, CMD
Dr. Stefanacci is a paid speaker for Merck, Sunovion, and Janssen, and an employee of The Access Group.

Phyllis C. Zee, MD, PhD
Dr. Zee is a paid consultant for Sanofi, Eisai, Jazz, Philips, and Harmony Biosciences and a stockholder of Teva and Express Scripts.

The following contributors have returned disclosure forms indicating that they (and/or their spouses/partners) have no affiliation with, or financial interest in, any commercial interest that may have direct interest in the subject matter of their chapters/questions:

Emaad M. Abdel-Rahman, MD, PhD, FASN
Melinda Gail Abernethy, MD, MPH
Susan E. Aiello, DVM, ELS
Kathleen M. Akgün, MD, MS
Cathy A. Alessi, MD, AGSF
Neil B. Alexander, MD
Naomi B. Anker, MD
Alicia I. Arbaje, MD, MPH, PhD
Kyrollis Attalla, MD
Priscilla F. Bade, MD, FACP, CMD
Sharon Baranoski, MSN, CWCN, APN-CCNS, FAAN
Kevin Barley, MD
Lisa C. Barry, PhD, MPH
Judith L. Beizer, PharmD, BCGP, FASCP, AGSF
Rachelle Bernacki, MD, MS, AGSF, FAAHPM
Sarah D. Berry, MD, MPH
Kecia-Ann Blissett, DO
Michael Bogaisky, MD, MPH
Marie Boltz, PhD, GNP-BC, FGSA, FAAN
Emily A. Bowen, MD
Cynthia M. Boyd, MD, MPH
Sharon A. Brangman, MD, FACP, AGSF
Cynthia J. Brown, MD, MSPH, AGSF
Maciej S. Bukowski, PhD, FACN, FTOS
Daniel C. Butler, MD
Laura K. Byerly, MD
Debra L. Bynum, MD, MMEL
Johanna A. Cabassa, MD
Elizabeth Capezuti, PhD, RN, FAAN
Thomas V. Caprio, MD, MPH, MS, AGSF
Deirdre M. Carolan, PhD, ANP-BC, GNP-BC, FAANP
Jarrod A. Carrol, MD
Mirnova E. Ceïde, MD
Sujana S. Chandrasekhar, MD, FACS
Susan Charette, MD
Pei Chen, MD
Victoria Chima, MD, MPH
Natsurang Chongkrairatanakul, MD, ABIM
Colleen Christmas, MD, FACP
Carolyn Clevenger, RN, DNP, AGPCNP-BC, FAANP
Jason A. Cohen, MD
Jessica Colburn, MD
Leo M. Cooney, Jr, MD
Grace A. Cordts, MD, MPH, MS
Jason Costa, MD
Lenise A. Cummings-Vaughn, MD, CMD
Ian M. Deutchki, MD
Kumar Dharmarajan, MD, MBA
Danielle J. Doberman, MD, MPH, HMDC
John A. Dodson, MD, MPH, FACC
Catherine E. Dubeau, MD
Clark DuMontier, MD
Robert Eckles, DPM, MPH
Jerome Epplin, MD, AGSF
Elisabeth Erekson, MD, MPH, FACOG, FACS
Manuel A. Eskildsen, MD, MPH, CMD, AGSF
Michelle T. Fabian, MD
Timothy W. Farrell, MD, AGSF
Neal S. Fedarko, PhD
Luigi Ferrucci, MD, PhD
Mary Ann Forciea, MD, MACP
Daniel E. Forman, MD, FAHA, FACC

Jonathan M. Flacker, MD, AGSF
Kathleen T. Foley, PhD, OTR/L, FAOTA
Kevin T. Foley, MD, FACP, AGSF
Elizabeth Galik, PhD, CRNP, FAAN, FAANP
Angela Gentili, MD
JoAnn A. Giaconi, MD
Thomas M. Gill, MD
Suzanne M. Gillespie, MD, RD, CMD, AGSF
Michael Godschalk, MD
Jane M. Grant-Kels, MD, FAAD
Lisa J. Granville, MD, FACP, AGSF
Shelly L. Gray, PharmD, MS, AGSF
David A. Gruenewald, MD, FACP
Elizabeth N. Harlow, MD
G. Michael Harper, MD, AGSF
Scott Hebert, MD
Kevin T. Hendler, DDS, FASGD, DABSCD, FICD
Timothy J. Holahan DO, CMD
Victoria Hornyak, PT, DPT, GCS
Lee A. Jennings, MD, MSHS
Peter Jin, MD
Karin A. Johnson, OD, DO
Deirdre Johnston, MB BCh BAO, MRCPsych
Manisha Juthani-Mehta, MD
Sarah H. Kagan, PhD, RN
Fran E. Kaiser, MD, AGSF, FGSA
Kathleen M. Kan, MD
Philip O. Katz, MD
Gary J. Kennedy, MD
Laurie Kennedy-Malone, PhD, GNP-BC, FAANP, FGSA
Anne Kenny, MD
Rashmi Khadilkar, MD
Sana F. Khan, MD
Douglas P. Kiel, MD, MPH
Tia Kostas, MD
Lawrence R. Krakoff, MD
Stephen Krieger, MD, FAAN
Michael L. Krol, MD
Mark S. Lachs, MD, MPH
Melinda S. Lantz, MD
Paul C. LaStayo, PT, PhD, CHT
June C. Lee, DO
Sei J. Lee, MD, MAS
Susan W. Lehmann, MD
Jeffrey M. Levine, MD, AGSF, CWSP
Milta Oyola Little, DO, CMD
Daphne Lo, MD, MAEd
Vera P. Luther, MD, FACP, FIDSA
William L. Lyons, MD, AGSF
Allison Magnuson, DO
Ronald J. Maggiore, MD
Una E. Makris, MD, MSc
Elizabeth Mann, MD
Edward R. Marcantonio, MD, SM
Robin Marcus, PT, PhD, OCS
Stephen A. McCullough, MD
Sarah McGee, MD, MPH
Daniel T. McGovern, MD
Matthew K. McNabney, MD, AGSF
Diana V. Messadi, DDS, MMSc, DMSc
Isuzu Meyer, MD
Leigh Ann Mike, PharmD, BCPS, BCGP
Rachel K. Miller, MD
Brianna Morgan, MSN, AGPCNP-BC

Daniel L. Murman, MD, MS, FAAN
Aman Nanda, MD, AGSF, CMD
Ian Neel, MD
Judith Neugroschl, MD
Tyson A. Oberndorfer, MD, MS
Cynthia X. Pan, MD, FACP, AGSF
Manisha Parulekar, MD, FACP, AGSF, CMD
Vyjeyanthi S. Periyakoil, MD
Thomas T. Perls, MD, MPH, AGSF, FGSA
Edgar Pierluissi, MD
Margaret Pisani, MD, MPH
Jane F. Potter, MD, FACP, AGSF
James S. Powers, MD, AGSF
Pradeep S. Prasad, MD, MBA
Barbara Resnick, PhD, CRNP, FAAN, AGSF
Thomas M. Reske, MD, PhD, FACP, CMD
Bernardo J. Reyes, MD
Michael W. Rich, MD, AGSF, FACC
Katherine Ritchey, DO, MPH
Dalia Ritter
Josette A. Rivera, MD
Christopher K. Rogers, MPH
Scott A. Roof, MD
Tony Rosen, MD, MPH
Theresa A. Rowe, DO, MS
Matthew Leo Russell, MD, MSc
Ayman Samman Tahhan, MD
Arunima Sarkar MD, FACP, CMD
Paul Scalzo, BS
J. William Schleifer, MD
Mara A. Schonberg, MD, MPH
Jean-Pierre Schuster, MD
Himanshu S. Sharma, MD
Priya Sharma, MD, FRCPC
Win-Kuang Shen, MD
Andrea N. Sherman, MS
Mark J. Simone, MD, AGSF
Nina J. Solenski, MD
Rainier Patrick Soriano, MD
Margarita Sotelo, MD
Amir E. Soumekh, MD
Niharika Suchak, MBBS, MHS, FACP, AGSF
Winnie Suen, MD, MSc, AGSF
Dennis H. Sullivan, MD, AGSF
Amy Swift, MD
Zaldy S. Tan, MD, MPH
Kristen Thornton, MD, FAAFP, AGSF, CWSP
S.P.J. (Bas) van Alphen, PhD
Jessie VanSwearingen, PhD, PT, FAPTA
Camille P. Vaughan, MD, MS
Taya Varteresian, DO, MS
Elizabeth K. Vig, MD, MPH
Jeremy D. Walston, MD
Andrew Warren, MB, BS, DPhil
Michael R. Wasserman, MD, CMD
Amy M. Westcott, MD, CMD, FAAHPM
Christina R. Whitehouse, PhD, CRNP, CDE
Eric Widera, MD
Supakanya Wongrakpanich, MD
L. Pilar Wyman
Rebecca L. Wysoske, MD
Fariba S. Younai, DDS
Michi Yukawa, MD, MPH, AGSF
Raymond Yung, MD
Valerie Zamudio, MD

INDEX

NOTE: References followed by *t* and *f* indicate tables and figures, respectively. Numbers preceded by Q indicate question numbers and critiques.

A-a (alveolar-arterial) gradient, 380
AAA. *See* Abdominal aortic aneurysm
AARP (American Association of Retired Persons), 37–38, 39*t*
Abaloparatide, 268*t*, 269–270
Abandonment, 89
Abatacept, 488
ABC (Aging Brain Care) Program, Q77
Abdominal aortic aneurysm (AAA), 404
    indications for repair, 405
    screening for, 62*t*, 66–68
Abdominal ultrasonography, 62*t*
ABI (ankle-brachial index), 239, 404, 505
Abiraterone, 582*t*, 588
Abnormal Involuntary Movement Scale (AIMS), 333
Abscesses, 479, 539–540
Abstinence, 344, 350, 351
Abuse. *See* Mistreatment
ACA (Affordable Care Act). *See* Patient Protection and Affordable Care Act
Acamprosate, 349*t*, 350
Acarbose, 564*t*
ACC. *See* American College of Cardiology
Accountable care organizations (ACOs), 21, 173
Acculturation, 45
Accumulation theories of aging, 7
ACE (Acute Care for Elders), 135–136
ACE inhibitors. *See* Angiotensin-converting enzyme inhibitors
Acetaminophen
    adverse effects of, Q3
    for delirium, 298, 300*t*
    for fibromyalgia, 495–496
    for OA-related pain, 486
    for persistent pain, 121–122
    for postsurgical pain, 105
    for sleep issues, 312
Acetylcholinesterase inhibitors, 251*t*, 252
N-Acetylcysteine, 387
Achalasia, 423, 424
Aclidinium, 384–385, 384*t*
Acne rosacea, 361
ACOG (American College of Obstetricians and Gynecology), 447
ACOs (accountable care organizations), 21, 173
ACP. *See* Advance care planning; American College of Physicians
ACPA (anti-cyclic citrullinated peptide/protein antibodies), 487
Acquired immunodeficiency syndrome (AIDS), 538–539, Q107
    nursing-home care, 160
    treatment and care, 52

ACR. *See* American College of Rheumatology
ACR (albumin/creatinine ratio), 436
Acral lentiginous melanoma, 370, 370*f*
Acromioclavicular disease, 477
ACS (acute coronary syndromes), 390, 393–394
ACSM. *See* American College of Sports Medicine
ACTH (adrenocorticotropic hormone), 551, 551*t*
ACTH (adrenocorticotropic hormone) stimulation test, 552, 553
Actinic cheilitis, 368
Actinic keratoses, 368, 369*f*
Actinobacillus, 398, 536–537
Action tremor, 512–513
Active listening, 115
Active surveillance, 460–462, 460*t*, 461*t*
Activities of daily living (ADLs), 26–27
    Barthel ADL Index, 145*t*, 148
    instrumental, 27, 148, 577
Activity Measure for Post Acute Care (AM-PAC), 145*t*
Activity therapy, 292
Acupuncture, 85–86, 88
    for fibromyalgia, 495
    for low back pain, Q92
    for pain, 121
Acute adrenal insufficiency, 553
Acute back pain, 482
Acute bacterial prostatitis, 463
Acute care, 161. *See also* Hospital care
Acute Care for Elders (ACE), 135–136
Acute colonic pseudo-obstruction, 434
Acute confusional state, 294
Acute coronary syndromes (ACS), 390, 393–394
Acute functional decline, 28
Acute inflammatory demyelinating polyneuropathy (AIDP), 515
Acute interstitial nephritis (AIN), 441
Acute ischemic stroke, 519–520
Acute kidney injury (AKI), 435, 440–443
Acute leukemia, 576
Acute mental status change, 294
Acute myeloid leukemia (AML), 572, 589
Acute olecranon bursitis, Q122
Acute pain, 117
Acute rehabilitation, Q93
Acute tubular necrosis (ATN), 441
Acute urinary retention (AUR), 457
Acute viral conjunctivitis, Q117
Acyclovir, 366
ADA (American Diabetes Association), 66, 558, 561, 562

Adacel® (Tdap vaccine), Q64
Adalimumab, 488
ADAMTS 13, 571
Adaptive behavioral difficulties, 355
Adaptive methods, 155, 157–158
Adaptive servo-ventilation (ASV), 307
Addictions, 123, 344–351, Q78, Q112
    treatment of, 348–351, 349*t*
Adenocarcinoma, 451
Adenomas, 551–552, 554, 585–586
ADEPT (Advanced Dementia Prognostic Tool), 32*t*, 33, Q26
ADEs. *See* Adverse drug events
Adhesive capsulitis (frozen shoulder), 477
Adjustment disorders, 338–339
ADLs. *See* Activities of daily living
Ado-trastuzumab emtansine (TDM-1), 581, 582*t*
Adrenal androgens, 554–555
Adrenal cortex disorders, 553–555
Adrenal crisis, 553
Adrenal incidentalomas, 554, 554*t*
Adrenal insufficiency, 542, 553
Adrenal neoplasms, 554
Adrenalectomy, 554
α-Adrenergic agonists, 188*t*, 212, 226*t*
β-Adrenergic agonists, 382, 384–385, 384*t*, 385*t*
α-Adrenergic antagonists or blockers
    for BPH, 456, 456*t*, 457
    and falls, 251*t*
    for HTN, 420
    and incontinence, 226*t*
β-Adrenergic antagonists. *See* β-Blockers
Adrenocortical adenomas, 554
Adrenocorticotropic hormone (ACTH), 551, 551*t*
Adrenocorticotropic hormone (ACTH) stimulation test, 552, 553
ADRs (adverse drug reactions), 81
ADT (androgen-deprivation therapy), 263*t*, 587–588
Adult day care, 168, 170*t*, 283, Q101
Adult foster care, 171
Adult Protective Services (APS), 89, 94, 95, 167, Q17, Q25
Advance care planning (ACP), 15–16, 28–29, Q52, Q65
    cultural aspects, 47–48
    nursing-home care, 163–164
Advance directives, 11, 15, 163, 220, Q52, Q65
    recommendations for, 63*t*, 67*t*–68*t*, 73
Advanced Dementia Prognostic Tool (ADEPT), 32*t*, 33, Q26

Adverse drug events (ADEs), 81, 81*t*, 328. *See also specific drugs*
    in-hospital, 127
Adverse drug reactions (ADRs), 81
Aerobic activity recommendations, 55–56
Aerobic exercise, 86, 262, 323–324. *See also* Exercise
Aerobic exercise training, Q21
AF. *See* Atrial fibrillation
Afatinib, 582*t*
Afferent pupillary defects, 185
Affordable Care Act (ACA). *See* Patient Protection and Affordable Care Act
Aflibercept (VEGF Trap-Eye), 189–190, 582*t*
AFO (ankle and foot orthosis), 157
Afrezza (inhaled insulin), 565*t*
African Americans. *See* Black or African Americans
African plum, 87
Age-associated financial vulnerability, Q17
Age-based life expectancy, 31
Age-related changes, 213–214
    in anterior pituitary function, 551
    in antidiuretic hormone, 436
    in auditory system, 193
    in body composition, 213
    in bone formation, 261
    bone remodeling and bone loss, 261
    in calcium homeostasis, 547, 547*t*
    cardiovascular, 390, 391*t*
    in circulating hormone levels, 543*t*
    in eating, 222
    in endocrine system, 542
    in energy requirements, 213
    of eye, 186*t*
    in female sexuality, 469–470
    in fluid needs, 214
    in GI tract, 423
    in hematopoietic stem cells, 567
    in immune function, 525, 526*t*
    in kidney, 435, 436*t*, Q48, Q69
    in lower urinary tract, 226–227
    in macronutrient needs, 213
    in male sexuality, 465
    in micronutrient needs, 214
    normal aging, 8, 9*t*
    in oral tissues, 372, 373*t*
    in organ systems, 8, 9*t*, 10*t*
    pathologies, 8, 10*t*
    in pharmacodynamics, 77*t*, 78–79, 579–580, 579*t*
    in pharmacokinetics, 76–78, 77*t*, 579–580, 579*t*
    physiologic, 8, 9*t*
    in pituitary function, 551
    in PTH, 547, 547*t*
    pulmonary, 380
    in salivary function, 374–375
    in salivary glands, 372, 373*t*
    in sexuality, 465
    in skin, 360, Q45
    in sleep, 304–305, 305*t*
    in smell, 376–377
    in swallowing, 222
    in taste, 376–377
    in teeth, 372, 373*t*
    in testosterone, 555
Age-related macular degeneration (ARMD), 185, 186*t*, 189–190
Age-related visual impairment, Q10
Agency for Health Care Policy and Research (AHCPR), 351, 384
Aggression, 292–293, 356, Q44
Aging
    cancer and, 575
    concerns about, 53
    definition of, 5
    demography of, 1–4, 1*f*, Q118
    global trends, 1–2, 1*f*
    hematopoietic stem cells and, 567
    homeostenosis and, 8–10
    normal, 8, 9*t*
    photoaging, 360
    theories of, 5–8
    US trends, 2–4
Aging and Disability Resource Centers, 168
Aging Brain Care Medical Home, 176
Aging Brain Care (ABC) Program, Q77
Agitated delirium, 299–300, 301*t*
Agitation
    in Alzheimer disease, Q44, Q67
    Cohen-Mansfield Agitation Inventory (CMAI), 285
    in dementia, 284–285, 292–293, Q32, Q44
    intermittent, 292–293
    pain-related, 120
    in Parkinson disease, Q60
Agoraphobia, 326, 329*t*
AGS. *See* American Geriatrics Society
Agudath Israel of America, Q65
AHA. *See* American Heart Association
AIDP (acute inflammatory demyelinating polyneuropathy), 515
AIDS (acquired immunodeficiency syndrome), 538–539, Q107
    nursing-home care, 160
    treatment and care, 52
AIMS (Abnormal Involuntary Movement Scale), 333
AIN (acute interstitial nephritis), 441
Air-bone gap, Q13
Air conduction tests, Q13
Akathisia, 513
AKI (acute kidney injury), 435, 440–443
Alanine aminotransferase, 562
Albiglutide, 564*t*
Albumin, 215
Albumin/creatinine ratio (ACR), 436
Albuminuria, 436
Albuterol, 384–385
Albuterol sulfate, 384*t*
Alcohol
    and delirium, 300*t*
    and HF, 408
    and incontinence, 226*t*
    nutrient interactions, 215*t*
    and risk of osteoporosis, 262, 262*t*
Alcohol detoxification, 349*t*, 350
Alcohol intoxication, 335, 344
Alcohol-related dementia, 347–348, 355
Alcohol use disorders, 346, Q78
    and Alzheimer disease, Q72
    at-risk drinking, 346, 349*t*, 350, Q78
    binge drinking, 344, 345
    counseling interventions for, 63*t*, 70
    diagnostic criteria for, Q78
    heavy drinking, 346
    low-risk or moderate use, 344–345
    mental health problems, 347–348
    problem drinking, 349*t*, 350
    problems associated with, 346–347
    recommended upper limit of, 344
    screening for, 348
    in transgender adults, 53
    treatment of, 349–351, 349*t*, Q112
Alcohol Use Disorders Identification Test (AUDIT), 70
Alcohol withdrawal, 335, 350
Alcoholics Anonymous, 350, Q112
Alcoholics Victorious, 350
Aldosterone antagonists
    for ACS, 393
    for HF, 407, 409, 411, 412–413
    for HTN, 420
Aldosteronism, primary, 554
Alendronate, 267–268, 268*t*, 549, 550
ALFs (assisted-living facilities), 160, 162, 170–171, 170*t*
Alfuzosin, 456, 456*t*
Algorithm for Falls Risk Assessment and Interventions (CDC), 252, 253*f*
Aliskiren, 420, Q89
Alkaline phosphatase, 550, 551
Allergic conjunctivitis, 187*t*, 188, Q117
Allergic disease, 382–383
Allopurinol, 489
Alogliptin, 564*t*
Alosetron, 432
α-Adrenergic agonists, 188*t*, 212, 226*t*
α-Adrenergic antagonists or blockers
    for BPH, 456, 456*t*, 457
    and falls, 251*t*
    for HTN, 420, 421
    and incontinence, 226*t*
α-Interferon, 581
Alprostadil, 468*t*, 469
ALS (amyotrophic lateral sclerosis), 515–516
Alteplase (rt-PA), 520
Altered mental status, 294
Alternative medicine, 85. *See also* Complementary and integrative medicine (CIM)
Alternative Payment Models (APMs), 22
Alveolar-arterial (A-a) gradient, 380
Alzheimer disease (AD), 272, 507
    agitation in, Q44, Q67

Behavioral Pathology in Alzheimer Disease Rating Scale (BEHAVE-AD), 285
caregiver burden, Q41
CIM for, 87
delirium and, 296
dementia associated with, 87
diagnosis reporting, 276
diagnostic features and treatment of, 277t
differential diagnosis of, 276, 277
disease management, 176
in Down syndrome, 354, 355, Q94
drug therapy for, Q15
etiology of, 273
familial, 273
gait abnormalities, 246
general progression of, 278t
personality changes in, 336
protective factors for, 273, 274t
with REM sleep behavior disorder, Q68
risk factors for, 273, 274t, Q72
Alzheimer's Association, 39t, 280, 283, Q22
AM-PAC (Activity Measure for Post Acute Care), 145t
AMA. See American Medical Association
Amantadine, 300t, 510, 532–533
Amaurosis fugax, 518
Ambulance services, 19t
Ambulatory blood pressure monitoring, 417
Ambulatory electrocardiographic monitoring, 210, 211t
American Academy of Family Practitioners, 216
American Academy of Ophthalmology, 185
American Academy of Otolaryngology–Head and Neck Surgery, 380–381
American Association of Clinical Endocrinologists, 269
American Association of Retired Persons (AARP), 37–38, 39t
American Association of Sex Educators, Counselors, and Therapists, 471
American Board of Internal Medicine Choosing Wisely® Recommendations. See Choosing Wisely® Recommendations
American Cancer Society, 458, Q56
online resources and tools, 39t
recommendations for screening, 65
American College of Cardiology (ACC), 562
cardiac risk assessment for noncardiac surgery, 98, 99f
guidelines for preoperative cardiac assessment, 98
recommendations for screening, 69
American College of Chest Physicians, 133

American College of Obstetricians and Gynecology (ACOG), 447
American College of Physicians (ACP), 100, 101
recommendations for HIV screening, 467
recommendations for screening for prostate cancer, 458–459
American College of Rheumatology (ACR), Q38
classification criteria for gout, 488–489
provisional classification criteria for polymyalgia rheumatica, 490–491
American College of Sports Medicine (ACSM)
Exercise Management for Chronic Diseases and Disabilities, 58–59
recommendations for physical activity, 56, 57, 58–59
American College of Surgeons, 98
American Diabetes Association (ADA), 66, 558, 561, 562
American Dietetic Association, 216
American Geriatrics Society (AGS), 60
Beers Criteria®, 80, 80t, 127, 427, 471
Clinician's Guide to Assessing and Counseling Older Drivers, 28, 73
definition of person-centered care, 173, 174t
guidelines for care of older adults with diabetes mellitus, 560
guidelines for falls prevention, 256
guidelines for persistent pain management, 486–487
guidelines for prevention and management of postoperative delirium, 302t, 303
Multimorbidity GEMS Mobile App, 34
recommendations for alcohol use screening, 70
recommendations for preventing falls, 71, 252, 257, 259
American Heart Association (AHA), 562, Q39
cardiac risk assessment for noncardiac surgery, 98, 99f
guidelines for preoperative cardiac assessment, 98
online resources and tools for caregivers, 39t
recommendations for dental treatment of older adults, 378
recommendations for physical activity, 56, 58
recommendations for screening, 69
recommendations for treatment of acute ischemic stroke, 520
American Indian and Alaska Natives, 3, 219, 575

American Medical Association (AMA), 28, 134
American Psychiatric Association, 49, 350
American Psychological Association (APA), 39t
American Society of Anesthesiologists (ASA), 98, 98t
American Society of Clinical Oncology, 578–579
American Stroke Association, 39t
American Urogynecologic Association, 451
American Urological Association International Prostate Symptom Score, 455
recommendations for prostate cancer risk stratification and treatment, 460, 460t
recommendations for prostate cancer screening, 458–459
Amiloride, 80t, 439t
Aminobisphosphonates, 550
Aminoglycosides, 539
Amiodarone, 251t, 394, 401, 412
Amitriptyline, 300t
AML (acute myeloid leukemia), 572, 589
Amlodipine, Q16, Q37, Q89
Amoxicillin, 378t, 539
Ampicillin, 539
Amputation, 152–153, Q104
Amylin analogues, 564t
Amyloid precursor protein (APP), 273
Amyloidosis, 443
Amyotrophic lateral sclerosis (ALS), 515–516
Amyotrophy, diabetic, 515
Anabolic agents, 219
Anakinra, 488
Anal cancer, 50, 581
Analgesia. See Pain management
Analgesics
and delirium, 300t
and incontinence, 226t
medications to avoid, 124
misuse, 345
for myelopathy, 516
narcotic, 215, 226t
nonopioid, 121, 124
for OA-related pain, 486
opioid, 105
for postsurgical pain, 105
Andexanet, 389, 401
Androgen ablation, 461t, 463
Androgen deficiency, Q87
Androgen deprivation, 461t, 463
Androgen-deprivation therapy (ADT), 263t, 587–588
Androgen replacement therapy, 467, 556
Androgens, adrenal, 554–555
Anemia, 567–571, Q73
of chronic disease, 569–570, 569f
CKD-associated, 444–445

classification of, 568, 568t
evaluation of, 567–570, 569f
hemolytic, 442, 568t, 570–571
hypoproliferative, 568t
iron-deficiency, 432, 433, 568–569, 569f, 570
and rehabilitation, 148
Aneurysms
abdominal aortic (AAA), 62t, 66–68, 404
cerebral, 523
intracranial, 523
Angina pectoris, 328, 393
Angiodysplasia, 433
Angiography
computed tomography, Q99
coronary, 395
renal, 439, 440
Angioplasty
carotid artery, 521–522
renal artery, 440
Angiotensin-converting enzyme (ACE) inhibitors
for ACS, 393, 394
adverse events, 410, 420
for chronic CAD, 395–396
for HF, 409, 410, 410t, 412–413
for HTN, 419–420, 419t
and hyperkalemia, 438, 439t
and incontinence, 226t
for PAD, 405
for prevention of cardiovascular disease, 561
for RAS, 440
Angiotensin-receptor blockers (ARBs)
for ACS, 393, 394
for chronic CAD, 396
for HF, 409, 410–411, 410t, 412–413
for HTN, 419–420, 419t
and hyperkalemia, 438, 439t
for PAD, 405
for prevention of cardiovascular disease, 561
for RAS, 440
Angular cheilitis, 375, 376t
Anhedonia, 317
Ankle and foot orthosis (AFO), 157
Ankle-brachial index (ABI), 239, 404, 505
Ankle problems, 497, 505–506
Annual Wellness Visit (AWV), 24, 67t–68t, 71, 72, 73, Q7
Anorectal manometry, 430
Anorexia, 112–113, Q42
Anserine bursitis, 480
Antabuse reaction, 349t
Antacids, 112t, 215t, 527
Antagonistic pleiotropy theory of aging, 5
Antalgic gait, 245t, 246
Anterior ischemic optic neuropathy, 191–192
Anterior pituitary disorders, 551–553
Anterior pituitary hormones, 551, 551t
Anterior uveitis, 186t

Anthracyclines, 579t
Anthraquinones, 579t
Anthropometrics, 214
Anti-cyclic citrullinated peptide/protein antibodies (anti-CCP or ACPA), 487
Anti-TNF agents, 365
Anti-VEGF therapy, 189–190, 191
Antiandrogens, 292, 461t, 463, 473
Antianxiety agents, 340
Antiarrhythmics
for ACS, 394
adverse events, 335
for AF, 401
and falls, 252
for tachy-brady syndrome, 404
Antibiotic stewardship, 162–163
Antibiotics
for COPD exacerbation, 385, 385t
de-escalation of, 527
drug interactions, 527
for endocarditis, 372, 378, 378t, 398, 537, 537t, Q18
for foot ulcers, 506
for IBS, 432
for infections, 527
minimal criteria for initiation in long-term care, 525, 527, 528t
nutrient interactions, 215t
for osteomyelitis, 538
for PDIs, 537
for pneumonia, 531–532
for prostatitis, 463, 464
for rhinosinusitis, 381
for UTIs, 533–534
Antibodies, monoclonal, 580–581, 582t
Antibody-drug conjugates, 581
Anticholinergics
adverse events, 230
for COPD, 384–385, 384t, 385t
and delirium, 298, 300t
for drug-induced movement disorders, 513
for dystonia, 512
and falls, 251t
and incontinence, 226t
for nausea, 112t
for PD motor symptoms, 510
Anticoagulation therapy
for ACS, 393–394
adverse events, 81
for AF, 521
cessation before surgery, 99–100, 100t
for chronic CAD, 395
direct oral anticoagulants (DOACs), 401, 403t
for HF, 412
for ICH, 523
for nephrotic syndromes, 442
novel oral anticoagulants (NOACs), 521
perioperative, 98–100
for stroke prevention, 401, 403t, 521
for VTE, 388, 389

Anticonvulsants
and delirium, 300t
for fibromyalgia, 495–496
for inappropriate sexual behavior, 473
for persistent pain, 124
and risk of osteoporosis, 263t
to stabilize mood in mania and bipolar depression, 320–321, 322t
Antidepressants
adverse events, 288–289
for alcohol use disorders, 349t, 350, Q112
for anxiety disorders, 329
and delirium, 300t
for dementia, 282
for depression, 115, 319–320, 320t
for depressive features in dementia, 288–289, 288t
and falls, 251–252, 251t
for fibromyalgia, 495–496
for headaches, 517
for IBS, 432
and incontinence, 226t
indications to start, 317, 318t
interventions for preventing falls with, 258t
for migraine, 517
for neuropathic pain, 515
for persistent pain, 124
for personality disorders, 340, Q57
for psychotic symptoms in mood disorders, 334
sedating, 312, 313t, 314
for sexual dysfunction, 472t
tricyclic, 226t, 251t, 288–289, 288t, 300t, 314, 320t, 432, 514–515, 517
Antidiarrheal medications, 430
Antidiuretic hormone (ADH), 320, 436, 437
Antidiuretic hormone (ADH) receptor antagonists, 437
Antiepileptic drugs, 508
Antifungals, 504
Antihistamines
for asthma symptoms, 383
and delirium, 300t
drug interactions, 527
and falls, 251t
for nausea, 112t
sedating, 310, 315
Antihypertensives
drug interactions, 527
interventions for preventing falls with, 258t
for prevention of cardiovascular disease, 561
for renal artery stenosis, 440
Antimanic medications, 334
Antimicrobial management. *See* Antibiotics
Antimuscarinics, 232
and falls, 251t

for LUTS in BPH, 457
for UI, 227t, 230
Antineoplastic agents, 335
Antioxidants, 241
Antiparkinsonian agents, 300t
Antiplatelet therapy
for ACS, 394
adverse events, 81
for chronic CAD, 395
dual antiplatelet therapy (DAPT), 394, 395
for ICH, 523
for PAD, 405
perioperative, 99
for stroke prevention, 521
Antipsychotics
adverse events, 81, 332–333, 335t
for agitation, Q32
for bipolar depression, 321
black-box warnings, 291
for delirium, 299–300, 300t, 301t
for dementia, 282
dosing, 332–333, 335t
and falls, 251–252, 251t
for inappropriate sexual behavior, 292, 473
and incontinence, 226t
interventions for preventing falls with, 258t
for personality disorders, 340
for psychotic depression, 320
for psychotic symptoms in dementia, 284, 290–291, 290t, 334
for psychotic symptoms in mood disorders, 334
second-generation, 81, 282, 290–291, 300t, 321, 335, Q32, Q67
sedating, 314
to stabilize mood in mania and bipolar depression, 321, 322t
Antiretroviral therapy, 538–539
Antisecretory medications, 112, 113t
Antisocial personality disorder, 337t, 338, 339, 340
Antispasmodic medications, 112, 113t, 432
Antisynthetase syndrome, 494
Antithrombin deficiency, 572
Antithrombotics, 393–394
Antiviral agents, 335
Anxiety, 325, Q19
Anxiety disorders, 325–330, Q113
features of anxious or fearful behaviors, 337t
generalized anxiety disorder (GAD), 327, 329, 329t
illness anxiety disorder, 340, 342t
management of, 87, 329–330, 329t, 350
and medical disorders, 328, 329t
social anxiety disorder (social phobia), 326–327, 329t
AOA (Older Americans Act), 168
Aortic regurgitation (AR), 397–398, 400t

Aortic sclerosis, Q76
Aortic stenosis (AS), 390, 397, 400t
Aortic valve replacement, 390, 398
APA (American Psychological Association), 39t
Apathetic, avolitional syndrome, 336
Apathetic thyrotoxicosis, 545
Aphonia, psychogenic, Q28
Aphthous ulcers, 375, 376t
Apidra (insulin glulisine), 565t
Apixaban, Q9
for AF, 401
Beers Criteria® for, 80t
for stroke prevention, 401, 403t, 521
for VTE, 388–389
APMs (Alternative Payment Models), 22
Apolipoprotein E gene (APOE), 273
APP (amyloid precursor protein), 273
Appendicitis, 539–540
Appetite loss, Q42
Appetite stimulants, 219
Applied behavioral analysis, 356
Apps for mobile devices, 34, 106, 192, 195
Aprepitant, 112t
APS (Adult Protective Services), 94, 95, 167
Aqueous outflow facilitators, 188t, 191
Aqueous suppressants, 188t, 191
AR (aortic regurgitation), 397–398, 400t
ARBs. See Angiotensin-receptor blockers
Arch disorders, 498
Arcus senilis, 186t
Area Agencies on Aging (AAAs), 39t, 41, 167–168, 283, Q85
Arformoterol, 384t
Arginine, 241
Aripiprazole
for depression, 320t
dosing and adverse events, 291, 335t
for psychosis in dementia, 290, 290t
to stabilize mood in mania and bipolar depression, 322t
ARMD (age-related macular degeneration), 185, 186t, 189–190
ARNIs (ARB + neprilysin inhibitors), 409, 410–411, 410t
Aromatase inhibitors, 263t, 580, 584
Aromatherapy, 292, 330
Arrhythmias, 398–404
syncope due to, 207, 208t
Arsenic trioxide, 582t
Arterial insufficiency, 505
Arterial wounds, 242
Arteriosclerotic parkinsonism, 246
Arteriovenous malformation, 433
Arthritis
of elbow, 478
of foot, 506
gouty, 489
of hand, 478, 485, 486f

of hip, 479, 485
of knee, 480, 485, 486f, Q38
osteoarthritis, 477, 479, 480, 485–487, 486f, Q38, Q96
psoriatic, 365
rheumatoid, 476, 481, 487–488, 506
of shoulder, 155
of wrist, 478
Arthritis Foundation, 120, 486
Arthrocentesis, 490
Arthroplasty, 151–152, 155
Artificial feeding, 220
Artificial sphincter, 231
Artificial tears, 188, 494
AS (aortic stenosis), 390, 397, 400t
ASA (American Society of Anesthesiologists), 98, 98t
ASB (asymptomatic bacteriuria), 525, 533, 534–535
Ascites, 82
Asenapine, 290t, 335t
Asian Americans, Q80, Q126
burning mouth syndrome, 376
cancer, 575
CVD mortality rates, 390
nursing-home population, 159
osteoporosis, 260
population projections, 219, 575
poverty rates, 3
urinary incontinence, 225
Aspiration, 223
Aspiration pneumonia, 147–148, 222, 223, 377–378
Aspiration pneumonitis, 222
Aspirin sensitivity, 383
Aspirin therapy
for ACS, 393, 394
for AF, 401
for chronic CAD, 395
for DM, 561
for ET, 573
for GCA, 492
for PAD, 405
perioperative, 99
preventive, 73–74, 401, 521, 561
Assessment, 24–29. See also Screening
of anxiety, 325
audiologic, 195–196
of behavioral disturbances in dementia, 285–287
Berg Balance Test, 254
Breast Cancer Risk Assessment Tool, 74
brown-bag evaluation, 83
of cancer patients, 574, 577–578
cardiac risk assessment for noncardiac surgery, 98, 99f
caregiver, 39t, 41
Chemotherapy Risk Assessment Scale for High-Age Patients (CRASH), 578
Clinical Assessment of Driving-Related Skills (CADReS), 73

Clinician's Guide to Assessing and Counseling Older Drivers (AGS), 28, 73
cognitive, 25–26, 67*t*, 559, Q23, Q75
comprehensive eye examination, 185
comprehensive geriatric assessment (CGA), 71, 148, 176, Q27
Confusion Assessment Method (CAM), 127, 294–295
Confusion Assessment Method for the Intensive Care Unit (CAM-ICU), 295
daily evaluation of hospitalized patients, 130
of decisional capacity, 13–14, 14*t*
of delirium, 294–295
depression, 559
driving, 27–28, 63*t*, 73, 280
executive function testing, 26
falls risk assessment, 63*t*, 252, 253*f*, 254–255
fracture risk assessment model (FRAX™), 68, 260, 262–263, 265, 265*t*
of frailty, 182–183
functional, 26–28, 145*t*, 275, 559
Functional Assessment of Cancer Therapy, 583
Functional Assessment Scale, 33
of gait, 254
General Practitioner Assessment of Cognition, 72
Health in Aging Caregiver Self-Assessment Questionnaire, 39*t*
health risk assessment (HRA), 67*t*
of hearing loss, 195
of hip, 148
in home care, 167
home-hazard, 256, 258*t*
on hospital admission, 130, 131*t*
of hospitalized older patients, 130
kidney, 435–436
life space, 27
of lower back pain, 481, 481*t*
medication, 25
Mini-Cog Assessment Instrument for Dementia, 26, 72, 130, 274, 275*t*
Mini-Nutritional Assessment (MNA), 216, 216*t*, 578
Mini-Nutritional Assessment–Short Form, 213
Mini–Mental State Examination (MMSE), 26, 275*t*, 578
Montreal Cognitive Assessment (MoCA), 26, 130, 274, 275*t*, Q91
of nutrition, 214–217
of older drivers, 27–28
oral, 378–379
of oropharyngeal dysphagia, 223
Outcome and Assessment Information Set (OASIS), 145, 165

Patient Health Questionnaire (PHQ-2), 26, 72, 317
Patient Health Questionnaire (PHQ-9), 26, 317–318, 318*t*
Performance-Oriented Mobility Assessment (POMA), 27, 247, 254
of persistent pain, 118–119
physical, 25, 92–93
of physical activity, 58
preoperative, 97–102, Q114
of pressure injuries, 236–237, Q11
psychological, 26, 93
psychosocial, 559
of quality of life, 28–29, 28*t*
of sedentarism, 58
Short Form-36 Health Survey (SF-36), 28
Simplified Nutrition Assessment Questionnaire, 216
Sinai Abbreviated Geriatric Evaluation (SAGE), 102
skin, 237–238
St. Louis University Mental Status (SLUMS) examination, 26, 274, 275*t*
St. Thomas's Risk Assessment Tool (STRATIFY), 255
systematic, 130, 131*t*
Timed Up and Go (TUG) test, 27, 247
of UI, 231–232
vertebral fracture assessment (VFA), 265, 266*t*
vision testing, 63*t*, 72, 185
Assessment instruments, 145*t*
Assisted-living facilities (ALFs), 160, 162, 170–171, 170*t*, Q27, Q101
Assisted ventilation, 387
Assistive devices, 155, 258*t*, 485–486
Assistive listening devices, 197, 199, 199*t*
Asthma, 380, 381, 382–383
Asthma action plans, 382, 382*t*
Astigmatism, 189
ASV (adaptive servo-ventilation), 307
Asymptomatic bacteriuria (ASB), 525, 533, 534–535
At-risk drinking, 346, 349*t*, 350, Q78
At-risk use, 344
Atenolol, 420–421, Q3
Atezolizumab, 582*t*, 588
Atherosclerotic disease
  cerebral, 521–522
  guidelines for cholesterol treatment, 562
  renovascular, 439–440
  risk factors for, 559
Atherosclerotic renal artery stenosis, 422
ATN (acute tubular necrosis), 441
Atorvastatin, 393, 395
ATP-binding cassette subfamily A member 7 gene (*ABCA7*), 273

Atrial fibrillation (AF), 390, 399–402, 404, Q26
  management of, 394, 399–402, 408, 521
Atrial flutter, 394, 402
Atrial tachycardia, 402
Atrioventricular block, 403, 405*t*
Atrioventricular-nodal reentrant tachycardia, 402
Atrioventricular reentrant tachycardia, 402
Atrophic vaginitis, Q97
Atrophy
  endometrial, 454
  multiple system, 511
  urethral mucosal, 449
  urogenital, 448, 449
  vaginal, 449, 470, 471, 555
  vulvovaginal, 449, 471
Atrophy, tubular, Q48
Atropine eye drops, 114
Attenuated delirium, 295
Attenuated varicella-zoster vaccine, 530–531
Audiologic assessment, 195–196
Audiometry, Q13, Q66
Audiometry screening, 63*t*, 72, 195
AUDIT (Alcohol Use Disorders Identification Test), 70
AUDIT-C, 348
Auditory hallucinations, 334
Auditory system changes, 193
AUR (acute urinary retention), 457
Autism spectrum disorders, 356, Q51
Auto-titrating PAP (autoPAP), 307
Autoimmune hemolysis, 571
Autoimmune skin conditions, 360–365
Autolytic debridement, 239
Automatisms, 507
Automobile accidents, 27
Autonomic dysfunction, 511, Q71, Q76
Autonomic neurologic testing, 211*t*
Autonomy, 11, 13
AutoPAP (auto-titrating PAP), 307
Avanafil, 468–469, 468*t*
Avelumab, 582*t*, 588
Avoidant personality disorder, 337*t*, 338, 340
AWV (Annual Wellness Visit), 24, 67*t*–68*t*, 71, 72, 73, Q7
Axitinib, 582*t*
Ayurvedic medicine, 85
Azathioprine, 364, 387, 493, 495
Azithromycin, 378*t*
Azotemia, prerenal, 440–441

B-CAM, 295
B-type natriuretic peptide (BNP), 408
Back disease, 479, 480–482
Back pain, 480–482
  conditions causing, 481, 481*t*, 482–484
  treatment of, 85–86, 124, Q83, Q92
Back problems, 475
Baclofen, 335, 512, 513

Bacteremia, 531
Bacterial conjunctivitis, Q117
Bacterial endocarditis, 378, 378t, Q18
Bacterial keratitis, 187
Bacterial meningitis, 539
Bacterial prostatitis, 463, 464
Bacterial vaginosis, 449–450, Q1
Bacteriuria, 232
    antibiotic prophylaxis of, 535
    asymptomatic, 525, 533, 534–535
    urinary catheter-associated, 129–130
Baker cyst, 480
Balance assessment, 27
    Berg Balance Scale (Test), 247, 254
Balance impairment, 258t
Balance screening, 63t
Balance training, 55, 57, 256–257, 258t, 392, Q40
Balanced Budget Act of 1997 (BBA 97), 144, 161
BAP (bone alkaline phosphatase), 550
Barbiturates, 300t
Barium esophagography, Q49
Barthel ADL Index, 145t, 148
Basaglar (insulin glulisine), 565t
Basal cell carcinoma, 369, 369f, 451, Q30
Baseline activity, 56
Basilar artery stenosis, Q71
Bathing, 312
Bazedoxifene, 268t, 270
BBA 97 (Balanced Budget Act of 1997), 144, 160
Beclomethasone diproprionate, 384t
Bed alarms, Q108
Bed bugs, 368
Bed rails, Q108
Bed rest, Q92
Bedsores. *See* Pressure injuries
Beers Criteria® (AGS), 80, 80t, 127, 427, 471
BEHAVE-AD (Behavioral Pathology in Alzheimer Disease Rating Scale), 285
Behavior(s)
    adaptive, 355
    anxious or fearful, 337t
    challenging, 353
    compulsive, 327
    dramatic, emotional, or erratic, 337t, 340
    inappropriate sexual behavior (ISB), 473
    odd or eccentric, 337t
    pain behaviors in cognitively impaired, 120, 120t
    self-injurious, 354, 355, 356
Behavioral disturbances
    in delirium, 298t, 299–300
    in dementia, 284–293, 288t, Q32, Q44, Q53
    with intellectual disability, 355–356
    management of, 287–293, 288t, 299–300
    manic-like features of, 289, 289t

Behavioral health management, 324
Behavioral interventions. *See also* Cognitive-behavioral therapy
    for aggression or agitation, 292
    for dementia care, 287, 287t
    dialectical behavior therapy, 339, Q57
    for frailty, 184
    for insomnia, 291, 292t, 311–312
    to reduce urine culture ordering and overtreatment of ASB, 534–535
    for UI, 229–230, 231–232, Q4
Behavioral Pathology in Alzheimer Disease Rating Scale (BEHAVE-AD), 285
La belle indifférence, Q28
Bell's palsy (facial nerve palsy), 539
Benazepril, 410t
Bendamustine, 589
Beneficence, 11, 13
Bengay (menthol and methylsalicylate), 121t
Benign growths, 368
Benign paroxysmal positional vertigo (BPPV), 202, 205–206, Q99
Benign prostatic hyperplasia (BPH), 455–457, Q86
    management of, 31t, 87, 456, 456t, Q89
Benzodiazepines
    for alcohol detoxification, 349t, 350
    for anxiety disorders, 329, 329t, 350, Q113
    chronic use of, 314–315
    and delirium, 298, 300t, 303
    and falls, 251–252, 251t
    for insomnia, 311, 313t, 314, 347
    interventions for preventing falls with, 258t
    long-acting, 350
    long-term use, 345, 346, 347, 348
    for nausea, 112t
    problem use, 344
    for RLS, 514
    for sleep problems, 308, 310
Benzoyl peroxide, 361–362
Benztropine, 300t, 333
Bereavement, 317, Q112
Bereavement care, 108
Berg Balance Scale (Test), 247, 254
Bernard-Soulier syndrome, 571–572
β-Adrenergic agonists, 382, 384–385, 384t, 385t
β-Blockers
    for ACS, 393, 394
    adverse events, 188t, 335
    for AF, 399, 408
    for anxiety disorders, 329t
    for chronic CAD, 396
    for essential tremor, 513
    for HF, 409, 410, 410t, 413
    for HTN, 419t, 420–421
    and hyperkalemia, 439t
    for inappropriate sexual behavior, 473
    for migraine, 517

    perioperative, 100
    for prevention of cardiovascular disease, 561
    for vasovagal syncope, 212
    for ventricular arrhythmias, 402
β-Carotene, 219
β-Lactam/β-lactamase, 526
β-Lactam/β-lactamase antibiotics, 531–532
β-Blockers, Q3
Bevacizumab, 189–190, 580, 582t, 586
Bi-level positive-airway pressure (biPAP), 307, 516
Biceps tendonopathy and tendon rupture, 477
Biguanides, 563, 564t
Bile acid sequestrants, 432
Biliary disease, 427–428
Binge drinking, 344, 345
Bio-identical compounded hormonal preparations, 449
Bioavailability, 76
Biofeedback therapy, 429, 430
Biologic therapy, 239
    for cancer, 574, 580–581
    for psoriasis, 365
    for RA, 488
    safety issues, 85
Biology, 5–10, 575, Q55, Q103
BiPAP (bi-level positive-airway pressure), 307, 516
Bipolar depression, 316, 318–319, 321, 322t
Bipolar disorder, 318–319, Q33
Bisexual men, 50, 51–52. *See also* Lesbian gay bisexual transgender (LGBT) health
Bisexual women, 51, 52, Q124. *See also* Lesbian gay bisexual transgender (LGBT) health
Bismuth subsalicylate, Q9
Bisoprolol, 396, 410, 410t
Bisphosphonates, 590, Q74
    adverse events, 267–269, 378
    for bone pain, 463
    for humoral hypercalcemia of malignancy, 550
    for hyperparathyroidism, 549
    for MGUS, 590
    for osteoporosis, 260, 267–269, 268t, 445
    for Paget disease of bone, 550
    for persistent pain, 124
Bivalirudin, 393
Black hairy tongue, 376
Black or African Americans
    advance care planning, Q52
    cancer, 574, 575
    CKD, 443
    CVD mortality rates, 390
    diabetes mellitus, 558
    HTN, 419–420
    hypertension, 416
    life expectancy, 2
    mobility aids for, 156

multiple myeloma, 590
nursing-home population, 159
osteoporosis, 260
pain management, Q80, Q83
periodontitis, 373
population projections, 219, 575
poverty rates, 4, Q118
prostate cancer, 458
risk factors for depression, 316
vitamin D deficiency, 548
Bladder cancer, 65, 581, 588
Bladder diaries, 229
Bladder lift, Q1
Bladder neck slings, 231
Bladder obstruction, 227
Bladder outlet obstruction, 232, 441
Bladder relaxants, Q15
Bladder training, 229
Bleeding
gastrointestinal, 432–433, Q9
hypertensive bleeds, 522
vaginal, 449, 453–454, 454t
Bleeding diatheses, 571
Bleeding disorders, 572
Bleomycin, 590
Blepharitis, 187–188, 187t
Blepharochalasis, 185
Blepharoptosis, 185
Blindness, 185
Blood glucose screening, 62t
Blood loss, 571
Blood pressure. *See also* Hypertension
diastolic, 416, 418
screening, 62t
systolic, 416, 418
Blood pressure management, 561, Q37
guidelines for, 561
lag time to benefit, 31t
to prevent ICH, 523
targets in hypertension, 439
Blood pressure monitoring
ambulatory, 417
home, 421
indirect or cuff, 417
Blood transfusions, 19t
BMD. *See* Bone mineral density
BMI (body mass index), 70, 214
BNP (B-type natriuretic peptide), 408
Board and care, 170t
BODE Index, 32t, 33, Q26
Body composition changes, 213
Body language, 44
Body mass index (BMI), 70, 214
Body size classification, 214
Body weight, 57
Bodywork services, 85
Bone, 8, 9t, 10t, 261
Bone alkaline phosphatase (BAP), 550
Bone densitometry, Q2
Bone disease, 479
adynamic, 445
Paget disease of bone, 196, 550–551
renal, 445
Bone infections, 538

Bone loss, 261. *See also* Osteoporosis
Bone marrow failure, 570
Bone metastasis, 463
Bone mineral density (BMD), 264
diagnostic criteria for osteoporosis, 260
indications for, 264
recommendations for, 68, 264
serial measurement, 270
WHO definitions, 260, 261t
Bone remodeling, 261
Bone-specific alkaline phosphatase (BSAP), 550, 551
Bone spurs, 500
Bone turnover, 261, 265–266
Boostrix® (Tdap vaccine), Q64
Borderline personality disorder, 337t, 338, 339, 340
Bordetella pertussis, Q64
Bortezomib, 579t, 580, 582t, 590
Bosutinib, 582t
Botulinum toxin, 231, 360, 512
Bouchard nodes, 485
Bowel incontinence, 358t, 430
Bowel obstruction, 111–112, 113t
BPH. *See* Benign prostatic hyperplasia
BPPV (benign paroxysmal positional vertigo), 202, 205–206, Q99
Brachytherapy, 461t, 462, 466
Bracing, Q38
Braden Scale, 31, 237
Bradyarrhythmias, 399, 402–404, 405t
Bradycardia, 402–403, 405t
Bradykinesia, 509, 510
Brain cancer, 581
Brain imaging, 275–276, Q99
Brain injury, traumatic (TBI), 552, Q72
Brain natriuretic peptide: N-terminal prohormone of (NT-proBNP), Q14
Brain tumors, 337
Breast cancer, 583–584, Q125
characteristics of, 576
incidence rates, 574
metastatic, 584
prevention of, 74
risk in older lesbian and bisexual women, 51
screening for, 31t, 61, 578–579
therapy for, 88, 580, 581, 584
Breast Cancer Risk Assessment Tool, 74
Breast self-examination (BSE), 61
Breathing disorders, sleep-related, 306–307
Breathlessness, 113–114
Brentuximab, 580, 582t
Brexpiprazole, 290t
Bridging integrator 1 gene *(BIN1)*, 273
Brief interventions, 348–350, 349t
Bright light, 310, 312, 312t
Brimonidine, 188t
British Geriatrics Society (BGS), 252, 256, 257, 259
Bromocriptine, 564t
Bronchitis, chronic, 385t
Bronchodilators, inhaled, 380, 384–385, 384t, 385t

Brown-bag review, 83, 297
BSAP (bone-specific alkaline phosphatase), 550, 551
BSE (breast self-examination), 61
Budesonide, 384t
Bulbocavernosus reflex, 228
Bulking agents, 430, 432, Q96
Bullous pemphigoid, 363–364, 363f
Bumetanide, 411
Bundled Payments for Care Improvement initiative, 21
Bunions, 499t
Buprenorphine, 349t, 350–351
Bupropion, 288, 288t, 320t, 321, 351, Q33
Burch operation (colposuspension), 231
Bureau of Consumer Protection, 93
Burning mouth syndrome, 376
Bursitis
anserine, 480
olecranon, 478, Q122
trochanteric, 479
Buspirone, 319, 329, 329t
Butorphanol, 124
Bypass surgery, 396–397, Q114

C-reactive protein (CRP), 392, 487
CA-UTIs (catheter-associated urinary tract infections), 129–130, 534–535
Cabazitaxel, 582t
Cabergoline, 552
CABG (coronary artery bypass graft) surgery, 396–397, Q114
Cabozantinib, 582t
Cachexia, 112–113
CAD. *See* Coronary artery disease
CADReS (Clinical Assessment of Driving-Related Skills), 73
Caffeine, 259t
CAGE (Cut down, Annoy, Guilt, Eye-opener) questionnaire, 70, 348
Calcaneal spur, 499t
Calcitonin, 268t, 270
Calcium
abnormalities in CKD, 445
coronary artery content, 392
dietary intake, 266
disorders of metabolism of, 547–551
drug interactions, 215t
foods that contain, 266, 267t
homeostasis changes, 547, 547t
Calcium-channel antagonists (CCAs)
for ACS, 394
adverse events, 215, 378
for chronic CAD, 396
for HTN, 419–420, 419t
and incontinence, 226t
for migraine, 517
for prevention of cardiovascular disease, 561
and UI, 231
Calcium deficiency, 262
Calcium hydroxylapatite, 360

Calcium pyrophosphate dihydrate deposition disease (CPPD), 480, 487, 490
Calcium supplements
	for hyperparathyroidism, 548, 549
	for osteoporosis, 262, 262t, 266–267
	preventive, 63t, 74, 548, 550–551, Q2, Q63
Caloric requirements, 241
Calorie supplements, Q88
CAM (Confusion Assessment Method), 127, 294–295
Canadian Study of Health and Aging, Q109
Canagliflozin, 263t, 564t
Canalith repositioning procedure, 205–206
Cancer, 574
	advanced, Q42
	anal, 50, 581
	assessment of, 574, 577–578
	back pain due to, 481
	biologic therapies for, 580–581
	biology of, 575
	bladder, 65, 581, 588
	brain, 581
	breast, 31t, 51, 61, 74, 574, 576, 581, 583–584, Q125
	cervical, 51, 64, 581
	characteristics of, 576
	chemotherapy for, 574, 579–580, 579t, Q119
	CIM for, 88
	colon, 31t, 431, 574, 575, 585–586, Q119
	colorectal, 61–64, 574, 581, 586, Q56
	end-stage, Q42
	endometrial, 453–454
	esophageal, 581, 587, Q49
	ethnic differences in, 574–575
	gastric, 587
	guidelines for assessment and treatment of, 577
	head and neck, 581, Q29
	hormonal therapy for, 580
	immunotherapy for, 574, 580–581
	incidence rates, 574
	lung, 65, 574, 581, 584–585
	management of, 576–583, 590
	metastatic, Q74, Q125
	oral, 65, 376, Q29, Q74
	ovarian, 65
	pancreatic, Q126
	prevalence of, 575–576
	prognostic indices, 32, 32t
	prostate, 50, 65–66, 455, 457–463, 574, 581, 587–588, Q74
	quality-of-life issues, 583
	radiation therapy for, 574, 581
	recommendations for, 590
	rectal, 586
	renal cell, 581, 588–589
	risk in older gay and bisexual men, 50
	risk in older lesbian and bisexual women, 51
	skin, 65, 360, 369–370, Q30
	surgery for, 574, 581–583
	targeted therapies for, 580–581
	terminal, Q42
	thyroid, 65, 546–547
	treatment options, 578
	of vulva, 450, 451
Cancer pain, 121, 122
Cancer screening, 31t, 578–579, Q7, Q56
	counseling on, 74–75
	recommendations for, 60–65, 62t, 75
	tests, 60–65
	in transgender older adults, 51
Candesartan, 410t, 412–413, 440
Candidiasis
	esophageal, Q49
	oral, 375, 376t
	skin, 367
	vulvovaginal, 449
Canes, 155–156, 157t, Q47
Canker sores, 376t
Cannabinoids, 88, 112t
Cannabis (marijuana), 86t, 88, 335, 345
CAP (community-acquired pneumonia), 531–532, Q69
Capecitabine, 580, 582t, 587
Capsaicin, 121, 121t, 486
Capsaicin cream, 364, 514
Capsicum frutescens (cayenne), 86
Capsulitis, 499t
Captopril, 410t
Carbamazepine
	adverse events, 508, Q120
	for alcohol detoxification, 349t
	for behavioral disturbances in dementia with manic-like features, 289, 289t
	for dementia, 282
	for persistent pain, 124
	for personality disorders, 340
	to stabilize mood in mania and bipolar depression, 322t
Carbidopa-levodopa. See Levodopa-carbidopa
Carbon dioxide (CO_2) laser therapy, 449
Carbonic anhydrase inhibitors, 188t
Carboplatin, 582t, 588
Cardiac arrest, in-hospital (IHCA), 133
Cardiac arrhythmias, 398–404
	syncope due to, 207, 208t
Cardiac assessment, preoperative, 97–100
Cardiac asthma, 381
Cardiac ischemia, Q76
Cardiac rehabilitation (CR), 153–154, 397, 409
Cardiac resynchronization therapy (CRT), 413
Cardiac risk assessment, 98, 99f
Cardiac stress testing, 98, 210, 395
Cardiac syncope, 207, 208t, 209, 210t
Cardiobacterium, 398, 536–537
Cardioembolic events: prevention of, 401–402, 403t
Cardioembolic stroke, 519
Cardiology, 406
Cardiotoxicity, 581, 582t
Cardiovascular diseases and disorders, 390–406
	in centenarians, Q103
	with developmental disabilities, 358t
	epidemiology of, 390, 391t
	in lesbian and bisexual women, Q124
	management of, 86–87, 102–103
	and periodontal disease, 377, 378
	prevalence of, 390, 391t
	prevention of, 31t, 73–74, 561
	risk factors, 50, 391–392
	screening for, 69
	shared decision making in, 405–406
	and syncope, Q76
	in transgender older adults, 51
Cardiovascular events, 444
Cardiovascular Health Study, Q109
Cardiovascular system
	age-related changes in, 9t, 10t, 390, 391t
	indications for perioperative revascularization, 98, 99t
	perioperative therapy to reduce complications, 98–100
	preoperative assessment and management of, 97–100
Care Area Assessments, 220
Care plans, 36
Care transitions, 139–142, 301–302
Care Transitions Intervention®, Q85
Caregiver burden, Q41, Q77
Caregivers, 37–38, 40
	assessment of, 39t, 41
	communication with, 141–142
	education of, 279–280
	family caregivers, 37, 38, Q22
	for LGBT patients, Q90
	relationship between older adults and, 94
	resources and tools for, 39t–40t
	support for, 40, 279–280, 292
	training for, Q77
Caregiving, 37–41
	informal, 37, 38, Q22
	observations that should raise concern, 90, 91t
	risk factors for elder abuse, 89–90, 91t
Carers, 37
Carfilzomib, 582t
Caring for Older Adults and Caregivers at Home (COACH), Q77
Carotid artery angioplasty and stenting (CAS), 521–522
Carotid artery intima-media thickness, 392

Carotid artery stenosis, 69, 521–522
Carotid endarterectomy (CEA), 521–522
Carotid sinus hypersensitivity, 258t
Carotid sinus massage, 211t, 402–403
Carotid sinus syndrome, Q76
Carotid ultrasound, 392
Carpal tunnel syndrome, 478
Carvedilol
    for chronic CAD, 396
    for HF, 410, 410t
    for HTN, 421
CAS (carotid artery angioplasty and stenting), 521–522
CASCADE (Choices, Attitudes, and Strategies for Care of Advanced Dementia at the End-of-Life), 106
Case managers, 146, 147t
Casuistry, 11
Cataract surgery, 257, 259t
Cataracts, 186t, 188–189, Q10
Catechol-*O*-methyltransferase (COMT) inhibitors, 510
Catheter ablation, 401, 402
Catheter-associated urinary tract infections (CA-UTIs), 129–130, 534–535
Catheter care, 232–233
Catheters, 129–130, 232–233
Cavus deformity, 498
Cayenne *(Capsicum frutescens)*, 86
CBE (clinical breast examination), 61
CBT. *See* Cognitive-behavioral therapy
CBT-I (cognitive-behavioral therapy for insomnia), 87–88, 311–312, 312t, Q43, Q81
CCAs. *See* Calcium-channel antagonists
CCM (chronic care management), 177–178
CCRCs (continuing-care retirement communities), 171, Q101
CCTP (Community Care Transitions Program), 141
CDC. *See* Centers for Disease Control and Prevention
CDI (*Clostridium difficile* infection), 425, 540
CEA (carotid endarterectomy), 521–522
Cefotaxime, 531, 539
Ceftazidime, 539
Ceftriaxone, 531, 539
Celecoxib, 427
Celiac disease, 69, 430, 569
Centenarians, Q55, Q103
Center for Medicare and Medicaid Innovations (CMMI), 21
Centers for Disease Control and Prevention (CDC), 486
    Algorithm for Falls Risk Assessment and Interventions, 252, 253f
    recommendations for HIV screening, 467
Centers for Medicare and Medicaid Services (CMS)
    Bundled Payments for Care Improvement initiative, 21
    chronic care codes, Q77
    Hospital Compare, 136–137
    Hospital Readmissions Reduction Program, 414
    Medicare Learning Network, 23
    Medicare Prescription Drug Plan Finder, 16, 22
    Nursing Home Compare tool, 22, 39t, 234
    quality measures for nursing homes, 161–162
    Quality Payment Program (QPP), 22
    reimbursement strategies, Q95
    Risk-Standardized-Readmission Rates (RSRR), 137
Central nervous system (CNS) infections, 539
Central nervous system (CNS) medications, 345
Central retinal artery occlusion, 186t, 187
Central retinal vein occlusion, 186t
Central sleep apnea, 306–307
Cephalexin, 378t
Cephalosporins, 531–532
Cerebellar ataxia, 246
Cerebral aneurysms, 523
Cerebral palsy, 357
Cerebrovascular disease, 507, 518–519, 521, 524
Certificate of Terminal Illness, 107
Certolizumab, 488
Cerumen impaction, 195
Cervical cancer
    radiation therapy for, 581
    risk in older lesbian and bisexual women, 51
    screening for, 64, 578–579
Cervical disc disease, 476
Cervical disc displacement, 476
Cervical myelopathy, 248
Cervical radiculopathy, 476
Cervical stenosis, 476
Cetuximab, 582t, 587
Cevimeline, 375, 494
CGA (comprehensive geriatric assessment), 71, 148, 176, Q27
CGIC-PF (Clinical Global Impression of Change in Physical Frailty), 182–183
CHA_2DS_2-VASc score, 401–402
$CHADS_2$ score, 31, 401–402
Chair alarms, Q108
Chair yoga, 486
Chalazion, 187t
Chaplains on Hand, 39t
Charles Bonnet syndrome, 192, 335
Cheilectomy, 500
Chemical colitis, 429–430
Chemical restraints, 299
Chemoprophylaxis, 63t, 73–74
Chemosensory perception, oral, 376–377
Chemotherapy, 574, 579–580, 579t
    for breast cancer, 584
    for colon cancer, 586
    for colorectal cancer, 586
    for gastric cancer, 587
    for ITP, 571
    for lung cancer, 585
    for MDS, 573
    for non-Hodgkin lymphoma, 589
    for prostate cancer, 461t, 463, 587–588
    and risk of osteoporosis, 263t
Chemotherapy, adjuvant, Q119
Chemotherapy-induced nausea and vomiting (CINV), 88, Q96
Chemotherapy Risk Assessment Scale for High-Age Patients (CRASH) Score, 578
Cherry angiomas, 368
Chest radiography, 408, Q69
Children's Health Insurance Program (CHIP), 21
Chinese Americans, Q126
Chinese medicine, 85
Chiropractic services, 85
Chlamydia trachomatis, 463
Chlorambucil, 589
Chlorthalidone, 420
"Choice Act" (Veterans Access, Choice and Accountability Act of 2014), 22
Choices, Attitudes, and Strategies for Care of Advanced Dementia at the End-of-Life (CASCADE), 106
Cholangitis, 427–428
Cholecalciferol. *See* Vitamin D_3
Cholecystitis, 427–428, 539–540
Cholesterol, 215
Cholesterol screening, 62t
Cholesterol treatment, 562
Cholestyramine, 111, 432
Cholinesterase inhibitors (ChIs)
    adverse events, 215
    for dementia, 281, 355
    for inappropriate sexual behavior, 473
    and incontinence, 226t
    for PD nonmotor symptoms, 511
    for psychotic symptoms, 334
Chondrocalcinosis, 490, 491f
Chondroitin, 85
Choosing Wisely® Recommendations
    for acute back pain, 482
    for behavioral problems in dementia, 293
    for cancer screening, 579
    for cardiology, 406
    for colorectal cancer screening, 64
    for coronary artery disease, 406
    for delirium, 137, 303
    for dementia, 283
    for diabetes mellitus, 566
    for DM, 192
    for eating and feeding, 137
    for feeding and swallowing, 220, 224

for gastroenterology, 434
for heart failure/device therapy, 415
for heart transplantation, 415
for hospice, 116
for hospital care, 137
for hypertension, 422
for infectious diseases, 541
for mechanical circulatory support, 415
for musculoskeletal pain, 484
for nephrology, 446
for oncology, 590
for osteoporosis, 271
for pain management, 125
for palliative care, 111, 116
for perioperative care, 105
for peripheral arterial disease, 406
for pharmacotherapy, 84
for prevention, 75
for prostate disease, 464
for rheumatology, 496
for sleep issues, 315
for stroke and cerebrovascular disease, 524
for syncope, 212
for urinary incontinence, 233
for valvular heart disease, 406
for visual loss, 192
Chorea, 512
Choroidal neovascularization (CNV), 189–190
Christian Scientists, Q65
Chronic adrenal insufficiency, 542, 553
Chronic bacterial prostatitis, 464
Chronic benzodiazepine use, 314–315
Chronic bronchitis, 385t
Chronic care, Q77
Chronic care management (CCM), 177–178
Chronic coronary artery disease, 394–397
Chronic cough, 381, 381t, 383t
Chronic diarrhea, 430–431
Chronic disease
  age-related, 8, 10t
  anemia of, 569–570, 569f
Chronic dislocated metatarsal phalangeal joint, 498–500
Chronic hospitalization, 141
Chronic hypnotic use, 314–315
Chronic inflammation: anemia of, 569f
Chronic inflammatory demyelinating polyradiculoneuropathy (CIDP), 515
Chronic kidney disease (CKD), 435, 443–445, Q73
  Beers Criteria® for medications that should be avoided or have dosage reduced in, 80, 80t
  recommendations for, 446
  screening for, 69, 443
  staging of, 443, 444f
Chronic Kidney Disease Epidemiologic Collaboration (CKD-EPI), 101, 435
Chronic leg ulcers, 360, 365

Chronic low back pain, 120, 124
Chronic lymphocytic leukemia (CLL), 571, 589
Chronic myeloid leukemia (CML), 573
Chronic myeloproliferative neoplasms, 573
Chronic obstructive pulmonary disease (COPD), 380, 383–386
  anxiety and, 328
  diagnostic criteria for, 380, 383t
  GOLD guidelines for, 383–384, 383t
  inhaled bronchodilators and corticosteroids for, 384–385, 384t
  prognostic indices, 32–33, 32t
  screening for, 69, 384
  therapy for, 384–385, 384t, 385t
Chronic pain, 117, 495, Q36. See also Persistent pain
Chronic pain syndromes with developmental disabilities, 357, 358t
Chronic prostatitis, 455
Chronic subdural hematoma, 523
Chronic traumatic encephalopathy, 355
Chronic venous insufficiency, 365
Chronic wounds, 235, 241, 242, 242t
CIDP (chronic inflammatory demyelinating polyradiculoneuropathy), 515
Cilostazol, 405
CIM (complementary and integrative medicine), 85–88
Cimetidine, 80t, 112t, 466
Cinacalcet, 549
CINV (chemotherapy-induced nausea and vomiting), 88, Q96
Ciprofloxacin, 431, Q97
Circadian rhythm sleep disorders, 308–309, 312
Circulatory support, mechanical, 413–414
Circumduction, 245t
Cisplatin, 579–580, 579t, 582t, 588
Citalopram, 288, 288t
  adverse events, Q67, Q102
  for agitation and psychosis, Q67
  for alcohol use disorder, Q112
  for anxiety disorders, 325, 329
  for dementia-related agitation, Q44
  for depression, 319, 320t
  for depression or anxiety, Q60
CKD. See Chronic kidney disease
CKD-EPI (Chronic Kidney Disease Epidemiologic Collaboration), 101, 435
Clarithromycin, 378t
Claw toe, 500
Clindamycin, 378t
Clinical Assessment of Driving-Related Skills (CADReS), 73
Clinical breast examination (CBE), 61

Clinical feasibility, 35–36
Clinical Global Impression of Change in Physical Frailty (CGIC-PF), 182–183
Clinical management, 34
Clinical practice guidelines (CPGs), 34
Clinician's Guide to Assessing and Counseling Older Drivers, 28, 73
Clinker theory, 7
CLL (chronic lymphocytic leukemia), 571, 589
Clobetasol propionate, 450
Clock-drawing test, 26, 72
Clomipramine, 329t
Clonazepam, 124, 309
Clonidine, 421, 448–449
Clopidogrel
  for ACS, 393–394
  for chronic CAD, 395
  for PAD, 405
  for stroke prevention, 401, 521
Clostridium difficile infection (CDI), 425, 540
Clotting disorders, 572
Clotuzumab, 590
Clozapine
  and delirium, 300t
  dosing and adverse events, 291, 335t
  for PD nonmotor symptoms, 334, 511
  for psychosis in dementia, 290–291, 290t, Q32
Clubbing, 387
Clusterin gene *(CLU)*, 273
CMAI (Cohen-Mansfield Agitation Inventory), 285
CML (chronic myeloid leukemia), 573
CMMI (Center for Medicare and Medicaid Innovations), 21
CMS. See Centers for Medicare and Medicaid Services
CNV (choroidal neovascularization), 189–190
COACH (Caring for Older Adults and Caregivers at Home), Q77
Coagulation disorders, 571–572. See also Anticoagulation
Cobimetinib, 582t
Cocaine, 335, 345
Cochlear implants, 200–201, 200t
Cockcroft-Gault equation, 78, 101, 435
Coconut oil, 87
Cocooning, Q64
Code of Federal Regulations, 161
Code status discussions, 133
Codman pendulum exercise, 155
Coenzyme Q_{10}, 86–87, 86t
Cognitive assessment, 25–26, 559, Q23, Q75
  Medicare wellness visits, 67t
  Mini-Cog Assessment Instrument for Dementia, 26, 72, 130, 274, 275t

Mini–Mental State Examination (MMSE), 26, 275t
Montreal Cognitive Assessment (MoCA), 26, 130, 274, 275t, Q91
screening instruments for, 274, 275t
St. Louis University Mental Status (SLUMS) examination, 26, 274, 275t
Cognitive-behavioral therapy (CBT), 115
for alcohol use disorders, 349t, Q112
for anxiety disorders, 325, 329–330, 329t, Q113
for bereavement disorder, Q112
for chronic benzodiazepine use, 314–315
for depression, 323
for fibromyalgia, 495
for insomnia, 87–88, 311–312, 312t, Q43, Q81
for pain, 120
for personality disorders, 339
for preventing falls, 258t
psychotherapy, Q57
for sexual dysfunction, 472t
for somatic symptom disorders, 343
Cognitive-behavioral therapy for insomnia (CBT-I), 87–88, 311–312, 312t, Q43, Q81
Cognitive dysfunction, postoperative (POCD), 297, Q91
Cognitive enhancers, 281–282
Cognitive history, 274, 274t
Cognitive impairment, 578
CIM for, 87
in dementia, 278t, 279
in ED patients, 134
and falls, Q62
in hospitalized patients, 130–132, 131t
interventions for, 130–132, 131t
interventions for preventing falls, 257, 258t
mild, 87
in nursing-home population, 159
oral care in, 379
pain assessment and treatment in, 118, 120
pain behaviors in, 120, 120t
pain management in, Q80
postoperative cognitive dysfunction (POCD), 297, Q91
postoperative decline, 104, 397
screening for, 63t, 72
and sexual consent, 473
substance-induced, 344, 347–348
UTIs in, 534
Cognitive reconditioning, 298t
Cognitive restructuring, 330
Cognitive retraining, 150
Cognitive training, 279
Cogwheel phenomenon, 509
Cohen-Mansfield Agitation Inventory (CMAI), 285

Cohousing, senior, 170
Colchicine
Beers Criteria® for, 80t
for CPPD, 490
for gout, 489
nutrient interactions, 215t
Colesevelam, 564t
Colestipol, 432
Colitis
C difficile, 540
chemical, 429–430
ischemic, 433
microscopic, 430–431
pseudomembranous, 540
Collagen, 231
Collagen-containing products, 239, 240t
Collagenous colitis, 430–431
Colon: disorders of, 429–434
Colon cancer, 431, 585–586
incidence rates, 574
prevalence of, 575
screening for, 31t, 62t, 578–579, Q56
therapy for, 88, Q119
Colonic adenomas, 585–586
Colonic angiodysplasia, 433
Colonic ischemia, 433–434
Colonic polyps, 585–586
Colonic pseudo-obstruction, acute, 434
Colonic secretagogues, 429
Colonoscopy, 62t, 64, 434, 585, 586, Q56
Color Doppler ultrasonography, Q110
Colorectal cancer, 581, 586, Q56
incidence rates, 574
metastatic, 586
screening for, 61–64, 62t
Colpocleisis, 453
Colposuspension (Burch operation), 231
Comfort measures, Q45
Comfrey root extract *(Symphytom officinale L.)*, 86
Communication
addressing the healthcare provider, 43
addressing the patient, 42–43
asking about sexual orientation and gender identity, 50
body language, 44
code status discussions, 133
disclosure, 46, Q126
discussing death, 107
discussing serious news, 108–109, Q126
with hearing-impaired people, 196, 197t
key techniques, 43
patient-clinician, 24–25
with patients, Q52, Q65, Q126
preferred terms for cultural or religious identity, 42
of prognosis, 33
between providers, Q95
respectful nonverbal communication, 44

SPIKES framework for delivering difficult news, 33, 109, 110t
strategies to enhance, 196, 197t
teach-back method, 43
tips for communicating with older patients in ways that are respectful and effective, 25
in transitional care, 141–142
unspoken challenges, 46
Community-acquired pneumonia (CAP), 531–532, Q69
Community-based care, 165–172, 170t
Community Care Transitions Program (CCTP), 141
Community-dwelling older Americans, 253f
Community Living Centers (VA), 159–160
Community resources, Q85, Q101
Comorbidity, 146–148, Q55, Q57, Q119. *See also* Multimorbidity (multiple morbidity)
Compassionate Care Program, 115
Complementary and integrative medicine (CIM), 85–88
Complex bereavement disorder, persistent, 317
Complex regional pain syndrome (CRPS), 119
Comprehensive eye examination, 185
Comprehensive geriatric assessment (CGA), 71, 148, 176, Q27
Comprehensive Primary Care Plus (CPC+), 21
Compression, intermittent pneumatic, 389
Compulsions, 327
Computed tomography (CT), 431, 434
low-dose, 65
Computed tomography angiography, Q99
COMT (catechol-*O*-methyltransferase) inhibitors, 510
Concierge practice, 19
Concurrent care, 108, 115
Conduction disturbances, 403, 405t
Conductive hearing loss, 194, Q13
Confusion, Q102
Confusion Assessment Method (CAM), 127, 294–295
B-CAM, 295
CAM-Severity (CAM-S), 295
4AT, 295
3D-CAM, 127, 295
Confusion Assessment Method for the Intensive Care Unit (CAM-ICU), 295
Congestive heart failure, Q104
Conjunctivitis, 187t, 188, Q117
Conn syndrome, 439
Consciousness
altered level of, 295
sudden loss of, 207, 208t
Consent
attitudes regarding, 46

informed consent, 13–14
sexual, 472–473
Consequentialism, 11
Conservative care, 446, 460–462
Conservator of finances, Q17
Constipation, 429–430
    with developmental disabilities, 358t
    IBS with (IBS-C), 432
    IBS with alternating constipation and diarrhea (IBS-M or IBS mixed), 432
    irritable bowel syndrome with (IBS-C), 432
    opioid-induced, 110–111, 123, Q96
    postoperative, 103
    in terminal illness, 110–111
Constraint-induced movement therapy, 150
Consultation
    ethics, 11–12
    outpatient, 176
Consumer Financial Protection Bureau, 93
Continuing-care retirement communities (CCRCs), 171, Q101
Continuous positive-airway pressure (CPAP), 307, 386–387
Contrast sensitivity, Q10
Conversion disorder, 340, 342t, Q28
COPD. *See* Chronic obstructive pulmonary disease
Copper, 215t
Corneal ulcers, 186t, 187, 188
Coronary angiography, 395
Coronary artery bypass graft (CABG) surgery, 396–397, Q114
Coronary artery calcium content, 392
Coronary artery disease (CAD), 392–393
    chronic, 394–397
    diagnosis of, 394–395, 408
    management of, 394–395, 408
    recommendations for, 406
    revascularization for, 396–397
Coronary revascularization, 98, 99t
Coronary stents, 100
Corticobasal degeneration, 511
Corticosteroids. *See also* Glucocorticoids
    adverse events, 335
    for asthma, 382
    for bowel obstruction, 112
    for COPD, 384–385, 384t, 385t
    for CPPD, 490
    for hemolytic anemia, 571
    high-dose, 530
    for idiopathic pulmonary fibrosis, 387
    inhaled, 380, 382, 384–385, 384t, 385t
    for nausea, 112t
    for neuropathic pain, 124
    ophthalmic, 188
    for osteoarthritis, 480
    for pain, 124
    perioperative, 104
    for PMR, 491
    for SLE, 493
    stress doses, 104
    for vulvar lesions, 450–451
Corticotropin-releasing hormone (CRH), 551
Cortisol, 551
Cosmetic surgery, 360
Costs
    of assisted-living residences, 171
    of assistive listening devices, 199, 199t
    of caregiving, 38
    of dementia care, 272
    exercise benefits, 56
    of health care, 18–23
    of hearing aids, 199, 199t
    of nursing-home care, 160
    of pressure ulcers, 234
    of preventive measures, 62t–63t
    related to HF, 407
    related to UI, 225–226
Cosyntropin, 553
Cough
    chronic, 381, 381t, 383t
    in terminal illness, 114
Councils on Aging, 283
Counseling
    for cancer screening and preventive health, 74–75
    family counseling, 300–301
    healthy lifestyle counseling, 63t, 70–71
    Medicare wellness visits, 67t
    multicultural, 220
    nutrition, 70, 220
    for physical activity, 55, 57
    for STI prevention, 70–71
CPAP (continuous positive-airway pressure), 307, 386–387
CPC+ (Comprehensive Primary Care Plus), 21
CPGs (clinical practice guidelines), 34
CPPD (calcium pyrophosphate dihydrate deposition disease), 480, 487, 490
CR. *See* Cardiac rehabilitation
CR (cardiac rehabilitation), 153–154, 397, 409
Cranberry products, 535, Q97, Q123
CRASH (Chemotherapy Risk Assessment Scale for High-Age Patients) Score, 578
Creatinine, 436
Creatinine clearance, 78, 435
CRH (corticotropin-releasing hormone), 551
Crohn disease, 430
Cross-over toe deformity, 498–500, 498f
CRP (C-reactive protein), 392, 487
CRPS (complex regional pain syndrome), 119
CRT (cardiac resynchronization therapy), 413
Crutches, 156
Cryoprecipitate, 571

Cryotherapy, 588
Cryptogenic stroke, 519, 522
CSA (central sleep apnea), 306–307
CT (computed tomography), 431, 434
    low-dose, 65
Cultural aspects of care, 13, 42–48, Q65, Q83, Q126
    alcohol use, 346
    and mistreatment, 91
    nutritional care, 219–220
    palliative care, 106–107
Cultural competence, 42
Cultural identity, 42
CURB-65 score, 525
Curcumin, 85, 86t
Cushing syndrome, 439, 554
Cutaneous horn, 368
CVD. *See* Cardiovascular disease
Cyclooxygenase-2 inhibitors, 122, 489
Cyclophosphamide, 364, 488, 579t, 589
Cyclosporine, 335, 378, 493, 494
Cyclosporine A, 187
Cyproheptadine, 219
Cystitis, 533
Cystocele, 451, 452
Cysts, epidermal inclusion, 503
Cytochrome P450, 77t
Cytokine-modulating agents, 219
Cytosine arabinoside, 579t

D-dimer, 388
D2S2 (Decision Support and Discharge Screening) tool, Q93
Dabigatran
    for AF, 401
    Beers Criteria® for, 80t
    overdose, Q9
    for stroke prevention, 401, 403t, 521
    for VTE, 388–389
Dabrafenib, 370, 582t
Dacarbazine, 590
Daily evaluation, 130
Dakin's solution (hypochlorite), 240t
Danazol, 571
Dance, 258t, 279
Dapagliflozin, 564t
DAPT (dual antiplatelet therapy), 394, 395
Daptomycin, 532
Daratumumab, 590
Darifenacin, 227t
Dasatinib, 582t
DASH diet (Dietary Approaches to Stop Hypertension), 86
Day care, 168, 170t, 283
Day hospitals, 168
DBP (diastolic blood pressure), 416, 418
DBS (deep brain stimulation), 513
DDAVP (vasopressin), 231
DDIs (drug-drug interactions), 80, 81
De-escalation, 527
De Quervain tenosynovitis, 478
Death
    overall care near, 106
    physician-assisted, 16

Debridement, 239, Q11
Decision making, Q126
  approaches to, 11–12, 46
  in cardiovascular disease, 405–406
  cultural aspects, 42–48, 106–107
  deontological/rights-based
      approach, 11
  end-of-life, 16–17, 46
  ETHNICS mnemonic, 45
  about institutionalization, 167
  sample ethical dilemmas, 12t
  shared, 13, 405–406
  supported, 357
  surrogate, 14–15, 15t
Decision Support and Discharge
    Screening (D2S2) tool, Q93
Decisional capacity, 11, 13–14
  assessment of, 13–14, 14t
  for sexual consent, 472–473
DEED (Discharge of Elderly from the
    Emergency Department) program,
    140
Deep brain stimulation (DBS), 513
Deep-tissue pressure injury (DTPI), 235,
    236, Q70
Deep venous thrombosis (DVT), 380,
    387–389
  prophylaxis in hospitalized
      patients, 132–133
  risk assessment, 133
Defense of Marriage Act (DOMA), 54
Degenerative joint disease, 358t
Dehydration, 214, 411
Dehydroepiandrosterone (DHEA),
    554–555
  for dyspareunia, 471, 472t
  safety issues, 86t
  supplements, 542, 555
Dehydroepiandrosterone sulfate
    (DHEA-S), 554–555
Delirium, 294–303, 331
  agitated, 299–300, 301t
  attenuated, 294, 295
  definition of, 276
  diagnosis of, 294–295, Q28, Q58
  differential diagnosis of, 276, 294–
      295
  features of, Q58
  guidelines for prevention and
      management of, 302t, 303
  in hospitalized patients, 127, 137
  management of, 298–303, 298t,
      300t, 301t, Q12, Q60, Q102
  personality changes in, Q53
  postoperative, 104, 297, 302t, 303
  preoperative, 101–102
  prevention of, Q6
  psychotic symptoms in, 333
  quiet, 295
  recommendations for, 137, 303
  in rehabilitation, 148
  reversible causes of, 296, 296t
  risk factors for, 296, 296t, Q6, Q58
  in terminal illness, 113
DELIRIUM mnemonic for reversible
    causes of delirium, 296t

Delusional disorder, 333
Delusions, 319, Q54
  antipsychotic medications for,
      290–291, 290t
  definition of, 331
  in dementia, 289–291, 290t
  due to medical conditions, 334
  grandiose, 334
  management of, 332, 333
  mood-congruent, 331, 333–334
  paranoid, 331
  of poverty, 334
  somatic, 319, 333
Dementia, 272–283, 508
  advanced, Q59
  Advanced Dementia Prognostic
      Tool (ADEPT), 32t, 33, Q26
  aggression or agitation in, 292–293,
      Q32
  alcohol-related, 347–348, 355
  of Alzheimer disease, 87
  behavioral disturbances in, 284–
      293, Q32, Q44, Q53
  behavioral interventions for, 287,
      287t
  CIM for, 87
  delirium and, 296
  delusions in, 289–291, 290t
  depression in, 284, 287–289, 288t
  diagnostic features of, 276, 277t
  disease management, 176
  drug interactions, 82
  frontotemporal, 272, 273, 277–279,
      277t, 286–287, 336, Q68
  gait abnormalities, 244, 246
  general progression of, 276, 278t
  hallucinations in, 289–291, 290t
  HIV-associated, 538–539
  in hospitalized patients, 130–132
  inappropriate sexual behavior in,
      292, 473
  and incontinence, 226
  with intellectual disability, 354–
      355, Q94
  Lewy body, 272, 273, 277, 277t,
      286–287, 331, 334, 511
  manic-like behavioral syndromes
      in, 285, 289, 289t
  mild or moderate, Q75
  Mini-Cog Assessment Instrument
      for Dementia, 26, 72, 130,
      274, 275t
  mood disturbances in, 287–289
  in nursing-home population, 159
  oral care in, 379
  pain management in, Q80
  Parkinson disease, 273, 277t
  personality changes in, 336
  prognostic indices, 32t, 33
  protective factors for, 273, 274t
  psychologic signs of, Q32
  psychosis in, 285, 290t
  psychotic symptoms in, 334
  recommendations for, 283, 293
  and rehabilitation, 148

  resources for, 282–283
  risk factors for, 273, 274t, Q72
  screening for, 72
  and sexual consent, 472–473
  sleep changes in, 309
  sleep disturbances in, 291–292
  treatment of, 277t, 279–283, Q94
  and urinary incontinence, 226
  vascular, 244, 272, 277, 277t
Dementia Screening Questionnaire for
    Individuals with Intellectual
    Disabilities (DSQIID), 355
Demographics
  of aging, 1–4, 1f, Q118
  of alcohol use, 346
  of nursing-home population, 159
  rural, Q8
Denosumab, 268t, 269, 550
Dental abscesses, 375
Dental anatomy, 372, 373f
Dental caries, 372, 375, 376t
Dental dams, 52
Dental decay, 372, 375
Dental/oral conditions with
    developmental disabilities, 358t
Dental pulp changes, 372, 373t
Dental services, 19t
Dental surgery, 379, 537
Dental treatment, 378, 537
Dentistry, 372–379, Q29, Q74
Denture sores, 374
Denture stomatitis, 375
Dentures, 372, 374
Deontological/rights-based approach, 11
Dependence
  alcohol, Q78
  nicotine, 351
  opioid, 350–351
  physical, 122–123
  psychological, 123
Dependent personality disorder, 337t,
    338, 339, 340
Depression, 316–324
  bipolar, 316, 318–319, 321–322,
      322t, Q33
  CIM for, 87
  in CKD, 445
  in dementia, 284, 288
  with developmental disabilities,
      358t
  differential diagnosis of, 276
  Geriatric Depression Scale (GDS),
      26, 132, 318
  in hospitalized patients, 131t, 132
  indications to start antidepressant
      therapy based on PHQ-9, 317,
      318t
  in insomnia, 305–306
  interventions for, 31t, 131t, 132,
      323–324
  interventions for preventing falls,
      258t
  with marked anxiety, 328
  minor, 316, 319, 323
  in nursing-home population, 159

pharmacotherapy for, 288–289, 288t, 319–320
prescriber response guidelines based on PHQ-9 and the STAR*D studies, 317, 318t
recommended preventive measures for, 63t
and rehabilitation, 148
screening for, 63t, 72, 211t, 317–318, Q7, Q75, Q121
with severe anxiety, 329t
in stroke, Q100
suicidal, 317–318, 319, Q36
in terminal illness, 114–115
Depression assessment, 559
Depressive personality disorder, 336
Dermatitis
atopic, 362, 362f
eczematous, 362, 362f
neurodermatitis, 362, 450
seborrheic, 360–361, 361f
stasis, 360, 365
Dermatofibromas, 503
Dermatology, 360–371, Q3, Q30, Q95. *See also* Skin problems
Dermatomyositis, 494–495
Desensitization, graded, 330
Desipramine, 288, 288t
Desvenlafaxine, 288t
DETERMINE checklist, 216
Detoxification, 349t, 350
Detrusor overactivity (DO), 226, 227
Detrusor underactivity, 227
Deutetrabenazine, 512
Developmental disabilities, 352–359, Q51, Q94
comorbidities, 357, 358t
Device therapy, 413–414, 415
Devil's claw *(Harpagophytum procumbens)*, 86
DEXA (dual energy x-ray absorptiometry), 62t, 264, 265, Q98
Dexamethasone, 112t, 551, 590
Dexamethasone suppression tests, 554
Dextroamphetamine, 115
Dextromethorphan, Q44
Dextromethorphan-quinidine, 293
DHA (docosahexaenoic acid), Q39
DHEA (dehydroepiandrosterone), 554–555
for dyspareunia, 471, 472t
safety issues, 86t
supplements, 542, 555
DHEA-S (dehydroepiandrosterone sulfate), 554–555
Diabetes mellitus (DM), 558–566
and cardiovascular risk, 391
etiology of, Q61
and foot, 505–506
and incontinence, 226
interventions for, 560–563
management of, 31t, 104, 559–560, Q31
and periodontal disease, Q29
pharmacologic agents for, 562–563, 564t

postoperative, 104
recommendations for, 192, 195, 566
and rehabilitation, 148
screening for, 62t, 66
self-management of, 558, 560–561, Q31
type 1, 558
type 2, 66, 558, 562, 563, Q98
Diabetic amyotrophy, 515
Diabetic foot ulcers, 242
Diabetic nephropathy, 442
Diabetic neuropathy, 124, 507, 514–515
Diabetic retinopathy, 190–191
Diagnosis-related groups (DRGs), 128, 165
Diagnostic and Statistical Manual of Mental Disorders, 4th edition, Text Revision (DSM IV-TR), 336
Diagnostic and Statistical Manual of Mental Disorders, Fifth Edition (DSM-5), 272, 284, 325, 327
criteria for bipolar disorder type 1 and type 2, 318
criteria for delirium, 294
criteria for depression, 316, 317
criteria for intellectual disability, 352
criteria for personality disorders, 336–337
criteria for somatic symptom disorders, 340
criteria for substance use disorder, 344
Diagnostic interventions, 30, 31t
Dialectical behavior therapy, 339, Q57
Dialysis, 445, 446
Diarrhea
chronic, 430–431
IBS with (IBS-D), 432
IBS with alternating constipation and diarrhea (IBS-M or IBS mixed), 432
infectious, 540
postobstructive, 434
postoperative, 103
in terminal illness, 111
Diastolic blood pressure (DBP), 416, 418
Diastolic heart failure, 407
Diazepam, 350
DIC (disseminated intravascular coagulation), 571
Diclofenac, 121, 121t, 486
Dicyclomine, 231
Diet(s), Q84
altered consistencies, 223
and cancer, 88
for chronic CAD, 395
for CKD, 445
for DM, 559, 561
FODMAP diet (fermentable oligo-, di- and monosaccharides and polyols), 432
for gout, 489

for HF, 409
for HTN, 419
for IBS, 432
Mediterranean diet, 86, 184, Q84
Modified Diet in Renal Disease (MDRD) formula, 101, 435
sodium restriction, 409, 419
for syncope, 212
Dietary Approaches to Stop Hypertension (DASH diet), 86
Dietary Guidelines for Americans, 70
Dietary Reference Intakes (DRIs), 214
Dietary supplements, 85, 218–219, 414
for cancer, 88
for depression, 87
for pressure ulcers, 241
safety issues, 85, 86t
Dietitians, 146, 147t
Diffuse large B-cell lymphoma, 589
Diffuse peritonitis, 431
Digestive system, 9t, 10t
Digit quinti varus, 499t
Digital hearing aids, 199, 199t
Digital rectal examination (DRE), 456, 459
Digitalis, 439t
Dignity therapy, 115
Digoxin
for ACS, 394
adverse events, 215, 412
for AF, 399
drug interactions, 527
and falls, 252
for HF, 412–413
nutrient interactions, 215, 215t
Dihydropyridines, 215, 394
Diltiazem, 394, 399
Diphenhydramine
adverse events, 310
and delirium, 300t
for insomnia, 315
for nausea, 111, 112t
Diphenoxylate/atropine, 430
Diplopia, 185, 187, 187t
Dipyridamole, 521
Direct oral anticoagulants (DOACs), 401, 403t
Direct thrombin inhibitors, 389
Disabilities of the Arm, Shoulder, and Hand Outcome Measure, 154
Disability
excess, 346–347
functional, 159
hospital-associated, 126–127
International Classification of Functioning, Disability, and Health (ICF) (WHO), 143
preclinical, 26
Disc displacement, 476, 482t
Discharge destinations, 141
Discharge medication regimen, 141
Discharge of Elderly from the Emergency Department (DEED) program, 140
Discharge planning/summary, Q85, Q93

Disclosure, 46, Q126
DISCUS (Dyskinesia Identification System Condensed User Scale), 333
Disease management, 175–176, 324
Disease-modifying anti-inflammatory drugs (DMARDs), 487–488
Disinhibited impulsive syndrome, 336
Dislocation, metatarsal phalangeal joint, 498–500, 499*t*
Disopyramide, 401
Disorganized thinking, 295
Disseminated intravascular coagulation (DIC), 571
Distraction techniques, 292
Disulfiram, 349*t*, 350, Q112
Diuretic resistance, Q104
Diuretics
    adverse events, 81, 411
    and falls, 252
    for HF, 411, 413, Q21
    for HTN, 419–420, 419*t*
    for hyperkalemia, 439
    for hypervolemia, 438
    for hyponatremia, 437
    loop, 226*t*, 411, 420, 437, 438
    nutrient interactions, 215*t*
    potassium-sparing, 438
    for prevention of cardiovascular disease, 561
    thiazide, 411, 419–420, 437
Divalproex sodium
    for behavioral disturbances in dementia, 289, 289*t*, Q32
    for personality disorders, 340
    to stabilize mood in mania and bipolar depression, 321, 322*t*
Diverticular disease, 431
Diverticulitis, 431, 539–540
Diverticulosis, 431
Dix-Hallpike test, 205, 246, Q99, Q121
Dizziness, 202–206
    classification of, 202–204, 203*t*
    functional, Q121
    mixed, 202, 203*t*, 204
    terminology for, Q99
DM. *See* Diabetes mellitus
DM-1 (emtansine), 581
DMARDs (disease-modifying anti-inflammatory drugs), 487–488
DO (detrusor overactivity), 226, 227
Do-not-hospitalize orders, 163–164
Do-not-resuscitate (DNR) orders, 163, Q125, Q126
DOACs (direct oral anticoagulants), 401, 403*t*
Docetaxel, 461*t*, 463, 582*t*, 588
Docosahexaenoic acid (DHA), Q39
Doctrine of double effect, 16
Documentation
    asthma action plans, 382, 382*t*
    Durable Power of Attorney (DPOA) documents, 11, 14, 15, 163–164
    for house calls, 166, Q115

Medical Orders for Life-Sustaining Treatment (MOLST), 16
Medical Orders for Scope of Treatment (MOST), 16
of mistreatment, 95
Physician Orders for Life-Sustaining Treatment (POLST), 16, 109
Physician Orders for Scope of Treatment (POST), 16
of pressure injuries, 236–237, Q11
wound, 237
Docusate sodium, 429
Dofetilide, 401
DOMA (Defense of Marriage Act), 54
Domestic activity, 56
Donepezil
    adverse events, Q19
    for Alzheimer disease, 291, Q15
    for dementia, 281, 355, Q94, Q100
Dopamine agonists
    adverse events, 552
    and delirium, 300*t*
    for hyperprolactinemia, 552
    for PD motor symptoms, 510–511
    for RLS, 514
Dopamine antagonists, 112*t*, 512
Dopaminergic agents, 335
Doppler ultrasonography, Q99, Q110
Dorzolamide, 188*t*
Double effect doctrine, 16
Down syndrome, 354, 355, 356, 357, Q94
Doxazosin, 421, 456, 456*t*, Q89
Doxepin, 300*t*, 313*t*, 314
Doxorubicin, 579*t*, 582*t*, 589, 590
Doxycycline, 188, 539
DPOA (Durable Power of Attorney) documents, 11, 14, 15, 163–164
DPP-4 enzyme inhibitors, 563, 564*t*
Dramatic, emotional, or erratic behaviors, 337*t*, 340
DRE (digital rectal examination), 456, 459
Dressings
    for chronic wounds, 241
    for foot ulcers, 505–506
    for pressure injuries, 239, 240*t*, 241, Q45
DRGs (diagnosis-related groups), 128, 165
Drinking. *See* Alcohol
DRIs (Dietary Reference Intakes), 214
Driving, night, Q10
Driving accidents: risk factors for, 27
Driving assessment, 27–28, 280
    Clinician's Guide to Assessing and Counseling Older Drivers (AGS), 28, 73
    recommendations for, 63*t*, 73
Driving evaluation, Q23
Dronabinol, 88, 112*t*, 219, Q42
Dronedarone, 401
Drop arm sign, 477
Droxidopa, 511

Drug abuse, 53, 344, 345–346. *See also* Substance abuse
Drug-disease interactions, 82
Drug-drug interactions (DDIs), 80, 81
Drug holidays, 269
Drug-induced esophageal injury, 426
Drug-induced hyponatremia, Q19
Drug-induced lupus erythematosus, 493
Drug-induced movement disorders, 511, 512–513
Drug-induced myopathy, 515
Drug-induced nausea and vomiting, Q96
Drug-induced parkinsonism, 511, 512
Drug-nutrient interactions, 215, 215*t*
Drug regimen review, 83
Drug resistance, 526, 532, 534, 539
Drugs. *See also* Pharmacotherapy; *specific drugs*
    absorption of, 76–77, 77*t*
    antiepileptic, 508
    to avoid in older adults, 124–125
    Beers Criteria® for, 80, 80*t*
    in CKD, 444
    classes associated with increased risk of falls, 251–252, 251*t*
    clearance of, 78
    discontinuing, 83
    distribution of, 77, 77*t*
    elimination of, 77*t*, 78
    half-life of, 78
    hydrophilic, 77
    lipophilic, 77
    Medicare Prescription Drug Plan Finder (CMS), 16, 22
    metabolism of, 77–78, 77*t*
    preventing falls with, 256, 258*t*
    to reduce or eliminate in management of delirium, 298, 300*t*
    to stabilize mood in mania and bipolar depression, 320–321, 322*t*
    that can cause or worsen UI, 226, 226*t*
    that can increase risk of osteoporosis, 262*t*, 263*t*
    that cause hyperkalemia, 438, 439*t*
    that interfere with gustation (taste) and olfaction (smell), 376–377, 377*t*
Dry eye, 186*t*, 187–188, 187*t*
Dry mouth, 374–375, 378
Dry weight, 409
DSQIID (Dementia Screening Questionnaire for Individuals with Intellectual Disabilities), 355
DTPI (deep tissue pressure injury), 235, 236, Q70
Dual antiplatelet therapy (DAPT), 394, 395
Dual eligibles, 20–21, 168, 169, Q22
Dual energy x-ray absorptiometry (DEXA or DXA), 62*t*, 264, 265, Q98
Dual tasking, 247

Dulaglutide, 564t
Duloxetine (Cymbalta)
    for anxiety, 329
    Beers Criteria® for, 80t
    for depression, 320t
    for depressive features in dementia, 288t
    for fibromyalgia, 495–496
    for neuropathic pain, 124, 514–515
    for OA-related pain, 486
    for persistent pain, 124
    for UI, 231
Dupuytren contractions, 479
Durable medical equipment, 19t, 155
Durable Power of Attorney (DPOA) documents, 11, 14, 15, 163–164
Durvalumab, 588
Dutasteride, 456–457, 456t
DVT (deep venous thrombosis), 380, 387–389
Dysequilibrium, 202, 203t, 204
Dyskinesia, 508–509, 510
Dyskinesia Identification System Condensed User Scale (DISCUS), 333
Dyslipidemia, 391, 582t
Dysnatremias, 436
Dyspareunia, 449, 470–471, 472t
Dyspepsia, 426
Dysphagia, 222–223
    esophageal, 222, 223, 423–424, Q49, Q116
    oropharyngeal, 223, 423, 424, Q116
    after stroke, 150
Dyspnea, 380, 381, 383t, 386
    severe, 385t, 386
    in terminal illness, 113–114
Dysproteinemias, 441–442, 443
Dystonia, 508–509, 512

E-Care Diary, 39t
Ears, 9t, 10t
EASI (Elder Abuse Suspicion Index), 90
Eastern Cooperative Oncology Group (ECOG) performance status, 32, 577
Eating changes, 222
Eccentric behaviors, 337t
Echinacea, 86t
Echocardiography, 210, 211t, 392, 398
    transesophageal (TEE), 398, 537
Echocardiography, transesophageal, Q18
ECOG (Eastern Cooperative Oncology Group) performance measures, 577
Ectropion, 185, 186t
Eczema, 362, 362f, 504
ED (erectile dysfunction), 465–467
Edaravone, 516
Edema
    macular, 190
    pitting, 487, 488
Eden Alternative, 163
Edentulism, 373–374

Edoxaban
    for AF, 401
    Beers Criteria® for, 80t
    for stroke prevention, 401, 403t, 521
    for VTE, 388–389
Educational attainment, 3
EEG (electroencephalography), 211t, Q75
EFFECT Heart Failure Mortality Prediction Model, 32, 32t
eGFR (estimated glomerular filtration rate), 78, 435, Q14
EGSYS (Evaluation of Guidelines in Syncope Study) score, 209, 210t
EHRs (electronic health records), Q93
Eicosapentaenoic acid (EPA), Q39
Eikenella, 398, 536–537
Ejaculatory dysfunction, 456
Ejection fraction, Q14
Elbow pain, 477–478, Q122
Elder Abuse Suspicion Index (EASI), 90
Elder Financial Protection Network, 93
Elder Justice Roadmap, 89, 95
Elder mistreatment. See Mistreatment
Eldercare Locator, 39t
Electrocardiography (ECG)
    ambulatory monitoring, 210, 211t
    in HF, 408
    implantable loop recorders, 210, 211t
    preoperative, 98
    screening, 69
    in syncope, 209, 210, 211t
Electroconvulsive therapy
    for depression in terminally ill, 115
    for depressive features of behavioral disturbances in dementia, 288
    for major depressive disorder and mania, 323
    for psychotic depression, 320
Electroencephalography (EEG), 211t, Q75
Electrolyte disorders, 103
Electromyography (EMG), 514
Electronic health records (EHRs), Q93
Electrophysiologic studies (EPS), 210, 211t
Elotuzumab, 590
Emergencies, hypertensive, 421
Emergency department (ED) care, 134–135, 135t
    Discharge of Elderly from the Emergency Department (DEED) program, 140
EMG (electromyography), 514
Emotion-oriented psychotherapy, 279
Emotional behaviors, 337t
Emotional/psychological abuse, 89, 90t
Empagliflozin, 564t
Employment, 4
Empty can sign, 477
Empty sella syndrome, 552–553
Emtansine (DM-1), 581

Enalapril, 410t, Q37
Encephalopathy, 294, 337, 355
End-of-life care
    advance care planning, 15–16, Q52
    controversial procedures, 16–17
    cultural aspects of, 46, 48, 106–107
    financing, 18
    for HF, 415
    palliative care, 109–115
    patient preferences, 15–16, Q65
    for terminal illness, Q42
    transitions of care, 160
End-stage cancer, Q42
End-stage renal disease (ESRD), 33, 445–446
Endocarditis
    antimicrobial prophylaxis for, 378, 378t, 537, 537t
    bacterial, 378, 378t, Q18
    infective, 372, 378, 378t, 398, 536–537
    native-valve, 398
Endocrine disorders, 104, 542–543
Endocrine myopathy, 515
Endocrine Society, 470
Endocrine system, 9t, 10t, 436t, 542
Endocrine theory of aging, 7
Endocrinology, 542–557, Q87, Q102
Endometrial cancer, 453–454, 580
Endometrium, atrophic, 454
Endoscopy, 426, 427, Q49
Endovascular thrombectomy, 520
Endurance exercise training, 154
Enemas, 429–430
Energetics theories of aging, 7
Energy intake, 214
Energy requirements, 213
Enhanced primary care, 174–175
Enoxaparin, 80t, 393
Entacapone, 510
Entecavir, 488
Enterocele, 451
Enterococcus, Q18
Entrapment syndrome, 499t
Entropion, 185, 186t
Environmental modifications
    for behavioral disturbances, 292
    for delirium, 298t
    for dementia, 280
    home care, 167
    for preventing falls, 256, 258t
    for rehabilitation, 155, 157–158
    for sleep disorders, 309–310
Enzalutamide, 582t, 588
Enzymatic debridement, 239
EORTC Quality of Life Questionnaire Core, 583
EPA (eicosapentaenoic acid), Q39
Epidermal inclusion cysts, 503
Epidural hematoma, 522–523
Epigenetic theory of aging, 6–7
Epilepsy, 336–337, 507–508, Q75
Eplerenone, 411, 420, 439t
Epley maneuver, 205–206

Epothilones, 582*t*
ePrognosis, 31, Q26
Eprosartan, 410*t*
EPS (electrophysiologic studies), 210, 211*t*
Equinovarus, 245*t*
Equinus deformity, 498, 499*t*
Erectile dysfunction (ED), 457, 465–467, Q34, Q87
    causes of, 465–466, 466*t*
    evaluation of, 467–468
    treatment options for, 468–469, 468*t*
Erectile physiology, 465–467
Ergotamines, 517
Eribulin, 582*t*
Erlotinib, 582*t*
Erratic behaviors, 337*t*
Error catastrophe theory of aging, 7
Erythromycin, 230, 361–362
Erythroplakia, 376
Erythropoiesis, ineffective, 568*t*, 570
Erythropoiesis-stimulating agents (ESAs), 444, 446, Q73
Erythropoietin, 568, 590
ESAs (erythropoiesis-stimulating agents), 444, 446, Q73
ESBLs (extended spectrum β-lactamase–producing gram-negative rods), 526
Eschar, 239
Escherichia coli, 463, 540
Escitalopram, 288*t*, 320*t*
Eskenazi Health, Q77
Eskimos, 219
Esophageal cancer, 581, 587
Esophageal candidiasis, Q49
Esophageal carcinoma, Q49
Esophageal dysphagia, 222, 223, 423–424, Q49, Q116
Esophageal manometry, Q49
Esophagitis, pill, 426
Esophagus: disorders of, 423–426
ESRD (end-stage renal disease), 33, 445–446
Essential thrombocythemia (ET), 571, 573
Essential tremor (ET), 513
Estazolam, 312
Estimated glomerular filtration rate (eGFR), 78, 435, Q14
Estradiol vaginal cream, Q1
Estrogen deficiency, 261–262
Estrogen-progestin therapy, 549
Estrogen therapy
    for atrophic vaginitis, Q97
    for exposed vaginal mesh, Q1
    for female sexual dysfunction, 471, 472*t*
    for incontinence, 226*t*, 231
    for menopausal symptoms, 447
    for osteoporosis, 268*t*, 270
    for vaginal atrophy, 449, 470
    for vasomotor symptoms, 448
Eszopiclone, 313–314, 313*t*

ET (essential thrombocythemia), 571, 573
ET (essential tremor), 513
Etanercept, 488, 492
Ethambutol, 536
Ethical issues, 11–17, 12*t*, Q17, Q126
    in home care, 167
    related to nutritional status, 220
Ethics consultation, 11–12
Ethnic differences
    in cancer incidence and mortality, 574–575
    in depression, 316
    in urinary incontinence, 225
Ethnic minorities, 2, 575, Q80, Q83
ETHNICS mnemonic, 45
Etoposide, 579*t*, 580
European Guidelines on Cardiovascular Disease Prevention, 561
European League Against Rheumatism (EULAR)
    classification criteria for gout, 488–489
    provisional classification criteria for polymyalgia rheumatica, 490–491
European Society for Microbiology, 534
Euthanasia, 16–17
Evaluation of Guidelines in Syncope Study (EGSYS) score, 209, 210*t*
Everolimus, 582*t*, 589
Evidence, 35
Evolutionary theories of aging, 5
Executive dysfunction, 316, 318
Executive function testing, 26
Exenatide, 563, 564*t*
Exercise, 298
    aerobic, Q21
    for behavioral disturbances, 287
    benefits of, 392, Q38
    for cancer, 88
    for cardiovascular disease, 86
    for chronic CAD, 395
    counseling for, 63*t*, 70
    for dementia, 279, 287
    for depression, 323–324
    for DM, 558, 559
    for DVT, 389
    for fall prevention, Q24, Q40, Q82
    for fatigue in SLE, 493
    for frailty, Q88
    for gait disorders, 248
    for HF, 409
    home, 59
    for HTN, 419
    inspiratory muscle training, Q114
    integrating into daily life, 58
    for low fitness or low functional ability, 59
    for neck pain, 476
    for OA-related pain, 480, 486
    for osteoporosis, 266
    for PAD, 404–405
    for pain, 120
    pelvic floor muscle (Kegel), 472*t*, Q4

    pelvic muscle exercises (PMEs), 229–230
    for polymyositis, 494–495
    for preventing falls, 256–257, 258*t*, 259
    recommendations for, 55–57, 58, 86
    to reduce risk of osteoporosis, 262
    relative exercise intensity, 55
    shoulder exercises, 155
    for sleep problems, 312
    total body preoperative exercise, 248
    for urinary incontinence, Q4
    vestibular rehabilitation therapy (VRT), 205
Exercise capacity, Q21
Exercise intensity, 55, 56*t*
Exercise Management for Chronic Diseases and Disabilities (ACSM), 58–59
Exercise prescription, Q31
Exercise stress tests, 210, 395
Exercise training, 154
Exercise volume, 55, 56*t*
Exostoses, 375
Expanded In-home Services for the Elderly Program, 168
Expectant or conservative management, 460–462
Exploitation, financial, 89, 90*t*, 93, Q17, Q105
Exposure with response prevention, 330
Extended spectrum β-lactamase–producing gram-negative rods (ESBLs), 526
External beam radiation therapy, 461*t*, 462
Extracellular fluid volume
    depletion, 437
    normal, 437
    overload, 437
Eye conditions, 185–187, 187*t*, Q117
    inflammatory conditions, 493–494
    that require immediate referral, 185–187, 186*t*
    treatment of, 187*t*
Eye drops, 188*t*, 191
Eyes
    age-related changes, 9*t*, 10*t*, 186*t*
    comprehensive examination of, 185

F-tags, 161, 231, 232
Faces Pain Scale, 118
Facial nerve palsy (Bell's palsy), 539
Facial volume restoration, 360
Factitious disorder, 340, 342*t*
Factor Xa inhibitors, 389, 401
Fair process, 134
Faith/spiritual beliefs, 46
Falls, 250–259
    assessment of, Q2
    in hospitalized patients, 128–129, 131*t*

interventions for, 128–129, 131t, 504–505, Q47, Q82, Q108
medication classes associated with increased risks, 251–252, 251t
prevention of, 57, 71, 251, 252, 253f, 255–259, 258t–259t, Q24, Q40, Q82, Q108
risk assessment, 63t, 71, 252, 253f, 254–255
risk factors, 250–252, 258t–259t, 259, 504–505, Q62
risk reduction, 252, 253f, 255t, Q24, Q63
screening for, 253f, 254–255
Famcyclovir, 366
Familial Alzheimer disease, 273
Families, 279–280
  fictive kin, 46
  of LGBT older adults, 53
  resources for, 22
Family Caregiver Alliance, 39t
Family caregivers, 37, 38, 272, Q22
Family counseling, 300–301
Family education, 298t
Famotidine, 80t, 112t
Fasting blood glucose, 542
Fatalism, 220
FDA (Food and Drug Administration), 347
Fearful behaviors, 337t
Febuxostat, 489
Fecal bulking agents, 430
Fecal DNA testing, 585
Fecal impaction, 429–430
Fecal incontinence, 430
  with developmental disabilities, 358t
Fecal microbiota transplantation (FMT), 540
Fecal occult blood testing (FOBT), 61, 64, 432, 585
  recommendations for, 62t
Fecal softeners, 429, Q96
Federal health care spending, 18
Federal Trade Commission (FTC), 93
Fee-for-service (FFS) care
  Medicare, 18–19, 19t, 22, 137
  private plans, 19
  readmissions, 137
Feeding, 223–224
  artificial, 220
  hand, 224
  recommendations for, 137, 220, 224
  tube, 223–224
Feeding, hand, Q59
Feeding assistance, 298, 298t
Feeding difficulties, Q49, Q59
Feeding problems, 224
Feeding tubes, 220, 223–224, Q59
Female sexual dysfunction, 469–470
  evaluation of, 470–471
  treatment of, 470–471
Female sexuality, 469–471
Femoral fractures, Q70

Femoral hernia, 479
Femoral neck fracture, 151
Femoral neuropathy, 479
FE_{Na} (fractional excretion of sodium), 440
Fermentable oligo-, di- and monosaccharides and polyols (FODMAP diet), 432
Ferric gluconate, 569
Ferrous gluconate, 569
Ferrous sulfate, 569, Q9
Fesoterodine, 227t, 230, Q4
Festination, 245t
FEV_1 (forced expiratory volume in 1 second), 380
Fever
  evaluation of, 541t
  in frail, older residents, 525, 526–527, 527t
  in older adults, 526–527
  in older long-term care residents, 526–527
Fever of uncertain etiology, Q18
Fever of unknown origin (FUO), 540–541, 541t
FFS care. See Fee-for-service care
Fiber, dietary, 213
Fiber-bulking agents, 432
Fiber supplements, 429
Fibrinogen, 571
Fibrinolytic therapy, 394
Fibromyalgia, 118–119, 119t, 495–496
  nonopioid treatment of, 124
FICA (faith and belief, importance, community, and address in care), 47
Fictive kin, 46
Fidaxomicin, 540
FIM (Functional Independence Measure), 145, 145t
Financial assessment, 93
Financial exploitation, 89, 90t, 93, Q17, Q105
Financial security challenges, 53–54
Financial vulnerability, age-associated, Q17
Financing, Q20, Q78
  for assisted living, 171
  conservator of finances, Q17
  costs of hearing aids, 199, 199t
  for end-of-life care, 18
  for health care, 18–23
  for home-health care, 18
  for house calls, 166
  for nursing-home care, 160
  for outpatient care, 18, 20
  for rehabilitation services, 144–146, 144t
Finasteride, 456–457, 456t, 473
  for BPH, 31t
  lag time to benefit, 31t
Find A Lawyer (National Academy of Elder Law Attorneys), 39t
Fine-needle aspiration (FNA), 547
Firearms, 317–318

Fish, fatty, 87
Fitness, low, 59
"Five A's" method of smoking cessation, 351, 384
Flashes, 187t
Flat foot, 498
Flavor enhancement, 377
Flavoxate, 231
Flecainide, 401
Flexibility activity recommendations, 56–57
Flexible medication times, 309–310
Flexible sigmoidoscopy, 61
Floaters, 185, 186t, 187, 187t
Floating the heels, 238
Flu. See Influenza
Fludarabine, 589
Fludrocortisone, 212, 259t, 511, 553
Fluid needs, 214
Fluid replacement, 428–429
Fluid restriction, 409, 437
Fluoride, 372
Fluoroquinolones, 532, 534
Fluorouracil, 579t, 582t, 586, 587
Fluoxetine, 230, 287–288, 288t
Flutamide, 463
Fluticasone, 384t
FMT (fecal microbiota transplantation), 540
FNA (fine-needle aspiration), 547
FOBT. See Fecal occult blood testing
Focal segmental glomerulosclerosis (FSGS), 443
FODMAP diet (fermentable oligo-, di- and monosaccharides and polyols), 432
Folate, 215t
Folate deficiency, 569f, 570
Folic acid, 218–219
Follicle-stimulating hormone (FSH), 551t
Follicular lymphoma, 589
Folstein Mini–Mental State Examination (MMSE), 26, 275t
Fondaparinux, 393
  Beers Criteria® for, 80t
  for thromboprophylaxis, 133
  for VTE prophylaxis, 389
Food and Nutrition Board, Institute of Medicine, 213, 214
Foods, calcium-containing, 266, 267t
Foot care, 497, Q50
Foot diseases and disorders, 497
  arthritis, 506
  associated deformities, 498–502
  common deformities, 497–503, 499t
  in diabetes mellitus, 505–506
  interventions for preventing falls, 256
  nail disorders, 504
  peripheral arterial disease, 506
  skin lesions, 503
  skin problems, 503–504
  surgical considerations for deformities, 502–503

systemic diseases, 505–506
treatment strategies for, 502–503
Foot drop, 245t, 246
Foot slap, 245t
Foot ulcers, 242, 505
Footwear, Q82
for preventing falls, 256, 258t
recommended shoe characteristics, 254, 254f
shoe terms, 503t
shoes, 258t, 502
Forced expiratory volume in 1 second (FEV_1), 380
Forced vital capacity (FVC), 380
Formality, 42–43
Formoterol fumarate, 384t
Fosinopril, 410t, Q9
Foster care, 171
400-meter walk test, 247
Fractional carbon dioxide (CO_2) laser therapy, 449
Fractional excretion of sodium (FE_{Na}), 440
Fracture risk assessment model (FRAX™), 68, 260, 262–263, 265, 265t
Fracture Risk Assessment tool (FRAX®), Q2
Fractures
diagnosis of, 262–266
femoral, Q70
fragility, 260
of hip, 150–151, 260–261
low-trauma, 260
prediction of, 262–266
prevention of, Q2, Q63
risk factors for, 262–263, 262t
sacral fractures, 481, 481t, 482t, 483
secondary causes of, 263–264
of shoulder, 155
vertebral, 265, 271
vertebral compression fractures, 271, 475, 481, 481t, 482t, 483
Fragile X syndrome, 353, 354, 357
Fragility fracture, 260
FRAIL scale, 182
Frailty, 180–184
assessment of, 102, 182–183
and cardiovascular disease, 392
causes of, 182
cycle of, 181, 181f
fever in frail, older residents of long-term care facilities, 525, 526–527, 527t
in HIV, 538
hypertension in, 421–422
management of, 183, Q88
pre-frailty, 392
preoperative, 102
screening for, 182, Q109
Frailty Index, 179
FRAX™ (fracture risk assessment model), 68, 260, 262–263, 265, 265t

Free radical theory of aging, 6
Free T_3 test, 545
Free T_4 test, 545
Free water deficit, 438
Freezing of gait, 246
Frequency-volume charts, 229
Fresh frozen plasma, 571
Frontal lobe disease, 246
Frontal lobe injury, 336
Frontotemporal dementia (FTD), Q68
behavioral disturbances in, 286–287
diagnostic features and treatment of, 277t
differential diagnosis of, 277–279
epidemiology of, 272
etiology of, 273
personality changes in, 336
Frontotemporal lobar degeneration, Q53
Frozen shoulder (adhesive capsulitis), 477
FSGS (focal segmental glomerulosclerosis), 443
FSH (follicle-stimulating hormone), 551t
FTD. See Frontotemporal dementia
Functional Activities Questionnaire, 275t
Functional Ambulation Classification scale, 247
Functional Assessment of Cancer Therapy, 583
Functional Assessment Scale, 33
Functional decline, Q75
Functional dizziness, Q121
Functional Independence Measure (FIM), 145, 145t
Functional neurologic symptom disorder, 342t
Functional reach test, 254
Functional status
acute decline, 28
assessment of, 26–28, 145t, 275, 559
with developmental disabilities, 358t
impairments in hospitalized patients, 131t
International Classification of Functioning, Disability, and Health (ICF) (WHO), 143
interventions for, 131t
low fitness or low functional ability, 59
of nursing-home population, 159
performance-based assessment of, 247
postoperative decline, 397
preoperative assessment and management of, 102
Fungal infections, 504
FUO (fever of unknown origin), 540–541, 541t
Furosemide, 215, 411, Q14, Q37
Futility, 134
FVC (forced vital capacity), 380

GABAergic agents, 226t
Gabapentin (Neurontin, Gralise, Horizant)
for alcohol detoxification, 349t
Beers Criteria® for, 80t
for depressive features in dementia, 288t
for essential tremor, 513
and incontinence, 226, 226t
for insomnia, 292
for menopausal vasomotor symptoms, 448–449
for neuropathic pain, 514–515
for persistent pain, 124
for RLS, 308, 514
GAD (generalized anxiety disorder), 327, 329, 329t
Gait abnormalities, 244, 245t
antalgic gait, 245t, 246
freezing of gait, 246
idiopathic, 245
"senile" gait disorder, 245
steppage gait, 245t
Trendelenburg gait, 245t, 246
Gait and balance screening, 63t, 247
Gait apraxia, 246
Gait assessment, 254
Gait disorders, 244, 507
interventions to reduce, 247–249
rehabilitation of, 248
Gait disturbances, Q62
Gait evaluation, 211t
Gait impairment, 27, 244–249
conditions that contribute to, 10, 244–245
interventions for preventing falls, 258t
Gait instability, Q69
Gait speed, 27, 55, 247, Q46, Q109
Gait training, 256–257, 258t
Galantamine, 281, 291, 355, Q94
Gall stones, 427–428
Gambling, 351
Gammopathy, monoclonal, of uncertain significance (MGUS), 590
Gastric cancer, 587
Gastroenterology, 423–434
infections, 539–540
postoperative management, 103–104
Gastroesophageal reflux disease (GERD), 358t, 424–426, 434
Gastrointestinal bleeding, 432–433, Q9
Gastrointestinal obstruction, 111–112
Gastrostomy
contraindications to, 224
percutaneous endoscopic, 223–224
Gastrostomy tube placement, 223–224
Gay men, 50, 51–52, 53. See also Lesbian gay bisexual transgender (LGBT) health
GCA (giant cell arteritis), 186–187, 186t, 187t, 491–492, 517, Q110
GDS (Geriatric Depression Scale), 26, 72, 132, 318, Q75
Gefitinib, 582t

GEM (geriatric evaluation and management) units, 135, 176
Gemcitabine, 579t, 580, 588
Gender differences
　cultural aspects, 46–47
　in drug metabolism, 78
　in urinary incontinence, 225
Gender identity, 50
General Practitioner Assessment of Cognition, 72
Generalized anxiety disorder (GAD), 327, 329, 329t
Generalized Anxiety Disorder-7, 325
Genetic damage, 5–6
Genetic disorders, 357
Genetics, 261
GENEVA tool, 133
Genitourinary syndrome of menopause, 447, 449, 470, 555
Genu recurvatum, 245t
Geographic distribution of older adults, 3
Geographic tongue, 375
"Geographical Practices Cost Indices," 165–166
GERD (gastroesophageal reflux disease), 424–426, 434
Geriatric approach, 174, 174t
Geriatric assessment, comprehensive, Q27
Geriatric Depression Scale (GDS), 26, 72, 132, 318, Q75
Geriatric EDs, 134–135
Geriatric evaluation and management (GEM) units, 135, 176
Geriatric Resource Nurse (GRN) Model, 136
Geriatric Resources for Assessment and Care of Elders (GRACE) teams, 175
Geriatric specialty care, 176–178
Geriatrics in Primary Care model, 173–176
GFI (Groningen Frailty Indicator), Q109
GFR. See Glomerular filtration rate
GH. See Growth hormone
GHRH (growth hormone regulating hormone), 551t
Giant cell arteritis (GCA), 186–187, 186t, 187t, 491–492, 517, Q110
Gingival enlargement, 378
Gingivitis, 373, 376t
Ginkgo biloba
　for dementia, 281–282
　for memory complaints, 87
　for mild cognitive impairment, 87
　safety issues, 86t
Glanzmann thrombasthenia, 571–572
Glare sensitivity, Q10
Glaucoma, 188, 191
　angle-closure, 186, 186t, 187t
　eye drops for, 188t, 191
　screening for, 72, 185
　signs and symptoms of, 186t
　treatment of, 187t
Gleason grading system, 459–460

Glenohumeral joint osteoarthritis, 477
Glimepiride, 564t
Glioblastoma, 581
Glipizide, 563, 564t
Global aging trends, 1–2, 1f
Global Initiative for Chronic Obstructive Lung Disease (GOLD), 383–384, 383t
Glomerular disease, 442–443
Glomerular filtration rate (GFR), 101, 435, 444
　age-related changes in, 78, 436t
　estimated (eGFR), 78, 435, Q14
Glomerulonephritis (GN), 442
Glomerulosclerosis, Q48
Glomerulosclerosis, focal segmental, 443
Glossitis, migratory, 375
GLP-1 (glucagon-like peptide 1) receptor agonists, 563, 564t
Glucocorticoid-induced osteoporosis, 263–264, 263t
Glucocorticoids
　for adrenal insufficiency, 553
　for asthma symptoms, 383
　for dermatomyositis, 495
　for GCA, 492
　for gout, 489
　for leukemia, 589
　for OA-related pain, 486
　for polymyositis, 495
Glucosamine, 86t
Glucose screening, 62t
α-Glucosidase inhibitors, 563, 564t
Gluten-sensitive enteropathy, 433
Glyburide, 563, 564t
Glycemic control, 562
　lag time to benefit, 31t
　medications for, 562–563
Glycoprotein IIb/IIIa inhibitors, 393–394
Glycopyrrolate
　for bowel obstruction, 113t
　for COPD, 384t
　for loud respirations, 114
GnRH (gonadotropin-releasing hormone) agonists, 263t, 587
GO-FAR (Good Outcome Following Attempted Resuscitation) calculator, 32t, 133
Goiter, toxic multinodular, 545
Gold, 488
GOLD (Global Initiative for Chronic Obstructive Lung Disease), 383–384, 383t
Golfer's elbow, 478
Golimumab, 488
Gonadotropin-releasing hormone (GnRH) agonists, 263t, 587
Gonadotropin-secreting adenomas, 552
Good Outcome Following Attempted Resuscitation (GO-FAR) calculator, 32t, 133
Gottron papules, 494
Gout, 480, 488–489

GRACE Team Care™, 175
Graded desensitization, 330
Grading of Recommendations Assessment, Development and Evaluation (GRADE) Working Group, 35
Grandiose delusions, 334
Granisetron, 112t
Granulocyte colony-stimulating factor, 579t
Granulocyte-macrophage colony-stimulating factor, 579t
Graves disease, 545, 546
Green House Model, 163
Green tea, 87
Grief and bereavement, 108
GRN (Geriatric Resource Nurse) Model, 136
Groin pain, 479
Groningen Frailty Indicator (GFI), Q109
Group homes, 171
Growth hormone (GH), 551t
Growth hormone (GH)-secreting tumors, 552
Growth retardation, 358t
Guardianship, 357
Guided Care, 140, 174–175
Guillain-Barré syndrome, 515
Gum boils (parulis), 375, 376t
Gustatory dysfunction
　age-related changes, 376–377
　medications that cause, 376–377, 377t
　nonpharmacologic causes of, 377, 377t
Gynecology, 447–454, Q1, Q4

H_2-receptor antagonists
　adverse events, 215
　and delirium, 298, 300t
　drug interactions, 527
　for GERD, 425
　for nausea, 112t
HAART (highly active antiretroviral therapy), 538
HACEK (*Haemophilus, Actinobacillus, Cardiobacterium, Eikenella,* and *Kingella*) organisms, 398, 536–537
Haemophilus, 398, 536–537
Haemophilus influenzae type b immunization, 529t
Haemophilus influenzae type B vaccine, Q64
Haglund deformity, 499t
Hair, 360
Hairy tongue, 376
Halachic Living Will, Q65
HALE (healthy life expectancy), 2–3
Half-life, 78
Hallucinations, 333
　antipsychotic medications for, 290–291, 290t
　auditory, 334
　definition of, 331

in dementia, 289–291, 290t
due to medical conditions, 334
isolated, 335
visual, 192, 333, 334, 335
Hallus valgus, 500
Hallux abducto valgus, 498f, 499t
Hallux limitus, 499t, 500
Hallux rigidus, 499t
Hallux valgus, 499t
Halo sign, Q110
Haloperidol, Q12, Q60
for agitated delirium, 299–300, 301t
for chorea, 512
dosing and adverse events, 335t
for nausea, 111, 112t
for psychosis in dementia, 290, 290t
Hammertoe deformities, 499t, 500–501
Hand feeding, 224, Q59
Hand-foot syndrome, 582t
Hand osteoarthritis, 485, 486f
Hand pain, 478–479
Hand washing, 540
Handoffs, 139
Handovers, 139
Harpagophytum procumbens (devil's claw), 86
Harris Hip Questionnaire, 145t, 148, 151
HAS-BLED score, 402
Hawthorn extract, 86–87
Hayflick's limit, 6
HD (Huntington disease), 273, 508–509, 512
Head and neck cancer, 581, Q29
Head injury, 338, 552, Q72
Head/neck squamous cell carcinoma, 581
Head-thrust test, 205
Headaches, 507, 516–517
Healers, 46
Healing
caloric requirements, 241
chronic wounds, 235
Pressure Ulcer Scale for Healing, 237
products that promote, 239
protein requirements, 241
Healing touch, 85
Health beliefs, 45
Health care
attitudes toward North American health services, 45
Bundled Payments for Care Improvement initiative, 21
costs of, 18–23
coverage of, 18–23
federal spending on, 18
financing of, 18–23
GRACE team model, 175
Health care expenditures, 4
Health care insurance, Q90
Health care proxy, 73
Health in Aging Caregiver Self-Assessment Questionnaire, 39t

Health insurance
coverage for older Americans, 4, 18–23, 19t
coverage for rehabilitation, 144–146
long-term care insurance, 21
trends in, 4
Health literacy, 42, 43
Health Maintenance Organizations (HMOs), 19t
Health Professional Shortage Areas, Q95
Health risk assessment (HRA), 67t
Healthcare providers
addressing, 43
primary, 165–166
response guidelines based on PHQ-9 and STAR*D studies, 317, 318t
role in home care, 165–166
Healthy life expectancy (HALE), 2–3
Healthy lifestyle counseling, 63t, 70–71
Hearing, 193
Hearing aids, 194–195, 197–199
caring for, 199–200
costs of, 199, 199t
digital, 199, 199t
styles of, 197–198, 198t
Hearing Handicap Inventory for the Elderly—Screening Version (HHIE-S), 195, Q66
Hearing loss, 193–201
assessment of, 25
conductive, 194, Q13
evaluation of, 195–196, Q66
indications for medical evaluation of, 195, 196t
mixed, Q13
recommended preventive measures for, 63t, 72
screening for, 63t, 72, 195
sensorineural, 194, Q13
treatment of, 196–201
Heart, 9t, 10t
Heart disease
and rehabilitation, 148
valvular, 397–398, 400t, 406, 408
Heart failure, 407–415
classification of, 411, 411t
congestive, Q104
EFFECT Heart Failure Mortality Prediction Model, 32, 32t
end-of-life care for, 415
management of, 408–414, 409t, 410t, Q35, Q37
prognostic indices, 32, 32t
with renal failure, Q14
Seattle Heart Failure Model, 32, 32t
Heart-healthy diet, Q84
Heart rate abnormalities, 257
Heart transplantation, 413–414, 415
Heart valve disease, 397–398, 400t, 406
Heartburn, 424
Heat/cold therapy, 121
Heat therapy, Q92

Heat treatment, 516
Heavy-chain deposition disease, 442
Heavy drinking, 346
Heberden nodes, 485
Heel pain, 501–502
Heel pressure ulcers, 235–236
prevention strategies, 238
Heel spur, 499t
Height measurement, 62t, 70
Helicobacter pylori infection, 426, 427
HELP (Hospital Elder Life Program), 136, 302
HELP (Hospitalized Elderly Longitudinal Project), 106
Hemangioma, 503
Hematologic malignancies, 589–590
Hematology, 567–573, Q6, Q73
Hematoma
epidural, 522–523
subdural, 522–523
Hematopoietic stem cells (HSCs), 567
Hematuria, 440
Hemiplegia, 244
Hemodialysis, 445
Hemoglobin A_{1c}, Q87
Hemoglobin A_{1c} (HbA$_{1c}$), 558, 563
Hemoglobin electrophoresis, 568
Hemoglobinopathies, 568
Hemolytic anemia, 442, 568t, 570–571
Hemolytic uremic syndrome (HUS), 442, 571
Hemophilia, 572
Hemorrhage
intracerebral, 522–523
intracranial, 522–523
subarachnoid, 523
subconjunctival, 187t, 188
Hemorrhagic bursitis, Q122
Hemorrhagic stroke, 522–523
Heparin
and hyperkalemia, 439t
LMWH (low-molecular-weight heparin), 99–100, 100t, 133, 388–389
and risk of osteoporosis, 263t
for thromboprophylaxis, 133
unfractionated, 133, 388, 389, 393
for VTE, 388–389
Heparin-induced thrombocytopenia, 571
Hepatitis A vaccine, 529t
Hepatitis B screening, 62t, 69
Hepatitis B vaccine, 529t
Hepatitis B virus, Q64
Hepatitis C, 539
Hepatitis C screening, 62t, 69, 539
Hepatocellular carcinoma, 581
Hepcidin, 570
Herbal medicines, 85
for cancer, 88
cannabis and cannabinoids, 88
for low back pain, 85–86
for menopausal vasomotor symptoms, 448–449
safety issues, 85
sleeping agents, 315

Hernia, 479
  femoral, 479
  inguinal, 479
Herpes simplex, oral, 375, 376t
Herpes simplex dendriform corneal ulcers, 188
Herpes simplex keratitis, 187, 187t
Herpes zoster (shingles), 187t, 188, 365–367, 366f
Herpes zoster ophthalmicus
  signs and symptoms of, 186t, 188
  treatment of, 187t, 188
Herpes zoster vaccine, 528, 530–531
  immunization schedule for adults ≥65 years old, 529t
  Medicare benefits, 530
  recommendations for, 62t, 73
HF. See Heart failure
HGH (human growth hormone), 219
HHIE-S (Hearing Handicap Inventory for the Elderly—Screening Version), 195, Q66
HHRGs (home-health–related groups), 165
HHS (U.S. Department of Health and Human Services), 56
High-grade squamous intraepithelial lesion (HSIL), 451
High T_4 syndrome, 545
Highly active antiretroviral therapy (HAART), 538
Hip disease, 479, 482t
Hip fracture, 150–151, 260–261
Hip joint assessment, 145t, 148
Hip osteoarthritis, 485, 486–487
Hip pain, 490
Hip protectors, 151, Q63
Hip surgery
  rehabilitation after, 248
  total hip and knee arthroplasty, 151–152
Hispanic Americans, Q118
  cancer, 575
  caregivers, 37
  CKD, 443
  CVD mortality rates, 390
  diabetes mellitus, 558
  hypertension, 416
  life expectancy, 2
  mobility aids for, 156
  nursing-home population, 159
  periodontitis, 373
  population projections, 219, 575
  poverty rates, 3
  urinary incontinence, 225
History of immigration or migration, 44
History of traumatic experiences, 44
Histrionic personality disorder, Q57
  features of, 337t
  long-term course, 339
HIV (human immunodeficiency virus) infection, 538–539, Q29, Q90, Q107
  in LGBT older adults, 51

  nursing-home financing for care for those with, 160
  prevention of, 539
  prophylaxis in, 538
  risk in older gay and bisexual men, 51
  risk in older lesbian and bisexual women, 52
  risk in transgender people, 52
  screening for, 70–71, 467
  treatment and care, 52
HMOs (Health Maintenance Organizations), 19t
Hoarding disorder, 327
Hodgkin lymphoma, 576, 581, 589–590
Home and Family Caregiving Resource Center (AARP), 39t
Home blood pressure monitoring, 421
Home care, 165–167, Q27, Q35, Q93
  Expanded In-home Services for the Elderly Program, 168
  fee-for-service, 18
  financing, 18
  interventions for preventing falls, 255t, 256
  for LGBT older adults, 53
  Medicare benefits, 19t, 145–146, 165, 166, Q79
  pressure ulcers in, 234
  preventing falls, 255t, 256
  rehabilitation services, 144t, 145–146
  skilled care, 171, 171t
  technologic innovations, 169
  transition from hospital to, 140
  virtual home visits, 170
Home-delivered meals, 218
Home exercise, 59
Home-hazard assessment, 256, 258t
Home health agencies, 165
Home health aides, 166
Home Health Compare tool, 165
Home health nursing, Q35
Home-health–related groups (HHRGs), 165
Home hospitals, 136, 169
Homeopathy, 85
Homeostasis, 542
Homeostenosis, 8–10
Homosexuality, 50
Hormonal regulation
  influences in men, 262
  screening tests for hypersecretion, 554, 554t
Hormone replacement therapy (HRT)
  for menopausal vasomotor symptoms, 447, 448, 454
  strategies for risk reduction, 448
Hormone supplements, Q88
Hormone therapy
  for breast cancer, 580, 584
  for cancer, 580
  for endometrial cancer, 580
  for erectile dysfunction, 469
  for female sexual dysfunction, 470–471, 472t

  for hyperparathyroidism, 549
  for incontinence, 226t
  for osteoporosis, 268t, 269–270
  preventive, 63t, 74
  for prostate cancer, 461t, 580
  testosterone replacement therapy, 556–557
  testosterone supplementation, 542, 555, 556–557, 556t
  for UI, 231
Horse chestnut seed, 86–87
Hospice, 106, 107–108, Q79, Q125
  for ESRD, 446
  issues on the horizon, 115–116
  Medicare benefits, 19t, 20, 22, 108, Q79, Q125
  new models, 115
  recommendations for, 116
  services, 107, 108t
Hospice in a Minute app, 106
Hospital-acquired pneumonia, 532
Hospital-acquired pressure ulcers, 129, 131t, 234
Hospital-associated disability, 126–127
Hospital-at-home care, 136
Hospital care, 126–138
  day hospitals, 168
  delirium management in, Q12
  discharge planning/summary, Q85, Q93
  flexible medication times, 309–310
  geriatric EDs, 134–135
  geriatric evaluation and management (GEM) units, 135, 176
  hazards and opportunities commonly overlooked in, 130, 131t
  home hospitals, 169
  interventions for lowering risk of falls in, 255t
  Medicare benefits, 19t
  post-hospital syndrome, 139
  recurrent hospitalization, 414
  rehabilitation hospitals, 144–145, 144t
  systematic assessment in, 130, 131t
  transition to home from, 140
  transition to SNFs from, 141
Hospital Compare, 136–137
Hospital Elder Life Program (HELP), 136, 302
Hospital Readmissions Reduction Program, 414
Hospitalization, chronic, 141
Hospitalized Elderly Longitudinal Project (HELP), 106
Hospitalized patients
  alcohol use, 346
  assessment of, 130
  daily evaluation, 130
  management of, 130–135
  models of care for, 135–136
  sleep disturbances in, 309–310
Hot flushes, 448–449

Hounsfield units (HU), 554
House calls, 166, Q115
Housing, 53, 170, 171
Housing and Urban Development programs, 171
HPA (hypothalamic-pituitary-adrenal) axis, 551
HPV (human papillomavirus), Q29, Q107
HPV (human papillomavirus) testing, 64
HRA (health risk assessment), 67t
HRT. *See* Hormone replacement therapy
HSCs (hematopoietic stem cells), 567
HSDD (hypoactive sexual desire disorder), 470
HSIL (high-grade squamous intraepithelial lesion), 451
Humalog (insulin lispro), 565t
Humalog mix (insulin lispro protamine suspension and insulin lispro), 565t
Human growth hormone (HGH), 219
Human immunodeficiency virus (HIV) infection. *See* AIDS; HIV infection
Human papillomavirus (HPV), Q29, Q107
Human papillomavirus (HPV) testing, 64
Humoral hypercalcemia of malignancy, 548t, 549–550
Humulin R (insulin), 565t
Huntington disease (HD), 273, 508–509, 512
Huperzine, 87
HUS (hemolytic uremic syndrome), 442, 571
Hutchinson sign, 188, 366
Hutchison sign, 370
Hyaluronic acid, 360, 480, 486
Hydralazine, 411–412, 421
Hydroaerobics, 120
Hydrocephalus, normal-pressure (NPH), 244, 248
Hydrochlorothiazide, Q9, Q86, Q89
Hydrocodone, 121
Hydrocortisone, 553
Hydromorphone, 121, 122
Hydrophilic drugs, 77
Hydrotherapy, 239, 495
Hydroxychloroquine, 488, 493
Hydroxyurea, 573
Hydroxyzine, 112t
Hyoscyamine, 113t, 114, 231
Hyperadrenocorticoidism, 553–554
Hyperbaric oxygen, 242
Hypercalcemia, 542, 548–550, 548t
Hypercalciuria, idiopathic, 263t
Hypercortisolism, 439
Hyperglycemia
 management of, 562–563, 564t, 565
 perioperative, 104
Hypericum perforatum (St. John's wort), 86t, 87
Hyperkalemia, 438–439, 439t
Hyperkinetic movement disorders, 512–514

Hyperlipidemia, 69
Hypernatremia, 438
Hyperparathyroidism
 differential diagnosis of, 548–549, 548t
 indications for parathyroid surgery, 549, 549t
 primary, 263t, 548–549, 548t
 secondary, 262, 548
Hyperprolactinemia, 551–552
Hypersexuality, 292
Hypertension, 416–422, Q16, Q37, Q89
 blood pressure targets, 439
 cancer treatment-induced, 581, 582t
 and cardiovascular risk, 391
 CIM for, 86–87
 mineralocorticoid, 439
 pseudohypertension, 417
 recommendations for, 62t, 422
 refractory or resistant, 421
 screening for, 66
 secondary, 417, 439–440
 special considerations, 421–422
 treatment of, 417–421, 419f, 419t
 white-coat, 417
Hypertensive bleeds, 522
Hyperthyroidism, 543, 545–546
 circulating hormone levels in, 543t
 subclinical, 543t, 545
Hypertonic saline, 437
Hypervolemia, 438
Hypnotherapy, 85
Hypnotics
 chronic use of, 314–315
 and delirium, 300t
 and falls, 251–252, 251t
 and incontinence, 226t
 interventions for preventing falls with, 258t
 misuse, 345
 for sleep problems, 311, 312
Hypoactive sexual desire disorder (HSDD), 470
Hypoadrenocorticoidism, 553
Hypocalcemia, 550–551
Hypochondriasis, 341
Hypoglycemia, 564–565
Hypoglycemics, 81
Hypogonadism, 263t, Q87
 male, 466t, 467, 469, 555
Hypomania, 318
Hyponatremia, 436–437
 hypervolemic, Q102
 hypovolemic, Q102
 medication-induced, Q19
 with normal extracellular fluid volume, 437
 secondary to SIADH, Q69
 severe or symptomatic, 437
 treatment of, 437
 with volume depletion, 437
 with volume overload, 437
Hypopituitarism, 552–553
Hypoproliferative anemia, 568t

Hypotension. *See* Postural (orthostatic or postprandial) hypotension
Hypothalamic-pituitary-adrenal (HPA) axis, 551
Hypothyroidism, 543–544
 circulating hormone levels in, 543t
 screening for, 66
 secondary, 543t, 544
 subclinical, 66, 543–544, 543t
Hypoventilation, 387
Hypovolemia, 438
Hypoxis rooperi, 87

IADLs (instrumental activities of daily living), 27, 148, 577
Ibandronate, 267–268, 268t
Ibrutinib, 582t, 589
IBS. *See* Irritable bowel syndrome
Ibuprofen, 122
ICD-9 (International Classification of Diseases), 165
ICD-10 (International Classification of Diseases), 284
ICDs (implantable cardiac defibrillators), 413–414, 415, Q21
ICF (International Classification of Functioning, Disability, and Health), 143
ICH (intracerebral hemorrhage), 522–523
Idarucizumab, 389, 401, Q9
Idelalisib, 582t, 589
Identification of Seniors at Risk (ISAR), 134, 135t
Identity
 cultural or religious, 42
 gender, 50
Idiopathic myelofibrosis (IMF), 573
Idiopathic pulmonary fibrosis (IPF), 387
Idiopathic thrombocytopenic purpura (ITP), 571
IFIS (intraoperative floppy iris syndrome), 456
IGRAs (interferon gamma release assays), 535, 536
IHCA (in-hospital cardiac arrest), 133
IL-2 (interleukin-2), 581, 589
Illicit drug use, 345, 346
Illness anxiety disorder, 340, 342t
Iloperidone
 dosing and adverse events, 335t
 for psychosis in dementia, 290t
ILRs (implantable loop recorders), 210, 211t
Imagery, 329
Imaging
 abdominal ultrasonography, 62t
 brain imaging studies, 275–276
 of gait impairment, 247
 in mistreatment, 93
Imatinib, 582t
IMF (idiopathic myelofibrosis), 573
Imipramine, 231, 300t
Immigration history, 44
Immigration status, 44

Immobility, 131*t*
Immune system, 8, 9*t*, 10*t*, 525, 526*t*
Immune theory of aging, 7
Immunizations, 62*t*, 73, 528–531, Q64
 for hospitalized patients, 130, 131*t*
 interventions for, 131*t*
 recommendations for, 73
 schedule for adults ≥65 years old, 529*t*
Immunoglobulin, intravenous, 495, 515, 571
 for MGUS, 590
Immunosenescence, 7, 525
Immunosuppressive therapy, 530
Immunotherapy
 for cancer, 574, 580–581
 for colon cancer, 586
 for radiculopathy, 515
 toxicities of, 581, 582*t*
IMPACT (Improving Mood—Promoting Access to Collaborative Treatment), 175–176
Implantable cardiac defibrillators (ICDs), 413–414, 415, Q21
Implantable hemodynamic monitoring, 414
Implantable loop recorders (ILRs), 210, 211*t*
Implants
 cochlear, 200–201, 200*t*
 osseointegrated, 200
IMPROVE tool, 133
Improving Mood—Promoting Access to Collaborative Treatment (IMPACT), 175–176
IMRT (intensity-modulated radiation therapy), 581
In-hospital cardiac arrest (IHCA), 133
Inactivated subunit zoster vaccine, 530
Inappropriate sexual behavior (ISB), 292, 473
Inattention, 295
Incidentalomas
 adrenal, 554, 554*t*
 pituitary, 552
Inclusion body myositis, 494
Income, 3
Incontinence, Q4, Q15
 with developmental disabilities, 358*t*
 fecal, 430
 and rehabilitation, 147
 urinary, 63*t*, 71–72, 225–233
Indacaterol maleate, 384*t*
Indapamide, 418
Independence at Home Demonstration project, 166
Indigenous healing practices, 85
Indomethacin, 489
Ineffective erythropoiesis, 568*t*, 570
Infection control, 379, 532
Infections
 antimicrobial management of, 527
 back pain due to, 481, 481*t*, 482*t*
 bacterial endocarditis, Q18
 bone and joint, 538
 of central nervous system, 539
 diagnosis and management of, 526–527
 fungal, 504
 gastrointestinal, 539–540
 HIV, Q29, Q90, Q107
 HIV and AIDS, 52, 538–539
 latent tuberculosis (LTBI), 71
 postoperative, 187
 predisposition to, 525–526
 presentation of, 527
 in pressure ulcers, 241
 prosthetic device (PDIs), 537
 sexually transmitted, 51, 70–71, Q107
 skin problems, 365–368
 surveillance definitions of, 527, 528*t*
 tuberculosis, 71
 urinary tract (UTIs), 533–535, Q97, Q123
 vulvovaginal, 449–450
Infectious diarrhea, 540
Infectious diseases, 525–541
 recommendations for, 541
Infectious Diseases Society of America (IDSA)
 Guidelines for Management of Adults with Hospital-Acquired and Ventilator-Associated Pneumonia, 532
 guidelines for treatment of CAP, 531–532
 International Clinical Practice Guidelines, 534
 Primary Care Guidelines for Management of Persons Infected with HIV, 530
Infectious syndromes, 531–540
Infective endocarditis, 398, 536–537
 antibiotics for, 372, 378, 378*t*, 537, 537*t*
Inferior vena cava filter, 389
Infestations, 365–368
Inflammation
 anemia of, 569–570, 569*f*
 vulvovaginal, 449–450
Inflammatory skin conditions, 360–365
Infliximab, 488
Influenza, 532–533
Influenza vaccine, 130, 131*t*, 528
 immunization schedule for adults ≥65 years old, 529*t*
 recommendations for, 62*t*, 73, 532
Informal caregiving, 37, 38, Q22
Informed consent, 13–14
Ingrown nails, 504
Inguinal hernia, 479
INH (isoniazid), 536
Inhaled bronchodilators and corticosteroids, 380, 382, 384–385, 384*t*, 385*t*
Inhalers, 385–386
Initial Preventive Physical Examination (IPPE), 67*t*–68*t*, 69–70, 71, 72

Injectable agents
 for diabetes, 563, 564*t*, 565*t*
 insulin preparations, 563, 565*t*
Injury. *See also specific types of injury*
 preventing, 73
Inpatient Rehabilitation Facility (IRF) Prospective Payment System, 144–145
INR (international normalized ratio), Q9
Insomnia, 87–88, 305–306
 behavioral interventions for, 291, 292*t*, 311–312
 cognitive-behavioral therapy for insomnia (CBT-I), Q43, Q81
 epidemiology of, 304
 management of, 291–292, 310–315, Q43, Q81
 pharmacotherapy for, 282, 312–314, 313*t*, 347
Insomnia disorder, 305
Inspiratory muscle training, preoperative, Q114
Institute of Medicine
 Dietary Reference Intakes (DRIs), 214
 Food and Nutrition Board, 213, 214
 The Mental Health and Substance Use Workforce for Older Adults: In Whose Hands?, 346
 recommendations for cognitive health, 72
 recommended dietary allowances (RDAs), 214
Institutional mistreatment, 94–95
Institutionalization decisions, 167
Instrumental activities of daily living (IADLs), 27, 148, 577
Insulin aspart (NovoLog), 565*t*
Insulin degludec (Tresiba), 565*t*
Insulin degludec and insulin aspart (Ryzodeg 70/30), 565*t*
Insulin detemir (Levemir), 565*t*
Insulin glargine (Lantus, Toujeo, Basaglar), 565*t*
Insulin glulisine (Apidra), 565*t*
Insulin lispro (Humalog), 565*t*
Insulin lispro protamine suspension and insulin lispro (Humalog mix), 565*t*
Insulin therapy
 adverse events, 81
 for diabetes, 563, 564–565, 564*t*
 and falls, 251*t*
 preparations, 565*t*
Insurance coverage, 18–23, 19*t*
Integrative medicine, 85. *See also* Complementary and integrative medicine
Intellectual disability, 352–359, Q51, Q94
 developmental disabilities with, 357, 358*t*
Intensity-modulated radiation therapy (IMRT), 581
Intensive care
 Confusion Assessment Method for the Intensive Care Unit (CAM-ICU), 295
 of critically ill, 133–134

INTERACT (Interventions to Reduce Acute Care Transfers), 140, 161
Interdisciplinary team approach, 41
Interferon, 335, 581, 589
Interferon gamma release assays (IGRAs), 535, 536
Interleukin-2 (IL-2), 581, 589
Interleukin-6 (IL-6), 492
Intermittent clean catheterization, 232
Intermittent pneumatic compression, 389
International Classification of Diseases, 353
International Classification of Diseases (ICD-9), 165
International Classification of Diseases (ICD-10), 284
International Classification of Functioning, Disability, and Health (ICF), 143
International Clinical Practice Guidelines, 534
International Continence Society, 451
International Myeloma Working Group, 590
International normalized ratio (INR), Q9
International Prostate Symptom Score, 455
International Society of Clinical Densitometry, 265, 266t
Interpersonal therapy, 323
Interpreters, 43–44
Interstitial fibrosis, Q48
Interstitial nephritis, acute, 441
Intertrigo, 362–363, 363f
Interventions to Reduce Acute Care Transfers (INTERACT), 140, 161
Intra-abdominal abscess, 539–540
Intra-articular steroids, 489, 490
Intra-articular viscosupplementation therapy, 486–487
Intracerebral hemorrhage (ICH), 522–523
Intracranial aneurysms, 523
Intracranial hemorrhage, 522–523
Intracranial saccular aneurysms, 523
Intraoperative floppy iris syndrome (IFIS), 456
Intravenous fluids, 428–429
Intravenous immunoglobulin (IVIG), 495, 515, 571
for MGUS, 590
Invasive mechanical ventilation, 385t
Iodine, radioactive, 546, 547
IPF (idiopathic pulmonary fibrosis), 387
Ipilimumab, 370, 581, 582t
IPPE (Initial Preventive Physical Examination), 67t–68t, 69–70, 71, 72
Ipratropium bromide
adverse events, 215
for COPD, 384–385, 384t, 385t
Irbesartan, 410t, 412–413

IRF (Inpatient Rehabilitation Facility) Prospective Payment System, 144–145
Iris prolapse, 456
Iron deficiency, 444–445, 513, 569
Iron-deficiency anemia, 432, 433
differential diagnosis of, 570
evaluation of, 568–569, 569f
Iron malabsorption, 569
Iron supplements, 433, Q73
Iron therapy, Q73
for anemia, 444–445, 568, 569
drug interactions, 215t
preparations, 568
for RLS, 514
Irrigation, 239
Irritable bowel syndrome (IBS), 431–432
with alternating constipation and diarrhea (IBS-M or IBS mixed), 432
with constipation (IBS-C), 432
with diarrhea (IBS-D), 432
recommendations for, 434
ISAR (Identification of Seniors at Risk), 134, 135t
ISB (inappropriate sexual behavior), 292, 473
Ischemia, cardiac, Q76
Ischemic bowel, 539–540
Ischemic optic neuropathy, 186–187, 186t, 191–192
Ischemic stroke, 518–522
acute, 519–520
prevention of, 520–522
Isoniazid (INH), 215t, 536
Isosorbide dinitrate, 411–412
Isosorbide mononitrate, 396, 413
Isotonic saline, 437
Isotretinoin, 361
Itching, Q3
ITP (idiopathic thrombocytopenic purpura), 571
Ivermectin, 367
IVIG (intravenous immunoglobulin), 495, 515, 571
for MGUS, 590
Ixabepilone, 582t
Ixasomib, 582t

Jaeger cards, 25, 132
Janeway lesions, Q18
Jaw: osteonecrosis of, 268–269, 372, 378, Q29, Q74
Jehovah's Witnesses, 13, Q65
Jejunostomy, percutaneous endoscopic, 223–224
Jewish Health Care Proxy, Q65
Jimmo v. Sebelius, 145
Joint Commission on Accreditation of Healthcare Organizations, 47, 116
Joint disease, degenerative, 358t
Joint infections, 538
Joint National Committee (JNC-8), 561
Joint Principles of the PCMH, 173, 174t

Joint replacement
hip replacement, 248
knee replacement, 248
rehabilitation after, 248
total hip and knee arthroplasty, 151–152
Justice, 11, 13

Kaposi sarcoma, recurrent, Q29
Karnofsky Performance Status, 32, 577
Kava, 315
Kayexalate (sodium polystyrene), 439
KDIGO (Kidney Disease: Improving Global Outcomes) CKD Work Group 2012 Guidelines, 443, 444f
KDOQI (Kidney Disease Outcomes Quality Initiative), 443
Kegel (pelvic floor muscle) exercises, 472t, Q4
Keratitis, bacterial, 187–188
Keratitis sicca, 187
Keratoconjunctivitis sicca, 493
Keratotic lesions, 503
Ketoconazole, 230
"Kicking CAUTI: The No Knee-Jerk Antibiotics Campaign," 534–535
Kidney(s), Q48, Q69
age-related changes, 10t, 78, 435, 436t, Q48, Q69
assessment of, 101, 435–436
preoperative management of, 101
Kidney Disease: Improving Global Outcomes (KDIGO) CKD Work Group 2012 Guidelines, 443, 444f
Kidney Disease Outcomes Quality Initiative (KDOQI), 443
Kidney diseases and disorders
acute kidney injury (AKI), 435, 440–443
Beers Criteria® for medications that should be avoided or have dosage reduced in, 80, 80t
chronic kidney disease (CKD), 80, 80t, 435, 443–445, Q73
drug interactions, 82
end-stage renal disease (ESRD), 33, 445–446
impaired kidney function, 78, 82
intrinsic renal disease, 441–443
metabolic disorders, 436–439
Modified Diet in Renal Disease (MDRD) formula, 101, 435
postoperative management of, 103
prognostic indices, 33
recommendations for, 446
renal cell cancer, 581, 588–589
vascular disease, 442
volume disorders, 436–439
Kidney failure, Q14
Kidney transplantation, 445–446
Kingella, 398, 536–537
Knee osteoarthritis, 480, 485, 486, 486f, Q38
nonopioid treatment of, 124

Knee pain, 480, 490
Knee replacement
    rehabilitation after, 248
    total hip and knee arthroplasty, 151–152
Koebner phenomenon, 365
Kyphoplasty, 271

Labetalol, 421
Labor force participation, 3
Laboratory testing
    for clotting disorders, 572
    in endocrine disorders, 542–543
    in falls, 255
    in gait impairment, 247
    Medicare benefits, 19t
    in mistreatment, 92–93
    in osteoporosis, 263, 263t
    in syncope, 211t
Lactose intolerance, 432
Lacunar stroke, Q106
Lag time to benefit, 30, 31t
Lamivudine, 488
Lamotrigine, 508, Q33
    for behavioral disturbances in dementia with manic-like features, 289, 289t
    for bipolar depression, 321, 322t
    for personality disorders, 340
Language, 43
    body language, 44
    preferred terms for cultural or religious identity, 42
Language therapy, 150
Lansoprazole, 112t
Lantus (insulin glargine), 565t
Lapatinib, 582t
Larval therapy, 239
Laryngoscopy, nasopharyngeal, 223
Laser therapy
    for esophageal cancer, 587
    fractional CO_2, 449
    for telangiectasias, 362
Laser trabeculoplasty, 191
Latanoprost, 188t
Latent tuberculosis infection (LTBI), 71
Lateral epicondylitis, 478
Latinos, 220
Law/ethics, Q17, Q126
Laxatives
    for constipation, 429
    nutrient interactions, 215t
    osmotic, 429
    polyethylene glycol, 429
    saline, 429
    stimulant, 429
LDCT (low-dose computed tomography), 65
LDL-C testing, direct, 69
LEAP (Lower Extremity Amputation Prevention) program, 505
Lee-Schonberg index, 32t, 75
Leflunomide, 488
LeFort colpocleisis, 453
Left ventricular assist devices (LVADs), 414

Left ventricular ejection fraction (LVEF), 408
Left ventricular mass, 392
Leg amputation, 152–153, Q104
Leg-length discrepancies, 246
Leg pain, 479–480
Leg ulcers, 242, 360, 365
Legal issues, 11–17, Q17, Q126
    in home care, 167
    related to nutritional status, 220
Legislation, 161–163
Lenalidomide, 579–580, 582t, 590
Length of stay, 160
Lentigo maligna, 369, Q30
Lenvatinib, 582t
Lesbian gay bisexual transgender (LGBT) health, 49–54
    caregivers, Q90
    end-of-life care, 107
    long-term care, 53, 473–474
Lesbian women, 51, 52, 53, Q124. See also Lesbian gay bisexual transgender (LGBT) health
Lesser metatarsal phalangeal joint dislocation, 499t
Leukemias, 589
    acute, 576
    acute myeloid (AML), 572, 589
    chronic lymphocytic (CLL), 571, 589
    chronic myeloid (CML), 573
Leukoplakia, 376
Leukotriene inhibitors, 383
Leukotriene-receptor antagonists, 382
Leuprolide acetate, 292
Levalbuterol, 384t
Level I screen, 216
Level II screen, 216
Levemir (insulin detemir), 565t
Levetiracetam, 80t, 508
Levodopa-carbidopa, 215t
    adverse events, Q71
    and delirium, 300t
    for multiple system atrophy, 511
    for PD motor symptoms, 510
    for PLMD, 308
    for progressive supranuclear palsy, 512
    for RLS, 308, 514
Levofloxacin, 532
Levothyroxine supplementation, 542, 544
Levothyroxine suppressive therapy, 547
Lewy body, 509
Lewy body dementia, 331, 334, 511
    behavioral disturbances in, 286–287
    diagnostic features and treatment of, 277t
    differential diagnosis of, 277
    epidemiology of, 272
    etiology of, 273
LGBT older adults. See Lesbian gay bisexual transgender (LGBT) health
LH (luteinizing hormone), 551t

LHRH (luteinizing hormone-releasing hormone) agonists, 461t, 463, 473
Liability, 167
Libido, decreased, 470, 471, 472t
Lice, 367–368
Lichen planus, 450–451
Lichen sclerosus, 450
Lichen simplex chronicus, 362, 363f, 450
Lid abnormalities, 185, 186t
Lid ectropion or entropion, 185, 186t
Lid malposition/exposure, 187–188, 187t
Lidocaine, 394
Lidocaine patch, 121, 121t, 514
Life expectancy, 1–2, 2–3
    age-based, 31
    estimation of, 75
    healthy life expectancy (HALE), 2–3
    quartile tables, 31, 31t
Life space assessment, 27
Lifestyle modification
    for BPH, 456, 456t
    for cancer, 88
    for DM, 558, 559
    for gout, 489
    healthy lifestyle counseling, 63t, 70–71
    for HTN, 419
    for UI, 229
Lifestyle modifications, Q51
Lifitegrast, 494
Light-chain or heavy-chain deposition disease, 442
Light therapy, 310, 312, 312t
Limb movements
    periodic limb movements disorder (PLMD), 307–308
    periodic limb movements during sleep (PLMS), 307–308, 513, 514
    restless legs syndrome, 307–308
Limb pain, phantom, 153
Linaclotide, 432
Linagliptin, 564t
Linezolid, 532
Lipid-binding resins, 215t
Lipid control, 31t
Lipid-lowering therapy, 527
Lipid management, 561–562
Lipohyalinosis, 518
Lipophilic drugs, 77
Liraglutide, 564t
Lisinopril, 410t, Q19
Listening, active, 115
Listening devices, 197
    costs of, 199, 199t
Listeria, 539
Literacy, 43
Lithium
    for behavioral disturbances in dementia with manic-like features, 289, 289t
    for bipolar depression, 321

for personality disorders, 340
to stabilize mood in mania and bipolar depression, 321, 322t
Living arrangements, 2, 3
Living wills, 11, 15, 163
Lixisenatide, 564t
LMWH (low-molecular-weight heparin)
perioperative, 99–100, 100t
for thromboprophylaxis, 133
for VTE, 388–389
Long lie, 250
Long-term care, 170t, Q11, Q79. *See also* Assisted-living facilities; Nursing-home care
competencies for attending physicians in, 161, 162t
fever in frail, older residents, 525, 526–527, 527t
fever in older residents, 526–527
hypertension in, 421–422
interface with acute care, 161
for LGBT older adults, 53, 473–474
managed long-term care programs (MLTC), 169
minimum criteria for initiation of antibiotic therapy in, 525, 527, 528t
oral hygiene in, 379
pneumonia in, 532
pressure ulcers in, 234
sexuality in, 471–473
sleep in, 310
tuberculosis in, 535
UI in, 231–232
UTIs in, 534
wound care in, 241
Long-term care insurance, 21
Long-term care ombudsman, 96
Loop diuretics
for HF, 411
for HTN, 420
for hypervolemia, 438
for hyponatremia, 437
and incontinence, 226t
Loperamide, 430, 432
LOPS (Loss of Protective Sensation) program, 505
Lorazepam, Q44, Q60
for agitated delirium, 301t
for anxiety disorders, 329
for detoxification and stabilization, 350
for nausea, 111, 112t
Losartan, 410t
Loss of appetite, 106, 112–113, Q42
Loss of consciousness, Q71
Loss of consciousness, sudden, 207, 208t
Loss of Protective Sensation (LOPS) program, 505
Louse infestations, 367–368
Low back pain, 119, 481
assessment of, 481, 481t
nonspecific, 483–484
physical examination of, 481–482, 482t
treatment of, 85–86, 120, 124, Q92
Low-dose computed tomography (LDCT), 65
Low-molecular-weight heparin (LMWH)
perioperative, 99–100, 100t
for thromboprophylaxis, 133
for VTE, 388–389
Low T_3 syndrome, 544
Low T_4 syndrome, 544
Low-vision aids, 192
Low-vision rehabilitation, 192
Lower extremities: innervation of, 482, 482t
Lower Extremity Amputation Prevention (LEAP) program, 505
Lower extremity wounds, 242
Lower urinary tract
age-related changes in, 226–227
pathophysiology in UI, 227
Lower urinary tract symptoms (LUTS), 225, 455
LTBI (latent tuberculosis infection), 71
Lubiprostone, 111, 429
Lubricant ointments, 185
Lubrication, decreased, 470–471, 472t
Lumbar spinal stenosis, 248, 475, 481, 481t, 482–483, 482t
Lumbar spine disease, 479
Lumbar supports, Q92
Lumpectomy, 584
Lung cancer, 584–585
chemotherapy for, 580, 585
CIM for, 88
immunotherapy for, 581
incidence rates, 574
radiation therapy for, 581
screening for, 62t, 65, 578–579
Lung disease
chronic obstructive pulmonary disease (COPD), 328, 383–386
with developmental disabilities, 358t
restrictive lung disorders, 387
Lung transplantation, 387
Lupus erythematosus
drug-induced, 493
late-onset, 492–493
Lurasidone
dosing and adverse events, 335t
for psychosis in dementia, 290t
LUT. *See* Lower urinary tract
Luteinizing hormone (LH), 551t
Luteinizing hormone-releasing hormone (LHRH) agonists, 461t, 463, 473
LUTS (lower urinary tract symptoms), 225, 455
LVADs (left ventricular assist devices), 414
LVEF (left ventricular ejection fraction), 408
Lyme disease, 539
Lymphocytic colitis, 430–431
Lymphomas, 575, 581, 589–590
diffuse large B-cell, 589
follicular, 589
Hodgkin, 576, 581, 589–590
non-Hodgkin, 571, 589

M-spike, 570
M2 inhibitors, 532
MA. *See* Medicare Advantage
MACRA (Medicare Access and CHIP Reauthorization Act of 2015), 18, 22
MACRA Value-Based Programs, 23
Macrocytic anemia, 570
Macrolides, 361, 532
Macronutrient guidelines, 213
Macronutrient needs, 213
Macroprolactinemia, pituitary, 551–552
Macular degeneration, age-related (ARMD), 185, 186t, 189–190
Macular edema, diabetic, 190
Maggot debridement therapy, 239
MAGI (modified adjusted gross income), 21
Magnesium, 215t
Magnesium hydroxide, 429
Magnetic resonance imaging (MRI), 408, 516, Q99
Magnetic resonance pulmonary angiography, 388
Magnetic stimulation, repetitive transcranial (rTMS), 323
Major depressive disorder, 316
diagnosis of, 317
electroconvulsive therapy for, 323
screening for, 317
treatment of, 319
without mania but with hypomania, 318
Malabsorption, iron, 569
Malassezia furfur, 361
Male hypogonadism, 466t, 467, 469, 555
Male sexuality, 465–469
Malignancy
hematologic malignancies, 589–590
humoral hypercalcemia of, 548t, 549–550
Malignant melanoma, 451
Mallet toe, 500
Malnutrition, 70, 213
Mammography, 61, 62t
Managed long-term care programs (MLTC), 169
Mania
DSM-5 criteria for, 318
electroconvulsive therapy for, 323
hypomania, 318
late-onset, 318
medications to stabilize mood in, 322t
pharmacotherapy for, 320–321, 322t
Manic-like behavioral syndromes
in dementia, 285, 289
mood stabilizers for, 289, 289t
treatment of, 289

Manipulation therapy, 85–86
Marche a petits pas, 246
Marijuana *(Cannabis)*, 88, 334, 345
    safety issues, 86*t*
Marital status, 2, 3
Marrow failure, 570
Martel sign, 489
MASD (moisture-associated skin damage), 238
Massage, 85–86, 88, 516
    carotid sinus, 402–403
    for low back pain, Q92
    for pain, 121
MAST (Michigan Alcoholism Screening Test)—Geriatric Version, 348
Material exploitation, 89, 90*t*
Maximizing Independence at Home (MIND at Home), Q77
Maze procedure, 401
MCD (minimal change disease), 443
McGill Pain Questionnaire, 118
MCI (mild cognitive impairment), 87
MCV (mean corpuscular volume), 568
MDRD (Modified Diet in Renal Disease) formula, 101, 435
MDROs (multidrug resistant organisms), 526, 532, 534
MDS. *See* Minimum Data Set
MDS (myelodysplastic syndromes), 569*f*, 570, 572–573
Meals-on-Wheels, 283
Mean corpuscular volume (MCV), 568
Mechanical circulatory support, 413–414, 415
Mechanical debridement, 239
Mechanical ventilation, 385*t*
Mechanic's hands, 494
Meclizine, 112*t*
Medicaid, 18, 20–21
    assisted-living benefits, 171
    benefits for LGBT older adults, 54
    continuing-care retirement community benefits, 171
    day care benefits, 168
    dual eligibles, 20–21, 168, 169, Q22
    expansion of, 22
    federal spending, 18
    hearing aid benefits, 199
    hospice benefits, 107, Q125
    long-term care benefits, Q79
    primary care physician reimbursements, 22
    self-direction programs, Q22
    spousal impoverishment benefits, 473
Medicaid Home and Community-Based Services waiver, 175
Medical cannabis, 88
Medical decision making, Q126
Medical devices, 239
    prosthetic device infections (PDIs), 537
Medical directors, 162
    roles and functions, 164*t*

Medical ethics, 13
Medical homes, 175
Medical interpreters, 43–44
Medical-legal interface, 95–96
Medical marijuana, 88
Medical Orders for Life-Sustaining Treatment (MOLST), 16
Medical Orders for Scope of Treatment (MOST), 16
Medical savings accounts (MSAs), 19*t*
Medicare, 4
    ACA changes, 21–22
    ACO programs, 21
    Annual Wellness Visit (AWV), 24, 67*t*–68*t*, 71, 72, Q7
    cardiac rehabilitation benefits, 153–154
    care venues, 141
    chronic care management (CCM), 177–178
    cochlear implant benefits, 200, 201
    continuing-care retirement community benefits, 171
    day hospital benefits, 168
    dermatology benefits, Q95
    diabetes self-management training benefits, 560–561
    dual eligibles, 20–21, 168, 169, Q22
    federal spending, 18
    fee-for-service (FFS), 18–19, 19*t*, 22, 137
    "Geographical Practices Cost Indices," 165–166
    hearing aid benefits, 199
    herpes zoster vaccine benefits, 530
    home health care benefits, 19*t*, 145–146, 165, 166, Q79
    Home Health Compare tool, 165
    hospice benefits, 19*t*, 20, 22, 108, Q79, Q125
    house-call benefits, 166, Q115
    Initial Preventive Physical Examination (IPPE), 67*t*–68*t*, 69–70, 71, 72
    key features, 18, 19*t*
    Loss of Protective Sensation (LOPS) program, 505
    mobility-related device benefits, 155
    nursing facility benefits, Q93
    nursing-home care benefits, 19*t*, 160
    nursing services benefits, 166
    Part A, 18–19, 19*t*, 20, 144–145, 144*t*, Q79, Q125
    Part B, 18–19, 19*t*, 71, 144, 144*t*, 146, 560–561, Q79
    Part C, 18, 19*t*, 20. *See also* Medicare Advantage (MA)
    Part D, 18, 19, 19*t*, 20, 21–22, 530
    post-acute care benefits, Q79
    prescription drug benefits, 18, 19*t*, 21–22
    preventive care benefits, 19, 19*t*, 60, 71, 72

    primary care physician reimbursements, 22
    private contracts, 19
    prospective payment system (PPS), 160, 165
    prospective reimbursement, 145
    Quality Payment Program (QPP), 22
    readmissions, 137
    rehabilitation benefits, 143–146, 144*t*, Q79
    reimbursement for house calls, Q115
    requirements for rehabilitation sites, 144*t*
    skilled-nursing-facility benefits, 144*t*, 145–146, 160
    spousal impoverishment benefits, 473
    state assistance offices, 16
    subacute rehabilitation benefits, Q79
    telemedicine benefits, Q95
    "Welcome to Medicare" visits, 24, 69–70, 71, Q31
Medicare Access and CHIP Reauthorization Act of 2015 (MACRA), 18, 22
Medicare Administrative Contractors, 18
Medicare Advantage (MA), 18, 19*t*, 20
    Compassionate Care Program, 115
Medicare carriers, 19
Medicare Health Maintenance Organizations (HMOs), 19*t*
Medicare Learning Network, 23
Medicare Prescription Drug Plan Finder, 16, 22
Medicare SELECT, 20
Medicare & You Annual Guide, 22
Medicated urethral system for erection (MUSE), 468*t*, 469
Medication assessment, 25
Medication-induced parkinsonism, 511, 512
Medication-induced psychotic disorder, 334–335
Medication reconciliation, Q85
Medication review, 83, 346
    brown-bag evaluation, 83
    for delirium, 297
    discharge medication regimen, 141
    for DM, 559
    on hospital admission, 131*t*
    in nursing-home care, 162
    for preventing falls, 256, 258*t*
Medications. *See* Drugs; Pharmacotherapy; *specific medications*
Medigap, 18, 19–20
Meditation, 85, 88, 495
    for Alzheimer disease, 88
Mediterranean diet, 86, 184, Q84
Medline Plus, 39*t*
Medroxyprogesterone, 292
Megestrol, 219, 553, Q42

Meglitinides, 563, 564t
Melanoma, 369–370, 370f, 503, Q30
    acral lentiginous, 370, 370f
    immunotherapy for, 581
    malignant, 451
    nodular, 370
    superficial spreading, 370
    vulvar, 451, 451f
Melatonin
    safety issues, 86t
    for sleep disorders, 87–88, 292, 308–309, 315
Melatonin receptor agonists, 313t, 314
Memantine, 281, 355
    adverse events, Q19
    for dementia, Q94, Q100
Membranous nephropathy, 444
Memory Impairment Screen, 72
Memory problems. *See* Cognitive impairment; Dementia
Memory retraining, 279
Men's health
    alcohol use, 346
    benign prostatic hyperplasia, 87
    CAD in, 392
    cancer, 574
    cardiovascular disease, 390, 391t
    centenarians, Q103
    ejaculatory dysfunction, 456
    erectile dysfunction, 457, 465–467, 467–468, Q34, Q87
    gay and bisexual men, 50
    hormonal influences, 262
    indications for osteoporosis screening, 264
    labor force participation, 3
    life expectancy, 2, 31, 31t
    marital status and living arrangements, 3
    population projections, 2
    poverty rates, 3, Q118
    prostate disease and cancer, 88, 455–464, 587–588
    recommendations for calcium intake, 266
    recommendations for macronutrient intake, 213
    recommendations for osteoporosis screening, 264
    recommendations for vitamin D intake, 266
    schizophrenia, 331
    sexual dysfunction, 465–469, 466t
    testosterone supplementation for, 555, 556t
    UTIs, 533, 534
Men who have sex with men (MSM), 50, 51–52. *See also* Bisexual men; Gay men; Lesbian gay bisexual transgender (LGBT) health
Mendelson syndrome, 223
Ménière disease, 198, 202, Q13
Meningitis, bacterial, 539
Meningococcal vaccination, 529t
Meniscal disease, 480

Menopausal symptoms, 448–449, 555
Menopause, 447, 448, 449, 470, 555
The Mental Health and Substance Use Workforce for Older Adults: In Whose Hands? (IOM), 346
Mental health problems, 347–348
    acute mental status change, 294
    in aging adults with intellectual disability, 353, 354–356
    diagnosis and treatment of, 356
    in LGBT older adults, 52
    rehabilitation and, 148
Menthol and methylsalicylate (Bengay), 121t
Meperidine, 300t
Merit-based Incentive Payment System (MIPS), 22
Mesh, vaginal, 453, Q1
Metabolic disorders, 436–439
Metabolic encephalopathy, 294
Metabolism
    age-associated changes in, 77–78, 77t
    of drugs, 77–78, 77t
    preoperative assessment and management of, 101
Metal stents, 587
Metastatic breast cancer, 584, Q125
Metastatic colorectal cancer, 586
Metastatic prostate cancer, 461t, 463, Q74
Metatarsal phalangeal joint dislocation, 498–500, 499t
Metatarsalgia, 499t
Metformin
    for diabetes, 562–563
    for DM, 559, 564t
    nutrient interactions, 215t
Methadone
    for opioid use disorders, 349t, 350–351
Methicillin-resistant *Staphylococcus aureus* (MRSA), 526, 532
Methimazole, 546
Methotrexate, 488, 492, 493, 495, 579t
    and osteoporosis, 263t
Methylcellulose, 430
Methylnatrexone, 110–111, 123
Methylphenidate, 115, 288
    for depression, 319, 320t
Methylprednisolone, Q110
    for dermatomyositis, 495
    for PMR, 491
    for polymyositis, 495
Metoclopramide
    for nausea, 112t
Metolazone, 411, Q104
Metoprolol, Q37
    adverse events, 335
    for chronic CAD, 396
    for HF, 410, 410t
Metronidazole, Q97
    for *C difficile* infection, 540
    for diverticulitis, 431
    for rosacea, 361–362

Metronidazole gel, 242
Mexican Americans, 260–261
mFI (Modified Frailty Index), 179
MGUS (monoclonal gammopathy of uncertain significance), 590
Michigan Alcoholism Screening Test (MAST)—Geriatric Version, 348
Micro-prolactinomas, pituitary, 552
Microalbuminuria, 436
Microangiopathy, thrombotic, 442
Microcytic anemia, 570
Micrographia, 509
Micronutrient needs, 214
Micronutrient supplements, 218–219
Microscopic colitis, 430–431
Micturition syncope, Q111
Middle cerebral artery stroke, Q100
Midodrine, 259t, 511
Miglitol, 564t
Migraine headaches, 516, 517
Migration history, 44
Migratory glossitis, 375
Mild cognitive impairment (MCI), 87
Mild diverticulitis, 431
Million Hearts initiative, 154
Milnacipran (Savella), 495–496
MIND at Home (Maximizing Independence at Home), Q77
Mind-body interventions, 85
    for cancer, 88
    for cardiovascular disease, 86
    for depression and anxiety disorders, 87
    for neurocognitive disorders, 87
Mineral oil, 215t
Mineralocorticoid hypertension, 439
Mineralocorticoid replacement, 553
Mini-Cog Assessment Instrument for Dementia, 26, 72, 130, 274, 275t
Mini-Nutritional Assessment (MNA), 216, 216t, 578
Mini-Nutritional Assessment–Short Form (MNA-SF), 213, 216
Minimal change disease (MCD), 444
Mini–Mental State Examination (MMSE), 26, 275t, 578
Minimum Data Set (MDS), 161–162, 179, 231
    definition of significant weight loss, 214
    sections related to nutritional status, 220
Minor depression, 319
Minority individuals, 575, Q80, Q83
    population projections, 2, 42
    risk factors for depression in, 316
Minoxidil, 421
Miotics, 188t
MIPS (Merit-based Incentive Payment System), 22
Mirabegron, 227t, 230–231, Q15
Mirror therapy, 150
Mirtazapine
    for depression, 320t
    for depressive features in dementia, 288, 288t

for erectile dysfunction, Q87
for essential tremor, 513
for insomnia, 282, 313t, 314
for sleep disturbances in dementia, 292
for undernutrition, 219
Misoprostol, 122, 426
Mistreatment, 89–96
 emotional/psychological abuse, 89, 90t
 financial exploitation, 89, 90t, 93, Q17, Q105
 indications of, 90, 91t
 observations that should raise concern, 90, 91t
 physical abuse, 89, 90t, 92, 92t
 risk factors for, 89–90, 91t
 safety issues, Q25
 screening for, 72–73, 90, 92, 92t
 sexual abuse, 89, 90t, 92–93, 92t
 signs of abuse, 92, 92t
 types of elder abuse and neglect, 89, 90t
Mistreatment history, 90–92, 91t
Mitochondrial DNA (mtDNA) theory of aging, 6
Mitomycin C, 579t
Mitral regurgitation (MR), 397, 398, 400t
Mitral stenosis (MS), 397, 398, 400t
Mixed dementia, 272
Mixed pain syndromes, 119
Mixed UI, 225, 227, 229–230
MLTC (managed long-term care programs), 169
MMSE (Mini–Mental State Examination), 26, 275t, 578
MNA (Mini-Nutritional Assessment), 216, 216t, 578
MNA-SF (Mini-Nutritional Assessment–Short Form), 213, 216
Mobility aids, 155–156, 155–157, 157t, 248–249
Mobility assessment
 activities of daily living (ADLs), 26
 Performance-Oriented Mobility Assessment (POMA), 27, 247, 254
MoCA (Montreal Cognitive Assessment), 26, 130, 274, 275t, Q91
Modified adjusted gross income (MAGI), 21
Modified Diet in Renal Disease (MDRD) formula, 101, 435
Modified Frailty Index (mFI), 179
Moexipril, 410t
Moisture-associated skin damage (MASD), 238
Moisture balance, 239
MOLST (Medical Orders for Life-Sustaining Treatment), 16
Mometasone furoate, 384t
Monoamine oxidase (MAO)-B inhibitors, 510
Monoclonal antibodies, 580–581, 582t

Monoclonal gammopathy of uncertain significance (MGUS), 590
Montreal Cognitive Assessment (MoCA), 26, 130, 274, 275t, Q91
Mood-congruent delusions, 331, 333–334
Mood disorders, 316–324
 with developmental disabilities, 358t
 psychotic symptoms in, 333–334
Mood disturbances, 287–289
Mood stabilizers
 for alcohol detoxification, 349t
 for behavioral disturbances in dementia with manic-like features, 289, 289t
 for bipolar depression, 321
 for mania, 320–321
 for personality disorders, 340
Moral distress, 11, 17
Morbidity, multiple, Q55, Q57, Q119
Morpheaform basal cell carcinoma, 369
Morphine, 121, 122, 393
Morse Fall Scale, 255
Morton foot, 499t
Morton neuroma, 501
MOST (Medical Orders for Scope of Treatment), 16
Motor neuron disease, 515–516
Motor planning, Q62
Motor vehicle collisions, Q23
Motorized scooters and wheelchairs, 156–157
Mouse trapping, 479
Mouth cancer, 65
Movement disorders, 507, 508–514
Moxifloxacin, 532
MPNs (myeloproliferative neoplasms), 572, 573
MR (mitral regurgitation), 397, 398, 400t
MRI (magnetic resonance imaging), 408, 516, Q99
MRSA (methicillin-resistant *Staphylococcus aureus*), 526, 532
MS (mitral stenosis), 397, 398, 400t
MSAs (medical savings accounts), 19t
MSM (men who have sex with men), 50, 51–52. *See also* Bisexual men; Gay men; Lesbian gay bisexual transgender (LGBT) health
Multicultural nutrition counseling, 220
Multidrug resistant organisms (MDROs), 526, 532, 534
Multifocal atrial tachycardia, 402
Multimorbidity (multiple morbidity), 34–36, 35t, Q55, Q57, Q119. *See also* Comorbidity
Multimorbidity GEMS Mobile App (AGS), 34
Multinodular goiter, toxic, 545
Multiple myeloma, 441–442, 443, 590
Multiple sclerosis, 337
Multiple system atrophy, 511
Multivitamin supplements, 63t, 74, Q84

Muscle energy techniques, 85–86
Muscle relaxants, 251t, 512
Muscle-strengthening activity recommendations, 55, 56
Musculoskeletal diseases and disorders, Q38, Q92
 CIM for, 85–86
 regional complaints, 476–484
 and rehabilitation, 148
Musculoskeletal pain, 475–484
Musculoskeletal system, 8, 9t, 10t
MUSE (medicated urethral system for erection), 468t, 469
Music therapy, 287, 292, 330
Mutation accumulation theory of aging, 5
Mutism, Q28
My Plate for Older Adults (USDA), 220
Myalgias, 562
Mycobacterium tuberculosis, 535
Mycophenolate mofetil, 493
Mycoplasma genitalium, Q107
Myelodysplasia, 570
Myelodysplastic syndromes (MDS), 569f, 570, 572–573
Myelofibrosis, idiopathic (IMF), 573
Myeloma, 441–442, 443
Myelopathy, 514–515, 516
Myeloproliferative neoplasms (MPNs), 572, 573
Myelotoxicity, chemotherapy-related, 579–580, 579t
Myocardial infarction, 392–393, Q76
 indications for permanent pacemaker implantation, 403, 405t
 TIMI score, 31
Myofascial pain, 118–119
Myofascial pain syndrome, 119t, 121
Myopathy, 515
Myopia, 189
Myositis, 494–495
MyPlate (USDA), 213

N-terminal pro-BNP (NT-proBNP), 408
N-terminal prohormone of brain natriuretic peptide (NT-proBNP), Q14
Nab-paclitaxel, 579t, 582t
Nabilone, 88
NAC (National Alliance of Caregiving), 37–38, 39t
Nadolol, 513
Nail disorders, 504
Nails, ingrown, 504
Nalbuphine, 124
Naloxegol, 110–111
Naloxone, 124, Q96
Naloxone overdose, 346
Naltrexone, 349t, 350, Q112
Narcissistic personality disorder, 337t, 339, 340
Narcotics
 adverse events, 215
 and incontinence, 226t

misuse, 345
  for OA-related pain, 486
Narcotics Anonymous, 350
Nasal pillows, 386–387
Nasopharyngeal laryngoscopy, 223
Nateglinide, 564t
National Academies, 213
National Academy of Elder Law Attorneys, 39t
National Adult Day Services Association, 39t
National Adult Protective Services Association, 95
National Alliance of Caregiving (NAC), 37–38, 39t
National Association of Area Agencies on Aging, 168
National Center for Complementary and Integrative Health (NCCIH), 85
National Center on Elder Abuse, 95
National Comprehensive Cancer Network (NCCN), 462, 577
National Council on Aging, Inc., 59, 216
National Heart, Lung and Blood Institute, 562
National Highway Traffic Safety Administration, 28
National Hospice and Palliative Care Organization, 107
National Institute on Aging (NIA), 25, 39t
National Institutes of Health (NIH)
  guidelines regarding body size classification based on BMI, 214
  online resources and tools for caregivers, 39t
  Stroke Scale, 149, 519, 519t
National Kidney Foundation (NKF)
  guidelines for CKD, 443, 444f
  Kidney Disease Outcomes Quality Initiative (KDOQI), 443
  online calculator, 435
  recommendations for CKD screening, 443
National Osteoporosis Foundation (NOF), 68, 260, 264
National PACE Association (NPA), 169, 178
National Pressure Ulcer Advisory Panel (NPUAP), 235, 236, 236t, 238
National Resource Center on LGBT Aging, 474
National Transitions of Care Coalition, 142
Native Americans
  burning mouth syndrome, 376
  cancer incidence, 575
  CKD, 443
  CVD mortality rates, 390
  population projections, 575
Native Hawaiians and Other Pacific Islanders
  CVD mortality rates, 390
  life expectancy, 2

population projections, 219, 575
poverty rates, 3
Native-valve endocarditis, 398
Natural products, 85, 86t
Naturopathy, 85
Nausea and vomiting
  drug-induced, 88, 123, Q96
  medications for nausea, 112t
  postoperative nausea, 103–104
  in terminal illness, 111
NBRAs (nonbenzodiazepine-benzodiazepine receptor agonists), 313–314
NCCIH (National Center for Complementary and Integrative Health), 85
NCCN (National Comprehensive Cancer Network), 462, 577
NCD. See Neurocognitive disorder
Nd:YAG (neodymium-yttrium-aluminum-garnet) laser, 587
Nebivolol, 413, Q89
Neck dystonia, 512
Neck pain, 476
Negative-pressure wound therapy (NPWT), 239–241, 242
Neglect, 89, 90t. See also Mistreatment
  psychological, 93
  risk factors for, 89–90, 91t
  self-neglect, 94
  signs of, 92, 92t
Neisseria gonorrhea, 463
Neodymium-yttrium-aluminum-garnet (Nd:YAG) laser, 587
Neoplasia
  adrenal, 554
  myeloproliferative neoplasms, 572, 573
  vulvar, 451
Neostigmine, 434
Nephrectomy, 588
Nephritic syndromes, 442
Nephritis, acute interstitial, 441
Nephrolithiasis, 440
Nephrology, 435–446, Q48, Q69
Nephropathy, membranous, 444
Nephrotic-range proteinuria, 442–443
Nephrotic syndromes, 442–443
Neprilysin inhibitors, 409, 410–411, 410t
Nerve conduction studies, 514
Nervous system, 9t, 10t
Netardusil, 188t
Neuraminidase inhibitors, 533
Neurocognitive disorder (NCD), 272, 284
  CIM for, 87–88
  differential diagnosis of, 277
  HIV-associated, 538–539
Neurodermatitis, 362, 450
Neurogenic orthostatic hypotension, Q71
Neuroimaging, 275–276, Q75
Neurokinin-1 receptor antagonists, 112t
Neurologic diseases and disorders, 87, 507, 518–522

Neurologic testing, 210–211, 211t, 282–283
Neurology, 507–517, Q75
Neuromas, 501
Neuromuscular disorders, 514–516
Neuropathic pain, 119, 119t, 121, 124, 514–515
Neuropsychiatric concerns, preoperative, 101–102
Neuropsychiatric Inventory (NPI), 285
Neurosyphilis, 539
Neuroticism, 341
Never events, 128–130
Nevus, atypical, Q30
New York Heart Association (NYHA) classification of heart failure, 411, 411t, Q14
NIA. See National Institute on Aging
Niacin, 215t
NICHE (Nurses Improving Care of Health System Elders), 136
Nicotine dependence, 349t, 351
Nicotine replacement, 349t, 351
NIFTP (noninvasive follicular thyroid neoplasms with papillary-like nuclear features), 547
Night driving, Q10
NIH. See National Institutes of Health
NIH Stroke Scale (NIHSS), 149, 519, 519t
Nilotinib, 582t
Nintedanib, 387
Nitrates, 396, 411–412
Nitrofurantoin, 534
Nitroglycerin, 393
Nivolumab, 370, 581, 582t, 588
Nizatidine, 80t
NKF. See National Kidney Foundation
NOACs (novel oral anticoagulants), 521
Nociceptive pain, 119, 119t
Nocturia, 227, 231
Nocturnal oxygen therapy, Q21
Nodular basal cell carcinoma, 369
Nodular melanoma, 370
Nodular thyroid disease, 546–547
NOF (National Osteoporosis Foundation), 260
Non-Hodgkin lymphoma, 571, 589
Nonadherence to medication regimens, 25, 83–84, 581
Nonbenzodiazepine-benzodiazepine receptor agonists (NBRAs), 313–314
Nongonococcal urethritis, Q107
Noninvasive follicular thyroid neoplasms with papillary-like nuclear features (NIFTP), 547
Nonmaleficence, 11, 13
Non–small-cell lung cancer (NSCLC), 581, 584–585
Non–ST-elevation myocardial infarction (NSTEMI), Q76
Nonsteroidal anti-inflammatory drugs (NSAIDs)
  adverse events, 81, 215, 426–427

for CPPD, 490
and falls, 252
gastric complications, 426–427
for gout, 489
for headaches, 517
and hyperkalemia, 438, 439t
and incontinence, 226t
for OA-related pain, 486
for persistent pain, 122
for secondary OA, 550–551
for SLE, 493
and UI, 231
Nonthyroidal illness syndromes, 544
Nonverbal communication, 44
Nordic diet, Q84
Normal-pressure hydrocephalus (NPH), 244, 248
North American Menopause Society, 471
Nortriptyline, 288, 288t, 320t
Novel oral anticoagulants (NOACs), 521
Novolin 70/30 (isophane insulin and regular insulin injectable), 565t
Novolin R (insulin), 565t
NovoLog (insulin aspart), 565t
NPA (National PACE Association), 169
NPH (normal-pressure hydrocephalus), 244, 248
NPH insulin (Humulin, Novolin), 565t
NPI (Neuropsychiatric Inventory), 285
NPUAP (National Pressure Ulcer Advisory Panel), 235, 236, 236t, 238
NPWT (negative-pressure wound therapy), 239–241, 242
NSAIDs. *See* Nonsteroidal anti-inflammatory drugs
NSCLC (non–small-cell lung cancer), 581, 584–585
NSTEMI (non–ST-elevation myocardial infarction), Q76
NT-proBNP (N-terminal prohormone of brain natriuretic peptide), Q14
Numeric Rating Scale, 118
Nummular or coin-shaped eczema, 362, 362f
Nurse practitioners
in home care, 166
rehabilitation team role, 146, 147t
Nurses Improving Care of Health System Elders (NICHE), 136
Nursing, 171, 171t, Q35
Nursing facilities
CMS 5-star rating system, 161
medical directors of, 162
regulations, 161–163
sexual activity policy, 472–473
special-care units, 163
staffing patterns, 160–161
Nursing-home care, 159–172, 170t
discharge planning for, Q93
fall prevention in, Q108
falls risk in, 250
interventions for lowering risk of falls in, 255t
Interventions to Reduce Acute Care Transfers (INTERACT), 140
involuntary weight loss in, 217
Medicare benefits, 19t, 160, Q93
oral hygiene in, 379
pain management, Q80
population, 3, 159
pressure injuries in, 234, Q10
Quality Assurance and Performance Improvement (QAPI) programs, 162–163
recommendations for preventing falls, 259
risk factors for placement in, Q41
sexuality in, 471–473
sleep in, 310
standards of care, 220
unacceptable weight loss in, 220
urinary incontinence in, 231–232
venues of care, 141
Nursing Home Compare (CMS), 22, 39t, 234
Nutrition, 213–221, Q84
for cancer, 88
for CKD, 445
drug-nutrient interactions, 215, 215t
for hospitalized patients, 128, 131t
interventions, 131t, 218–219
for pressure ulcers, 239, 241
to reduce risk of osteoporosis, 262
rehabilitation care, 146
risk factors for poor status, 215–216, 216t
under-nutrition, 70, 217, 219
Nutrition assessment, 25, 214–217
screening evaluations, 70
threshold to trigger, 220
Nutrition counseling, 70, 220
Nutrition Screening Initiative, 216
Nutritional screening, 70
Nutritional supplements, 218–219, 299, 514–515, Q39, Q84
for pressure ulcers, 241
safety issues, 85
Nutritional support, Q5
NW-CALMS mnemonic for cognitive history, 274, 274t
NYHA (New York Heart Association) classification of heart failure, 411, 411t, Q14

OA. *See* Osteoarthritis
OASIS (Outcome and Assessment Information Set), 145, 165
Obergefell v. Hodges, 54, 473
Obesity, 217–218, Q38, Q87
activity recommendations for, 55, 57
cardiovascular risk, 391–392
definition of, 392, 548
drug interactions, 82
recommendations for, 70
Obinutuzumab, 589
OBRA (Omnibus Budget Reconciliation Act), 94–95, 159, 161–162, 220
Observation, 90
Obsessions, 327
Obsessive-compulsive disorder (OCD), 327, 329, 329t, 330, 337t, 339
treatment of, 340
Obstruction
acute colonic pseudo-obstruction, 434
bowel, 111–112, 113t
gastrointestinal, 111–112
Obstructive pulmonary disease, chronic (COPD). *See* Chronic obstructive pulmonary disease (COPD)
Obstructive sleep apnea (OSA), 306, 307, 309–310, 386–387
screening for, 69
Obstructive uropathy, 441
Occupational activity, 56
Occupational therapy (OT)
for dementia, 283
for OA-related pain, 486
for preventing falls, 258t
rehabilitation team role, 145, 146, 147t
for shoulder rehabilitation, 154–155
OCD (obsessive-compulsive disorder), 327, 329, 329t, 330
Octreotide, 112t, 113t
Ocular lubricant ointments, 185
Ocular surface tumors, 187
Odd or eccentric behaviors, 337t
Odynophagia, 424
Ofatumumab, 589
Office visits, 24
Ogilvie syndrome, 434
1,25(OH)$_2$D levels, 547–548, 547t
25(OH)D levels, 547–548, 547t
Olanzapine
for agitated delirium, 299–300, 301t
for depression, 320
dosing and adverse events, 291, 333, 335t
for psychosis in dementia, 290, 290t
to stabilize mood in mania and bipolar depression, 322t
Old-age dependency ratio, 2
Older Adult Oncology guidelines (NCCN), 577
Older Americans Act (AOA), 168, 218, 283
Olecranon bursitis, 478, Q122
Olfactory dysfunction, 376–377, 377t
Oligometastatic disease, 586
Olmesartan, 410t
Olodaterol, 384t
Omalizumab, 383
Omega-3 fatty acids, 86t, 87, Q39
Omeprazole, 112t
Omnibus Budget Reconciliation Act (OBRA), 94–95, 159, 161–162, 220

OnabotulinumtoxinA, Q4
Oncology, 574–590. *See also* Cancer
Oncology Care Model, 115
Ondansetron, 112t
Onychocryptosis, 504
Onychomycosis, 504, Q50
Operative therapy. *See also* Surgical care
    iatrogenic complications, 102
    perioperative care, 97–105
    postoperative management, 102–105
    preoperative assessment and management, 97–102
Ophthalmic corticosteroids, 188
Ophthalmoplegia, Q117
Opioid Action Plan (FDA), 347
Opioid dependence, 349t, 350–351
Opioid-induced constipation, 110–111, Q96
Opioids
    adverse effects, 81, 123–124, 215, 335, Q96
    and delirium, 298, 300t
    for dyspnea, 114
    and falls, 251t
    for fibromyalgia, 495–496
    misuse, 344, 345
    for moderate to severe pain, 122
    for neuropathic pain, 515
    for OA-related pain, 486, Q96
    for persistent pain, 121
    for postsurgical pain, 105
    for RLS, 514
    special considerations for, 122–123
Optic neuropathy, ischemic, 186–187, 186t, 191–192
Optimizing therapies and care plans, 36
Oral appliances, 307
Oral assessment, 378–379
Oral cancer, Q29, Q74
Oral diseases and disorders, 372–379
    cancer, 65, 376
    candidiasis, 375, 376t
    with developmental disabilities, 358t
    lesions, 375–376, 376t
Oral dysphagia, 222
Oral health, 372–379
Oral hygiene, 372, 379
Oral nutrition, 218–219
Oral squamous cell carcinoma, Q74
Oral tissues, 372, 373t
Orchiectomy, 461t, 463
Orexin receptor antagonists, 314
Organ systems, 8, 9t, 10t
Oropharyngeal dysphagia, 223, 423, 424, Q116
Orthoses
    for foot disorders, 502
    for gait disorders, 248–249
    for osteoarthritis, 485–486
    for rehabilitation, 155, 157–158
Orthostasis, Q76
Orthostatic hypotension. *See* Postural (orthostatic or postprandial) hypotension

Orthotics, Q38
Orthotists, 146, 147t
OSA. *See* Obstructive sleep apnea
Oseltamivir, 533
Osimertinib, 582t
Osler nodes, Q18
Osmotic laxatives, 429
Ospemifene, 449, 471, 472t
Osseointegrated implants, 200
Osteitis fibrosis cystica, 445
Osteoarthritis (OA), 485–487
    activity recommendations for, 55
    of glenohumeral joint, 477
    of hand, 478, 486f
    of hip, 479, 485, 486–487
    interventions for preventing falls, 258t
    of knee, 124, 480, 485, 486, 486f, Q38
    secondary, 550–551
    of shoulder, 155
    treatment of, 85, 124, Q38, Q96
Osteolytic hypercalcemia, local, 548–549, 548t
Osteomyelitis, 538
Osteonecrosis: of jaw, 268–269, 372, 378, Q29, Q74
Osteopathic manipulation, 85
Osteopenia, 261t, 266, 358t, Q98
Osteophytes, 485
Osteoporosis, 260–271, 445
    definition of, 260, 261t
    with developmental disabilities, 358t
    diagnosis of, 260, Q2
    laboratory testing in, 263, 263t
    pharmacologic options for, 267–270, 268t
    prevention of, 260, 266–270, 491
    risk factors for, 261–262, 262–263, 262t, Q98
    sacral fractures of, 481, 481t, 482t, 483
    screening for, 62t, 68, 260, 264
    secondary, 260, 263–264, 263t
    vertebral compression fractures of, 481, 483
OT. *See* Occupational therapy
Otago Exercise Program, 257
Otoscopy, pneumatic, Q66
Outcome and Assessment Information Set (OASIS), 145, 165
Outpatient care
    Medicare benefits, 19t, 20
    patient selection for interventions, 178–179
    rehabilitation services, 144t, 146
    for substance abuse, 350
    systems of care, 173–179
Outpatient consultation, 176
Ovarian cancer, 65
Overactive bladder, 225
Overprescribing, 79–80, 79t, 83
Overweight, 57, 392, Q38
Oxaliplatin, 580, 582t, 586, 587

Oxandrolone, 219
Oxazepam, 329
Oxcarbazepine, 508
Oxybutynin
    and delirium, 300t
    for incontinence, 227t, 230, 232, Q15, Q86
Oxycodone, 122, Q96
Oxygen, hyperbaric, 242
Oxygen therapy
    for ACS, 393
    for COPD, 385t, 386
    for dyspnea, 114
    nocturnal, Q21
    for ventilatory disorders, 387

P_2Y_{12} inhibitors, 393–394, 395
PACE (Program of All-Inclusive Care for the Elderly), 21, 168–169, 178, Q20, Q27
PACE Innovation Act, 169
Pacemakers, 212
    indications for, 403, 405t
    and preventing falls, 257, 258t
Pacific Islanders. *See* Native Hawaiians and Other Pacific Islanders
Paclitaxel, 579t, 580, 582t, 588
PAD. *See* Peripheral arterial disease; Physician aid-in-dying
Padua Prediction Score, 133
Paget disease of bone, 196, 550–551
Pain
    acute, 117
    back pain, 480–482, 482t, Q83, Q92
    burning mouth syndrome, 376
    chronic, 117, 121, 357, 358t, 495, 497, Q36
    in cognitively impaired adults, 120, 120t
    definition of, 117
    dyspareunia, 470–471, 472t
    elbow pain, 477–478, Q122
    fibromyalgia, 495–496
    gait abnormalities, 246
    in groin, 479
    hand and wrist pain, 478–479
    heel pain, 501–502
    hip pain, 490
    knee pain, 480, 490
    leg pain, 479–480
    low back pain, 85–86, 481t, 482t, 483–484, Q92
    lumbar spinal stenosis, 475
    mixed or unspecified, 119
    musculoskeletal, 475–484
    myofascial, 118–119, 119t, 121
    neck pain, 476
    neuropathic, 119, 119t, 121, 124, 514–515
    nociceptive, 119, 119t
    OA-related, 480, 486
    persistent, 117, 121–122, 486–487
    phantom limb pain, 153
    shoulder, 476–477

somatic, 119, 119t
thigh pain, 479–480
total pain, 117
types of, 119, 119t
visceral, 119, 119t
vulvar, 450
Pain Assessment in Advanced Dementia (PAINAD), 118
Pain Disability Scale, 118
Pain disorder (somatic pain), 119, 119t, 340
Pain intensity scales, 118–119
Pain Ladder (WHO), 121
Pain management, 117–125, Q92
in cancer, 122, 463
in debridement, 239
for delirium, 298t
guidelines for, 486–487
in minorities, Q80, Q83
in nursing home residents, Q80
in osteoarthritis, 486–487, Q38, Q96
patient-controlled analgesia, 105
pharmacologic therapy, 105, 121–122, 121t
in post-herpetic neuralgia, 366–367
postoperative, 105
recommendations for, 125
in terminal illness, 110
topical agents, 121, 121t
in vertebral compression fractures, 271
Pain maps, 118
PAINAD (Pain Assessment in Advanced Dementia), 118
Painful diabetic neuropathy, 507
Painful diverticulosis, 431
Palbociclib, 582t
Paliperidone, 290t, 291, 335t
Palliative care, 106–116, Q42, Q45, Q52
for COPD and dyspnea, 386
for frailty, 184
for LGBT older adults, 53
services, 107, 108t
of wounds, 242, 242t
Palliative Performance Scale, 32, 32t
Palliative Prognostic Score, Q26
Palliative sedation, 16
Palsy, progressive supranuclear (PSP), 511–512
PAMA (Protecting Access to Medicare Act of 2014), 141
Pamidronate, 550
PAMORAs (peripherally acting mu-opioid antagonists), 110–111
Pancreatic cancer, Q126
Pancreatitis, 428–429
Panhypopituitarism, 552
Panic attacks, 325–326
Panic disorder, 325–326, 329, 329t, 330
Panitumumab, 582t, 587
Pantoprazole, 112t
PaO$_2$, 380
PAP (positive-airway pressure), 306–307

auto-titrating PAP (autoPAP), 307
bi-level (biPAP), 307, 516
continuous (CPAP), 307, 386–387
Pap smear, 62t
Papaverine, 468t, 469
Paranoid delusions, 331
Paranoid personality disorder, 337t, 339, 340
Paraprotein, 570
Parathyroid disorders, 547–551
Parathyroid hormone (PTH)
age-related changes in, 547, 547t
and CKD, 445
secondary hyperparathyroidism, 262
Parathyroid hormone analogues, 268t, 269–270
Parathyroid hormone-related peptide (PTHrp), 549–550
Parathyroid surgery, 549, 549t
Parkinson dementia, 273, 277t
Parkinson disease (PD), 507, 509–511
agitation in, Q60
dysphagia in, Q116
gait abnormalities, 244, 246
interventions for, Q47
interventions for preventing falls, 258t
nonmotor symptoms of, 511
psychotic symptoms of, 334
rapid eye movement (REM) sleep behavior disorder in, Q68
Parkinson disease dementia, 273, 277t
Parkinson drugs, 251t
"Parkinson-plus" syndromes, 511–512
Parkinsonian syndromes, 246, 511–512
Parkinsonism, 246, 509, 511, 512
Paronychia, 504
Paroxetine
adverse events, Q19, Q87
for depression, 287–288
for depressive features in dementia, 288t
for vasomotor symptoms, 448
Parulis, 375, 376t
Parvovirus infection, 570
Passive-aggressive personality disorder, 336
Past medical history, 131t
Patellar taping, Q38
Patellofemoral pain, 480
Patent foramen ovale (PFO), 522
Patient-centered medical homes (PCMHs), 173, 174t
Patient-clinician communication, 24–25
Patient-controlled analgesia, 105
Patient education
cultural appropriate nutrition materials, 220
for delirium, 298t
for diabetes, 560–561, Q31
for fibromyalgia, 495
in intellectual and developmental disability, Q51
for persistent pain, 120, Q80

for preventing falls, 257
for sexual dysfunction, 471
Patient Health Questionnaire (PHQ-9), 26, 317–318
indications to start antidepressant therapy based on, 317, 318t
initial two questions (PHQ-2), 26, 72, 317
prescriber response guidelines based on, 317, 318t
Patient preferences, 34–35, Q126
advance care planning, 15–16, Q65
code status discussions, 133
cultural aspects, 48
formality, 42–43
preferred terms for cultural or religious identity, 42
Patient Protection and Affordable Care Act (ACA), 18, 20, 21–22, 137, 140, 162, 414, 531
Community Care Transitions Program (CCTP), 141
Independence at Home Demonstration project, 166
Patient safety. See Safety
Patient Self-Determination Act (PSDA), Q126
Patiromer, 439
Pazopanib, 582t, 589
PCI (percutaneous coronary intervention), 394, 396–397
PCMHs. See Patient-centered medical homes
PCV13 (pneumococcal conjugate vaccine), 73, 529, 529t
PD-1 (programmed death receptor-1) inhibitors, 581
PDIs (prosthetic device infections), 537
PDL-1 (programmed death ligand-1) inhibitors, 581
PE (pulmonary embolism), 380, 387–389
Peak expiratory flow meters and inhalers, 386
Pediculosis capitis, 367–368
Pediculosis corporis, 367–368
Pediculosis pubis, 367–368
Pelvic examination, 65, 228, 447–448
Pelvic floor disorders, 451–453
Pelvic floor muscle (Kegel) exercises, Q4
Pelvic floor physical therapy, 430
Pelvic floor retraining, 429
Pelvic muscle exercises (PMEs), 229–230
Pelvic organ prolapse, 447, 451–452, 452f, Q4
Pelvic Organ Prolapse Quantification (POPQ), 451
Pelvic reconstruction, 453
Pembrolizumab, 370, 581, 582t
Penicillamine, 488
Penicillin, extended-spectrum, 539
Penile-brachial pressure index, 467–468

Penile prosthesis, 468t, 469
Penile revascularization, 469
Pentamidine, 439t
Pentoxifylline, 405
Peptic ulcer disease (PUD), 427
Percutaneous coronary intervention (PCI), 394, 396–397
Percutaneous endoscopic gastrostomy or jejunostomy, 223–224
Percutaneous tibial nerve stimulation, Q4
Performance-based functional assessment, 247
Performance-Oriented Mobility Assessment (POMA), 27, 247, 254
Perindopril, 410t, 412–413, 418
Periodic limb movements disorder (PLMD), 307–308
Periodic limb movements during sleep (PLMS), 307–308, 513, 514
Periodontal anatomy, 372, 373f
Periodontal disease, 373, 376t
　and cardiovascular disease, 377, 378
　diabetes-related, Q29
Periodontal ligament, 373
Periodontitis, 372, 373, 378
Periodontium, 373
Perioperative care, 97–105, Q91, Q114
Peripheral arterial disease (PAD), 390, 404–405
　and foot, 506
　and pressure injuries, 242
　recommendations for, 406
　screening for, 69
　and thigh pain, 479–480
Peripheral neuropathy, 246, 507, 514–515
Peripheral polyneuropathy, 514
Peripheral vascular disease, 148
Peripherally acting mu-opioid antagonists (PAMORAs), 110–111
Peritoneal dialysis, 445
Peritonitis, 431
Permethrin cream, 367
Perphenazine, 112t, 290t, 335t
Persistent complex bereavement disorder, 317
Persistent pain, 117
　assessment of, 118–119
　management of, 121–122, 124, 486–487
Person-centered care, 173, 174, 174t
Personal care attendants, 166
Personal sound amplification systems, 199, 199t
Personality changes, 336, Q53
Personality disorders, 336–340, 337t, Q28, Q57
Pertussis vaccine, Q64
Pertuzumab, 582t
Pes anserine, 480
Pes cavus, 498
Pes plano valgus, 498
Pes planus, 498

Pessaries, 231, 452–453, 453f
PFFS (private FFS) plans, 19–20, 19t
PFO (patent foramen ovale), 522
pH, vaginal, 449
Phalen maneuver, 478
Phantom limb pain, 153
Pharmacists, 82, 146, 147t
Pharmacodynamics
　age-associated changes in, 77t, 78–79, 579–580, 579t
　chemotherapy issues, 579–580, 579t
Pharmacokinetics
　age-associated changes in, 76–78, 77t, 579–580, 579t
　chemotherapy issues, 579–580, 579t
Pharmacotherapy, 76–84. *See also specific drugs*
　for addiction treatment, 349t
　adverse events, 81, 328, Q15
　for agitated delirium, 301t
　for alcohol use disorders, 350–351
　for anxiety, 328–329, 329t, 330, Q113
　for bipolar depression, 321–322, 322t
　for bipolar disorder, 319
　for BPH, 456–457, 456t
　for centenarians, Q103
　for constipation, 429
　for delirium, 296, 298, 298t, 299–300, 300t
　for dementia, 280–282
　for depression, 287–289, 288t, 319–320
　for depressive features in dementia, 287–289, 288t
　for diabetes, 562–563, 564t
　flexible medication times, 309–310
　for frailty, 183
　for glycemic control, 562–563
　for HF, 409–412, 412–413
　for HTN, 419–421, 419t
　inappropriate prescribing, 79–80, 79t
　inappropriate use, 344
　for incontinence, 230–231
　for insomnia, 312–313, 312–314, 313t
　for mania, 320–321, 322t
　Medicare benefits, 18, 19t, 21–22
　medications to avoid, 124–125
　nonadherence to regimens, 83–84, 581
　optimizing, 36, 79–81
　for osteoporosis, 267–270, 268t
　for pain, 105, 121–122, 121t
　for PD motor symptoms, 510–511
　for persistent pain, 121–122
　polypharmacy, 36
　potentially inappropriate medications (PIMs), 79–80
　prescribing cascade, 81, Q15
　prescription medication misuse, 344, 345–346

　principles of prescribing, 82–83, 82t
　recommendations for, 84
　for schizophrenia and schizophrenia spectrum syndromes, 332–333
　for somatic symptom and related disorders, 336
　suboptimal, 127–128, 131t
　for substance abuse, 350–351
　for undernutrition syndromes, 219
　for urge-predominant UI, 227t
Pharyngeal dysphagia, 222–223
Phenobarbital, 300t, 508
Phentolamine, 468t, 469
Phenytoin, 215, 215t, 300t, 378, 508
Phenytoin toxicity, 77
Phlebotomy, 573
PHN (post-herpetic neuralgia), 117, 124, 188, 366–367
Phobia
　social (social anxiety disorder), 326–327, 329t
　specific, 326, 329t
　treatment strategies for, 329t, 330
Phonation impairment, Q28
Phosphatidylinositol-binding clathrin assembly protein gene *(PICALM)*, 273
Phosphodiesterase inhibitors
　for BPH, 456t, 457
　for COPD, 385, 385t
　for erectile dysfunction, 467, 468–469
　for HFpEF, 413
　for PAD, 405
Phosphorus, 445
Photoaging, 360
Photodynamic therapy, 587
Photographs, 237
PHQ-2 (Patient Health Questionnaire), 26, 72, 317
PHQ-9 (Patient Health Questionnaire), 26, 317–318, 318t
Physical abuse, 89, 90t, 92, 92t
Physical activity, 55–59, Q24, Q40. *See also* Exercise
　for behavioral disturbances, 292
　for cardiovascular disease, 86, 392
　for constipation, 429
　counseling for, 57, 63t, 70
　for dementia, 279
　for DM, 561
　for fibromyalgia, 495
　for HF, 409
　for HTN, 419
　for OA-related pain, 486
　for pain, 120
　for sleep issues, 312
2008 Physical Activity Guidelines for Americans (HHS), 56
Physical assessment, 25, 92–93
Physical dependence, 122–123
Physical disability
　excess, 346–347
　International Classification of Functioning, Disability, and Health (ICF) (WHO), 143

Physical examination
   clinical breast examination (CBE), 61
   digital rectal examination, 456, 459
   eye examination, 185
   gynecologic, 447–448
   on hospital admission, 130, 131t
   Initial Preventive Physical Examination (IPPE), 67t–68t, 69–70, 71, 72
   of lower back pain, 481–482, 482t
   in mistreatment, 92–93
   in musculoskeletal pain, 475
   in osteoporosis, 264
   pelvic examination, 228, 447–448
   with UI, 228
Physical restraints, Q108
Physical status, 98, 98t
Physical therapy (PT)
   for delirium, 298t
   for dementia, 283
   for gait disorders, 248
   for myelopathy, 516
   for OA-related pain, 486
   for PD, 509
   pelvic floor, 430
   for preventing falls, 257, 258t, Q24
   rehabilitation team role, 145, 146, 147t
Physician aid-in-dying (PAD), 16
Physician assistants, 146, 147t, 166
Physician-assisted death, 16
Physician-assisted suicide, 16
Physician Orders for Life-Sustaining Treatment (POLST), 16, 109
Physician Orders for Scope of Treatment (POST), 16
Physicians
   home health care role, 165–166
   Medicare payments, 19t
   rehabilitation team role, 146, 147t
Physiologic theories of aging, 5–8
Pill esophagitis, 426
Pilocarpine, 187t, 188t, 375, 494
Pimavanserin, 290t, 291, 334
   dosing and adverse events, 335t
   for PD nonmotor symptoms, 511
PIMs (potentially inappropriate medications), 79–80
Pink eye, 188
Pioglitazone, 564t
Pirbuterol, 384t
Pirfenidone, 387
Pitting edema, 487, 488
Pituitary adenomas, 551–552
Pituitary gland disorders, 551–553
Pituitary gland hormones, 551, 551t
Plantar fasciitis, 499t, 501–502
Plantar verruca, 503
Plaque, 373
Plasma cell dyscrasias, 441–442
Plasma exchange, 515, 571
Plasmapheresis, 571
Platelet disorders, 571–572
Platinum, 582t, 586, 587

PLMD (periodic limb movements disorder), 307–308
PLMS (periodic limb movements during sleep), 307–308, 513, 514
PMDs (power mobility devices), 156–157
PMEs (pelvic muscle exercises), 229–230
PMR (polymyalgia rheumatica), 487, 488, 490–491, Q110
Pneumatic compression, intermittent, 389
Pneumatic otoscopy, Q66
Pneumococcal conjugate vaccine (PCV13), 73, 529, 529t
Pneumococcal pneumonia, 223
Pneumococcal polysaccharide vaccine (PPSV23), 73, 529, 529t
Pneumococcal vaccine, 528–529, 532
   in hospitalized patients, 130, 131t
   immunization schedule for adults ≥65 years old, 529t
   recommendations for, 62t, 73
Pneumocystis pneumonia prophylaxis, 491
Pneumonia, 531–532
   aspiration, 147–148, 222, 223, 377–378
   community-acquired, 531–532, Q69
   follow-up chest radiography after, Q69
   pneumococcal, 223
   postoperative, Q114
   and rehabilitation, 147–148
   surveillance definition of, 528t
Pneumonitis, aspiration, 222
POCD (postoperative cognitive dysfunction), 297, Q91
Pocket talkers, 43
Podagra, 488
Podiatry, 497–506
Poikiloderma, 360
Point of service (POS) plans, 19t
POLST (Physician Orders for Life-Sustaining Treatment), 16, 109
Poly-l-lactic acid, 360
Polycythemia vera (PV), 573
Polyethylene glycol, 429
Polymyalgia rheumatica (PMR), 487, 488, 490–491, Q110
Polymyositis, 494–495, 515
Polypharmacy, 25, 36, 79–80, 211, Q88, Q109
Polyps, colonic, 585–586
Polysomnography, 305
POMA (Performance-Oriented Mobility Assessment), 27, 247, 254
Pomalidomide, 582t
Ponatinib, 582t
Popeye sign, 477
Popliteal cyst, 480
POPQ (Pelvic Organ Prolapse Quantification), 451
Population projections, 1–2, 1f

POS (point of service) plans, 19t
Positional vertigo, benign paroxysmal (BPPV), 202, 205–206, Q99
Positioning, 238
Positive-airway pressure (PAP), 306–307
   auto-titrating PAP (autoPAP), 307
   bi-level (biPAP), 307, 516
   continuous (CPAP), 307, 386–387
POST (Physician Orders for Scope of Treatment), 16
Post-acute care, Q79
Post-herpetic neuralgia (PHN), 117, 124, 188, 366–367
Post-hospital syndrome, 139
Postacute care, 145t, 160
Postdiuretic sodium retention, Q104
Posterior tibial tendon dysfunction, 501
Posterior uveitis, 186t, 187
Postobstructive diarrhea, 434
Postoperative cognitive decline, 104, 397
Postoperative cognitive dysfunction (POCD), 297, Q91
Postoperative delirium, 297, 302t, 303
Postoperative infections, 187
Postoperative management, 102–105
Postprandial hypotension. See Postural (orthostatic or postprandial) hypotension
Posttraumatic stress disorder (PTSD), 328, 329, 329t
Postural (orthostatic or postprandial) hypotension, 201, 207, 211–212
   interventions for preventing falls, 256, 259t
   in long-term care residents, 422
   neurogenic, Q71
   in Parkinson and Parkinson-plus syndromes, 511
   treatment of, Q16, Q63, Q82
Postvoid residual (PVR), 225, 229
Potassium balance disorders, 438–439
Potassium excretion, 436t
Potassium-sparing diuretics, 438
Potassium supplements, 215, 215t, 419
Potentially inappropriate medications (PIMs), 79–80
Poverty: delusions of, 334
Poverty rates, 3, 53–54, Q118
Power mobility devices (PMDs), 156–157
PPD (purified-protein derivative) skin tests, 535, 536
PPIs. See Proton-pump inhibitors
PPOs (preferred provider organizations), 19t
PPS (prospective payment system), 160, 165
PPSV23 (pneumococcal polysaccharide vaccine), 73, 529, 529t
PR. See Pulmonary rehabilitation
Pra (Probability of Repeated Admission) Questionnaire, 178
Pramipexole, 308, 511, 514
Pramlintide, 564t

Prasterone, 449, 471
Prasugrel, 393–394
Prazosin, 329t, 456, 456t
Pre-frailty, 392
Prealbumin, 215
Preclinical disability, 26
Prednisolone, 385t, 553
Prednisone
    for adrenal insufficiency, 553
    for dermatomyositis, 495
    for giant cell arteritis, 492, Q110
    for gout, 489
    for nausea, 112t
    for non-Hodgkin lymphoma, 590
    for PMR, 491
    for polymyositis, 495
    for rheumatoid arthritis, 488
Preferred behavior programs, 356
Preferred provider organizations (PPOs), 19t
Pregabalin
    Beers Criteria® for, 80t
    for essential tremor, 513
    for fibromyalgia, 495–496
    and incontinence, 226t
    for neuropathic pain, 514–515
    for persistent pain, 124
    for RLS, 514
Prehabilitation, 135, 184, 248
Preoperative assessment and management, 97–102
Preoperative exercise, total body, 248
Prerenal azotemia, 440–441
Presbycusis, 194, Q13
Presbyesophagus, 222
Presbyopia, 189
Prescribing
    Beers Criteria® for, 80, 80t
    inappropriate, 79–80, 79t
    optimizing, 36, 79–81
    principles of, 82–83, 82t
Prescribing cascade, 81, Q15
Prescription drugs. See Drugs; Pharmacotherapy
Presenilin 1 (PS1), 273
Presenilin 2 (PS2), 273
Pressure injuries, 234–243
    assessment of, 236–237, Q11
    Braden Scale, 31, 237
    deep-tissue, 235, 236, Q70
    documentation of, 236–237, Q11
    dressings for, 239, 240t, 241
    hospital-acquired, 129, 131t, 234
    palliative care approach to, Q45
    prevention of, 129, 131t, 237–238, Q11
    and rehabilitation, 147
    risk factors for, 237–238
    staging, 235, 236t, Q5
    treatment of, 238–241, Q5, Q11, Q45, Q95
    unstageable, 235, 236t
Pressure Sore Status Tool, 237
Pressure stockings, 259t
Pressure Ulcer Scale for Healing, 237

Presyncope, 202, 203t
Prevention, 60–75. See also Screening
    of aspiration pneumonia, 147–148
    aspirin therapy, 73–74
    available health measures, 60, 62t–63t
    of cardiovascular disease, 561
    of CDI, 540
    counseling on, 74–75
    of diabetes mellitus, 558–559
    endocarditis prophylaxis, 378, 378t, 537, 537t
    of falls, 71, 251, 253f, 255–259, 258t–259t
    of frailty, 184
    of hip fracture recurrence, 151
    of HIV, 539
    of hypocalcemia, 550–551
    Initial Preventive Physical Examination (IPPE), 67t–68t, 69–70, 71, 72
    injury, 73
    lag time to benefit, 30, 31t
    Medicare benefits, 19, 19t, 60, 71, 72
    of migraine headache, 517
    of mistreatment, 89
    of osteoporosis, 260, 266–270, 491
    physical activity benefits for, 55
    Pneumocystis pneumonia prophylaxis, 491
    of pneumonia, 532
    of pressure ulcers, 129, 131t, 237–238
    recommendations for, 75
    recommended measures, 60, 62t–63t
    of stroke, 150, 401–402, 520–522
    of UTIs, 535
    of venous thromboembolism, 131t, 132–133
    "Welcome to Medicare" visits, 24, 69–70, Q31
Preventive services plan, 67t
Primary care
    comprehensive geriatric assessment (CGA) in, 176
    enhanced, 174–175
    Geriatrics in Primary Care model, 173–176
    GRACE team model, 175
Primary Care Guidelines for Management of Persons Infected with HIV, 530
Primary providers, 165–166
Primidone, 300t, 513
Principlism, 11
PRISMA 7, Q109
Prisms, Q82
Private contracts, 19
Private FFS (PFFS) plans, 19–20, 19t
Private insurance, 4
Proanthocyanidins, 535, Q123
Probability of Repeated Admission Questionnaire (Pra), 178

Probenecid, 80t, 489
Probiotics, 85, 432, 540
Problem drinking, 349t, 350
Problem-solving therapy, 323
Problem substance use, 344
Procainamide, 401
Prochlorperazine, 112t, Q96
Progesterone, 448
Prognosis, 30–33, 35
Prognostic indices, 31–32, 32t, Q26
Prognostication, 30–33, Q14, Q26
Program at Home (VA), 169
Program of All-Inclusive Care for the Elderly (PACE), 21, 168–169, 178, Q20, Q27
Programmed death ligand-1 (PDL-1) inhibitors, 581
Programmed death receptor-1 (PD-1) inhibitors, 581
Progressive supranuclear palsy (PSP), 511–512
Prokinetic agents, 112t
Prolactin, 551–552, 551t
Prolactinomas, 552
Prolapse
    iris, 456
    pelvic organ, 447, 451–452, 452f, Q4
    vaginal, 451–452, 452f, 453
Promethazine, 112t
Prompted voiding, 230, 231–232
Propafenone, 401
Propantheline, 231
Propranolol, 513, 517
Proprioceptive deficits, 246
Propulsion, 245t
Propylthiouracil, 546
Prospective payment system (PPS), 160, 165
Prostaglandin analogues, 122
Prostaglandins, 188t
Prostate: transurethral vaporization of, 456t, 457
Prostate cancer, 457–463, 587–588
    advanced/metastatic, 461t, 463
    CIM for, 88
    incidence of, 457–458, 574
    localized, 460–462, 460t, 461t, 462
    locally advanced, 461t, 462–463
    management of, 460–462, 461t, 462–463
    risk in older gay and bisexual men, 50
    risk stratification, 460, 460t
    screening for, 65–66, 458–459, 556–557, 578–579
    therapy for, 455, 460, 460t, 580, 581, 587–588
Prostate cancer, metastatic, Q74
Prostate disease, 455–464
Prostate-specific antigen (PSA) testing, 455, 458–459
    recommendations for, 62t, 64–65
Prostatectomy
    open, 456t, 457

radical, 460, 460t, 461t, 462
total, 464
Prostatic hyperplasia, benign. See Benign prostatic hyperplasia (BPH)
Prostatism, 455
Prostatitis, 455, 463–464
Prostheses, penile, 468t, 469
Prosthetic device infections (PDIs), 537
Prosthetic rehabilitation, 155
Prosthetists, 146, 147t
Proteasome inhibitors, 582t
Protecting Access to Medicare Act of 2014 (PAMA), 141
Protein: recommendations for daily intake, Q5
Protein excretion: measures of, 436
Protein gap, 570
Protein modification theory, 7
Protein requirements, 213, 241
Protein supplements, Q88
Proteinuria, 436, 442–443
Prothrombin, 572
Proton-pump inhibitors (PPIs), 486
adverse events, 215
Beers Criteria® for, 427
drug interactions, 527
for GERD, 424–426
for nausea, 112t
nutrient interactions, 215t
and osteoporosis, 263t
for persistent pain, 122
for PUD, 427
Provider-sponsored organizations (PSOs), 19t
Pruritus, 364, Q3
PS1 (presenilin 1), 273
PS2 (presenilin 2), 273
PSA (prostate-specific antigen) testing, 455, 458–459
recommendations for, 62t, 64–65
PSDA (Patient Self-Determination Act), Q126
Pseudo-obstruction, acute colonic, 434
Pseudocyesis, 342t
Pseudogout, 490
Pseudohyperkalemia, 438
Pseudohypertension, 417
Pseudomembranous colitis, 540
Pseudomonas, 539
Pseudothrombophlebitis, 480
Psoas abscess, 479
Psoralen with UVA light (PUVA), 365
Psoriasis, 364–365, 364f
PSOs (provider-sponsored organizations), 19t
PSP (progressive supranuclear palsy), 511–512
Psychiatric disorders, 87, 353, 354–356
Psychoactive medications, 256, 282
Psychogenic aphonia, Q28
Psychogenic ED, 466, 466t, 469
Psychogenic neurologic symptom disorder, 342t
Psychologic assessment, 26
Psychological abuse, 89, 90t, 93

Psychological assessment, 93
Psychological dependence, 123
Psychological neglect, 93
Psychologists, 146, 147t
Psychosis
antipsychotic medications for, 290–291, 290t, Q67
in dementia, 285, 290–291, 290t
late-onset, 331
Psychosocial assessment, 559
Psychosocial functioning, 323–324
Psychostimulants, 115
Psychotherapy
for abstinence, 350
for alcohol use disorders, 349t
for anxiety disorders, 325, 329–330
for bipolar disorder, 319
cognitive-behavioral, Q57
for depression, 319, 323, 324
emotion-oriented, 279
for personality disorders, 339
for sexual dysfunction, 472t
for somatic symptom and related disorders, 336
Psychotic depression, 319, 320
Psychotic disorders, 334–335
Psychotic symptoms, 331, 333–335
Psychotropic medications, 256, 339–340
Psyllium, 432
PT. See Physical therapy
PTH. See Parathyroid hormone
PTHrp (parathyroid hormone-related peptide), 549–550
Ptosis, 185, 186t
PTSD (posttraumatic stress disorder), 328, 329, 329t
Public reporting, 212
Published prognostic indices, 31–32
Published studies, 31
PubMed Health, 39t
PUD (peptic ulcer disease), 427
Pulmonary diseases, 380–389
chronic obstructive pulmonary disease (COPD), 32–33, 69, 328, 380, 383–386
with developmental disabilities, 358t
guidelines for risk assessment and perioperative management of, 100–101
Pulmonary embolism (PE), 380, 387–389
Pulmonary fibrosis, idiopathic, 387
Pulmonary rehabilitation, 154, 385t, 386
Pulmonary system, 9t, 10t, 380
Pulmonary thromboembolism, recurrent, 389
Pulmonology, 380–389
Pulsed lavage, 239
Pumpkin seed extracts, 87
Punctal plugs, 494
Pupillary defects, afferent, 185
Pure red cell aplasia, 570
Purified-protein derivative (PPD) skin tests, 535, 536

PUVA (psoralen with UVA light), 365
PV (polycythemia vera), 573
PVD (peripheral vascular disease), 148
PVR. See Postvoid residual
Pyelonephritis, 534
Pyrazinamide, 536
Pyridostigmine, 212
Pyuria, 535

Qi gong, 85
QPP (Quality Payment Program), 22
Quality Assurance and Performance Improvement (QAPI) programs, 162–163
Quality of care, 161–163
Quality of life, 28–29, 28t, 583
Quality Payment Program (QPP), 22
Quetiapine
for agitated delirium, 299–300, 301t, Q44, Q60
dosing and adverse events, 291, 333, 335t
for Parkinson disease and hallucinations, 334
for psychosis in dementia, 290, 290t
to stabilize mood in mania and bipolar depression, 322t
Quinapril, 410t
Quinidine, 401, 412, Q44

RA. See Rheumatoid arthritis
Racial or ethnic minorities, 2, 575, Q80, Q83
Radiation therapy. See also specific diseases and disorders
for cancer, 574, 581
for esophageal cancer, 587
external beam, 461t, 462
intensity-modulated, 581
for macroprolactinoma, 552
for MGUS, 590
for non-Hodgkin lymphoma, 589
postoperative, after lumpectomy, 584
for prostate cancer, 460, 460t, 461t, 462, 463
Radiculopathy, 515
Radioactive iodine (RAI) therapy, 546, 547
Radioactive iodine uptake (RAIU) testing, 545
Radiofrequency ablation, 588
Radiography, chest, 408, Q69
Radium, 463
RAI (radioactive iodine) therapy, 546, 547
RAIU (radioactive iodine uptake) testing, 545
Raloxifene, 268t, 270
Ramelteon, 313t, 314
Ramipril, 410t
Ramping technique, 386–387
Ramsay Hunt syndrome, 366
Ramucirumab, 582t

Randomized controlled trials (RCTs), 60
Ranibizumab, 189–190
Ranitidine, 80t, 112t, 466, Q102
RANKL (receptor activator of nuclear factor kappa-B ligand), 262
RANKL inhibitor, 268t, 269
Ranolazine, 396
Rapid eye movement (REM) sleep behavior disorder (RBD), 309, Q68
RAS (renal artery stenosis), 422, 439–440
Rasagiline, 510
Rate of living theory of aging, 7
Rational Recovery, 350
Raynaud phenomenon, 494
RBD (REM sleep behavior disorder), 309, Q68
RCTs (randomized controlled trials), 60
RDAs (recommended dietary allowances), 214
RDW (red cell distribution width), 570
Re-Engineered Discharge intervention, Q85
REACH (Resources for Enhancing Alzheimer's Caregivers Health), Q77
REACH II, Q77
REACH VA, Q77
Receptor activator of nuclear factor kappa-B ligand (RANKL), 262
Recombinant tissue-plasminogen activator (rt-PA), 520
Recommended dietary allowances (RDAs), 214
Rectal cancer, 586
Rectocele, 451
Red cell aplasia, pure, 570
Red cell distribution width (RDW), 570
Red eye, 185, 187–188, 187t, Q117
5α-Reductase inhibitors, 455, 456–457, 456t
Reflex syncope, 208, 211–212
Reflux, gastroesophageal, 358t, 424–426, 434
Refractive error, 188–189
Refusal of treatment, 13
Regorafenib, 582t, 587
Rehabilitation, 143–158, Q5, Q47
　acute, Q93
　cardiac, 153–154, 397, 409
　of gait disorders, 248
　after joint replacement, 248
　low-vision, 192
　Medicare benefits, Q79
　prehabilitation, 135, 184, 248
　pulmonary, 154, 385t, 386
　sites of care, 143–146, 144t
　teams and roles, 146, 147t
　vestibular rehabilitation therapy (VRT), 205
Rehabilitation Engineering and Assistive Technology Society of North America Wheelchair Service Guide, 156
Rehabilitation hospitals, 144–145, 144t

Relative exercise intensity, 55
Relaxation therapy, 85, 88, 312t, Q81
Relaxation training, 329t, 330
Religious advance directives, Q65
Religious beliefs, 46, 47
Religious identity, 42
REM sleep behavior disorder (RBD), 309, Q68
Reminiscence therapy, 279, 292
Remitting seronegative symmetrical synovitis with pitting edema (RS3PE) syndrome, 487, 488
Renal angiography, 439, 440
Renal artery angioplasty, 440
Renal artery disease, 439–440
Renal artery stenosis (RAS), 422, 439–440
Renal bone disease, 445
Renal cell cancer, 581, 588–589
Renal failure, Q14
Renal function, Q48, Q69
Renal insufficiency, 82
Renal replacement therapy, 445
Renin inhibitors, 412–413, 420
Renovascular disease, 439–440
Repaglinide, 564t
Reperfusion therapy, 394
Repetitive transcranial magnetic stimulation (rTMS), 323
Reset osmostat, 437
Resident Assessment Protocols, 220
Resistance training, 55, 258t
Resources for Enhancing Alzheimer's Caregivers Health (REACH), Q77
Respectful nonverbal communication, 44
Respiration, loud, 114
Respiratory depression, opioid-induced, 124
Respiratory diseases and disorders
　preoperative assessment and management of, 100–101
　pulmonary diseases, 380–389
Respiratory failure, 133
Respiratory symptoms and complaints, 380–381
Respiratory system. See Pulmonary system
Respite care, 170t, 283
Restless legs syndrome (RLS), 307–308, 513–514
Restraints, 293, 299, 303
Restrictive lung disorders, 387
Retinal detachment, 184–185, 186t
Retinal tears, 186t
Retinal vein occlusion, 187
Retinopathy, diabetic, 190–191
Retropulsion, 245t
Revascularization
　for chronic CAD, 396–397
　for PAD, 405
　penile, 469
Review of systems on hospital admission, 130, 131t
Revised Cardiac Risk Index, 98

RF (rheumatoid factor), 487
Rhabdomyolysis, 562
Rheumatoid arthritis (RA), 476, 481, 487–488
　of feet, 506
　of shoulder, 155
Rheumatoid factor (RF), 487
Rheumatology, 485–496, Q110
Rhinopyma, 362
Rhinosinusitis, 380–381, 382–383
Rhythm abnormalities, 257
Ribociclib, 582t
Rifampin, 536
Rifaximin, 432
Rights-based approach, 11
Rigidity, 509
Riluzole, 516
Rimantadine, 532
Rinne test, Q66
Risedronate, 267–268, 268t, 269
Risk-Standardized-Readmission Rates (RSRR), 137
Risperidone
　for agitated delirium, 299–300, 301t, Q32
　for chorea, 512
　dosing and adverse events, 291, 333, 335t
　for psychosis in dementia, 290, 290t
　to stabilize mood in mania and bipolar depression, 322t, Q33
Rituximab, 488, 495, 571, 581, 589
Rivaroxaban
　for AF, 401
　Beers Criteria® for, 80t
　for stroke prevention, 401, 403t, 521
　for VTE, 388–389
Rivastigmine, 281, 355, 511, Q94
RLS (restless legs syndrome), 307–308, 513–514
Roflumilast, 385, 385t
Rollators, 156, 157t
Rolling assessment, 24
Romberg test, 246
Ropinirole, 308, 511, 514
Rosacea, 361–362, 361f
Rosalynn Carter Institute for Caregiving, 39t
Rosiglitazone, 563, 564t
Rosuvastatin, 395, Q120
Rotator cuff arthropathy, 155
Rotator cuff tendonopathies and tears, 475, 477
Rotavirus, Q64
Rotigotine, 511, 514
Rowland test, 134, 135t
RS3PE (remitting seronegative symmetrical synovitis with pitting edema) syndrome, 487, 488
RSRR (Risk-Standardized-Readmission Rates), 137
rt-PA (recombinant tissue-plasminogen activator), 520

Index 769

rTMS (repetitive transcranial magnetic stimulation), 323
Runciman test, 134, 135t
Rural communities, Q8
Ruxolitinib, 573
Rye pollen, 87
Ryzodeg 70/30 (insulin degludec and insulin aspart), 565t

S-adenosylmethionine (SAM-e), 85, 86t, 87
Saccular aneurysms, intracranial, 523
Sacral fractures, 481, 481t, 482t, 483
Sacral nerve neuromodulation, 231
Sacubitril with valsartan, 409, 410–411, 410t
Safe Return, 280
Safety, 73, Q25
    attention to, 280
    of CIM therapies, 85
    and dementia, 280
    of dietary supplements, 85, 86t
    of natural products, 85
    preventing injury, 73
    in transitions, 139–140
SAGE (Services and Advocacy for LGBT Elders), 474
SAGE (Sinai Abbreviated Geriatric Evaluation), 102
SAGE National Resource Center, 40t
SAGECAP, 40t
SAGECare Credential, 474
SAH (subarachnoid hemorrhage), 523
Salicylates, 122, 215t
Saline, 437
Saline laxatives, 429
Saliva substitutes, 375
Salivary function, 374–375
Salivary glands, 372, 373t
Salix alba (white willow bark), 86
Salmeterol, 384–385, 384t
Salmonella, 540
Salsalate (Disalcid), 122
SAM-e (S-adenosylmethionine), 85, 86t, 87
SAMHSA (Substance Abuse and Mental Health Services Administration), 351
SAP (serum alkaline phosphatase), 550, 551
Sarcoma, 451, 581
Sarcopenia, 182, 222, 380, 577
Sarcopenic obesity, 217–218
Sarcoptes scabiei var *hominis*, 367
SAVR (surgical aortic valve replacement), 390, 398
Saw palmetto *(Serenoa repens)*, 86t, 87, 457
Saxagliptin, 564t
SBP (systolic blood pressure), 416, 418
Scabies, 367
SCALE (skin changes at life's end), Q45
Scheduled toileting, 298t
Schema therapy, 339, Q57
Schizoaffective disorder, 331

Schizoid personality disorder, 332, 337t, 339
Schizophrenia and schizophrenia spectrum syndromes, 331–333, Q51, Q54, Q67
Schizophrenia-like psychoses, 331, 332
Schizotypal personality disorder, 337t, 339
Schloendorff vs. Society of NY Hospital, 13
Schonberg 5- and 9-year index, 32t
Sciatica, 481t, 483
Scissoring, 245t
Scleritis, 186t, 187
Scooters, 156–157, 157t
Scopolamine, 112t, 113t
Score Hospitalier d'Evaluation du Risque de Perte d'Autonomie (SHERPA), 134, 135t
Screening, 66–70
    for alcoholism, 348
    for anxiety, 325
    for cancer, 31t, 51, 60–65, 74–75, 578–579, Q56
    for caregiver burden, Q41
    for CKD, 443
    for cognitive impairment, 63t, 274, 275t
    criteria for recommending, 60
    Dementia Screening Questionnaire for Individuals with Intellectual Disabilities (DSQIID), 355
    for depression, 63t, 211t, 317–318, Q7, Q75, Q121
    ED risk-screening tools, 134, 135t
    for frailty, 182, Q109
    gait and balance, 63t
    for glaucoma, 72, 185
    for hearing loss, 63t, 195
    for hepatitis C, 539
    for HIV, 467, Q107
    for hormone hypersecretion in adrenal incidentalomas, 554, 554t
    lag time to benefit, 31t
    for mistreatment, 72–73, 90, 92, 92t
    nutrition, 70, 214–217
    for osteoporosis, 260, 264
    PHQ-9 questions, 317–318
    physical activity, 57
    for prostate cancer, 458–459, 556–557
    recommendations for, 60, 62t, 75
    for risk of falls, 254–255
    for STIs, 470
    for substance use disorders, 348
    in transgender older adults, 51
    for UI, 63t, 228, 231
    for vitamin D deficiency, 218
Seattle Heart Failure Model, 32, 32t
Seborrheic dermatitis, 360–361, 361f
Seborrheic keratoses, 368, 368f
Section 8, Housing and Urban

Development programs, 171
Sedating antidepressants, 312, 313t, 314
Sedating antihistamines, 310, 315
Sedating antipsychotics, 314
Sedation, palliative, 16
Sedative/hypnotics
    chronic use, 314–315
    and falls, 251–252, 251t
    and incontinence, 226t
    for insomnia, 312, 313t
    interventions for preventing falls with, 258t
    misuse, 345
    for sleep problems, 311
Sedentarism, 58
Seizures, 507, Q75
    antiepileptic drugs for, 508
    with developmental disabilities, 357, 358t
    signs and symptoms of, 207, 208t, Q71
Selective estrogen-receptor modulators (SERMs)
    for menopausal vasomotor symptoms, 449
    for osteoporosis, 268t, 270
    for sexual dysfunction, 471, 472t
Selective norepinephrine-reuptake inhibitors (SNRIs)
    for anxiety disorders, 329, 329t
    for depression, 320t
    for depressive features in dementia, 288t
    for menopausal vasomotor symptoms, 448–449
Selective serotonin-reuptake inhibitors (SSRIs)
    adverse events, 215, Q19, Q87, Q102
    for alcohol abuse, 350
    for anxiety disorders, 325, 329, 329t, Q113
    for depression, 31t, 318, 319, 320t
    for depressive features in dementia, 287–288, 288t
    and falls, 251t, 252
    lag time to benefit, 31t
    for menopausal vasomotor symptoms, 448–449
Selegiline, 510, Q120
Self-assessment, caregiver, 39t
Self-care, 26
Self-injurious behavior, 354, 355, 356
Self-management, Q31
Self-neglect, 94
Self-prayer, 85
Self-reported health, Q109
"Senile" gait disorder, 245
Senior cohousing, 170
Senior health clinics (SHCs), 176–177
Senior housing, Q101
Senior villages, 170
Senna, Q96
Sensorineural hearing loss, 194, Q13
Sensory deprivation, 298t

Sensory impairment
  with developmental disabilities, 358*t*
  hearing loss, 193–201
  in hospitalized patients, 131*t*, 132
  interventions for, 131*t*, 132
  and rehabilitation, 148
  smell dysfunction, 376–377, 377*t*, 509
  taste dysfunction, 376–377, 377*t*
  vision loss, 185–192
Sepsis, 134, 531
Septic bursitis, Q122
Sequenced Treatment Alternatives to Relieve Depression (STAR*D), 318*t*
Serenoa repens (saw palmetto), 86*t*, 87, 457
Serious Illness Care Program, 108
SERMs. *See* Selective estrogen receptor modulators
Serotonin antagonists, 112*t*, 432
Serotonin-release assay, 571
Serotonin syndrome, 320, 321*t*
Sertraline
  for anxiety disorders, 325
  for depression, 320, 320*t*, Q100
  for depressive features in dementia, 287–288, 288*t*
Serum alkaline phosphatase (SAP), 550, 551
Services and Advocacy for LGBT Elders (SAGE), 474
Sex-education programs, 292
Sex hormone-binding globulin (SHBG), Q87
Sex hormones, 261–262
Sex therapy, 468*t*, 471
Sexual abuse, 89, 90*t*, 92–93, 92*t*
Sexual activity, 70–71, 465
  inappropriate sexual behavior (ISB), 292, 473
  in long-term care, 472–473
Sexual consent, 472–473
Sexual desire disorders, 470
Sexual dysfunction
  counseling for, 63*t*
  in older men, 465–469, 466*t*, Q34, Q87
  in older women, 465, 469–470, 470–471, 472*t*
Sexual health of LGBT older adults, 51–52
Sexual orientation, 50, 473–474
Sexual risk, 51–52
Sexuality, 465–474
Sexually transmitted infections (STIs)
  counseling for, 70–71
  in LGBT older adults, 51
  screening for, 470, Q107
SF-36 (Short Form-36 Health Survey), 28, 148
SGLT2 (sodium glucose co-transporter 2) inhibitors, 226*t*, 263*t*, 563, 564*t*
SGR (Sustainable Growth Rate), 22

Shared decision-making, 13, 405–406
Sharp debridement, 239
SHBG (sex hormone-binding globulin), Q87
SHCs (senior health clinics), 176–177
Sheltered housing, 171
SHERPA (Score Hospitalier d'Evaluation du Risque de Perte d'Autonomie), 134, 135*t*
Shigella, 540
Shingles (herpes zoster), 117, 186*t*, 188, 365–367, 366*f*
  vaccine against, 62*t*, 73, 528, 529*t*, 530
Shingrix, 73
Shoe terms, 503*t*
Shoes, 254, 254*f*, 258*t*, 502
Shopping cart sign, 483
Short Brief Michigan Alcoholism Screening Test-Geriatric Version (SMAST), 70
Short Form-36 Health Survey (SF-36), 28, 148
Shoulder arthritis, 155
Shoulder arthroplasty, 155
Shoulder fractures, 155
Shoulder pain, 476–477
Shoulder rehabilitation, 154–155
SIADH (syndrome of inappropriate antidiuretic hormone), 320, 437, Q19, Q69, Q102
Sick sinus syndrome, 399, 404
Side-lying test, 205
Sight problems. *See* Visual loss
Sigmoidoscopy, 61, Q56
Sildenafil, 387
  for dysphagia, 424
  for erectile dysfunction, 467, 468, 468*t*, Q87
  for HF, 413
Silodosin, 456, 456*t*
Simplified Nutrition Assessment Questionnaire, 216
Sinai Abbreviated Geriatric Evaluation (SAGE), 102
Sinusitis, 380–381
Sitagliptin, 564*t*
Sitaxsentan, 413
Sites of care, 141
Sitz marker study, 429
6-minute walk test, 247
Sjögren syndrome, 374–375, 493–494
Skeletal system, 9*t*, 10*t*
Skeleton loading, 262
Skilled-nursing facilities (SNFs), 19*t*, Q93
  CMS 5-star rating system, 161
  Medicare benefits, 144*t*, 145–146, 160
  transitions from hospital to, 141
Skin, 8, 9*t*, 10*t*, 360, Q45
Skin assessment, 237–238
Skin changes at life's end (SCALE), Q45
Skin failure, 235

Skin problems
  autoimmune conditions, 360–365
  benign growths, 368
  cancer, 65, 360, 369–370, Q30
  dermatology, 360–371
  on foot, 497, 503–504
  infections, 365–368, 528*t*
  infestations, 365–368
  inflammatory conditions, 360–365
  lesions, 503
  moisture-associated skin damage (MASD), 238
  tears, Q11
  toxicities of cancer treatment agents, 581, 582*t*
SLE (systemic lupus erythematosus), 443, 492–493
Sleep attacks, 511
Sleep hygiene, 291, 298*t*
Sleep issues, 304–315
  age-related changes, 304–305, 305*t*
  in dementia, 291–292, 292*t*, 309
  in hospitalized patients, 128, 131*t*, 309–310
  interventions for, 131*t*, 291, 292*t*, 311–312, 312*t*
  management of, 87–88, 291–292, 310–315, Q43, Q81
  measures to improve sleep hygiene, 311, 311*t*
  obstructive sleep apnea (OSA), 306, 307, 309–310, 386–387
Sleep-related breathing disorders, 306–307
Sleep restriction, 312*t*, Q81
Sleeping medications, 310, 315
Slings, 231
SLUMS (St. Louis University Mental Status) examination, 26, 274, 275*t*
Small-cell lung cancer, 581, 585
Small molecular inhibitors, 580
SMAST (Short Brief Michigan Alcoholism Screening Test-Geriatric Version), 70
Smell dysfunction, 376–377, 377*t*, 509
Smoking, 347
Smoking cessation, 88, 350, 380
  and cardiovascular risk, 391
  CIM for, 88
  for COPD, 384, 385*t*
  for DM, 561
  "Five A's" method, 351, 384
  for HF, 408
  for PAD, 404
  preoperative, Q114
  to prevent pneumonia, 532
  to prevent stroke, 521
  to reduce risk of osteoporosis, 262, 262*t*
Smoking cessation counseling, 63*t*, 70
Snellen charts, 25
SNFs. *See* Skilled-nursing facilities
SNPs (special needs plans), 19*t*
SNRIs. *See* Selective norepinephrine-reuptake inhibitors

Social anxiety disorder (social phobia), 326–327, 329t
Social assessment, 26
Social behavior, inappropriate, Q53
Social conditions, 357
Social history, 130, 131t
Social phobia (social anxiety disorder), 326–327, 329t
Social Services Block Grant programs, 171
Social support(s), 53
Social workers, 146, 147t, 283
Socially detached personality, 332
Society for Healthcare Epidemiology of America, 534
Sodium, 436
Sodium balance disorders, 438
Sodium conservation, 436t
Sodium excretion, 436t, 440
Sodium glucose co-transporter 2 (SGLT2) inhibitors, 226t, 263t, 563, 564t
Sodium polystyrene (Kayexalate), 439
Sodium restriction, 409, 419
Sodium retention, postdiuretic, Q104
Soft-tissue augmentation, 360
Soft-tissue infections, 528t
Solifenacin, 227t, 230
Somatic delusions, 319, 333
Somatic pain (pain disorder), 119, 119t, 340
Somatic symptom and related disorders, 336, 340–343, 342t, Q28
Somatization disorder, 341
Somatoform disorder, undifferentiated, 341
Sorafenib, 580, 582t
Sotalol, 401
Space-occupying pessaries, 452
Spasmodic torticollis, 512
Spasticity, 148, 246
Special-care units, 163
SPECIAL mnemonic for palliative care of wounds, 242t
Special needs plans (SNPs), 19t
Specialty care, geriatric, 176–178
Speech impairment, 358t
Speech therapy, 145, 146, 147t, 150
SPIKES framework for delivering difficult news, 33, 109, 110t
Spinal cord dysfunction, 516
Spinal deformities, 358t
Spinal manipulation, 85–86
Spinal stenosis, 476
Spine osteoarthritis, 485
Spirituality, 46, 47, 107, Q65
Spironolactone
    Beers Criteria® for, 80t
    for HF, 411, 412–413
    for HTN, 419t, 420
    and hyperkalemia, 439t
Splenectomy, 571, 589
Squamous cell carcinoma, 369
    oral, 376t, Q29, Q74
    of skin, Q30
    of vulva, 450, 451

Squamous hyperplasia, 450
SSI (Supplemental Security Income), 171
SSRIs. See Selective serotonin-reuptake inhibitors
St. Andrew's Sexual Behaviour Assessment, 473
St. John's wort *(Hypericum perforatum)*, 86t, 87
St. Louis University Mental Status (SLUMS) examination, 26, 274, 275t
St. Thomas's Risk Assessment Tool (STRATIFY), 255
ST-elevation myocardial infarction (STEMI), 393
Stabilization, 350
Staffing patterns, 160–161
Staphylococcus, Q18
Staphylococcus aureus, 398, 536–537, 538, Q18
    methicillin-resistant (MRSA), 526, 532
STAR*D (Sequenced Treatment Alternatives to Relieve Depression), 318t
Stasis dermatitis, 360, 365
State Medicare assistance offices, 16
State Veterans Homes, 159–160
Statin therapy
    for ACS, 393
    for cardiovascular disease, 31t, 69
    for chronic CAD, 395
    lag time to benefit, 31t
    recommendations for, 69, 562
    for stroke prevention, 521
    toxicity, 494
Stem cell/progenitor cell theory of aging, 7–8
Stem cells, hematopoietic, 567
STEMI (ST-elevation myocardial infarction), 393
Stenson's papillae, 375
Stenting, 422, 440
    for BPH, 456t, 457
    carotid artery angioplasty and, 521–522
    coronary stents, 100
    for esophageal cancer, 587
Steppage gait, 245t
Stimulant laxatives, 429
Stimulus control, 312t
Stinging nettle, 87
STIs. See Sexually transmitted infections
Stomach disorders, 426–429
Stomatitis, denture, 375
Stool softeners, 429, Q96
STOPP/START Criteria, 127
STRATIFY (St. Thomas's Risk Assessment Tool), 255
Strength training, 256–257, 258t, 262, 392, Q40
Streptococci viridans, 398, 536–537
Streptococcus bovis, Q18
Streptococcus pneumoniae, 539

Streptococcus viridans, Q18
Streptomycin, 536
Stress incontinence, 225, 227
    management of, 229–230, 231
    in nursing-home residents, 232
Stress management, 88
Stress-reduction techniques, 419
Stress tests, 98, 210, 395
Stress urinary incontinence, Q4
Stroke
    associated with AF, 399
    cardioembolic, 519
    cryptogenic, 519, 522
    fatality rate, 518
    hemorrhagic, 522–523
    incidence of, 518
    ischemic, 518–522
    lacunar, Q106
    management of, 149–150
    middle cerebral artery, Q100
    NIH Stroke Scale, 149, 519, 519t
    prevention of, 150, 401–402, 403t, 520–522, Q106
    recommendations for, 524
    rehabilitation after, 148–150
    risk factors for, 520–521
Stroke Impact Scale, 145t, 148
Strontium, 463
Subacute rehabilitation, Q79
Subarachnoid hemorrhage (SAH), 523
Subclinical depression, 319
Subclinical hyperthyroidism, 543t, 545
Subclinical hypothyroidism, 543–544, 543t
Subconjunctival hemorrhage, 187t, 188
Subdural hematoma, 522–523
Suboptimal care transitions, 139
Substance Abuse and Mental Health Services Administration (SAMHSA), 351
Substance-induced psychotic disorders, 334–335
Substance use disorders, 344–345, 345–346
    in LGBT older adults, 52–53
    risk factors for, 346–347, 347t, 348
    treatment of, 63t, 348–350, 348–351
Subsyndromal depression, 319
Suicidal depression, 317–318, 319, Q36
Suicide, 317–318
    in LGBT older adults, 52
    physician-assisted, 16
Sulfamethoxazole, 534
Sulfasalazine, 488
Sulfonylureas, 563, 564t
Sumatriptan, 517
Sunitinib, 580, 582t, 588
Sunscreens, 360
Superficial basal cell carcinoma, 369
Superficial spreading melanoma, 370
Supplemental Security Income (SSI), 171
Supplements, 218–219, Q84
    for cancer, 88

for depression, 87
for pressure ulcers, 241
safety issues, 85, 86t
Support pessaries, 452, 453f
Support surfaces, 238
Supported decision making, 357
Supraventricular arrhythmias, 399, 402
Supraventricular tachyarrhythmias, 394
Supraventricular tachycardia, 398–399, 404
Surgical aortic valve replacement (SAVR), 390, 398
Surgical care. *See also specific diseases and disorders; specific procedures*
  bypass surgery, 396–397, Q114
  for cancer, 574, 581–583
  cardiac risk assessment for, 98, 99f
  cosmetic, 360
  dental, 379, 537
  iatrogenic complications, 102
  parathyroid, 549, 549t
  pelvic reconstruction, 453
  perioperative care, 97–105
  postoperative cognitive decline, 104
  postoperative cognitive dysfunction (POCD), 297, Q91
  postoperative delirium, 297, 302t, 303
  postoperative management, 102–105, Q114
  preoperative assessment and management, 97–102, Q114
  total hip and knee arthroplasty, 151–152, 486
  trans-sphenoidal, 552
Surgical co-management, 136
Surrogate decision-making, 14–15, 15t
Surveillance, 460–462, 460t, 461t
Sustainable Growth Rate (SGR), 22
Suvorexant, 314, Q43
Swallowing, 220, 222–223, 224, Q49, Q59
Swinging flashlight test, 185
Symphytom officinale L. (comfrey root extract), 86
Symptom Severity score, 495
Syncope, 207–212
  cardiac, 207, 208t, 209, 210t
  causes of, 207, Q76
  diagnostic evaluation of, 209–211, 211t
  indications for permanent pacemaker implantation, 403, 405t
  micturition, Q111
  predictors of, 209, 210t
  presyncope, 202
  recurrent, Q71
  signs and symptoms of, 207, 208t
  vasovagal, 207–208, 208t, 212, Q76
Syndrome of inappropriate antidiuretic hormone (SIADH), 320, 437, Q19, Q69, Q102

Synthetic somatostatin analogues, 112t
Syphilis, 71, 539
Systematic assessment, 130, 131t
Systemic lupus erythematosus (SLE), 443, 492–493
Systems review, 130, 131t
Systolic blood pressure (SBP), 416, 418
Systolic heart failure, 407

T-score, 260, 264, 265
T_3. *See* Triiodothyronine
T_4. *See* Thyroxine
Tachy-brady syndrome, 404
Tachyarrhythmias, 394, 404
Tachycardia
  atrial, 402
  atrioventricular reentrant, 402
  AV-nodal reentrant, 402
  supraventricular, 398–399, 404
  ventricular, 402
Tadalafil
  for BPH, 456t, 457
  for ED, 468–469, 468t
Tai chi, 85
  for Alzheimer disease, 87
  for frailty, 184
  for pain, 120
  for preventing falls, 57, 256, 257, 258t, Q63
  recommendations for, 70
  to reduce risk of osteoporosis, 262
  for sleep disorders, 87–88
Tailor's bunion, 499t
Tamoxifen, 580
Tamsulosin, 456, 456t, Q86, Q120
Tapentadol (Nucynta), 124, 515
Taping, patellar, Q38
Tardive dyskinesia (TD), 333, 508–509, 513
Tardive dystonia, 513
Target theory of genetic damage, 5–6
Targeted therapies, 580–581, 588–589
Tarsal tunnel syndrome, 499t
Task-specific training, 247
Taste dysfunction, 376–377, 377t
TAVR (transcatheter aortic valve replacement), 390, 398
Taxanes, 580, 582t
TB (tuberculosis), 535–536
TBI (traumatic brain injury), 552, Q72
TCAs. *See* Tricyclic antidepressants
TD (tardive dyskinesia), 333, 508–509, 513
Td/Tdap (tetanus, diphtheria, acellular pertussis) vaccine, 73, 529t, 531
Tdap (tetanus, diphtheria, and pertussis) vaccine (Boostrix® or Adacel®), Q64
TDM-1 (ado-trastuzumab emtansine), 581, 582t
Teach-back method, 43
Teams
  GRACE Team Care™, 175
  home care approach, 165–166
  rehabilitation teams, 146, 147t

Tears, artificial, 494
Technology, in-home, 169
TEE (transesophageal echocardiography), 398, 537, Q18
Teeth, 372, 373f, 373t
Telangiectasias, 362, 433
Telecoil, 198
Telemedicine, 169–170, 324, Q95
Telephone quit lines, 63t
Telmisartan, 410t
Telomere theory of aging, 6
Telomeres, 575–576
Temazepam, 312, 313t
Temporal arteritis, 517
Temporal artery biopsy, Q110
Temporal lobe dysplasia, Q71
Temporal lobe epilepsy, 336–337
Temsirolimus, 582t
Tender points, 119
Tennis elbow, 478
Tenosynovitis, 499t
TENS (transcutaneous electrical nerve stimulation), 121, 154–155
Terazosin, 456, 456t
Teriparatide, 268t, 269–270
Terminal illness, 109–115, Q36, Q42
Terminology
  glossary of gait abnormalities, 245t
  preferred terms for cultural or religious identity, 42
  shoe terms, 503t
Testosterone, 555–557, 568
Testosterone deficiency, 555–556
Testosterone replacement therapy, 555, 556–557
Testosterone supplementation, 542, 555, 556–557, 556t
Testosterone therapy (TT), 469, Q87
Tetanus: vaccine against, 62t
Tetanus, diphtheria, acellular pertussis (Td/Tdap) vaccine, 73, 529t, 531, Q64
Tetrabenazine, 512, 513
Tetracyclines, 361
Thalassemia minor, 570
Thalidomide, 582t
The Arc, 357
Theophylline
  adverse events, 215, 382
  for asthma or COPD, 382, 385, 385t
  drug interactions, 527
Theories of aging, 5–8
Therapeutic interventions: lag time to benefit, 30, 31t
Thiamine supplements, 411
Thiazide diuretics, 252, 411, 419, 437
Thiazolidinediones, 226t, 263t, 563, 564t
Thigh pain, 479–480
Thinking problems. *See* Cognitive impairment
Thioglitazone, 226
Thought disorder, 331
3D-CAM (Confusion Assessment Method), 127, 295

Index **773**

Thrombectomy, endovascular, 520
Thrombocythemia, essential (ET), 571, 573
Thrombocytopenia, 442, 571
Thrombocytosis, 571
Thromboembolic events, 448
Thromboembolism, venous (VTE), 99–100, 100t, 387–389
Thrombolysis in myocardial infarction (TIMI) score, 31
Thrombopoietin-receptor agonists, 571
Thromboprophylaxis, 100, 131t, 132–133
Thrombotic microangiopathy, 442
Thrombotic thrombocytopenic purpura (TTP), 442, 571
Thrush, 375
Thyroid disorders, 65, 358t, 543–547
Thyroid hormone replacement, 263t, 544
Thyroid hormone requirements, 544
Thyroid scans, 546–547
Thyroid-stimulating hormone (TSH, thyrotropin), 66, 542, 551, 551t, 568
    age-related changes in, 543, 543t
    screening test, 62t
Thyroid ultrasonography, 546–547, 547t
Thyrotoxic myopathy, 515
Thyrotoxicosis, 545
Thyrotropin (thyroid-stimulating hormone), 66, 542, 551, 551t
    age-related changes in, 543, 543t
    screening test, 62t
Thyroxine (T_4), 543, 543t, 544, 545
Thyroxine (T_4) replacement therapy, 544
Thyroxine (T_4) supplementation, 544
TIAs (transient ischemic attacks), 520, Q99, Q106
Tibial nerve stimulation, percutaneous, Q4
Tibialis posterior dysfunction, 499t, 501
Ticagrelor, 393–394
Tilt-table testing, 210, 211t, Q121
Timed Up and Go (TUG) test, 27, 71, 204, 247, Q109
TIMI (thrombolysis in myocardial infarction) score, 31
Timolol, 188t
Tinel test, 478
Tinnitus, 194
Tiotropium bromide, 384–385, 384t, 385t
Tipiracil, 587
Tissue plasminogen activator (tPA), recombinant, 520
Tizanidine, 517
TKIs (tyrosine kinase inhibitors), 573, 582t
TMP (trimethoprim), 215t, 439t
TMP-SMX (trimethoprim-sulfamethoxazole), 534, Q3
Tobacco cessation, 88. See also Smoking cessation
Tocilizumab, 488, 492

α-Tocopherol (vitamin E), 215t, 282
α-Tocopherol (vitamin E) supplements, 219
Toe nails, Q50
Tofacitinib, 488
Toileting, scheduled, 298t
Tolerance, 122–123
Tolterodine, 227t, 230, Q15
Tongue
    black hairy, 376
    geographic, 375
Tooth extraction, incomplete, Q74
Toothlessness, 373–374
Topiramate, 349t, 508, 513, 517
Torsemide, 411
Torticollis, spasmodic, 512
Torus (tori), 375, 376t
Total body preoperative exercise, 248
Total hip and knee arthroplasty, 151–152, 486
Total pain, 117
Toujeo (insulin glargine), 565t
Toxic encephalopathy, 294
Toxic multinodular goiter, 545
Toxic myopathy, 515
Toxic nodular thyroid disease, 545, 546
Toxicity
    of cancer treatment agents, 581, 582t
    chemotherapy, 579–580, 579t
    statin therapy, 494
TPA (tissue plasminogen activator), recombinant, 520
Trabecular bone scans, Q98
Tradition, 45
Training BIG program, 509
Tramadol
    adverse effects of, Q3
    Beers Criteria® for, 80t
    for fibromyalgia, 495
    for neuropathic pain, 515
    for OA-related pain, 486
    for persistent pain, 124
Trametinib, 370
Trandolapril, 410t
Trans-sphenoidal surgery, 552
Transcatheter aortic valve replacement (TAVR), 390, 398
Transcranial magnetic stimulation, 150
Transcranial magnetic stimulation, repetitive (rTMS), 323
Transcutaneous electrical nerve stimulation (TENS), 121, 154–155
Transdermal lidocaine patch, 121, 121t, 514
Transdermal rotigotine patch, 511
Transesophageal echocardiography (TEE), 398, 537, Q18
Transfer dysphagia, 423
Transfer skills impairment, 258t
Transfers, 139
Transgender adults, 49, 51, 52
Transient ischemic attacks (TIAs), 520, Q99, Q106
Transitional care, 140–141, 140t, Q35, Q85

Transitional Care Model, Q85
Transitions of care, 139–142
    in delirium, 301–302
    at end-of-life, 160
Transplantation
    fecal microbiota (FMT), 540
    heart, 413–414, 415
    kidney, 445–446
    lung, 387
Transportation activity, 56
Transposable element activation theory of aging, 6
Transurethral incision of the prostate (TUIP), 456t, 457
Transurethral resection of the prostate (TURP), 456t, 457, 464
Transurethral vaporization of prostate, 456t, 457
Trastuzumab, 581, 582t
Trauma
    history of traumatic experiences, 44
    posttraumatic stress disorder (PTSD), 328, 329, 329t
Traumatic brain injury (TBI), 552, Q72
Traumatic encephalopathy, chronic, 355
Traumatic ulcers, oral, 376, 376t
Trazodone
    for depressive features in dementia, 288t
    for insomnia, 282, 313t, 314, Q43
    for sleep disturbances in dementia, 292
Treatment decisions. See Decision making
Treatment plans, 36
Tremetinib, 582t
Tremors, 508–509, 512–513
Trendelenburg gait, 245t, 246
Trends, 1–2, 1f, 2–4
Tresiba (insulin degludec), 565t
Tretinoin, 360, 361
Triage Risk Stratification Tool (TRST), 134, 135t
Triamcinolone, 364, 450
Triamterene, 80t, 439t
Tricyclic antidepressants (TCAs), 432
    adverse events, 288–289
    and delirium, 300t
    for depression, 320t
    for depressive features in dementia, 288t
    for depressive features of behavioral disturbances in dementia, 288
    and falls, 251t
    for headaches, 517
    and incontinence, 226t
    for insomnia, 314
    for migraine, 517
    for neuropathic pain, 514–515
    for persistent pain, 124
Trifluridine eye drops, 188
Trifluridine/tipiracil, 587
Trigger finger, 479
Trigger points, 119

Triggering receptor expressed on myeloid cells 2 gene *(TREM2)*, 273
Trihexyphenidyl, 333, 510, 511, 513
Triiodothyronine (T_3), 543, 543*t*, 544, 545
Triiodothyronine (T_3) thyrotoxicosis, 545
Trimethoprim (TMP), 215*t*, 439*t*
Trimethoprim-sulfamethoxazole (TMP-SMX), 534, Q3
Triple therapy, 395
Triptans, 517
Trisalicylate, 122
Trochanteric bursitis, 479
Trospium, 227*t*, 230
TRST (Triage Risk Stratification Tool), 134, 135*t*
Truth telling, 14
TSH (thyroid-stimulating hormone), 551, 551*t*, 568
TST (tuberculin skin test), 535, 536*t*
TT (testosterone therapy), 469, Q87
TTP (thrombotic thrombocytopenic purpura), 442, 571
Tube feeding, 223–224, Q59
Tuberculin skin test (TST), 535, 536*t*
Tuberculosis (TB), 71, 535–536
Tubular atrophy, Q48
Tubular necrosis, acute (ATN), 441
Tubulointerstitial disease, 441–442
TUG (Timed Up and Go) test, 27, 71, 204, 247, Q109
TUIP (transurethral incision of the prostate), 456*t*, 457
Tumor, regional node, metastasis (TNM) staging system, 460
Tumors
  back pain due to, 481, 481*t*, 482*t*
  ocular surface, 187
Tuning fork test, Q66
Turn en bloc, 245*t*
Turning and positioning, 238
Turning schedules, Q5
TURP (transurethral resection of the prostate), 456*t*, 457, 464
Tyrosine kinase inhibitors (TKIs), 573, 582*t*

Ubiquinone, 86–87
UI. *See* Urinary incontinence
Ulcers
  aphthous ulcers, 375, 376*t*
  chronic leg ulcers, 360, 365
  corneal, 186*t*, 187, 188
  foot ulcers, 505
  peptic ulcer disease, 427
  pressure injuries, 234–243
  traumatic, oral, 376, 376*t*
  venous ulcers, 365
Ulnar neuropathy, 478
Ultrasound
  abdominal, 62*t*
  carotid, 392
  thyroid, 546–547, 547*t*
Ultraviolet (UV) light therapy, 364, 365
Umeclidinium, 384–385, 384*t*

Under-nutrition, 70, 217, 219
Underprescribing, 79*t*, 80–81
Underweight, 392
United States, 2–4
University of Pennsylvania Smell Identification Test (UPSIT), 509
Unspoken challenges, 46
Up and Go test, 254
Upper endoscopy, Q49
UPSIT (University of Pennsylvania Smell Identification Test), 509
Ureteral obstruction, 441
Urethral mucosal atrophy, 449
Urethral sphincter support, impaired, 227
Urethritis, nongonococcal, Q107
Urge incontinence, 225, Q4, Q15
  with DO, 227
  minimally invasive procedures for, 231
  therapy for, 227*t*, 229–230
Urgencies, hypertensive, 421
Urgency, urinary, Q4, Q15
Urinary catheter use, 129–130
Urinary incontinence (UI), 225–233
  comorbid conditions, 226
  with developmental disabilities, 358*t*
  medications that can cause or worsen, 226, 226*t*
  mixed UI, 225, 227, 229–230, Q4
  screening for, 63*t*, 71–72, 228, 231
  stress UI, 225, 227, 229–230, 231, 232, Q4
  urge UI, 225, 227, 227*t*, 229–230, 231, Q4, Q15
Urinary protein excretion: measures of, 436
Urinary retention, 457, Q86
Urinary system, 9*t*, 10*t*
Urinary tract infections (UTIs), 533–535, Q97, Q123
  catheter-associated (CA-UTIs), 129–130, 534–535
  guidelines for diagnosis of, 528*t*, 534
  surveillance definition of, 528*t*
Urinary tract obstruction, 441
Urine collection, 24-hour, 436
Urine culture ordering, 534–535
Urine dipsticks, 436
Urodynamic testing, 229, Q86
Urogenital atrophy, 448, 449
U.S. Department of Agriculture (USDA), 213, 220
U.S. Department of Health and Human Services (HHS), 56, 70, 171
U.S. Department of Veterans Affairs (VA). *See* Veterans Affairs
U.S. Multi-Society Task Force on Colorectal Cancer, Q56
U.S. Preventive Services Task Force (USPSTF), 57, 60
  indications for osteoporosis screening, 264

  recommendations for aspirin use, 74
  recommendations for BMD testing, 264
  recommendations for breast cancer prevention, 74
  recommendations for cancer screening, 65
  recommendations for CKD screening, 443
  recommendations for colorectal cancer screening, 64, Q56
  recommendations for depression screening, 72
  recommendations for hepatitis B screening, 69
  recommendations for hepatitis C screening, 69, 539
  recommendations for HIV screening, 70
  recommendations for LTBI screening, 71
  recommendations for lung cancer screening, 65
  recommendations for preventing falls, Q40
  recommendations for prostate cancer screening, 458–459
  recommendations for statin therapy, 69
  recommendations for STI screening, 71
  recommendations for sustained weight loss, 70
USDA (U.S. Department of Agriculture), 213, 220
USPSTF. *See* U.S. Preventive Services Task Force
Uterine prolapse, 452*f*
Uterovaginal prolapse, 451
Utilitarianism/consequentialism, 11
UTIs. *See* Urinary tract infections
Uveitis, 186*t*, 188

V2-receptor antagonists, 437
Vaccinations, 525, 528–531, Q64
  hepatitis A, 529*t*
  hepatitis B, 529*t*
  herpes zoster, 62*t*, 73, 528, 529*t*, 530–531
  for hospitalized patients, 130, 131*t*
  immunization schedule for adults ≥65 years old, 529*t*
  influenza, 62*t*, 73, 130, 528, 529*t*, 532
  meningococcal, 529*t*
  pneumococcal, 62*t*, 73, 130, 131*t*, 528–529, 529*t*, 532
  tetanus, 62*t*
  tetanus, diphtheria, acellular pertussis (Td/Tdap), 73, 529*t*, 531
  zoster, 366
Vacuum-assisted erection devices, 469
Vacuum devices, 468*t*

Vaginal atrophy, 449, 470, 471, 555
Vaginal bleeding, 449, 453–454, 454t
Vaginal mesh, 453, Q1
Vaginal pH, 449
Vaginal prolapse, 451–452, 452f, 453
Vaginitis, atrophic, Q97
Vaginosis, bacterial, Q1
Valacyclovir, 366
Valbenazine, 333, 513
Valerian, 315
Valerian root, 87
Valgus position, 499t
Validation therapy, 292
Valproic acid (valproate, divalproex), 282, 508, 517, Q33
Valsartan, 410, 410t
Valsartan with sacubitril, 409, 410–411, 410t
Value-Based Programs (MACRA), 23
Values, 11, 12t
Valvular heart disease, 397–398, 400t, 406, 408
Vancomycin, 532, 539, 540
Vancomycin-resistant enterococci (VRE), 526
Vandetanib, 582t
Vardenafil, 467, 468–469, 468t
Varenicline, 349t, 351
Varicella zoster virus (VZV), 365–366
Varicella-zoster virus (VZV) vaccine, 366, 528, 530–531
    immunization schedule for adults ≥65 years old, 529t
    recommendations for, 62t, 73
Varus position, 499t
Vascular dementia, 244, 272, 277, 277t
Vascular disease
    cardiovascular disease, 390–406
    in kidneys, 442
        peripheral vascular disease, 148
        renovascular disease, 439–440
Vascular ectasia, 433
Vascular endothelial growth factor (VEGF) inhibitors, 189–190, 580, 582t
Vascular insufficiency, 479
Vascular parkinsonism, 511
Vasculature, 8, 9t, 10t
Vasodilators, 421
Vasomotor symptoms, 448
Vasopressin (DDAVP), 231
Vasovagal syncope, 207–208, 208t, 212, Q76
VDE (videofluoroscopic deglutition examination), 222, 223
VDRL (Venereal Disease Research Laboratory) test, 539
VEGF (vascular endothelial growth factor) inhibitors, 189–190, 580, 582t
Vemurafenib, 370, 582t
Venereal Disease Research Laboratory (VDRL) test, 539
Venetoclax, 582t
Venlafaxine (Effexor)
    for anxiety disorders, 329
    for depression, 319, 320t
    for depressive features in dementia, 288, 288t
    for persistent pain, 124
Venous insufficiency, 360, 365
Venous thromboembolic disease (VTED), 387–389
Venous thromboembolism (VTE), 99–100, 100t, 387–389
Venous thrombosis prophylaxis, 100
    in hospitalized patients, 131t, 132–133
Venous ulcers, 365
Ventilation, 307, 385t, 387
Ventilation/perfusion scans, 388
Ventilatory disorders, 387
Ventricular arrhythmias, 399, 402
Ventricular tachycardia, 402
Venues for care, 141
Verapamil, 394
    adverse events, 396
    for AF, 399
    drug interactions, 412
    for migraine, 517
Verbal Descriptor Scale, 118
Vertebral compression fractures, 271, 475, 481, 481t, 482t, 483
Vertebral fracture assessment (VFA), 265
Vertebral fracture management, 271
Vertebrobasilar syndrome, Q71
Vertebroplasty, 271, 483
Vertigo, 202, 203t
    benign paroxysmal positional vertigo (BPPV), 202, 205–206, Q99
VES-13 (Vulnerable Elders Survey-13), 179
Vestibular rehabilitation therapy (VRT), 205
Veterans, 107
Veterans Access, Choice and Accountability Act of 2014 ("Choice Act"), 22
Veterans Administration (VA), 159–160, 169
Veterans Affairs, Department of (VA)
    Community Living Centers (VA), 159–160
    guidelines for rehabilitation after stroke, 149, 150
    hearing aid benefits, 199
    hospice benefits, 108
    medical benefits, 22, 54
    palliative care services, 107
    Surgical Quality Improvement Program, 101
Veterans Health Administration (VHA), Q77, Q125
VFA (vertebral fracture assessment), 265
Videofluoroscopic deglutition examination (VDE), 222, 223
Videofluoroscopy, 150, Q116
Vilanterol, 384t
Vilazodone, 288t
VIN (vulvar intraepithelial neoplasia), 451
Vinblastine, 582t, 590
Vinca alkaloids, 582t
Vincristine, 579t, 582t, 589
Vinorelbine, 579t, 580, 582t
Viral conjunctivitis, 187t, 188, Q117
Viridans streptococci, 398, 536–537
Virtual home visits, 170
Virtual reality, 150
Visceral pain, 119, 119t
    referred, 481, 482t
Viscosupplementation therapy, 486–487
Vision, Q10
Vision services, 19t
Vision testing, 63t, 72, 185, Q10
Visual hallucinations, 192, 333, 334, 335
Visual imagery, 330
Visual loss, 185–192, Q10
    assessment of, 25
    interventions for preventing falls, 257, 259t
    red eye, Q117
    screening for, 63t, 72
    signs and symptoms requiring immediate referral, 185–187, 186t
    sudden decrease in vision, 185, 187t
VitalTalk, 108
Vitamin A, 215t, 219
Vitamin B_1, 215t
Vitamin B_2, 215t
Vitamin B_6, 215t
Vitamin B_6 supplements, 218–219
Vitamin B_{12}, 215t
Vitamin B_{12} deficiency, 569f, 570
Vitamin B_{12} supplements, 218–219
Vitamin C supplements, 569
Vitamin D, Q120
    dietary sources, 266
    drug interactions, 215t
    preventive, 63t, 71, 74
    RDIs for adults, 266
Vitamin D deficiency, 262, 542, 547–548, 549, 550
    in hospitalized patients, 128
    screening for, 218
Vitamin D insufficiency, 266–267
Vitamin D supplements, 218, 542
    for frailty, Q88
    for hyperparathyroidism, 549
    for osteoporosis, 266–267
    to prevent falls, 71, 258t, Q24
    to prevent fractures, Q2
    to prevent hypocalcemia, 550–551
    recommendations for, 71, 74
Vitamin D_2 supplements, 548
Vitamin D_3 (cholecalciferol) supplements, 262, 548, Q24
Vitamin E (α-tocopherol) supplements, 215t, 219, 282
Vitamin K, 215t, 522

Vitamin K replacement, 572
Vitamin therapy, 63*t*, 74, Q84
Volume depletion, 437
Volume overload, 437
Voluntary stopping of eating and drinking (VSED), 17
Vomiting. *See* Nausea and vomiting
von Willebrand disease (vWD), 572
Vortioxetine, 288*t*, 320*t*
VRE (vancomycin-resistant enterococci), 526
VRT (vestibular rehabilitation therapy), 205
VSED (voluntary stopping of eating and drinking), 17
VTE (venous thromboembolism), 99–100, 100*t*, 387–389
VTED (venous thromboembolic disease), 387–389
Vulnerability, 180, 183, Q17
Vulnerable Elders Survey-13 (VES-13), 179
Vulvar disorders, 450–451, 451*f*
Vulvar intraepithelial neoplasia (VIN), 451
Vulvectomy, radical, 451
Vulvodynia, 450
Vulvovaginal atrophy, 449, 471
Vulvovaginal infection and inflammation, 449–450
vWD (von Willebrand disease), 572
VZV (varicella zoster virus), 365–366
VZV (varicella-zoster virus) vaccine, 528, 530–531
   immunization schedule for adults ≥65 years old, 529*t*
   recommendations for, 62*t*, 73

Walkers, 156, 157*t*, Q47
Walking, 86, Q62
   for DVT, 389
   400-meter walk test, 247
   limitations in, 244
   pulmonary rehabilitation, 154
   to reduce risk of osteoporosis, 262
   rehabilitation, 150
   6-minute walk test, 247
Walter 1-year index, 32*t*
Warfarin therapy
   for ACS, 394
   adverse events, 81
   for AF, 395, 401
   cessation before surgery, 99–100, 100*t*
   for chronic CAD, 395
   drug interactions, 527, 534
   for HF with AF, 412
   for stroke prevention, 401, 521
   for VTE, 388–389
Watchful waiting, 460–462, 461*t*
Watchman device, 402
Water aerobics, 120
Water balance disorders, 436–438
We Honor Veterans program, 107
Weber test, Q66
Weight loss, Q38
   anorexia, 112–113
   for chronic CAD, 395
   for DM, 558, 559
   for gout, 489
   for HTN, 419
   involuntary, 217, 217*t*, 577
   for pain management, 485
   recommendations to promote, 70
   significant, 214
   for UI, 229
   unacceptable, 220
   for ventilatory disorders, 387
Weight management, 57, 409
Weight screening, 62*t*, 70
Wellspring Model, 163
Wernicke-Korsakoff syndrome, Q68
Wheelchairs, 156, 157*t*
Wheezing, 381
Whipple disease, 430
Whisper-voice test, 25, 72
White Americans
   cancer, 575
   caregivers, 37
   CVD mortality rates, 390
   diabetes mellitus, 558
   life expectancy, 2
   nursing-home population, 159
   osteoporosis, 260
   periodontitis, 373
   population projections, 2, 575
   poverty rates, 3, Q118
   urinary incontinence, 225
White-coat hypertension, 417
White willow bark *(Salix alba)*, 86
WHO. *See* World Health Organization
Widespread Pain Index, 495
Widower's syndrome, 466, 466*t*
Withdrawal, alcohol, 335, 344, 350
Women's health
   adrenal insufficiency, 555
   alcohol use, 346
   breast cancer, 583–584
   cancer, 574, 583–584
   cardiovascular disease, 390, 391*t*
   caregivers, 37
   centenarians, Q103
   colonic adenomas, 586
   coronary artery disease, 393
   diabetes, Q98
   drug metabolism, 78
   estrogen deficiency, 261–262
   fecal incontinence, 429
   female sexuality, 469–471
   gynecologic diseases and disorders, 447–454
   history and physical examination, 447–448
   hypertension, 416
   indications for osteoporosis screening, 264
   labor force participation, 3
   lesbian and bisexual women, 51, Q124
   life expectancy, 2, 31, 31*t*
   marital status and living arrangements, 2, 3
   population projections, 2
   poverty rates, 4, Q118
   preventive hormone therapy, 63*t*
   recommendations for BMD testing, 264
   recommendations for calcium intake, 266
   recommendations for macronutrient intake, 213
   recommendations for vitamin D intake, 266
   schizophrenia, 331, 332
   sexual dysfunction, 465, 469–470, 470–471, 472*t*
   sexuality, 465
   stroke, 518
   temporal arteritis, 517
   urinary incontinence, 71–72, 225–226
   urinary tract infections, 533
   vertebral compression fractures, 475, 483
Word-finding difficulty, Q106
World Health Organization (WHO)
   BMD definitions, 260, 261*t*
   definition of osteoporosis, 260, 261*t*
   fracture risk assessment model (FRAX™), 68, 260, 262–263, 265, 265*t*
   healthy life expectancy (HALE), 2–3
   International Classification of Functioning, Disability, and Health (ICF), 143
   International Prostate Symptom Score, 455
   Pain Ladder, 121
   recommendations for prostate cancer grading, 460
Wound bed preparation, 239
Wound care, 234–243, Q45
   palliative care, 242, 242*t*
   treatment modalities, 239, 240*t*
Wound documentation, 237
Wound healing, 235, 237, 241, Q5
Wrist pain, 478–479, 490, 491*f*
Writer's cramp, 512

Xerophthalmia, 493–494
Xerosis, 362, 364, 504
Xerostomia, 493–494

Yoga, 85
   for Alzheimer disease, 87
   for cancer, 88
   for flexibility, 57
   for pain, 120, 486
   for preventing falls, 258*t*

Z-drugs, 252
Z-score, 264, 383
Zaleplon, 292, 313–314, 313*t*, Q43
Zanamivir, 533
Zarit Burden Interview, 41
Zika virus, Q107

Zinc, 215t, 241
Ziprasidone, 290t, 291, 301t, 335t
Zoledronic acid, 267–268, 268t, 550
Zolpidem, 78
    and delirium, 300t
        for insomnia, 313–314, 313t, Q43
        for sleep disturbances in dementia, 292
Zostavax, 73
Zoster sine herpete, 366